a LANGE medical book

D0149027

CURRENT
Diagnosis &
Treatment
in Cardiology

second edition

Edited by

Michael H. Crawford, MD
Professor of Medicine
Mayo Medical School
Rochester, Minnesota
Consultant in Cardiovascular Diseases
Mayo Clinic
Scottsdale, Arizona

Lange Medical Books/McGraw-Hill
Medical Publishing Division

New York   Chicago   San Francisco   Lisbon   London
Madrid   Mexico City   Milan   New Delhi   San Juan
Seoul   Singapore   Sydney   Toronto

The **McGraw·Hill** Companies

CURRENT Diagnosis & Treatment in Cardiology, Second Edition

3 4 5 6 7 8 9 0 DOC/DOC 0 9 8 7 6 5 4

ISBN: 0-8385-1473-1

ISSN: 1079-1051

Notice

Medicine is an ever-changing science. As new research and clinical experience broaden our knowledge, changes in treatment and drug therapy are required. The authors and the publisher of this work have checked with sources believed to be reliable in their efforts to provide information that is complete and generally in accord with the standards accepted at the time of publication. However, in view of the possibility of human error or changes in medical sciences, neither the authors nor the publisher nor any other party who has been involved in the preparation or publication of this work warrants that the information contained herein is in every respect accurate or complete, and they disclaim all responsibility for any errors or omissions or for the results obtained from use of the information contained in this work. Readers are encouraged to confirm the information contained herein with other sources. For example and in particular, readers are advised to check the product information sheet included in the package of each drug they plan to administer to be certain that the information contained in this work is accurate and that changes have not been made in the recommended dose or in the contraindications for administration. This recommendation is of particular importance in connection with new or infrequently used drugs.

This book was set in Adobe Garamond by Rainbow Graphics, Inc.
The editors were Isabel Nogueira and Nicky Panton.
The production supervisor was Richard Ruzycka.
The cover designer was Mary McKeon.
The text was designed by Eve Siegel.
The index was prepared by Jerry Ralya.

R.R. Donnelley was printer and binder.

This book is printed on acid-free paper.

Contents

Authors

Imran Afridi, MD, FACC
Attending Cardiologist, North Texas Cardiovascular
  Associates and Methodist Hospital of Dallas, Texas
Aortic Regurgitation

Masood Akhtar, MD
Clinical Professor of Medicine, University of
  Wisconsin Medical School, Milwaukee Clinical
  Campus; Aurora Sinai Medical Center and St.
  Luke's Medical Center, Milwaukee, Wisconsin
llandis@hrtcare.com
Ventricular Tachycardia

Mohammed Zaher Akkad, MD
Attending Physician, Division of Cardiology, Harper
  Hospital, Detroit, Michigan
Myocarditis

Kathleen M. Allen, MD
Assistant Professor of Medicine, Division of
  Cardiology, The University of New Mexico School
  of Medicine, Albuquerque
kmallen@salud.unm.edu
Coronary Revascularization

Richard W. Asinger, MD
Professor of Medicine, University of Minnesota
  Medical School-Minneapolis; Director, Division
  of Cardiology, Department of Medicine,
  Hennepin County Medical Center, Minneapolis,
  Minnesota
asing001@umn.edu
Chronic Anticoagulation for Cardiac Conditions

Alvin S. Blaustein, MD
Associate Professor of Medicine, Baylor College of
  Medicine; Chief, Cardiology Section and Director,
  Non-invasive Laboratory, Veterans Affairs Medical
  Center, Houston, Texas
blaustein.alvins@med.va.gov
Evaluation and Treatment of the Perioperative Patient

Syed W. Bokhari, MD
Fellow, Cardiovascular Diseases, Division of
  Cardiology, UCI Medical Center, Orange,
  California
sbokhari@uci.edu
Heart Disease in Pregnancy

Robert J. Bryg, MD
Chief, Division of Cardiology; Associate Chairman of
  Medicine, University of Nevada School of
  Medicine, Reno, Nevada
nevsimbob@aol.com
Mitral Stenosis

Christopher S. Cadman, MD, FACC
Assistant Professor of Medicine & Director,
  Arrhythmia Service, University of New Mexico
  School of Medicine, Veterans Administration
  Medical Center, Albuquerque, New Mexico
Syncope

Blase A. Carabello, MD
Professor of Medicine, Veterans Affairs Medical
  Center, Houston, Texas
blaseanthony.carabello@med.va.gov
Aortic Stenosis

Enrique V. Carbajal, MD
Assistant Clinical Professor of Medicine, University of
  California, San Francisco Medical Education
  Program; Assistant Chief, Cardiology Section,
  Veterans Affairs Central California Health Care
  System, Fresno, California
enrique.carbajal@med.va.gov
Congestive Heart Failure

John D. Carroll, MD
Professor of Medicine, University of Colorado Health
  Sciences Center, Denver, Colorado
john.carroll@uchsc.edu
Restrictive Cardiomyopathies

Edmond W. Chen, MD
Cardiology Fellow, Division of Cardiology, University
  of California, San Francisco
Cardiac Tumors

Peter C. Chien, MD
Assistant Professor of Medicine, New York
  Medical College; Director Adult Primary Care
  Center, Westchester Medical Center, Valhalla,
  New York
peterchien71@hotmail.com
Lipid Disorders

Kuang-Yuh Chyu, MD, PhD
Assistant Professor-in-Residence, Department of
  Medicine, University of California, Los Angeles;
  Staff Cardiologist, Cedars-Sinai Medical Center,
  Los Angeles, California
Unstable Angina

Michael H. Crawford, MD
Professor of Medicine, Mayo Medical School;
  Consultant in Cardiovascular Diseases, Mayo
  Clinic, Scottsdale, Arizona
crawford.michael@mayo.edu
*Approach to Cardiac Disease Diagnosis; Chronic
  Ischemic Heart Disease; Aortic Stenosis; Mitral
  Regurgitation; Restrictive Cardiomyopathies*

Prakash C. Deedwania, MD
Chief, University of California, San Francisco School
  of Medicine, Cardiology Section, Veterans Affairs
  Central California Health Care System
deed@ucsfresno.edu
Congestive Heart Failure

John P. DiMarco, MD, PhD
Professor of Medicine, Cardiovascular Division,
  Department of Medicine, University of Virginia
  Health System, Charlottesville
jdimarco@virginia.edu
Sudden Cardiac Death

John A. Elefteriades, MD
Professor & Chief, Section of Cardiothoracic Surgery,
  Yale University School of Medicine, New Haven,
  Connecticut
john.elefteriades@yale.edu
Thoracic Aortic Aneurysms

Michael D. Faulx, MD
Fellow, Division of Cardiology, Case Western Reserve
  University and University Hospitals of Cleveland,
  Ohio
mdf8@po.cwru.edu
Tricuspid and Pulmonic Valve Disease

Elyse Foster, MD
Professor of Clinical Medicine & Anesthesia,
  University of California, San Francisco; Director,
  Echocardiography Laboratory and Adult
  Congenital Heart Disease Service, Cardiology
  Division, Department of Medicine, Moffitt-Long
  Hospital, San Francisco, California
foster@medicine.ucsf.edu
Congenital Heart Disease in Adults

William H. Frishman, MD, MACP
Barbara & William Rosenthal Professor of Medicine;
  Chairman of Medicine & Professor of
  Pharmacology, New York Medical College; Chief
  of Medicine, Westchester Medical Center,
  Valhalla, New York
william_frishman@nymc.edu
Lipid Disorders

Samuel Z. Goldhaber, MD
Associate Professor of Medicine, Harvard Medical School;
  Director, Venous Thromboembolism Research Group
  & Director, Anticoagulation Service, Brigham and
  Women's Hospital, Boston, Massachusetts
sgoldhaber@partners.org
Pulmonary Embolic Disease

Nora Goldschlager, MD
Professor of Clinical Medicine, University of
  California, San Francisco; Director, Coronary
  Care Unit, ECG Department and Pacemaker
  Clinic, San Francisco General Hospital
ngoldschlager@medsfgh.ucsf.edu
Conduction Disorders & Cardiac Pacing

William F. Graettinger, MD, FACC, FACP, FCCP
Professor & Vice-Chairman, Department of
  Medicine, University of Nevada School of
  Medicine; Chief, Medical Service, Veterans Affairs
  Sierra Nevada Health Care System, Reno, Nevada
williamg@unr.edu
Systemic Hypertension

Brian D. Hoit, MD
Professor of Medicine, Case Western Reserve
    University and University Hospitals of Cleveland,
    Ohio
bdh6@po.cwru.edu
Tricuspid and Pulmonic Valve Disease

Allan S. Jaffe, MD
Professor of Medicine & Consultant, Divisions of
    Cardiology and Laboratory Medicine, Mayo
    Clinic, Rochester, Minnesota
jaffe.allan@mayo.edu
Acute Myocardial Infarction

Samer S. Kabbani, MD, FACC
Assistant Professor of Medicine, Cardiology Unit,
    University of Vermont College of Medicine,
    Burlington
samer.kabbani@vtmednet.org
Pericardial Diseases

Peter R. Kowey, MD
Professor of Medicine, Jefferson Medical College,
    Philadelphia, Pennsylvania; Chief of Cardiology,
    Lankenau Hospital and Main Line Health System,
    Wynnewood, Pennsylvania
Supraventricular Arrhythmias

Martin M. LeWinter, MD
Professor of Medicine & Director, Heart Failure Unit
    University of Vermont College of Medicine,
    Burlington
martin.lewinter@vtmednet.org
Pericardial Diseases

Roger Marinchak, MD
Clinical Professor of Medicine, Thomas Jefferson
    University School of Medicine, Philadelphia,
    Pennsylvania; Clinical Electrophysiologist, The
    Heart Group and Lancaster General Hospital,
    Lancaster, Pennsylvania
ramarinchak@pol.net
Supraventricular Arrhythmias

Wayne L. Miller, MD, PhD
Associate Professor of Medicine, Consultant, Division
    of Cardiovascular Medicine, Mayo Clinic and
    Foundation, Rochester, Minnesota
miller.wayne@mayo.edu
Acute Myocardial Infarction

J.V. Nixon, MD, FACC
Professor of Medicine & Cardiology; Director,
    Echocardiography Laboratories and the Heart
    Station, Medical College of Virginia at Virginia
    Commonwealth University, Richmond
jnixon@hsc.vcu.edu
The Athlete's Heart

John B. O'Connell, MD
Professor & Chairman, Department of Internal
    Medicine, Wayne State University School of
    Medicine, Detroit, Michigan
jo'connell@intmed.wayne.edu
Myocarditis

Rita F. Redberg, MD, MSc, FACC
Associate Professor of Medicine & Director, Women's
    Cardiovascular Services, Division of Cardiology,
    University of California, San Francisco Medical
    Center
redberg@medicine.ucsf.edu
Cardiac Tumors

Cheryl L. Reid, MD
Associate Professor of Medicine; Director, Noninvasive
    Cardiology, University of California, Irvine
c2reid@uci.edu
Heart Disease in Pregnancy

Carlos A. Roldan, MD
Associate Professor of Medicine, Cardiology Division,
    Veterans Affairs Medical Center and University of
    New Mexico, Albuquerque
carlos.roldan2@med.va.gov
Connective Tissue Diseases and the Heart

Melvin M. Scheinman, MD
Professor of Medicine, Division of Cardiology,
    University of California San Francisco
scheinman@medicine.ucsf.edu
Atrial Fibrillation

Pravin Shah, MD, MACC
Clinical Professor of Medicine, Loma Linda
    University School of Medicine, Loma Linda,
    California; Medical Director Non-Invasive
    Cardiac Imaging and Academic Programs, Hoag
    Heart Institute, Newport Beach, California
pshah@hoaghospital.org
Hypertrophic Cardiomyopathies

Prediman K. Shah, MD, FACC
Shapell and Webb Chair & Director, Division of
    Cardiology and Atherosclerosis Research Center,
    Cedars-Sinai Medical Center;
Professor of Medicine, University of California, Los
    Angeles
Unstable Angina

Bruce K. Shively, MD
Associate Professor of Medicine & Director, Adult
    Echocardiography, Oregon Health Science
    University, Portland
shivelyb@ohsu.edu
Infective Endocarditis

Helge U. Simon, MD
Cardiology Fellow, University of Cincinnati Medical
    Center & the Veterans Affairs Medical Center,
    Cincinnati, Ohio
husimon@massmed.org
Evaluation and Treatment of the Perioperative Patient

Chad Stoltz, MD
Cardiology Fellow, Department of Cardiovascular
    Medicine, University of Wisconsin School of
    Medicine, Madison
Mitral Stenosis

Robert A. Taylor, MD
Assistant Professor of Medicine, University of New
    Mexico Health Sciences Center
rtaylor@salud.unm.edu
Pulmonary Hypertension

Richard D. Taylor, MD
Staff Cardiologist & Director, Arrhythmia
    Management Program, Division of Cardiology,
    Hennepin County Medical Center, Minneapolis,
    Minnesota
richard.taylor@co.hennepin.mn.us
Chronic Anticoagulation for Cardiac Conditions

Nikola Tede, MD, FAAP
Pediatric Cardiologist, California Pacific Medical
    Center, San Francisco; Clinical Faculty,
    Department of Pediatrics/Cardiology, University
    of California, San Francisco
Congenital Heart Disease in Adults

Craig Timm, MD
Associate Professor of Internal Medicine, University
    of New Mexico Health Sciences Center,
    Albuquerque
ctimm@salud.unn.edu
Cardiogenic Shock

B. Sylvia Vela, MD
Associate Professor of Clinical Medicine, University
    of Arizona Health Sciences Center; Program
    Director, Phoenix Citywide Endocrinology
    Fellowship, Carl T. Hayden Veterans Affairs
    Medical Center, Phoenix, Arizona
sylvia.vela@med.va.gov
Endocrinology and the Heart

Barry M. Weinberger, DO
Clinical Electrophysiologist, Attending Community
    Medical Center, Toms River, New Jersey
Supraventricular Arrhythmias

Jorge A. Wernly, MD
W. Sterling Edwards Professor & Chief, Division of
    Thoracic and Cardiovascular Surgery, University
    of New Mexico Health Sciences Center,
    Albuquerque
jwernly@salud.unm.edu
Thoracic Aortic Dissection

Laura F. Wexler, MD
Associate Dean, Student Affairs & Admissions;
    Professor of Medicine, Division of Cardiology,
    University of Cincinnati College of Medicine,
    Cincinnati, Ohio
wexler1@ucmail.uc.edu
Evaluation and Treatment of the Perioperative Patient

William A. Zoghbi, MD, FACC
Professor of Medicine, Baylor College of Medicine;
    Director, Echocardiography Laboratory, The
    Methodist DeBakey Heart Center, Houston, Texas
wzoghbi@bcm.tmc.edu
Aortic Regurgitation

Preface

Current Diagnosis & Treatment in Cardiology is designed to be a concise discussion of the essential knowledge needed to diagnose and manage cardiovascular diseases. *Current Diagnosis & Treatment in Cardiology* cannot be considered a condensed textbook because detailed pathophysiologic discussions are omitted; there are no chapters on diagnostic techniques; and rare or obscure entities are not included. Also, it is not a cardiac therapeutics text because diagnostic techniques, prevention strategies, and prognosis are fully discussed.

INTENDED AUDIENCE

Current Diagnosis & Treatment in Cardiology is designed to be a quick reference source in the clinic or on the ward for the experienced physician. Cardiology fellows will find that it is an excellent review for Board examinations. Also, students and residents will find it useful to review the essentials of specific conditions and to check the current references included in each section for further study. Nurses, technicians, and other health care workers who provide care for cardiology patients will find *Current Diagnosis & Treatment in Cardiology* a useful source for all aspects of heart disease care.

COVERAGE

The 37 chapters in *Current Diagnosis & Treatment in Cardiology* cover the major disease entities and therapeutic challenges in cardiology. There are chapters on major management issues in cardiology such as pregnancy and heart disease, the use of anticoagulants in heart disease, and the pre-operative evaluation of heart disease patients. Each section is written by experts in the particular area, but has been extensively edited to insure a consistent approach throughout the book and the kind of readability found in single-author texts.

Since the first edition the book has grown somewhat. Each chapter has been thoroughly revised and the references updated. Also, there are three new chapters in areas that have increased in importance in the last 5 years: coronary revascularization, atrial fibrillation, and aortic aneurysms.

My hope is that the book is found useful and improves patient care. Also, I hope it is an educational tool that improves knowledge of cardiac diseases. Finally, I hope it stimulates clinical research in areas where our knowledge is incomplete.

Michael H. Crawford, MD
Scottsdale, Arizona
November 2002

Approach to Cardiac Disease Diagnosis

Michael H. Crawford, MD

General Considerations

The patient's history is a critical feature in the evaluation of suspected or overt heart disease. It includes information about the present illness, past illnesses, and the patient's family. From this information, a chronology of the patient's disease process should be constructed. Determining what information in the history is useful requires a detailed knowledge of the pathophysiology of cardiac disease. The effort spent on listening to the patient is time well invested because the cause of cardiac disease is often discernible from the history.

A. COMMON SYMPTOMS

1. Chest pain—Chest pain is one of the cardinal symptoms (Table 1–1) of ischemic heart disease, but it can also occur with other forms of heart disease. The five characteristics of ischemic chest pain, or angina pectoris, are

- Anginal pain usually has a substernal location but may extend to the left or right chest, the shoulders, the neck, jaw, arms, epigastrium and, occasionally, the upper back.
- The pain is deep, visceral, and intense; it makes the patient pay attention but is not excruciating.

Table 1–1. Common symptoms of potential cardiac origin.

Chest pain or pressure
Dyspnea on exertion
Paroxysmal nocturnal dyspnea
Orthopnea
Syncope or near syncope
Transient neurologic defects
Edema
Palpitation
Cough

Many patients describe it as a pressure-like sensation.
- The duration of the pain is minutes, not seconds.
- The pain tends to be precipitated by exercise or emotional stress.
- The pain is relieved by resting or taking sublingual nitroglycerin.

2. Dyspnea—A frequent complaint of patients with a variety of cardiac diseases, dyspnea is ordinarily one of four types. The most common is exertional dyspnea, which usually means that the underlying condition is mild because it requires the increased demand of exertion to precipitate symptoms. The next most common is paroxysmal nocturnal dyspnea, characterized by the patient awakening after being asleep or recumbent for an hour or more. This symptom is caused by the redistribution of body fluids from the lower extremities into the vascular space and back to the heart, resulting in volume overload; it suggests a more severe condition. Third is orthopnea, a dyspnea that occurs immediately on assuming the recumbent position. The mild increase in venous return (caused by lying down) before any fluid is mobilized from interstitial spaces in the lower extremities is responsible for the symptom, which suggests even more severe disease. Finally, dyspnea at rest suggests severe cardiac disease.

Dyspnea is not specific for heart disease, however. Exertional dyspnea, for example, can be due to pulmonary disease, anemia, or deconditioning. Orthopnea is a frequent complaint in patients with chronic obstructive pulmonary disease and postnasal drip. A history of "two-pillow orthopnea" is of little value unless the reason for the use of two pillows is discerned. Resting dyspnea is also a sign of pulmonary disease. Paroxysmal nocturnal dyspnea is perhaps the most specific for cardiac disease because few other conditions cause this symptomatology.

3. Syncope and presyncope—These signs (lightheadedness, dizziness, etc) are important symptoms of a reduction in cerebral blood flow. These symptoms are nonspecific and can be due to primary central nervous system disease, metabolic conditions, dehydration, or inner-ear problems. Because brady- and tachyarrhythmias are important cardiac causes, a history of palpitations preceding the event is significant.

4. Transient central nervous system deficits— Deficits such as transient ischemic attacks (TIAs), suggest emboli from the heart or great vessels or, rarely, from the venous circulation through an intracardiac shunt. A TIA should prompt the search for cardiovascular disease. Any sudden loss of blood flow to a limb also suggests a cardioembolic event.

5. Fluid retention—These symptoms are not specific for heart disease but may be due to reduced cardiac function. Typical symptoms are peripheral edema, bloating, weight gain, and abdominal pain from an enlarged liver or spleen. Decreased appetite, diarrhea, jaundice, and nausea and vomiting can also occur from gut and hepatic dysfunction due to fluid engorgement.

6. Palpitation—Normal resting cardiac activity usually cannot be appreciated by the individual. Awareness of heart activity is often referred to by patients as palpitation. Among patients there is no standard definition for the type of sensation represented by palpitation, so the physician must explore the sensation further with the patient. It is frequently useful to have the patient tap the perceived heartbeat out by hand. Commonly, unusually forceful heart activity at a normal rate (60–100 bpm) is perceived as palpitation. More forceful contractions are usually the result of endogenous catecholamine excretion that does not elevate the heart rate out of the normal range. A frequent cause of this phenomenon is anxiety. Another frequent sensation is that of the heart stopping transiently or of the occurrence of isolated forceful beats or both. This sensation is usually caused by premature ventricular contractions and the patient either feels the compensatory pause or the resultant more forceful subsequent beat or both. Occasionally, the individual feels the ectopic beat and refers to this phenomenon as "skipped" beats. The least frequent sensation reported by individuals, but the one most linked to the term *palpitation* is rapid heart rate that may be regular or irregular and is usually supraventricular in origin.

7. Cough—Although cough is usually associated with pulmonary disease processes, cardiac conditions that lead to pulmonary abnormalities may be the root cause of the cough. A cardiac cough is usually dry or nonproductive. Pulmonary fluid engorgement from conditions such as heart failure may present as cough. Pulmonary hypertension from any cause can result in cough. Finally, angiotensin-converting enzyme inhibitors, which are frequently used in cardiac conditions, can cause cough.

B. History

1. The present illness—This is a chronology of the events leading up to the patient's current complaints. Usually physicians start with the chief complaint and explore the patient's symptoms. It is especially important to determine the frequency, intensity, severity, and duration of all symptoms; their precipitating causes; what relieves them; and what aggravates them. Although information about previous related diseases and opinions from other physicians are often valuable, it is essential to explore the basis of any prior diagnosis and ask the patient about objective testing and the results of such testing. A history of prior treatment is often revealing because medications or surgery may indicate the nature of the original problem. A list should be made of all the patient's current medications, detailing the dosages, the frequency of administration, whether they are helping the patient, any side effects, and their cost.

2. Antecedent conditions—Several systemic diseases may have cardiac involvement. It is therefore useful to search for a history of rheumatic fever, which may manifest as Sydenham's chorea, joint pain and swelling, or merely frequent sore throats. Other important diseases that affect the heart include metastatic cancer, thyroid disorders, diabetes mellitus, and inflammatory diseases such as rheumatoid arthritis and systemic lupus erythematosus. Certain events during childhood are suggestive of congenital or acquired heart disease; these include a history of cyanosis, reduced exercise tolerance, or long periods of restricted activities or school absence. Exposure to toxins, infectious agents, and other noxious substances may also be relevant.

3. Atherosclerotic risk factors—Atherosclerotic cardiovascular disease is the most common form of heart disease in industrialized nations. The presenting symptoms of this ubiquitous disorder may be unimpressive and minimal, or as impressive as sudden death. It is therefore important to determine from the history whether any risk factors for this disease are present. The most important are a family history of atherosclerotic disease, especially at a young age; diabetes mellitus; lipid disorders such as a high cholesterol level; hypertension; and smoking. Less important factors include a lack of exercise, high stress levels, the type-A personality, and truncal obesity.

4. Family history—A family history is important for determining the risk for not only atherosclerotic cardiovascular disease but for many other cardiac diseases as well. Congenital heart disease, for example, is more common in the offspring of parents with this condition, and a history of the disorder in the antecedent family or siblings is significant. Other genetic diseases, such as neuromuscular disorders or connective tissue disorders (eg, Marfan's syndrome) can affect the heart. Acquired diseases such as rheumatic valve disease can cluster in families because of the spread of the streptococcal infection among family members. The lack of a history of hypertension in the family might prompt a more intensive search for a secondary cause. A history of atherosclerotic disease sequelae such as limb loss, strokes, and heart attacks may provide a clue to the aggressiveness of an atherosclerotic tendency in a particular family group.

Physical Findings

A. PHYSICAL EXAMINATION

The physical examination is less important than the history in patients with ischemic heart disease, but it is of critical value in patients with congenital and valvular heart disease. In the latter two categories, the physician can often make specific anatomic and etiologic diagnoses based on the physical examination. Certain abnormal murmurs and heart sounds are specific for structural abnormalities of the heart. The physical examination is also important for confirming the diagnosis and establishing the severity of heart failure, and it is the only way to diagnose systemic hypertension because this diagnosis is based on elevated blood pressure recordings.

1. Blood pressure—Proper measurement of the **systemic arterial pressure** by cuff sphygmomanometry is one of the keystones of the cardiovascular physical examination. We recommend that the brachial artery be palpated and the diaphragm of the stethoscope be placed over it, rather than merely sticking the stethoscope in the antecubital fossa. Current methodologic standards dictate that the onset and disappearance of the Korotkoff sounds define the systolic and diastolic pressures, respectively. Although this is the best approach in most cases, there are exceptions. For example, in patients in whom the diastolic pressure drops to near zero, the point of muffling of the sounds is usually recorded as the diastolic pressure. Because the diagnosis of systemic hypertension involves repeated measures under the same conditions, the operator should record the arm used and the position of the patient to allow reproducible measurements to be made on serial visits.

If the blood pressure is to be taken a second time, the patient should be in another position, such as standing, to determine any orthostatic changes in blood pressure. Orthostatic changes are a very important physical finding, especially in patients complaining of transient central nervous system symptoms, weakness, or unstable gait. The technique involves having the patient assume the upright position for at least 90 s before taking the pressure to be sure that the maximum orthostatic effect is measured. Although measuring the pressure in other extremities may be of value in certain vascular diseases, it provides little information in a routine examination beyond palpating pulses in all the ex-

tremities. Keep in mind, in general, that the pulse pressure (the difference between systolic and diastolic blood pressures) is a crude measure of left ventricular stroke volume. A widened pulse pressure suggests that the stroke volume is large; a narrowed pressure, that the stroke volume is small.

2. Peripheral pulses—When examining the peripheral pulses, the physician is really conducting three examinations. The first is an examination of the cardiac rate and rhythm, the second is an assessment of the characteristics of the pulse as a reflection of cardiac activity, and the third is an assessment of the adequacy of the arterial conduit being examined. The pulse rate and rhythm are usually determined in a convenient peripheral artery, such as the radial. If a pulse is irregular, it is better to auscultate the heart; some cardiac contractions during rhythm disturbances do not generate a stroke volume sufficient to cause a palpable peripheral pulse. In many ways, the heart rate reflects the health of the circulatory system. A rapid pulse suggests increased catecholamine levels, which may be due to cardiac disease, such as heart failure; a slow pulse represents an excess of vagal tone, which may be due to disease or athletic training.

To assess the characteristics of the cardiac contraction through the pulse, it is usually best to select an artery close to the heart, such as the carotid. Bounding high-amplitude carotid pulses suggest an increase in stroke volume and should be accompanied by a wide pulse pressure on the blood pressure measurement. A weak carotid pulse suggests a reduced stroke volume. Usually the strength of the pulse is graded on a scale of 1 to 4, where 2 is a normal pulse amplitude, 3 or 4 is a hyperdynamic pulse, and 1 is a weak pulse. A low-amplitude, slow-rising pulse, which may be associated with a palpable vibration (thrill), suggests aortic stenosis. A bifid pulse (beating twice in systole) can be a sign of hypertrophic obstructive cardiomyopathy, severe aortic regurgitation, or the combination of moderately severe aortic stenosis and regurgitation. A dicrotic pulse (an exaggerated, early, diastolic wave) is found in severe heart failure. Pulsus alternans (alternate strong and weak pulses) is also a sign of severe heart failure. When evaluating the adequacy of the arterial conduits, all palpable pulses can be assessed and graded on a scale of 0 to 4, where 4 is a fully normal conduit, and anything below that is reduced, including 0—which indicates an absent pulse. The major pulses routinely palpated on physical examination are the radial, brachial, carotid, femoral, dorsalis pedis, and posterior tibial. In special situations, the abdominal aorta and the ulnar, subclavian, popliteal, axillary, temporal, and intercostal arteries are palpated. In assessing the abdominal aorta, it is important to make note of the width of the aorta because an increase suggests an abdominal aortic aneurysm. It is particularly important to palpate the abdominal aorta in older individuals because abdominal aortic aneurysms are more prevalent in those older than 70. An audible bruit is a clue to significantly obstructed large arteries. During a routine examination, bruits are sought with the bell of the stethoscope placed over the carotids, abdominal aorta, and femorals at the groin. Other arteries may be auscultated under special circumstances, such as suspected temporal arteritis or vertebrobasilar insufficiency.

3. Jugular venous pulse—Assessment of the jugular venous pulse can provide information about the central venous pressure and right-heart function. Examination of the right internal jugular vein is ideal for assessing central venous pressure because it is attached directly to the superior vena cava without intervening valves. The patient is positioned into the semiupright posture that permits visualization of the top of the right internal jugular venous blood column. The height of this column of blood, vertically from the sternal angle, is added to 5 cm of blood (the presumed distance to the center of the right atrium from the sternal angle) to obtain an estimate of central venous pressure in centimeters of blood. This can be converted to millimeters of mercury (mm Hg) with the formula:

$$mm\ Hg = cm\ blood \times 0.736.$$

Examining the characteristics of the right internal jugular pulse is valuable for assessing right-heart function and rhythm disturbances. The normal jugular venous pulse has two distinct waves: *a* and *v;* the former coincides with atrial contraction and the latter with late ventricular systole. An absent *a* wave and an irregular pulse suggest atrial fibrillation. A large and early *v* wave suggests tricuspid regurgitation. The dips after the *a* and *v* waves are the *x* and *y* descents; the former coincide with atrial relaxation and the latter with early ventricular filling. In tricuspid stenosis the *y* descent is prolonged. Other applications of the jugular pulse examination are discussed in the chapters dealing with specific disorders.

4. Lungs—Evaluation of the lungs is an important part of the physical examination: Diseases of the lung can affect the heart, just as diseases of the heart can affect the lungs. The major finding of importance is rales at the pulmonary bases, indicating alveolar fluid collection. Although this is a significant finding in patients with congestive heart failure, it is not always possible to distinguish rales caused by heart failure from those caused by pulmonary disease. The presence of pleural fluid, although useful in the diagnosis of heart failure, can be due to other causes. Heart failure most commonly causes a right pleural effusion; it can cause effusions on both sides but is least likely to cause isolated left pleural effusion. The specific constellation of dullness at the left base with bronchial breath sounds suggests an increase in heart size from pericardial effusion (Ewart's sign) or another cause of cardiac enlargement; it is thought to be due to compression by the heart of a left lower lobe bronchus.

When right-heart failure develops or venous return is restricted from entering the heart, venous pressure in the abdomen increases, leading to hepatosplenomegaly and eventually ascites. None of these physical findings is specific for heart disease; they do, however, help establish the diagnosis. Heart failure also leads to generalized fluid retention, usually manifested as lower extremity edema or, in severe heart failure, anasarca.

5. Cardiac auscultation—Heart sounds are caused by the acceleration and deceleration of blood and the subsequent vibration of the cardiac structures during the phases of the cardiac cycle. To hear cardiac sounds, use a stethoscope with a bell and a tight diaphragm. Low-frequency sounds are associated with ventricular filling and are heard best with the bell. Medium-frequency sounds are associated with valve opening and closing; they are heard best with the diaphragm. Cardiac murmurs are due to turbulent blood flow, are usually high-to-medium frequency, and are heard best with the diaphragm. Low-frequency atrioventricular valve inflow murmurs, such as that produced by mitral stenosis, are best heard with the bell, however. Auscultation should take place in areas that correspond to the location of the heart and great vessels. Such placement will, of course, need to be modified for patients with unusual body habitus or an unusual cardiac position. When no cardiac sounds can be heard over the precordium, they can often be heard in either the subxiphoid area or the right supraclavicular area.

Auscultation in various positions is recommended because low-frequency filling sounds are best heard with the patient in the left lateral decubitus position, and high-frequency murmurs, such as that of aortic regurgitation, are best heard with the patient sitting.

a. Heart sounds—The **first heart sound** is coincident with mitral and tricuspid valve closure and has two components in up to 40% of normal individuals. There is little change in the intensity of this sound with respiration or position. The major determinant of the intensity of the first heart sound is the electrocardiographic PR interval, which determines the time delay between atrial and ventricular contraction and thus the position of the mitral valve when ventricular systole begins. With a short PR interval, the mitral valve is widely open when systole begins, and its closure increases the intensity of the first sound, as compared to a long PR-interval beat when the valve partially closes prior to the onset of ventricular systole. Certain disease states, such as mitral stenosis, also can increase the intensity of the first sound.

The **second heart sound** is coincident with closure of the aortic and pulmonic valves. Normally, this sound is single in expiration and split during inspiration, permitting the aortic and pulmonic components to be distinguished. The inspiratory split is due to a delay in the occurrence of the pulmonic component because of a decrease in pulmonary vascular resistance, which prolongs pulmonary flow beyond the end of right ventricular systole. Variations in this normal splitting of the second heart sound are useful in determining certain disease states. For example, in atrial septal defect, the second sound is usually split throughout the respiratory cycle because of the constant increase in pulmonary flow. In patients with left bundle branch block, a delay occurs in the aortic component of the second heart sound, which results in reversed inspiratory splitting; single with inspiration, split with expiration.

A **third heart sound** occurs during early rapid filling of the left ventricle; it can be produced by any condition that causes left ventricular volume overload or dilatation. It can therefore be heard in such disparate conditions as congestive heart failure and normal pregnancy. A **fourth heart sound** is due to a vigorous atrial contraction into a stiffened left ventricle and can be heard in left ventricular hypertrophy of any cause or in diseases that reduce compliance of the left ventricle, such as myocardial infarction.

Although third and fourth heart sounds can occasionally occur in normal individuals, all other extra sounds are signs of cardiac disease. Early ejection sounds are due to abnormalities of the semilunar valves, from restriction of their motion, thickening, or both (eg, a bicuspid aortic valve, pulmonic or aortic stenosis). A midsystolic click is often due to mitral valve prolapse and is caused by sudden tensing in midsystole of the redundant prolapsing segment of the mitral leaflet. The opening of a thickened atrioventricular valve leaflet, as in mitral stenosis, will cause a loud opening sound (snap) in early diastole. A lower frequency (more of a knock) sound at the time of rapid filling may be an indication of constrictive pericarditis. These early diastolic sounds must be distinguished from a third heart sound.

b. Murmurs—Systolic murmurs are very common and do not always imply cardiac disease. They are usually rated on a scale of 1 to 6, where grade 1 is barely audible, grade 4 is associated with palpable vibrations (thrill), grade 5 can be heard with the edge of the stethoscope, and grade 6 can be heard without a stethoscope. Most murmurs fall in the 1–3 range, and murmurs in the 4–6 range are almost always due to pathologic conditions; severe disease can exist with grades 1–3 or no cardiac murmurs, however. The most common systolic murmur is the crescendo/decrescendo murmur that increases in intensity as blood flows early in systole and diminishes in intensity through the sec-

ond half of systole. This murmur can be due to vigorous flow in a normal heart or to obstructions in flow, as occurs with aortic stenosis, pulmonic stenosis, or hypertrophic cardiomyopathy. The so-called innocent flow murmurs are usually grades 1–2 and occur very early in systole; they may have a vibratory quality and are usually less apparent when the patient is in the sitting position (when venous return is less). If an ejection sound is heard, there is usually some abnormality of the semilunar valves. Although louder murmurs may be due to pathologic cardiac conditions, this is not always so. Distinguishing benign from pathologic systolic flow murmurs is one of the major challenges of clinical cardiology. Benign flow murmurs can be heard in 80% of children; the incidence declines with age, but may be prominent during pregnancy or in adults who are thin or physically well trained. The murmur is usually benign in a patient with a soft flow murmur that diminishes in intensity in the sitting position and neither a history of cardiovascular disease nor other cardiac findings.

The **holosystolic,** or **pansystolic,** murmur is almost always associated with cardiac pathology. The most common cause of this murmur is atrioventricular valve regurgitation, but it can also be observed in conditions such as ventricular septal defect, in which an abnormal communication exists between two chambers of markedly different systolic pressures. Although it is relatively easy to determine that these murmurs represent an abnormality, it is more of a challenge to determine their origins. Keep in mind that such conditions as mitral regurgitation, which usually produce holosystolic murmurs, may produce crescendo/decrescendo murmurs, adding to the difficulty in differentiating benign from pathologic systolic flow murmurs.

Diastolic murmurs are always abnormal. The most frequently heard diastolic murmur is the high-frequency decrescendo early murmur of aortic regurgitation. This is usually heard best at the upper left sternal border or in the aortic area (upper right sternal border) and may radiate to the lower left sternal border and the apex. This murmur is usually very high frequency and may be difficult to hear. Although the murmur of pulmonic regurgitation may sound like that of aortic regurgitation when pulmonary artery pressures are high, it is usually best heard in the pulmonic area (left second intercostal space parasternally). If structural disease of the valve is present with normal pulmonary pressures, the murmur usually has a midrange frequency and begins with a slight delay after the pulmonic second heart sound. Mitral stenosis produces a low-frequency rumbling diastolic murmur that is decrescendo in early diastole, but may become crescendo up to the first heart sound with moderately severe mitral stenosis and sinus rhythm. The murmur is best heard at the apex in the left lateral decubitus position with the bell of the stethoscope. Similar findings are heard in tricuspid stenosis, but the murmur is loudest at the lower left sternal border.

A **continuous murmur** implies a connection between a high- and a low-pressure chamber throughout the cardiac cycle, such as occurs with a fistula between the aorta and the pulmonary artery. If the connection is a patent ductus arteriosus, the murmur is heard best under the left clavicle; it has a machine-like quality. Continuous murmurs must be distinguished from the combination of systolic and diastolic murmurs in patients with combined lesions (eg, aortic stenosis and regurgitation).

Traditionally, the origin of heart murmurs was based on five factors: (1) their timing in the cardiac cycle, (2) where on the chest they were heard, (3) their characteristics, (4) their intensity, and (5) their duration. Unfortunately, this traditional classification system is unreliable in predicting the underlying pathology. A more accurate method, **dynamic auscultation,** changes the intensity, duration, and characteristics of the murmur by bedside maneuvers that alter hemodynamics.

The simplest of these maneuvers is observation of any changes in murmur intensity with normal respiration because all right-sided cardiac murmurs should increase in intensity with normal inspiration. Although some exceptions exist, the method is very reliable for detecting such murmurs. Inspiration is associated with reductions in intrathoracic pressure that increase venous return from the abdomen and the head, leading to an increased flow through the right heart chambers. The consequent increase in pressure increases the intensity of right-sided murmurs. These changes are best observed in the sitting position, where venous return is smallest, and changes in intrathoracic pressure can produce their greatest effect on venous return. In a patient in the supine position, when venous return is near maximum, there may be little change observed with respiration. The ejection sound caused by pulmonic stenosis does not routinely increase in intensity with inspiration. The increased blood in the right heart accentuates atrial contraction, which increases late diastolic pressure in the right ventricle, partially opening the stenotic pulmonary valve and thus diminishing the opening sound of this valve with the subsequent systole.

Changes in position are an important part of normal auscultation; they can also be of great value in determining the origin of cardiac murmurs (Table 1–2). Murmurs dependent on venous return, such as innocent flow murmurs, are softer or absent in upright positions; others, such as the murmur associated with hypertrophic obstructive cardiomyopathy, are accentuated by reduced left ventricular volume. In physically capable individuals, a rapid squat from the standing position is often diagnostically valuable because it suddenly increases venous return and left ventricular volume and accentuates flow murmurs but diminishes the murmur of hypertrophic obstructive cardiomyopathy. The stand-squat maneuver is also useful for altering the timing of the midsystolic click caused by mitral valve prolapse during systole. When the ventricle is small during standing, the prolapse occurs earlier in systole, moving the midsystolic click to early systole. During squatting, the ventricle dilates and the prolapse is delayed in systole, resulting in a late midsystolic click.

Valsalva's maneuver is also frequently used. The patient bears down and expires against a closed glottis, in-

Table 1–2. Differentiation of systolic murmurs based on changes in their intensity from physiologic maneuvers.

Maneuver	Origin of Murmur					
	Flow	TR	AS	MR/VSD	MVP	HOCM
Inspiration	– or ↑	↑	–	–	–	–
Stand	↓	–	–	–	↑	↑
Squat	↑	–	–	–	↓	↓
Valsalva	↓	↓	↓	↓	↑	↑
Handgrip/TAO	↓	–	–	↑	↑	↓
Post–PVC	↑	–	↑	–	–	↑

AS = aortic stenosis; Flow = innocent flow murmur; HOCM = hypertrophic obstructive cardiomyopathy; MR = mitral regurgitation; MVP = mitral valve prolapse; PVC = premature ventricular contraction; TAO = transient arterial occlusion; TR = tricuspid regurgitation; VSD = ventricular septal defect; ↑ or ↓ = change in intensity of murmur; – = no consistent change.

creasing intrathoracic pressure and markedly reducing venous return to the heart. Although almost all cardiac murmurs decrease in intensity during this maneuver, there are two exceptions: (1) The murmur of hypertrophic obstructive cardiomyopathy may become louder because of the diminished left ventricular volume. (2) The murmur associated with mitral regurgitation from mitral valve prolapse may become longer and louder because of the earlier occurrence of prolapse during systole. When the maneuver is very vigorous and prolonged, even these two murmurs may eventually diminish in intensity. Therefore, the Valsalva maneuver should be held for only about 10 s, so as not to cause prolonged diminution of the cerebral and coronary blood flow.

Isometric hand grip exercises have been used to increase arterial and left ventricular pressure. These maneuvers increase the flow gradient for mitral regurgitation, ventricular septal defect, and aortic regurgitation; the murmurs should then increase in intensity. Increasing arterial and left ventricular pressure increases left ventricular volume, thereby decreasing the murmur of hypertrophic obstructive cardiomyopathy. If the patient is unable to perform isometric exercises, **transient arterial occlusion** of both upper extremities with sphygmomanometers can achieve the same increases in left-sided pressure.

Noting the changes in murmur intensity in the heart beat following a premature ventricular contraction, and comparing these to a beat that does not, can be extremely useful. The premature ventricular contraction interrupts the cardiac cycle, and during the subsequent compensatory pause, an extralong diastole occurs, leading to increased left ventricular filling. Because of this, the murmurs of hypertrophic cardiomyopathy and mitral valve prolapse decrease in intensity, and murmurs caused by the flow of blood out of the left ventricle increase in intensity. There is usually no change in the intensity of the murmur of typical mitral regurgitation because blood pressure falls during the long pause and increases the gradient between the left ventricle and the aorta, allowing more forward flow. This results in the same amount of mitral regurgitant flow as on a normal beat with a higher aortic pressure and less forward flow. The increased volume during the long pause goes out of the aorta rather than back into the left atrium. Unfortunately, there is no reliable way of inducing a premature ventricular contraction in most patients; it is fortuitous when a physician is present for one. Atrial fibrillation with markedly varying cycle lengths produces the same phenomenon and can be very helpful in determining the origin of murmurs.

Various rapid-acting pharmacologic agents have been used to clarify the origin of cardiac murmurs. A once-popular bedside pharmacologic maneuver was the inhalation of amyl nitrite. Because this produces rapid vasodilatation and decreases in blood pressure, it diminishes the murmurs of aortic and mitral regurgitation and ventricular septal defect and increases systolic flow murmurs (eg, those caused by aortic stenosis and hypertrophic obstructive cardiomyopathy). Although patients never liked the unpleasant odor of amyl nitrite, it became a popular recreational drug in the 1970s; its popularity has since waned. Other pharmacologic maneuvers have occasionally been used to clarify the origin of a murmur. These include the infusion of synthetic catecholamines to increase blood pressure, isoproterenol to increase the heart rate, and intravenous β-blockers to decrease the heart rate. With the ready availability of echocardiography, these more invasive interventions have also diminished in popularity.

Crawford MH: Examination of the Heart. Part 2: Inspection and Palpation of Venous and Arterial Pulses. American Heart Association, 1990.

Grewe K, Crawford MH, O'Rourke RA et al: Differentiation of cardiac murmurs by dynamic auscultation. Curr Probl Cardiol 1988;13:675.

Schlant RC, Hurst JW: Examination of the Heart. Part 3: Examination of the Precordium: Inspection and Palpation. American Heart Association, 1990.

Shaver JA, et al: Examination of the Heart. Part 4: Auscultation of the heart. American Heart Association, 1990.

Silverman ME: Examination of the heart. Part 1: The clinical history. The American Heart Association, 1990.

B. DIAGNOSTIC STUDIES

1. Electrocardiography—Electrocardiography (ECG) is perhaps the least expensive of all cardiac diagnostic tests, providing considerable value for the money. Modern electrocardiogram-reading computers do an excellent job of measuring the various intervals between waveforms and calculating the heart rate and the left ventricular axis. These programs fall considerably short, however, when it comes to diagnosing complex ECG patterns and rhythm disturbances, and the test results must be read by a physician skilled at ECG interpretation.

Analysis of cardiac rhythm is perhaps the ECG's most widely used feature; it is used to clarify the mechanism of an irregular heart rhythm detected on physical examination or that of an extremely rapid or slow rhythm. The ECG is also used to monitor cardiac rate and rhythm; Holter monitoring and other continuous-ECG monitoring devices allow assessment of cardiac rate and rhythm on an ambulatory basis. ECG radio telemetry is also often used on hospital wards and between ambulances and emergency rooms to assess and monitor rhythm disturbances. There are two types of ambulatory ECG recorders: continuous recorders that record all heart beats over 24 or more hours and intermittent recorders that can be attached to the patient for weeks for months and then activated to provide brief recordings of infrequent events. In addition to analysis of cardiac rhythm, ambulatory ECG recordings can be used to detect ST-wave transients indicative of myocardial ischemia and certain electrophysiologic parameters of diagnostic and prognostic value. The most common use of ambulatory ECG monitoring is the evaluation of symptoms such as syncope, near-syncope, or palpitation for which there is no obvious cause and cardiac rhythm disturbances are suspected.

The ECG is an important tool for rapidly assessing **metabolic and toxic disorders** of the heart. Characteristic changes in the ST-T waves indicate imbalances of potassium and calcium. Drugs such as procainamide and the tricyclic antidepressants have characteristic effects on the QT and QRS intervals at toxic levels. Such observations on the ECG can be life-saving in emergency situations with comatose patients or cardiac arrest victims.

Chamber enlargement can be assessed through the characteristic changes of left or right ventricular and atrial enlargement. Occasionally, isolated signs of left atrial enlargement on the ECG may be the only diagnostic clue to mitral stenosis. Evidence of chamber enlargement on the ECG usually signifies an advanced stage of disease with a poorer prognosis than that of patients with the same disease but no discernible enlargement.

The ECG is an important tool in managing **acute myocardial infarction.** In patients with chest pain that is compatible with myocardial ischemia, the characteristic ST-T-wave elevations that do not resolve with nitroglycerin (and are unlikely to be the result of an old infarction) become the basis for thrombolytic therapy or primary angioplasty. Rapid resolution of the ECG changes of myocardial infarction after reperfusion therapy has prognostic value and identifies patients with reperfused coronary arteries.

Evidence of **conduction abnormalities** may help explain the mechanism of bradyarrhythmias and the likelihood of the need for a pacemaker. Conduction abnormalities may also aid in determining the cause of heart disease. For example, right bundle branch block and left anterior fascicular block are often seen in Chagas' cardiomyopathy, and left-axis deviation occurs in patients with a primum atrial septal defect.

A newer form of electrocardiography is the signal-averaged, or high-resolution, electrocardiogram. This device markedly accentuates the QRS complex so that low-amplitude afterpotentials, which correlate with a propensity toward ventricular arrhythmias and sudden death, can be detected. The signal-averaged ECG permits a more accurate measurement of QRS duration, which also has prognostic significance of established value in the stratification of risk of developing sustained ventricular arrhythmias in postmyocardial infarction patients, patients with coronary artery disease and unexplained syncope, and patients with nonischemic cardiomyopathy.

2. Echocardiography—Another frequently ordered cardiac diagnostic test, echocardiography is based on the use of ultrasound directed at the heart to create images of cardiac anatomy and display them in real time on a television screen or oscilloscope. Two-dimensional echocardiography is usually accomplished by placing an ultrasound transducer in various positions on the anterior chest and obtaining cross-sectional images of the heart and great vessels in a variety of standard planes. In general, two-dimensional echocardiography is excellent for detecting any anatomic abnormality of the heart and great vessels. In addition, because the heart is seen in real time, this modality can assess the function of cardiac chambers and valves throughout the cardiac cycle.

Transesophageal echocardiography (TEE) involves the placement of smaller ultrasound probes on a gastroscopic device for placement in the esophagus behind the heart; it produces much higher resolution images of posterior cardiac structures. TEE has made it possible to detect left atrial thrombi, small mitral valve vegetations, and thoracic aortic dissection with a high degree of accuracy.

The older analog echocardiographic display referred to as M-mode, motion-mode, or time-motion mode, is currently used for its high axial and temporal resolution. It is superior to two-dimensional echocardiography for measuring the size of structures in its axial direction, and its 1/1000-s sampling rate allows for the resolution of complex cardiac motion patterns. Its many disadvantages, including poor lateral resolution and the inability to distinguish whole heart motion from the motion of individual cardiac structures, have relegated it to a supporting role.

Doppler ultrasound can be combined with two-dimensional imaging to investigate blood flow in the heart and great vessels. It is based on determining the change in frequency (caused by the movement of blood in the given structure) of the reflected ultrasound compared with the transmitted ultrasound, and converting this difference into flow velocity. Color-flow Doppler echocardiography is most frequently used. In this technique, frequency shifts in each pixel of a selected area of the two-dimensional image are measured and converted into a color, depending on the direction of flow, the velocity, and the presence or absence of turbulent flow. When these color images are superimposed on the two-dimensional echocardiographic image, a moving color image of blood flow in the heart is created in real time. This is extremely useful for detecting regurgitant blood flow across cardiac valves and any abnormal communications in the heart.

Because color-flow imaging cannot resolve very high velocities, another Doppler mode must be used to quantitate the exact velocity and estimate the pressure gradient of the flow when high velocities are suspected. Continuous-wave Doppler, which almost continuously sends and receives ultrasound along a beam that can be aligned through the heart, is extremely accurate at resolving very high velocities such as those encountered with valvular aortic stenosis. The disadvantage of this technique is that the source of the high velocity within the beam cannot always be determined but must be assumed, based on the anatomy through which the beam passes. When there is ambiguity about the source of the high velocity, pulsed-wave Doppler is more useful. This technique is range-gated such that specific areas along the beam (sample volumes) can be investigated. One or more sample volumes can be examined and determinations made concerning the exact location of areas of high-velocity flow.

Two-dimensional echocardiographic imaging of dynamic left ventricular cross-sectional anatomy and the superimposition of a Doppler color-flow map provide more information than the traditional left ventricular cine-angiogram can. Ventricular wall motion can be interrogated in multiple planes, and left ventricular wall thickening during systole (an important measure of myocardial viability) can be assessed. In addition to demonstrating segmental wall motion abnormalities, echocardiography can estimate left ventricular volumes and ejection fraction. In addition, valvular regurgitation can be assessed at all four valves with the accuracy of the estimated severity equivalent to contrast angiography.

Doppler echocardiography has now largely replaced cardiac catheterization for deriving hemodynamics to estimate the severity of valve stenosis. Recorded Doppler velocities across a valve can be converted to pressure gradients by use of the simplified Bernoulli equation (pressure gradient = $4 \times$ velocity^2). Cardiac output can be measured by Doppler from the velocity recorded at cardiac anatomic sites of known size visualized on the two-dimensional echocardiographic image. Cardiac output and pressure gradient data can be used to calculate the stenotic valve area with remarkable accuracy. A complete echocardiographic examination including two-dimensional and M-mode anatomic and functional visualization, and color-, pulsed-, and continuous-wave Doppler examination of blood flow provides a considerable amount of information about cardiac structure and function. A full discussion of the usefulness of this technique is beyond the scope of this chapter, but individual uses of echocardiography will be discussed in later chapters.

Unfortunately, echocardiography is not without its technical difficulties and pitfalls. Like any noninvasive technique, it is not 100% accurate. Furthermore, it is impossible to obtain high-quality images or Doppler signals in as many as 5% of patients—especially those with emphysema, chest wall deformities, and obesity. Although TEE has made the examination of such patients easier, it does not solve all the problems of echocardiography. Despite these limitations, the technique is so powerful that it has moved out of the non-invasive laboratory and is now frequently being used in the operating room, the emergency room, and even the cardiac catheterization laboratory, to help guide procedures without the use of fluoroscopy.

3. Nuclear cardiac imaging—Nuclear cardiac imaging involves the injection of tracer amounts of radioactive elements attached to larger molecules or to the patient's own blood cells. The tracer-labeled blood is concentrated in certain areas of the heart, and a gamma ray detection camera is used to detect the radioactive emissions and form an image of the deployment of the tracer in the particular area. The single-crystal gamma camera produces planar images of the heart, depending on the relationship of the camera to the body. Multiple-head gamma cameras, which rotate around the patient, can produce single-photon emission computed tomography, displaying the cardiac anatomy in slices, each about 1-cm thick.

a. Myocardial perfusion imaging—The most common tracers used for imaging regional myocardial blood-flow distribution are thallium-201 and the technetium-99m-based agents, sestamibi and teboroxime. Thallium-201, a potassium analog that is efficiently extracted from the bloodstream by viable myocardial cells, is concentrated in the myocardium in areas of adequate blood flow and living myocardial cells. Thallium perfusion images show defects (a lower tracer concentration) in areas where blood flow is relatively reduced and in areas of damaged myocardial cells. If the damage is from frank necrosis or scar tissue formation, very little thallium will be taken up; ischemic cells may take up thallium more slowly or incompletely, producing relative defects in the image.

Myocardial perfusion problems are separated from nonviable myocardium by the fact that thallium eventually washes out of the myocardial cells and back into the circulation. If a defect detected on initial thallium imaging disappears over a period of 3–24 h, the area is presumably viable. A persistent defect suggests a myocardial scar. In addition to detecting viable myocardium and assessing the extent of new and old myocardial infarctions, thallium-201 imaging can also be used to detect myocardial ischemia during stress testing (see item 5. Stress Testing) as well as marked enlargement of the heart or dysfunction. The major problem with thallium imaging is photon attenuation because of chest wall structures, which can give an artifactual appearance of defects in the myocardium.

The technetium-99m-based agents take advantage of the shorter half-life of technetium (6 h; thallium

201's is 73 h); this allows for use of a larger dose, which results in higher energy emissions and higher quality images. Technetium-99m's higher energy emissions scatter less and are attenuated less by chest wall structures, reducing the number of artifacts. Because sestamibi undergoes considerably less washout after the initial myocardial uptake than thallium does, the evaluation of perfusion versus tissue damage requires two separate injections. Teboroxime, on the other hand, undergoes rapid washout after its initial accumulation in the myocardium, and imaging must be completed within 8 min after injection. It is used to detect rapid changes in the patient's status caused by dynamic changes in coronary patency that are produced by progression of the disease or the effects of treatment.

In addition to detecting perfusion deficits, myocardial imaging with the single-photon emission computed tomography (SPECT) system allows for a three-dimensional reconstruction of the heart, which can be displayed in any projection on a monitor screen. Such images can be formed at intervals during the cardiac cycle to create an image of the beating heart, which can be used to detect wall motion abnormalities and derive left ventricular volumes and ejection fraction. Matching wall motion abnormalities with perfusion defects provides additional confirmation that the perfusion defects visualized are true and not artifacts of photon attenuation. Also, extensive perfusion defects and wall motion abnormalities should be accompanied by decreases in ejection fraction.

b. Radionuclide angiography—Radionuclide angiography is based on visualizing radioactive tracers in the cavities of the heart over time. Radionuclide angiography is usually done with a single gamma camera in a single plane, and only one view of the heart is obtained. The most common technique is to record the amount of radioactivity received by the gamma camera over time and plot it. Although volume estimates by radionuclide angiography are not as accurate as those obtained by other methods, the ejection fraction is quite accurate. Wall motion can be assessed in the one plane imaged, but the technique is not as sensitive as other imaging modalities for detecting wall motion abnormalities.

Of the two basic techniques for performing radionuclide angiography, the oldest is the first-transit technique. This requires injecting a bolus of technetium-99m and observing its movement through the venous system into the right heart, pulmonary circulation, and finally to the left heart and the aorta. Because the sampling rate is relatively short in relation to the ECG R-R interval, it is possible to sample at least one cardiac cycle in each chamber of the heart. By determining the change in radioactivity over time, it is possible to measure the stroke volume or ejection fraction for each ventricle or chamber. The more popular radionuclide angiographic technique is multiple-gated ac-

quisition (MUGA), or equilibrium-gated blood pool, radionuclide angiography. In this approach, technetium-99m is used to label the patient's own red blood cells, which remain within the vascular space, allowing imaging studies to be acquired for several hours. Imaging acquisition is synchronized with the R wave of the ECG, so that the lower amounts of radioactivity generated from this equilibrium technique can be accumulated from beat to beat. Once enough counts are collected in each phase of the cardiac cycle, the camera computer generates a composite cardiac cycle, with the final time/activity curve and imaging representing a composite of approximately 200 heart beats. MUGA is well suited for exercise stress testing because one injection of isotope can be used for both the resting and the exercise studies. Because many heart beats must be collected, imaging during exercise must be done during steady-state periods, when no marked fluctuations are present in heart rate. One limitation of the technique is that sudden beat-to-beat changes in left ventricular performance are obscured by the averaging technique. Because ischemic heart disease often results in such changes, the exercise MUGA has lost favor as a technique for detecting ischemic heart disease, since its sensitivity is not as high as other techniques. Currently, the major use of MUGA is to assess left ventricular performance (ejection fraction), especially in patients with technically inadequate echocardiograms.

4. Other cardiac imaging

a. Plain-film chest radiography—Plain-film chest radiography is used infrequently now for evaluating cardiac structural abnormalities because of the superiority of echocardiography in this regard. The chest x-ray film, however, has no equal for assessing pulmonary anatomy and is very useful for evaluating pulmonary venous congestion and hypoperfusion or hyperperfusion. In addition, abnormalities of the thoracic skeleton are found in certain cardiac disorders and radiographic corroboration may help with the diagnosis. Detection of intracardiac calcium deposits by the x-ray film or fluoroscopy is of some value in finding coronary artery, valvular, or pericardial disease.

b. Computed tomographic scanning—Computed tomography (CT) has been applied to cardiac imaging, but the image suffers because of the motion of the heart. Computed tomography has done a better job with evaluating the thoracic aorta and the pericardium, which are less mobile than the heart. Both these structures are more accurately evaluated with magnetic resonance imaging (MRI), however. Electron beam computed tomography (EB-CT) solves some of the motion problems and can be used more successfully for cardiac imaging. The major application of this newer technology to date has been the detection of small amounts of coronary artery calcium as an indicator of atherosclerosis in the coronary arterial tree. Although this technique has tremendous potential, its actual clinical utility, compared with other standard approaches is controversial.

c. Magnetic resonance imaging—Magnetic resonance imaging (MRI) probably has the most potential as a technique for evaluating cardiovascular disease. It is excellent for detecting aortic dissection and pericardial thickening and assessing left ventricular mass. Newer computer analysis techniques have solved the problem of myocardial motion and can be used to detect flow in the heart, much as color-flow Doppler is used. In addition, regional molecular disturbances can be created that place stripes of a different density in either the myocardium or the blood; these can then be followed through the cardiac cycle to determine structural deformation (eg, of the left ventricular wall) or the movement of the blood. When its full potential is reached, MRI might well compete successfully, in terms of image quality and information obtained, with Doppler echocardiography. Unfortunately, MRI studies take a long time to perform and are not readily done in sick patients who need a bedside evaluation; it is not likely to replace echocardiography in the near future.

d. Positron emission tomography—Positron emission tomography (PET) is a technique using tracers that simultaneously emit two high-energy photons. A circular array of detectors around the patient can detect these simultaneous events and accurately identify their origin in the heart. This results in improved spatial resolution, compared with single-photon emission computed tomography. It also allows for correction of tissue photon attenuation, resulting in the ability to accurately quantify radioactivity in the heart. PET scanning can be used to assess myocardial perfusion and myocardial metabolic activity separately by using different tracers coupled to different molecules. Most of the tracers developed for clinical use require a cyclotron for their generation; the cyclotron must be in close proximity to the PET imager because of the short half-life of the agents. Agents in clinical use include oxygen-15 (half-life 2 min), nitrogen-13 (half-life 10 min), carbon-11 (half-life 20 min) and fluorene-18 (half-life 110 min). These tracers can be coupled to many physiologically active molecules for assessing various functions of the myocardium. Because rubidium-82, with a half-life of 75 s, does not require a cyclotron and can be generated on-site, it is frequently used with PET scanning, especially for perfusion images. Ammonia containing nitrogen-13 and water containing oxygen-15 are also used as perfusion agents. C-11-labeled fatty acids and ^{18}F fluorodeoxyglucose are common metabolic tracers used to assess myocardial viability, and acetate containing carbon-11 is often used to assess oxidative metabolism.

The main clinical uses of PET scanning involve the evaluation of coronary artery disease. It is used in perfusion studies at rest and during pharmacologic stress (exercise studies are less feasible). In addition to a qualitative assessment of perfusion defects, PET allows for a calculation of absolute regional myocardial blood flow or blood flow reserve. PET also assesses myocardial viability, using the metabolic tracers to detect metabolically active myocardium in areas of reduced perfusion. The presence of viability imply that returning perfusion to these areas would result in improved function of the ischemic myocardium. Although many authorities consider PET scanning the gold standard for determining myocardial viability, it has not been found to be 100% accurate. Thallium reuptake techniques and echocardiographic and MR imaging of wall-thickening characteristics have proved equally valuable for detecting myocardial viability in clinical studies.

5. Stress testing—Stress testing in various forms is most frequently applied in cases of suspected or overt ischemic heart disease (Table 1–3). Because ischemia represents an imbalance between myocardial oxygen supply and demand, exercise or pharmacologic stress increases myocardial oxygen demand and reveals an inadequate oxygen supply (hypoperfusion) in diseased coronary arteries. Stress testing can thus induce detectable ischemia in patients with no evidence of ischemia at rest. It is also used to determine cardiac reserve in patients with valvular and myocardial disease. Deterioration of left ventricular performance during exercise or other stresses suggests a diminution in cardiac reserve that would have therapeutic and prognostic implications. Although most stress test studies use some technique (Table 1–4) for directly assessing the myocardium, it is important not to forget the symptoms of angina pectoris or extreme dyspnea: light-headedness or syncope can be equally important in evaluating patients. Physical findings such as the development of pulmonary rales, ventricular gallops, murmurs, peripheral cyanosis, hypotension, excessive increases in heart rate, or inappropriate decreases in heart rate also have diagnostic and prognostic value. It is therefore important that a symptom assessment and physical examination always be done before, during, and after stress testing.

Table 1–3. Indications for stress testing.

Evaluation of exertional chest pain
Assess significance of known coronary artery disease
Risk stratification of ischemic heart disease
Determine exercise capacity
Evaluate other exercise symptoms

Table 1–4. Methods of detecting myocardial ischemia during stress testing.

Electrocardiography
Echocardiography
Myocardial perfusion imaging
Position emission tomography
Magnetic resonance imaging

Table 1–5. Types of stress tests.

Exercise
 Treadmill
 Bicycle
Pharmacologic
 Adenosine
 Dipyridamole
 Dobutamine
 Isoproterenol
Other
 Pacing

Electrocardiographic monitoring is the most common cardiac evaluation technique used during stress testing; it should be part of every stress test in order to assess heart rate and detect any arrhythmias. In patients with normal resting ECGs, diagnostic ST depression of myocardial ischemia has a fairly high sensitivity and specificity for detecting coronary artery disease in symptomatic patients if adequate stress is achieved (peak heart rate at least 85% of the patient's maximum predicted rate, based on age and gender). Exercise ECG testing is an excellent low-cost screening procedure for patients with chest pain consistent with coronary artery disease, normal resting ECGs, and the ability to exercise to maximal age- and gender-related levels.

A **myocardial imaging** technique is usually added to the exercise evaluation in patients whose ECGs are abnormal or, for some reason, less accurate. It is also used for determining the location and extent of myocardial ischemia in patients with known coronary artery disease. Imaging techniques, in general, enhance the sensitivity and specificity of the tests but are still not perfect, with false-positives and -negatives occurring 5–10% of the time.

Which adjunctive myocardial imaging technology to choose depends on the quality of the tests, their availability and cost, and the services provided by the laboratory. If these are all equal, the decision should be based on patient characteristics. For example, echocardiography might be appropriate for a patient suspected of developing ischemia during exercise profound enough to depress segmental left ventricular performance and worsen mitral regurgitation. On the other hand, in a patient with known three-vessel coronary artery disease and recurrent angina after revascularization, perfusion scanning might be the best test to determine which coronary artery is producing the symptoms.

Choosing the appropriate form of stress is also important (Table 1–5). Exercise, the preferred stress for increasing myocardial oxygen demand, also simulates the patient's normal daily activities and is therefore highly relevant clinically. There are essentially only two reasons for not choosing exercise stress, however: the patient's inability to exercise adequately because of physical or psychologic limitations; or the chosen test cannot be performed readily with exercise (eg, PET

scanning). In these situations, pharmacologic stress is appropriate.

6. Cardiac catheterization—Cardiac catheterization is now mainly used for the assessment of coronary artery anatomy by coronary angiography. In fact, the cardiac catheterization laboratory has become more of a therapeutic than a diagnostic arena. Once significant coronary artery disease is identified, a variety of catheter-based interventions can be used to alleviate the obstruction to blood flow in the coronary arteries. At one time, hemodynamic measurements (pressure, flow, oxygen consumption) were necessary to accurately diagnose and quantitate the severity of valvular heart disease and intracardiac shunts. Currently, Doppler echocardiography has taken over this role almost completely, except in the few instances when Doppler studies are inadequate or believed to be inaccurate. Catheter-based hemodynamic assessments are still useful for differentiating cardiac constriction from restriction, despite advances in Doppler echocardiography. Currently, the catheterization laboratory is also more often used as a treatment arena for valvular and congenital heart disease. Certain stenotic valvular and arterial lesions can be treated successfully with catheter-delivered balloon expansion.

Myocardial biopsy is necessary to treat patients with heart transplants and is occasionally used to diagnose selected cases of suspected acute myocarditis. For this purpose, a biotome is usually placed in the right heart and several small pieces of myocardium are removed. Although this technique is relatively safe, myocardial perforation occasionally results.

7. Electrophysiologic testing—Electrophysiologic testing uses catheter-delivered electrodes in the heart to induce rhythm disorders and detect their structural basis. Certain arrhythmia foci and structural abnormalities that facilitate rhythm disturbances can be treated by catheter-delivered radiofrequency energy (ablation) or by the placement of various electronic devices that monitor rhythm disturbances and treat them accordingly through either pacing or internally delivered defibrillation shocks. Electrophysiologic testing and treatment now dominate the management of arrhythmias; the test is more accurate than the surface ECG for diagnosing many arrhythmias and detecting their substrate, and catheter ablation and electronic devices have been more successful than pharmacologic approaches at treating arrhythmias.

8. Test selection—In the current era of escalating health-care costs, ordering multiple tests is rarely justifiable, and the physician must pick the one test that will best define the patient's problem. Unfortunately, cardiology offers multiple competing technologies that often address the same issues, but only in a different way. The following five principles should be followed when considering which test to order:

- What information is desired? If the test is not reasonably likely to provide the type of information needed to help the patient's problem, it should not be done, no matter how inexpensive and easy it is to obtain. At one time, for example, routine preoperative ECGs were done prior to major noncardiac surgery to detect which patients might be at risk for cardiac events in the perioperative period. Once it was determined that the resting ECG was not good at this, the practice was discontinued, despite its low cost and ready availability.

- What is the cost of the test? If two tests can provide the same information and one is much more expensive than the other, the less expensive test should be ordered. For example, to determine whether a patient's remote history of prolonged chest pain was a myocardial infarction, the physician has a choice of an ECG or one of several imaging tests, such as echocardiography, resting thallium-201 scintigraphy, and the like. Because the ECG is the least expensive test, it should be performed for this purpose in most situations.

- Is the test available? Sometimes the best test for the patient is not available in the given facility. If it is available at a nearby facility and the patient can go there without undue cost, the test should be obtained. If expensive travel is required, the costs and benefits of that test versus local alternatives need to be carefully considered.

- What is the level of expertise of the laboratory and the physicians who interpret the tests? For many of the high-technology imaging tests, the level of expertise considerably affects the value of the test. Myocardial perfusion imaging is a classic example of this. Some laboratories are superlative in producing tests of diagnostic accuracy. In others, the numbers of false-positives and -negatives is so high as to render the tests almost worthless.

Therefore, even though a given test may be available and inexpensive and could theoretically provide essential information, if the quality of the laboratory is not good, an alternative test should be sought.

- What quality of service is provided by the laboratory? Patients are customers, and they need to be satisfied. If a laboratory makes the patients wait a long time, if it is tardy in getting the results to the physicians, or if great delays occur in accomplishing the test, choose an alternative lab (assuming, of course, that alternatives are available). Poor service cannot be tolerated.

Many other situations and considerations affect the choice of tests. For example, a young patient with incapacitating angina might have a high likelihood of having single-vessel disease that would be amenable to catheter-based revascularization. It might be prudent to take this patient directly to coronary arteriography with an eye toward diagnosing and treating the patient's disease in one setting for maximum cost-effectiveness. This approach, however, presents the risk of ordering an expensive catheterization rather than a less-expensive noninvasive test if the patient does not have significant coronary disease. If an assessment of left ventricular global performance is desirable in a patient known to need coronary arteriography, the assessment could be done by left ventricular cine-angiography at the time of cardiac catheterization. This would avoid the extra expense of echocardiography if it was not otherwise indicated. Physicians are frequently solicited to use the latest emerging technologies, which often have not been proved better than the standard techniques. It is generally unwise to begin using these usually more expensive methods until clinical trials have established their efficacy and cost-effectiveness.

Akhtar M: AHA Examination of the heart (Part 5)—The electrocardiogram. American Heart Association, 1990.

Cain M et al: ACC Expert consensus document: Signal-averaged electrocardiography. J Am Coll Cardiol 1996;27:238–249.

Cheitlin M, Albert JS, Armstrong WF et al: ACC/AHA guidelines for the clinical application of echocardiography: Executive summary—A report of the American College of Cardiology/American Heart Association task force on practice guidelines (Committee on Clinical Application of Echocardiography). J Am Coll Cardiol 1997;29:862–879.

Crawford MH, Berstein SJ, Deedwania PC et al: ACC/AHA guidelines for ambulatory electrocardiography: A report of the American College of Cardiology/American Heart Association task force on practice guidelines (Committee to Revise the Guidelines for Ambulatory Electrocardiography). J Am Coll Cardiol 1999;34:912–948.

Gibbons RJ, Balady GJ, Beasley JW et al: ACC/AHA guidelines for exercise testing: Executive summary: A report of the American College of Cardiology/American Heart Association task force on practice guidelines (Committee on Exercise Testing). Circulation 1997;96:345–354.

Grundy SM, Pasternak R, Greenland P et al: ACC/AHA scientific statement: Assessment for cardiovascular risk by use of multiple-risk-factor assessment equations; A statement for healthcare professionals from the American Heart Association and the American College of Cardiology. J Am Coll Cardiol 1999;34:1348–1359.

O'Rourke R, Brundage BH, Froelicher VF et al: ACC/AHA expert consensus document: American College of Cardiology/American Heart Association expert consensus document on electron-beam computed tomography for the diagnosis and prognosis of coronary artery disease. J Am Coll Cardiol 2000;36:326–340.

Ritchie JL, Bateman TM, Bonow RO et al: ACC/AHA task force report: Guidelines for clinical use of cardiac radionuclide imaging; report of the American college of Cardiology/American Heart Association task force on assessment of diagnostic and therapeutic cardiovascular procedures (Committee on Radionuclide Imaging), developed in collaboration with the American Society of Nuclear Cardiology. J Am Coll Cardiol 1995;25:521–547.

Scanlon PJ, Faxon DP, Audet AM et al: ACC/AHA practice guidelines: ACC/AHA guidelines for coronary angiography: A report of the American College of Cardiology/American Heart Association task force on practice guidelines (Committee on Coronary Angiography); Developed in collaboration with the Society of Cardiac Angiography and Interventions. J Am Coll Cardiol 1999;33:1756–1824.

Schlant RC, Adolph RJ, DiMarco JP et al: ACC/AHA guidelines for electrocardiography: A report of the American College of Cardiology/American Heart Association Task Force on Assessment of Diagnostic and Therapeutic Cardiovascular Procedures (Committee on Electrocardiography). J Am Coll Cardiol 1992;19:473–481.

Zipes DP, DiMarco JP, Gillette PC et al: ACC/AHA Task Force Report: Guidelines for clinical intracardiac electrophysiological and catheter ablation procedures; a report on the American College of Cardiology/American Heart Association Task Force on Practice Guidelines (Committee on Clinical Intracardiac Electrophysiologic and Catheter Ablation Procedures), developed in collaboration with the North American Society of Pacing and Electrophysiology. J Am Coll Cardiol 1995;26:555–573.

Lipid Disorders

2

Peter C. Chien, MD & William H. Frishman, MD

ESSENTIALS OF DIAGNOSIS

- *Total serum cholesterol greater than 200 mg/dL on two samples at least 2 weeks apart*
- *LDL cholesterol greater than 100 mg/dL*
- *HDL cholesterol less than 40 mg/dL*
- *Triglycerides greater than 200 mg/dL*

General Considerations

In recent years, a great deal of emphasis has been placed on the relationship between elevated serum cholesterol levels—especially low-density lipoprotein cholesterol (LDL-C)—and the incidence of coronary artery disease (CAD). Hyperlipidemia represents a public health epidemic that continues to parallel the increased prevalence of obesity and is intimately im-plicated in the development of CAD. It is estimated that approximately 100 million American adults have total serum cholesterol levels in excess of 200 mg/dL and more than 12 million adults would qualify for lipid-lowering therapy by current national standards. Lowering LDL levels through diet and medication has been shown to reduce the progression of CAD and CAD mortality. According to the Framingham study, a 10% decrease in cholesterol level is associated with a 2% decrease in incidence of CAD morbidity and mortality.

A. LIPOPROTEINS

The major circulatory forms of cholesterol, cholesterol ester and triglyceride, are both insoluble in water; to circulate in an aqueous environment they combine with phospholipids and proteins in complexes known as lipoproteins. The protein components of these com-plexes, *apoproteins,* play an important role in the inter-action between cell surface lipases and the lipoprotein receptors necessary for lipid catabolism. The six major classes of lipoproteins are listed in Table 2–1.

Table 2–1. Lipoprotein classes and composition.

| Lipoprotein | Density (water = 1.000) | Composition (Weight %) | | | |
		C	TG	Protein	Major Apoprotein
Chylomicron	0.940	5	85–90	1–2	B-48, E, C-11
VLDL	0.940–1.006	20	60–70	5–10	B-100, E, C-11
Chylomicron remnant	1.006–1.019	30	30	15–20	B–48, E
VLDL remnant (IDL)	1.006–1.019	30	30	15–20	B-100, E
LDL	1.019–1.063	50–60	4–8	20	B-100
HDL	1.063–1.210	15–20	2–7	45–55	A-1, A-11

C = cholesterol; TG = triglyceride; VLDL = very low-density lipoprotein; IDL = intermediate-density lipoprotein; LDL = low-density lipoprotein; HDL = high-density lipoprotein.

Source: Reproduced, with permission, from Frishman WH et al: Lipids and lipoproteins: Atherosclerotic risk and management. In Frishman WH, ed: Medical Management of Lipid Disorders: Focus on Prevention of Coronary Artery Disease. Armonk, NY: Futura, 1992.

1. Lipoprotein metabolism—Lipoprotein metabolism can be divided into exogenous and endogenous pathways, as shown in Figure 2–1.

a. Exogenous pathway—The exogenous pathway is mainly responsible for absorption of dietary fat in the postprandial state and its subsequent distribution to the tissues. It begins with the absorption of dietary cholesterol and free fatty acids in intestinal microvilli, where they are converted to cholesterol esters and triglycerides, respectively, and packaged into chylomicrons that are secreted into the lymphatic system and enter the systemic circulation. In the capillaries of adipose tissue and muscle, the chylomicrons interact with an enzyme, lipoprotein lipase, which cleaves core triglycerides into mono- and diglycerides and free fatty acids that are taken up by surrounding tissue. Triglyceride hydrolysis reduces the core size of the chylomicron, resulting in an excess of surface components that are transferred to high-density lipoprotein (HDL). The remaining particle, a chylomicron remnant, is greatly reduced in size; it contains approximately equal amounts of cholesterol and triglycerides, and it acquires atherogenic potential.

The chylomicrons are rapidly removed from the circulation by the liver in a receptor-mediated process.

The cholesterol can also be secreted, as bile acids, into the bile.

b. Endogenous pathway—The endogenous pathway delivers cholesterol and triglyceride to the tissues in the fasting state. It begins with the synthesis and secretion of very-low-density lipoprotein (VLDL) by the liver. This triglyceride-rich lipoprotein, which is smaller than the chylomicron, also interacts with lipoprotein lipase in the capillaries, adipose tissue, and muscle. Triglycerides within the core of the particle are cleaved and taken up by the surrounding fat and muscle; the redundant surface components are transferred to the HDL fractions. The remaining particle (VLDL remnant, or intermediate-density lipoprotein [IDL]), is a smaller lipoprotein, similar to the chylomicron remnant in its lipid composition and atherogenic potential. Approximately 50% of VLDL remnants are removed by the liver through the LDL receptor, which recognizes apoprotein E or the VLDL remnant. The highly atherogenic LDL contains mostly cholesterol ester and only one apoprotein, B-100. Its function is the delivery of cholesterol to tissues that require it (gonads, adrenals, rapidly dividing cells). The liver also plays a role in removing LDL from the blood via the LDL receptor. Two thirds of LDL is removed in this fashion; the re-

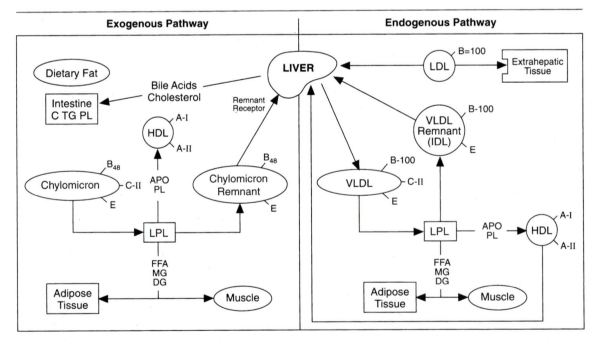

Figure 2–1. Exogenous and endogenous pathways of lipoprotein metabolism. C = cholesterol; TG = triglyceride; MG = monoglyceride; DG = diglyceride; FFA = free fatty acid; LPL = lipoprotein lipase; APO = apolipoprotein; PL = phospholipids. Reproduced, with permission, from Mitchel Y: Evaluation and treatment of lipid disorders. Prac Diabetol 1987;6:6.

mainder is removed by a non-LDL-receptor-mediated pathway in Kupffer cells, smooth muscle cells, and macrophages. It is believed that this mode of LDL uptake contributes to the development of foam cells and atherosclerosis. HDL, which seems to exert a protective effect against the development of atherosclerosis, is synthesized in both the liver and intestine and receives components during the lipoprotein lipase reaction. HDL is composed of approximately 50% protein (apoprotein A-I, A-II) and 20% cholesterol and comprises two major subfractions in the blood: HDL_2 and HDL_3. The latter is a small, dense particle that is believed to be the precursor of the larger cholesterol-enriched HDL_2. The transfer of surface components during the lipoprotein lipase reaction is felt to be important in the formation of HDL_2 and HDL_3. HDL_2 is believed to exert its protective effect through its participation in reverse cholesterol transport (picking up cholesterol from the cells involved in the atherosclerotic process and delivering them to the liver for excretion). HDL levels are higher in premenopausal women than in men, contributing to the lower incidence of CAD in women. There has been recent interest in cholesterol ester transfer protein, which is involved with the enzyme lecithin cholesterol acyl transferase in driving the reverse cholesterol transport process in moving cholesterol from peripheral tissues into plasma and then back into the liver.

B. Lipoprotein(a)

Lipoprotein(a), a variation of LDL, is formed by two components: an LDL-like particle with apoprotein B-100 and a hydrophilic protein moiety known as *apoprotein(a)*, which has a close structural homology with plasminogen. It may cause a perturbation in the thrombolytic system by binding to and displacing plasminogen from binding sites on fibrin, fibrinogen, and cell surfaces. It inhibits plasminogen activation by tPA through stearic hindrance of tPA-binding sites.

Accumulation of lipoprotein(a) has been found in atherosclerotic lesions, and it is now believed to be an atherogenic lipoprotein. Elevated plasma levels greater than 30 mg/dL in humans appear to be associated with an increased risk for the development of CAD, with a rate of occurrence estimated to be two to five times greater than in normal controls. Lipoprotein(a) is thought to be inherited by autosomal codominance. Some studies restrict identification of lipoprotein(a) as a risk factor for CAD only in the setting of elevated plasma LDL levels. Others have found the condition to be an independent risk factor. Diet, age, sex, smoking, body mass index, and apoprotein E polymorphism have not been found to correlate with plasma levels of lipoprotein(a). Increased lipoprotein(a) levels have been noted in patients with diabetes mellitus or nephrotic syndrome and immediately following myocardial in-

farction. In other studies, no changes have been observed in lipoprotein(a) levels in patients with acute myocardial infarction or unstable angina. Of the hypolipidemic interventions, niacin, neomycin, and extracorporeal removal of cholesterol have been shown to affect elevated lipoprotein(a) levels. Estrogen and fenofibrate may also reduce lipoprotein(a) levels.

C. Lipoproteins and Atherosclerosis

Current concepts in atherosclerosis suggest that oxidation of LDL is involved in its pathogenesis. It is hypothesized that the critical role of oxidized LDL in atherogenesis is due to its rapid uptake by the foam cells lining the arterial intima, which are thought to have macrophage-like properties. The LDL is then oxidized, exerting a chemotactic effect on monocytes, leading to more uptake of LDL and thus to the formation of the atherosclerotic plaque. The endothelial cells and smooth muscles can also oxidize LDL.

Support for this lipid oxidation hypothesis comes from evidence that antioxidants such as vitamin E inhibit formation of lesions in hypercholesterolemic rabbits. Observations in some population studies also show an association between low plasma vitamin E levels and CAD incidence. However, clinical trials have not substantiated a reduction in the rates of fatal or nonfatal myocardial infarction with daily vitamin E use.

Clinical Findings

A. History

A history of lipid disorders should be sought in all routine evaluations and in patients with suspected or overt cardiovascular disease. Many individuals already know they have high cholesterol levels from screening tests performed at shopping malls, in other physicians' offices, or during prior hospitalization. A family history of premature cardiovascular disease is also useful. A history compatible with overt cardiovascular disease, especially in a young man or a premenopausal woman is highly suggestive of a lipoprotein disorder. In addition, a history or symptoms of other diseases associated with lipoprotein abnormalities (eg, diabetes mellitus, hypothyroidism, end-stage renal disease) should be sought (Table 2–2). Other risk factors for CAD should also be identified because they multiply the risk caused by lipid disorders (Table 2–3).

B. Physical Examination

Most individuals with lipid disorders have no specific physical findings. Depending on the duration and severity of the lipid disorder, they may have overt evidence of lipid deposition in the integument that follows certain phenotypes (I–V), as originally proposed by Frederickson and Lees. Eruptive xanthomas occur

Table 2–2. Some acquired causes of hyperlipidemia.

Condition	Liproprotein Accumulating	Lipid Phenotype	HDL Level
Diabetes			
Type 1 DM	Chylomicron, VLDL	↑TG	↓
Type 2 DM	VLDL	↑TG	↓
Obesity	VLDL	↑TG	– or ↓
Alcohol	VLDL	↑TG	– or ↑
Oral contraceptives	VLDL	↑TG	– or ↑
Hypothyroidism	LDL	↑C	–
Nephrotic syndrome	VLDL, LDL	↑TG, ↑C	– or ↑
Renal failure	VLDL, LDL	↑TG, ↑C	– or ↓
Primary biliary cirrhosis	LDL	↑C	
Acute hepatitis	VLDL	↑TG	

C = cholesterol; DM = diabetes mellitus; HDL = high-density lipoprotein; LDL = low-density lipoprotein; TG = triglyceride; VLDL = very low-density lipoprotein.

↑ = increase; ↓ = decrease; – = no change.

Source: Reproduced, with permission, from Frishman WH et al: Lipids and lipoproteins: Atherosclerotic risk and management. In Frishman WH, ed: Medical Management of Lipid Disorders: Focus on Prevention of Coronary Artery Disease. Armonk, NY: Futura, 1992.

when triglyceride levels are high; they are seen in types I (increased chylomicrons caused by lipoprotein lipase deficiency), IV (familial combined hyperlipidemia), and V (familial hypertriglyceridemia). Tendon xanthomas are characteristic of type II (familial hypercholesterolemia) patients, who can also have tuberous xanthomas and xanthelasma; the latter, however, is nonspecific and can be found in individuals with normal lipid levels. Palmar and tuberoeruptive xanthomas are characteristic of type III (familial dysbetalipoproteinemia).

C. LABORATORY ASSESSMENT

The Expert Panel Report of the National Cholesterol Education Program on Detection, Evaluation, and Treatment of High Blood Cholesterol in Adults (NCEP) suggests that a fasting lipid profile should be obtained in all adults 20 years of age or older at least once every 5 years. Without a family history of premature CAD or a history of familial hyperlipidemia, cholesterol screening should not be done routinely in children. Cholesterol values in the general pediatric population may not always predict the future development of hypercholesterolemia in adults.

For many years clinicians depended on total cholesterol and triglyceride measurements to determine specific patient treatment regimens. More sophisticated lipoprotein measurements were available only in re-

search facilities. Recent advances have made lipoprotein subclass and apoprotein determinations available from many clinical laboratories.

LDL-C has been shown to be a more accurate predictor of CAD risk than is total-C. Low levels of HDL-C and the subfractions HDL_2 and HDL_3 have also been shown to be more powerful than total-C in predicting CAD. Levels of plasma apoproteins are also accurate predictors of CAD risk. It is controversial whether increases in plasma apoprotein B levels (the major apoprotein of LDL) and decreases in levels of apoproteins A-I and A-II (the major apoproteins of HDL) are better predictors of increased coronary risk than are total-C, HDL-C, LDL-C, or the ratio of total-C to HDL-C.

Nonetheless, a patient's risk of CAD can be adequately estimated by an accurate total-C measurement and a calculated LDL-C determination. (Mean serum cholesterol and calculated LDL-C values for various population groups have been reported on by the National Center for Health Statistics.)

Serum total-C levels can be measured at any time of day in the nonfasting state because total-C concentrations do not vary appreciably after eating. Patients who are acutely ill, losing weight, or pregnant or who recently had a myocardial infarction or stroke should be studied at a later time because cholesterol levels may be suppressed. Venipuncture should

Table 2–3. Risk factors that modify LDL-cholesterol goals[a]

Major risk factors (exclusive of LDL-C)	
Cigarette smoking	
Hypertension (blood pressure ≥140/90 mm Hg or on antihypertensive medication)	
Low HDL-C (<40 mg/dL)[b]	
Family history of premature CAD (CAD in male first-degree relative <55 years; CAD in female first-degree relative <65 years)	
Age (men ≥45 years; women ≥55 years)	
Categories of risk	**LDL goal (mg/dL)**
CAD and CAD risk equivalents	<100
Multiple (2+) risk factors	<130
0–1 risk factor	<160

[a] Diabetes is regarded as a CAD risk equivalent.

[b] HDL cholesterol ≥60 mg/dL counts as a "negative" risk factor; its presence removes one risk factor from the total count.

LDL = low-density lipoprotein; HDL = high-density lipoprotein; CAD = coronary artery disease.

Source: Adapted, with permission, from Expert Panel on Detection, Evaluation and Treatment of High Blood Cholesterol in Adults: Executive summary of the Third Report of the NCEP Expert Panel on Detection, Evaluation and Treatment of High Blood Cholesterol in Adults (Adult Treatment Panel III). JAMA 2001;285:2487 (Tables 3, 4 combined).

be carried out in patients who have been in the sitting position for at least 5 min, with the tourniquet applied for the briefest time possible. The blood may be collected as either serum or plasma. The National Cholesterol Education Program has established guidelines for standardization of lipid and lipoprotein measurements because of the great variations in accuracy at different laboratories that have been reported. The recommendation is that intralaboratory precision and accuracy for cholesterol determinations be no more than 3%. In a recent study assessing compact chemical analyzers for routine office determinations, some of the machines tested were shown to have accuracy and precision above the older (1988) target of 5% variance. A rapid capillary blood (fingerstick) methodology for cholesterol measurement is currently under development and evaluation.

LDL-C measurements are usually indirectly derived from the following formula:

$$\text{LDL–C (mg/dL)} = \text{Total–C (mg/dL)} - \text{HDL–C (mg/dL)} - \text{triglyceride (mg/dL)} \div 5$$

When using this formula with mm/L units, divide the triglyceride value by 2.3.

A reliable direct method for measuring LDL-C is needed because the accuracy of indirect estimates of LDL-C reflects measurements of total-C, HDL-C, and triglycerides, each of which contributes some degree of imprecision. Because triglyceride values are influenced by food, the patient should fast for at least 12 h before blood is taken for the LDL-C determination. If the triglyceride values are higher than 4.52 mm/L (> 400 mg/dL), the LDL-C value will be even less accurate. Direct measurement of LDL in a specialized laboratory, using ultracentrifugation, may be necessary when significant hypertriglyceridemia persists despite fasting.

Tests are now available for specific apolipoproteins. These tests have proven to be accurate predictors of cardiovascular risk in various research studies. Unfortunately, until more is known about their utility in clinical practice, they should not be used in routine clinical management.

Davis CE, Rifkind BM, Brenner H, et al: A single cholesterol measurement underestimates the risk of coronary heart disease. An empirical example from the Lipid Research Clinics Mortality Follow-Up Study. JAMA 1990;264:3044.

Expert Panel on Detection, Evaluation, and Treatment of High Blood Cholesterol in Adults: Executive summary of the third report of the National Cholesterol Education Program (NCEP) expert panel on detection, evaluation, and treatment of high blood cholesterol in adults (Adult Treatment Panel III). JAMA 2001;285:2486.

Frishman WH, Zimetbaum P: Lipid-lowering drugs. In: Frishman WH, Sonnenblick EH, eds. *Cardiovascular Pharmacotherapeutics.* New York: McGraw Hill, 1997:399.

Frishman WH: Medical Management of Lipid Disorders: Focus on Prevention of Coronary Artery Disease. Mt. Kisco: Futura Publishing, 1992.

Lauer RM, Clarke WR: Use of cholesterol measurements in childhood for the prediction of adult hypercholesterolemia. The Muscatine Study. JAMA 1990;264:3034.

Virtamo J, Rapola JM, Ripatti S et al: Effect of vitamin E and beta-carotene on the incidence of primary nonfatal myocardial infarction and fatal coronary heart disease. Arch Intern Med 1998;158:668.

Treatment

A. RATIONALE FOR TREATMENT

The rationale of treatment of hyperlipidemia is based on the hypothesis that abnormalities in lipid and lipoprotein levels are risk factors for CAD and that changes in blood lipids can decrease the risk of disease and complications. Levels of plasma cholesterol and LDL have consistently been shown to directly correlate with the risk of CAD. Since the promulgation of the previous NCEP (Adult Treatment Panel II) guidelines, the results of numerous studies involving the primary and secondary prevention of CAD with 3-hydroxy-3-methylglutaryl coenzyme A (HMG-CoA) reductase inhibitors have been reported. These trials have overwhelmingly demonstrated a significant reduction in CAD events, CAD mortality, and mortality from all other causes, in addition to ameliorating LDL-C, HDL-C, and triglyceride levels. Data from the West of Scotland Coronary Prevention Study and from the Air Force/Texas Coronary Atherosclerosis Prevention Study have provided cogent evidence that primary prevention of CAD in hypercholesterolemic individuals reduces the incidence of coronary events and, in the former study, death from cardiovascular events. Secondary prevention trials such as the Scandinavian Simvastatin Survival Study (4S) and Long-Term Intervention with Pravastatin in Ischemic Disease (LIPID) study have revealed that lowering LDL cholesterol levels can retard the progression of coronary atherosclerosis and reduce CAD events, CAD mortality, and cerebrovascular events. These compelling data have prompted a more aggressive approach to the treatment of hyperlipidemia, culminating in the new NCEP (Adult Treatment Panel III [ATP III]) guidelines (Table 2–4). Although ATP III maintains attention to intensive treatment of patients with CAD, its major new focus is on primary prevention in patients with multiple risk factors (Table 2–5).

Epidemiologic studies and clinical trials are consistent in supporting the observation that for individuals with serum cholesterol levels in the 6.47–7.76 mm/L (250–300 mg/dL) range, each 1% reduction in serum cholesterol would yield about a 2% reduction in the rate of combined morbidity and mortality from coronary heart disease. The absolute magnitude of these benefits would even be greater in those individuals having other risk factors for CAD, such as cigarette smoking and hypertension. These risk relationships are the basis for recommending lower cholesterol cutpoints and goals for those who are at high risk for developing coronary heart disease.

Recent meta-analyses have indicated that triglycerides are an independent risk factor for the development of CAD. In addition, serum triglyceride levels are inversely related to HDL levels, and a reduction in triglyceride levels is associated with a rise in HDL. Raising HDL may protect against CAD, therefore providing an additional rationale for treating hypertriglyceridemia.

Downs JR, Clearfield M, Weis S et al: Primary prevention of acute coronary events with lovastatin in men and women with average cholesterol levels: results of AFCAPS/TexCAPS. JAMA 1998;279:1615.

The Long-Term Intervention with Pravastatin in Ischemic Heart Disease (LIPID) Study Group: Prevention of cardiovascular

Table 2–4. ATP III classification of LDL, total and HDL cholesterol (mg/dL).

LDL cholesterol	
<100	Optimal
100–129	Near or above optimal
130–159	Borderline high
160–189	High
≥190	Very high
Total cholesterol	
<200	Desirable
200–239	Borderline high
≥240	High
HDL cholesterol	
<40	Low
≥60	High

ATP = adult treatment panel; HDL = high-density lipoprotein; LDL = low-density lipoprotein.

Source: Reprinted, with permission, from Expert Panel on Detection, Evaluation and Treatment of High Blood Cholesterol in Adults: Executive summary of the Third Report of the NCEP Expert Panel on Detection, Evaluation and Treatment of High Blood Cholesterol in Adults (Adult Treatment Panel III). JAMA 2001; 285:2487.

events and death with pravastatin in patients with coronary artery disease and a broad range of initial cholesterol levels. N Engl J Med 1998;339:1357.

Scandinavian Simvastatin Survival Study Group: Randomized trial of cholesterol lowering in 4444 patients with coronary heart disease: The Scandinavian Simvastatin Survival Study (4S). Lancet 1994;344:1383.

Shepherd J, Cobbe SM, Ford I et al: Prevention of coronary heart disease with pravastatin in men with hypercholesterolemia. N Engl J Med 1995;333:1301.

B. TREATMENT GUIDELINES

1. Hypercholesterolemia—The NCEP has classified all adult patients into those with desirable cholesterol values (5.17 mm/L [<200 mg/dL]), borderline high blood cholesterol values (5.17–6.18 mm/L [200–239 mg/dL]), and high blood cholesterol values (6.21 mm/L [≥240 mg/dL]) (see Table 2–4). LDL-C values of <2.58 mm/L (100 mg/dL) are considered optimal; those between 2.58 and 3.36 mm/L (100–129 mg/dL) are near optimal; those between 3.36 and 4.11 mm/L (130–159 mg/dL) are borderline high; those between 4.13 and 4.88 mm/L (160–189 mg/dL) are high; and those greater than or equal to 4.91 mm/L (190 mg/dL)

Table 2–5. New features of ATP III.

Focus on multiple risk factors
Raises persons with diabetes without CAD, most of whom have multiple risk factors, to the risk level of CAD risk equivalent
Uses Framingham projections of 10-year absolute CAD risk (ie, the percent probability of having a CAD event in 10 years) to identify certain patients with multiple (2+) risk factors for more intensive treatment
Identifies persons with multiple metabolic risk factors (metabolic syndrome) as candidates for intensified therapeutic lifestyle changes
Modifications of lipid and lipoprotein classification
Identifies LDL cholesterol <100 mg/dL as optimal
Raises categorical low HDL cholesterol from <35 mg/dL to <40 mg/dL because the latter is a better measure of a depressed HDL
Lowers the triglyceride classification cutpoints to give more attention to moderate elevations
Support for implementation
Recommends a complete lipoprotein profile (total, LDL and HDL cholesterol and triglycerides) as the preferred initial test, rather than screening for total cholesterol and HDL alone
Encourages use of plant stanols/sterols and viscous (soluble) fibers as therapeutic dietary options to enhance lowering of LDL cholesterol
Presents strategies for promoting adherence to therapeutic lifestyle changes and drug therapies
Recommends treatment beyond LDL lowering for persons with triglycerides ≥200 mg/dL

ATP = Adult Treatment Panel; CAD = coronary artery disease; HDL = high-density lipoprotein; LDL = low-density lipoprotein.
Source: Reprinted, with permission, from Expert Panel on Detection, Evaluation and Treatment of High Blood Cholesterol in Adults: Executive summary of the Third Report of the NCEP Expert Panel on Detection, Evaluation and Treatment of High Blood Cholesterol in Adults (Adult Treatment Panel III). JAMA 2001; 285; 2487.

are very high. HDL-C values of less than 1.03 mm/L (40 mg/dL) are considered to be low, and those greater than or equal to 1.54 mm/L (60 mg/dL) are considered to be high.

The NCEP recommends an approach in adults based on LDL-cholesterol levels (Figure 2–2, Table 2–6). Management should always begin with dietary intervention, as outlined in Table 2–7. When response to diet is inadequate, the NCEP recommends the addition of pharmacologic therapy (Figure 2–3).

2. Hypertriglyceridemia—Non-HDL cholesterol, comprising LDL and VLDL, is a secondary treatment goal in patients with hypertriglyceridemia (levels > 200 mg/dL). The non-HDL cholesterol goal is set at 30 mg/dL higher than the LDL target level. Triglyceride values of less than 1.69 mm/L (150 mg/dL) are regarded as optimal; those from 1.69 to 2.25 mm/L (150–199 mg/dL) are borderline high; those from 2.26 to 5.64 mm/L (200–499 mg/dL) are high; and values greater than or equal to 5.65 mm/L (500 mg/dL) are considered to be very high. A link between plasma triglycerides and disease is most apparent in patients

with severe hypertriglyceridemia with chylomicronemia. These patients are prone to abdominal pain and pancreatitis. Both changes in lifestyle (control of weight, increased physical activity, restriction of alcohol, restriction of dietary fat to 10–20% of total caloric intake, reduction of high carbohydrate intake) and drug therapy are often required.

Much of hypertriglyceridemia (2.82–5.65 mm/L [250–500 mg/dL]) is due to various exogenous or secondary factors (see Table 2–2), which include alcohol, diabetes mellitus, hypothyroidism, obesity, chronic renal disease, and drugs. Changes in lifestyle or treatment of the primary disease process may be sufficient to reduce triglyceride levels.

Patients with high triglycerides that is familial in origin (type IV) are not at risk for premature CAD. Caloric restriction and increased exercise should be instituted as first-line therapies. Patients with familial combined hyperlipoproteinemia often have mild hypertriglyceridemia and are at risk of premature coronary heart disease. These patients should have dietary treatment first, followed, if necessary, by drugs. Patients with high triglycerides and clinical manifestations of

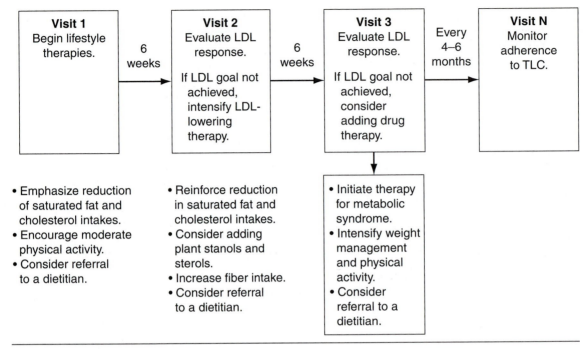

LDL = low-density lipoprotein.

Figure 2–2. Model of steps in therapeutic lifestyle changes (TLC). Reprinted, with permission, from: Expert Panel on Detection, Evaluation and Treatment of High Blood Cholesterol in Adults: Executive summary of the Third Report of the NCEP Expert Panel on Detection, Evaluation and Treatment of High Blood Cholesterol in Adults (Adult Treatment Panel III). JAMA 2001; 285; 2491 (Fig. 1).

Table 2–6. LDL cholesterol goals and cutpoints for therapeutic lifestyle changes (TLC) and drug therapy in different risk categories.

Risk Category	LDL Goal (mg/dL)	LDL Level at Which to Initiate TLC (mg/dL)	LDL Level at Which to Consider Drug Therapy (mg/dL)
CHD or CHD risk equivalents (10-y risk >20%)	<100	≥100	≥130 (100–129 drug optional)[a]
2+ risk factors (10-y risk ≤20%)	<130	≥130	10-y risk 10–20%: ≥130
			10-y risk <10%: ≥160
0–1 risk factor[b]	<160	≥160	≥190 (160–189 LDL-lowering drug optional)

CHD = coronary heart disease; LDL = low-density lipoprotein.

[a] Some authorities recommend use of LDL lowering drugs in this category if an LDL cholesterol level of <100 mg/dL cannot be achieved by TLC. Others prefer use of drugs that primarily modify triglycerides and HDL, eg, nicotinic acid or fibrate. Clinical judgement also may call for deferring drug therapy in this subcategory.

[b] Almost all people with 0–1 risk factor have a 10-y risk <10%; thus, 10-y risk assessment in people with 0–1 risk factor is not necessary.

Source: Reprinted, with permission, from Expert Panel on Detection, Evaluation and Treatment of High Blood Cholesterol in Adults: Executive summary of the Third Report of the NCEP Expert Panel on Detection, Evaluation and Treatment of High Blood Cholesterol in Adults (Adult Treatment Panel III). JAMA 2001;285; 2490.

Table 2–7. Nutrient composition of the therapeutic lifestyle changes (TLC) diet.

Nutrient	Recommended Intake
Saturated fat[a]	<7% of total calories
Polyunsaturated fat	Up to 10% of total calories
Monounsaturated fat	Up to 20% of total calories
Total fat	25–35% of total calories
Carbohydrate[b]	50–60% of total calories
Fiber	20–30 g/day
Protein	Approximately 15% of total calories
Cholesterol	<200 mg/day
Total calories[c]	Balance energy intake and expenditure to maintain desirable body weight and prevent weight gain.

[a] *Trans* fatty acids are another LDL-raising fat that should be kept at a low intake.
[b] Carbohydrates should be derived predominantly from foods rich in complex carbohydrates, including grains, especially whole grains, fruits, and vegetables.
[c] Daily energy expenditure should include at least moderate physical activity (contributing approximately 200 kcal/day).

Source: Reprinted, with permission, from Expert Panel on Detection, Evaluation and Treatment of High Blood Cholesterol in Adults: Executive summary of the Third Report of the NCEP Expert Panel on Detection, Evaluation and Treatment of High Blood Cholesterol in Adults (Adult Treatment Panel III). JAMA 2001; 285: 2490.

CAD can be treated as though they have familial combined hyperlipoproteinemia.

3. Low serum HDL cholesterol—A low serum HDL cholesterol level has emerged as the strongest single lipoprotein predictor of coronary heart disease. Although clinical trials suggest that raising HDL will reduce the risk of CAD, the evidence is insufficient at this time to specify the goal of therapy. The major causes of reduced serum HDL-C are shown in Table 2–8. Clearly, attempts should be made to raise low HDL-C by nonpharmacologic means. When a low HDL is associated with an increased VLDL, therapeutic modification of the latter should be considered, but attempts to raise HDL levels by drugs when there are no other associated risk factors cannot be justified.

4. Coronary artery disease—
a. Myocardial infarction—Numerous trials have demonstrated the efficacy of employing HMG-CoA reductase inhibitors in the primary and secondary prevention of CAD. Lipid-lowering agents especially bene-

fit hypercholesterolemic patients at the greatest risk for coronary events—those with CAD and CAD equivalents, such as diabetes mellitus, symptomatic cerebrovascular disease, abdominal aortic aneurysm, and peripheral vascular disease. The NCEP now classifies these conditions as tantamount to having established CAD because of their high prevalence of overt and subclinical atherosclerosis. The goal LDL for CAD and its equivalents is less than 2.6 mm/L (100 mg/dL), and dietary modification should be implemented in patients exceeding this target level, with concurrent initiation of drug therapy also being a consideration. Patients should obtain a fasting lipid profile within 24 h of the onset of an acute coronary syndrome or several weeks after the event because LDL levels may remain depressed and yield spurious results. It is recommended that drug therapy be initiated whenever a patient is hospitalized and found to have an LDL-C above 100 mg/dL.

b. Coronary artery bypass grafts—Progressive atherosclerosis has been identified as the single most important cause of occlusion of saphenous vein coronary artery grafts; it is found in approximately two thirds of grafts within 10 years. Low HDL-C, high LDL-C, and high apolipoprotein B are the most significant predictors of atherosclerotic disease in grafts. Many investigators believe that internal mammary artery bypass grafting is the coronary bypass procedure of choice because atherosclerosis progresses less rapidly with these grafts than with saphenous veins. Moreover, lipid-lowering therapy may improve the patency of bypass grafts. The Coronary Artery Bypass Graft Trial demonstrated that aggressive LDL reduction as compared to moderate LDL reduction attenuated the progression of atherosclerosis in saphenous vein coronary artery bypass grafts. It also concluded that low-dose warfarin was ineffective in achieving this end-point.

c. Coronary angioplasty—Restenosis after successful coronary angioplasty has been observed in 25–40% of patients undergoing this procedure. Restenosis after angioplasty appears to result from intimal smooth muscle cell proliferation. Placement of coronary stents has reduced angioplasty restenosis rates, CAD events, and the need for repeat revascularization procedures. Stent patency may be improved with the subsequent administration of glycoprotein IIb/IIIa inhibitors and other antiplatelet agents, such as aspirin and clopidogrel, along with HMG-CoA reductase inhibitors.

5. Diabetes mellitus—Although elevated triglycerides, low HDL-C, or both are common in patients with diabetes, clinical trial data support the identification of LDL-C as the primary focus of therapy. Diabetes is designated a CAD risk equivalent in ATP III, and the LDL goal should be below 100 mg/dL.

6. Metabolic syndrome—Factors that characterize the metabolic syndrome are abdominal obesity, dyslipi-

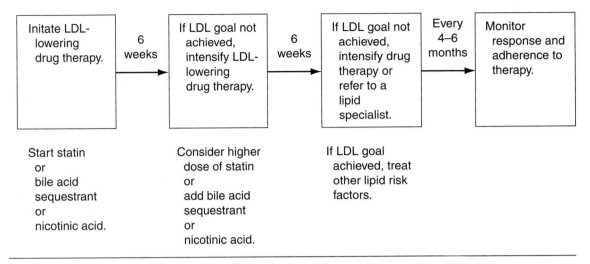

LDL = low-density lipoprotein.

Figure 2–3. Progression of drug therapy in primary prevention. Reprinted, with permission, from: Expert Panel on Detection, Evaluation and Treatment of High Blood Cholesterol in Adults: Executive summary of the Third Report of the NCEP Expert Panel on Detection, Evaluation and Treatment of High Blood Cholesterol in Adults (Adult Treatment Panel III). JAMA 2001; 285; 2492 (Fig. 2).

demia (elevated triglycerides, small dense LDL particles, low HDL-C), raised blood pressure, insulin resistance, and prothrombotic and proinflammatory states. ATP III recognizes this syndrome as a secondary target of risk reduction therapy after the primary target, LDL-C.

Ballantyne CM, Herd A, Ferlic LL et al: Influence of low HDL on progression of coronary artery disease and response to fluvastatin therapy. Circulation 1999;99:736.

Table 2–8. Major causes of reduced serum HDL-cholesterol.

Cigarette smoking
Obesity
Lack of exercise
Androgenic and related steroids
    Androgens
    Progestational agents
    Anabolic steroids
β-Adrenergic-blocking agents
Hypertriglyceridemia
Genetic factors
Primary hypoalphalipoproteinemia

Source: Reproduced, with permission, from Frishman WH et al: Lipids and lipoproteins: Atherosclerotic risk and management. In Frishman WH, ed: Medical Management of Lipid Disorders: Focus on Prevention of Coronary Artery Disease. Armonk, NY: Futura, 1992.

Erbel R, Haude M, Hopp HW et al: Coronary artery stenting compared with balloon angioplasty for restenosis after initial balloon angioplasty. N Engl J Med 1998;339:1672.

Pitt B, Waters D, Brown WV et al: Aggressive lipid-lowering therapy compared with angioplasty in stable coronary artery disease. N Engl J Med 1999;341:70.

The Post Coronary Artery Bypass Graft Trial Investigators: The effect of aggressive lowering of low density lipoprotein cholesterol levels and low-dose anticoagulation on obstructive changes in saphenous vein coronary artery bypass grafts. N Engl J Med 1997;336:153.

Stenestrand U, Wallentin L: Early statin treatment following acute myocardial infarction and 1-year survival. JAMA 2001;285: 430.

Syvanne M, Nieminen MS, Frick H et al: Association between lipoproteins and the progression of coronary and vein graft atherosclerosis in a controlled trial with gemfibrozil in men with low baseline levels of HDL cholesterol. Circulation 1998;98:1993.

Walter DH, Schachinger V, Elsner M et al: Effect of statin therapy on restenosis after coronary stent implantation. Am J Cardiol 2000;85:962.

C. NONPHARMACOLOGIC APPROACHES

1. Dietary modification—The NCEP recommends dietary modification as the first-line treatment for hyperlipidemia (see Table 2–7). It advises a diet that limits cholesterol intake to no more than 200 mg daily and fat intake of less than 30% of total calories, saturated fat constituting less than 7% of daily caloric intake. High intakes of saturated fat, cholesterol, and calories (in excess of body requirements) are implicated as causes for elevated plasma cholesterol. Current recommendations for dietary modification are founded largely on both population-based observational studies and smaller, controlled dietary trials.

Saturated, polyunsaturated, and monounsaturated fats are thought to raise, lower, and have no effect on serum cholesterol, respectively. It has been postulated that monounsaturated fats (eg, olive oil, rapeseed oil), which consist mainly of oleic acid, lower serum cholesterol as much as do polyunsaturated fats, which consist mainly of linoleic acid. The monounsaturated fats offer the added benefit of maintaining heart-protective HDL-C levels. One randomized trial involving post-myocardial infarction patients suggested that intake of *n*-3 polyunsaturated fatty acids reduced nonfatal myocardial infarction, cerebrovascular accidents, and mortality rates as compared with vitamin E and placebo. However, the study was limited by relatively high drug discontinuation rates. The favorable effects of polyunsaturated fat on serum cholesterol have been counterbalanced by evidence that high intake not only tends to lower HDL levels but may promote gallstone formation.

Trans-fatty acids are formed by commercial hydrogenation processes, which harden polyunsaturate-rich marine and vegetable oils. In the United States, consumption of dietary *trans*-fatty acids averages about 8–10 g/d, or approximately 6–8% of total daily fat intake, much of it in the form of margarine. Lipid profiles are known to be adversely affected by a high *trans*-fatty-acid diet, which depresses mean HDL-C levels and elevates mean LDL-C levels. Patients at increased risk of atherosclerosis should therefore limit their intake of this type of fat.

Stearic acid, which contributes substantially to the fatty acid composition in beef and other animal products, has been found to be as effective as oleic acid (monounsaturated fat) in lowering plasma cholesterol, when either one replaced palmitic acid (saturated fat). These findings have implications for the use of lean beef as a meat choice in a lipid-lowering diet.

The ATP III also emphasizes the use of plant stanols and sterols and viscous (soluble) fiber as therapeutic dietary options to enhance the lowering of LDL-C.

Clearly, research remains equivocal on certain key issues: the most effective macronutrient composition of a lipid-lowering diet and the relationship of exogenous cholesterol to serum lipid levels.

DeLorgeril M, Salen P, Martin J-L et al: Mediterranean diet, traditional risk factors, and the rate of cardiovascular complications after myocardial infarction. Circulation 1999;99:779.

Denke MA: Dietary prescriptions to control dyslipidemias. Circulation 2002;105:132.

GISSI-Prevenzione Investigators: Dietary supplementation with *n*-3 polyunsaturated fatty acids and vitamin E after myocardial infarction: Results of the GISSI-Prevenzione trial. Lancet 1999;354:447.

Von Schacky C, Angerer P, Kothny W et al: The effect of dietary w-3 fatty acids on coronary atherosclerosis: A randomized, double blind, placebo controlled trial. Ann Intern Med 1999;130:554.

2. Exercise—Daily physical activity is recommended as an adjunct to dietary modification for the initial treatment of hyperlipidemia. Cross-sectional and prospective studies have provided evidence suggesting that increased physical activity reduces the risk of morbidity and mortality from CAD. An independent relationship between exercise and fitness, and the level of total-C, HDL, LDL, and triglycerides has yet to be established definitively, however. The effects of exercise on plasma lipids and lipoproteins may be a consequence of changes in body weight, diet, or medication use.

It thus appears that individuals with high total cholesterol, LDL, and triglyceride levels and those with low HDL levels can show favorable changes in these parameters with physical training (both endurance and resistance). A randomized, controlled trial examined dietary modification and aerobic exercise with controls and concluded that the combination of diet and exercise reduced LDL levels but not HDL levels. Moreover, diet or exercise alone did not significantly alter LDL levels. What still needs to be defined, however, is the intensity, duration, and frequency of exercise necessary to benefit patients.

Stampfer MJ, Hu FB, Manson JE et al: Primary prevention of coronary heart disease through diet and lifestyle. N Engl J Med 2000;343:16.

Stefanik ML, Mackey S, Sheehan M et al: Effects of diet and exercise in men and postmenopausal women with low levels of HDL cholesterol and high levels of LDL cholesterol. N Engl J Med 1998;339:12.

D. Pharmacologic Treatment

1. Lipid-lowering drugs—

a. Bile acid sequestrants—The bile acid-binding resins cholestyramine, colestipol, and colesevelam are primarily used as second-line therapy and in combination with other agents to treat hypercholesterolemia without concurrent hypertriglyceridemia (Tables 2–9 and 2–10). The Lipid Research Clinics Coronary Primary Prevention Trial demonstrated a reduction in myocardial infarctions and CAD deaths in hypercholesterolemic men without CAD using cholestyramine.

(1) Mode of action—These agents bind bile acids in the intestinal lumen, interrupting the enterohepatic circulation of bile acids, which are subsequently excreted in the feces. Increased synthesis of bile acids from endogenous cholesterol is then stimulated, resulting in the depletion of the hepatic cholesterol pool. This, in turn, leads to a compensatory increase in the biosynthesis of cholesterol and in the number of specific high-affinity LDL receptors on

Table 2–9. The four major classes of lipid-modifying drugs.

Drug Class	Mechanism of Action	Metabolic Effects	Plasma Lipoproteins		
			LDL	HDL	VLDL
Bile-acid sequestrants	Interruption of enterohepatic circulation of bile salts leading to increased hepatic bile acid synthesis and enhanced LDL receptor activity	Increased LDL clearance through the LDL receptor	↓↓↓	↑	→↓
Nicotinic acid	Inhibition of adipose tissue lipolysis and reduction of free fatty acid flux to liver	Decreased VLDL and LDL synthesis; decreased clearance of HDL	↓↓↓	↑↑↑↑	↓↓↓↓
Fibric acid derivatives	Increased lipoprotein lipase activity; reduced hepatic VLDL and apolipoprotein B production; ? increased LDL receptor activity	Increased VLDL catabolism; increased synthesis of HDL	↓	↑↑	↓↓↓↓
HMG-CoA reductase inhibitors	Competitive inhibitors of early stage in cholesterol synthesis leading to increased LDL receptor activity	Enhanced LDL clearance through the LDL receptor	↓↓↓↓	↑	↓

Source: Adapted, with permission, from Betteridge DJ: Combination drug therapy for dyslipidaemia. Curr Opin Lipidology 1993;4:50.

the liver cell membrane. The increased number of high-affinity LDL receptors expressed on hepatocytes stimulates an enhanced rate of LDL catabolism from plasma and thereby lowers the concentration of this lipoprotein.

(2) Clinical use—With their interruption of the enterohepatic circulation of bile acids and consequent stimulation of endogenous LDL biosynthesis, bile acid resins may have a synergistic effect with concomitant administration of HMG-CoA reductase inhibitors.

Table 2–10. Therapeutic options for treatment of primary dyslipidemias.

Dyslipoproteinemia	Drug Therapy		
	First-Line Agents	Second-Line Agents	Combination Therapy
Familial lipoprotein lipase deficiency	None	None	None
Heterozygous familial hypercholesterolemia	Reductase inhibitors, resins, nicotinic acid	Fibrates	Resins + reductase inhibitors, resin + nicotinic acid, resins + fibrates
Familial combined hyperlipidemia	Fibrates, nicotinic acid	Reductase inhibitors	Reductase inhibitors + nicotinic acid Reductase inhibitors + fibrates Reductase inhibitors + resins
Remnant particle disease (type III, dysbetalipoproteinemia)	Fibrates, nicotinic acid	Reductase inhibitors	Reductase inhibitors + nicotinic acid Reductase inhibitors + fibrates
Familial hypertriglyceridemia	Fibrates, nicotinic acid	Reductase inhibitors	Fibrates + nicotinic acid/ reductase inhibitors
Polygenic hypercholesterolemia	Resins, reductase inhibitors	Fibrates	

Source: Adapted, with permission, from Betteridge DJ: Combination drug therapy for dyslipidaemia. Curr Opin Lipidology 1993; 4:51.

They are indicated as adjunct therapy to reduce serum cholesterol in patients with primary hypercholesterolemia. Their use should be preceded by dietary therapy, which should address both the specific type of hyperlipoproteinemia in the patient and the patient's body weight, because obesity has been shown to be a contributing factor in hyperlipoproteinemia. Resin use can cause a 5–20% increase in VLDL levels, hence, it should be restricted to hypercholesterolemic patients with only slightly increased triglyceride levels. The increase in VLDL seen with resin use usually starts during the first few weeks of therapy and disappears 4 weeks after the initial rise. It is thought that excessive increases in the VLDL particles may blunt the LDL-lowering effect of the drug by competitively binding the upregulated LDL receptors on the hepatocyte. The resins should, therefore, not be used in patients whose triglyceride levels exceed 3.5 mmol/L unless they are accompanied by a second drug with triglyceride-lowering effects; some suggest not using resins if the triglyceride level exceeds 2.5 mmol/L. A general rule of thumb is that the LDL concentration is seldom raised if the triglyceride level exceeds 7 mmol/L, and bile acid resin treatment would not be effective in this setting.

Cholestyramine and colestipol are powders that must be mixed with water or fruit juice before ingestion and are taken in two or three divided doses with or just after meals. Colestipol is also available in tablet form for greater ease of administration. Colesevelam is a newer bile acid resin, which may have fewer adverse effects and drug interactions than older resins due to its novel structure and higher affinity for bile acids. It should be noted that bile acid sequestrants can decrease absorption of some antihypertensive agents, including thiazide diuretics and propranolol. As a general recommendation, all other drugs should be administered either 1 h before or 4 h after the bile acid sequestrant. The cholesterol-lowering effect of 4 g of cholestyramine appears to be equivalent to 5 g of colestipol. The response to therapy is variable in each individual, but a 15–30% reduction in LDL cholesterol may be seen with colestipol (20 g/day), cholestyramine (16 g/day), or colesevelam (3.8 g/day) treatments. The fall in LDL concentration becomes detectable 4–7 days after the start of treatment, and approaches 90% of maximal effect in 2 weeks. The initial dose should be 4 g of cholestyramine, 5 g of colestipol, or 1.88 g of colesevelam twice a day, and if there is an inadequate response, the dosage can be titrated upward accordingly. Using more than the maximum dosage does not increase the antihypercholesterolemic effect of the drug appreciably, but because it does increase side effects, it decreases compliance. Because resins are virtually identical in action, the choice is based on potential drug interactions and patient preference, specifically taste and the ability to tolerate the ingestion of bulky material.

If resin treatment is discontinued, cholesterol levels return to pretreatment levels within a month. In patients with heterozygous hypercholesterolemia who have not achieved desirable cholesterol levels on resin-plus-diet therapy, the combination therapy of bile acid resins and HMG-CoA reductase inhibitors or nicotinic acid can further lower serum cholesterol, triglyceride, and LDL levels and increase serum HDL concentration.

(3) Side effects—The side effects of bile acid resins include constipation, gastrointestinal irritation or bleeding, cholelithiasis, liver function test abnormalities, myalgias, dizziness, vertigo, and anxiety.

b. Fibric acid derivatives—Fibric acid derivatives are a class of drugs that inhibit the production of VLDL while enhancing VLDL clearance, as a result of the stimulation of lipoprotein lipase activity. These drugs reduce plasma triglycerides and concurrently raise HDL-C levels. Their effects on LDL-C are less marked and more variable. The Helsinki Heart Study demonstrated not only decreased triglycerides, decreased LDL-C and increased HDL-C in men treated with gemfibrozil, but also a decrease in the number of myocardial infarctions compared with placebo.

(1) Mode of action—These drugs increase the activity of the enzyme lipoprotein lipase, enhancing the catabolism of VLDL and triglycerides and promoting the transfer of cholesterol to HDL. VLDL production also appears to be decreased. Gemfibrozil has a more pronounced inhibiting effect on VLDL synthesis than clofibrate. Because gemfibrozil and clofibrate reduce LDL-C concentrations by less than 10%, they cannot be considered first-line agents for the treatment of hypercholesterolemia.

(2) Clinical use—It is well established that fibric-acid derivatives are first-line therapy to reduce the risk of pancreatitis in patients with very high levels of plasma triglycerides. Results from the Helsinki Heart Study have also suggested that hypertriglyceridemic patients with low HDL values can derive a cardioprotective effect from gemfibrozil. A Veterans Administration study found that gemfibrozil confers a significant risk reduction in major cardiovascular events in patients with established CAD and low HDL levels as their primary lipid disorder. However, it is not currently recommended to treat isolated low HDL levels with pharmacologic intervention.

The newer generation of fibric acid derivatives, such as fenofibrate, may decrease total cholesterol and LDL levels to a greater extent than gemfibrozil or clofibrate. Fenofibrate also reduces lipoprotein(a) levels and increases LDL size and buoyancy, as does nicotinic acid. These drugs should not be used as first-line therapy for hypercholesterolemic patients *unless* hypertriglyceridemia is present; type IIb hyperlipidemic patients would benefit from this therapy. HMG-CoA reductase inhibitors combined with fibric acid derivatives are excellent therapy for severe type IIb hyperlipidemia, however, creatine phosphokinase (CPK) values must be closely monitored. Nicotinic acid or bile acid resins plus gemfibrozil are also a reasonable combination for type IIb disease, but HDL levels may drop slightly with the latter combination.

(3) Side effects—The Side effects of fibric acid derivatives include cholelithiasis, gastrointestinal disturbance, myalgias from myositis, and liver function test abnormalities.

c. Nicotinic acid—Nicotinic acid, a water-soluble vitamin that, at doses much higher than those at which its vitaminic actions occur, lowers VLDL and LDL levels and increases HDL levels. It has been shown to reduce overall morbidity and mortality caused by coronary heart disease and to produce regression of some of the signs of atheroma.

(1) Mode of action—The mode of action of nicotinic acid is unknown and appears to be independent of the drug's role as a vitamin. One of its important actions is believed to be partial inhibition of free fatty acid release from adipose tissue. Experiments show that nicotinic acid inhibits the accumulation of cyclic-adenosinemonophosphate (AMP) stimulated by lipolytic hormones; the cAMP concentration controls the activity of triglyceride lipase and thus lipolysis. Nicotinic acid decreases the synthesis of VLDL and LDL by the liver and has been reported to increase the rate of triglyceride removal from the plasma as a result of increased lipoprotein lipase activity.

(2) Clinical use—Through its beneficial effects on VLDL-TG, LDL-C and HDL-C levels, nicotinic acid is indicated for most forms of hyperlipoproteinemia (types II, III, IV, and V) and for patients with depressed HDL. It is the most potent medication among lipid-lowering agents for the augmentation of HDL levels. It is also particularly useful for patients who have elevated plasma VLDL-TG levels as a part of their lipid profile. It is important to remember, however, that a diet low in cholesterol and saturated fats is the foundation of therapy for hyperlipoproteinemia.

Nicotinic acid is available in 100-, 125-, 250-, and 500-mg tablets as well as in a time-release form. The typical dosage is 3–7 g/day given in three divided doses. Therapeutic effects of the drug are usually not seen until the patient reaches a total daily dose of at least 3 g. A greater response may be attained with periodic increases to a maximum of 7–8 g/day, although the incidence of adverse effects also increases with higher doses. In general, it is best to use the lowest dose that will achieve the desired alterations in plasma lipoprotein levels.

(3) Side effects and contraindications—Unfortunately, many patients cannot tolerate therapeutic doses of nicotinic acid, whose primary side effects are cutaneous flushing and gastrointestinal disturbance, and

appropriate steps should be taken to minimize these untoward effects. Taking two aspirins 30 min before the nicotinic acid will reduce flushing; taking the nicotinic acid with meals can ameliorate dyspepsia.

Regardless of the dose, it is important to draw laboratory test samples at regular intervals to monitor potential adverse effects. These include assessment of liver function (bilirubin, alkaline phosphatase, and transaminase levels), uric acid levels, and serum glucose levels.

Nicotinic acid is contraindicated in patients with active peptic ulcer disease. Because the drug may also impair glucose tolerance, it is contraindicated in patients with poorly controlled diabetes. Nicotinic acid is also associated with reversible elevations of liver enzymes and uric acid and should not be used in patients with hepatic disease or a history of symptomatic gout.

Patients taking a time-release form of nicotinic acid have a lower incidence of flushing than do patients with unmodified nicotinic acid (this side effect is thought to be related to the rate of gastrointestinal absorption). This is outweighed, however, by the far greater incidence of gastrointestinal and constitutional symptoms experienced by patients on the time-release form. These include nausea, vomiting, diarrhea, fatigue, and impaired male sexual function. In addition, even with low doses, the time-release preparation may be associated with more hepatotoxicity, entailing greater alkaline phosphatase and transaminase elevations.

Other adverse effects of nicotinic acid include pruritus (which responds to aspirin), acanthosis nigricans, cardiac arrhythmias, gout, and myopathy.

d. Hepatic 3-methylglutaryl coenzyme A reductase inhibitors—These inhibitors (HMG-CoA) inhibit the conversion of HMG-CoA to mevalonic acid, a rate-limiting step in the synthesis of cholesterol in the liver and intestines, the two main sites for production of cholesterol in the body.

HMG-CoA reductase inhibitors produce the greatest reduction in levels of LDL cholesterol, the primary atherogenic lipoprotein, along with ameliorating HDL and triglyceride levels to a lesser extent. In modest daily doses, HMG-CoA reductase inhibitors reduce total and LDL-C at a rate of 15–50% and may reduce triglycerides by 10–30%. Although effective as monotherapy, HMG-CoA reductase inhibitors can be combined to good effect with bile acid sequestrants when a greater effect on cholesterol is required, or with fibric acid derivatives when an additive effect on triglyceride levels is desired. These combinations may, however, increase the risk of rhabdomyolysis.

(1) Mode of action—Most cholesterol that is endogenously produced is synthesized in the liver. HMG-CoA reductase inhibitors interrupt an early rate-limiting step in cholesterol synthesis: the conversion of HMG-CoA to mevalonic acid. Because the synthesis rates of LDL receptors are inversely related to the

amount of cholesterol in cells, the action of HMG-CoA reductase inhibitors reduces cholesterol synthesis and cellular concentrations of cholesterol and increases the expression of LDL receptors in the liver. Furthermore, because LDL receptors are responsible for clearing about two thirds to three quarters of plasma LDL (and associated cholesterol), HMG-CoA reductase inhibitors may promote the clearance of LDL as well as VLDL remnants. By reducing cholesterol synthesis, they may also interfere with the hepatic formation of lipoproteins. As cholesterol synthesis is maximal at night, it is recommended that HMG-CoA reductase inhibitors be given at bedtime.

(2) Clinical use—HMG-CoA reductase inhibitors have revolutionized the treatment of hyperlipidemia by their potency, efficacy, and tolerability and have evolved into first-line therapy for most forms of hyperlipidemia. Numerous studies with reductase inhibitors involving primary and secondary prevention of CAD have demonstrated a reduction in CAD events, CAD mortality, cerebrovascular events, and mortality from all other causes. Increased LDL receptor activity and decreased LDL synthesis are responsible for the hypocholesterolemic effect of the drug. This increase in LDL receptor activity occurs in response to a decrement in cholesterol synthesis by HMG-CoA reductase inhibition. LDL may be reduced by either its increased clearance from the plasma or its decreased production.

Reductase inhibitors exhibit pleiotropic effects beyond the lowering of LDL cholesterol levels. The reduction in coronary events and mortality rates is not solely attributable to the attenuation of atherosclerosis and improvement in vessel patency. They are postulated to possess antiinflammatory properties, contribute to coronary plaque stabilization, and improve endothelial cell function, conditions that are increasingly recognized as emerging areas of therapy for the treatment of coronary artery disease. They also reduce C-reactive protein levels, which are markers of inflammation and strong predictors of coronary events. One primary prevention trial suggested that pravastatin use may delay or prevent the development of diabetes mellitus, which is intimately linked to a constellation of multiple CAD risk factors known as the metabolic syndrome. Some studies have indicated that reductase inhibitors may prevent the onset of congestive heart failure, osteoporosis, and Alzheimer's disease as well.

(3) Side effects, drug interactions, and contraindications—HMG-CoA reductase inhibitors are contraindicated in pregnancy, lactation, hypersensitivity to the drugs, and active liver disease.

Immunosuppressive drugs, fibric acid derivatives, nicotinic acid, and erythromycin all may increase the risk of rhabdomyolysis. Concurrent use with warfarin (Coumadin) may potentiate the anticoagulant effect. Bile acid sequestrants decrease the bioavailability of the drug. ACE inhibitors may cause hyperkalemia when used with HMG-CoA reductase inhibitors. Digoxin tends to raise simvastatin levels.

Although the HMG-CoA reductase inhibitors are well tolerated, 10% of patients experience unwanted side effects. Although liver enzymes are elevated in 0.5–2% of patients, the patients are asymptomatic, and values may revert to normal on discontinuation of treatment. It is recommended that treatment be stopped if enzymes increase to a level three times that of normal.

Myositis, myalgia, and myopathy have been reported with increased creatine kinase levels in 5% of patients. Creatine kinase may increase further with the combined use of HMG-CoA reductase inhibitors with fibrates or nicotinic acid. Cerivastatin has been discontinued from production due to a high incidence of rhabdomyolysis and death, especially when combined with gemfibrozil. Although the question of cataract induction has been brought up with the use of these agents, clinical studies with lovastatin have not shown an increase in lens opacity. Recently cases of peripheral neuropathy have been described with these agents.

e. Estrogens and progestogens—Women are at increased risk of atherosclerosis after menopause. This is thought to be due to the lack of the protective effect of estrogen on lipoproteins. In this connection, several investigators have observed reductions in total-C and LDL in women taking exogenous estrogens compared with women not receiving any estrogen supplements. Exogenous estrogens can also produce modest elevations in HDL cholesterol (Table 2–11). There is, however, an increased risk of endometrial hyperplasia, possibly leading to endometrial cancer, with unopposed estrogen therapy. Therefore, in treating a postmenopausal woman with an intact uterus, it is advisable to add progesterone to offset the possible carcinogenic effect of estrogen on the uterus. By doing so, however, the beneficial effects on the lipoprotein profile induced by estrogens tend to be lost (Table 2–12).

The Heart Estrogen/Progestin Replacement Study concluded that hormone replacement therapy (HRT) for the secondary prevention of CAD did not confer a reduction in CAD events or CAD mortality rates overall in the 4.1-year average follow-up period. In addition, a higher rate of venous thromboembolism and gallbladder disease was noted in the patients taking HRT. A subsequent angiographic end-point study demonstrated no benefit with estrogen or the combination of estrogen and medroxyprogesterone on the progression of coronary atherosclerosis compared with placebo in postmenopausal women with established CAD. The Women's Health Initiative trial recently showed that the combination of a conjugated estrogen with methoxyprogesterone increased the rate of coronary events, strokes, breast cancers, and thromboembolic diseases despite significant reductions in LDL-C and HDL-C levels.

Table 2–11. Possible beneficial effects of estrogens in reducing the risk of coronary artery disease in postmenopausal women.

Favorable effect on LDL-cholesterol (possible increase of LDL receptors)

Elevation of HDL-cholesterol (HDL₂); inhibition of hepatic lipase

Direct effect (estrogen receptors) to prevent cholesterol deposition in vascular lesions

Prevention of vasoconstrictive actions of acetylcholine on atherosclerotic vessels

Interference with thromboxane effects on blood vessels

Increased production of prostacyclin from blood vessels

Source: Reproduced, with permission, from Frishman WH et al: Lipids and lipoproteins: Atherosclerotic risk and management. In Frishman WH, ed: Medical Management of Lipid Disorders: Focus on Prevention of Coronary Artery Disease. Armonk, NY: Futura, 1992.

Table 2–12. Effects of estrogens and progestogens on lipids and lipoproteins.

	Estrogen	Progestogen
Total cholesterol	↓	↑
LDL-cholesterol	↓	↑
HDL-cholesterol[a]	↑	↓
Triglycerides	↑	↓

[a] Major effect is on HDL₂ cholesterol; ↓ = decrease, ↑ = increase.

Source: Reproduced, with permission, from Frishman WH et al: Lipids and lipoproteins: Atherosclerotic risk and management. In Frishman WH, ed: Medical Management of Lipid Disorders: Focus on Prevention of Coronary Artery Disease. Armonk, NY: Futura, 1992.

2. Combination drug therapy—When treating patients with most severe genetic dyslipidemias, such as heterozygous familial hypercholesterolemia or familial combined hyperlipidemia, it is common for single-drug therapy to fail to achieve satisfactory plasma lipoprotein levels, even with HMG-CoA reductase inhibitors. In this setting, combination drug therapy is often successful in controlling plasma lipid levels (see Table 2–10). With less severe disorders, it is beneficial sometimes to use a combination of low-dose therapeutic agents with complementary effects rather than high doses of either agent alone in order to minimize their individual dose-related toxicities.

Common lipid-modifying agents to be used in combination regimens are the bile acid resins cholestyramine, colestipol, and colesevelam. They have the advantage of not being absorbed and thus cause fewer drug interactions. When the resins are used in full doses in combination with niacin, LDL-C levels are reduced 32–55% in patients with familial hyperlipidemia. Niacin is poorly tolerated by some patients, however, particularly because of its side effects. Recently a combination niacin–lovastatin formulation has become available for use in the treatment of hyperlipidemia.

Bile acid sequestrants can also be used in combination with fibric acid derivatives; some studies have shown an LDL-C reduction of 36–42%. Bile acid sequestrants and HMG-CoA reductase inhibitors used together are highly effective in lowering plasma LDL-C concentrations. A study of cholestyramine and lovastatin use in 62 patients showed a mean reduction in total-C of 48% and LDL-C levels of 59%.

The antifungal agent ketoconazole has an inhibitory effect on several enzymes linked to cytochrome P450. Large doses of this compound have been demonstrated to reduce total-C and LDL-C levels substantially, probably through inhibition of cholesterol synthesis at the demethylation-of-lanosterol step. The effects of low-dose ketoconazole (400 mg) alone and in combination with cholestyramine (12 g/day) have led to reductions in LDL-C levels of 22% and 31–41%, respectively.

Gotto AM Jr, Kuller LH: Eligibility for lipid-lowering drug therapy in primary prevention. How do the Adult Treatment Panel II and Adult Treatment Panel III guidelines compare? Circulation 2002;105:136.

Gupta EK, Ito MK: Lovastatin and extended-release niacin combination product. The fast drug combination for the treatment of hyperlipidemia. Heart Dis 2002;4(2):124.

Heart Protection Study Collaborative Group: MRC/BHF Heart Protection Study of cholesterol lowering with simvastatin in 20,536 high-risk individuals: A randomised placebo-controlled trial. Lancet 2002;360:7.

Herrington DM, Reboussin DM, Brosnihan KB et al: Effects of estrogen replacement on the progression of coronary-artery atherosclerosis. N Engl J Med 2000;343:522.

Hulley S, Grady D, Bush T et al: Randomized trial of estrogen plus progestin for secondary prevention of coronary heart disease on postmenopausal women. JAMA 1998;280:605.

The LIPID Study Group: Long-term effectiveness and safety of pravastatin in 9014 patients with coronary heart disease and average cholesterol concentrations: The LIPID trial follow up. Lancet 2002;359:1379.

Pasternak RC, Smith SC Jr, Bairey-Merz CN et al: ACC/AHA/NHLBI Clinical advisory on the use of safety stains. J Am Coll Cardiol 2002;40:567.

Rubins HB, Robins SJ, Collins D et al: Gemfibrozil for the secondary prevention of coronary heart disease in men with low levels of high-density lipoprotein cholesterol. N Engl J Med 1999;341:410.

Women's Health Initiative Investigators: Risks and benefits of estrogen plus progestin in healthy postmenopausal women. Principal results from the Women's Health Initiative Randomized Controlled Trial. JAMA 2002;288:321.

Chronic Ischemic Heart Disease

3

Michael H. Crawford, MD

ESSENTIALS OF DIAGNOSIS

- *Typical exertional angina pectoris or its equivalents*
- *Objective evidence of myocardial ischemia by electrocardiography, myocardial imaging, or myocardial perfusion scanning*
- *Likely occlusive coronary artery disease because of history and objective evidence of prior myocardial infarction*
- *Known coronary artery disease shown by coronary angiography*

General Considerations

For clinical purposes, patients with chronic ischemic heart disease fall into two general categories: those with symptoms related to the disease, and those who are asymptomatic. Although the latter are probably more common than the former, physicians typically see symptomatic patients more frequently. The issue of asymptomatic patients becomes important clinically when physicians are faced with estimating the risk to a particular patient who is undergoing some stressful intervention, such as major noncardiac surgery. Another issue is the patient with known coronary artery disease who is currently asymptomatic. Such individuals, especially if they have objective evidence of myocardial ischemia, are known to have a higher incidence of future cardiovascular morbidity and mortality. There is, understandably, a strong temptation to treat such patients, despite the fact that it is difficult to make an asymptomatic patient feel better, and some of the treatment modalities have their own risks. In such cases, strong evidence that longevity will be positively influenced by the treatment must be present in order for its benefits to outweigh its risks.

Pathophysiology & Etiology

In the industrialized nations, most patients with chronic ischemic heart disease have coronary atherosclerosis. Consequently, it is easy to become complacent and ig-

nore the fact that other diseases can cause lesions in the coronary arteries (Table 3–1). In young people, coronary artery anomalies should be kept in mind; in older individuals, systemic vasculitides are not uncommon. Today, collagen vascular diseases are the most common vasculitides leading to coronary artery disease, but in the past, infections such as syphilis were a common cause of coronary vasculitis. Diseases of the ascending aorta, such as aortic dissection, can lead to coronary ostial occlusion. Coronary artery emboli may occur as a result of infectious endocarditis or of atrial fibrillation with left atrial thrombus formation. Infiltrative diseases of the heart, such as tumor metastases, may also compromise coronary flow. It is therefore essential to keep in mind diagnostic possibilities other than atherosclerosis when managing chronic ischemic heart disease.

Myocardial ischemia is the result of an imbalance between myocardial oxygen supply and demand. Coronary atherosclerosis and other diseases reduce the supply of oxygenated blood by obstructing the coronary arteries. Although the obstructions may not be enough to produce myocardial ischemia at rest, increases in myocardial oxygen demand during activities can precipitate myocardial ischemia. This is the basis for using stress testing to detect ischemic heart disease. Some patients may develop transient increases in the degree of coronary artery obstruction as a result of platelet and thrombus formation or through increased coronary vasomotor tone. Although it is rare in the

Table 3–1. Nonatherosclerotic causes of epicardial coronary artery obstruction.

Fixed	Congenital anomalies
	Myocardial bridges
	Vasculitides
	Aortic dissection
	Granulomas
	Tumors
	Scarring from trauma, radiation
Transient	Vasospasm
	Embolus
	Thrombus in situ

United States, pure coronary vasospasm in the absence of atherosclerosis can occur and cause myocardial ischemia and even infarction. In addition, in the presence of other cardiac diseases, especially those that cause a pressure load on the left ventricle, myocardial oxygen demand may outstrip the ability of normal coronary arteries to provide oxygenated blood, resulting in myocardial ischemia or infarction. A good example would be the patient with severe aortic stenosis, considerable left ventricular hypertrophy, and severely elevated left ventricular pressures who tries to exercise. The manifestations of chronic ischemic heart disease thus have their basis in a complex pathophysiology of multiple factors that affect the myocardial oxygen supply and demand.

Clinical Findings

A. Clinical Milieu

Coronary atherosclerosis is more likely to occur in patients with certain risk factors for this disease (Table 3–2). These include advanced age, male gender or the postmenopausal state in females, a family history of coronary atherosclerosis, diabetes mellitus, systemic hypertension, high serum cholesterol and other associated lipoprotein abnormalities, and tobacco smoking. Additional minor risk factors include a sedentary lifestyle, obesity, high psychologic stress levels, and such phenotypic characteristics as earlobe creases, auricular hir-

---

Table 3–2. Risk factors for coronary heart disease.

Major independent risk factors
   Advancing age
   Tobacco smoking
   Diabetes mellitus
   Elevated total and low density lipoprotein cholesterol
   Low high-density lipoprotein cholesterol
   Hypertension
Conditional risk factors
   Elevated serum homocysteine
   Elevated serum lipoprotein (a)
   Elevated serum triglycerides
   Inflammatory markers (eg, C-reactive protein)
   Prothrombic factors (eg, fibrinogen)
   Small LDL particles
Predisposing risk factors
   Abdominal obesity
   Ethnic characteristics
   Family history of premature coronary heart disease
   Obesity
   Physical inactivity
   Psychosocial factors

---

sutism, and a mesomorphic body type. The presence of other systemic diseases—hypothyroidism, pseudoxanthoma elasticum, and acromegaly, for example—can accelerate a propensity to coronary atherosclerosis. In the case of nonatherosclerotic coronary artery disease, evidence of such systemic vasculitides as lupus erythematosus, rheumatoid arthritis, and polyarthritis nodosa should be sought. Although none of these risk factors is in itself diagnostic of coronary artery disease, the more of them are present, the greater the likelihood of the diagnosis.

B. Symptoms

The major symptom of chronic ischemic heart disease is angina pectoris, with a clinical diagnosis based on five features:

- The character of the pain is a deep visceral pressure or squeezing sensation, rather than sharp or stabbing or pinprick-like pain.

- The pain almost always has some substernal component, although some patients complain of pain only on the right or left, back, or epigastrium.

- The pain may radiate from the thorax to the jaw, neck, or arm. Arm pain in angina pectoris typically involves the ulnar surface of the left arm. Occasionally, the radiated pain may be more noticeable to the patient than the origin of the pain, resulting in complaints of only jaw or arm pain. These considerations have led some physicians to suggest that any pain between the umbilicus and the eyebrows should be considered angina pectoris until proven otherwise.

- Angina is usually precipitated by exertion, emotional upset, or other events that obviously increase myocardial oxygen demand, such as rapid tachyarrhythmias or extreme elevations in blood pressure.

- Angina pectoris is transient, lasting between 2 and 30 min. It is relieved by cessation of the precipitating event, such as exercise, or by the administration of treatment, such as sublingual nitroglycerin. Chest pain that lasts longer than 30 min is more consistent with myocardial infarction; pain of less than 2 min is unlikely to be due to myocardial ischemia.

For reasons that are unclear, some patients with chronic ischemic heart disease do not manifest typical symptoms of angina pectoris but have other symptoms that are brought on by the same precipitating factors and are relieved in the same way as angina. Because myocardial ischemia can lead to transient left ventricular dysfunction, resulting in increased left ventricular end-diastolic pressure and consequent pulmonary capillary pressure, the sensation of dyspnea can occur during episodes of myocardial supply-and-demand imbalance. Dyspnea may be the patient's only symptom during myocardial ischemia, or it may overshadow the chest pain in the patient's mind. Therefore, dyspnea out of proportion to the degree of exercise or activity can be considered an angina equivalent. Severe myocardial ischemia may lead to ventricular tachyarrhythmias manifesting as palpitations or even frank syncope. Severe episodes of myocardial ischemia may also lead to transient pulmonary edema, especially if the papillary muscles are involved in the ischemic myocardium and moderately severe mitral regurgitation is produced. The most dramatic result of myocardial ischemia is sudden cardiac death.

Patients with chronic myocardial ischemia can also present with symptoms caused by the effects of repeated episodes of ischemia or infarction. Thus, patients may present with the manifestations of chronic cardiac rhythm disorders, especially ventricular arrhythmias. They may present with chronic congestive heart failure, or they may have symptoms related to atherosclerosis of other vascular systems. Patients with vascular disease in other organs are more likely to have coronary atherosclerosis. Those with prior cerebral vascular accidents or symptoms of peripheral vascular disease may be so disabled by these diseases that their ability to either perceive angina or generate enough myocardial oxygen demand to produce angina may be severely limited.

C. PHYSICAL EXAMINATION

The physical examination is often not helpful in the diagnosis of chronic ischemic heart disease. This is because many patients with chronic ischemic heart disease have no physical findings related to the disease, or if they do, the findings are not specific for coronary artery disease. For example, a fourth heart sound can be detected in patients with chronic ischemic heart disease, especially if they have had a prior myocardial infarction; however, fourth heart sounds are very common in hypertensive heart disease, valvular heart disease, and primary myocardial disease. Palpation of a systolic precordial bulge can occur in patients with prior myocardial infarction, but this sign is not specific and can occur in patients with left ventricular enlargement from any cause. Other signs can also be found in cases of chronic ischemic heart disease, such as those associated with congestive heart failure or mitral regurgitation. Again, these are nonspecific and can be caused by other disease processes. Because coronary atherosclerosis is the most common heart disease in industrialized nations, any physical findings suggestive of heart disease should raise the suspicion of chronic ischemic heart disease.

D. DIAGNOSTIC STUDIES

1. Stress tests—Because angina pectoris or other manifestations of myocardial ischemia often occur during the patient's normal activities, it would be ideal to detect evidence of ischemia at that time. This can be done with ambulatory electrocardiogram (ECG). Under unusual circumstances, a patient may have spontaneous angina or ischemia in a medical facility, where it is possible to inject a radionuclide agent and immediately image the myocardium for perfusion defects. Detection of myocardial ischemia during a patient's normal activities, however, does not have as high a diagnostic yield as exercise stress testing does.

Of the various forms of exercise stress that can be used, the most popular is treadmill exercise, for several reasons: It involves walking, a familiar activity that often provokes symptoms. Because of the gravitational effects of being upright, walking requires higher levels or myocardial oxygen demand than do many other forms of exercise. In addition, walking can be performed on an inexpensive treadmill device, which makes evaluating the patient easy and cost-effective. Bicycling is an alternative form of exercise that is preferred by exercise physiologists because it is easier to quantitate the amount of work the person is performing on a bicycle than on a treadmill. Unfortunately, bicycle exercise does not require as high a level of myocardial oxygen demand as does treadmill walking. Thus, a patient may become fatigued on the bicycle before myocardial ischemia is induced, resulting in lower diagnostic yields. On the other hand, bicycle exercise can be performed in the supine position, which facilitates some myocardial ischemia detection methods such as echocardiography. In patients with peripheral vascular disease or lower limb amputations, arm and upper trunk rowing or cranking exercises can be substituted for leg exercise. Arm exercise has a particularly low diagnostic yield because exercising with the small muscle mass of the arms does not increase myocardial oxygen demand by much. Rowing exercises that involve the arms and the trunk muscles produce higher levels of myocardial oxygen demand that can equal those achieved with bicycle exercise—but not quite the levels seen with treadmill exercise. For these reasons, patients who cannot perform leg exercises are usually evaluated using pharmacologic stress testing.

There are two basic kinds of pharmacologic stress tests. One uses drugs, such as the synthetic catecholamine dobutamine, that mimic exercise; the other uses vasodilator drugs, such as dipyridamole and adenosine, that, by producing profound vasodilatation, increase heart rate and stroke volume, thereby raising myocardial oxygen demand. In addition, vasodilators may dilate normal coronary arteries more than diseased coronary arteries, augmenting any differences in regional perfusion of the myocardium, which can be detected by perfusion scanning. In general, vasodilator stress is preferred for myocardial perfusion imaging, and synthetic catecholamine stress is preferred for wall motion imaging.

2. Electrocardiography—Electrocardiography (ECG) is the most frequently used method for detecting myocardial ischemia because of its ready availability, low cost, and ease of application. The usual criterion for diagnosing ischemia is horizontal or down-sloping ST segment depression, achieving at least 0.1 mV at 80 ms beyond the J point (junction of the QRS and the ST segment). This criterion provides the highest values of sensitivity and specificity. Sensitivity can be increased by using 0.5 mV, but at the expense of lower specificity; similarly, using 0.2 mV increases the specificity of the test at the expense of lower sensitivity. Furthermore, accuracy is highest when ECG changes in the lateral precordial leads (V_4, V_5, V_6) are used instead of the inferior leads (II, III, aVF). In the usual middle-aged, predominantly male population of patients with chest pain syndromes, who have normal resting ECGs and can achieve more than 85% of their maximal predicted age-based heart rate during treadmill exercise, the preceding ECG criteria have a sensitivity and specificity of approximately 85%. If the resting ECG is abnormal, if the patient does not achieve 85% of maximum predicted heart rate, or if the patient is a woman, the sensitivity and specificity are lower and range from 70% to 80%. In an asymptomatic population with a low pretest likelihood of disease, sensitivity and specificity fall below 70%.

3. Myocardial perfusion scanning—This method detects differences in regional myocardial perfusion rather than ischemia per se; however, there is a high correlation between abnormal regional perfusion scans and the presence of significant **coronary artery occlusive lesions.** Thus, when coronary arteriography is used as the gold standard, the sensitivity and specificity of stress myocardial perfusion scanning in the typical middle-aged, predominantly male population with symptoms are approximately 85–95%. Testing an asymptomatic or predominantly female population would result in lower values. Failure to achieve more than 85% of the maximal predicted heart rate during exercise also results in lower diagnostic accuracy. Although treadmill exercise is the preferred stress modality for myocardial perfusion imaging, pharmacologically induced stress with dipyridamole or adenosine produces nearly as good results and is an acceptable alternative in the patient who cannot exercise. **Position emission tomography** with vasodilator stress also can be used to detect regional perfusion differences indicative of coronary artery disease.

4. Assessing wall motion abnormalities—Reduced myocardial oxygen supply results in diminishment and, if severe enough, failure of myocardial contraction. Using methods to visualize the left ventricular wall, a reduction in inward endocardial movement and systolic myocardial thickening is observed with ischemia. **Echocardiography** is an ideal detection system for wall motion abnormalities because it can examine the left ventricle from several imaging planes, maximizing the ability to detect subtle changes in wall motion. Five percent of the time (or less), the image may not be adequate to ensure a high degree of accuracy. In the 95% of patients who can be adequately imaged, however, the results with either exercise or pharmacologic stress are comparable to those of myocardial perfusion imaging and superior to the ECG stress test detection of ischemia. The preferred pharmacologic detection method with wall motion imaging is dobutamine because it directly stimulates the myocardium to increase contractility, as well as raising heart rate and blood pressure and increasing myocardial oxygen demand. In some laboratories, if the heart rate increase is not comparable to that usually achieved with exercise testing, atropine is added to further increase myocardial oxygen demand. **Magnetic resonance imaging** can also be used to assess left ventricular wall motion during pharmacologic stress, but there is relatively little experience with this technique.

5. Evaluating global left ventricular performance—Myocardial ischemia, if profound enough, results in a reduction in global left ventricular performance, which can be detected by either a decrease in left ventricular ejection fraction or a failure for it to increase during exercise; the latter is the normal response. Therefore, techniques such as **radionuclide angiography**, single-photon emission computed tomography (SPECT) left ventricular reconstruction, and echocardiography have been used for the detection of myocardial ischemia. Because fairly profound ischemia is required to depress global left ventricular function, this method has not been as sensitive as other techniques. Furthermore, myocardial disease can lead to an abnormal exercise ejection fraction response, which lowers the specificity of the test. In addition, age and female gender blunt the ejection fraction response to exercise, making the test less reliable in the elderly and in women. As a result, there is currently little enthusiasm for the use of exercise radionuclide angiography alone for detecting ischemic heart disease.

6. Evaluating coronary anatomy—
  a. Coronary angiography—Coronary angiography is the standard for evaluating the anatomy of the coronary artery tree. It is best at evaluating the large epicardial coronary vessels that are most frequently diseased in coronary atherosclerosis. Experimental studies

suggest that lesions that reduce the lumen of the coronary artery by 70% or more in area (50% in diameter) significantly limit flow, especially during periods of increased myocardial oxygen demand. If such lesions are detected, they are considered compatible with symptoms or other signs of myocardial ischemia. This assessment is known to be imprecise for several reasons, however. First, the actual cross-sectional area of the coronary artery at the point of an atherosclerotic lesion must be estimated from two-dimensional diameter measurements in several planes. When compared with autopsy findings, stenosis severity is usually found to have been underestimated by the coronary angiography. Second, the technique does not take into consideration that lesions in series in a coronary artery may incrementally reduce the flow to distal beds by more than is accounted for by any single lesion. Thus, a series of apparently insignificant lesions may actually reduce myocardial blood flow significantly. Third, the cross-sectional area is not actually measured routinely. It is instead referenced to a supposed normal segment of artery in terms of a percentage of stenosis or percentage of reduction in the normal luminal diameter or cross-sectional area. The problem with this type of estimate is that it is often difficult to determine what a normal segment of artery is, especially in patients with diffuse coronary atherosclerosis.

Quantitative coronary angiogram measurements are an improvement over this visual inspection technique, but they are not commonly used except in research projects. **Epicardial coronary artery anatomy** is a static representation at the time of the study. It does not take into consideration potential changes in coronary vasomotor tone that may occur under certain circumstances and further reduce coronary blood flow. In addition, coronary angiography does not adequately evaluate disease in the intramyocardial blood vessels; this may be important in some patients, especially insulin-dependent diabetics. In patients with pure vasospastic angina, the coronary arteries are usually normal or minimally diseased. To establish increased vasomotion as the cause of the angina, provocative tests have been used to induce coronary vasospasm in the cardiac catheterization laboratory. The most popular of these is an **ergonovine infusion,** which is reputed to produce focal vasospasm only in naturally susceptible arteries and not in normal coronary arteries, which usually exhibit only a uniform reduction in vessel diameter. Ergonovine infusion has some risks, however, in that the resultant coronary vasospasm may be difficult to alleviate and can be quite profound. In addition, not all patients with vasospastic angina may respond to this agent. Its use has diminished in favor of electrocardiographic monitoring during the patient's normal daily activities.

b. Other techniques—ECG or imaging evidence of old myocardial infarction is often presumed to indicate

that severe coronary artery stenoses are present in the involved vessel. Myocardial infarction, however, can occur as a result of thrombus on top of a minor plaque that has ruptured and occasionally from intense vasospasm or coronary emboli from the left heart. In these cases, coronary angiography would not detect significant (narrowing of more than 50% of the diameter) coronary lesions despite the evidence of an old myocardial infarction. Coronary artery imaging is therefore necessary because estimating the degree of stenosis from the presence of infarction is not accurate. The presence of inducible myocardial ischemia almost always correlates with significant coronary artery lesions. Under the right clinical circumstances, coronary angiography can often be avoided if noninvasive stress testing produces myocardial ischemia. Coronary angiography could then be reserved for patients who failed medical therapy and were being considered for revascularization, where visualizing the coronary anatomy is necessary.

Other imaging techniques have also had some success. Echocardiography, especially transesophageal, can often visualize the first few centimeters of the major epicardial coronary arteries, and magnetic resonance imaging (MRI) has also shown promise. At present, neither of these noninvasive imaging techniques has reached the degree of accuracy needed to replace contrast coronary angiography; however, technical improvements may change this in the future.

E. CHOOSING A DIAGNOSTIC APPROACH

Normally, noninvasive stress testing is performed first in the evaluation of suspected coronary atherosclerosis. There are several reasons for this: There is less risk with stress testing than with invasive coronary angiography. Mortality rates for stress testing average 1 per 10,000 patients, compared with 1 per 1000 for coronary angiography. The physiologic demonstration of myocardial ischemia and its extent forms the basis for the therapeutic approach irrespective of coronary anatomy. Mildly symptomatic patients who show small areas of ischemia at intense exercise levels have an excellent prognosis and are usually treated medically. Knowledge of the coronary anatomy is not necessary to make this therapeutic decision. In general, therefore, a noninvasive technique should be used to detect myocardial ischemia and its extent before considering coronary angiography, which is both riskier and more costly.

In patients whose profound symptoms with minimal exertion are almost certainly due to severe diffuse coronary atherosclerosis or left main obstruction and when the likelihood of needing revascularization is extremely high, it is prudent to proceed directly with coronary angiography. Anyone with severe unstable angina should receive coronary angiography because of the potential increased risk posed by stress testing. If this approach is not appropriate in a particular clinical setting, the physician might medicate the patient and perform careful stress testing after demonstrating a lack of symptoms on medical therapy. Patients with angina or evidence of ischemia in the early period after myocardial infarction are categorized as having unstable angina and probably should be taken directly to coronary angiography. The typical postinfarction patient who is not having recurrent ischemia, however, can usually be evaluated by stress testing and then a decision can be made about the advisability of coronary angiography. If the clinical situation is such that it is likely that noninvasive testing will be inaccurate or uninterpretable, coronary angiography should be performed. Left bundle branch block on the ECG, for example, not only renders the ECG useless for detecting myocardial ischemia but may also affect the results of myocardial perfusion imaging and wall motion studies. Noninvasive techniques have poor diagnostic accuracy in morbidly obese female patients who are unable to exercise. In general, patients whose medical conditions preclude accurate noninvasive testing are candidates for direct coronary angiography.

Which type of noninvasive testing to select is based on several factors. The most important of these is the type of information desired; second, certain characteristics of the patient, which may make one test more applicable than another. There is, for example, some evidence that wall motion imaging may be more accurate than perfusion scanning in women. On the other hand, perfusion scanning is more likely than echocardiographic imaging to provide adequate technical quality in obese individuals or those with chronic obstructive pulmonary disease. Cost is also an important consideration, and the ECG stress test is the least expensive. In most patients with a low-to-medium clinical pretest likelihood of disease, using the ECG stress test makes sense, especially because good exercise performance with a negative ECG response for ischemia indicates an excellent prognosis even if coronary artery disease is present. In the patient who is highly likely to have coronary artery disease, however, it is useful to not only confirm the presence of the disease but to document its extent. For this purpose, myocardial imaging techniques are better at determining the extent of coronary artery disease than is the ECG. It is also believed that myocardial perfusion scanning is somewhat better at identifying the coronary arteries involved in the production of ischemia than are techniques for detecting wall motion abnormalities.

Grundy SM, Pasternak R, Greenland P et al: Assessment of cardiovascular risk by use of multiple-risk-factor assessment equations: A statement for healthcare professionals from the American Heart Association and the American College of Cardiology. J of Am Coll Cardiol 1999;34:1348.

Kuntz KM, Fleischmann, Hunink MG et al: Cost-effectiveness of diagnostic strategies for patients with chest pain. Ann Intern Med 1999;130:709.

Lee TH, Boucher CA: Clinical practice. Noninvasive tests in patients with stable coronary artery disease. N Engl J Med 2001;344:1840.

Treatment

A. GENERAL APPROACH

Because myocardial ischemia is produced by an imbalance between myocardial oxygen supply and demand, in general, treatment consists of increasing supply or reducing demand—or both. Heart rate is a major determinant of myocardial oxygen demand, and attention to its control is imperative. Any treatment that accelerates heart rate is generally not going to be efficacious in preventing myocardial ischemia. Therefore, care must be taken with potent vasodilator drugs, which may lower blood pressure and induce reflex tachycardia. Furthermore, because most coronary blood flow occurs during diastole, the longer the diastole, the greater the coronary blood flow; and the faster the heart rate, the shorter the diastole.

Blood pressure is another important factor: Increases in blood pressure raise myocardial oxygen demand by elevating left ventricular wall tension, and blood pressure is the driving pressure for coronary perfusion. A critical blood pressure is required that does not excessively increase demand, yet keeps coronary perfusion pressure across stenotic lesions optimal. Unfortunately, it is difficult to tell in any given patient what this level of blood pressure should be, and a trial-and-error approach is often needed to achieve the right balance. Consequently, it is prudent to reduce blood pressure when it is very high, and it may be important to allow it to increase when it is very low. It is not uncommon to encounter patients whose myocardial ischemia has been so vigorously treated with a combination of pharmacologic agents that their blood pressure is too low to be compatible with adequate coronary perfusion. In such patients, withholding some of their medications may actually improve their symptoms. Although myocardial contractility and left ventricular volume also contribute to myocardial oxygen demand, they are less important than heart rate and blood pressure. Myocardial contractility usually parallels heart rate. Attention should be paid to reducing left ventricular volume in anyone with a dilated heart, but not at the expense of excessive hypotension or tachycardia because these factors are more important than volume for determining myocardial oxygen demand.

It is important to eliminate any aggravating factors that could increase myocardial oxygen demand or reduce coronary artery flow (Table 3–3). Hypertension and tachyarrhythmias are obvious factors that need to be controlled. Thyrotoxicosis leads to tachycardia and increases in myocardial oxygen demand. Anemia is a common problem that increases myocardial oxygen demand because of reflex tachycardia; it reduces oxygen supply by decreasing the oxygen-carrying capacity of the blood. Similarly, hypoxia from pulmonary disease reduces oxygen delivery to the heart. Heart failure increases angina because it often results in left ventricular dilatation, which increases wall stress, and in excess catecholamine tone, which increases contractility and produces tachycardia.

The long-term outlook for patients with coronary atherosclerosis must be addressed by reducing their risk factors for the disease. Once a patient is known to have atherosclerosis, risk-factor reduction should be fairly vigorous: If diet has not reduced serum cholesterol, strong consideration should be given to pharmacologic therapy because it has been shown to reduce cardiac events. Patients should be encouraged to exercise, lose weight, quit smoking, and try to reduce stress levels. Daily low-dose aspirin is important for preventing coronary thrombosis. The use of megadoses of vitamin E, β-carotene, and vitamin C should be discouraged in the patient with known coronary atherosclerosis because clinical trials have not demonstrated efficacy.

B. PHARMACOLOGIC THERAPY

1. Nitrates—Nitrates, which work on both sides of the supply-and-demand equation, are the oldest drugs used to treat angina pectoris (Table 3–4). These agents are now available in several formulations to fit the patient's lifestyle and disease characteristics. Almost all patients with known coronary atherosclerosis should carry sublingual nitroglycerin to abort acute attacks of angina pectoris. Nitrates work principally by providing more nitrous oxide to the vascular endothelium and the arterial smooth muscle, resulting in vasodilation.

Table 3–3. Factors that can aggravate myocardial ischemia.

Increased myocardial oxygen demand	Tachycardia
	Hypertension
	Thyrotoxicosis
	Heart failure
	Valvular heart disease
	Catecholamine analogues (eg, bronchodilators, tricyclic antidepressants)
Reduced myocardial oxygen supply	Anemia
	Hypoxia
	Carbon monoxide poisoning
	Hypotension
	Tachycardia

This tends to ameliorate any increased coronary vasomotor tone and dilate coronary obstructions. As long as blood pressure does not fall excessively, nitrates increase coronary blood flow. Nitrates also cause venodilation, reducing preload and decreasing left ventricular end-diastolic volume. The reduced left ventricular volume decreases wall tension and myocardial oxygen demand.

Sublingual nitroglycerin takes 30–60 s to dissolve completely and begin to produce beneficial effects, which can last up to 30 min. Although most commonly used to abort acute attacks of angina, the drug can be used prophylactically if the patient can anticipate its need 30 min prior to a precipitating event. Prophylactic therapy is best accomplished, however, with longer acting nitrate preparations. Isosorbide dinitrate and mononitrate are available in oral formulations; each produces beneficial effects for several hours. Large doses of these agents must be taken orally to overcome nitrate reductases in the liver. Liver metabolism of the nitrates can also be avoided with cutaneous application. Nitroglycerin is available as a topical ointment that can be applied as a dressing; it is also available as a ready-made, self-adhesive patch that delivers accurate continuous dosing of the drug through a membrane. Although the paste and the patches produce similar effects, the patches are more convenient for patients to use.

Sublingual nitroglycerin tablets are extremely small and difficult for patients with arthritis to manipulate. A buccal preparation of nitroglycerin is available, which comes in a larger, more easily manipulable tablet that can be chewed and allowed to dissolve in the mouth, rather than being swallowed. This achieves nitrate effectiveness within 2–5 min and lasts about 30 min, as do the sublingual tablets. An oral nitroglycerin spray, which may be easier to manipulate and more convenient for some patients, is also available.

The major difficulty with all long-acting nitroglycerin preparations is the development of tolerance to their effects. The exact reason for tolerance development is not clearly understood, but it may involve liver enzyme induction or a lack of arterial responsiveness because of local adaptive factors. Regardless of the mechanism, however, round-the-clock nitrate administration will lead to progressively increasing tolerance to the drug after 24–48 h. Because of this, nitroglycerin is usually taken over the 16-h period each day that corresponds to the time period during which most of the ischemic episodes would be expected to occur. For most patients, this means not taking nitrate preparations before bed and allowing the ensuing 8 h for the effects to wear off and responsiveness to the drug to be regained. This timing would have to be adjusted for patients with nocturnal angina. The difficulty with the 8-h overnight hiatus in therapy, however, is that the patient

Table 3–4. Common oral antianginal drugs.

Drug	Usual Dose	Comments; Adverse Effects
Nitrates		
Nitroglycerin	0.4–0.6 mg SL	Aborts acute attacks; headaches, hypotension
Nitroglycerin	1–3 mg buccal	Larger tablet for handicapped patients
Nitroglycerin	0.4 mg spray	More convenient than pills
Nitroglycerin	1/2–2 in of 2% ointment	Prophylactic therapy; tolerance a problem
Nitroglycerin	0.1–0.6 mg/h patches	Prophylactic therapy; tolerance a problem
Isosorbide dinitrate	10–60 mg tid	Need 8 h off q24h to avoid tolerance
Isosorbide mononitrate	20 mg bid	Take 7 h apart
Drug	**Daily Dosage (mg)**	**Comments; Adverse Effects**
Beta–Blockers		
Propranolol	160–320	CNS side effects—fatigue, impotence—common
Nadolol	80–240	Long half-life, noncardioselective
Timolol	10–45	Noncardioselective
Metaprolol	100–400	Cardioselective
Atenolol	50–200	Cardioselective
Acebutolol	400–1200	Cardioselective, some intrinsic sympathomimetic activity
Betaxolol	5–40	Cardioselective, long half-life
Bisoprolol	5–20	Cardioselective
Pindolol	5–40	Marked intrinsic sympathomimetic activity
Calcium Blockers		
Bepridil	200–400	May prolong QT interval
Diltiazem	120–360	Heart-rate lowering; low incidence of adverse effects
Verapamil	120–480	Heart-rate lowering; AV block, heart failure, constipation
Dihydroperidines		
Amlodipine	5–10	Least myocardial depression
Nifedipine	30–60	Hypotension, tachycardia
Nicardipine	60–120	Potent coronary vasodilator
Felodipine	5–20	High vascular selectivity
Isradipine	2.5–10	Potent coronary vasodilator
Nisoldipine	10–40	Similar to nifedipine

has little protection during the critical early morning wakening period—when ischemic events are more likely to occur. Patients should therefore take the ni- trate preparation as soon as they arise in the morning. For this reason, the nitroglycerin patches have a small amount of paste on the outside of the membrane that delivers a bolus of drug through the skin, which quickly elevates the patient's blood level of the drug. It is important that the patient be careful not to wipe this paste off the patch before applying it.

Nitrates, which are effective in preventing the development of angina as well as aborting acute attacks, are helpful in both patients with fixed coronary artery occlusions and those with vasospastic angina. Their potency, compared with other agents, is limited, however, and patients with severe angina often must turn to other agents. In such patients, nitrates can be excellent adjunctive therapy.

2. Beta-blockers—Beta-adrenergic blocking agents are highly effective in the prophylactic therapy of angina pectoris. They have been shown to reduce or eliminate angina attacks and prolong exercise endurance time in double-blind, placebo-controlled studies. They can be used around the clock because no tachyphylaxis to their effects has been found. Beta-blockers mainly work by lowering myocardial oxygen demand through decreasing heart rate, blood pressure, and myocardial contractility. As mentioned earlier, however, they also increase myocardial oxygen supply by increasing the duration of diastole through heart rate reduction. Currently, several β-blocker preparations are available, with one or more features that may make them more—or less—attractive for a particular patient.

Among these features is the agent's pharmacologic half-life, which ranges from 4 to 18 h. Various delivery systems have been developed to slow down the delivery of short-acting agents and prolong the duration of drug activity through sustained release or long-acting formulations. Note that the pharmacodynamic half-life of β-adrenergic blockers is often longer than their pharmacologic half-life, and drug effects can be detected for days after discontinuation of chronic β-blocker therapy.

Ideally, β-blockers should be titrated against the heart rate response to exercise because blunting of the exercise heart rate response is the hallmark of their efficacy. Adverse effects of β-blockers include such expected pharmacologic effects as excessive bradycardia, heart block, hypotension, and—in susceptible individuals—bronchospasm. This is less commonly found in the $β_1$-selective agents. Blocking $β_2$-peripheral vasodilatory actions may aggravate claudication in patients with severe peripheral vascular disease. Beta-adrenergic stimulation is also important for the gluconeogenic response to hyperglycemia in severely insulin-dependent diabetics. Although β-blockers may impair this response, the major problem with their use in insulin-dependent diabetics is that they block the warning signals of hypoglycemia (sweating, tachycardia, piloerection) to the patient. Because of their negative inotropic properties, β-blockers may also precipitate heart failure in patients with markedly reduced left ventricular performance.

Other side effects of β-blockers are less predictably related to their anti-β-adrenergic effects. Adverse central nervous system effects are especially troublesome and include fatigue, mental slowness, and impotence. These side effects are somewhat less common with agents that are less lipophilic, such as atenolol and nadolol. Unfortunately, it is these side effects that make many patients unable to tolerate β-blockers.

3. Calcium channel antagonists—Calcium channel antagonists theoretically work on both sides of the supply-and-demand equation. By blocking calcium access to smooth muscle cells, they produce peripheral vasodilatation and are effective antihypertensive agents. In the myocardium, they block sinus node and atrioventricular node function and reduce the inotropic state. They dilate the coronary arteries and increase myocardial blood flow. The calcium blockers available today produce a variable spectrum of these basic pharmacologic effects. The biggest group is the dihydroperidine calcium blockers, which are potent arterial dilators and thereby cause reflex sympathetic activation, which overshadows their negative chronotropic and inotropic effects.

A second major group of calcium blockers are the heart rate-lowering calcium blockers. Because these drugs have less peripheral vasodilatory action in individuals with normal blood pressure, they produce little reflex tachycardia. The average daily heart rate is usually reduced with these agents because their inherent negative chronotropic effects are not suppressed; negative inotropic effects are also more common with these agents. Hypertensive and normotensive individuals seem to have a different vascular responsiveness to calcium blockers; interestingly, in hypertensive individuals, they lower the blood pressure as well as do the dihydroperidine agents. The two most commonly used drugs in this class are diltiazem and verapamil. Diltiazem is more widely used because of its low side effect profile. Verapamil, which is an excellent treatment for patients with supraventricular arrhythmias, has potent effects on the arteriovenous (AV) node; this can cause excessive bradycardia and heart block in patients with angina pectoris. Verapamil is also more likely than diltiazem to precipitate heart failure, and it often produces troublesome constipation, especially in elderly individuals. All the calcium blockers can produce peripheral edema. This is due not to their negative inotropic effects but rather to an imbalance between the efferent and afferent peripheral arteriolar tone, which increases capillary hydrostatic pressure. Other adverse effects of these drugs are idiosyncratic and include gastrointestinal and dermatologic effects.

Calcium blockers are titrated to the patient's symptomatology because no physiologic marker of their effect corresponds well to the heart rate response to exercise with β-blockers. This makes choosing the appropriate dosage difficult, and many physicians increase the dose until some side effect occurs, and then they reduce it. The most common side effects are related to the pharmacologic effects of the drugs. With the dihydroperidines, vasodilatory side effects such as orthostatic hypotension, flushing, and headache, occur. Hypotension is less common with the heart rate-lowering calcium blockers, and their side effects are more related to cardiac effects such as excessive bradycardia. These drugs are very useful because they are excellent for preventing angina pectoris, lowering high blood pressure, and, in the case of the heart rate-lowering agents, controlling supraventricular arrhythmias.

4. Combination therapy—Although monotherapy is desirable for patient convenience and cost considerations, many patients, especially those with severe inoperable coronary artery disease, require more than one antianginal agent to control their symptoms. Because all antianginal agents have a synergistic effect in preventing angina, the initial choices should be for agents with complementary pharmacologic effects. For example, nitrates can be added to β-blocker therapy: Nitrates have an effect on dilating coronary arteries and increasing coronary blood flow, and their peripheral effects may increase reflex sympathetic tone and counteract some of the negative inotropic and chronotropic effects of the β-blockers. This has proved to be a highly effective combination. Similarly, combining a β-blocker with dihydroperidine drugs, when the β-blockers suppress the reflex tachycardia produced by the dihydroperidine, has also proved to be highly effective. Combinations of the heart rate-lowering calcium blockers and nitrates have also proved efficacious. Extremely refractory patients may respond to the combination of a dihydroperidine calcium blocker and a heart rate-lowering calcium blocker.

Combining a dihydroperidine calcium blocker and nitrates makes little sense, however, because of the high likelihood of producing potent vasodilatory side effects. This combination may excessively lower blood pressure to the point that coronary perfusion pressure is compromised and the patient's angina actually worsens. In fact, in as many as 10% of patients with moderately severe angina, both the nitrates and the dihydroperidine calcium blockers alone have been reported to aggravate angina. Although few corroborative data exist, this percentage is certainly higher with the combination of the two agents.

The most difficult cases often involve triple therapy, with a calcium blocker, a β-blocker, and a nitrate. Although there are few objective data on the benefits of this approach, it has proven efficacious in selected patients. The major problem with triple therapy is that side effects, such as hypotension, are increased, which often limits therapy.

Gibbons RJ, Chaterjee K, Daley J et al: ACC/AHA/ACP-ASIM Guidelines for the management of patients with chronic stable angina: A report of the American College of Cardiology/American Heart Association task force on practice guidelines (Committee on Management of Patients with Chronic Stable Angina). J Am Coll Cardiol 1999;3:2092.

Opie LH: Calcium channel antagonists in the treatment of coronary artery disease: fundamental pharmacological properties relevant to clinical use. Prog Cordiovasc Dis 1996;38:273.

Pitt B, Waters D, Brown WV et al. Aggressive lipid-lowering therapy compared with angioplasty in stable coronary artery disease. N Engl J Med 1999;341:70–76.

Thadani U: Management of stable angina pectoris. Prog Cardiovasc Dis1999;14:349–358.

C. Revascularization

1. Catheter-based methods—The standard percutaneous coronary intervention (PCI) is balloon dilatation with placement of a metal stent. Such treatment is limited to the larger epicardial arteries and can be complicated by various types of acute vessel injury, which can result in myocardial infarction unless surgical revascularization is immediately employed. Smaller arteries may be amenable to plain old balloon angioplasty (POBA), and large arteries with complicated lesions may be candidates for other forms of PCI. PCI requires intense antiplatelet therapy usually with aspirin and clopidogrel for a month to prevent stent thrombosis. After the stent has been covered with endothelium this risk is much less.

In the absence of acute complications, initial success rates for significantly dilating the coronary artery are > 85%, and the technique can be of tremendous benefit to patients—without their undergoing the risk of cardiac surgery. The principal disadvantage to PCI is restenosis, which occurs in about one-fourth of patients during the first 6 months. Repeat PCI can be as effective as initial PCI, but, again, the restenosis rate remains around one fourth; however, a second PCI can result in a long-term success. Although many agents are under intense investigation, there is currently no pharmacologic approach to preventing restenosis.

PCI is ideal for symptomatic patients with one or two discrete lesions in one or two arteries. In patients with more complex lesions or those with three or more vessels involved bypass surgery is preferable for several reasons. First, the restenosis risk is the same for each lesion treated by PCI, so that if enough vessels are worked on the risk of restenosis in one of them will approach 100%. Second, the ability to completely revascularize patients with multivessel disease is less with PCI compared with bypass surgery. Finally, clinical trials have shown that diabetics have better outcomes after bypass surgery relative to PCI.

2. Coronary artery bypass graft surgery—Controlled clinical trials have shown that coronary artery bypass graft (CABG) surgery can successfully alleviate angina symptoms in up to 80% of patients. These results compare very favorably with pharmacologic therapy and catheter-based techniques and can be accomplished in selected patients with less than 2% operative mortality rates. Although the initial cost of surgery is high, studies have shown it can be competitive with repeated angioplasty and lifelong pharmacologic therapy in selected patients.

The standard surgical approach is to use the saphenous veins, which are sewn to the ascending aorta and then, distal to the obstruction, in the coronary artery, effectively bypassing the obstruction with blood from the aorta. Although single end-to-side saphenous-vein-to-coronary-artery grafts are preferred, occasionally surgeons will do side-to-side anastomoses in one coronary artery (or more) and then terminate the graft in an end-to-side anastomosis in the final coronary artery. There is some evidence that although these skip grafts are easier and quicker to place than multiple single saphenous grafts, they may not last as long. The major problem with saphenous vein grafts is recurrent atherosclerosis in the grafts, which is often quite bulky and friable, and ostial stenosis, probably from cicatrization at the anastomotic sites. Although these problems can be approached with PCI and other interventional devices, the success rate of catheter-delivered devices to open obstructed saphenous vein grafts is not as high as that seen with native coronary artery obstructions, and many patients require repeat saphenous vein grafting after an average of about 8 years. It is believed that meticulous attention to a low-fat diet, cessation of smoking, and the ingestion of one aspirin a day (80–325 mg) will retard the development of saphenous vein atherosclerosis; some patients do well for 20 years or more after CABG.

There is now considerable evidence that arterial conduits make better bypass graft materials. The difficulty is finding large enough arteries that are not essential to other parts of the body. The most popular arteries used today are the internal thoracic arteries. Their attachment to the subclavian artery is left intact, and the distal end is used as an end-to-side anastomosis into a single coronary artery. If a patient requires more than two grafts, some surgeons, rather than using a saphenous vein, have employed the radial artery or abdominal vessels, such as the gastroepiploic. There are less data on these alternative conduits, but theoretically they would have the same advantages as the internal thoracic arteries in terms of graft longevity. Efforts at preventing bypass graft failure are worthwhile because the risk of repeat surgery is usually higher than that of the initial surgery. There are several reasons for this, including the fact that the patient is older, the scar tissue from the first operation makes the second one more difficult, and finally, any progression of atherosclerosis

in the coronary arteries makes finding good-quality insertion sites for the graft more difficult.

D. SELECTION OF THERAPY

Pharmacologic therapy is indicated when other conditions may be aggravating angina pectoris and can be successfully treated. For example, in the patient with coexistent hypertension and angina, it is often prudent to treat the hypertension and lower blood pressure to acceptable levels before pursuing revascularization for angina, because lowering the blood pressure will often eliminate the angina. For this purpose, it is wise to use antihypertensive medications that are also antianginal (eg, β-blockers, calcium channel blockers) rather than other agents with no antianginal effects (eg, angiotensin-converting enzyme (ACE) inhibitors, centrally acting agents). The presence of heart failure can also produce or aggravate angina, and this should be treated. Care must be taken in choosing antianginal drugs that they do not aggravate heart failure. For this reason, nitrates are frequently used in heart failure and angina because these drugs may actually benefit both conditions. Calcium channel blockers should be avoided if the left ventricular ejection fraction is below 35%, unless it is clear that the heart failure is episodic and is being produced by ischemia. In this situation, however, revascularization may be a more effective strategy. Beta-blockers can be effective, but they must be started at low doses and uptitrated carefully. Although beta blockers are now part of standard therapy for heart failure, there is little data on their use in patients with angina and reduced left ventricular performance. Finally, the presence of ventricular or supraventricular tachyarrhythmias may aggravate angina. Rhythm disorders also afford an opportunity for using dual-purpose drugs. The heart rate-lowering calcium blockers may effectively control supraventricular arrhythmias and also benefit angina. Beta-blockers can often be effective treatment for ventricular arrhythmias in patients with coronary artery disease and should be tried before other, more potent antiarrhythmics or devices are contemplated. Keep in mind that digoxin blood levels may be increased by concomitant treatment with calcium blockers. In addition, the combination of digoxin and either heart rate-lowering calcium blockers or β-blockers may cause synergistic effects on the AV node and lead to excessive bradycardia or heart block.

The major indication for revascularization of chronic ischemic heart disease is the failure of medications to control the patient's symptoms. Drug-refractory angina pectoris is the major indication for revascularization. Note that myocardial ischemia should be established as the source of the patient's symptoms before embarking on revascularization, lest one find out after revascularization that the symptoms were actually due to gastroesophageal reflux. Consequently, some form of stress testing that verifies the relationship between demonstrable ischemia and symptoms is advisable before performing any revascularization procedure.

In some other instances—patient preference, for example—revascularization therapy might be considered before even trying pharmacologic therapy. Some patients do not like the prospect of lifelong drug therapy and would rather have open arteries. Although this is a valid reason to perform revascularization, the physician must be careful that his or her own enthusiasm for revascularization as treatment does not pressure the patient into such a decision. Other candidates for direct revascularization are patients with high-risk occupations who cannot return to these occupations unless they are completely revascularized (eg, airline pilots).

Revascularization is preferred to medical therapy in managing certain types of coronary anatomy that are known (through clinical trials) to have a longer survival if treated with CABG rather than medically. Such lesions include left main obstructions of more than 50%, three-vessel disease, and two-vessel disease in which one of the vessels is the left anterior descending artery. Currently, left main stenoses are not effectively treated with catheter-based techniques, but two- and three-vessel coronary disease could potentially be treated by PCI. Clinical trials have shown equivalent long-term outcomes between PCI and CABG in patients with multivessel disease.

CABG is also recommended for patients with two- or three-vessel coronary artery disease and resultant heart failure from reduced left ventricular performance, especially if viable myocardium can be demonstrated. Because the tests for viable myocardium are not perfect, however, many physicians believe that all these patients should be revascularized in the hope that some myocardial function will return. This seems a prudent approach, given that donor hearts for cardiac transplantation are difficult to obtain—and many patients with heart failure and coronary artery disease improve following bypass surgery.

Surgery is also recommended when the patient has a concomitant disease that requires surgical therapy, such as significant valvular heart disease, heart failure in the presence of a large left ventricular aneurysm, or mechanical complications of myocardial infarction, such as a ventricular septal defect. In the presence of hemodynamic indications for repairing these problems, any significant coronary artery disease that is found should be corrected with bypass surgery at the same time.

The risk of bypass surgery in a given individual must also be considered because several factors can increase the risk significantly and might make catheter-based techniques or medical therapy more desirable. Age is always a risk factor for any major surgery, and CABG is no exception. Also, female gender tends to increase the risk of CABG, possibly because women are, on the average, smaller and have smaller arteries than men. Some data indicate that if size is the only factor considered, gender disappears as a risk predictor with CABG. Other medical conditions that may complicate the perioperative period (eg, obesity, lung disease, diabetes) also raise the risks of surgery. Another factor (discussed earlier) is whether this is a repeat bypass operation. The technical difficulties are especially troublesome when a prior internal thoracic artery graft has been placed because this artery lies right behind the sternum and can be easily compromised when opening the chest.

The choice between catheter-based techniques and CABG surgery is based on several considerations: Is it technically feasible to perform either technique with a good anticipated result? What does the patient wish to do? The patient may have a strong preference for one technique over the other. Again, the physician must be careful not to unduly influence the patient in this regard, lest it give the appearance of a conflict of interest. Consideration must also be given to factors that increase the risk of surgery. The most difficult decision involves the patient who is suitable for either surgery or a catheter-based technique. The few controlled, randomized clinical trials that have been done on such patients have shown equivalent clinical results with PCI and surgery in terms of mortality and symptom relief. Note that this is accomplished by PCI at the cost of repeated procedures in many patients. Despite the necessity for these repeated procedures, the overall cost of bypass surgery is higher over the short term. Unfortunately, the trials do not leave us with clear guidelines for choosing PCI or CABG in the patient who is a good candidate for either treatment; this continues to be a decision to be made by the physician and the patient on a case-by-case basis.

BARI Investigators: Five-year clinical and functional outcome comparing bypass surgery and angioplasty in patients with multivessel coronary disease. JAMA 1997;277:715.

BARI Investigators: Seven-year outcome in the bypass angioplasty revascularization investigation (BARI) by treatment and diabetic status. J Am Coll Cardiol 2000;35:122.

Eagle KA, Guyton RA, Davidoff R et al: ACC/AHA Guidelines for coronary artery bypass graft surgery; A report of the American College of Cardiology/American Heart Association task force on practice guidelines. J Am Coll Cardiol 1999;34:1262.

Henderson RA, Pocock SJ, Sharp SJ et al: Long-term results of RITA-1 trial; clinical and cost comparison of coronary angioplasty and coronary-artery bypass grafting. Randomised Intervention Treatment of Angina. Lancet 1998;352:1419.

Hlatky MA, Rogers WJ, Johnstone I et al: Medical care costs and quality of life after randomization to coronary angioplasty or coronary bypass surgery. By pass Angioplasty Revascularization Investigation (BARI) Investigators. N Engl J Med 1997;336;92.

King SB 3rd, Kosinski AS, Guyton RA et al: Eight-year mortality in the Emory angioplasty versus surgery trial (EAST). J Am Coll Cardiol 2000;35:116.

Pocock SJ, Henderson RA, Clayton T et al: Quality of life after coronary angioplasty or continued medical treatment for angina: three-year follow-up in the RITA-2 trial. J Am Coll Cardiol 2000;35:907.

Rodriguez A, Bernardi V, Navia J et al: Argentine randomized study: Coronary angioplasty with stenting versus coronary bypass surgery in patients with multiple-vessel disease (ERACI II): 30-day and one-year follow-up results. J Am Coll Cardiol 2001;37:51.

Goy JJ, Eeckhout A, Moret C et al: Five-year outcome in patients with isolated proximal left anterior descending coronary artery stenosis treated by angioplasty or left internal mammary artery grafting: A prospective trial. Circulation 1999;99: 3255.

Prognosis

There are two major determinants of prognosis in patients with chronic ischemic heart disease. The first is the clinical status of the patient, which can be semi-quantitated by the Canadian Cardiovascular Society's angina functional class system. In this system, class I is asymptomatic, II is angina with heavy exertion, III is angina with mild-to-moderate exertion, and class IV comprises patients who cannot perform their daily activities without getting angina or who are actually experiencing angina decubitus. The higher the Canadian class, the worse the prognosis. Prognosis can also be determined by exercise testing. If patients can exercise more than 9 min or into stage IV of the modified Bruce protocol, their prognosis is excellent. The presence of either angina or significant ischemic ST depression on the exercise test indicates a poor prognosis. In addition, when using perfusion scanning, the more extensive the perfusion abnormalities with exercise, the worse the prognosis. Left ventricular dysfunction with exercise, evidenced by a decrease or a failure to increase the ejection fraction on left ventricular imaging, or by significant lung uptake of thallium during stress perfusion imaging, also connotes a worse prognosis. Perhaps the most powerful predictor for future mortality is the resting left ventricular ejection fraction; values of less than 50% are associated with an exponential increase in mortality.

A second prognostic system is based solely on coronary anatomy. The more vessels involved, and the more severely they are involved, the worse the prognosis.

This observation has formed the anatomic basis for revascularization in patients with coronary artery disease. Although this approach has some appeal, it has never been proven that revascularization in asymptomatic patients improves their prognosis. Even in patients with left main and severe three-vessel disease, proof is lacking that prophylactic revascularization is of any value if the patients are asymptomatic. Theoretical considerations suggest that ischemia—even in the absence of angina—that can be demonstrated by stress testing or ambulatory ECG recordings would support a decision to revascularize based on anatomy and the presence of ischemia. Although this seems like a much stronger case for revascularization in an asymptomatic patient, such treatment has not been proven efficacious in clinical trials.

The simplicity of the coronary anatomy approach to prognosis has resulted in considerable clinical data on the longevity of patients with chronic ischemic heart disease. Patients with one-vessel coronary artery disease have about a 3% per year mortality rate, less if the vessel is the right or circumflex coronary artery and somewhat more if it is the left anterior descending artery. Patients with two-vessel disease have a 5% or 6% mortality rate per year; in patients with three-vessel disease, this increases to 6–8% a year. Patients with left main disease, with or without other coronary occlusions, have about an 8–12% yearly mortality rate. Similar data do not exist for the clinical classification of patients because of the complexities of determining risk by this approach. A positive treadmill exercise test, at a low workload, for either angina or ischemic ST changes connotes a yearly mortality rate of 5%. This is less if the patient exercised a long time and had good left ventricular function and no previous myocardial infarction. It is worse if the patient exercised only a very short time on the treadmill and had evidence of left ventricular dysfunction or a prior myocardial infarction. How much modern pharmacologic and revascularization therapy can influence these prognostic figures is unclear at present.

Hilton TC, Chaitman BR: The prognosis in stable and unstable angina. Cardiol Clin 1991;9:27.

Thaulow E, Erikssen J, Sandvik L et al: Initial clinical presentation of cardiac disease in asymptomatic men with silent myocardial ischemia and angiographically documented coronary artery disease (the Oslo Ischemia Study). Am J Cardiol 1993; 72:629.

Unstable Angina

4

Prediman K. Shah, MD & Kuang-Yuh Chyu, MD

ESSENTIALS OF DIAGNOSIS

- *New or worsening symptoms (angina, pulmonary edema) or signs (electrocardiographic [ECG] changes) of myocardial ischemia*
- *Absence or mild elevation of cardiac enzymes (creatinine kinase and its MB fraction or troponin I or T) without prolonged ST segment elevation on ECG*
- *Unstable angina and non-ST elevation MI (USA/ NSTEMI) are closely related in pathogenesis and clinical presentation and are therefore discussed as one entity in this chapter.*

General Considerations

A. BACKGROUND AND HISTORICAL PERSPECTIVE

Nearly 40 years ago, the term *intermediate coronary syndrome* was used to describe what is now known as the syndrome of unstable angina, which has also been given numerous other labels: preinfarction angina, status anginosus, crescendo angina, impending myocardial infarction (MI), coronary failure, acute coronary insufficiency, spasmodic angina, and atypical angina—all of which terms attest to the heterogeneity of its clinical presentation. In the current era, unstable angina is the admitting diagnosis for about 40–50% of all admissions to cardiac intensive care units.

B. CLINICAL SPECTRUM

Atherosclerotic coronary artery disease comprises a spectrum of conditions that ranges from a totally asymptomatic state at one end to sudden cardiac death at the other (Table 4–1). It is clear that coronary artery disease, the primary cause of mortality and morbidity in much of the industrialized world, takes its toll through such acute complications (unstable coronary syndromes) as unstable angina, myocardial infarction, acute congestive heart failure, and sudden cardiac death. Also known as acute ischemic syndromes, these

are the first clinical expressions of atherosclerotic coronary artery disease in 30–40% of patients with coronary artery disease.

C. PATHOPHYSIOLOGY

Angina pectoris is the symptomatic equivalent of transient myocardial ischemia, which results from a temporary imbalance in the myocardial oxygen demand and supply. Most episodes of myocardial ischemia are generally believed to result from an absolute reduction in regional myocardial blood flow below basal levels, with the subendocardium carrying a greater burden of flow deficit relative to the epicardium, whether triggered by a primary reduction in coronary blood flow or an increase in oxygen demand. As shown in Figure 4–1, the various acute coronary syndromes share a more-or-less common pathophysiologic substrate. The differences in clinical presentation result largely from the differences in the magnitude of coronary occlusion, the duration of the occlusion, the modifying influence of local and systemic blood flow, and the adequacy of coronary collaterals.

In patients with unstable angina, most episodes of resting ischemia occur without antecedent changes in myocardial oxygen demand but are triggered by primary and episodic reductions in coronary blood flow.

Worsening of ischemic symptoms in patients with stable coronary artery disease may be triggered by such obvious extrinsic factors such as severe anemia, thyrotoxicosis, acute tachyarrhythmias, hypotension, and drugs capable of increasing myocardial oxygen demand

Table 4–1. Clinical spectrum of atherosclerotic coronary artery disease.

Subclinical symptoms or asymptomatic
Stable angina
Unstable angina[a]
Acute myocardial infarction[a]
Acute pulmonary edema[a]
Sudden death[a]

[a] Acute unstable ischemic syndromes.

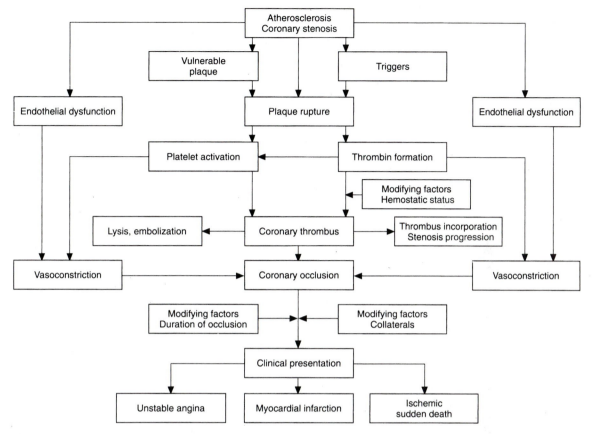

Figure 4-1. Schematic summarizing the current view of the key pathophysiologic events in acute coronary syndromes.

or coronary steal; in most cases, however, no obvious external trigger can be identified. In these patients— who constitute the majority—the evolution of unstable angina and its clinical complications is the outcome of a complex interplay involving coronary atherosclerotic plaque and resultant stenosis, platelet-fibrin thrombus formation, and abnormal vascular tone.

1. Unstable plaque—Several studies have shown that the atherosclerotic plaque responsible for acute unstable coronary syndromes is characterized by a fissure or rupture in its fibrous cap, most frequently at the shoulder region (junction of the normal part of the arterial wall and the plaque-bearing segment). These plaques tend to have relatively thin acellular fibrous caps infiltrated with foam cells or macrophages and eccentric pools of soft and necrotic lipid core (fatty gruel or pultaceous debris). Many clinical and angiographic studies suggest that plaque fissure leading to unstable angina or acute myocardial infarction may occur not only at sites of severe atherosclerotic stenosis, but even more commonly at minimal coronary stenoses. Serial

angiographic observations have shown that development from stable to unstable angina is associated with progression of atherosclerotic disease in 60–75% of patients. This may reflect ongoing episodes of mural thrombosis and incorporation into the underlying plaque. These and other studies have shown that coronary lesions initially occluding less than 75% of the coronary artery area are likely to progress and lead to unstable angina or myocardial infarction; lesions occluding more than 75% are likely to lead to total occlusion. The latter are less likely to lead to myocardial infarction, probably because of the possibility of collateral blood vessel development in more severely stenotic arteries. Furthermore, outward positive remodeling (Glagov effect) of coronary artery segments containing large atherosclerotic plaques may minimize luminal compromise and yet enhance vulnerability for plaque disruption.

Although the precise mechanisms are not known, several hypotheses explain the propensity of plaques to rupture. These include circumferential hemodynamic stresses related to arterial pulse and pressure, intraplaque hemorrhage from small intimal fissures, vasoconstriction, and the twisting and bending of arteries. Other possibilities are inflammatory processes that involve elaboration of matrix-degrading enzymes (collagenase, elastase, stromelysin) released by foam cells or macrophages and other mesenchymal cells in response to undefined stimuli (including, but not limited to, oxidized low-density lipoprotein [LDL]). An excess of matrix-degrading enzymatic activity may contribute to loss of collagen in the protective fibrous cap of the plaque, predisposing it to disruption. Similarly reduced synthesis of collagen, resulting from increased death of matrix-synthesizing smooth muscle cells by apoptosis (programmed cell death), may also contribute to plaque disruption. Intracellular pathogens, such as *Chlamydia pneumoniae, Helicobacter pylori,* cytomegalovirus (CMV), and immune activation have recently been shown to cause inflammatory responses in atherosclerotic plaques and are implicated as potential triggers for plaque rupture.

2. Dynamic obstruction—

a. Thrombosis—Plaque fissure or rupture initiates the process of mural—and eventually luminal—thrombosis by exposing platelets to the thrombogenic components of plaque (collagen, lipid gruel, and tissue factor, etc). This leads to platelet attachment, aggregation, platelet thrombus formation, and the exposure of tissue factor, an abundant procoagulant in the plaque, which interacts with clotting factor VII. The ensuing cascade of events results in the formation of thrombin, which contributes to further platelet aggregation, fibrin formation, and vasoconstriction; it may also play a role as a smooth muscle cell mitogen and chemoattractant for inflammatory cells. The magnitude of the thrombotic response may be further modulated by such local rheologic factors as the shear rate, as well as the status of local and circulating coagulability, platelet aggregability, and fibrinolysis. The superimposition of thrombus on a fissured atherosclerotic plaque can abruptly worsen the local coronary stenosis and lead to a sudden decrease in blood flow. In about 20% of acute coronary syndromes seen during autopsy, however, neither plaque fissure nor rupture can be found underlying thrombosis (plaque erosion). The mechanism of coronary thrombosis is unclear in these cases, but it might include severe stenosis and an enhanced prothrombic tendency of circulating blood.

b. Vasoconstriction—It has become increasingly clear that atherosclerosis is generally associated with a reduced vasodilator response, an increased vasoconstrictor response, or a paradoxical vasoconstrictor response to a variety of stimuli: flow changes, exercise, vasoactive substances (eg, acetylcholine, platelet aggregates, thrombin). This abnormal vasomotor response has been observed well before the development of full-blown atherosclerosis; it has also been seen in patients with risk factors for coronary artery disease but no overt atherosclerosis. The response has generally been attributed to endothelial dysfunction with enhanced inactivation or a reduction in the release of nitric oxide or related nitroso-vasodilators (eg, the relaxation factor produced by the normal endothelium). Some studies have also suggested other causes, such as enhanced sensitivity of the vascular smooth muscle, abnormal platelet function, and an increased release of endothelin (a vasoconstrictor peptide).

Braunwald E: Unstable angina, an etiologic approach to management. Circulation 1998;98:2219.

Ross R: Atherosclerosis—An inflammatory disease. N Engl J Med 1999;340:115.

Shah PK: Plaque disruption and thrombosis, potential role of inflammation and infection. Cardiol Clin 1999;17:271.

Clinical Findings

A. SYMPTOMS AND SIGNS

Unstable angina is a clinical syndrome characterized by symptoms of ischemia, which may include classic retrosternal chest pain or such pain surrogates as a burning sensation, feeling of indigestion, or dyspnea (Table 4–2). Anginal symptoms may also be felt primarily or as radiation in the neck, jaw, teeth, arms, back, or epigastrium. In some patients, particularly the elderly, dyspnea, fatigue, diaphoresis, light-headedness, a feeling of indigestion and the desire to burp or defecate, or nausea and emesis may accompany other symptoms—or may be the only symptoms. The pain of unstable angina typically lasts 15—30 min; it can last longer in some patients. The clinical presentation of unstable angina can take any one of several forms.

There may be an onset of ischemic symptoms in a patient who had been previously free of angina, with or

Table 4–2. Clinical presentation of unstable angina.

New onset of ischemic symptoms
At rest only
During exertion only
At rest and exertion
Intensification of previous ischemic symptoms
Increased frequency, severity, duration
Change in pattern (eg, symptoms at rest)
Recurrence of ischemic symptoms within 4–6 weeks after an acute myocardial infarction
Other
Recurrence of ischemia within 4–6 weeks following bypass surgery or coronary catheterization
Recurrent acute pulmonary edema
Prinzmetal's (variant) angina

without a history of coronary artery disease. If symptoms are effort-induced, they are often rapidly progressive, with more frequent, easily provoked, and prolonged episodes. Rest pain may follow a period of crescendo effort angina—or exist from the beginning.

Symptoms may intensify or change in a patient with antecedent angina. Pain may be provoked by less effort and be more frequent and prolonged than before. The response to nitrates may decrease and their consumption increase. The appearance of new pain at rest or with minimal exertion is particularly ominous. On the other hand, recurrent long-standing ischemic symptoms at rest do not necessarily constitute an acute ischemic syndrome.

Ischemic symptoms may recur shortly after (usually within 4 weeks) an acute myocardial infarction, coronary artery bypass surgery, or catheter-based coronary artery intervention.

In some patients, an acute unstable coronary syndrome may manifest itself as acute pulmonary edema or sudden cardiac death.

B. Physical Examination

No physical finding is specific for unstable angina, and when the patient is free of pain the examination may be entirely normal. During episodes of ischemia, a dyskinetic left ventricular apical impulse, a third or fourth heart sound, or a transient murmur of ischemic mitral regurgitation may be detected. Similarly, during episodes of prolonged or severe ischemia there may be transient evidence of left ventricular failure, such as pulmonary congestion or edema, diaphoresis, or hypotension. Arrhythmias and conduction disturbances may occur during episodes of myocardial ischemia.

C. Diagnostic Studies

Unstable angina is a common reason for admission to the hospital, and the diagnosis, in general, rests entirely on clinical grounds. In a patient with typical effort-induced chest discomfort that is new or rapidly progressive, the diagnosis is relatively straightforward, particularly (but not necessarily) when there are associated ECG changes. Often, however, the symptoms are less clear-cut. The pain may be atypical in terms of its location, radiation, character, and so on, or the patient may have had a single, prolonged episode of pain—which may or may not have resolved by the time of presentation. The physician should strongly suspect unstable angina, particularly in the presence of risk factors for or in the case of known coronary artery disease. When in doubt, it is safer to err on the side of caution and consider the diagnosis to be unstable angina until proven otherwise. Even though dynamic ST-T changes on the ECG make the diagnosis more certain, from 5% to 10% of patients with a compelling clinical history (especially middle-aged women) turn out to have angio-

graphically normal coronary arteries. In general, the more profound the changes, the greater the likelihood of an ischemic origin for the pain and the worse the prognosis.

1. ECG and Holter monitoring—Electrocardiographic abnormalities are common in patients with unstable angina. In view of the episodic nature of ischemia, however, the changes may not be present if the ECG is recorded during an ischemia-free period or the ischemia involves the myocardial territories (eg, the circumflex coronary artery territory) that do not show well on the standard 12-lead ECG. It is therefore not surprising that 40–50% of patients admitted with a clinical diagnosis of unstable angina have no electrocardiographic abnormalities on initial presentation. The ECG abnormalities tend to be in the form of transient ST segment depression or elevation and, less frequently, T wave inversion, flattening, peaking or pseudo-normalization (ie, the T wave becomes transiently upright from a baseline state of inversion). It must be emphasized, however, that a normal or unremarkable ECG in a patient with a compelling clinical history and an appropriate risk-factor profile should never be used to disregard the diagnosis of unstable angina.

Continuous Holter ambulatory ECG recording reveals a much higher prevalence of transient ST-T wave abnormalities, of which 70–80% are not accompanied by symptoms (silent ischemia). These episodes, which may be associated with transient ventricular dysfunction and reduced myocardial perfusion, are much more prevalent in patients with ST-T changes on their admission tracings (up to 80%) than in subjects without such changes. Frequent and severe ECG changes on Holter monitoring, in general, indicate an increased risk of adverse clinical outcome.

2. Angiography—More than 90–95% of patients with a clinical syndrome of unstable angina have angiographically detectable atherosclerotic coronary artery disease of varying severity and extent. The prevalence of single-, two-, and three-vessel disease is roughly equal, especially in patients older than 55 and those with a past history of stable angina. In relatively younger patients and in those with no prior history of stable angina, the frequency of single-vessel disease is relatively higher (50–60%). Left mainstem disease is found in 10–15% of patients with unstable angina. The minority of patients (5–10%) with angiographically normal or near normal coronary arteries may have noncardiac symptoms masquerading as unstable angina, the clinical syndrome X (ischemic symptoms with angiographically normal arteries and possible microvascular dysfunction), or the rare primary vasospastic syndrome of Prinzmetal (variant) angina. It should be recognized, however, that the majority of patients (even those with Prinzmetal's angina) tend to have a significant atherosclerotic lesion on which the spasm is superimposed. In general, the extent (number of vessels involved, location of lesions) and severity (the percentage of diameter-narrowing, the minimal luminal diameter, or the length of the lesion) of coronary artery disease and the prevalence of collateral circulation, as judged by traditional angiographic criteria, do not differ between patients with unstable angina and those with stable coronary artery disease. The morphologic features of the culprit lesions do tend to differ, however. The culprit lesion in patients with unstable angina tends to be more eccentric and irregular, with overhanging margins and filling defects or lucencies. These findings (on autopsy or in vivo angioscopy) represent a fissured plaque, with or without a superimposed thrombus. Such unstable features in the culprit lesion are detected more frequently when angiography is performed early in the clinical course.

3. Noninvasive tests—Any form of provocative testing (exercise or pharmacologic stress) is clearly contraindicated in the acute phase of the disease because of the inherent risk of provoking a serious complication. Several studies of patients who had been pain-free and clinically stable for more than 3–5 days, however, have shown that such testing, using electrocardiographic, scintigraphic, or echocardiographic evaluation may be safe. Provocative testing is used primarily to stratify patients into low- and high-risk subsets. Aggressive diagnostic and therapeutic interventions can then be selectively applied to the high-risk patients; the low-risk patients are treated more conservatively. In general, these studies have shown that patients who have good exercise duration and ventricular function, without significant inducible ischemia or ECG changes on admission, are at a very low risk and can be managed conservatively. On the other hand, patients with electrocardiographic changes on admission, a history of prior myocardial infarction, evidence of inducible ischemia, and ventricular dysfunction tend to be at a higher risk for adverse cardiac events and therefore in greater need of further and more invasive evaluation.

4. Other laboratory findings—Blood levels of myocardial enzymes are, by definition, not elevated in unstable angina; if they are elevated without evolution of Q waves, the diagnosis is generally a non-Q wave myocardial infarction (or non-ST elevation myocardial infarction, NSTEMI). This distinction is somewhat arbitrary, however.

There is evidence of elevated blood levels of biochemical inflammation markers (eg, C-reactive protein [CRP], serum amyloid A, fibrinogen) in patients presenting with USA/NSTEMI. An elevated blood level of CRP or serum amyloid A on admission is associated with a higher risk for early mortality, even in patients in whom classic myocardial damage marker (cardiac-spe-

cific troponins) is negative. Increased blood level of fibrinogen is also associated with increased rate of death or MI. The presence of such markers may be useful in risk stratification for clinical outcomes, however, their current roles in diagnosing USA/NSTEMI have not been established. It is also unclear whether treatment strategies based on these biochemical markers would alter clinical outcomes.

Morrow DA, Rafai N, Antman EM et al: C-reactive protein is a potent predictor of mortality independently of and in combination with troponin T in acute coronary syndromes: A TIMI 11A substudy. J Am Coll Cardiol 1998;31:1460.

Morrow DA, Rafai N, Antman EM et al: Serum amyloid A predicts early mortality in acute coronary syndromes: A TIMI 11A substudy. J Am Coll Cardiol 2000;35:358.

Toss H, Lindahl B, Siegbahn A et al: Prognostic influence of increased fibrinogen and C-reactive protein levels in unstable coronary artery disease. Circulation 1997;96:4204.

Differential Diagnosis

Conditions that simulate or masquerade as unstable angina include acute myocardial infarction, acute aortic dissection, acute pericarditis, pulmonary embolism, esophageal spasm, hiatal hernia, chest wall pain, and so on. Careful attention to the history, risk factors and objective findings of ischemia (transient ST-T changes and mild elevations of troponins in particular) remain the cornerstones for the diagnosis.

A. ACUTE MYOCARDIAL INFARCTION

Although myocardial infarction often produces more prolonged pain, the clinical presentation can be indistinguishable from that of unstable angina. As stated earlier, this distinction should be considered somewhat arbitrary because abnormal myocardial technetium-99m pyrophosphate uptake, mild creatine kinase elevations detected on very frequent blood sampling, and increases in troponin-T and I levels (released from necrotic myocytes) are observed in some patients with otherwise classic symptoms of unstable angina—which represents the severe end of the continuum of acute ischemic syndromes.

B. ACUTE AORTIC DISSECTION

The pain of aortic dissection is usually prolonged and severe. It frequently begins in or radiates to the back and tends to be relatively unrelenting and often tearing in nature; transient ST-T changes are rare. An abnormal chest x-ray film showing a widened mediastinum, accompanied by asymmetry in arterial pulses and blood pressure, can provide clues to the diagnosis of aortic dissection, which can be verified by bedside echocardiography (transesophageal, with or without transthoracic echocardiography), magnetic resonance imaging (MRI), computed tomography (CT) scanning, or aortography.

C. Acute Pericarditis

Acute pericarditis may be difficult to differentiate from unstable angina. A history of a febrile or respiratory illness suggests the former. The pain of pericarditis is classically pleuritic in nature and worsens with breathing, coughing, deglutition, truncal movement, and supine posture. A pericardial friction rub is diagnostic, but it is often evanescent, and frequent auscultation may be needed. Prolonged, diffuse ST elevation that is not accompanied by reciprocal ST depression or myocardial necrosis is typical of pericarditis. Leukocytosis and an elevated sedimentation rate are common in pericarditis but not in unstable angina. Echocardiography may detect pericardial effusion in patients with pericarditis; diffuse ventricular hypokinesis may imply associated myocarditis. Regional dysfunction, especially if transient, is more likely to reflect myocardial ischemia.

D. Acute Pulmonary Embolism

Chest pain in acute pulmonary embolism is also pleuritic in nature and almost always accompanied by dyspnea. Arterial hypoxemia is common, and the ECG may show sinus tachycardia with a rightward axis shift. Precordial ST-T wave abnormalities may simulate patterns of anterior myocardial ischemia or infarction. A high index of suspicion, combined with a noninvasive assessment of pulmonary ventilation-perfusion mismatch, evidence of lower extremity deep vein thrombosis, and possibly pulmonary angiography, is necessary to exclude the diagnosis.

E. Gastrointestinal Causes of Pain

Various gastrointestinal pathologies can mimic unstable angina. These include esophageal spasm, peptic ulcer, hiatal hernia, cholecystitis, and acute pancreatitis. A history compatible with those conditions, the response to specific therapy, and appropriate biochemical tests and imaging procedures should help clarify the situation. It should be noted that these abdominal conditions may produce ECG changes that simulate acute myocardial ischemia.

F. Other Causes of Chest Pain

Many patients present with noncardiac chest pain that mimics unstable angina, and sometimes no specific diagnosis can be reached. The pain may be musculoskeletal or there may be nonspecific changes on the ECG that increase the diagnostic confusion. In these patients, a definite diagnosis often cannot be reached despite careful clinical observation. When the pain has abated and the patient is stable, a provocative test for myocardial ischemia may help rule out ischemic heart disease. Although coronary angiography may provide evidence of atherosclerotic coronary artery disease, anatomic evidence does not necessarily prove an ischemic cause for the symptoms. In some patients acute myocarditis may also produce chest pain syndromes simulating unstable angina and acute myocardial infarction. Recreational drug use (cocaine and amphetamine) may also produce clinical syndromes of chest pain, sometimes related to drug-induced acute coronary syndrome precipitated by the vasoconstrictor and prothrombic effects of drugs.

Management

In treating unstable angina, the initial objective is to stratify patients for their short-term morbidity and mortality risks based on their clinical presentations (Figure 4–2). Following risk stratification, management objectives include eliminating episodes of ischemia and preventing acute myocardial infarction and death.

A. Initial Management

During this early in-hospital phase, therapy is primarily aimed at stabilizing the patient by stabilizing the culprit coronary lesion and thus preventing a recurrence of myocardial ischemia at rest and progression to myocardial infarction.

1. General measures—Patients whose history is compatible with a diagnosis of unstable angina should be promptly hospitalized—ideally, in an intensive or intermediate care unit. General supportive care includes bed rest with continuous monitoring of cardiac rate and rhythm and frequent evaluation of vital signs; relief of anxiety with appropriate reassurance and, if necessary, anxiolytic medication; treatment of associated precipitating or aggravating factors such as hypoxia, hypertension, dysrhythmias, heart failure, acute blood loss, and thyrotoxicosis. A 12-lead ECG should be repeated if it is initially unrevealing or if any significant change has occurred in symptoms or clinical stability. Serial cardiac enzyme evaluation should be performed to rule out an acute myocardial infarction

2. Specific drug therapy—

a. Nitrates—Nitrates are generally considered one of the cornerstones of therapy (Tables 4–3 and 4–4). They tend to relieve and prevent ischemia by improving subendocardial blood flow in the ischemic zone through their vasodilator actions, predominantly on the large epicardial vessels, including the stenotic segments and the coronary collaterals. Unlike acetylcholine and other endothelium-dependent vasodilators, nitrates produce their effects by directly stimulating cyclic guanosine monophosphate (GMP) in the vascular smooth muscle without requiring an intact or functional endothelium; hence their effects are generally well preserved in atherosclerosis. Reduction of left ventricular preload and afterload by peripheral vasodilator actions may contribute to the reduction of myocardial ischemia.

In the very acute phase, it is preferable to use intravenous nitroglycerin to ensure adequate bioavailability,

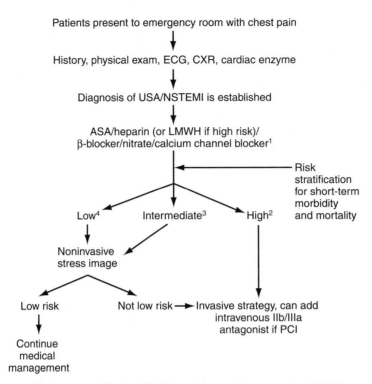

Patients present to emergency room with chest pain

History, physical exam, ECG, CXR, cardiac enzyme

Diagnosis of USA/NSTEMI is established

ASA/heparin (or LMWH if high risk)/
β-blocker/nitrate/calcium channel blocker[1]

Risk stratification for short-term morbidity and mortality

Low[4]   Intermediate[3]   High[2]

Noninvasive stress image

Low risk   Not low risk ⟶ Invasive strategy, can add intravenous IIb/IIIa antagonist if PCI

Continue medical management

[1] All patients should receive risk factor modification (lipid lowering, smoking cessation, BP/DM control, dietary counseling, exercise program, weight control)

[2] High risk features include accelerating ischemic symptoms in preceding 48 h, rest pain >20 min, presence of clinical congestive heart failure, advanced age (>75 years), new bundle-branch block or rest angina with transient ST-segment changes > 0.5 mm, sustained ventricular tachycardia or marked elevation of cardiac enzyme. (ACC/AHA guidelines for unstable angina. J Am Coll Cardiol 2000;36:970)

[3] Intermediate risk features include history of prior MI/PVD/CABG/CVA/aspirin use, resolved prolonged rest angina (>20 min), rest angina (<20 min) relieved with rest or sublingual NTG, age >70 years, T-wave inversion >2 mm, presence of pathologic Q wave, slightly elevated cardiac enzyme. (ACC/AHA guidelines for unstable angina. J Am Coll Cardiol 2000;36:970)

[4] Low risk features do not have the clinical features included in items 2 and 3 but have new-onset Canadian Cardiovascular Society (CCS) class III or IV angina in the past 2 weeks without prolonged (>20 min) rest angina, normal or unchanged ECG, normal cardiac enzyme. (ACC/AHA guidelines for unstable angina. J Am Coll Cardiol 2000;36:970)

Figure 4–2. Algorithm in risk stratification and management of USA/NSTEMI. ASA = acetyl salicylic acid; BP = blood pressure; CABG = coronary artery bypass grafting; CVA = cerebrovascular accident; CXR = chest x-ray film; DM = diabetes mellitus; ECG = electrocardiogram; LMWH = low-molecular-weight heparin; MI = myocardial infarction; PCI = percutaneous coronary intervention; PVD = peripheral vascular disease.

a rapid onset and cessation of action, and easy dose titratability. Oral, sublingual, transdermal, and transmucosal preparations are better suited for subacute and chronic use. To minimize the chances of abrupt hypotension, nitroglycerin infusion should be started at 20–30 μg/min and the infusion rate titrated according to symptoms and blood pressure. The goal is to use the lowest dose that will relieve ischemic symptoms without incurring side effects. The side effects of nitrates include hypotension, which should be meticulously avoided; reflex tachycardia associated with hy-

potension; occasional profound bradycardia, presumably related to vagal stimulation; headaches; and facial flushing. Rare side effects include methemoglobinemia, alcohol intoxication, and an increase in intraocular and intracranial pressure. Some studies have shown a nitroglycerin-induced decrease in the anticoagulant effect of heparin; these results have not been confirmed by others. More recent studies suggest that nitroglycerin may reduce the circulating levels of exogenously administered tissue plasminogen activator, possibly reducing its thrombolytic efficacy. Because

Table 4–3. Effects of medical therapy in unstable angina.

Therapy	Recurrent Ischemia	Progression to Acute Myocardial Infarction	Mortality
Nitrates	↓↓	?	?
Calcium blockers	↓↓	?*	?*
Beta-blockers	↓↓	↓?	↓?
Aspirin/clopidogrel	↓?	↓↓	↓↓
UFH/LMWH	↓↓	↓↓↓	↓↓↓
Thrombolytics	?	?	?

↓ = reduction in frequency; ? = benefit not clearly established; * = increased risk with nifedipine, decreased risk with diltiazem in non-Q/wave infarction in two studies.
LMWH = low-molecular-weight heparin; UFH = unfractionated heparin.

the magnitude of reduced arterial pressure that a patient can tolerate without developing signs of organ hypoperfusion varies, it is difficult to define an absolute cut-off point. A reasonable approach in normotensive subjects without heart failure is to maintain the arterial systolic blood pressure no lower than 100–110 mm Hg; in hypertensive patients, reduction below 120–130 mm Hg may be unwise.

Table 4–4. Mechanisms of action and adverse effects of drug therapy in unstable angina.

Agent	Myocardial Bloodflow	Myocardial Oxygen Demand	Vasoconstriction	Platelet Fibrin Thrombus	Adverse Effects
Nitrates	↑↑	↓↓	↓↓	↓?	Hypotension, reflex tachycardia, rarely bradycardia, headaches, increased intracranial and intraocular pressure, methemoglobinemia, alcohol intoxication, tolerance, decreased heparin effect not established.
Calcium blockers	↑↑	↓↓	↓↓	—	Hypotension, excessive bradyarrhythmias (verapamil, dilitiazem), increased heart rate (nifedipine), worsening heart failure, worsening ischemia from coronary steal (nifedipine).
Beta-blockers	↑	↓↓↓	?	?	Excessive bradyarrhythmias, worsening heart failure, increased bronchospasm.
Aspirin	↑↑↑*	?	?	↓↓↓	Gastritis or ulceration, bleeding, allergy
Heparin	↑↑↑*	?	?	↓↓↓	Bleeding, thrombocytopenia, rarely increased thrombotic risk, osteoporosis, increased K+.

↑ = increase; ↓ = decrease; ? = not established; * = increase or maintenance of coronary flow is due to prevention of thrombotic occlusion rather than to any direct vasodilator action.

Continuous and prolonged administration of intravenous nitroglycerin for more than 24 h may lead to the attenuation of both its peripheral and coronary dilator actions. This effect is due to the development of tolerance in some patients, presumably from depletion of sulfhydryl groups. Some studies show that this attenuation diminishes when sulfhydryl donors such as N-acetylcysteine are administered. At the present time, however, there is no easy and practical way to avoid or overcome this problem other than escalating the dose to maintain reduction in measurable endpoints (eg, the arterial blood pressure).

Although nitrates may reduce the number of both symptomatic and asymptomatic episodes of myocardial ischemia in unstable angina, no effect has yet been demonstrated on the incidence of myocardial infarction.

b. Antiplatelet and anticoagulant therapy—Coronary thrombosis had long been suspected as a culprit in the pathophysiology of unstable angina, and several observational studies published in the 1950s and 1960s reported on the beneficial effects of anticoagulation. The protective effects of aspirin (including the fact that taking a single aspirin had the same benefit as taking more than one) in coronary-prone patients were also described in the 1950s. The unequivocal benefits of antiplatelet and anticoagulant therapy in unstable angina were established only in the past decade, however, when several placebo-controlled randomized trials were completed.

1. Aspirin—Aspirin has been shown to reduce the risk of developing myocardial infarction by about 50% in at least four randomized trials. The protective effect of aspirin in unstable angina has been comparable, in the dosage range of 75–1200 mg/day. Low doses of aspirin (75–81 mg/day) are preferable because the gastrointestinal side effects are clearly lessened with lower doses. A lower dose should be preceded by a loading dose of 160–325 mg on the first day in order to initiate the antiplatelet effect more rapidly.

2. Ticlopidine and Clopidogrel—These two drugs are adenosine diphosphate (ADP) antagonists that are approved for antiplatelet therapy. They have been shown to be comparable to aspirin in reducing the risk of developing acute myocardial infarction in unstable angina. Because they are more expensive than aspirin and carry a 1% risk of agranulocytosis and rarely thrombotic thrombocytopenia purpura, ticlopidine and clopidogrel should be used only when a patient cannot tolerate aspirin due to hypersensitivity or major gastrointestinal side effects.

3. Unfractionated heparin and low-molecular-weight heparin—The protective effect of intravenous unfractionated heparin (UFH) in treating unstable angina has been demonstrated in randomized trials. During short-term use, the risk of myocardial infarction in unstable angina is reduced by about 90%, and ischemic episodes are reduced by about 70%.

Two studies have compared the relative benefits of intravenous heparin with those of aspirin alone or combined with heparin. Although both agents offer protection against the development of acute myocardial infarction in unstable angina, the studies show that heparin may be somewhat more effective in reducing both the risk of infarct development and the number of ischemic episodes. Aspirin and heparin together may not be superior to heparin alone, but aspirin does offer protection against rebound reactivation of acute ischemic syndromes shortly after short-term heparin therapy ends—a argument for their combined use in unstable angina. Because combined therapy may increase the risk of bleeding, only low-dose aspirin should be used.

Recently low-molecular-weight heparin (LMWH) was tested to examine its role as an alternative anticoagulation therapy to UFH in patients with USA/NSTEMI. Low-molecular-weight heparin has certain pharmacologically superior features to UFH: longer half-life, weaker binding to plasma protein, higher bioavailability with subcutaneous injection, more predictable dose response, less incidence of heparin-induced thrombocytopenia. Dalteparin has been shown to be superior to placebo and equivalent to UFH for acute, short-term treatment of USA/NSTEMI in reducing composite end-points in FRISC and FRIC trials, respectively. In FRISC II trial, dalteparin also lowered the risk of death or MI in patients receiving invasive procedures, especially in high-risk patients. In ESSENCE and thrombolysis in myocardial infarction (TIMI) 11B trials, enoxaparin modestly but significantly reduced the combined incidence of death, MI, or recurrent angina over UFH. This reduction is mainly due to a decrease of recurrent angina. Taken together, acute treatment with LMWH is as effective or marginally superior to UFH in USA/NSTEMI patients receiving aspirin,. However because LMWH is easier to use and does not require PTT monitoring, it is being increasingly preferred over UFH.

4. Glycoprotein IIb/IIIa receptor inhibitor—Activation of glycoprotein IIb/IIIa (GP IIb/IIIa) receptors leads to interaction of receptors with ligands such as fibrinogen followed by platelet aggregation. Several GP IIb/IIIa receptor antagonists have been developed to inhibit this agonist-induced platelet aggregation and tested in clinical trials. Current available intravenous IIb/IIIa receptor inhibitors are abciximab, a monoclonal antibody against receptor; nonpeptidic inhibitors, lamifiban and tirofiban and a peptidic inhibitor eptifibatide.

Four major randomized clinical trials (PRISM, PRISM-PLUS, PURSUIT and PARAGON) evaluated the efficacy of intravenous GP IIb/IIIa receptor inhibitors in reducing clinical events (death, MI, or refractory angina) in patients with USA/NSTEMI. Different inhibitors were tested in the trials (tirofiban in PRISM and PRISM-PLUS, eptifibatide in PURSUIT and lamifiban in PARAGON). Although patient population, experimental designs, angiographic strategies, and end-point measurement in these trials were different, these trials showed consistent, though small, reduction of short-term composite event rates in the management of the acute phase of USA/NSTEMI. However, the efficacy of these IIb/IIIa inhibitors in reducing short-term mortality is not as consistent if only death is considered as the clinical end-point. Subgroup analysis of these trials indicated that patients with high-risk features would benefit more from the use of IIb/IIIa inhibitors.

The efficacy of intravenous IIb/IIIa inhibitors in reducing clinical events in patients with USA/NSTEMI undergoing percutaneous coronary intervention (PCI) was also tested—abciximab in EPILOG and CAPTURE, tirofiban in RESTORE. These trials consistently showed a reduction of short-term clinical events (composite end-point of death, MI, urgent or repeat revascularization). The major benefit appears to be in nonfatal adverse events rather than mortality

At the present time there is no clinical role for oral GP IIb/IIIa antagonists such as xemilofiban, orbofiban, and sibrafiban because of lack of proven clinical benefit and increased risk of bleeding.

Thus, overall data suggest that intravenous GP IIb/IIIa inhibitor used judiciously, along with ASA and heparin, is beneficial in high-risk patients with UA/NSTEMI undergoing PCI,

c. Thrombolytic drugs—A number of trials have examined the role of thrombolytic therapy in unstable angina. Despite improved angiographic appearance of the culprit vessel following thrombolytic therapy, no clear-cut benefit over and above antiplatelet and anticoagulant therapy alone has been demonstrated. The precise reasons for this are unclear, especially because there is general agreement about the important pathophysiologic contribution of thrombus to unstable angina. It may well be that antiplatelet-anticoagulant therapy is so effective in itself that any additional benefits are difficult to demonstrate and adding thrombolytic therapy would reduce the risk-to-benefit ratio of the therapy. At this time, therefore, the routine use of thrombolytic therapy in unstable angina cannot be recommended.

d. Beta-blockers—Beta-blockers are commonly used in managing ischemic heart disease because they have been shown to reduce the frequency of both symptomatic and asymptomatic ischemic episodes in stable as well as unstable angina. The protective effects of β-blockers in ischemic heart disease are generally attributed to their negative chronotropic and inotropic effects, which reduce the imbalance of myocardial oxygen demand and supply. Their ability to reduce the risk of infarct development is less clear, but they do decrease reinfarction and mortality rates in postinfarction patients. The mechanism of their protective effect against reinfarction remains unexplained although it has been speculated that they reduce the risk of plaque rupture by reducing mechanical stress on the vulnerable plaque. It is also unclear whether β-blockers offer any additional benefit in unstable angina in patients who are already receiving nitrates and antiplatelet-anticoagulant therapy. At present, the use of β-blockers in patients with unstable angina should be considered an adjunctive therapy.

e. Calcium blockers—Calcium blockers are also frequently used in managing ischemic heart disease. Their beneficial effects in myocardial ischemia are generally attributed to their ability to improve myocardial blood flow by reducing coronary vascular tone and dilation of large epicardial vessels and coronary stenoses through an endothelium-independent action. They also reduce myocardial workload through their negative chronotropic and inotropic and peripheral vasodilator effects. Because exaggerated vasoconstriction may play a role in unstable angina, calcium blockers have been used in its management. In general, although calcium blockers have been shown to reduce the frequency of ischemic episodes in unstable angina, their protective effect against the development of acute myocardial infarction has not been definitively demonstrated. In fact, the use of such calcium blockers as nifedipine tends to increase the risk of ischemic complications in unstable angina. Such adverse effects may well be due to reflex tachycardia or coronary steal caused by the arteriole-dilating actions of some calcium blockers. The protective effects of the heart rate-slowing calcium blocker diltiazem have been reported in patients with a non-Q wave myocardial infarction and preserved ventricular function. As in the case of β-blockers, the additive benefits of calcium blockers in patients with unstable angina who are receiving nitrates and antithrombotic therapy have not been defined, and their use should also be considered an adjunct to such drugs.

Antman EM, McCabe CH, Gurfinkel EP et al: Enoxaparin prevents death and cardiac ischemic events in unstable angina/non-Q-wave myocardial infarction. Results of the thrombolysis in myocardial infarction (TIMI) 11B trial. Circulation 1999;100:1593.

Bertrand ME, Simoons ML, Fox KA et al: Management of acute coronary syndromes: Acute coronary syndromes without persistent ST segment elevation: Recommendations of the task force of the European society of Cardiology. Eur Heart J 2000;21:1406.

Braunwald E, Antman EM, Beasley JW et al: ACC/AHA guidelines for the management of patients with unstable angina and non-ST-segment elevation myocardial infarction: A report of the American College of Cardiology/American Heart Association Task Force on practice guideline (committee on the management of patients with unstable angina). J Am Coll Cardiol 2000;36:970.

CAPTURE investigators: Randomised placebo-controlled trial of abciximab before and during coronary intervention in refractory unstable angina: the CAPTURE study. Lancet 1997; 349:1429.

Chew DP, Bhatt DL, Sapp S et al: Increased mortality with oral platelet glycoprotein IIb/IIIa antagonists, a meta-analysis of phase III multicenter randomized trials. Circulation 2001; 103:201.

Cohen M, Demers C, Gurfinkel EP et al: A comparison of low molecular weight heparin with unfractionated heparin for unstable coronary artery disease. Efficacy and Safety of Subcutaneous Enoxaparin in Non-Q-Wave Coronary Events Study Group. N Engl J Med 1997;337:447.

EPILOG investigators: Platelet glycoprotein IIb/IIIa receptor blockade and low-dose heparin during percutaneous coronary revascularization. N Engl J Med 1997;336:1689.

Freeman MR, Langer A, Wilson RF et al: Thrombolysis in unstable angina. Randomized double-blind trial of t-PA and placebo. Circulation 1992;85:150.

FRISC II study group: Long-term low molecular mass heparin in unstable coronary artery disease: FRISC II prospective randomized multicenter study. Lancet 1999;354(9180):701.

FRISC study group: Low molecular weight heparin during instability in coronary artery disease, Fragmin during Instability in Coronary Artery Disease (FRISC) study group. Lancet 1996;347(9001):561.

Goodman SG, Cohen M, Bigonzi F et al: Randomized trial of low molecular weight heparin (enoxaparin) versus unfractionated heparin for unstable coronary artery disease, one-year results of the ESSENCE study. J Am Coll Cardiol 2000;36:693.

Kaul S, Shah PK: Low molecular weight heparin in acute coronary syndrome: Evidence for superior or equivalent efficacy compared with unfractionated heparin? J Am Coll Cardiol 2000;35:1699

Klein W, Buchwald M, Hillis SE et al: Comparison of low molecular weight heparin with unfractionated heparin acutely and with placebo for 6 weeks in the management of unstable coronary artery disease: Fragmin in unstable coronary artery disease study (FRIC). Circulation 1997;96(1):61.

PARAGON investigators: International, randomized, controlled trial of lamifiban (a platelet glycoprotein IIb/IIIa inhibitor), heparin, or both in unstable angina. Circulation 1998; 97:2386.

PRISM investigators: A comparison of aspirin plus tirofiban with aspirin plus heparin for unstable angina. The Platelet Receptor Inhibition in Ischemic Syndrome Management (PRISM) Study Investigators. N Engl J Med 1998;338:1498.

PRISM-PLUS investigators: Inhibition of the platelet glycoprotein IIb/IIIa receptor with tirofiban in unstable angina and non-Q-wave myocardial infarction. The Platelet Receptor Inhibition in Ischemic Syndrome Management in Patients Limited by Unstable Signs and Symptoms (PRISM-PLUS) study investigators. N Engl J Med 1998;338:1488.

PURSUIT investigators: Inhibition of platelet glycoprotein IIb/IIIa with eptifibatide in patients with acute coronary syndromes. N Engl J Med 1998;339:436.

RESTORE investigators: Effects of platelet glycoprotein IIb/IIIa blockade with tirofiban on adverse cardiac events in patients with unstable angina or acute myocardial infarction undergoing coronary angioplasty. Circulation 1997;96:1445.

RISC Group: Risk of myocardial infarction and death during treatment with low dose aspirin and intravenous heparin in men with unstable coronary artery disease. Lancet 1990;336:827.

Théroux P, Ouimet H, McCans J et al: Aspirin, heparin, or both to treat acute unstable angina. N Engl J Med 1988;319:1105.

Théroux P, Waters D, Lam J et al: Reactivation of unstable angina after the discontinuation of heparin. N Engl J Med 1992; 327:141.

Wallentin LC and the Research Group on Instability in Coronary Artery Disease in Southeast Sweden: Aspirin (75 mg/day) after an episode of unstable coronary artery disease: Long-term effects on the risk for myocardial infarction, recurrence of severe angina and the need for revascularization. J Am Coll Cardiol 1991;18:1587.

Williams DO, Topol EJ, Califf RM et al: Intravenous recombinant tissue-type plasminogen activator in patients with unstable angina pectoris. Results of a placebo-controlled randomized trial. Circulation 1990;82:376.

B. Definitive Management

1. Catheter-based interventions—Endovascular interventions such as percutaneous coronary angioplasty, atherectomy, and laser-assisted angioplasty are commonly performed in patients with unstable angina to reduce the critical stenosis in the culprit artery or in multiple coronary arteries. Although these interventions accomplish an acute reduction in the severity of stenosis (80–93%), in patients with unstable angina they carry a somewhat higher risk of acute complications, including death (0–2%), abrupt closure (0–17%), acute myocardial infarction (0–13%), and the need for urgent coronary artery bypass surgery (0–12%), than in patients with stable angina. The risk if especially great when the procedure is performed soon after the onset of symptoms, in the absence of prior treatment with heparin, or in the presence of an angiographically visible intracoronary thrombus. The 3–6-month restenosis rate with these interventions is 17–44%.

Several randomized clinical trials compared "early conservative" and "early invasive" strategies in treating patients with unstable angina. Earlier trials, such as TIMI IIIB and the Veterans Affairs non-Q wave infarction strategies in hospital (VANQUISH), did not show a beneficial role of early invasive strategy. In contrast, more recent trials such as FRISC II and TACTICS-TIMI 18 showed a reduction in nonfatal adverse events in USA/NSTEMI patients receiving early invasive treatment. Differences in patient characteristics, surgical mortality rates, and background antiischemic medications used may account for these conflicting results and thus it is difficult to reach a consensus recommendation when treating patients with USA/NSTEMI. Nevertheless, subgroup analysis from FRISC II and

TACTICS-TIMI 18 trials showed patients with high risk features such as older age, long-duration of ischemia, angina at rest, ST segment changes on ECG, positive cardiac enzymes, and high TIMI risk scores benefit more from early invasive strategy with revascularization.

2. Coronary artery bypass surgery—Randomized trials and observational series have shown that surgical myocardial revascularization in patients with unstable angina is relatively superior to medical therapy for controlling of symptoms and improving effort tolerance and ventricular function.

At the present time, surgical revascularization can be considered an appropriate option for patients with unstable angina who fail to stabilize with aggressive medical therapy or for whom angioplasty is unsuccessful or is followed by acute complications not amenable to additional catheter-based intervention. It is also applicable to patients who have severe multivessel or left mainstem coronary artery disease, particularly when left ventricular function is also impaired. Although multivessel angioplasty is performed in many centers, the bypass angioplasty revascularization investigation (BARI) trial showed CABG offered a lower repeat revascularization rate and a reduced instance of clinical angina compared with multivessel PTCA. BARI trial also revealed that CABG has a better long-term survival benefit compared with multivessel PTCA, especially in diabetic patients.

3. Intraaortic balloon counterpulsation—Intraaortic balloon counterpulsation is a useful adjunct in managing selected cases of unstable angina. It helps to maintain or improve coronary artery blood flow and myocardial perfusion by augmenting diastolic aortic pressure; at the same time, systolic unloading contributes to a reduction in ventricular wall tension and myocardial oxygen demand and an improvement in ventricular function. These beneficial effects on myocardial oxygen supply and demand help stabilize patients with recurrent myocardial ischemia and those with serious intermittent or persistent hemodynamic or electrical instability. Cardiac catheterization and revascularization can then be carried out with relative safety.

Intraaortic balloon counterpulsation (and the percutaneous method of insertion) carries a significant risk (as high as 35%) of vascular complications involving the lower extremities, especially in women, in patients older then 70 years, and in the presence of diabetes or aortoiliac disease. It should be viewed as a temporary stabilizing measure, pending definitive revascularization.

Anderson HV, Cannon CP, Stone PH et al: One-year results of the Thrombolysis in Myocardial Infarction (TIMI) IIIB clinical trial: A randomized comparison of tissue-type plasminogen activator versus placebo and early invasive versus early conservative strategies in unstable angina and non-Q wave myocardial infarction. J Am Coll Cardiol 1995;26:1643.

BARI Investigators: Seven-year outcome in the Bypass Angioplasty Revascularization Investigation (BARI) by treatment and diabetic status. J Am Coll Cardiol. 2000;35:1122.

Bentivoglio LG, Holubkov R, Kelsey SF et al: Short and long term outcome of percutaneous coronary angioplasty in unstable versus stable angina pectoris: A report of the 1985–1986 NHLBI PTCA registry. Cathet Cardiovasc Diagn 1991;23:227.

Boden WE, O'Rourke RA, Crawford MH et al: Outcomes in patients with acute non-Q-wave myocardial infarction randomly assigned to an invasive as compared with a conservative management strategy: Veterans Affairs non-Q-wave Infarction Strategies in Hospital (VANQUISH) Trial Investigators. N Engl J Med 1998;338:1785.

FRISC II investigators: Invasive compared with non-invasive treatment in unstable coronary artery disease: FRISC II prospective randomized multicenter study. Lancet 1999;354(9180):708.

Kamp O, Beatt KJ, DeFeyter PJ et al: Short-, medium- and long-term follow up after percutaneous transluminal coronary angioplasty for stable and unstable angina pectoris. Am Heart J 1989;117:991.

Morrison DA: Coronary angioplasty for medically refractory unstable angina within 30 days of acute myocardial infarction. Am Heart J 1990;120:256.

Szatmary LJ, Marco J, Fajadet J et al: The combined use of diastolic counterpulsation and coronary dilation in unstable angina due to multivessel disease under unstable hemodynamic conditions. Int J Cardiol 1988;19:59.

TACTICS-TIMI 18 investigators: Comparison of early invasive and conservative strategies in patients with unstable coronary syndromes treated with the glycoprotein IIb/IIIa inhibitor tirofiban. N Engl J Med 2001;344:1879.

Prognosis

The treatment of USA/NSTEMI has evolved rapidly over the past several years resulting in improved patient outcomes. It has been difficult to obtain an accurate and precise rate of adverse events because of the heterogeneous nature of the patient population and different designs and background medications used in clinical trials. However, it is clear that with the advancement of treatment strategies, clinical event rates for refractory angina, MI, and death have reduced substantially. For example, in patients who were not treated with aspirin and heparin, the rate of refractory angina, MI, and death was 23, 12, and 1.7%, respectively, within first week of treatment and the rates became 10.7, 1.6, and 0%, respectively, if the patients were treated with aspirin and heparin. With the addition of a IIb/IIIa receptor inhibitor, the rate for refractory angina, MI, or death was 10.6, 8.3, and 6.9%, respectively, at 6 months in the PRISM-PLUS trial. With the combination of early invasive strategy, IIb/IIIa inhibitor, heparin, and aspirin, the 6-month mortality rate decreased further to 3.3% in the TACTICS-TIMI 18 trial. Even with such decreases in the event rates, a substantial number of patients still continue to suffer from USA/NSTEMI and its complications due to the high prevalence of atherosclerosis. All patients should become acquainted with risk factor modification strategies, which include lipid lowering, smoking cessation, an exercise program, diabetes control, BP control, dietary counseling, and weight control. Recently, the use of angiotensin-converting enzyme inhibitors has also been shown to reduce atherothrombotic events in patients with coronary artery disease especially in presence of diabetes. With the advancement of therapies and risk factor modification, patients' short- and long-term outcomes can be further improved. A simple mnemonic—ABCDE (Table 4–5) summarizes the long-term risk-reducing approach for patients with unstable coronary artery disease.

Table 4–5. **ABCDE** approach for long-term risk reduction in patients with USA/NSTEMI.

A:	Antiplatelet therapy (aspirin, clopidogrel)
B:	Beta-blockers
	Blood pressure control
C:	Cholesterol-modifying medications (statins, fibrates, niacin)
	Converting enzyme inhibitors
	Cessation of smoking
D:	Dietary management (Mediterranean style diet, Ornish style low-fat diet)
E:	Exercise and weight control

Heart Outcomes Prevention Evaluation (HOPE) Study investigators: Effects of ramipril on cardiovascular and microvascular outcomes in people with diabetes mellitus: Results of the HOPE and MICRO-HOPE substudy. Lancet 2000;355:253.

PRISM-PLUS investigators: Inhibition of the platelet glycoprotein IIb/IIIa receptor with tirofiban in unstable angina and non-Q wave myocardial infarction. The Platelet Receptor Inhibition in Ischemic Syndrome Management in Patients Limited by Unstable signs and Symptoms (PRISM-PLUS) Study investigators. N Engl J Med 1998;338:1488.

TACTICS-TIMI 18 investigators: Comparison of early invasive and conservative strategies in patients with unstable coronary syndromes treated with the glycoprotein IIb/IIIa inhibitor tirofiban. N Engl J Med 2001;344:1879.

Théroux P, Oiumet H, McCans J et al: Aspirin, heparin, or both to treat acute unstable angina. N Engl J Med 1988;319:1105.

Acute Myocardial Infarction

Allan S. Jaffe, MD & Wayne L. Miller, MD

ESSENTIALS OF DIAGNOSIS

- *Evidence of myocardial injury*
- *Elevated marker protein such as troponin*
- *Evidence of acute myocardial ischemia*
- *Clinical symptoms and signs*
- *Characteristic ECG changes*
- *Cardiac imaging*

General Considerations

Acute myocardial infarction (AMI) is a clinical syndrome that results from an injury to myocardial tissue that is caused by an imbalance between myocardial oxygen supply and demand. The death of myocytes is generally confluent; this pattern of injury distinguishes infarction pathologically from other forms of myocardial injury, which tend to destroy myocytes more diffusely. Each year roughly 1.1 million people experience MI in the United States; even more, 6 million, are admitted for consideration of this diagnosis, and approximately 460,000 succumb to coronary-artery-related deaths.

Pathophysiology & Etiology

It is generally accepted that a prolonged imbalance between myocardial oxygen supply and demand leads to the death of myocardial tissue. Coronary atherosclerosis is an essential part of the process in most patients. Ischemic heart disease seems to progress through a process of plaque rupture that transiently increases the amount of luminal impingement by the stenotic lesion. Infarction may occur when the plaque ruptures and leads to thrombosis, erosion of the plaque causes thrombosis, or when cardiac work exceeds the ability of the narrowed coronary artery to supply nutritive perfusion. Recent work suggests that inflammation may play a pivotal role in the genesis of plaque rupture.

Greater numbers of acute infarctions occur during the early morning hours (from 6:00 AM to 12:00 noon) than any other time of the day, suggesting that perhaps the increased catecholamine secretion associated with awakening or circadian changes in coagulation common in the early morning (eg, increases in type-1 plasminogen activator inhibitor [PAI-1]) may induce platelet aggregation and lead to thrombus formation. Beta-blockers reduce this propensity and psychiatric depression shifts this pattern back 6 h—as it does with other circadian patterns. In keeping with this pattern, most infarctions do not appear to be induced by exertion. When severe exertion or severe emotional distress does occur, it appears to induce a window of vulnerability for roughly an hour or two after the acute event in susceptible individuals.

In general, patients with acute infarction tend to be males in their 50s and 60s, although infarction in elderly women in their 70s and older is now equally common. Indeed, acute infarction is now equal in incidence between women and men. Most often, those individuals have risk factors for the development of coronary artery disease, such as an increased cholesterol, diabetes, hypertension, cigarette smoking, a sedentary life-style, or a family history of early coronary artery disease. These risks are not present in all patients, however, and the absence of risk factors does not eliminate the possibility of infarction. This is especially true with the increasing prevalence of drug abuse. In patients who have AMI without apparent risk factors, an evaluation for the presence of novel risk factors, such as homocysteine, lipoprotein(a), small dense low-density lipoprotein (LDL), and markers of inflammation such as C-reactive protein and phospholipase A_2 is warranted.

A. TOTAL THROMBOTIC OCCLUSION

In many patients (roughly 50%), total thrombotic occlusion is superimposed on the atherosclerotic plaque. The occlusion is thought to develop in response to plaque rupture when the luminal diameter of the coronary artery is sufficiently reduced to initiate clot formation or if erosion of the plaque causes exposure of procoagulant factors. Procoagulant factors (such as tissue factor) reside within the plaque itself and the absence of counterbalancing antithrombotic factors (eg, heparin, tissue-factor-inhibitor) and fibrinolytic activities (tissue plasminogen activator [t-PA] and single-chain urokinase-type plasminogen activator) within the endothelial cells of the coronary artery can cause thrombosis. Total thrombotic occlusion occurs most commonly in proximal coronary arteries; its presence has been documented during the first 4 h after infarction in more than 85% of patients who present with ST segment elevation (Figure 5–1). Most patients who present in this manner subsequently develop Q waves. A similar type of myocardial insult occurs occasionally despite angiographically normal coronary arteries and is caused by emboli (eg, in patients with prosthetic valves or those with endocarditis), dissection of the coronary artery (most commonly in pregnant women), or on rare occasions, coronary vasospasm. It can also be caused by thrombosis in situ, the probable mechanism by which patients who have variant angina or who abuse cocaine can suffer acute infarction. In these cases, vasoconstriction secondary to endothelial dysfunction and a propensity to thrombosis is of sufficient magnitude and duration to cause thrombus formation. Oxygen consumption and possibly direct myocyte toxicity also increase with cocaine use. In addition, thrombosis in situ can apparently cause infarction among women who take estrogens (especially if they smoke).

B. Non-Q Wave Infarction

The remainder of infarctions occur generally in the absence of total thrombotic occlusion. The term **non-Q wave infarction** is used because the infarction is not associated with the development of new Q waves on the electrocardiogram. (This term is preferred to **nontransmural infarction** because no correlation has been found between Q waves and the presence of infarction through all levels of the ventricle). The frequency of this type of infarction is increasing because of the use of newer more sensitive and specific markers such as the troponins to detect small events.

Although, overall, the coronary anatomy of patients with non-Q wave infarctions is virtually identical to that of patients with Q wave infarctions, the incidence of documented total thrombotic occlusion during the initial 24 h after presentation with non-Q wave infarctions is only 29%.

Some clinicians believe that non-Q wave infarction is caused by small clots that dissolve prior to investigation, leaving only an open artery to be detected. Evidence for this includes an early rise in both the total and the MB isoenzyme of creatine kinase (CK_2) and the finding of contraction-band necrosis (a sign of calcium overload commonly seen after reperfusion). The rapidity of the rise and fall of marker proteins and the presence of contraction bands are related to coronary blood flow, however, and continued antegrade flow

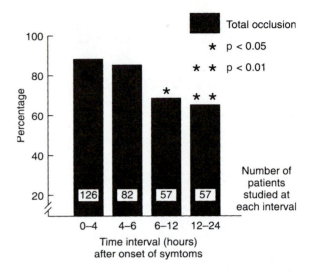

Figure 5–1. Incidence of total occlusion in patients with acute myocardial infarction. Reproduced, with permission, from DeWood MA, Spores J, Notske R et al: Prevalence of total coronary occlusion during the early hours of transmural myocardial infarction. N Engl J Med 1980;303:897.

could also be responsible. Because smaller infarctions also tend to have earlier times to peak CK concentrations, early enzyme peaking could represent a small infarction or the presence of antegrade coronary flow rather than spontaneous coronary recanalization.

Nonetheless, abundant data confirm that thrombosis is common in such patients if diagnosed by an elevated troponin level, especially if concomitant ST depression is present. There are other pathophysiologic possibilities for non-Q wave infarctions. An imbalance of myocardial oxygen supply and demand could be the result of a prolonged increase in myocardial work and oxygen consumption in the distribution of a coronary artery unable to increase its blood flow because of atherosclerosis or endothelial dysfunction. The coronary artery could also constrict abnormally and cause a similar imbalance. Small amounts of vasoconstriction can cause major changes in the cross-sectional area of a vessel since $A = \pi r^2$.

Patients with non-Q wave infarction and partial coronary occlusion are at increased risk for subsequent total occlusion and recurrent infarction during the hospital course and in the weeks and months following the event. After the first few days, although these infarctions are smaller, mortality rates increase more rapidly than in patients with Q wave infarctions because of the greater number of recurrent events. By 6 months, mortality rates are similar to those for patients with Q wave infarctions. However, it is now clear that invasive interventions such as stenting with the assistance of potent anticoagulant modalities such as IIB/IIIA antiplatelet agents and low-molecular-weight heparins (LMWH) can reduce these subsequent events.

Non-Q wave infarction is often seen when other medical illnesses coexist with ischemic heart disease. Pulmonary embolism, septic shock, severe anemia, or even great emotional distress can increase myocardial oxygen demand, reduce coronary perfusion pressure, or evoke paradoxical coronary artery responses and lead to non-Q wave infarction.

Regardless of the cause, the process of myocyte death occurs as a wavefront. It is clear that by 20 min after occlusion (in animal models and likely in humans) some myocytes have died. Then the infarction spreads, usually from the subendocardium toward the epicardium. In experimental animals, infarction is complete in 3–4 h, and it is difficult to save myocardium after that time. In human patients, the time window for myocardial salvage is less clear because the time of onset is more difficult to delineate. Some antegrade flow may occur in many coronary arteries from subtotal occlusion or transient constriction and relaxation of the affected vessel, or myocyte viability may be sustained by collateral perfusion from other vessels. There appears to be some time (in general, perhaps as long as 12 h, and in some patients possibly even longer) during which it may be possible to modify the extent of the myocardial injury by increasing blood flow to the infarct area.

DeWood MA, Sporess J, Notske R et al: Prevalence of total coronary occlusion during the early hours of transmural myocardial infarction. N Engl J Med 1980;303:897.

DeWood MA, Stifter WF, Simpson CS et al: Coronary angiographic findings soon after non-Q wave myocardial infarction. N Engl J Med1986;315:417.

Leor J, Poole WK, Kloner RA: Sudden cardiac death triggered by an earthquake. N Engl J Med 1996;334:413-19.

Libby P, Ridker PM, Maseri A: Inflammation and atherosclerosis. Circulation 2002;105:1135-43.

Muller JE, Stone PH, Turi ZG et al: Circadian variation in the frequency of onset of acute myocardial infarction. N Engl J Med 1995;313:1315-22.

Clinical Findings

The clinical presentations of patients with AMI vary. Although most patients have had chest discomfort prior to the onset of infarction, 20% or more have infarction as a first manifestation of ischemic heart disease; in 20–30% of patients, infarction may go unrecognized. Nonetheless, symptoms are generally present.

A. SYMPTOMS AND SIGNS

The most common and best symptom on which to base a consideration of MI is chest discomfort, usually described as "pressure," "dull," "squeezing," "aching," or "oppressive," although it may be described differently because of individual variability, differences in articulation or verbal abilities, or concomitant disease processes. The discomfort is usually in the center of the chest and may radiate to the left arm or the neck. In general, patients with ischemic chest pain tend to be still, but patients with infarction can be restless as well. The nature of the pain may lead patients to place a hand over the sternum (Levine's sign). These clinical signs and symptoms were originally defined in groups of males. It is now clear that women often have more disease symptoms or more atypical symptoms.

Patients with diabetes or hypertension also may have atypical presentations; a classic presentation in a diabetic is with abdominal pain that mimics the discomfort commonly associated with gallstones. Elderly patients often present with heart failure: by age 85, only 40% of patients will present with chest discomfort. Patients who present with symptoms compatible with ischemia, (paroxysms of dyspnea, for example) or atypical chest discomfort should have the diagnosis of MI considered. Patients can also present with discomfort that is sharper or that radiates to the back. These patients can have pericarditis alone, pericarditis induced by infarction, or a dissecting aortic aneurysm—with or without concomitant infarction.

Much has been made of the presence of associated symptoms and findings such as dyspnea, diaphoresis, nausea and vomiting, and the response of chest discomfort to antianginal agents. Although positive findings should evoke increased consideration of a diagnosis of ischemic heart disease, their absence is not definitive.

B. PHYSICAL EXAMINATION

The physical examination may vary tremendously, from markedly abnormal, with signs of severe congestive heart failure (CHF), to totally normal. In general, an S_4 sound is heard in patients with ischemic heart disease. Dyskinesis can be palpated in patients with larger infarctions. Signs of heart failure, such as neck vein distention, S_3 sounds, and rales, should be looked for specifically.

C. DIAGNOSTIC STUDIES

The diagnosis of infarction in patients with suspected acute ischemic heart disease requires evidence of myocardial necrosis. This finding usually depends on elevated molecular markers of cardiac injury.

1. Troponins are the markers of choice—They are significantly more sensitive than CK_2, and now with second- and third-generation assays, they have nearly absolute cardiac specificity. Absent analytic false-positives, one can be sure that the release of troponin is indicative of cardiac injury. However, because they are so sensitive, they detect cardiac insults that are nonischemic in nature (Table 5–1). Thus, the diagnosis of AMI requires clinical, electrocardiographic (ECG), or

Table 5–1. ESC/ACC definition of myocardial infarction.

Criteria for AMI
1. Typical rise and gradual fall (troponin) or more rapid rise and fall (CK-MB) of biochemical markers of myocardial necrosis with at least one of the following:
   a. Ischemic symptoms
   b. Development of pathologic Q waves on the ECG
   c. ECG changes indicative of ischemia (ST segment elevation or depression)
   d. Coronary artery intervention (eg, coronary angioplasty)

2. Pathologic findings of an AMI

Criteria for established MI
Any one of the following criteria satisfies the diagnosis for established MI:
1. Development of new pathologic Q waves on serial ECGs. The patient may or may not remember previous symptoms. Biochemical markers of myocardial necrosis may have normalized, depending on the length of time that has passed since the infarct developed.

2. Pathologic findings of a healed or healing MI

AMI = acute myocardial infarction; CK-MB = myocardial muscle creatinine kinase isoenzyme; ECG = electrocardiogram.

Source: Adapted, with permission, from J Am Coll Cardiol 2000;36:967.

other (eg, coronary angiographic) evidence of acute ischemia (see Table 5–1). Troponin is elevated between 4 and 6 h after onset of an AMI and remains elevated for 8–12 days. Thus, the late or retrospective diagnosis of AMI can be made with this marker, making the use of lactate dehydrogenase isoenzymes superfluous. Troponin elevations in patients with ST elevation at the time of admission presage a lower rate of recanalization regardless of reperfusion modality used and a worse prognosis. This may be, at least in part, because patients with elevations present later than those without elevations. Patients who present with ST depression also have a worse prognosis if troponin is elevated to any extent. Even minor elevations are of significance (Figure 5–2). This group also has a unique beneficial response to LMWH and IIb/IIIa agents. Patients at low risk for ischemic heart disease who present with chest pain have a high frequency of coronary artery disease if troponin is elevated. Because increases in troponin persist for up to 2 weeks after an acute event, if the initial troponin value is elevated, it may be of value to define a shorter-lived marker (eg, CK_2) if the cardiac injury is acute or has occurred in the days or weeks prior to presentation.

Coronary recanalization, whether spontaneous or induced pharmacologically or mechanically, alters the timing of all markers' appearance in the circulation. Because it increases the rapidity with which the marker is washed out from the heart, leading to rapid increases in plasma, the diagnosis of infarction can be made much earlier—generally within 2 h of coronary recanalization. Although patency can be approximated from the marker rise, distinguishing between thrombolysis in myocardial infarction (TIMI) II and TIMI III flow is not highly accurate. It should also be understood that peak elevations are accentuated, which must be taken into account if one wants to use peak values as a surrogate for infarct size.

2. Other molecular markers—The diagnosis of infarction requires increases in molecular markers of myocardial injury. Myoglobin release from injured myocardium occurs quite early and is very sensitive for detecting infarction. Unfortunately, it is not very specific because minor skeletal muscle trauma also releases myoglobin. Myoglobin is cleared renally, so even minor decreases in glomerular filtration rate lead to elevation. The other early marker advocated by some are isoforms of CK_2. This marker has comparable early sensitivity to myoglobin, but because it uses such sensitive criteria, it also has nearly similar specificity as well. The marker of choice in past years was the MB isoenzyme of creatine kinase (CK_2). A typical rising-and-falling pattern of CK_2 alone (in the proper clinical setting) was sufficient for the diagnosis of acute infarction. In the typical pattern of CK_2 release after infarction, the enzyme marker level exceeds the upper bound of the reference range within 6–12 h after the onset of infarction. Peak levels occur by 18–24 h and generally return to baseline within no more than 48 h. However, elevations can occur due to release of the enzyme from skeletal muscle. The lack of a rising-and-falling pattern should raise the suspicion that the release is from skeletal muscle, which is usually due to a chronic skeletal muscle myopathy. Elevations of CK_2 in patients with hypothyroidism (where clearance CK_2 is retarded) and those with renal failure (where clearance is normal because CK_2 is not cleared renally) have elevations caused, in part, by myopathy. The percentage of CK_2 with respect to total CK_2 is an unreliable criterion for the diagnosis of infarction.

3. Electrocardiography—Only a few ECG patterns have high specificity for infarction (Figure 5-3). In general, an upwardly concave elevation of the ST segment is considered diagnostic of acute myocardial injury, with a high degree of specificity. Patients with inferior infarction should all be evaluated with right-sided chest leads to determine if right ventricular (RV) infarction is present by detecting ST elevation in V_3R or V_4R. Patients with ST segment depression in V_1 and V_2 may have total circumflex occlusions, which can be un-

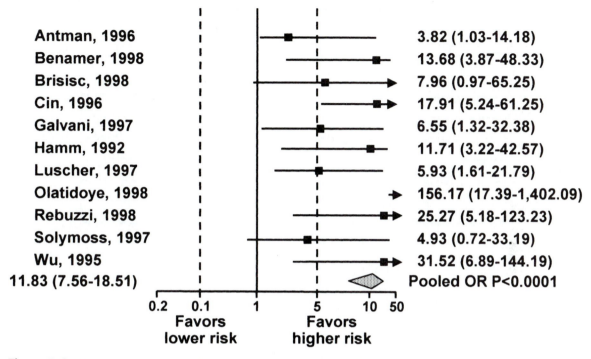

Antman, 1996	3.82 (1.03-14.18)
Benamer, 1998	13.68 (3.87-48.33)
Brisisc, 1998	7.96 (0.97-65.25)
Cin, 1996	17.91 (5.24-61.25)
Galvani, 1997	6.55 (1.32-32.38)
Hamm, 1992	11.71 (3.22-42.57)
Luscher, 1997	5.93 (1.61-21.79)
Olatidoye, 1998	156.17 (17.39-1,402.09)
Rebuzzi, 1998	25.27 (5.18-123.23)
Solymoss, 1997	4.93 (0.72-33.19)
Wu, 1995	31.52 (6.89-144.19)
11.83 (7.56-18.51)	Pooled OR P<0.0001

0.2 0.1 1 5 10 50

Favors lower risk   Favors higher risk

Figure 5–2. Prognosis in patients with acute coronary syndrome (ACS), elevated troponin, and no elevation of CK_2 (isoenzyme of creatinine kinase), Peto odds ratio (OR), and 95% confidence interval (fixed). Adapted, with permission, from Am Heart J 2000;140:917.

masked by the findings of ST segment elevation in the so-called posterior leads (V_7–V_9). The Q waves that tend to develop mark these patients as potential candidates for strategies designed to reduce the extent of infarction (discussed in the section on Implementation Reperfusion Strategies). Reperfusion accelerates the appearance of the Q waves often associated with this type of infarction. The electrocardiogram may not show typical changes, however, because of concomitant conduction disturbances (eg, left bundle branch block [LBBB]) that may mask the findings or because only ST depression, which is considered more nonspecific, is present. Without acute ST segment elevation or the development of new Q waves, no other ECG changes can be considered highly specific—and even these findings are not 100% specific. The ECG can even be totally normal. In the absence of an old ECG for comparison, any changes present should be presumed to be new. Although persistent or fixed changes are more characteristic of infarction, labile changes have a greater predictive value for the presence of ischemia for patients with elevated biomarkers thought to have non-Q wave MI, the presence of ST depression is a negative prognostic sign.

4. Imaging—Imaging can also be used to confirm the presence or absence of acute infarction, but it is rarely

used in modern practice. Infarct-avid imaging with technetium 99m pyrophosphate indium-111-labeled myosin or 99m sestamibi can be used. These techniques detect large AMIs well. With smaller infarctions, however, sensitivity is lost. In addition, with larger infarctions, a significant number (20–30%) of images will remain persistently positive for at least 6 months.

Echocardiography also may be helpful in detecting an AMI. Some researchers argue that the absence of regional abnormalities on the ECG is strong evidence against the presence of acute infarction. The sensitivity of echocardiography, however, is critically dependent on the quality of the views obtained; the absence of an abnormal ECG should not of itself be used to exclude the presence of ischemic heart disease. Furthermore, echocardiography cannot distinguish acute infarction from a persistent defect caused by an old myocardial injury. At present, therefore, it is diagnostically useful for AMI when the ECG and clinical history are equivocal. It is valuable in defining the presence of the complications of AMI.

Jaffe AS, Ravkilde J, Roberts R et al: It's time for a change to a troponin standard. Circulation 2000;102:1216-1220.

Menown IB, Allen B, Anderson JM et al: Early diagnosis of right ventricular or posterior infarction associated with inferior

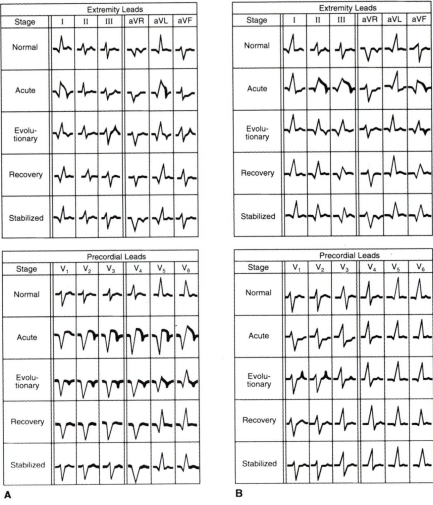

Figure 5–3. Typical evolution of the electrocardiographic changes of acute myocardial infarction. **A:** Anterior infarction. **B:** Inferior infarction. Reproduced, with permission, from Lipman BS, Dunn MI, Massie E: Clinical Electrocardiography. St. Louis: Mosby, 1984.

wall left ventricular acute myocardial infarction. Am J Cardiol 2000;85:934.

The Joint European Society of Cardiology/American College of Cardiology Committee: Myocardial infarction redefined: A consensus document for he redefinition of myocardial infarction. J Am Coll Cardiol 2000;36:959.

Treatment

Because myocardial damage progresses rapidly during the early hours, efforts during this critical period must be directed toward reducing myocardial oxygen demand and improving coronary blood supply to diminish the extent of myocardial damage. To be maximally effective, these interventions must be initiated as soon as possible: The reduction in benefit is very time-dependent, and patients who are treated within an hour fare significantly better than those treated later. Thus, prompt reperfusion therapy via primary angioplasty or thrombolytic therapy should be initiated in the absence of contraindications as early as possible in patients with ST elevation acute infarctions. It is now becoming clear that urgent treatment also reduces the morbidity associated with non-Q wave infarctions as well, especially if followed by definitive intervention on the infarct related artery.

A. EMERGENCY CARE AND PROTOCOLS

More than 85% of patients who present with ST elevation within 4 h of the onset of acute infarction have total thrombotic occlusion, thought to be caused by plaque rupture and subsequent development of an intramural coronary thrombus. The timely reestablishment of nutritive perfusion saves lives. This is best done, if possible, by primary angioplasty but if not available in <60 min (door to balloon time), thrombolytic agents should be used. The time window may not be the same for all patients, however. In some patients, collateral perfusion to the infarct zone extends this window; in others, there is only intermittent occlusion and transient recanalization prior to total occlusion, which may modify the time course of the infarction. It cannot be emphasized enough that the earlier treatment occurs the better (Figure 5–4). Although the magnitude of benefit varies for thrombolytic therapy, patients treated within 1 h of the onset of infarction (an impossibility if treatment requires 90 min to initiate) have up to a 50% reduction in mortality rates; those treated in the second hour have only half that benefit, and there is controversy about whether benefit occurs at all after 6 h. For primary angioplasty, this time dependence, especially after the first hour is less, but treatment during the initial 60–90 min is associated with profound benefit. The mortality rate for patients treated within 60–90 min of the onset of infarction in an outpatient trial of thrombolysis was 1%; for patients receiving identical treatment from 90 min to 3 h, the mortality rate was 10%. Emergency departments and hospitals must facilitate the way in which interventions aimed at coronary recanalization are implemented.

To this end, each hospital should have a plan that addresses each step in the identification, triage, and treatment of the patient who is a potential candidate for coronary recanalization.

It is starting to become clear that such a plan should be expanded, albeit with different therapies for patients with non-Q wave events as well. Such plans should include:

1. Activities that can be initiated by paramedics en route to the hospital—Paramedics can record and transmit 12-lead ECGs to the receiving facility; they can screen patients for indications for and contraindications to treatment with thrombolytic agents. In some emergency medical systems, thrombolytic therapy can safely be implemented by paramedics. Although the cost-effectiveness of initiating therapy in the field is unclear, screening by paramedics and the availability of a diagnostic ECG prior to arrival appear desirable.

2. Emergency room procedures—A triage plan should be developed to identify patients with chest discomfort compatible with ischemia and to facilitate rapid ECGs. Electrocardiograph machines should be available in all emergency facilities, with personnel trained to rapidly record 12-lead ECGs available at all times. The ECG must be read expeditiously by a physician. Although ECG screening by computer algorithms may be a reasonable adjunct, all computer systems do not perform equally well. The ultimate responsibility for interpretation of the ECG therefore resides with the physician. Emergency room physicians without a high level of expertise in this area should have readily available expert consultation (whether on-site or via electronic communications) to minimize delays in interpretation. This step should take no more than 5 min.

The first physician who sees the patient with chest discomfort and appropriate ECG changes should have

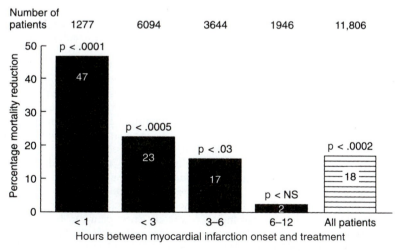

Figure 5–4. Time of treatment (postinfarction) and mortality rates associated with the use of thrombolytic agents. Adapted from Gruppo Italiano per lo Studio della Streptochinasi nell'Infarto Miocardico (GISSI): Effectiveness of intravenous thrombolytic treatment in acute myocardial infarction. Lancet 1986;1:397.

both the responsibility and the authority to initiate treatment. If there is a prospective plan to use primary angioplasty in patients with ST elevation events, this is the therapy of choice. If not or if there is delay, thrombolytic therapy should be given. For patients with non-Q wave events (those with elevated troponins), treatment with antiischemic agents such as nitrates and β-blockers and the use of heparin (LMWH is better) is called for, and if intervention is likely, IIB/IIIA agents should be initiated. Each hospital should develop a protocol to address the following issues:

- How many intravenous (IV) lines are necessary? One line must always be available in the event of an emergency and for infusion of medication to facilitate reperfusion (heparin, lytic agents, or IIB/IIIA agents). An additional line may be necessary for other medicines or for a heparin lock through which to draw blood.
- How much oxygen should be used routinely? This should be defined; blood gases are relatively contraindicated in this situation, oximetry is preferred.
- If primary angioplasty is the therapy of choice, prospectively detailed lines of communication must be established. If thrombolysis is the choice, the facility should know the thrombolytic agent of choice, and the dose for the routine patient. These should be decided by consensus. Instances in which an exception is necessary should be detailed, as should whom to call for consultation. The agent for routine use should, of course, be available in appropriate doses within the emergency department to facilitate rapid administration.
- Which medicines should be used adjunctively? Aspirin, heparin, nitroglycerin, β-blockers, and IIB/IIIA agents for the routine patient should be specified in advance—and should be immediately available in the emergency department.
- Which contraindications should preclude treatment?
- How will patients be moved rapidly from the treatment area to their ultimate destination in an intensive care unit?

B. GENERAL PROCEDURES

1. Intravenous line—An intravenous line should be placed immediately in any patient who is seriously considered to have suffered acute ischemia; this will provide access for the administration of pharmacologic agents should they be necessary and for emergency treatment should the need arise. The IV line should be large (18 gauge or greater); its patency should be maintained with an infusion of 5% dextrose in water, one-half normal saline, or normal saline solution.

2. Oxygen—Oxygen is appropriate for all patients with suspected AMI. Given the current aggressive approach toward anticoagulation and reperfusion in treating coronary heart disease, which often entails the use of potent anticoagulants or thrombolytic agents, blood gas determinations are not appropriate as a routine measure; oximetry is preferred. The empiric use of oxygen, usually via nasal prongs at 2–4 L/min, is recommended for all patients except those who have both normal oxygen saturations by oximetry or some reason to withhold oxygen (eg, a history of CO_2 retention). Even patients with severe chronic obstructive pulmonary disease who may be at risk for CO_2 retention should receive oxygen if systemic oxygenation is inadequate. Although supported by experimental data, the concern that supraphysiologic doses of oxygen may induce vasoconstriction and adverse effects has never been convincingly documented clinically.

3. Relief of discomfort—Relief of discomfort is a high priority.

a. Sublingual nitroglycerin—Unless contraindicated by hemodynamic abnormalities, sublingual nitroglycerin can be used to try to relieve chest discomfort and reverse ECG changes. A reversal of ECG changes is found most often in patients with patent infarct-related coronary arteries; it suggests that ischemia rather than infarction is present. Nitroglycerin must be given cautiously, however, especially to patients with inferior MI who may have RV infarction and who are prone to hypotension in response to this agent. A small subset of patients without RV infarction will also develop hypotension and an inappropriately slow heart rate after nitroglycerin. This is a vagally mediated phenomenon that has also been reported with morphine sulfate. Atropine (0.5 mg) is the treatment of choice in such cases.

b. Intravenous nitroglycerin—If patients have a beneficial response to sublingual nitroglycerin, it is reasonable to initiate treatment with IV nitroglycerin at a low dose (5–10 μg/min). Although this may relieve some of the chest discomfort in patients with acute infarction, it does not reduce the need for treatment with analgesics. Furthermore, reductions in blood pressure by more than 10% in normotensive patients are likely to be detrimental. Keeping the dose low and not expecting it to provide total relief of discomfort is recommended. This approach reduces the incidence of tolerance to the agent, which occurs in up to 25% of patients. Some physicians also use more potent vasodilators such as sublingual nifedipine to assess whether chest pain can be relieved and ECG changes reversed. Although these agents are effective, there is an associated incidence of marked hypotension that can cause detrimental cardiovascular effects. Calcium channel blockers are not recommended for routine administration.

c. Morphine sulfate—If the patient does not have a prompt response to sublingual nitroglycerin, morphine sulfate is the drug of choice. An IV dose of 2–4 mg and repeated as necessary and tolerated until chest discomfort is relieved is recommended. In addition to relieving pain, morphine sulfate reduces anxiety and the catecholamine secretion that occurs across the myocardial vasculature during acute infarction. As noted earlier, there is a small incidence of hypotension with an inappropriate heart-rate response that responds to atropine. Other analgesic agents used for the treatment of pain include meperidine and pentazocine.

d. Beta-blockers—Beta-blockers are commonly used to treat the chest discomfort associated with AMI in countries outside the United States. They have been shown to be effective, apparently because of both their membrane-stabilizing effects and their beneficial effects on myocardial oxygen supply and demand. Small doses of metoprolol (generally 5 mg), propranolol (1–3 mg IV) or esmolol (a loading dose of 250 mg/kg followed by 25–50 mg/kg/min, up to a maximum dose of 300 mg/kg/min) can be given as long as hemodynamic and electrical stability can be maintained. Although esmolol's efficacy in this area is not well established, it is rapidly metabolized by esterases in red cells and is the only agent with a brief duration of action. Beta-blockers may also be useful in reducing the extent of infarction and for secondary prevention (see section d. Adjunctive therapy).

e. Angiotensin-converting enzyme inhibitors—Patients with ST elevation infarction seem to benefit from the early initiation of treatment with angiotensin-converting enzyme inhibitors (ACEI) if blood pressure allows. This strategy improves ventricular remodeling acutely but is even more efficacious over the longer term

4. Activity—Bed rest, except for the patients who require the use of a bedside commode, is mandatory during the first 24 h; autonomic instability, hypotension, and arrhythmias are common. It was believed in years past that strict bed rest was appropriate for 7–10 days and that discharge should occur after approximately 2 weeks. It is now clear that it is less stressful and thus more beneficial medically if hemodynamically stable patients are allowed to sit in a chair and use a bedside commode after 24 h. In general, patients without complications remain in an intensive care unit for 2–3 days, during which time their activities are markedly restricted. On transfer out of the intensive care unit, they can gradually begin ambulation, and most patients without complications can be discharged as early as 4 days after infarction.

5. Diet—It generally has been recommended that patients with acute infarction avoid extremes of hot and cold, have no caffeine, and be maintained initially on a liquid diet. The rationale for this approach includes the presence of autonomic instability, concerns that caffeine might exacerbate arrhythmias, and fear that particulate matter could be aspirated in the event of cardiac arrest (which tends to occur early during the evolution of acute infarction). Although none of these concerns have been strictly validated, such restrictions are considered prudent. After the first day, if patients are stable, their diet can be advanced. Education to facilitate good eating habits and a reduction in fat intake can be initiated at that time.

6. Bowel care—Patients, especially those who are older and are put to bed-rest with a reduced oral intake, have a tendency to constipation. Given the autonomic instability indigenous to AMI, the reduction of straining when bowel movements occur is recommended. In general, the use of stool softeners such as docusate sodium in a once-a-day dose of 100 mg is adequate. Some degree of selection is appropriate; some patients are not in need of this treatment, whereas others require more potent treatment.

7. Sedation—If patients are excessively restless and no physical cause can be determined, sedation with small doses of a sedative-hypnotic agent such as diazepam is recommended. During the initial 24 h, the dosage should be the minimum required to relieve anxiety, and patients should be continually reassessed to ensure that what is being treated is anxiety and not an underlying complication of infarction.

8. Electrocardiographic monitoring—All patients with significant likelihood of AMI should be monitored electrocardiographically. Those with chest pain and ECG changes that are highly likely to be due to infarction should be hospitalized in an intensive care unit. Those deemed at less risk still require ECG monitoring in an environment where defibrillation is readily available. It is recommended that patients with uncomplicated acute infarction be monitored until discharge; patients with complications require longer periods of observation.

9. Heparin—Unless there are contraindications to its use or patients are receiving other anticoagulants, all patients should receive subcutaneous heparin, 5000 units every 12 h. This regimen has been shown to reduce the incidence of deep venous thrombi that occurs in as many as 24% of treated patients; it should reduce the frequency of pulmonary emboli as well. Although the studies documenting these effects were done at a time when long periods of bed rest were mandated, they are most likely still correct—at least in principle—and there is little morbidity associated with the relatively modest doses of heparin. Therefore, despite earlier ambulation, the use of subcutaneous heparin twice daily is still recommended. Most patients with ST segment elevation AMI or with non-Q wave AMI benefit from the use of therapeutic doses of heparin. Many still recommend unfractionated heparin to increase the activated partial thromboplastin time (aPTT) to 1½–2½ times. However, it is now clear that LMWH is more beneficial in large part because its effects are consistent in most patients, with the exception of those with renal dysfunction. The usual dose is 1 mg/kg (enoxaparin q12h or 120 units IV/kg q12h for dalteparin. Monitoring of coagulation parameters is not necessary.

Anonymous: Staffing and equipping emergency medical services systems: Rapid identification and treatment of acute myocardial infarction. National Heart Attack Alert Program Coordinating Committee Access to Care Subcommittee. Am J Emerg Med 1995;13:58.

Antman EM, Louwerneburg HW, Bears HF et al: Enoxaparin as adjunctive antithrombin therapy for ST-elevation myocardial infarction: Results of the ENTIRE-thrombolysis in myocardial infarction (TIMI) 23 trial. Circulation 2002;105:1642.

Every NR, Parsons LS, Hlatky M et al: A comparison of thrombolytic therapy with primary coronary angioplasty for acute myocardial infarction. Myocardial Infarction Triage and Intervention Investigators. N Engl J Med 1996;336:1253.

C. Recanalization Therapy

Prompt coronary recanalization clearly reduces infarct size and, in the long term, saves lives. The so-called open artery hypothesis also has additional benefits (see section 2. Implemantation of Reperfusion Strategies). At one time, there was legitimate controversy over whether coronary recanalization induced by mechanical means (angioplasty) was better, with lower mortality and morbidity rates, than that induced by thrombolysis in patients presenting with an ST elevation MI. Comparative studies indicate that the greater degree of coronary patency induced by angioplasty produces less residual ischemia and recurrent infarction. It is clear that patients whose vessels are open, with sluggish flow (TIMI II grade), have a substantially worse prognosis than do those whose vessels are widely patent with a normal (TIMI III grade) flow. Thus, because direct reperfusion of a coronary artery via mechanical means is more apt to induce TIMI grade III flow and, thus, better nutritive perfusion, it results in reduced mortality and morbidity. In general, patency rates with primary percutaneous coronary intervention (PCI) are in the range of 85–90%, whereas with thrombolysis, the rates are roughly 65% and recurrent events are more common. With modern advances, direct stenting appears to be by far the best approach. This is clearly the case for patients who present ≥1–1½ h after the onset of symptoms. The results with thrombolysis in early (<90 min) patients probably match the results of PCI. If intervention is delayed for more than 60 min, results are far less positive. Thus, unless PCI can be done immediately, treatment with thrombolytic agents should be initiated.

Similar data concerning the advantages of recanalization therapy are starting to emerge for those with non-Q wave infarction as well although the data are still controversial. However, both the FRISC 2 and Tactics TIMI 18 studies strongly suggest that the aggressive use of newer anticoagulants such as IIB/IIIA agents and LMWH along with urgent recanalization improve prognosis. Additional trials in this important area are ongoing.

1. Subsets of patients—
a. Inferior versus anterior myocardial infarction—The mortality rates associated with anterior ST elevation MI are at least twice those for ST elevation inferior MI, and patients with the former should be treated more aggressively. Specifically, recanalization therapy should be considered appropriate for as long as 12 h in patients with anterior MI. This is particularly true when the ST segment elevation is greater than 2 mm or when more than two anterior precordial leads are involved. Data from patients with inferior infarction suggest that those with marked ST elevation and especially those with ST depression in the right-sided anterior precordial leads (V_1–V_3) are at greatest risk. Such changes are associated with a larger area at risk for infarction and subsequent morbidity and mortality. In addition, patients with RV involvement benefit substantially from recanalization. Therefore, the site of infarction and the ECG changes must be factored in with the patient's age, hemodynamic stability, and other signs in determining the time during which treatment is appropriate.

b. Elderly patients—Elderly patients with acute ST elevation MI are at high risk for increased morbidity and mortality with thrombolytic agents. Indeed, some studies suggest that these agents have no benefit in this group. On the other hand, PCI is clearly beneficial. However, if PCI cannot be accomplished, individual decisions concerning the risk (which is substantial, especially in regard to intracranial bleeding) and the potential benefits must be balanced. Given the high (20–30%) mortality rate from ST elevation MI in the elderly, some increased risk may be reasonable.

c. Hypertension—Many studies of thrombolysis have been extremely cautious about enrolling patients with concurrent hypertension. In some studies, the presence of hypertension has been a demonstrable risk factor for bleeding; in others, this has not been the case. Although even patients with severe hypertension have been treated with beneficial results and no complications in some studies, definitive data are absent in this area. One important consideration is the ease with which blood pressure can be controlled. Transient hypertension that resolves quickly when pain is treated is less worrisome than that which requires treatment with vasodilators. The use of less aggressive dosing regimens and gentler anticoagulation may help to avoid morbidity when treating hypertensive patients. Again, PCI avoids many of these problems.

d. Prior cerebral vascular accidents—Initially, all patients with a history of cerebral vascular accidents were handled cautiously and were considered to have contraindications to the use of thrombolytic agents. It is now clear that this criterion is too rigid, and only cerebral vascular accidents that have occurred within the past 2 months and those associated with intracranial bleeding should be considered absolute contraindications.

2. Implementation of reperfusion strategies—Once the decision is made to treat a patient, treatment should be initiated promptly and the patient transferred to an intensive care unit. (Contraindications to the use of thrombolytic agents are contained in Table 5–2).

a. Urgent percutaneous coronary intervention—Recent data suggest that stenting with the use of clopidogrel for at least 4 weeks is the preferred modality of therapy. Although in one study, stenting appeared to present a possible initial early hazard, this was not observed in a subsequent study, and the frequency of subsequent ischemia and restenosis is clearly improved. The adjunctive use of LMWH is problematic because the only data concerning its use in this setting are preliminary. However, for enoxaparin, an initial IV dose of 30 mg appears optimal or dalteparin in a dose of 120 IU/kg subcutaneously.

b. Plasminogen activators—Plasmin, the key ingredient in the fibrinolytic system, degrades fibrin, fibrinogen, prothrombin, and a variety of other factors in the clotting and complement systems. This effect inhibits clot formation and can lead to bleeding. Patients with AMI and ST segment elevation have little evidence of spontaneous or intrinsic fibrinolysis, despite the intense thrombotic stimulus present. This may be due in part to increased levels of circulating PAI 1 in plasma or PAI-1 that is elaborated locally from platelets. The pharmacologic administration of plasminogen activators (Table 5–3) to such patients seems reasonable. Plasminogen activators can be administered intravenously or directly into the coronary artery. Although more rapid patency occurs with local administration, and lower doses can be used, given the need for early treatment, plasminogen activators are generally administered intravenously.

In addition to invoking fibrinolysis and inhibiting clotting by degrading clotting factors, all activators enhance clot formation. These effects seem greater with nonspecific activators such as streptokinase and urokinase and could partly explain why fibrin-specific activators such as t-PA open arteries more rapidly.

The enhancement of coagulation by plasminogen activators suggests an important role for the concomitant use of antithrombotic agents.

(1) Streptokinase—Streptokinase is derived from streptococcal bacteria and activates plasminogen indirectly, forming an activator complex with a slightly longer half-life than streptokinase alone (23 min versus 18 min after a bolus). Because it activates both circulating plasminogen and plasminogen bound to fibrin, both local and systemic effects occur; that is, circulating fibrinogen degrades substantially (fibrinogenolysis as well as fibrinolysis occurs).

Because antibodies to the streptococci exist in many patients, allergic reactions can occur; anaphylaxis is rare, however, and the use of steroids to avoid allergic reactions is no longer recommended. When streptokinase is administered intravenously, a large dose is necessary to overcome antibody resistance. Because a dose of 250,000 units will suffice in 90% of patients, the recommended dose of 1.5 million units over a 1-h period is generally more than adequate to overcome resistance. Patients who are known to have had a severe streptococcal infection or to have been treated with streptokinase within the preceding 5 or 6 months (or longer) should not receive the agent.

Rapid administration of streptokinase, even at the recommended dose, can cause a substantial reduction in blood pressure. Although this might be considered a potential benefit of the agent, it may also be detrimental. The rate of the infusion should therefore be reduced in response to significant hypotension, and the blood pressure should be monitored closely. Because streptokinase is more procoagulant than other thrombolytic agents, it should not be surprising that patients benefit to a greater extent from the concomitant use of potent antithrombins such as hirudin. However, in combination with IIB/IIIA agents, streptokinase seems to be associated with markedly increased bleeding rates.

(2) Urokinase—Urokinase is a direct activator of plasminogen. It has a shorter half-life than streptokinase (14 ± 6 min) and is not antigenic. Its effects on both circulating and bound-to-fibrin plasminogen are similar to those from streptokinase. It is therefore difficult to understand why IV doses of urokinase (2.0 million units as bolus or 3 million over 90 min) seem to induce coronary artery patency more rapidly than does streptokinase. There is substantial synergism between urokinase and t-PA.

(3) Tissue plasminogen activator—The initial human t-PA was made by recombinant DNA technology. The half-life in plasma was short (4 min) as a bolus but longer (46 min) with prolonged infusions. Despite the short half-life lytic activity persisted for many hours after clearance of the activator. Although t-PAs are considered "fibrin-specific," no activator is totally fibrin-specific, and fibrin specificity is lost at

Table 5–2. Contraindications to the use of thrombolytic agents.

Absolute
  Active internal bleeding
  Cerebrovascular accident within the past 2 months
  Known central nervous system neoplasm
  Recent severe trauma or major surgery within the past 2 weeks, especially with head trauma
  Pregnancy
  Severe hypertension (>180 mm Hg systolic or 110 mm Hg diastolic) that does not abate with relief of pain or pharmacologic
    treatment
  Prolonged CPR (>5–10 min), especially if intubation has occurred.
Major Relative
  Evidence of significant active internal bleeding within the past 2–4 weeks
  Suspected aortic dissection
  Cerebrovascular accident within the past 6 months
  Prolonged CPR (>5–10 min) within the past 2 weeks, especially with intubation
  Active malignancy
  Clearly positive hemoccult stool test
Relative
  Trauma or surgery (especially spinal or central nervous system) within the preceding 2 months
  Active peptic ulcer disease
  History of cerebrovascular accident, tumor, trauma, or CNS surgery
  CPR
  Hypertension (>180 mm Hg systolic or 110 mm Hg diastolic) that abates rapidly; persistent hypertension below these levels
  Known bleeding disorder; including that induced by pharmacologic agents (eg, aspirin, warfarin, dipyridamole)
  Severe hepatic or renal dysfunction
  Severe underlying life-threatening systemic illnesses
  Severe proliferative retinopathy in diabetic subjects
  Cardiogenic shock
  Invasive vascular procedure within the preceding 10 days
  Endocarditis

CPR = cardiopulmonary resuscitation; CNS = central nervous system.

higher doses. At clinical doses, however, less fibrinogen degradation took place than with nonspecific activators. Tissue plasminogen activator clearly opened coronary arteries more rapidly than nonspecific activators and this is likely why its use improved mortality rates. Bleeding was not less and there was a slight increase in the number of intracranial bleeds which was in part due to the need for dosage adjustment for lighter-weight patients.

The original regimen for the use of t-PA was 100 mg over 3 h: 10 mg as a bolus, followed by 50 mg over the first hour and 40 mg over the next 2 h. Patients who weighed less than 65 kg received 1.25 mg/kg over 3 h with 10% of the total dose given as a bolus. An alternative front-loaded regimen was found to be more effective and included an initial bolus of 15 mg, followed by 50 mg over 30 min and 35 mg over the next 60 min. Doses higher than 100 mg are associated with a higher incidence of intracranial bleeding.

(4) Reteplase—Over time a variety of t-PA variant molecules have been developed. This mutant, called reteplase, lacks several of the structural areas of the parent molecule (the finger domain, kringle 1, and the epidermal growth factor domain). It is less fibrin-specific (causes more systemic degradation of fibrinogen) than the parent molecule, and has a longer half-life. Accordingly, it is used as a double bolus of 10 units initially followed by a second bolus 30 min later. Initial studies suggested that such a regimen used with unfractionated heparin opened more coronary arteries faster than did t-PA. This led to a large trial (GUSTO III) that compared the activators and found no difference. If anything, the minor trends that were present, favored the parent molecule. Nonetheless, many have elected to use reteplase because of the convenience of the double bolus administration.

(5) Tenecteplase—Tenecteplase is also a mutant form of t-PA. It has substitutions in the kringle 1 and protease domains to increase its half-life, increase its fibrin specificity, and reduce its sensitivity to its native inhibitor (PAI-1). These effects were substantiated in clinical trials and initially it appeared that the agent

Table 5–3. Administration of plasminogen activators (FDA-approved agents only).

Agent	Dosage	Adjunctive Treatments
Streptokinase	1,500,000 units over 1 h	Aspirin, ± heparin
t-PA		
Standard	5 mg bolus, then 50 mg over 30 min and 35 mg over next 60 min	Aspirin, heparin, essential
Patients weighing less than 65 kg	1.25 mg/kg over 3 h, 10% of dose as initial bolus	
Urokinase	3,000,000 units over 1 h	Aspirin, ± heparin
r-PA	10 mg initial bolus, second 10-mg bolus after 30 min	Aspirin, heparin, essential
TNK	<60 kg: 30-mg bolus	
	60–70 kg: 35-mg bolus	
	71–80 kg: 40-mg bolus	
	81–90 kg: 45-mg bolus	
	>90 kg: 50-mg bolus	Aspirin, heparin essential

t-PA = tissue plasminogen activator; r-PA = reteplase; TNK = tenecteplase.

might be substantially superior to the parent molecule. However, in a direct comparison trial (Assent 2), using a 40-mg dose of tenecteplase, no differences in patient outcomes were observed with the possible exception of the group treated more than 4 h after the onset of symptoms. Nonetheless, because of the convenience of a single bolus dose, this agent is generally being used in preference to the parent molecule.

c. Combined thrombolysis and percutaneous coronary intervention—This combination approach has substantial promise. The early experience with coronary interventions after thrombolysis suggested substantial morbidity. Recent data using a half dose of thrombolytic agent (PACT) and studies using IIB/IIIA agents have suggested that now rapid serial thrombolysis and PCI can be accomplished without detriment and may in the long run permit the benefits of both modalities to be combined. This may be an important strategy for those patients living in areas where transport times or logistics make timely PCI impossible. Trials are ongoing to further test these strategies.

d. Adjunctive therapy—
(1) Aspirin—The ISIS II study showed that the combination of aspirin and streptokinase produced a greater reduction in mortality rates than did streptokinase or aspirin alone. Aspirin alone, however, in a dose of 162.5 mg, reduced mortality from acute infarction to almost the same extent as did streptokinase alone.

These impressive data have led to the use of aspirin in all patients with AMI. Such a posture is supported by strong experimental evidence that aspirin inhibits platelet aggregation and facilitates fibrinolysis. In general, chewable aspirin in a dose of 162.5–325 mg is recommended initially because its effects on platelets occur within 20 min.

(2) Heparin—Intravenous heparin, used with plasminogen activators, improves the rapidity with which patency is induced; it is essential for maintaining coronary patency, especially with t-PA type agents. Its use is less necessary after treatment with streptokinase, probably because of the anticoagulant effects of fibrinogen depletion and degradation products.

The standard dose of unfractionated heparin is usually a bolus of 5000 units, followed by a 1000-unit-per-hour infusion until the partial thromboplastin time (PTT) can be used to titrate a dose between 1.5 and 2 times the normal range. It has become clear that optimal titration of unfractionated heparin is problematic and that if the activated PTT is either too high or too low, some benefit is lost. For this reason, the use of LMWH is recommended. With the exception of patients with renal failure, a dose of 1 mg/kg for enoxaparin and 120 unit/kg for dalteparin provides for consistent reduction in anti-Xa levels and thus consistent anticoagulation. This is probably the reason that recent studies suggest it is more effective for the treatment of patients with AMI. In addition, because LMWH inhibits Xa activity predominantly, there is some suggestion that discontinuing it may be less problematic than is the case for unfractionated heparin, which has fewer effects on Xa and more direct effects (when combined with antithrombin 3) on thrombin itself. The ability to use the agent intravenously in the catheterization laboratory has not been a problem in regions where this strategy has been embraced.

(3) Beta-blockers—If given early, IV β-blockers have been shown to lower the risk of reinfarction in low-risk patients treated with thrombolytic agents. This provides a rationale for their use (metoprolol, 5 mg IV every 5 min for 3 doses, followed by 25–50 mg every 12 h orally; or propranolol, 0.1 mg/kg initially (IV), followed by 20–40 mg every 6 h) in patients receiving thrombolytic therapy. It is presumed but has not been proven that similar benefits accrue to patients treated with primary PCI. Contraindications to the use of β-blockers include rales more than one-third of the way up the posterior lung fields, systolic blood pressure of less than 100 mm Hg, a heart rate of less than 60 bpm, conduction disturbances, a history of chronic obstructive pulmonary disease or asthma, or a history of an adverse responses to β-blockers. Tachycardia should not be considered the result of increased adrenergic tone and should be treated with β-blockers until all possible physiologic causes can be excluded. This is particularly important with diabetic patients, in whom autonomic neuropathy can at times cause tachycardia. Once treat-

ment with β-blockers has been initiated, there will be some reason to discontinue the drug during the first 2–3 days for 20–30% of patients. This may be due to the evolution of infarction with the development of heart failure or to unanticipated complications of the drug (Table 5–4).

In general, β-blockers appear to induce most benefit in patients who reduce their degree of ST segment elevation in response to treatment. This is thought to be the marker of a patent infarct-related vessel and probably permits the agent to reach the infarct zone.

(4) Nitroglycerin—Sublingual nitroglycerin is usually administered immediately to patients with suspected AMI to assess resolution of ST elevation and relief of pain (discussed earlier). Intravenous nitroglycerin has been shown to reduce infarct size in patients not receiving reperfusion and to improve survival in patients with infarction and CHF. Its use during thrombolysis was presumed to induce similar benefit; however, the ISIS 4 trial failed to show any effect on subsequent morbidity and mortality. Therefore, the routine use of IV nitroglycerin is not recommended.

(5) Intravenous magnesium—Several small studies have documented a reduction in mortality rates after administration of IV magnesium (1–2 g over 1 h, followed by 8 g over 24 h) to patients presenting during the initial 24 h of acute infarction. ISIS 4, however, failed to demonstrate any benefit in morbidity or mortality with the routine use of IV magnesium. Therefore, because IV magnesium induces mild hypotension and

Table 5–4. Standard intravenous doses of commonly used agents in patients with acute myocardial infarction.

Agents	Dosage	Comments
Antiarrhythmics		
Lidocaine	Initial bolus of 1 mg/kg and 2 mg/min infusion, additional bolus doses to 3 mg/kg may be necessary.	For symptomatic arrhythmias and sustained ventricular tachycardia and ventricular fibrillation, not arrest
Procainamide	20 mg/min–1 g, then 2–4 mg/min drip	May cause hypotension, QRS or QT lengthening, or toxicity
Magnesium	1–2 g over 1–2 min or infusion of 8 g over 24 h	Observe for changes in heart rate, blood pressure
Amiodarone	15 mg/min × 10 min, then 1 mg/min × 6 h and 0.5 mg/min × 24 h	For refractory ventricular tachycardia, ventricular fibrillation and arrest
Beta-Blockers		
Esmolol	250 μg/kg IV loading dose, then 25–50 μg/kg/min to maximum dose of 300 μg/kg/min	Very short half-life

(continued)

Table 5–4. Standard intravenous doses of commonly used agents in patients with acute myocardial infarction. *(continued)*

Agents	Dosage	Comments
Beta-Blockers (continued)		
Metoprolol	5 mg q 5 min IV × 3 then 25–50 mg q12h orally	Long duration of action; may exacerbate heart failure
Propranolol	0.1 mg/kg over 5 mm IV, followed by 20–40 mg q6h orally	Long duration of action; may exacerbate heart failure
Calcium channel blockers		
Diltiazem	20–25 mg IV test dose, then 10–15 mg/h as needed; 90–120 mg tid orally	May exacerbate heart failure
Inotropes and Pressors		
Amrinone	Initial bolus of 0.75 mg/kg, then 5–10 mg/kg/min	May exacerbate ischemia
Dobutamine	Begin at 2.5 µg/kg/min and titrate to effect	Increases in heart rate >10% may exacerbate ischemia
Dopamine	Start at 2 µg/kg/min, titrate to effect	May exacerbate pulmonary congestion and ischemia
Norepinephrine	Start at 2 µg/min, titrate to effect	Temporizing treatment only
Vasodilators		
Nitroglycerin	Begin at 10 µg/min IV, titrate to effect	Avoid reducing blood pressure by >10% if normotensive, >30% if hypertensive
Nitroprusside	Begin at 0.1 µg/kg/min, titrate to effect	Mean dose 50–80 µg/kg/min
Nesiritide	2 µg/kg bolus followed by 0.01 µg/kg/min infusion, can increase by 0.005 to maximum infusion 0.03 µg/kg/min	Hold diuretics and other vasodilators. Keep blood pressure >100 systolic
Anticoagulants		
Unfractionated heparin	5000 unit bolus followed by 1000 U/h adjusted by a PTT	Less efficacious than LMWH
Enoxaparin	1 mg/kg SQ q12h, can give immediate 30 mg bolus intravenously if necessary	Hard to reverse effects; avoid in patients with renal failure
Dalteparin	120 IU/kg q12h.	Avoid in patients with renal failure
Abciximab	0.25 mg/kg followed by 0.125 µg/kg/min × 12 h, maximum time-24 h	Care necessary if renal failure; thrombocytopenia greater with repeated use
Eptifibatide	180 µg/kg bolus × 2 (30 min later) followed by 2 µg/kg/min for as long as 96 h for ACS, 24 h post PCI	Care necessary if renal failure
Tirofiban	0.4 µg/kg/min × 30 min followed by 0.1 µg/kg/min for up to 108 h for ACS, 12–19 h for PCI	Care necessary if renal failure
Clopidogrel	300 mg loading dose, then 75 mg/day × at least 1 month	TTP possible

ACS = acute coronary syndromes; LMWH = low-molecular-weight heparin; PCI = percutaneous coronary intervention; PTT = partial thromboplastin time.

bradycardia, its use cannot be recommended unless serum magnesium levels are shown to be low or other indications, such as torsade de pointes, are present.

(6) Calcium channel blockers—Dihydropyridine calcium channel blockers have shown to be detrimental in patients with AMI, probably because of a small but important incidence of severe hypotension. The data are inadequate to assess the risk or benefit of other calcium channel blockers. Although it is hoped that IV preparations may avoid adverse effects, allowing achievement of some of the benefits seen in experimental models, the use of calcium channel blockers cannot be recommended at this time.

(7) Lidocaine—Lidocaine was initially administered to patients receiving thrombolytic agents because of concern that coronary recanalization might exacerbate arrhythmias; However, recanalization reduces the incidence of such arrhythmias. In addition, recent analyses suggest the routine use of lidocaine may actually increase mortality rates. Accordingly, the use of prophylactic lidocaine is not recommended. The agent should be used if ventricular tachycardia (VT) or ventricular fibrillation (VF) occurs.

(8) IIB/IIIA agents—These agents bind to the platelet fibrinogen receptor and prevent platelet aggregation and activation. The initial agent in this group was abciximab, which is a chimeric antibody fragment to the receptor. Now both small peptide and nonpeptide competitive inhibitors of the receptor are available. These agents markedly inhibit hemostasis by both inhibiting hemostatic plug formation and reducing subsequent coagulation. They have not as yet been shown to be of benefit in patients with ST elevation AMI but are clearly efficacious in patients with non-Q wave events, especially if they undergo PCI. This is a group with an adverse long-term prognosis without intervention.

e. Complications—The most serious complication of treatment with thrombolytic agents is bleeding, particularly intracranial hemorrhage. Reduction in this dreaded complication is one of the very substantial benefits of catheter-based interventions. The mechanism of bleeding with thrombolytic agents is unclear but has been related to the efficacy of the agent, the concomitant use of antithrombotic agents such as heparin and aspirin, and the degree of hemostatic perturbation induced by the plasminogen activators. In most studies, the incidence of stroke and intracerebral bleeding has been slightly higher with t-PA type activators. This may be in keeping with the greater efficacy and rapidity of their effects. Although most bleeding occurs early during treatment, some can occur 24–48 h later, and vigilance even after the first few hours is important.

Bleeding may be of several types. Intracranial bleeding is by far the most dangerous because it is often fa-

tal. For most activators, the incidence of intracranial hemorrhage is less than 1%; it may be as high as 2–3% in elderly patients. Risk factors for intracranial bleeding include a history of cerebral vascular disease, hypertension, and age. These factors must be taken into account when determining whether a thrombolytic agent has an appropriate benefit-to-risk relationship. Changes in mental status require an immediate evaluation—clinical and computed tomography or magnetic resonance imaging. If bleeding is strongly suspected, heparin should be discontinued or reversed with protamine.

There also is a substantial incidence of nonhemorrhagic, probably thrombotic, stroke that may be partly due to dissolution of thrombus within the heart, followed by migration. The exact mechanisms of this phenomenon are unclear. In some studies, the excess of strokes with t-PA has been found to be related to this phenomenon and in others it has been due to an apparent increase in intracranial bleeding.

Bleeding outside the brain can occur in any organ bed and should be prevented whenever possible. The puncture of noncompressible arterial or venous vessels is relatively contraindicated in all cardiovascular patients: those with unstable angina one day may be candidates for thrombolytic treatment on the next. Blood gas determinations should therefore be avoided if possible and oximeters used instead in cardiovascular patients. It should be understood that central lines placed in cardiovascular patients pose a substantial risk should there be a subsequent need for a lytic agent. Foley catheters and endotracheal (especially nasotracheal) intubation can also predispose to significant hemorrhage. Bleeding should be watched for assiduously. If severe bleeding occurs while heparin is in use, it should be antagonized with protamine. In general, this and supportive measures are all that can be done. In some studies, there appears to be a slightly higher incidence of extracranial bleeding with nonspecific activators than with t-PA; this finding has not been consistent. In an occasional patient, who begins to bleed shortly after receiving the plasminogen activator, epsilon amino caproic acid, which changes the activation of plasminogen, may be useful. Otherwise, discontinuation of the drug and conservative local measures are all that can be done. If volume repletion is necessary, red blood cells are preferred to whole blood, and cryoprecipitate is preferred to fresh frozen plasma because they do not replenish plasminogen.

Allergic reactions related to the use of streptokinase are unusual but should be identified when they occur. Mild reactions such as urticaria can be treated with antihistamines; more severe reactions such as bronchospasm may require glucocorticoids or epinephrine.

Bleeding after primary PCI whether for ST elevation of non-Q wave AMI can also be substantial, particularly if IIB/IIIA agents are administered. The use of newer closure devices are touted by some but close observation is the key to minimizing bleeding from the catheter site. On occasion, platelet transfusions may be necessary.

3. Subsequent early management—Aggressive monitoring can help determine which patients have coronary recanalization in response to treatment and which do not. Conventional ECG monitoring for ST segments and arrhythmias and consideration of the presence or absence of chest pain are not particularly reliable for this purpose. In fact, increasing degrees of ST segment elevation during the first hour after treatment appear to be a sign of incipient recanalization.

Emergency cardiac catheterization and angioplasty are not indicated for the routine patient who has been successfully thrombolysed. However, patients with non-Q wave AMI who have been stabilized pharmacologically and who are candidates for intervention should have it performed promptly. Patients who suffer continuing or persistent chest discomfort, who have recurrent segment change, or who have difficult-to-treat hypotension and heart failure should be considered for cardiac catheterization.

D. Other Interventions

A variety of other interventions have been suggested throughout the years. These include the use of glucose, insulin, potassium, and hyaluronidase. Intraaortic balloon pumps have also been suggested, especially in patients with anterior infarction who might be deemed at risk for the development of severe heart failure. In general, none of these are recommended as routine measures. Perhaps the most promising of these is in the area of tight glucose control in diabetes. The DIGAMI study suggested an impressive benefit in early and late mortality and morbidity. With the availability of accurate glucose monitoring for point of care use, implementation of a strategy using rapid adjustments of IV insulin guided by hourly glucose measurements is likely to emerge as an important additional strategy.

Cannon CP, Weintraub WS, Demopoulos LA et al: TACTICS (Treat Angina with Aggrastat and Determine Cost of Therapy with an Invasive or Conservative Strategy)–Thrombolysis in Myocardial Infarction 18 Investigators. Comparison of early invasive and conservative strategies in patients with unstable coronary syndromes treated with the glycoprotein IIb/IIIa inhibitor tirofiban. New Engl J Med 2001;344:1879.

Malmberg K: Prospective randomized study of intensive insulin treatment on long term survival after acute myocardial infarction in patients with diabetes mellitus. DIGAMI (Diabetes Mellitus, Insulin Glucose Infusion in Acute Myocardial Infarction) Study Group. BMJ 1997;314:1512.

Ottani F, Galvan M, Nicolini FA et al: Elevated Cardiac Troponin Levels and the Risk of Adverse Outcome in Patients with Acute Coronary Syndromes. AMJ 2000;140:917.

Ross AM, Coyne KS, Reiner JS et al: A randomized trial comparing primary angioplasty with a strategy of short-acting thrombolysis and immediate planned rescue angioplasty in acute myocardial Infarction: The PACT trial. PACT investigators. Plasminogen-activator Angioplasty Compatibility Trial. J Am Coll Cardiol 1999;34:1954.

Stone GW, Grines CL, Cox DA et al: The Controlled Abciximab and Device Investigation to Lower Late Angioplasty Complications (CADILLAC) Investigators. Comparison of angioplasty with stenting, with or without abciximab, in acute myocardial infarction. N Engl J Med 2002; 346:957.

Wallentin L, Lagerquist B, Husted S et al: Outcome at 1 year after an invasive compared with a non-invasive strategy in unstable coronary-artery disease: The FRISC II invasive randomized trial. FRISC II Investigators. Fast Revascularization during Instability in Coronary Artery Disease. Lancet 2000;356:9.

E. Therapies at 6–72 Hours After Acute Myocardial Infarction

Optimal benefits in mortality rates and infarct size have been clearly demonstrated for early intervention with the establishment of TIMI-III flow in the infarct-related artery. Patients with symptoms of 6 h or less duration with ST segment elevation or new LBBB should be considered for immediate reperfusion therapy either with primary PCI or intravenous thrombolysis. The benefits of reperfusion therapy during the later phase of AMI (between 6 and 12 h) although having a less dramatic effect on improving postinfarction mortality rates, nonetheless have been demonstrated. Patients with ongoing angina, anterior infarctions, or persisting ST segment elevation present greater than 6 h after onset of symptoms are high-risk patients who will benefit even from late treatment in the absence of contraindications. The inverse association of coronary artery flow rate and death is confirmed in multiple studies of acute reperfusion and is the basis of the current approach to treatment. Optimal reperfusion therapy requires normal (TIMI grade III) epicardial and also normal myocardial perfusion. The mechanism of late benefit is unclear but has been discussed in terms of an open artery hypothesis. It has been suggested that the benefits from late intervention are associated with the presence of collateral circulation that preserves jeopardized myocardium and that this increases the time window during which thrombolytic therapy or percutaneous intervention can be beneficial. Stuttering or transient occlusion and reperfusion may also occur and therefore be a situation that allows the benefit of late reperfusion to be demonstrated. Additional considerations are the effects on ventricular remodeling and arrhythmias that may mediate late benefits of a patent infarct-related artery. Benefit in the 12–18-h post-MI period is less clear, but certainly those patients who remain at high risk with ongoing or stuttering angina and persistent ST segment elevation or combination of elevation and depression should still be considered for intervention. Such patients would be best served by a catheter-based intervention rather than thrombolytic therapy.

Once the diagnosis of AMI has been confirmed and appropriate reperfusion therapy has been undertaken, the patient should remain in an intensive care unit with telemetry monitoring. This should be followed by the early initiation of adjunctive therapy for stabilization during the early post-MI period as well as for long-term secondary prevention.

1. Beta-blocker therapy—Multiple randomized trials involving more than 50,000 patient have demonstrated a benefit of β-blocker therapy in AMI both for early and late cardiovascular mortality rates and reinfarction. The use of β-blocker therapy in ST segment elevation MI is well supported and is a class I indication by the ACC/AHA guidelines. Beta-blocker therapy is less well evaluated in patients with non-ST segment elevation and AMI, but most investigators would support its use in this setting. Currently the β-blocker therapy in this setting is a class IIA indication by ACC/AHA guidelines. Many of the β-blocker trials were performed in the prethrombolytic era, but more recent trials, such as the TIMI IIB study, which included approximately 1400 patients, randomized subjects to immediate intravenous metoprolol followed by oral metoprolol vs oral β-blocker begun postinfarction day 6. No statistically significant difference in mortality rates alone was detected, but there was a significant reduction in the combined rate of nonfatal infarction and recurrent ischemia in the immediate treatment group. The rate of death or reinfarction at 6 weeks was 5.4% in the immediate treatment group and 13.7% in the deferred treatment group (p =.007). Beta-blocker therapy after MI was also analyzed in approximately 202,000 patient by the Cooperative Cardiovascular Project. At hospital dismissal only 34% of patients were receiving β-blocker therapy, but these patients tended to have fewer risk factors for death than those not treated. Multivariate analysis to account for confounding factors demonstrated, however, that patients with uncomplicated infarction had a 40% reduction in mortality rate over 2 years and that the mortality rate was also reduced by 40% among patients with ST segment elevation infarctions. Additionally, high-risk patients, such as those who were elderly, had reduced LV systolic function (left ventricular ejection fraction <0.20) and those with diabetes and renal insufficiency, benefited even more from β-blocker therapy than others and often are left untreated. These findings suggests a benefit of secondary prevention with β-blockade both in high- as well as low-risk subgroups of patients and particularly in those patients previously considered to have contraindications to β-blockade, such as patients with diabetes, reduced LV systolic function, mild-to-moderate heart failure, and the elderly. Therapy should be titrated to reduce resting heart rate (Figure 5–5).

2. Angiotensin-converting enzyme inhibitors—Angiotensin-converting enzyme inhibitors are now reasonably well established as an important adjunctive therapy after AMI. The mechanism(s) by which such agents act to reduce mortality rates remains unclear, however, evidence supports that ACEIs alter the detrimental process of ventricular remodeling. The remodeling process is most significant in those patients with extensive anterior MIs; however, progressive remodeling and deterioration can occur in the absence of overt symptoms of CHF. Patients with Q wave MIs and impaired LV function should be treated with ACEIs early after hemodynamic stabilization tp improve long-term survival and reduce recurrent AMI (Figure 5–6). It is, therefore, reasonable to initiate ACEI therapy within the first 24 h if it has not been started acutely as long as no contraindications exists. Currently such use is a class I indication by the ACC/AHA guidelines. Both GISSI-3 and ISIS-4 trials demonstrated that one third of mortality rate reduction was attributable to therapy initiated within the first 24 h post-MI with beneficial

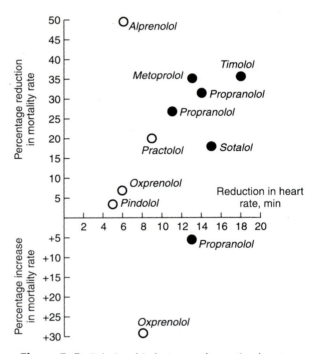

Figure 5–5. Relationship between the resting heart rate and the reduction in mortality. Closed circles indicate no intrinsic sympathomimetic activity (ISA); open circles indicate the presence of ISA. Reproduced, with permission, from Kjekshus JK: Importance of heart rate in determining beta-blocker efficacy in acute and long-term acute myocardial infarction intervention trials. Am J Cardiol 1986;57:43F.

effects demonstrated even better long after the acute setting. Therapy should be continued in patients who have high-risk features, such as reduced LV systolic function, evidence of clinical heart failure, significant mitral regurgitation, or hypertension.

The results of the recent HOPE trial further expanded the indications for ACEI therapy. This trial evaluated approximately 9300 high-risk patients who had evidence of vascular disease or diabetes plus additional cardiovascular risk factors. In a randomized trial design patients were assigned to ramipril, 10 mg qd orally or placebo for 5 years. The predetermined primary end-point of MI, stroke, or cardiovascular disease was significantly reduced (16% vs 18.6%, $p < .001$) in the ramipril group. The mechanism of action of the ACEIs includes antagonizing angiotensin II but also may have a benefit in plaque stabilization, vascular endothelial function, and limitation of smooth muscle cell proliferation. The results of the HOPE trial and other studies support a low threshold for ACEI use, particularly in patients at increased risks of cardiovascular events.

3. Lipid-lowering therapy—Lipid-lowering therapy has emerged as an important treatment in the secondary prevention of MI. Multiple secondary prevention trials have demonstrated reduction in mortality rates by

reducing cholesterol levels. Patients with AMI are considered by virtue of the MI itself to benefit from treatment regardless of the absolute cholesterol value. The addition of the noncholesterol-lowering properties of statins are of benefit and should be used. The Monitored Atherosclerosis Regression Study (MARS) as well as other angiographic trials of cholesterol-lowering therapies using statin drugs have demonstrated decreased rates of progression and modest regression of atheromatous disease in treated patients. The Scandinavian Simvastatin Survival Trial (4S) in which approximately 4400 patients with angina or prior MI were randomized to placebo or simvastatin demonstrated reduction of 42% mortality rate from coronary artery disease in the treated patients at 5-year follow-up. In the CARE study patients who had MIs and more typical total cholesterol levels, demonstrated at 5-year follow-up to have a 24% reduction in relative risk of death with pravastatin therapy.

Cholesterol-reduction therapy after AMI is being demonstrated to be a critical intervention for the treatment of patients with established coronary artery disease. The timing of initiation of drug therapy post-MI has not been clearly established, but initial studies with preliminary data suggests that early intervention probably within 72 h of presentation should be undertaken.

4. Antiplatelet/antithrombotic therapy—

a. Aspirin—Aspirin has been shown to be the single most cost-effective adjunctive therapy for acute coronary syndrome treatment. Aspirin decreases the mortality rate in MI and is currently a class I indication by the ACC/AHA guidelines. Patients who have bona fide aspirin allergy can be treated with clopidogrel or ticlopidine, which inhibit platelet aggregation by blocking the adenosine diphosphonate receptor and also IIb/IIIa receptor. In the ISIS-2 trial of approximately 17,000 patients with ST segment elevation MI, aspirin therapy produced a decrease in mortality rate of 23% compared with placebo. Secondary prevention benefits with aspirin have also been effective.

b. Heparin—Heparin has been a key adjunctive agent in the treatment of patients with MI. Unfractionated heparin acts to inhibit the thrombotic cascade by potentiating antithrombin III and also by a direct antithrombin effect.

c. Low-Molecular-Weight Heparin—Low-molecular-weight heparin administered by subcutaneous fixed-dose injection has a more predictable and longer duration of action than unfractionated heparin. Various LMWH differ in their ratio of factor Xa to antithrombin III inhibition, which accounts for differences observed in efficacy in acute coronary syndromes. The FRISC trial evaluated 1500 patients comparing dalteparin with placebo in aspirin-treated patients with

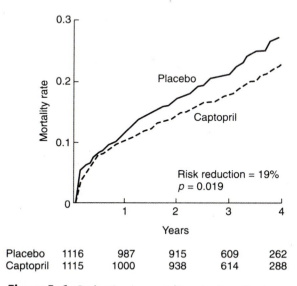

| Placebo | 1116 | 987 | 915 | 609 | 262 |
| Captopril | 1115 | 1000 | 938 | 614 | 288 |

Figure 5–6. Reduction in mortality rates in patients treated with captopril to alter the remodeling process seen after acute infarction. Reproduced, with permission, from Pfeffer MA et al: Left ventricular dysfunction after myocardial infarction—Results of the survival and ventricular enlargement trial. The SAVE Investigators. N Engl J Med 1992;327:669.

unstable angina or non-Q wave AMI. The investigators demonstrated an early reduction in death and recurrent MI (4.8% vs 1.8%), but this benefit was lost at 4 months after the event. In the meta-analysis of TIMI IIB and ESSENCE trials, use of enoxaparin resulted in a 20% reduction in combined end-point of death and ischemic events from 48 h through 43 days and without an increase in major hemorrhage (Table 5–5). Currently only short-term use (3–7 days) of enoxaparin is recommended in patients with ACS, especially those with elevated troponins and high-risk patients undergoing coronary intervention. The routine use of LMWH in AMI is not established and current ACC/AHA guidelines do not recommend use with percutaneous interventions. The results of ongoing trials, however, will most likely establish a role for LMWH as adjunctive therapy in AMI.

5. Calcium-channel blockers—Studies of calcium-channel blockers in AMI have in general failed to demonstrate any benefit. In a meta-analysis of 22 trials, no benefit to survival rates, infarct size or incidence of reinfarction was demonstrated. Two randomized trials evaluating secondary prevention with verapamil, DAVIT-1 and DAVIT-2, demonstrated benefit for death and re-

infarction rates when surviving patients were without evidence of heart failure. The CRIS trial demonstrated no benefit with verapamil therapy post-AMI.

The use of short-acting dihydropyridine calcium channel antagonists in the acute treatment of the postinfarct patients is not currently recommended. Both diltiazem and verapamil, however, have been shown to the reduce reinfarction rate slightly in patients who have had an MI with preserved LV systolic function. Therefore, selective use of calcium channel antagonists in such patients can be considered, but the generalized use of calcium channel blockers should be avoided in the early management (within 6 h) of AMI.

ACE Inhibitor Myocardial Infarction Collaborative Group: Indications for ACE inhibitors in the early treatment of acute myocardial infarction: Systematic overview of individual data from 100,000 patients in randomized trials. Circulation 1998;97:2202.

Antman EM, Cohen M, Radley D et al: Assessment of the treatment effect of enoxaparin for unstable angina/non-Q-wave myocardial infarction. TIMI IIB-Essence meta-analysis. Circulation 1999;100:1602.

Hennekens CH, Albert CM, Godfried SL et al: Adjunctive drug therapy of acute myocardial infarction—evidence from clinical trials. N Engl J Med 1996;335:1660.

Table 5–5. Meta-analysis of randomized trials of drug therapy administered during and after acute myocardial infarction.

Drug Class and Time Administered	Number of Trials	Number of Patients	Relative Risk of Death (95% CI)	p-Value
Beta-adrenergic antagonists				
During MI	29	28,970	0.87 (0.77–0.98)	0.02
After MI	26	24,298	0.77 (0.70–0.84)	<0.001
ACE inhibitors				
During MI	15	100,963	0.94 (0.89–0.98)	0.006
After MI, patients with left ventricular dysfunction	3	5,986	0.78 (0.70–0.86)	<0.001
Nitrates (during MI)	22	81,908	0.94 (0.90–0.99)	0.03
Calcium-channel blockers (during and after MI)	24	20,342	1.04 (0.95–1.14)	0.41
Antiarrhythmic drugs				
Lidocaine (during MI)	14	9,155	1.38 (0.98–1.95)	>0.05
Class I drugs (after MI)	18	6,300	1.21 (1.01–1.44)	0.04
Amiodarone (after MI)	9	1,557	0.71 (0.51–0.97)	0.03
Magnesium (during MI)	11	61,860	1.02 (0.96–1.08)	>0.05

Source: Reproduced, with permission, from Hennekens CH, Albert CM, Godfried SL et al: Adjunctive drug therapy of acute myocardial infarction—evidence from clinical trials. N Engl J Med 1996;335:1660.

ISIS-4 (Fourth International Study of Infarct Survival) Collaborative Group. ISIS-4: A randomized factorial trial assessing early oral captopril, oral mononitrate, and intravenous magnesium sulphate in 58,050 patients with suspected acute myocardial infarction. Lancet 1995;345:669.

LaRosa JC, He J, Vypputuri S et al: Effect of statins on risk of coronary disease: A meta-analysis of randomized controlled trials. JAMA 1999; 282:2340.

Vorchheimer DA, Badimon JJ, Fuster V et al: Platelet glycoprotein IIb/IIIa receptor antagonists in cardiovascular disease. JAMA 1999;281:1407.

Yusef S, Sleight P, Pogue J et al: Effect of an angiotensin-converting enzyme inhibitor, ramipril, on cardiovascular events in high-risk patients. The Heart Outcomes Prevention Evaluation Study Investigators. N Engl J Med 2000;342:145.

Complications of Myocardial Infarction

A. CHEST PAIN

Episodes of chest pain recur in up to 60% of patients after infarction. When chest discomfort recurs early (within 24 h of MI), the discomfort usually reflects the process of completing the infarction. Chest discomfort may reflect the effects of ongoing ischemia or recurrent infarction. In this situation prompt reassessment and treatment is critical. Patients with hemodynamic compromise in association with new ECG changes in the distribution other than that of the infarct-related artery are at significant risk and require prompt attention, often including coronary angiography with catheter-based intervention.

In those patients who were treated initially with reperfusion therapy and have recurrent chest pain, prompt evaluation is needed to assess the adequacy of anticoagulation and the possibility of reocclusion of the culprit coronary artery. Adequacy of adjunctive therapy in the setting of recurrent chest pain is necessary, and often adjustments in drug doses are required. Occasionally short-term use of IV nitroglycerin and IV β-blockers are required to quiet the ischemic episode. In this setting glycoprotein IIb/IIIa inhibitors should be considered if no contraindications are present. In patients with non-Q wave MIs, recurrent chest pain is a marker of significant risk for reinfarction, especially if transient ST segment and T wave changes are noted or if persistent ST segment depression is associated with the initial presentation. Prompt coronary angiography and PCI is often required in this setting.

B. HYPERTENSION

Uncontrolled hypertension in the setting of AMI is poorly tolerated and produces the unwanted effect of significantly increasing myocardial work. In the absence of ischemic CHF or AMI, hypertension is best treated with IV nitroprusside. Nitroprusside is an arterial vasodilator and is usually started at a dose of 0.1 µg/kg/min and titrated to reduce blood pressure to the range of 130–140 mm Hg systolic pressure.

Intravenous nitroglycerin can be best employed in the presence of ischemic CHF with hypertension. Nitroglycerin initiated at 5–10 µg/min and titrated to effect has arterial vasodilating effects; however, they are less potent than those for nitroprusside. Its benefit in the setting of heart failure is its reduction of preload and stroke volume; however, it may induce increased myocardial work. Adequacy of cardiac filling and cardiac output must be closely monitored.

An additional agent that is beneficial in this setting is IV esmolol, a β-blocker agent with a short half-life that permits rapid dose response to changing hemodynamic conditions. Another agent, labetalol, can be used when α-blocking properties are required in conjunction with β-blocker capability. Both esmolol and labetalol can be titrated to a desired effect. Subsequent oral β-blocker therapy is important in the setting of patients with known hypertension after infarction, particularly those patients who have experienced an anterior wall infarction. Adequate blood pressure control as part of a secondary prevention regimen is necessary.

C. CONGESTIVE HEART FAILURE

In general there is greater urgency in treating patients with CHF during the early phases of AMI because such patients often have multivessel disease and are at increased risk of recurrent infarction and increased infarct size. A high-degree of suspicion and close monitoring are key to anticipating this complication of AMI. Echocardiography has been the technique of choice in evaluating such patients from a perspective of both valvular and myocardial function. Swan-Ganz pulmonary artery catheterization can also be used to aid diagnosis and to assess ongoing management. Killip and Kimball originally (1967) described the outcome of LV failure occurring with AMI. They developed a clinical classification scheme to assess prognosis of patients with no evidence of heart failure to those in frank cardiogenic shock (Table 5–6). In patients with mild CHF characterized by rales present in at least 50% of lung fields or an S_3 gallop, the in-hospital mortality rate was approximately 17%. Those patients with pulmonary edema had an in-hospital mortality rate of 38%, and those who developed cardioshock had in-hospital mortality rate in excess of 75%. With the development of newer treatment strategies, particularly reperfusion therapy, these risks have been reduced but nonetheless remain substantial.

Management strategies depend on the clinical history of the patient. Patients with new-onset acute CHF are typically euvolemic and benefit from nitrate therapy for ischemia. These patients in general should not receive diuretics initially because diuretic therapy

Table 5–6. Killip classification.

Class	Features	Patients (%)	Hospital Mortality Rates (%)
1	No signs of CHF	33	6
2	S_3, gallop, rales, radiographic CHF	38	17
3	Pulmonary edema	10	38
4	Cardiogenic shock	19	81

CHF = congestive heart failure.
Source: Data from Killip T, Kimball JT: Treatment of myocardial infarction in a coronary care unit: A two-year experience with 250 patients. Am J Cardiol 1967;20:457.

often complicates their clinical course with the development of hypotension. Additionally, reduced respiratory effort, reduced heart rate, and normalization of oxygen saturation are central to early clinical management. Nitroglycerin is often the best agent to use for ischemia in patients with CHF; however, in some instances the hemodynamic profile provided by nitroprusside may be desirable. There is, however, an issue of nitroprusside exacerbating ischemia by inducing a coronary steal phenomenon. Nitroprusside in this setting would be a second-line therapy. Nesiritide (recombinant BNP) infusion has demonstrated hemodynamic and neurohormonal benefits in the management of acute heart failure. The use of natriuretic peptides in acute heart failure is being explored and may limit LV remodeling effects of AMI. Intravenous ACEI therapy should not be used in this setting until hemodynamic stability is achieved. Hypotension is a complicating factor because it reduces coronary perfusion and may lead to further ischemia. Low-dose dobutamine, starting at 2.5 µg/kg/ min can be used to achieve hemodynamic benefit. Also, phosphodiesterase inhibitors can be considered although their vasodilating effects may limit their inotropic benefit in patients with significant hypotension. The use of Swan-Ganz catheterization monitoring is controversial, and no randomized controlled data support their use as a first-line recommendation in the management of CHF with AMI. However, Swan-Ganz monitoring can be beneficial in verifying diagnosis, and its use in the early phases of management may allow rapid titration of parenteral therapy.

Once hemodynamic stabilization has been achieved, which is generally within the first 6–12 h, initiation of oral agents is appropriate. Drugs of choice in this setting are ACEIs, which improve cardiac performance, have beneficial effects on ventricular remodeling, and have been demonstrated not only to reduce morbidity but also to reduce mortality rates in patients with CHF. Oral β-blocker therapy should also be initiated early in the treatment of these patients, however, this should be done in a stepwise fashion in relation to ACEI therapy to avoid hypotensive effects.

D. CARDIOGENIC SHOCK

Cardiogenic shock is a clinical syndrome characterized by peripheral hypoperfusion and hypotension refractory to volume repletion. This occurs secondary to inadequate cardiac output resulting from severe LV dysfunction. Approximately 7% of patients with AMI develop cardiogenic shock, and at the time of the development of the Killip classification (1967) such patients experienced an approximately 80% in-hospital mortality rate. A trend toward increased in-hospital survival, however, occurred in the mid to late 1990s and can be correlated with more aggressive application of reperfusion therapies.

Goals for therapy for cardiogenic shock include hemodynamic stabilization to ensure adequate oxygenation of perfused tissue and prompt assessment for reversible causes of the cardiogenic shock. Positive inotropes are often the first drug to be considered, and because dobutamine reduces central pressures, it is often used initially. Dopamine may worsen pulmonary congestion but in the setting of hypotension is often used with dobutamine to increase peripheral resistance. The effects of dopamine are therefore modulated by the vasodilating action of dobutamine. The use of vasodilators can also be considered for their ability to fine-tune peripheral resistance and perfusion and thus allow adequate blood flow and oxygenation. Hemodynamic monitoring with balloon-tip pulmonary artery catheter allows prompt access to valuable hemodynamic information. Forrester and colleagues (1976) developed hemodynamic criteria related to pulmonary artery wedge pressure and cardiac output, which allowed risk profiles to be developed for subsets of patients with AMI. Goals of hemodynamic monitoring in this setting are to adjust the volume status to bring pulmonary wedge pressure into the range of 16–20 mm Hg and optimize coronary output with inotropic agents, vasodilators, or both, as needed. Additionally, severely hypotensive patients benefit with intraaortic balloon pumping or use of ventricular assist devices. Such interventions, however, often have only a temporary stabilizing benefit and with prolonged use may have significant risk of complication.

The results of several studies suggest that mortality rates are reduced in cardiogenic shock with prompt reperfusion therapy. The GUSTO-1 trial analyzed approximately 1320 patients with shock and assessed those patients who were revascularized within 30 days and compared them to patients who received nonrevascularization therapy. This multivariate analysis suggests that revascularization is independently associated with reduced 1-year mortality rates and that the in-hospital mortality rate is reduced to nearly 50%. More recently randomized trial data have been reporting results on revascularization in AMI complicated by cardiogenic shock. In this trial by Hickman and colleagues 302 patients were randomly assigned to early revascularization or initial medical stabilization. The primary end-point was death at 30 days from all causes, and the secondary end-point was 6-month survival. Results demonstrated a nonsignificant 9% mortality rate reduction at 30 days; however, the 6-month mortality rate was significantly lower in the revascularization group (50.3% vs 63.1%, $p = .027$). Subgroup analysis of interactions suggested that only patients younger than 75 benefited from the early revascularization strategy. Although the 17% relative reduction in the 30-day mortality rate did not reach statistical significance secondary to sample size, it nonetheless is important clinically to the extent that revascularization produced results that very favorably compared with the benefits achieved by fibrinolytic therapy or primary angioplasty in nonshock patients with AMI.

Although cardiogenic shock continues to produce high mortality rates in patients with AMI, the aggressive application of current reperfusion therapies have reduced those rates, and results of randomized controlled trials promise to further improve our clinical approaches to the management of heart failure.

E. ACUTE MITRAL VALVE REGURGITATION

The development of acute severe mitral valve regurgitation occurs in approximately 1% of patients with AMI and contributes to 5% of deaths. Mitral regurgitation occurs as a result of papillary muscle rupture most commonly involving the posterior medial papillary muscle because its singular blood vessel supply is derived from the posterior descending coronary artery. In contrast, the anterior lateral papillary muscle much less commonly ruptures because it has a dual blood supply derived from the left anterior descending and circumflex coronary arteries. Rupture of the papillary muscle may be complete or partial with the development of a

failed mitral valve leaflet. Pulmonary edema usually ensues rapidly and usually occurs within 2–7 days after inferior infarction. The intensity of associated murmur varies depending on the extent of unobstructed flow back into the left atrium. If severe regurgitation is present, no murmur may be audible. As a result, a high degree of suspicion is needed to promptly diagnose inferior wall infarction. Two-dimensional echocardiography can be used to demonstrate the partial or completely ruptured papillary muscle head and the flail segment of the mitral valve. Typically hyperdynamic LV function is demonstrated, and its occurrence in severe CHF should prompt the diagnosis. The treatment of choice is to stabilize the patient hemodynamically with the use of IV vasodilators and possibly intraaortic balloon counterpulsation. The basis of successful outcome, however, is prompt emergency surgery. The operative mortality rate in this setting can be up to 10%, but this affords most opportunity for survival. Mitral valve repair with reimplantation of the severed papillary muscle is the preferred technique as an alternative to mitral valve replacement. The mortality rate is unacceptably high in the absence of prompt surgery.

Ischemic mitral regurgitation without papillary muscle rupture occurs in up to 50% of patients with acute inferior wall MI. In those patients who develop severe CHF symptoms, hemodynamic compensation needs to be undertaken and could include the use of intraaortic balloon pump for adequate afterload reduction. Treatment of ischemia in this setting may include reperfusion therapy with PCI, IV vasodilator therapy, and mechanical support. Once the acute phase of the infarction is past, resolution of the severe mitral regurgitation may occur, which would then avoid a need for surgery.

F. ACUTE VENTRICULAR SEPTAL RUPTURE

Rupture of the ventricular septum has been reported to occur in up to 3% of AMIs and contributes to about 5% of deaths. Typically half of ventriculoseptal defects (VSDs) occur in anterior wall MIs, often in patients with their first infarction, with peak incidence occurring 3–7 days after initial infarction. Findings associated with VSD can be confused with acute mitral regurgitation because both can result in hypotension, severe heart failure, and prominent murmur. However, the diagnosis of VSD should be suspected clinically when a new pansystolic murmur is noted. Generally, the murmur is most prominent along the left sternal border and may have an associated thrill. Prompt surgical intervention is recommended, which, if successful, can reduce the mortality rate from nearly 100% to below 50%. The 30-day mortality rate reported by the GUSTO-1 database investigators in patients who developed periinfarction VSD was 74%. In those patients selected for surgical repair versus ongoing medical management, the 30-day mortality rate was 47% versus 94%, respectively. Patients surviving the initial 30 days after infarction demonstrated an excellent 1-year survival rate.

G. CARDIAC RUPTURE

Rupture of the free wall of the left ventricle occurs in approximately 1–3% of patients with acute infarction and accounts for up to 15% of periinfarction deaths. The incidence of free wall rupture has decreased in the fibrinolytic era but may occur as early as within the first 48 h of infarction. Fifty percent of ruptures occur within the first 5 days of infarction and 90% within the first 2 weeks. Rupture may be due to expansion of the periinfarct zone, with thinning of the infarcted wall occurring in response to increased stress. The paradoxical motion of the infarcted segment at the margin of the infarcted zone may also contribute stress, resulting in muscle rupture. Electrocardiographic changes of myocardial ischemia often do not herald the onset of rupture, and, not uncommonly, the presentation is that of rest with electromechanical dissociation. Prompt intervention at that time may include echocardiography with pericardiocentesis, intraaortic balloon pump placement, and urgent cardiac catheterization with anticipation of immediate surgery. Unfortunately, all too often signs of cardiac rupture are not present until acute hemodynamic decompensation occurs. This then requires immediate intervention for any possibility of preventing death.

H. PERICARDITIS

Pericarditis is common in patients with AMI, particularly in the course of transmural infarctions. In general, the larger the area of infarction, the more likely pericarditis will develop. Pericarditis may be clinically silent or may be associated with a pericardial rub, description of pleuritic chest pain by the patient or pericardial effusion as suggested by chest radiograph or two-dimensional echocardiography. The associated chest discomfort, classically described as being relieved by sitting up, may also be associated with a description of shortness of breath and epigastric discomfort with inflammation of the contiguous diaphragm. Pericardial rubs are most commonly heard when the patient is seated with held inspiration. Late pericardial inflammation occurring 2 weeks to 3 months after MI is termed Dressler's syndrome and most likely reflects an autoimmune mechanism. This is often associated with large serosanguinous pleural and pericardial effusions, and those who die from this syndrome develop tamponade. The treatment of choice in this setting is aspirin, NSAIDs, or colchicine, and in some instances steroids may be necessary. The use of steroids, however, is not advocated because of the high frequency of relapse when steroid therapy is discontinued. Echocardiographic assessment

is appropriate as a follow-up tool in these patients to determine the extent of effusion if present and to exclude tamponade or the possibility of partial myocardial rupture. If possible, NSAIDs should be avoided in patients with ischemic heart disease, particularly those with evidence of acute infarction. Agents such as indomethacin inhibit new collagen deposition and, therefore, may impair the healing process necessary for stabilization of the infarcted region. This may, in a small number of patients, contribute to the development of myocardial rupture. When used in cases refractory to aspirin, NSAIDs should be used for the shortest time possible and tapered as rapidly as possible.

I. RIGHT VENTRICULAR INFARCTION

Right ventricular involvement in acute inferior wall MI is common. Hemodynamically significant RV dysfunction, however, is uncommon, occurring in relatively few patients with RV infarction. Substantial RV infarction contributing to hemodynamic compromise occurs in up to 20% of patients with inferior and posterior infarction. These patients often clinically demonstrate hypotension and elevated jugular venous pressure but clear lung fields in the setting of acute inferior wall infarction. ST segment elevation in right-sided leads (V_3R or V_4R), RV wall motion abnormalities on echocardiography help confirm the diagnosis of RV involvement. With RV infarction, the right ventricle becomes noncontractile, and cardiac output is maintained by increased excursion of the septum into the right ventricle. The incidence of high-grade AV block is also increased in patients with RV infarction.

The prognosis of patients with RV infarction is generally good, especially with recanalization therapy and supportive care. If reperfusion is not possible, the stunned right ventricle tends to resolve its dysfunction. Support entails IV fluid administration and, on some occasions, the use of dobutamine-positive inotropic therapy, and occasionally AV sequential pacing is required. Aggressive volume resuscitation was at one time considered the cornerstone of therapy in these patient, however, overhydration can lead to peripheral and pulmonary edema. Therefore, caution needs to be practiced in fluid management in RV infarction. Early treatment with IV diuretics may lead to hypotension and confound patient presentation and, therefore, lead to overzealous fluid repletion. Patients who display the development of shock despite supportive treatment may benefit from catheter-based intervention (angioplasty and stenting) of the occluded right coronary artery. The balance between the extent of RV and LV dysfunction, however, determines long-term outcome.

J. CONDUCTION DISTURBANCES

The presence of a conduction disturbance is associated with increased in-hospital and long-term mortality rates. The prognostic significance and management of these disturbances may vary with the location of the infarction, the type of conduction disturbance, associated clinical findings, and the extent of hemodynamic compromise. Patients whose conduction disturbances result in bradycardias and produce hemodynamic compromise generally require transvenous pacing. Bradycardias, especially those associated with inferior infarction, can often be treated with atropine. Recurrent episodes, however, warrant insertion of a pacemaker. Often ventricular pacing to provide a back-up rate is all that is required. A need for improved hemodynamics may be a reason to consider AV sequential pacing.

1. Anterior ST elevation myocardial infarction— The highest risk conduction disturbances occur in these patients. Abnormalities are present early after the onset of infarction and are usually the result of extensive infarction producing pump failure; treatment with a pacemaker may not improve the prognosis. Conduction disturbances in this circumstance are generally RBBB, with or without concomitant fascicular block. Right bundle branch block without fascicular block may have the same incidence of progression to complete heart block (20–40%) as does an RBBB with fascicular block. Patients with RBBB and a fascicular block with anterior MI should undergo placement of transarterial pacing and be observed for evidence of progression to complete heart block warranting permanent transvenous pacing.

Left bundle branch block is most often a chronic manifestation of hypertension and myocardial dysfunction rather than an acute abnormality. In a setting of AMI, however, it is often difficult to determine whether the LBBB is new. Recommendations have been to use pacemakers for patients with LBBB known to be new; this approach has also been advocated for patients with RBBB. Given the present availability of external pacemakers, these issues appear to be less critical.

In the absence of the signs and symptoms of hemodynamic instability or evidence of the progression to heart block, it is reasonable to observe patients with RBBBs or LBBBs and to use external pacing if conduction disturbances develop. Once such a disturbance develops, a transvenous pacemaker is indicated, and it is likely that AV sequential devices would be of benefit.

2. Inferior myocardial infraction— Conduction disturbances with acute inferior MI are often less critical, but they do suggest a poorer prognosis. The conduction disturbances that commonly occur represent involvement of the AV node and usually include first-degree (Wenckebach) AV block, Mobitz II second-degree AV block with narrow QRS complexes, and complete heart block with a junctional rhythm. Conduction disturbances are more common in patients with RV in-

farction. If hemodynamic stability is maintained, patients with these conduction disturbances do not require pacemakers, they often respond to the administration of atropine (0.5 mg IV). If hemodynamic compromise occurs in association with either Wenckebach block or a junctional rhythm, however, or if any arrhythmia requires treatment with more than one dose of atropine, a transvenous pacemaker is warranted. Large initial or total doses of atropine can lead to tachycardia with exacerbation of ischemia and, at times, VT or VF. For patients with RV infarction and hemodynamic compromise associated with the loss of atrial kick, an AV sequential pacemaker is recommended. In general, hemodynamically significant conduction disturbances occur in patients with inferior infarction early during the evolution of infarction; late conduction disturbances are usually well tolerated. Some of these conduction disturbances respond to an IV infusion of 250 mg of aminophylline.

3. Mobitz II second-degree AV block— Mobitz II second-degree AV block or complete heart block with a wide QRS complex are both absolute indications for transvenous pacemaker insertion. Such disturbances can occur from electrolyte abnormalities or conduction system disease, but they are most often associated with hemodynamic abnormalities caused by bradycardia. The use of temporary AV sequential pacing may benefit patients who have hemodynamic abnormalities; these patients are also likely to require permanent pacing (see the section, Prognosis, Risk Stratification & Management).

K. Other Arrhythmias

1. Sinus tachycardia— Sinus tachycardia occurs in up to 25% of patients with AMI. It is a marker of physiologic stress (pain, anxiety, hypovolemia) and often indicates the presence of CHF. In some patients, such as those with RV infarction, it may represent relative or absolute volume depletion. In general, although tachycardia increases myocardial oxygen consumption and can exacerbate ischemia, it should not be treated as a discrete entity. The proper approach is to treat the underlying physiologic drive. It may be unwise to block a tachycardia that is compensating for the increased cardiac work required, for example, by sepsis. Accordingly, β-blockers should be used only once if it is clear that no underlying abnormality is inducing the tachycardia or that the underlying abnormality (eg, hyperthyroidism) is amenable to such treatment. Making this determination may require hemodynamic monitoring.

2. Supraventricular tachycardia— Paroxysmal supraventricular tachycardia,, atrial flutter, and atrial fibrillation can all occur with AMI. Atrial fibrillation is by far the most common arrhythmia and is often associated with the presence of high atrial filling pressures.

The presence of supraventricular tachycardia should lead to consideration of CHF as a cause. A complete differential diagnosis, including conditions such as hyperthyroidism, pulmonary embolism, pericarditis, and drug-induced arrhythmias, is appropriate. Paroxysmal supraventricular tachycardia should be treated immediately because of the high likelihood in this setting that the tachycardia will induce ischemia. Adenosine in bolus doses of 6–12 mg IV is the initial approach of choice and often terminates the tachycardia. If it does not, cardioversion should be considered prior to other treatment, unless the PSVT terminates and restarts recurrently. Prolonged pharmacologic management before cardioversion may complicate the procedure, and the delay may induce toxicity if the heart rate is rapid, even in the absence of overt hemodynamic compromise. For recurrent or once-terminated PSVT (depending upon the mechanisms of the tachycardia; see Chapter 19), small doses of digitalis, diltiazem, verapamil, or a class I antiarrhythmic agent are reasonable choices for maintenance—as long as the indications and contraindications for each of these agents are kept in mind.

Atrial flutter and atrial fibrillation are generally markers of CHF. Frequently the diagnosis of flutter or fibrillation is made after administration of adenosine; once diagnosed, control of the ventricular response is critical. This can generally be accomplished with digitalis, verapamil, or diltiazem in conventional doses (see Chapter 20) once the CHF is treated. Intravenous diltiazem is effective in an emergency situation, usually with an initial test dose of 20–25 mg. If the response is favorable, a titrated dose of 10–15 mg/h should be used. Intravenous diltiazem should be used cautiously in patients with AMI and CHF. Cardioversion is indicated if a rapid ventricular response persists; the ventricular rate is difficult to control; or there are signs of hypotension, CHF, or recurrent ischemia. In general, PSVT and atrial flutter require 100 J as the initial shock energy; atrial fibrillation, 200 J.

Arrhythmias that recur after transient reversion in response to pharmacologic maneuvers or cardioversion require additional treatment. Treatment of the underlying initiating stimulus is critical. Beta-blockers can also be used to control the ventricular response acutely or for maintenance.

3. Ventricular arrhythmias—The incidence of postinfarct malignant ventricular arrhythmias in patients with AMI appears to be diminishing, perhaps because of the use of reperfusion therapy. It also is conceivable that interventions such as IV β-blockers have also contributed to this decline. Because of the diminishing incidence of VT and fibrillation in patients with acute infarction—as well as an unfavorable benefit-risk ratio—the use of prophylactic lidocaine is not recommended. Although prophylactic lidocaine reduces the incidence of VF, it is associated in many series with an increase in cardiac death (Figure 5–7), possibly because it abolishes ventricular escape rhythms in patients who may also be prone to bradycardia. Because warning arrhythmias, once considered progenitors of VF, do not appear to be highly predictive, it is recommended that only symptomatic arrhythmias and VT be indications for the administration of lidocaine.

Lidocaine is the drug of choice for treating symptomatic arrhythmias and sustained VT; it should be administered as an initial bolus of 1 mg/kg. A 2 mg/min drip is usually started concurrently. Because an infusion takes a substantial time to produce therapeutic levels, if arrhythmias persist, additional boluses of 0.5 mg/kg, every 8–12 min to a maximum dose of 3 mg/kg can be given. The loading dose should be reduced in patients who are older than 65, and the maintenance infusion reduced in those with hepatic disease or those with CHF, in whom the volume of distribution is reduced.

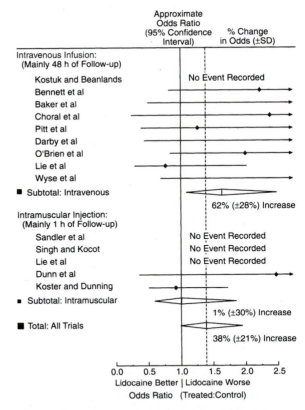

Figure 5–7. Meta-analysis of the trial of prophylactic lidocaine suggesting increased mortality rates in treated patients. Reproduced, with permission from MacMahon S et al: Effects of prophylactic lidocaine in suspected acute myocardial infarction. An overview of results from the randomized, controlled trials. JAMA 1988;260:1910.

Because the half-life of lidocaine changes after 24 h of a constant infusion, the dose must be reduced to maintain therapeutic but nontoxic blood levels. Lidocaine should be continued until the patient is hemodynamically stable and without ischemia. It can then be discontinued and treatment with agents for secondary prevention initiated. If arrhythmias are still present at that time, electrophysiologic evaluation should be considered.

If lidocaine does not relieve the symptoms or the arrhythmias, patients can be treated with IV procainamide. The initial loading dose is 1 g, at no more than 50 mg/min, followed by a 2–6 mg/min drip. The infusion rate should be reduced if hypotension occurs; this effect is due to procainamide's α-adrenergic effects. If successful, the drug is continued until the patient is hemodynamically stable; it can then be tapered after initiation of treatment with secondary-prevention agents and an assessment made in terms of long-term risk stratification. Occasional cases will be refractory to these agents and require IV amiodarone to control ventricular arrhythmias. Because of its long half-life in patients and its toxicity, this is not the first-line agent. Hypotension and CHF can be induced during the acute administration of amiodarone as a result of its negative inotropic effects. Amiodarone should therefore be used only if patients can be followed by a clinician with long-term experience with the agent. On rare occasions, a pacemaker may need to be placed in the left ventricle to compete with or overdrive-suppress malignant ventricular arrhythmias. This is usually reserved for rhythms refractory to pharmacologic therapy and can on occasion be life-saving. The ventricular pacemaker is generally set at 90–110 bpm—or whatever rate is necessary to suppress the ventricular arrhythmias.

Accelerated idioventricular rhythm occurs in up to 40% of patients and can in some instances be a marker of reperfusion. This rhythm is generally thought to be benign and is usually not treated.

Pulseless VT and VF should be treated as they are in any other patient with cardiac arrest.

L. Mural Thrombi

Patients with AMI are at risk for the development of endocardial thrombi for a variety of reasons. Left ventricular thrombus develops in up to 40% of patients with anterior wall infarction but uncommonly in inferior infarcts. Large areas of dyskinesis with poor flow are prone to develop clots. Because there may be a return in contractility in the borders of the infarcted zone during the remodeling process, it could paradoxically be that patients with larger infarctions tend to develop clots more readily, but those with somewhat smaller ones tend to have them result in emboli more frequently. It has been recommended that all patients with an anterior wall MI receive anticoagulation during hospitalization and for 3–6 months thereafter. If anticoagulation is not used routinely, echocardiographic evaluation for the presence of mural thrombi is recommended. Because short-term anticoagulation until the ventricle is remodeled might well be adequate for most patients, the value of long-term (3 months or more) anticoagulation is unclear. In the absence of contraindications, it is probably worthwhile to use heparin during hospitalization and subsequently to use warfarin for 3 months for patients with anterior infarction. Because it has not been established whether low doses of warfarin are as effective as larger doses in inhibiting LV mural thrombi, only full doses (an INR 2.0–2.5) is recommended. Old mural thrombi in patients with prior infarction and severe ventricular dysfunction are less prone to clot propagation than are fresh thrombi, and routine anticoagulation for these patients is not substantial. Anticoagulation may be valuable for some of these patients for other reasons, such as atrial fibrillation. Patients with inferior or non-Q wave infarctions require anticoagulation only if mural thrombi are detected during noninvasive evaluation. Some clinicians use echocardiographic criteria to select patients who should be treated; others would treat any thrombus detected.

Mural thrombi can form in the atrium as well as in the ventricle. Atrial fibrillation is common in patients with CHF; in the setting of atrial fibrillation, stagnation of blood in the atrial appendage leads to a high incidence of clots. This condition can be established only with TEE, but it may explain the high incidence of emboli in patients with paroxysmal atrial fibrillation. Accordingly, patients with atrial fibrillation should receive anticoagulation, not only because of their increased incidence of thrombus but because it appears that emboli can be prevented in this group with reasonably modest doses of anticoagulants (goal INR 2.0–2.5). Anticoagulation is discussed in depth in Chapter 28.

Patients with CHF and AMI are at increased risk for pulmonary emboli because of deep venous thrombosis in the calf and thigh. This may be prevented by the use of warfarin. An argument can be made to consider the use of warfarin in any patient with acute infarction who has had no contraindications for several months. Because aspirin was withheld in some studies, it is unclear whether it offers similar benefits, which would allow it to be substituted for warfarin.

M. Aneurysm and Pseudo-Aneurysms

Large areas of infarction tend to thin and bulge paradoxically. These large dyskinetic areas eventually form discrete aneurysms with defined borders. In general, treatment involves the same principles as those for patients with heart failure: vasodilatation and adequate control of filling pressures to reduce pulmonary congestion. Often patients with large dyskinetic areas will have a component of heart failure. If severe heart failure can be managed over time, an aneurysm may form that will then be amenable to surgical resection.

Occasionally, while aneurysms are forming, a myocardial rupture will occur. A small amount of rupture can become tamponaded by the pericardium, leading to what is known as a pseudo-aneurysm. Pseudo-aneurysms, which tend to have narrow necks and are not lined with endocardium, function like aneurysms in that they fill with blood during ejection, reducing systolic performance. In addition to reducing stroke volume and leading to increases in ventricular volume as a compensatory response with concomitant increases in pulmonary congestion, pseudo-aneurysms are prone to rupture. The larger the pseudo-aneurysm, the greater the possibility of rupture. Accordingly, the diagnosis of pseudo-aneurysm usually leads to relatively prompt surgery. Although pseudo-aneurysms can occur with both anterior and inferior MIs, true aneurysms are rare in the inferior-posterior distribution. A large aneurysmal dilatation is therefore more apt to be a pseudo-aneurysm in inferior-posterior location.

N. Dissecting Aortic Aneurysm

Dissection of a coronary artery in association with acute dissection of the ascending thoracic aorta can occur. Dissection of the right coronary artery is more common, but any coronary artery can be involved. The presence of infarction can obscure the diagnosis of aortic dissection. Pain that radiates to the left shoulder, is tearing or ripping, or occurs in association with severe hypertension is suggestive. Specific mention of the signs and symptoms of aortic dissection and their presence or absence should be elicited as part of every history and physical examination in all patients with suspected acute infarction particularly elderly patients with a history of hypertension. Close scrutiny of the proximal aorta by chest radiograph and TEE in any patient with heart failure or severe hypertension that is difficult to control is likely to unmask the diagnosis when concomitant dissection is present. Initial therapy is with nitroprusside for vasodilatation and IV β-blockers (either esmolol or metoprolol) to blunt the rapidity of the upstroke of systolic ejection. In general, aortic dissection with involvement of the coronary artery requires surgical repair once hemodynamic stabilization is achieved.

Bowers TR, O'Neil WW, Grines C et al: Effect of reperfusion on biventricular function and survival after right ventricular infarction. N Engl J Med 1998;338:933.

Crenshaw BS, Granger CB, Birnbaum Y et al: Risk factors, angiographic patterns, and outcomes in patients with ventricular septal defect complicating acute myocardial infarction. GUSTO-I (Global Utilization of Streptokinase and TPA for Occluded Coronary Arteries) Trial Investigators. Circulation 2000;101:27.

Fornecter JS, Diamond G, Chatterjee K: Medical therapy of acute MI by application of hemodynamic subsets. N Engl J Med 1976;295:1356.

Goldberg RJ, Zevallos JC, Yarzebski J et al: Prognosis of acute myocardial infarction complicated by complete heart block. The Worcester Heart Attack Study. Am J Cardiol 1992;69:1135.

Goldberg RJ, Samad NA, Yarzebski J et al: Temporal trends in cardiogenic shock complicating acute myocardial infarction. N Engl J Med 1999; 340:1162.

Hochman JS, Sleeper LA, Webb JG et al: Early revascularization in acute myocardial infarction complicated by cardiogenic shock. N Engl J Med 1999;341:625.

Sugiura T, Iwasaka T, Takehana K et al: Clinical investigation: Factors associated with pericardial effusion in acute Q wave myocardial infarction. Circulation 1990;81:477.

Welch PJ, Page RL, Hamdan MH et al: Management of ventricular arrhythmias. A trial-based approach. J Am Coll Cardiol 1999;34:621.

Yeo TC, Malout JF, Reeder GS et al: Clinical characteristics and outcome in postinfarction pseudoaneurysm. Am J Cardiol 1999;84:592.

Prognosis, Risk Stratification, and Management

A. Risk Predictors

1. Infarction size—Infarction size is an important determinant of long-term risk: the larger the infarction, the poorer the long-term prognosis. This association is easy to demonstrate in patients with first infarctions. In patients with multiple infarctions, the cumulative amount of damage is predictive. Measures that estimate cumulative infarct size (eg, ejection fraction; sestamibi scanning) provide important prognostic information. Nonetheless, the presence of an adverse prognosis does not, in and of itself, mandate a more aggressive therapeutic approach, however, ACEI and β-blockers are important adjunctive therapies.

2. Infarction type—In patients with non-ST segment elevation, infarctions are more prone to recurrent episodes of chest discomfort and infarction than are patients with ST elevation infarctions. Patients with ST segment elevation infarctions have an adverse short-term prognosis and should be considered for immediate reperfusion therapy; they often manifest arrhythmias that, especially in association with a low ejection fraction, are an important marker of an adverse prognosis. Often these are the patients who have CHF during hospitalization for acute infarction. Their prognosis is worse than that of patients without heart failure, even if the ejection fraction appears reasonably well preserved.

3. Malignant arrhythmias—Many patients who suffer malignant arrhythmias during evolution of the infarction are also at increased risk. The one exception appears to be patients with primary VF (ie, VF with no complication of infarction). It has not been demonstrated (except for the GISSI-1 investigation) that primary VF has an adverse prognostic effect.

B. RISK ASSESSMENT

Advanced age (>65 years), prior MI, anterior location of infarction, postinfarction angina, non-ST elevation MI, mechanical complications of infarction, CHF, and the presence of diabetes all suggest higher risk for reinfarction or death in the 6 months following infarction. These patients require aggressive risk stratification prior to hospital discharge after infarction.

1. Myocardial ischemia—Patients with recurrent ischemia during hospitalization are generally considered unstable because of the adverse prognosis associated with recurrent angina following MI. The extent to which brief or solitary episodes fit this definition is unclear. To date there is no evidence that such minor episodes adversely affect the prognosis or that mechanical interventions improve morbidity or mortality rates. For patients with multiple episodes of recurrent chest discomfort, or ischemia in a distribution distant from the current infarction, however, cardiac catheterization is recommended to permit consideration of PCI.

In patients without complications, who are not receiving reperfusion therapy, treadmill stress tests provide additional prognostic information. Thallium or sestamibi scintigraphy add to the sensitivity and specificity of this analysis. Nuclear or echocardiographic imaging can be used in patients whose ECGs cannot be interpreted because of drug effects, resting ST-T wave changes, or conduction disturbances. Patients who are unable to exercise may benefit from pharmacologic stress tests, such as dobutamine echoes, dipyridamole, adenosine, or dobutamine nuclear stress imaging. The inability to exercise is in itself a marker of poor prognosis.

Patients who have received thrombolytics or PCI and have not had recurrent episodes of chest discomfort constitute a very low-risk group for which the ability of any stress testing method to predict events is significantly reduced. Generally, however, patients who have been treated with thrombolytic agents and have evidence of ischemia undergo invasive study. Those without evidence of ischemia do well long-term without catheterization.

The evidence that the prognosis of patients with non-ST elevation infarction is adequately determined by stress testing is controversial and in part depends on the nature of the stress procedure, perhaps including whether patients exercise rigorously enough. There is some suggestion that because most stress tests during acute hospitalization tend to be submaximal, a maximal stress test 6–8 weeks after the infarction is most appropriate for thorough risk stratification.

2. Ventricular function—Patients with complications of infarction or any findings of CHF should have a noninvasive evaluation of ventricular function during their acute hospitalization. Assuming the absence of intercurrent events, one evaluation of ventricular function generally suffices.

In the absence of such an assessment, a stress echocardiogram can provide information concerning both ischemia and ventricular performance. Advocates believe that the combination of these parameters is important; detractors argue that the evaluation of ischemia is less complete than can be accomplished with radionuclide scintigraphy.

The evaluation of some patients with poor ventricular function may also require determining the presence of viable but dysfunctional myocardium (stunned or hibernating regions). Sophisticated metabolic studies using positron emission tomography seem to have the most promise for delineating the regions apt to improve with revascularization; however, they are not widely available for routine use. The response of dysfunctional regions may also be evaluated with dobutamine echocardiography (improved function is thought to be predictive of viable myocardium) or delayed thallium imaging (delayed uptake suggests viability).

3. Arrhythmias—Patients who have VT or recurrent episodes of VF after the first day require further evaluation. Evaluation is mandatory for patients who have recurrent arrhythmias without easily remediable causes, especially sustained VT, which generally requires invasive EPS. Although treadmill- and Holter-guided therapy are equivalent in some studies, the use of invasive EPS to select and titrate antiarrhythmic agents or choose a mechanical device provide one approach. Recent data suggest that if the ejection fraction is <0.35 and VT is present that implantable cardioverter defibrillators save lives.

At present it is unclear how to manage less severe arrhythmias, which may include frequent ectopy or nonsustained VT. Signal-averaged ECG can be used in such patients; although a negative study is reassuring, the sensitivity of the procedure for detecting risk is inadequate.

Patients who have had bradycardias often require pacemakers. Long-term pacemakers improve the prognosis for patients who have developed complete heart block via a mechanism involving bundle branch block. Some clinicians advocate pacing for patients who had transient complete heart block without the development of bundle branch blocks (those with inferior MI and narrow QRS complexes), but supportive data are not conclusive. There also is controversy concerning the use of pacemakers in patients with conduction disturbance such as RBBB and anterior fascicular block, who may (or may not) have had transient Mobitz II second-degree AV block; the benefits of pacing have yet to be established.

C. RISK MANAGEMENT

Patients with recurrent ischemia, severe ventricular arrhythmias, reduced ejection fraction (<0.40), or evidence of severe ischemia during stress testing require cardiac catheterization. Although, in general, treatment is guided by anatomic considerations and their relationship to a long-term prognosis, the ability to predict—from the anatomy—which vessels are apt to be involved in subsequent events is poor. Furthermore it is unclear that mechanical interventions will reduce the incidence of infarction or death except in well-defined subsets of patients (eg, those with left main disease, proximal three-vessel disease, and a reduced ejection fraction).

1. Risk factor modification—Central to the patient's in-hospital treatment is the identification of factors that increase the risk for progression of coronary artery disease. These include the traditional risk factors for atherosclerosis: hypertension, diabetes, smoking, cholesterol abnormalities, family history, and a sedentary life-style. Attempts to modify the diet, stop smoking, and increase exercise, should begin once the patient has left the intensive care unit. Although such efforts will vary with each patient, a structured program should be in placed with active follow-up of patients to ensure some level of success.

Recent statin therapy trials support aggressive reduction in cholesterol for the regression of atherosclerosis (in reality the retardation of the development of new lesions), therefore, a very aggressive approach toward the reduction of LDL cholesterol and increases in high-density lipoprotein is justified early (within the first 24–48 h) in postinfarction management. Patients with LDL cholesterol of more than 100 mg/dL should be treated (see Chapter 2).

2. Secondary prevention—Beta-blockers should be given to all patients who have had acute ST and non-ST elevation MIs with or without reperfusion therapy. Patients with CHF tend to benefit most with gradual titration of dose.

Although secondary-prevention trials with aspirin have not indicated statistically significant benefits, most studies do show a trend toward improvement, and meta-analysis supports the concept that aspirin improves prognosis after acute infarction. Whether this benefit is synergistic with the effects of β-blockers is unclear. Nonetheless, it appears reasonable to start patients on low doses of aspirin (81–325 mg/day) after AMI and to continue it long-term.

Long-term treatment with ACEIs is recommended for patients at risk for ventricular remodeling and the sequelae associated with that process. In general, this includes patients with ejection fractions of less than 0.45. Given results of recent trials, even patients with a low normal ejection fraction, after infarction should be considered for ACEI treatment, particularly with an anterior MI.

The long-term use of digitalis in patients with acute infarction and normal sinus rhythm remains controversial. It is clear that digitalis has hemodynamic benefits in patients with CHF, whether or not they are treated with ACEIs. Therefore, if digitalis is essential for improved hemodynamic performance, it should be used at low dose (0.125 mg/day after loading). Digitalis in association with other agents is also indicated for control of ventricular response in patients with atrial fibrillation.

3. Rehabilitation—Studies of exercise rehabilitation have been confounded by the fact that individuals who participate in such programs generally have favorable risk factor and psychologic profiles that lessen their risk of recurrent events. It has been argued that the improved prognosis of such patients is related to these initial characteristics—and not to the effects of exercise training. Nonetheless, exercise training clearly improves peripheral muscle efficiency, and intense long-term physical training (5 days a week for at least 9 months) has been shown to reduce the development of cardiac ischemia. Therefore, exercise rehabilitation programs are recommended whenever possible for postinfarction patients.

The amount of exercise prescribed must obviously be based on the patient's heart rate and blood pressure. These should be monitored as the patients start to walk during the convalescent phase in the hospital, and marked increases (eg, blood pressure more than 140/90 mm Hg) should be avoided. The patient's rehabilitation activity schedule should be reduced if this level of hypertension occurs. This may also indicate the treatment with β-blockers or ACEIs to reduce the labile hypertensive response. In any event , the response of blood pressure and heart rate to exercise must be monitored. Phase II of the program begins at hospital dismissal and generally continues for 8–12 weeks. Objectives should include further patient education, risk factor modification, and gradual resumption of normal work and recreational activities.

4. Psychologic factors—It is now clear that as many as 20–25% of patients with AMI meet formal clinical criteria for depression. It also appears that this is an adverse prognostic feature and that such patients have increased morbidity and mortality rates. Although there is some argument that this is so, because these patients have more severe disease, this hypothesis has not been supported by recent studies. It may well be that whatever leads to depression is negatively synergistic with underlying coronary artery disease, as suggested by the increase in catecholamines in such patients. Regardless of the mechanism, however, careful consideration of the presence or absence of depression in patients is recommended. Psychologic consultation should be sought for patients suspected of depression and treatment initiated to improve both the quality of the individual's life and—to the extent that there is an interaction with ischemic heart disease—the prognosis. Because tricyclics initially liberate catecholamines and may thereby induce adverse effects, drug treatment has previously been thought to be problematic in cardiovascular patients. On the other hand, these agents have membrane-stabilizing effects that may reduce the propensity to arrhythmias and it is believed that the potential for risk has been exaggerated. Newer agents that antagonize serotonin as their primary mode of action may (at least in theory) be safer, but cognitive therapy has also been shown to be effective.

Antman EM, Cohen M, Bernik PJL et al: The TIMI risk score for unstable angina/non-ST elevation MI. A method for prognostication and therapeutic decision making. JAMA 2000; 284:835.

Dorn J, Naughton J, Imamura D et al: Results of a multicenter randomized clinical trial of exercise and long-term survival in myocardial infarction patients: The National Exercise and Heart Disease Project (NEHDP) Circulation 1999;100: 1764.

Fielding R: Depression and acute myocardial infarction. A review and reinterpretation. Soc Sci Med 1991;32:1017.

Hochman JS, Tamis JE, Thompson TD et al: Sex, clinical presentation and outcome in patients with acute coronary syndrome. Global Use of Strategies to Open Occluded Coronary Arteries in Acute Coronary Syndromes IIb Investigators. N Engl J Med 1999;341:226.

Reeder GS, Gibbons RJ: Acute myocardial infarction: Risk stratification in the thrombolytic era. Mayo Clin Proc 1995;70:87.

Cardiogenic Shock

Craig Timm, MD

ESSENTIALS OF DIAGNOSIS

- *Tissue hypoperfusion, depressed mental status, cool extremities, urine output less than 30 mL/h*
- *Hypotension: systolic blood pressure less than 80 mm Hg*
- *Cardiac index less than 2.2 L/min/m²*
- *Pulmonary artery wedge pressure more than 18 mm Hg*

General Considerations

Although overall mortality from coronary artery disease and myocardial infarction continues to decline, mortality from cardiogenic shock—which is caused primarily by acute myocardial infarction—continues at a very high rate in medically treated patients. The initial development of coronary care units and rapid cardioversion or defibrillation of life-threatening ventricular arrhythmias, followed by risk-factor modification and such major advances as thrombolytic therapy and emergency revascularization, have contributed significantly to the successful care of the acute myocardial infarction patient. To understand the reasons for the continued high mortality rates in cardiogenic shock patients, it is important to understand the pathophysiology of cardiogenic shock and to examine the optimal treatment strategies that may improve mortality rates. In a strict sense, cardiogenic shock syndrome develops as a result of cardiac muscle failure (either right or left ventricle) that causes inadequate cardiac output. The cardiovascular system can contribute in a number of other ways to the development of shock: hypovolemia, mechanical problems, nonischemic valve lesions, arrhythmias, and abnormalities of diastolic filling. Although the primary focus of this chapter is cardiogenic shock that is due to muscle failure, there is also some discussion of other mechanical causes associated with acute myocardial infarction.

A number of definitions have been proposed; although they differ in some ways, there is general agreement that both hemodynamic and clinical parameters should be included. The hemodynamic criteria include a systolic blood pressure less than 80 mm Hg (less than 90 mm Hg if the patient is on pressors, inotropic agents, or intraaortic balloon pumping) and cardiac index less than 2.2 L/min/m². Clinical criteria require that signs of decreased peripheral perfusion be present, including cool clammy skin, cyanosis, altered mental status, and diminished urine output (less than 30 mL/h). The common denominator of the clinical findings is that they reflect a failure of tissue perfusion. Oxygen delivery is insufficient to sustain aerobic metabolism and therefore lactic acidosis is a metabolic consequence, regardless of the cause.

Using a combination of clinical and hemodynamic measurements means that fewer patients with only some symptoms (eg, low blood pressure but no signs of diminished tissue perfusion, or normal blood pressure with altered mental status or diminished urine output) are given an inappropriate diagnosis of shock.

Etiology

The most common cause of cardiogenic shock is acute myocardial infarction and is due to the loss of a large amount of myocardium. The incidence of shock in acute myocardial infarction is between 5% and 10%, and the mortality rate is extremely high in medically treated patients, ranging between 70% and 100%, a figure unchanged over the last several decades. Cardiogenic shock may occur in a patient with a massive first infarction, or it may occur with a smaller, recurrent infarction in a patient with an already substantially infarcted myocardium.

Mechanical complications of acute myocardial infarction can cause shock; ventricular septal rupture, papillary muscle rupture or dysfunction, and myocardial rupture are all associated with cardiogenic shock. Right ventricular infarction in the absence of significant left ventricular infarction or dysfunction can cause shock. Hypovolemia or hypovolemic shock, although distinct from cardiogenic shock by definition, may be an important contributor to the development of shock in acute myocardial infarction.

Refractory tachyarrhythmias or bradyarrhythmias, usually in the setting of left ventricular dysfunction, are occasionally a cause of shock, which can occur with either ventricular or supraventricular arrhythmias.

Cardiogenic shock may occur as the end-stage, final common pathway for any progressive myocardial dysfunction, including ischemic heart disease and idiopathic, hypertrophic, and restrictive cardiomyopathies.

Pathophysiology

In cardiogenic shock resulting from acute myocardial infarction, dysfunction of a large enough quantity of myocardium (if in the left ventricle, approximately 40% must be infarcted) occurs to prevent the heart from meeting its minimum work requirements as a pump. The initial event is obstruction of a coronary artery, usually the left anterior descending coronary artery in first infarctions, but it can be any artery when previous infarctions have caused significant cumulative myocardial damage. The obstruction decreases the oxygen supply, resulting in myocardial ischemia, which in turn leads to diminished myocardial contractility and impaired left ventricular function. The ensuing drop in cardiac output and blood pressure leads to decreased coronary perfusion, resulting in further ischemia and additional deterioration in left ventricular function. This process of ischemia leading to myocardial dysfunction leading to further ischemia and so on has been appropriately termed a vicious cycle. Prolonged serum enzyme elevations, rather than the characteristic rise and fall seen in acute myocardial infarction, also suggest a protracted, stuttering course. Evidence for this vicious cycle is also found in autopsy studies that show infarct extension at the edges of an infarct in addition to discrete, remote infarctions throughout the ventricle.

The majority of patients with shock in acute myocardial infarction have extensive coronary disease. In patients dying of cardiogenic shock, more than two thirds have severe three-vessel coronary artery disease.

Early studies of acute myocardial infarction identified clinical and hemodynamic subsets that had prognostic significance. The Killip classification is based on clinical subsets, as shown in Table 6–1. The Forrester classification uses hemodynamic instead of clinical subsets (Table 6–2). Although the Killip and Forrester subsets have somewhat different definitions, they very clearly establish the point that progressive worsening of left ventricular function, whether measured by clinical or by hemodynamic parameters, is associated with a poorer prognosis. The pathophysiology of cardiogenic shock in acute infarction complicated by mechanical problems is somewhat different. Acute severe mitral regurgitation from papillary muscle or chordal rupture markedly diminishes cardiac output, leading to pulmonary edema. The sympathetic nervous system response to cardiac failure results in increased afterload and a further increase in the regurgitant fraction, another example of a disastrous vicious cycle causing cardiogenic shock.

Rupture of the myocardial free wall resulting in shock, a rare complication of acute myocardial infarction, generally occurs within 4–7 days and may account for 10–30% of all deaths from acute infarction. Acute bleeding into a relatively nondistendible pericardial space leads rapidly to pericardial tamponade and cardiovascular collapse.

Rupture of the ventricular septum with formation of a ventricular septal defect has an incidence of 2–4% in acute myocardial infarction. A large ventricular septal defect causes significant left-to-right shunting and right ventricular volume overload. As with acute mitral regurgitation, the sympathetic nervous system response results in increased afterload, thereby shunting a larger fraction of the cardiac output across the interventricular septum. Pulmonary congestion develops as a consequence of the right ventricular volume and pressure overload. Diminished forward car-

Table 6–1. Killip classification.

Class	Features	Patients (%)	Hospital Mortality Rates (%)
1	No signs of CHF	33	6
2	S_3, gallop, rales, radiographic CHF	38	17
3	Pulmonary edema	10	38
4	Cardiogenic shock	19	81

CHF = congestive heart failure.

Source: Data taken, with permission, from Killip T, Kimball JT: Treatment of myocardial infarction in a coronary care unit: A two-year experience with 250 patients. Am J Cardiol 1967;20:457.

Table 6–2. Forrester classification.

Forrester Class	Hemodynamics		Patients %	Mortality %
	PCW	CI		
1.	<18	>2.2	25	3
2.	>18	>2.2	25	9
3.	<18	<2.2	15	23
4.	>18	<2.2	35	51

CI = cardiac index, L/min/m²; PCW = pulmonary capillary wedge pressure, mm Hg.
Source: Reprinted, with permission, from Forrester JS et al: Medical therapy of acute myocardial infarction by applications of hemodynamic subsets. New Engl J Med 1976;295:1356.

diac output from the left ventricle leads to depression of blood pressure and the diminished tissue perfusion characteristic of shock.

Right ventricular infarction occurs in 10–20% of patients with inferior myocardial infarctions and may be a cause of cardiogenic shock. The degree of left ventricular function is variable and shock can occur even in the absence of left ventricular dysfunction. Failure of the right ventricle leads to diminished right ventricular stroke volume, which results in a decreased volume of blood returning to the left ventricle (preload). Markedly diminished left ventricular filling pressure, even with normal left ventricular contractility, causes decreased systemic cardiac output.

As noted earlier, a variety of arrhythmias can contribute to the development of shock. A sustained arrhythmia, that is, one that does not culminate in ventricular fibrillation and sudden death, is generally a cause of shock only in the already compromised ventricle. Atrial and ventricular tachyarrhythmias are associated with both a greatly diminished time for ventricular filling in diastole and loss of the atrial contribution to diastolic filling. The diminished preload causes decreased volume available for forward output and, by the Frank-Starling relationship for ventricular performance, diminished contractility. These factors, superimposed on an already impaired left ventricle, may be enough to result in cardiogenic shock.

Bradyarrhythmias do not generally result in diastolic filling abnormalities, although (as with tachyarrhythmias) loss of atrial systole may be a factor. The major problem here is diminished forward cardiac output caused by the slow heart rate. Because total cardiac output is a function of heart rate and stroke volume, a markedly decreased heart rate, especially with left ventricular dysfunction and reduced stroke volume, may result in shock.

Many forms of heart disease can result in an end-stage dilated and congested cardiomyopathy. These include hypertensive heart disease; ischemic heart disease; restrictive, idiopathic, and toxic cardiomyopathies; and cardiomyopathy secondary to endocrine disease. In all cases, the inexorable progression of myocardial disease, accompanied by the effects of volume and pressure overload, can ultimately lead to inadequate cardiac output and shock.

Chatterjee K: Pathogenesis of low output in right ventricular infarction. Chest 1992;102(Suppl 2):590S.

Hollenberg SM, Kavinsky CJ, Parrillo JE: Cardiogenic Shock. Ann Intern Med 1999;131(1):47.

Clinical Findings

Approximately half the patients destined to develop shock will present initially with shock; the other half will develop cardiogenic shock after admission to the hospital.

A. HISTORY

The symptoms and signs that precede the development of cardiogenic shock depend on the cause. Patients with acute myocardial infarction will generally have the typical history of acute-onset chest pain, possibly in the setting of known coronary artery disease. The mechanical complications of acute myocardial infarction all tend to occur several days to a week following the infarction. They may be heralded by chest pain, but they more commonly present abruptly as acute pulmonary edema or cardiac arrest. Patients with arrhythmias may have a history of symptoms, such as palpitations, presyncope, syncope, or a sensation of skipped beats, that suggest this cause. The patient may appear obtunded and lethargic as a result of decreased central nervous system perfusion. Regardless of the cause, however, by the time shock develops, the patient may be unable to give any useful history. Family members may be able to help by identifying any previous history of heart disease and providing the history of the present illness.

B. PHYSICAL EXAMINATION

1. Vital signs—Blood pressure is less than 90 mm Hg systolic in patients on pressors and less than 80 mm Hg in the untreated patient. Heart rate is commonly elevated from sympathetic stimulation, and the respiratory rate is generally increased as a result of pulmonary congestion.

2. Chest—The chest examination in most cases shows diffuse rales. Patients with right ventricular infarction or those who are hypovolemic may have less evidence of pulmonary congestion.

3. Cardiovascular system—Neck veins are commonly elevated, although they may be normal in hypovolemic patients. The apical impulse is displaced in patients with dilated cardiomyopathy, and the intensity of heart sounds is diminished in pericardial effusion or tamponade. A gallop rhythm, especially a third heart sound suggesting significant left ventricular dysfunction, may be present. A mitral regurgitation or ventricular septal defect murmur can help in establishing these causes. Patients with significant right heart failure may have such signs (on abdominal examination) as liver enlargement, a pulsatile liver in the presence of significant tricuspid regurgitation, or ascites in long-standing right heart failure.

4. Extremities—Peripheral pulses will be diminished, and peripheral edema may be present. Cyanosis and cool extremities are indicative of diminished tissue perfusion. Profound peripheral vasoconstriction can result in livido reticularis on the abdomen.

C. DIAGNOSTIC STUDIES

The diagnosis of cardiogenic shock is a clinical diagnosis based on hypotension and evidence of peripheral hypoperfusion. Information gathered from history, physical examination, and laboratory data—especially hemodynamic monitoring—will corroborate the diagnosis and give valuable information as to its cause. It must be stressed, however, that shock in general and cardiogenic shock in particular are clinical syndromes that are diagnosed by clinical criteria.

1. Electrocardiography—The electrocardiogram (ECG) is often helpful in distinguishing between causes of cardiogenic shock. Patients with coronary disease and acute myocardial infarction may show evidence of both old and new infarctions. Right-sided chest leads in patients with inferior myocardial infarctions can detect the presence of right ventricular infarction (ST elevation in V_4R). Although the ECG readily aids in the diagnosis of arrhythmias contributing to cardiogenic

shock, it is often not precise when shock is caused by problems other than acute infarction or arrhythmia.

2. Chest radiograph—The chest radiograph shows cardiomegaly and evidence of pulmonary congestion or edema in patients with severe left ventricular failure. Ventricular septal defect or mitral regurgitation associated with acute infarction will lead to pulmonary congestion but not necessarily cardiomegaly, however, particularly in patients suffering a first infarction. Findings of pulmonary congestion may be less prominent—or absent—in the case of predominantly right ventricular failure or hypovolemia.

3. Echocardiography—The noninvasive nature and ready availability of two-dimensional and Doppler echocardiography make these techniques suitable for immediate assessment of the patient in shock and a tremendous benefit in the bedside diagnosis and treatment of many types of heart disease. Information obtained by echocardiography includes assessment of right and left ventricular function (global as well as segmental), valvular function (stenosis or regurgitation), right ventricular pressures; and detection of shunts (eg, ventricular septal defect with left-to-right shunting), pericardial fluid, or tamponade. The echocardiogram is especially helpful in diagnosing the mechanical complications of myocardial infarction.

4. Hemodynamic monitoring—The use of Swan-Ganz catheters to measure pulmonary artery and pulmonary capillary wedge pressure (PCWP) is generally very useful, if not essential, in establishing the diagnosis and cause of cardiogenic shock and in planning and monitoring therapy. Patients with cardiogenic shock as a result of severe left ventricular failure have, by definition, elevation of the PCWP. The presence of a wedge pressure higher than 18 mm Hg in a patient with acute myocardial infarction indicates adequate intravascular volume. Patients with primarily right ventricular failure or significant hypovolemia may have normal or reduced PCWP. The presence of a large v wave on the PCWP tracing implies significant mitral regurgitation.

The value of hemodynamic monitoring lies in its ability to assist in optimizing the ventricular function and thereby tissue perfusion. The Frank-Starling relationship of cardiac performance (measured by cardiac output, stroke work, or stroke volume) as a function of filling pressure demonstrates that the performance of the heart will increase as filling pressure increases—up to a point. In the failing heart, this point is eventually reached where no further increases in performance are gained by additional increases in preload—the "flat" part of the curve. Serial measurements of cardiac performance and left ventricular filling pressure indicate the optimal preload (ie, the lowest preload at which cardiac work is optimized).

Monitoring of hemodynamic parameters also allows calculation of the afterload (systemic vascular resistance [SVR]), defined by the following equation:

$$SVR = \frac{(\text{mean arterial pressure} - \text{central venous pressure}) \times 80}{\text{cardiac output}}$$

Minimizing afterload is important because increasing afterload mimics the effect of decreased contractility, resulting in diminished cardiac output.

Right-side filling pressures (central venous or right atrial pressure) are commonly normal, except in the case of right ventricular infarction, pericardial tamponade, or preexisting pulmonary disease.

Hemodynamic definitions of cardiogenic shock, as noted previously, include a cardiac index less than 2.2 L/min/m². Cardiac index is preferred to cardiac output as a measure because it normalizes the cardiac output for body size. Small patients may be incorrectly diagnosed with shock if cardiac output alone is used.

5. Oxygen saturation—Venous O_2 saturation may be helpful in two ways. The arteriovenous difference in oxygen content, which is a useful indicator of cardiac output, increases as more oxygen is extracted from the blood in the setting of low cardiac output. Serial determinations are especially useful in monitoring a patient's course and response to therapy.

Oxygen saturations obtained while placing the Swan-Ganz catheter may also be helpful in diagnosing a ventricular septal defect. The shunting of oxygenated blood from the left ventricle to the right ventricle results in an oxygen saturation step-up when comparing venous oxygen saturation from the venae cavae with that obtained in the pulmonary artery.

Treatment

A. GENERAL

Although some general therapeutic considerations are applicable to all patients in cardiogenic shock, treatment is most effective when the cause is identified. In many situations, this identification allows rapid correction of the underlying problem. In fact, survival in most forms of shock requires a quick, accurate diagnosis. The patient is so critically ill that only prompt, directed therapy can reverse the process. It is clear that the already high mortality rates in cardiogenic shock are even higher in patients for whom treatment is delayed. Therefore, although measures aimed at temporarily stabilizing the patient may provide enough time to start definitive therapy, potentially life-saving treatment can be carried out only when the cause is known (Table 6–3).

Table 6–3. Management of cardiogenic shock.

Clinical diagnosis of shock established
Intubation, ventilation, oxygen supplementation
Swan-Ganz catheter
  PCW less than 18: administer fluids
  PCW 18 or higher: administer inotropic agents
ECG, echocardiogram
  No MI: use hemodynamic management
  Acute MI: go to cardiac catheterization, intra-aortic balloon pump, coronary angioplasty, or bypass surgery
  MI with mechanical complications: use intraaortic balloon pump, emergency surgery

PCW = pulmonary capillary wedge pressure; ECG = electrocardiogram; MI = myocardial infarction.

B. MECHANICAL COMPLICATIONS

Acute mitral regurgitation secondary to papillary muscle dysfunction or rupture or to ventricular septal defect is a true emergency when associated with cardiogenic shock. The only effective therapy for these catastrophes is surgical repair. If the patient is to survive, all efforts must be made to get the patient to the operating room as soon as possible after the diagnosis is made. Pharmacologic agents and intraaortic balloon pumping (see section "Circulatory support devices") are useful as temporizing measures only and should not delay surgical treatment.

Patients with ventricular free-wall rupture rarely survive if the rupture is massive and results in shock and pericardial tamponade. As is true with the other major mechanical problems, emergency surgical correction is the only hope for survival.

C. RIGHT VENTRICULAR INFARCTION

Cardiogenic shock may occur with right ventricular infarction and no or only minimal left ventricular dysfunction. The probability for long-term survival is excellent if the diagnosis is made promptly and appropriate treatment instituted. Hemodynamic data suggesting right ventricular dysfunction out of proportion to left ventricular dysfunction and ST elevation in lead V_4R are most helpful in establishing the diagnosis. Initial treatment is fluid resuscitation to increase right ventricular preload and output. Significant amounts of fluid (1–2 L or more) may be required to develop an adequate preload for the failing ventricle. Inotropic agents are usually necessary when the right ventricular failure is so profound that shock continues despite adequate volume administration. Vasodilators may be helpful in some circumstances, diminishing the right ventricular afterload, which would theoretically improve the cardiac output. Vasodilators such as nitroprusside, which affect both the arterial and venous systems, may actually decrease preload, however—to the point that right ventricular output is unchanged.

Patients with right ventricular infarction are dependent on atrial contraction. As a result, single-chamber ventricular pacing may be inadequate in patients who require pacing, and atrioventricular sequential pacing is required to improve cardiac output.

D. ARRHYTHMIAS

Arrhythmias contributing to cardiogenic shock are readily recognized with ECG monitoring and should be promptly treated. Tachyarrhythmias (ventricular tachycardia and supraventricular tachycardias) should be treated with electrical cardioversion. Bradyarrhythmias may respond to pharmacologic agents (atropine, isoproterenol) in some circumstances, but external or transvenous pacing may be required.

E. ACUTE MYOCARDIAL INFARCTION

In patients with cardiogenic shock caused by a large amount of infarcted or stunned myocardium, it has become increasingly clear that the only treatment that can decrease mortality is revascularization, with either coronary angioplasty or coronary artery bypass surgery (discussed later). A number of pharmacologic and nonpharmacologic measures may be helpful in stabilizing the patient prior to cardiac catheterization or surgery.

1. Ventilation-oxygenation—Because respiratory failure usually accompanies cardiogenic shock, every effort should be made to ensure adequate ventilation and oxygenation. Adequate oxygenation is essential to avoid hypoxia and further deterioration of oxygen delivery to tissues. The majority of patients with cardiogenic shock require mechanical ventilation with supplemental oxygen. Hypoventilation can lead to respiratory acidosis, which could exacerbate the metabolic acidosis caused by tissue hypoperfusion. Acidosis worsens cardiac function; it also makes the heart less responsive to inotropic agents.

2. Fluid resuscitation—Although hypovolemia is not the primary defect in cardiogenic shock, a number of patients may be relatively hypovolemic when shock develops following myocardial infarction. The causes of decreased intravascular volume include increased hydrostatic pressure and the increased permeability of blood vessels. Note that the physical examination may not always be helpful in determining the adequacy of left ventricular filling pressure. Furthermore, because the central venous pressure correlates poorly with PCWP in shock, it may not be useful, especially with a single reading. These facts underscore the importance of hemodynamic monitoring with a pulmonary artery catheter for an accurate assessment of left ventricular

filling pressure. The optimal filling pressure is higher in patients with shock because the left ventricle is operating on a depressed function curve (less stroke volume for any given filling pressure). Generally, a PCWP of 18–22 mm Hg is considered adequate; further increases will lead to pulmonary congestion without a concomitant gain in cardiac output. Fluid resuscitation, when indicated by low or normal PCWPs, should be undertaken in boluses of 200–300 mL saline, followed by reassessment of hemodynamic parameters, especially cardiac output and PCWP.

3. Inotropic agents—A variety of drugs are available for intravenous administration to increase the contractility of the heart. Because the heart is operating on a markedly depressed Frank-Starling curve, a positive inotropic agent may improve the hemodynamic status significantly.

a. Digoxin—Although digoxin benefits patients with chronic congestive heart failure, it is of less benefit in cardiogenic shock because of its delayed onset of action and relatively mild potency (compared with other available agents).

b. Beta-adrenergic agonists—**Dopamine** is an endogenous catecholamine with qualitatively different effects at varying doses. At low doses (less than 4 μg/kg/ min) it predominantly stimulates dopaminergic receptors that dilate various arterial beds, the most important being the renal vasculature. Intermediate doses of 4–6 μg/kg/min cause β_1-receptor stimulation and enhanced myocardial contractility. Further increases in dosage lead to prominent α-receptor stimulation (peripheral vasoconstriction) in addition to continued β_1 stimulation. Dopamine improves cardiac output, and its combination of cardiac stimulation and peripheral vasoconstriction may be especially beneficial as initial treatment of hypotensive patients in cardiogenic shock.

Dobutamine is a synthetic sympathomimetic agent that differs from dopamine in two important ways: It does not cause renal vasodilation, and it has a much stronger β_2 (arteriolar vasodilation) effect. The vasodilatory effect may be deleterious in the hypotensive patients because a further drop in blood pressure may occur. On the other hand, many patients with cardiogenic shock experience excessive vasoconstriction and inappropriately elevated afterload as a result of the natural sympathetic discharge or of treatment with inotropic agents, such as dopamine, that also have prominent vasoconstrictor effects. In such patients, the combination of cardiac stimulation and decreased afterload with dobutamine may improve cardiac output without a loss of arterial pressure.

Isoproterenol is also a synthetic sympathomimetic agent. It has very strong chronotropic and inotropic effects, resulting in a disproportionate increase in oxygen consumption and ischemia. It is therefore not generally recommended for cardiogenic shock except for bradyarrhythmias responsive to its chronotropic effect.

Norepinephrine has even stronger α and β_1 effects than dopamine and may be beneficial when a patient continues to be hypotensive despite large doses of dopamine (more than 20 μg/kg/min). Because of the intense peripheral vasoconstriction that occurs, perfusion of other vascular beds such as the kidney, extremities, and mesentery may be compromised. Therefore, norepinephrine cannot be used for any extended time unless plans are made for definitive treatment. Beta-adrenergic agonists, which are extremely useful agents for improving the circulatory state of patients with cardiogenic shock, can also have adverse effects. Their ability to increase cardiac output is accompanied by an increased oxygen demand from enhanced contractility, a faster heart rate, and increased blood pressure—which can be harmful to the already ischemic myocardium. In addition, β-agonists can precipitate serious ventricular or atrial tachyarrhythmias.

c. Phosphodiesterase inhibitors—The intracellular mediator of β-adrenergic-receptor stimulation is cyclic adenosine monophosphate (cAMP), produced by adenylate cyclase after stimulation of the receptor. Cyclic-AMP in turn increases calcium influx into the cell, thereby increasing contractility. The phosphodiesterase inhibitors, such as milrinone and amrinone, inhibit the breakdown of cAMP by phosphodiesterase, prolonging its effect on cardiac contractility. These agents also act on cAMP produced at sites of β_2 stimulation to prolong the vasodilatory effects. Phosphodiesterase inhibitors appear to have no advantage over the β-agonists in patients with cardiogenic shock.

4. Vasodilators—Vasodilation (especially of the arterioles to reduce afterload) is often necessary because of the increased levels of catecholamines and resultant peripheral vasoconstriction. Vasodilators are also useful in patients who require the enhanced contractility of β_1 stimulation by an adrenergic agonist, even though the associated vasoconstriction (especially with dopamine) may inappropriately increase the afterload. In addition, the preload may be inappropriately high in many patients; here, a venodilator will be beneficial in reducing filling pressure (preload).

a. Nitroprusside—Nitroprusside is a direct-acting vascular smooth muscle relaxant, with a balanced effect (vasodilation of both the arterial and venous beds). It is commonly used in combination with an inotropic agent. Doses begin as low as 0.25–0.5 μg/kg/min and may go as high as 8–10 μg/kg/min. Even though nitroprusside is a very short-acting drug, hypotension is a common side effect, and close arterial pressure monitoring is required.

b. Phentolamine—Phentolamine is an α-antagonist that acts predominantly on arterial α receptors to produce vasodilation. It is not commonly used because of the tachycardia induced by the release of cardiac norepinephrine stores.

c. Nitroglycerin—Nitroglycerin is primarily a venodilator, although it may have some arterial effects at high doses. Its benefits arise from a decrease in pulmonary congestion and, through its coronary vasodilatory effects, a decrease in myocardial ischemia. It is not commonly used in cardiogenic shock, however, unless coronary vasospasm is thought to be contributing to myocardial ischemia.

5. Circulatory support devices—Among the mechanical devices developed to assist the left ventricle until more definitive therapy can be undertaken, the intraaortic balloon pump (IABP) has been in use the longest and is the most well studied.

The IABP is placed in the descending aorta via the femoral artery. Its inflation and deflation are timed to the cardiac cycle (generally synchronized with the ECG). The balloon inflates in diastole immediately following aortic valve closure. The augmentation of diastolic pressure (to a level higher than systolic pressure) increases coronary perfusion as well as that of other tissues. The balloon deflates at the end of diastole, immediately before left ventricular contraction, abruptly decreasing the afterload and improving left ventricular ejection.

Indications for use of the IABP include shock from severe ischemia, severe ventricular failure (especially when used as a bridge to cardiac transplant), ventricular septal rupture, and mitral regurgitation. In both ventricular septal rupture and mitral regurgitation, the principal benefit is caused by the decreased afterload as the balloon deflates. This results in a larger fraction of the left ventricular volume being ejected into the aorta rather than into the left atrium (mitral regurgitation) or the right ventricle (ventricular septal rupture).

The complication rate, especially vascular damage, is significant because of the large catheter size. As a result, the IABP is contraindicated in patients with significant peripheral vascular disease. In selected cases the balloon can be placed in the descending thoracic aorta from an axillary cut-down. It must be remembered that although these devices can clearly improve hemodynamics in the short term, they cannot improve survival by themselves, reaffirming the importance of definitive treatment.

A number of other circulatory support devices have been developed in recent years. A percutaneous cardiopulmonary bypass device with large-bore catheters placed in the right atrium and the femoral artery is capable of creating flow rates of 3–5 L/min. Prosthetic left ventricles and various surgically placed left ventricular assistance devices have also been used in patients with cardiogenic shock as a bridge to cardiac transplant. Although anecdotal reports of their benefits are encouraging, none has yet been subjected to controlled studies for comparison with IABP.

6. Revascularization—Revascularization is the only definitive therapy shown to decrease mortality in patients who develop cardiogenic shock following myocardial infarction. Early, primarily retrospective, studies of coronary angioplasty or coronary artery bypass graft surgery (CABG) reported survival rates of 60–80% in revascularized patients compared with 0–30% survival rate with medical therapy alone. More recently the multicenter, randomized SHOCK (Should We Emergently Revascularize Occluded Coronaries for Cardiogenic Shock) trial showed a trend toward improved survival at 30 days in patients randomized to revascularization (either angioplasty or CABG). The survival benefit for revascularization became significant at 6 months, a benefit that persisted at 1 year. Of note, patients 75 years of age and older had worse survival rates with revascularization, a finding that was also seen in earlier nonrandomized studies. Many experts believe that the SHOCK trial was underpowered to show a mortality difference at 30 days and, based on the 6 month and 1 year data, now recommend emergency revascularization for patients with cardiogenic shock complicating acute myocardial infarction.

   a. Coronary angioplasty—Studies of coronary angioplasty in cardiogenic shock have consistently found that older patients (65 years of age or older) do not appear to benefit from coronary angioplasty. It is also noteworthy that although the likelihood of survival appears to be much improved in patients with successful coronary angioplasty, it remains very low—around 20%—in those with failed angioplasty. Whether these patients should be offered any further CABG surgery is unclear at this time. Future research will be aimed at identifying patients at high risk for failed coronary angioplasty and determining any preferable alternatives.

   b. Coronary artery bypass graft surgery—Emergency CABG has also been studied in patients with cardiogenic shock caused by acute myocardial infarction. As with coronary angioplasty, the studies are generally retrospective but also show an improved survival rate (60–80%) over patients treated medically. These benefits appear to be more consistent in trials reflecting post-1980 improvements in surgical techniques. Again, as in coronary angioplasty, elderly patients do not appear to benefit from CABG.

7. Thrombolytic therapy—Thrombolytic therapy is considered a reperfusion strategy comparable to coronary angioplasty for decreasing mortality rates in acute myocardial infarction patients without cardiogenic shock. It would seem logical that patients in cardiogenic shock might also benefit from thrombolytic therapy. This benefit, however, has not been realized. Analysis of survival data for thrombolytic trials of patients with cardiogenic shock have consistently shown mortality rates in the 70–80% range—no different from those treated conservatively. Thrombolysis has been less successful in patients with cardiogenic shock; the rates of reperfusion are lower. It has been suggested that the low flow state present in shock may explain this lack of benefit in that adequate cardiac output appears to be necessary for successful thrombolysis. If the patient is not a candidate for angioplasty or CABG, however, or if revascularization is not immediately available, there appears to be no harm from thrombolytic therapy—and it may succeed in some cardiogenic shock patients.

8. Other medical therapies—Platelet IIb/IIIa inhibitors have been studied extensively in recent years in the setting of acute coronary syndromes and with percutaneous coronary interventions. A retrospective analysis of one such trial showed that patients randomized to the IIb/IIIa inhibitor eptifibatide had a significant 50% absolute risk reduction for mortality at 30 days. This finding will need to be verified in future trials designed to prospectively evaluate the efficacy of IIb/IIIa inhibitors in cardiogenic shock.

Bates ER, Topol EJ: Limitations of thrombolytic therapy for acute myocardial infarction complicated by congestive heart failure and cardiogenic shock. J Am Coll Cardiol 1991;18:1077.

Gacioch GM, Ellis SG, Lee L et al: Cardiogenic shock complicating acute myocardial infarction: The use of coronary angioplasty and the integration of the new support devices into patient management. J Am Coll Cardiol 1992;19:647.

Goldenberg IF: Nonpharmacologic management of cardiac arrest and cardiogenic shock. Chest 1992;102(Suppl 2):596S.

Hasdai D, Harrington RA, Hochman JS et al: Platelet glycoprotein IIb/IIIa blockade and outcome of cardiogenic shock complicating acute coronary syndromes without persistent ST-segment elevation. J Am Coll Cardiol 2000;36:685.

Hasdai D, Topol, EJ, Califf RM et al: Cardiogenic shock complicating acute coronary syndromes. Lancet 2000;356:749.

Hibbard MD, Holmes Dr Jr, Bailey KR et al: Percutaneous transluminal coronary angioplasty in patients with cardiogenic shock. J Am Coll Cardiol 1992;19:639.

Hochman JS, Sleeper LA, Webb JG et al: Early revascularization in acute myocardial infarction complicated by cardiogenic shock. N Engl J Med 1999;341(9):625.

Lee L, Erbel R, Brown TM et al: Multicenter registry of angioplasty therapy of cardiogenic shock: Initial and long-term survival. J Am Coll Cardiol 1991;17:599.

McGhie AI, Goldstein RA: Pathogenesis and management of acute heart failure and cardiogenic shock: Role of inotropic therapy. Chest 1992;102(Suppl 2):626S.

Moosvi AR, Khaja F, Villanueva L et al: Early revascularization improves survival in cardiogenic shock complicating acute myocardial infarction. J Am Coll Cardiol 1992;19:907.

Prognosis

Although the prognosis for patients with cardiogenic shock is improving with emergency revascularization, shock still represents a major cause of mortality in acute myocardial infarction. The early reports of less than 30% survival in medically treated patients are being supplanted by survival figures of 60–80% following successful revascularization. It should be noted that these figures may reflect selection bias for patients likely to do better, and that if revascularization fails, the likelihood of survival continues to be very poor.

Coronary Revascularization

Kathleen M. Allen, MD

General Considerations

Coronary revascularization is indicated in a broad spectrum of patients who have been identified to have physiologically significant coronary artery disease (CAD). A noninvasive or invasive assessment, generally driven by a clinical syndrome, leads to a diagnosis of clinically significant CAD. When a noninvasive evaluation is done, a cardiac catheterization is necessary to define the patient's anatomy and formulate an approach for revascularization. Three methods are currently used for revascularizing patients with CAD: percutaneous coronary intervention (PCI), coronary artery bypass grafting (CABG), and myocardial revascularization. Myocardial revascularization has two subtypes: transmyocardial (TMR), which is surgical, and percutaneous (PMR). The modality of choice requires careful evaluation of the patient, including clinical syndrome and coronary anatomy.

Background and Historical Perspective

The first cardiac catheterization was performed in 1929 by Werner Forssmann of Germany who was interested in identifying a workable method of giving intracardiac medications. He threaded a catheter into his own left basilic vein and proceeded to advance the catheter into the right atrium. An x-ray film was taken to confirm its position.

In 1941, André Frédéric Cournand and Dickinson Woodruff Richards again took interest in the cardiac catheter but this time as a diagnostic tool. They investigated the use of right-heart catheters and pressure measurements. They expanded this to include diagnostic assessment of congenital and rheumatic conditions. Forssman, Cournand, and Richards were jointly awarded the 1956 Nobel Prize in physiology or medicine for their contributions to the science of cardiac catheterization. The use of cardiac catheters quickly advanced, and many discoveries were made that enhanced our understanding of coronary pathophysiology. They became valuable tools in the diagnosis of congenital and acquired heart disease.

Over the years, the use of catheters evolved to include therapeutic interventions. In the late 1950s and early 1960s Sones and Judkins performed the first selective coronary angiography. In the late 1960s, catheters were used to unclog peripheral arteries, and the procedure was named percutaneous transluminal coronary angioplasty (PTCA). These procedures were initially performed on peripheral vessels. The technique remained cumbersome and often resulted in complications. The technique evolved however, and equipment was miniaturized to access and treat coronary arteries. Andreas Gruentzig in Switzerland performed the first coronary angioplasty in 1974 on a 37-year-old man with a high-grade proximal left anterior descending lesion. Follow-up angiography at 1 month and years later revealed a patent angioplasty site.

The technology of coronary catheterization and angioplasty has evolved quickly since the 1970s. The use of rotational atherectomy, directional atherectomy, excisional atherectomy, laser angioplasty, thrombectomy, intravascular ultrasound, intracoronary stents, and other catheter devices for treating atherosclerosis are considered components of the current PCI armamentarium. These devices serve to ablate, pulverize, excise, smash, extract, or trap atherosclerotic plaque and debris. Because coronary devices traumatize the vessel wall, adjunctive pharmacologic therapy to prevent arterial thrombosis has become an important facet in coronary revascularization. These new technologies have revolutionized the field of interventional cardiology and broadened the armamentarium available for addressing CAD.

The number of percutaneous interventions has grown exponentially since 1977. More than 1,000,000 procedures have been performed worldwide, over half a million of which were done in the United States. New technology such as stents and brachytherapy have expanded the indications for PCI by decreasing complications and facilitating intervention on increasingly difficult lesions. Stents have revolutionized PCI and are now used in approximately 60–80% of percutaneous interventions. They can be used alone or in conjunction with other modalities such as atherectomy, radiation, and thrombectomy. Sufficient data is available to support the use of stenting in a number of patient subsets. These data have been extrapolated to include a wide variety of coronary artery and bypass graft lesions. The wide use of stenting has resulted in another conundrum—restenosis. Some progress has been made in preventing restenosis. Both brachytherapy and drug-coated stents are promising developments for dealing with in-stent restenosis as well as limiting restenosis in the future.

Indications for Coronary Revascularization

Coronary revascularization is indicated in a broad spectrum of clinical scenarios. They range from acute myocardial infarction (MI) to a stable clinical syndrome, to asymptomatic cases. Each time a revascularization procedure is considered the risks of the procedure must be weighed against its potential benefit. A wealth of information is available based on clinical trial data, which sought to evaluate various treatment strategies.

The initial simplicity and associated low morbidity of PCI compared with surgery is always attractive; however, the limitations of PCI must be taken into account. Subgroups of patients, including those with multivessel CAD and diabetes mellitus or impaired left ventricular function, have been shown to benefit from surgical revascularization or CABG.

In those patients with CAD who are asymptomatic or have mild symptoms, a noninvasive approach with attention to antianginal therapy and aggressive risk factor modification must be considered.

The following recommendation for coronary revascularization is based on the ACC/AHA guidelines for PCI.

Asymptomatic or Mild Angina

The majority of patients who are symptomatic or who have only mild angina can be treated medically. A subset of these patients may have one or more significant lesions in one or more coronary arteries suitable for PCI with a high likelihood of success and low risk for complications. Such lesions must involve a significant area of myocardium judged to be at risk. The patient's lifestyle and career (eg, pilot, bus driver) may also play a role in the decision. There should be evidence of myocardial ischemia by stress testing, stress nuclear imaging, stress echocardiography, or physiologic assessment. The diabetic patient may be at higher risk of restenosis or procedural difficulty and must be considered to be in a different category.

Moderate or Severe Angina

Patients who have moderate or severe angina usually fall within the Canadian Cardiovascular Society (CCS) class II–IV. These patients are often on a medical regimen and continue to have angina despite maximal medical therapy. Cases with one or more significant lesions in one or more coronary arteries suitable for PCI are strongly indicative for percutaneous intervention. These lesions should be surgically approachable as assessed by the angiographer and subtend a moderate to large area of myocardium at risk. The following criteria help determine which lesions put the patient at high risk as defined by greater than 3% mortality at 1 year. These patients will benefit most from revascularization.

- High risk treadmill score
- Stress-induced large perfusion defect
- Stress-induced perfusion defects of moderate size
- Stress-induced multiple perfusion defects with left ventricle dilation or increased lung uptake (thallium-201)
- Echocardiographic wall motion abnormality with stress involving greater than two wall segments
- Stress echo evidence of extensive ischemia

Other patients who benefit from percutaneous revascularization in the setting of unstable angina include prior bypass patients who have either saphenous vein grafts or arterial conduits, which are amenable to percutaneous revascularization.

Ryan TJ et al: Guidelines for percutaneous transluminal coronary angioplasty. Angioplasty J Am Coll Cardiol 1993;22:2033.

Smith SC et al: ACC/AHA Guidelines for Percutaneous Coronary Intervention (Revision of the 1993 PTCA Guidelines). J Am Coll Cardiol 2001;37:2216.

Equipment

Since the advent of PCI, vast improvements have been made in catheter design and operator technique. Early equipment was rather primitive. The first guide catheters were made of Teflon, which is not malleable. Balloon catheters were bulky and difficult to maneuver. These restrictions markedly limited the spectrum of lesions considered approachable by PCI. Current guide catheters are formed from several different layers, which improves torqueability, stability, and shape formation. Many preformed guide catheter shapes allow for entry into a wide variety of anatomically challenging coronary ostia.

The balloon dilatation catheters have also evolved. They are amazingly sleek, small catheters with tapered tips that make it possible to maneuver through incredibly tortuous and severely stenotic lesions. These balloons are passed over guidewires to the area of stenosis.

The standard diameter of the guidewires is 0.0009–0.018 in. The tip of the guidewire is shapeable or comes with a preformed J. The wires range from floppy to stiff. The wire itself can be coated with a hydrophilic coating that makes it slippery, thereby facilitating passage through severe or even total occlusions.

The imaging quality of cardiac catheterization laboratories has also improved markedly. We are capable of visualizing structures more efficiently and with less radiation. Industry has developed high-resolution fluoroscopy, digital subtraction, and on-line qualitative coronary analysis. All of these advances have improved cineangiographic imaging and interpretation.

Technique

Patients receive an antiplatelet agent, such as aspirin, clopidogrel, or ticlopidine, prior to the beginning of the procedure. There is evidence that giving a loading dose of clopidogrel or ticlopidine can decrease complications, and many centers begin these agents 2–3 days prior to the procedure. The use of these agents has markedly decreased the rate of acute and subacute thrombosis. Additional evidence suggests that clopidogrel may also benefit patients with acute coronary syndromes by decreasing recurrent ischemic events. Access to the arterial system can be obtained using the femoral, radial, or brachial arteries. The first access site commonly used was the brachial artery. It is now standard to use the femoral artery, and preformed catheters are made with this approach in mind. The radial artery offers an alternative that allows earlier patient ambulation. The chosen access site is anesthetized with a local anesthetic. Access to the arterial system is via the percutaneous approach. A sheath is placed in the artery, and catheters are passed through this sheath and advanced to the coronary ostia. The catheters are attached to a manifold for continuous pressure monitoring and injection of contrast material. The sheaths used for PCI range from 6 to 9 French in diameter (2.0–3.0 mm). The guide is positioned in the ostia of the coronary artery, and angiograms are taken in several radiographic pro-

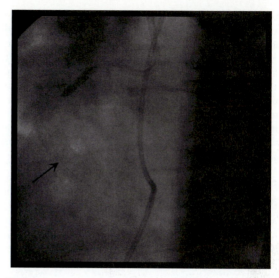

Figure 7–1. Coronary guidewire positioned in a right coronary artery with an inflated angioplasty balloon positioned at the site of a coronary stenosis.

jections to visualize the culprit lesion. Intravenous heparin is given to achieve adequate anticoagulation during the procedure.

A guidewire is then maneuvered past the stenosis under fluoroscopic guidance (Figure 7–1). Once a stable guidewire position is achieved, a balloon catheter is passed over the wire to the lesion. The size of the balloon generally approximates the size of the vessel and the length of the lesion. The balloon is then inflated at the site of the lesion under fluoroscopy until the balloon is fully expanded (Figure 7–2). If the result is in-

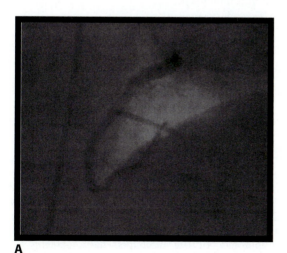

A

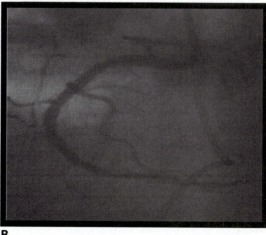

B

Figure 7–2. Right coronary artery **A:** before and **B:** after angioplasty.

adequate, more balloon inflations, a larger balloon, or another device may be used. A coronary stent is placed in approximately 60–80% of vessels that undergo angioplasty. Ample data support the use of coronary stenting, which results in less subsequent acute closure and recurrent angina. After the procedure the patient is observed for recurrent ischemia, vascular complications, renal insufficiency, and arrhythmias. Patients are maintained on aspirin therapy indefinitely. The patient should receive follow-up as needed and should be counseled on the need for risk factor modification.

Risks of Cardiac Catheterization and Revascularization

A number of procedural complications can occur during a cardiac catheterization and PCI. Extensive analysis of a large patient database revealed the following:

- Death (< 0.2%)
- Cerebral vascular accident (< 0.5%)
- MI (< 0.5%)
- Emergency CABG (< 0.7%)
- Arrhythmias, including ventricular tachycardia, ventricular fibrillation, atrial arrhythmia, heart block, and asystole (< 1%)
- Vascular injury, including hemorrhage at puncture site, retroperitoneal bleed, thrombosis, hematoma, dissection, arteriovenous fistula, and pseudoaneurysm (< 1%). Vascular complications are more frequent when using a brachial approach. This does not seem to be the case with the radial approach.
- Cardiac perforation or tamponade (< 0.1%)
- Infection (< 1.0%)
- Contrast reaction (< 2–5%)
- Nephrotoxicity (5%)
- Vasovagal reactions (< 0.5%)

Certain patient subsets are at higher risk for complications:

- Known or suspected left main disease
- Severe three-vessel CAD
- Severe valvular heart disease
- Congestive heart failure
- Severely impaired left ventricular function (< 35%)
- Diabetes
- Age older than 75 years
- Unstable coronary syndrome
- Acute MI
- Prior cerebrovascular accident
- Renal insufficiency
- Peripheral vascular disease

- Obesity
- Uncontrolled hypertension

Noto TJ, Johnson LW, Krone R et al: Cardiac Cath 1990: A report of the Registry of the Society for Cardiac Angiography and Interventions, Cathet Cardiovasc Diagn 1991;24:75.

Procedural Outcomes

Lesion morphology has been divided into three distinct groups based on the characteristics of the lesion. The classification of the lesion directly translates into the likelihood of a successful procedure.

Type A (high success rate > 85%)
Discrete < 10 mm
Concentric
Readily accessible
Nonangulated < 45° angle
Smooth contour
Little or no calcification
Less than total occlusion
No major sidebranch involvement
Absence of thrombus

Type B (moderate success rate 60–85%)
Tubular 10–20 mm in length
Eccentric
Moderate tortuosity of proximal segment
Moderately angulated segment 45–90° angle
Irregular contour
Moderate to heavy calcification
Total occlusion less than 3 months old
Ostial location
Bifurcation lesion
Thrombus present

Type C (low success rate < 60%)
Diffuse 20 mm in length
Excessive tortuosity of proximal segment
Extreme angulation > 90°
Total occlusion > 3 months old
Inability to protect major sidebranches
Degenerated vein graft with friable lesions

Acute vessel closure, a sudden closure of the vessel during or after PCI, can occur in 3–8% of cases. Acute closure can be the result of an uncovered luminal dissection, thrombus formation, or intramural hematoma formation. The advent of coronary stenting and adjunctive therapy (ticlopidine, clopidogrel, and platelet glycoprotein IIb/IIIa inhibitors) have markedly decreased the incidence of acute closure. A number of clinical trials have shown that the use of IIb/IIIa inhibitors has reduced acute closure and recurrent events by as much as 30% in a broad spectrum of patients. If a procedure is unsuccessful and the patient's health is compromised, emergent CABG may be necessary.

In addition to the lesion characteristics the clinical presentation of the patient also factors into procedural success. The unstable patient with ongoing pain or hemodynamic instability has a higher complication rate. This is true in unstable coronary syndromes as well as in cases of acute MI. Operator and institutional experience and volume also positively or negatively affect outcome. Current ACC/AHA guideline recommend that PCI be performed by operators with a minimum of 75 procedures per year in a center that performs at least 400 procedures a year.

Topol EJ: Textbook of Interventional Cardiology, Philadelphia: WB Saunders, 1999.

Restenosis

Angioplasty is believed to relieve a coronary stenosis by various mechanisms, including plaque compression, plaque fracture, and arterial stretch. The act of inflating a balloon inside the artery may be considered traumatic and sets off an inflammatory response that ultimately leads to tissue proliferation. The balloon can denude the arterial intima, disrupt the plaque, and expose subendothelial elements. With balloon angioplasty elastic recoil is often the mechanism by which recurrent symptoms occur. When an intracoronary stent has been placed, the mechanism is usually neointimal hyperplasia. Restenosis is defined as a recurrent stenosis of at least 50% at the site of a prior PCI.

The majority of patients who undergo PCI have immediate relief of their symptoms. Patients that remain symptom-free for 6–12 months are considered to be outside the period for restenosis. The incidence of restenosis varies widely and can range from 8% to 60%, depending on lesion characteristics and procedural success. The mortality rate at 1 year is less than 3%. Vigorous research is ongoing in hopes of discovering a way to reduce or treat restenosis. A number of agents have undergone clinical or animal trials but have not proven efficacious. These include aspirin, IIb/IIIa inhibitors, ticlopidine, prostacyclin analogs, warfarin, enoxaparin, calcium channel blockers, colchicine, corticosteroids, lovastatin, and fish oil.

The use of stents has markedly reduced the rate of restenosis, but this technique has brought with it a new challenge, in-stent restenosis (ISR). ISR has subsequently triggered a whole new direction in PCI, the prevention of ISR. The use of radiation to treat ISR has proven very effective, reducing subsequent restenosis by up to 60% in comparison with conventional treatment. Plaque ablation or fracture within the stent has also

been promising using atherectomy catheters and cutting balloons. The latest technology being investigated is the drug-eluting stent, in which antiproliferative drugs, such as sirolimus, and paclitaxel, are bound to stents and appear to prevent the neointimal proliferation. Initial trials reveal restenosis rates as low as 2–3% over 6 months.

Repeat angioplasty in patients with restenosis is usually symptom-driven. These patients may be prone to another recurrence of restenosis. Multiple restenoses may be an indication for a CABG operation in select patients.

Technology

1. Atherectomy—The FDA has approved three atherectomy devices: rotational atherectomy, directional atherectomy, and transluminal extraction catheters.

a. Rotational atherectomy—This device consists of an elliptically shaped, diamond-tipped catheter on the end of a long, flexible driveshaft that tracks along a central guidewire. The burr rotates at speeds of up to 200,000 rpm. Burr sizes range from 1.25 to 2.5 mm in diameter. The patient receives a continuous infusion or a "cocktail" consisting of calcium channel blockers and nitrates to prevent vasospasm during the rotational atherectomy. The rotating catheter is advanced over the wire through the stenosis and ablates the plaque. Several slow passes are performed to ensure adequate plaque ablation. Several burrs of increasing size may be used to achieve an adequate result. Rotational atherectomy is followed by a low-pressure balloon inflation. Rotational atherectomy can be used as the primary modality or in conjunction with other modalities such as stents. The debris is microscopic and is cleared by the reticuloendothelial system. Rotational atherectomy is indicated in severely calcified lesions, diffuse disease, ostial sidebranch lesions, undilatable lesions, chronic total occlusions, and ISR. Contraindications to rotational atherectomy include thrombus and degenerated vein grafts.

b. Directional atherectomy—Directional atherectomy (DCA) is an over-the-wire cutting and retrieval system. The prototype consists of a metal housing that contains a cutter and acts as a retrieval chamber. A balloon is adjacent to the metal housing. Directional atherectomy was designed to cut and remove obstructive atheroma with directional control. The catheter is advanced over the wire to the site of stenosis with the cutting window oriented in the direction of greatest plaque burden. The balloon is then inflated, pushing the cutting window up against the plaque. A motor drive unit attached to the end of the catheter shaft allows the operator to advance the cutter at speeds of up to 2000 rpm. Slow advancement allows for gentle cutting and removal of the tissue protruding into the metal housing. Eight to ten passes are made, and the catheter is removed. Depending on whether the plaque is concentric or eccentric, the housing can be rotated to facilitate plaque removal. The complication rate is similar to that for balloon angioplasty. Indications include eccentric lesions and ostial lesions. The vessel must be of suitable size to accommodate the directional atherectomy catheter. Several trials have compared DCA with balloon angioplasty. The CAVEAT trial found DCA had better initial outcomes with higher procedural success rates, but with more in-hospital complications. No difference was noted in target vessel revascularization or event-free survival.

c. Transluminal extraction catheter—The transluminal extraction catheter (TEC) is another over-the-wire cutting and extraction system. The system consists of a dome-shaped cutting head with two stainless steel blades attached to the end of a flexible catheter. The catheter is attached to a battery-powered motor drive unit and to a vacuum bottle for aspiration of debris. A switch on the motor drive activates the cutting and aspiration, and a lever on the top of the unit allows forward movement of the unit. During extraction, warm saline is infused under pressure to create a solution of blood and tissue. TEC is indicated in degenerated vein grafts and in thrombus-laden arteries.

The use of both TEC and DCA has markedly decreased with the advent of stenting and other new modalities. These devices still have a niche, but few operators perform adequate numbers of procedures to remain facile with these techniques.

Stents

The use of intracoronary stents has been proven to decrease clinical and angiographic restenosis. As a result, stents have become the mainstay of PCI, being used in 60–80% of procedures performed. The Magic Wallstent was the first to undergo clinical evaluation in trials that began in 1986. The initial trials were feasibility studies and proved very promising. The Palmaz-Shatz (P-S) stent was simultaneously developed and studied. These first stents were made of stainless steel (P-S stent) or cobalt alloys with a platinum core (Wallstent). The designs differed radically. The Wallstent was self-expanding, and the P-S stent was balloon-expandable. Stent design has continued to be modified, with over 60 intracoronary stents currently available worldwide in multiple designs, materials, and characteristics. This is now the era of second- and third-generation stents. The popularity of stents exploded when the revolutionary STRESS and BENESTENT trials were published. These landmark trials compared balloon angioplasty with and without stents and showed that stents significantly reduced the inci-

dence of angiographic restenosis in large, de novo lesions.

The design, material, or mode of delivery can classify stents. Designs vary and include slotted tubes, coils, and mesh. Different materials used include stainless steel, nitinol, tantalum, and platinum. Stents can be either self-expanding or balloon-expandable. Radioactive stents are being studied in hopes they will diminish ISR. Current research and design is geared toward drug-eluting stents in the hopes of reducing ISR. Promising drugs include sirolimus and paclitaxel.

Although initial trials were directed at a select group of patients with short de novo lesions in large arteries, current research continues to assess the utility of stents in many patient subgroups. Stents have been shown efficacious in almost all patient subsets, including those undergoing multivessel procedures, those with long lesions, diabetics, and women. Adjunctive drug therapy has also improved outcomes. The use of antiplatelet agents and IIb/IIIa inhibitors has nearly eradicated acute and subacute thrombosis and has decreased target vessel revascularization by up to 30%. When possible, patients are given a loading dose with an antiplatelet agent up to 3 days before their PCI. The majority of stents used today are mounted on a balloon. The stent on the balloon is advanced over a guidewire to the lesion. The balloon is then inflated and expands the stent. The size of the stent is chosen by the operator to be the estimated diameter and length of the lesion. Stents come in many diameters and lengths. High-pressure balloon inflations of 12–16 atm are standard to ensure adequate stent deployment. During their PCI with stenting most patients receive a IIb/IIIa inhibitor. They are maintained on aspirin indefinitely and receive ticlopidine or clopidogrel for 2–4 weeks.

The initial indication for stenting was suboptimal angioplasty or threatened closure. This has now been expanded to include a broad spectrum of other symptoms. The ACC/AHA has published a recent guideline directed at identifying those patients who would benefit from stenting.

Thrombectomy Devices

One FDA approved thrombectomy device is currently in use. This catheter-based, over-the-wire device consists of a cap, which is open on one side. Heparinized flush is rapidly infused into the artery at the area of thrombosis and the design creates a Venturi effect, which vacuums the solution along with pulverized thrombus into the catheter. Initial data supports the use of the thrombectomy device in saphenous vein grafts and in acute MI or other situations where a large thrombus burden may exist.

Lasers

A laser source is transmitted through a fiberoptic cable to the end of an angioplasty balloon. The energy is transmitted from the fiber to the plaque, thereby melting and ablating the plaque. Current lasers employ various wavelengths, including ultraviolet (excimer) and infrared (holmium). The laser is advanced over a guidewire to the stenosis. The laser is then activated, and the tissue is ablated. Lasers have been used in a wide spectrum of patients. Their true niche seems to be chronic total occlusions and transmyocardial revascularization. The success rate for total occlusions was improved from 69% with conventional angioplasty to between 86 and 90% with laser. Laser angioplasty has a steep learning curve,, and complication rates, particularly perforations, have been high. Highly experienced operators perform laser angioplasty in a few centers.

Myocardial laser revascularization, which includes TMR (surgical transmyocardial revascularization), DMR (percutaneous directed myocardial revascularization), and PMR (percutaneous myocardial revascularization), is based on the concept that small channels in areas with myocardial ischemia will spur angiogenesis and provide direct delivery of oxygenated blood to the ischemic territory. The laser is used to create channels in the area of ischemia that is deemed viable. Anywhere from 10 to 20 channels are made, percutaneously or surgically, in the ischemic territory. This procedure has been used in those patients for whom revascularization via traditional methods in contraindicated. Initial clinical trials appeared promising; however, recent data reveal that the procedure conferred no benefit over aggressive medical therapy.

Modified Balloons

1. Cutting balloons—A cutting balloon is a conventional angioplasty balloon with either three or four longitudinal blades on its surface. As the balloon is inflated these blades act to score the plaque and create "controlled" dissections that serve to allow for arterial expansion and remodeling. Some positive results have been reported for patients with ISR and for ostial lesions. The risk of arterial perforation in these patients is slightly greater, and care must be taken to select an appropriate patient population.

Physiologic Assessment

Angiography is limited in its ability to assess plaque characteristics and physiologic significance. An important adjunct to percutaneous interventions has been the advent of physiologic assessment. These physiologic assessments can be used to either decide on the physiologic significance of a lesion or guide a percutaneous intervention to maximize the procedural outcome. Coronary anatomy can be physiologically assessed in a number of ways.

Intravascular Ultrasound

Intravascular ultrasound (IVUS) uses high-frequency transducers to visualize and characterize arterial composition. The most commonly used catheter consists of a number of transducers arranged circumferentially around the tip of a catheter, which transmit a 360° image. The catheter can be advanced over a guidewire and then be pulled back manually or via a mechanical pullback device. These images visualize the inner surface of the artery; the intima, media, and adventitia are identifiable. IVUS has markedly increased our understanding of plaque morphology and arterial remodeling. It has become evident that we frequently underestimate the plaque burden in an artery. An artery may look angiographically normal yet have layered plaque circumferentially around the entire lumen. Additionally, plaque is highly visible, and ultrasound can easily identify its characteristics, a feature that may assist in device selection. IVUS can be instrumental in defining adequate and optimal stent deployment. It is indicated to treat patients with borderline anatomy, to size vessels, to ensure adequate angioplasty results, and to identify calcified lesions. A new indication is in the treatment of ISR. It can assess whether the previously deployed stent was properly sized and deployed and identify any proximal or distal problems.

Doppler Wires

Doppler wires employ the measurement of blood velocity using the Doppler principle. Piezoelectric crystals adhering to the end of a coronary guidewire measure coronary blood flow proximal and distal to a stenosis and compare the blood velocity, thereby determining the physiologic significance of the lesion. The wire, which can range from 0.014 to 0.018 in. in diameter, is passed to the area of stenosis. A potent vasodilator such as adenosine is used to create a hyperemic response. Coronary flow reserve (CFR) is the ratio of hyperemic to basal blood flow. An impaired hyperemic response corresponds to a physiologically significant lesion. Doppler wires are useful in assessing the physiologic significance of a borderline angiographic stenosis. A number of clinical trials have also verified their utility in assessing the adequacy of a percutaneous intervention by assessing CFR before and after angioplasty. Several trials looked at the use of flow reserve to guide angioplasty. With the guided PCI, the operators were able to decrease recurrent events.

Flow Wires

Fractional flow reserve is the ratio of the distal coronary pressure to the aortic pressure measured during maximal hyperemia. A wire with a miniaturized pressure transducer is advanced beyond the occlusion; the pressure is then compared with aortic pressure. The pressure wire, like the Doppler wire, can be used to make therapy decisions in cases of moderate lesions and to assess angiographic results.

Angioscopy

Angioscopy was the first method to facilitate direct visualization of coronary artery lumens. The angioscopy catheter is a miniaturized flexible catheter equipped with fiberoptic imaging. These catheters are advanced into coronary arteries over a guidewire, which allows the area of interest to be visualized. Angioscopy is useful in defining thrombus and plaque characteristics. The initial work done in saphenous vein grafts was important in visualizing the diffuse, friable nature of these grafts.

Columbo A, Ferraro M, Itoh A et al: Results of coronary stenting for restenosis. J Am Coll Cardiol 1996;28:830.

Fishman DL, Leon MB, Baim DS et al: A randomized comparison of coronary stent placement and balloon angioplasty is the treatment of coronary artery disease. Stent Restenosis Study investigators. N Engl J Med 1994;331:496.

Holmes D: Coronary artery stents. J Am Coll Cardiol 1998:32;1471.

Ryan TJ, Bauman WB, Kennedy JW et al: Guidelines for percutaneous transluminal coronary angioplasty. Angioplasty J Am Coll Cardiol 1993;22:2033.

Surreys PW, de Haegere P, Kiemeneij F et al: A comparison of balloon expandable stent implantation with balloon angioplasty in patients with coronary artery disease. Benestent Study Group. N Engl J Med 1994;331:489.

Topol EJ: Textbook of Interventional Cardiology, Philadelphia: WB Saunders, 1999.

CORONARY ARTERY BYPASS GRAFTING

Surgical revascularization has become a mainstay in the treatment of patients with CAD. It preceded percutaneous revascularization and has had a remarkable success in alleviating symptoms and improving lifestyle and has improved the mortality rate in select patients. A large number of clinical trials comparing PCI with CABG have defined which patient subsets will benefit most from PCI versus CABG. The number of patients undergoing CABG has grown exponentially and will likely exceed 500,000 a year in the United States.

Background and Historical Perspective

Alexis Carrel pioneered the first use of a conduit to bypass a stenotic coronary artery. He used canine models to construct the first aortocoronary anastomosis. In conjunction with Charles Lindbergh, he subsequently developed a heart-lung bypass machine. Charles Gibbons used this system on a patient in the 1950s and further developed this technology. William Mustard probably performed the first coronary bypass operation using a carotid-coronary bypass graft. In 1958, Longmire performed a number of endarterectomies as a method to relieve coronary stenosis. He used an internal thoracic artery (ITA) to salvage a failed coronary endarterectomy. Debakey and Garrett had a similar experience and used a saphenous vein graft (SVG) to rescue a failed endarterectomy. It was about this time that The Vineberg procedure was devised using an ITA to directly anastomose to the myocardium.

The first planned CABG using an end-to-end anastomosis and cardiopulmonary bypass was performed at Duke University in 1962 by David Sabiston. The technique was further advanced by the work of Favaloro and Sones, who demonstrated that SVGs were feasible conduits for bypassing a number of coronary stenoses. The use of the ITA slowly followed that of SVGs. Data soon confirmed using the ITA as a conduit for the left anterior descending artery demonstrated improved survival. By the 1970s, CABG was the accepted method of revascularization for CAD. Several large clinical trials comparing CABG with medical therapy strongly favored CAGB in selected patients, demonstrating a subsequently improved quality of life and improved mortality benefits. Improvements in technique and new technology have continued to advance the science of coronary artery surgery.

Indications

CABG is indicated for symptom relief as well as mortality benefit. The American College of Cardiology has formulated a set of guidelines that define those patients who will likely benefit from this type of revascularization. In all cases, the advantages and disadvantages of percutaneous revascularization versus surgical revascularization must be considered.

1. Asymptomatic or mild angina—For patients who are asymptomatic or who have only mild angina, there must be compelling evidence that revascularization will improve the mortality probability. A large area of myocardium must be at risk or a significant area of ischemia must be evident on noninvasive tests. For instance:

- Significant left main stenosis
- Left main equivalent defined as significant proximal left anterior descending (LAD) and significant proximal circumflex disease
- Triple-vessel disease, especially if left ventricular function is impaired and the ejection fraction (EF) is less than 50%

2. Stable angina—In cases of stable angina, the indication for CABG must be based on the likelihood that survival will be prolonged and that symptoms will be relieved and the quality of life improved. Medical therapy must be instituted and maximized. Risk factor modification is mandated. Trials evaluating CABG in this subset of patients with stable angina found that the patients with severe proximal LAD or multivessel disease showed the most benefit from surgical revascularization. Other factors, which tip the scales toward surgery, include diabetes mellitus and impaired left ventricular function. Indications include:

- Significant left main stenosis
- Left main equivalent defined as significant proximal LAD and significant proximal circumflex disease
- Triple-vessel disease, especially if left ventricular function is impaired and the EF is less than 50%
- Two-vessel disease, including proximal LAD with an EF of less than 50%, or documented ischemia on noninvasive testing
- One- or two-vessel disease without proximal LAD and high-risk criteria on noninvasive testing (see PCI section)
- Refractory angina despite maximal medical therapy

3. Unstable angina—The use of revascularization in this cases of unstable angina is driven by survival benefit as well as symptom relief. The indications are the same as for stable angina; however, the timing of surgery must be considered. A number of studies evaluating CABG did subgroup analyses, which indicated that patients with an unstable syndrome and those patients who had a non-ST elevation MI had a worse outcome than stable patients did. If possible, it is prudent to stabilize patients with medical therapy and allow them to "cool off" before scheduling surgery. Those with refractory symptoms should undergo revascularization as soon as possible.

4. ST elevation myocardial infarction—Patients undergoing an ST elevation MI receive thrombolytic therapy or undergo percutaneous intervention in order to reestablish blood flow to the infarct-related artery. Some patients referred for cardiac catheterization at the time of MI are not deemed candidates for percutaneous intervention. These include patients with severe left main disease, severe three-vessel disease, severe valvular disease or a mechanical complication of MI such as papillary muscle rupture, free wall rupture, or acute ventricular-septal defect. The decision to perform surgery must be made with the knowledge that the patient has adequate targets and conduits. The patient must have failed alternative therapy, such as medical management, thrombolysis, or percutaneous intervention. Like

PCI, the risks of CABG in the throes of an MI are higher than in a stable patient.

Another subset of patients who may benefit from surgical revascularization are those who meet the previously cited criteria and who, additionally, are in cardiogenic shock. As discussed in the PCI section, patients with cardiogenic shock benefit from early revascularization compared with medical management, showing improved survival rates at 6 months.

Eagle K, Guyton R: ACC/AHA guidelines for coronary artery bypass surgery. J Am Coll Cardiol 1999;34:1262.

Technique

Median sternotomy with cardiopulmonary bypass is the standard approach to bypass surgery. A newer technique, which allows for surgery "off-pump," permits the surgeon to operate on the beating heart without putting the patient on cardiopulmonary bypass (CPB). Additionally, different access to the heart has become possible with approaches via right or left thoracotomy.

Cardiopulmonary bypass requires cannulation of large vessels for drainage of systemic venous blood into the CPB machine that then returns to the circulation via an arterial conduit, the distal descending aorta, or the femoral artery. The cannulae remove unoxygenated blood from the venous drainage system and pool it in a venous reservoir. A heat exchanger allows temperature regulation of the blood. The blood is sent through filters that do not permit particles larger than 40 μm to pass through, thereby preventing air or atheroembolization. The blood is then passed through an oxygenator and returns to the arterial system to circulate through the body.

Two important issues in CPB relate to two of its physiologic effects: the exposure of blood to artificial surfaces, such as cannulae and membrane oxygenators, and the loss of the normal pulsatile flow of the blood.

The massive, repetitive exposure of blood to artificial surfaces causes an inflammatory response with complement activation, increased capillary permeability, and the release of many humoral markers. A large dose of steroids added to the priming solution used for the pump offsets this response to some degree. This exposure also results in physical damage to the blood cells, resulting in platelet damage, prolongation of the coagulation profile, and fibrinolysis. Pulmonary effects include surfactant consumption and pulmonary sequestration of blood cells. About 5% of patients will develop adult respiratory distress syndrome to some degree.

Two types of blood pumps are used for CPB. Both provide nonpulsatile flow, which results in redistribution of blood flow from the normal pattern, thereby affecting the renal, splanchnic, and mesenteric beds. This may result in impaired renal function and intestinal ischemia. Pumps that electronically pulse the blood have been developed and have reduced the effects of nonpulsatile flow; however; this does not fully mimic normal pulsatile blood flow, and impaired renal function is not infrequent.

Myocardial protection is achieved by cooling the heart. Experiments have shown the heart can tolerate interruption of coronary blood flow for 15 to 20 min at mild hypothermia. To achieve this cooling of the heart, a cardioplegic solution is infused into the coronary arteries. Some surgeons are intermittently using cardioplegia while doing the anastomoses to minimize the length of ischemic time.

Once the heart is on CPB, conduits are identified. The conduits used can be arterial or venous. The common arterial conduits include the ITAs, the radial artery, and the gastroepiploic artery. Veins are harvested from the legs. There is ample evidence that the ITAs have superior long-term patency compared with SVGs, resulting in improved survival. Multiple arterial conduits can be used, but the additional harvesting time and higher infection rate, especially in diabetics, does not seem to justify the outcome unless no other conduits are available. Thus, the left ITA is used for the left anterior descending coronary artery conduit, with vein grafts being used for other coronary arteries.

A new approach to cardiac surgery is called minimally invasive direct coronary bypass, or MIDCAB. A MIDCAB is a CABG performed on the beating heart without the need for cardiopulmonary bypass. The surgery can be done via a small intercostal incision or a partial sternotomy. The most common target and conduit is the left ITA anastomosed to the LAD artery. The major advantage is the elimination of the risk of CPB, such as thromboembolic events and renal dysfunction.

Clinical Trials

In the 1970s and 1980s the focus of clinical trials was to determine which patients would benefit from surgery versus medical therapy. The current guidelines have incorporated these data into the guidelines for PCI and CABG. The 1990s focused on PCI versus CABG. Several clinical trials have compared percutaneous and surgical techniques. The patient populations in these groups have varied widely, so care must be taken when comparing the data. These trials have been instrumental in formulating clinical strategies for revascularization. It is important to realize that the technical aspects of both PCI and CABG have changed drastically, so the trials done in the 1990s may not be applicable in the current milieu.

In reviewing the various clinical trials, attention must be paid to the number of patients in the trial. The number of patients in the trial must be adequate to achieve statistical significance in evaluating endpoints. The therapy chosen must be instituted. Follow-up must be long enough to detect a survival benefit for either group, and the results must be generalizable to other similar patients. All of the large randomized trials comparing the revascularization strategies lack one or more of these criteria.

CABG versus medical therapy was evaluated by three large randomized trials: the Veteran's Administration Cooperative Study (VA Study), the European Coronary Surgery Study, and the Coronary Artery Surgery Study (CASS). Inclusion criteria for these trials varied. Yusef and colleagues performed a meta-analysis of seven randomized trials that compared medical versus surgical therapy. A total of 2649 patients were evaluated, the majority of whom came from the three aforementioned trials. The 30-day mortality rate was 3.2% overall. Initial surgical revascularization resulted in a statistically significant decrease in mortality at 5, 7, and 10 years. Those subsets that most benefited included patients with left main disease, triple-vessel disease, one- or two-vessel disease including the LAD, depressed left ventricular function, and those felt to have a high-risk profile. Recall that the medical and surgical treatments used are not those used today. CABG improves survival rates in the aforementioned subsets considered to be at moderate to high risk when compared with medical therapy.

The major clinical trials comparing angioplasty and surgery include BARI, EAST, GABI, Toulouse, RITA, ERACI, MASS, Lausanne, CABRI, SOS.

Three of these trials addressed single-vessel left anterior descending CAD: RITA, Lausanne, and MASS. Both the Lausanne and MASS trials targeted the proximal LAD. The RITA trial had a larger number of patients (456) than the Lausanne and MASS trials and included patients with unstable angina. All three trials revealed good outcomes for both groups with a statistically significant mortality benefit for either group. The PCI group had a greater need for repeat revascularization as well as a higher incidence of angina. The MASS trial also included a medical therapy arm, and both revascularization strategies proved superior to medical therapy in single-vessel proximal LAD disease with good left ventricular function.

The next group of trials addressed multivessel CAD and included a subset of the RITA group, ERACI, GABI, EAST, CABRI, and BARI. These patients represent an extremely heterogeneous group. They differed in risk factor profile, lesion character, clinical presentation, and left ventricular function, among other variables. It is important to keep these differences in mind when evaluating these data.

The largest of the these trials is the BARI trial, which also had a large registry that followed the outcomes of eligible patients who were not randomized and were referred for PCI or CABG based on the judgment of their physicians. The BARI trial enrolled 1792 patients with multivessel CAD to either angioplasty or surgery. The primary endpoint was mortality from all-causes at 5 years. Over 25,000 patients were screened. Besides the 1792 patients randomized, an additional 2013 patients were deemed eligible but not randomized. A registry of these patients was kept, and much additional data has been gleaned. Exclusion criteria included left main stenosis of > 50% or need for emergent revascularization. An unstable coronary syndrome was present in > 64% of patients. A subgroup analysis done at 5 years did not reveal a survival advantage for any of the following: stable versus unstable coronary syndrome, left ventricular dysfunction, two- or three-vessel disease, or lesion type. However, diabetics who had CABG had a statistically significant survival benefit over those who underwent PCI; this was limited to the patients who received an internal thoracic artery to their LAD. The need for repeat revascularization was significantly higher in the PCI group. EAST and CABRI had similar overall outcomes with no survival benefit for either revascularization strategy, but a lower recurrence of symptoms and repeat revascularization.

The above-mentioned trials have become dated because they do not integrate the latest technology available, including the use of intracoronary stents and antiplatelet agents. The use of stents has markedly decreased the need for repeat revascularization procedures. Three recently published trials, SOS, ARTS, and ERACI II, address the use of stents in conjunction with angioplasty compared with surgery. The stent or surgery (SOS) trial was designed to compare PCI supported by stent implantation with surgery for angina. Patients were randomized to either percutaneous intervention with stenting or CABG. Other therapy was state of the art. Mean follow-up was 2 years, with all patients having at least 1 year follow-up. The average number of vessels revascularized was 2.7 for PCI and 2.25 for the CABG group. Death and MI rates were approximately equal at 2 years (9.5%). The restenosis rate was only 17% at 1 year, which is about half that of earlier balloon angioplasty trials. The surgical mortality rate was also extremely low, < 1%. Both of these statistics imply improved outcomes for both PCI and CABG with improvements in technique, technology, and medical therapy. The Argentine Randomized Study Optimal Coronary Balloon Angioplasty and Stenting vs. Coronary Bypass Surgery in Multiple Vessel Disease (ERACI II) also compared PCI and stenting with CABG in 440 patients. The primary comparisons used major adverse cardiac events (defined as death, MI, and repeat revascularization) at 30 days, 1, 3, and 5 years after randomization. At 30 days only 3.6% of PCI patients had a major adverse cardiac event compared with

12.3% of CABG patients. At 18 months, 96.9% of PCI patients were alive compared with 92.5% of CABG patients. Like the other studies comparing PCI and CABG, the PCI patients required more repeat revascularization than the CABG patients, but this has been markedly decreased with the advent of stents. Stents have helped to equalize the circumstances by decreasing the need for repeat revascularization.

PCI and CABG are both effective means of revascularization. Although CABG has higher initial complications, including death, this technique clearly has a lower rate of recurrent angina and need for repeat revascularization. However, stents and adjunctive therapies have markedly narrowed the gap between these approaches. In addition, improved medical therapy and risk factor modification will likely decrease or slow the progression of disease. It is probable that we will see a combined approach using the best of both revascularization techniques in the future.

Argentine randomized study: Coronary angioplasty with stenting versus coronary bypass surgery in patients with multiple-vessel disease (ERACI II) 30 day and one year results. J Am Coll Cardiol 2001;37:51.

Bypass Angioplasty Revascularization Investigation (BARI) Investigators. Comparison of coronary bypass surgery with angioplasty in patients with multivessel disease. N Engl J Med 1996;335:217.

Carrie D, Elbaz M, Puel J et al: Five year outcome after coronary angioplasty versus bypass surgery in multivessel coronary artery disease: Results from the French Monocentric Study. Circulation 1997:96 Suppl II:1.

Coronary angioplasty versus coronary artery bypass surgery: The Randomized Intervention Treatment of Angina (RITA) trial. Lancet 1993;341:573.

First year results of CABRI (coronary Angioplasty versus Bypass Revascularization Investigation): CABRI trial participants. Lancet 1995;346:1179.

Goy JJ, Eeckout E, Burand B et al: Coronary angioplasty versus left internal mammary grafting for isolated proximal left anterior descending artery stenosis. Lancet 1994;343:1449.

Hamm CW, Reimers J, Ischinger T et al: A randomized study of coronary angioplasty compared with bypass surgery in patients with symptomatic multivessel coronary disease. German Angioplasty Bypass Surgery Investigation (GABI). N Engl J Med 1994;331:1037.

Hueb WA, Belloti G, de Oliveira SA et al: The Medicine, Angioplasty of Surgery Study (MASS): A prospective, randomized trial of medical therapy, balloon angioplasty of bypass surgery for single proximal left anterior descending stenosis. J Am Coll Cardiol 1995;26:1600.

King SB, Lembo NJ, Weintraub WS et al: A randomized trial comparing coronary angioplasty with coronary bypass surgery: Emory Angioplasty versus Surgery Trial (EAST). N Engl J Med 1994;331:1044.

Rodriguez A, Boullon F, Perez-Balino N et al: Argentine randomized trial of percutaneous transluminal coronary angioplasty versus coronary artery bypass surgery in multivessel disease (ERACI): In hospital results and 1-year follow-up: ERACI Group. J Am Coll Cardiol 1993;22:1060.

Aortic Stenosis

Blase A. Carabello, MD & Michael H. Crawford, MD

ESSENTIALS OF DIAGNOSIS

- *Angina pectoris*
- *Dyspnea (left ventricular heart failure)*
- *Effort syncope*
- *Systolic ejection murmur radiating to the carotid arteries*
- *Carotid upstroke delayed in reaching its peak and reduced in amplitude (parvus et tardus)*
- *Echocardiography shows thickened, immobile aortic valve leaflets*
- *Doppler echocardiography quantifies increased transvalvular pressure gradient and reduced valve area*

General Considerations & Etiology

Aortic stenosis is the narrowing of the aortic valve orifice, caused by failure of the valve leaflets to open normally. This reduction in orifice area produces an energy loss as laminar flow is converted to a less efficient turbulent flow, in turn increasing the pressure work that the left ventricle must perform in order to drive blood past the narrowed valve. The concentric left ventricular hypertrophy that develops as a major compensatory mechanism helps the left ventricle cope with the increased pressure work it must perform. These factors—turbulence, energy loss, and hypertrophy—constitute the pathophysiologic underpinnings for the patient's symptoms. The disease is confirmed through history and physical examination, Doppler echocardiography, and cardiac catheterization.

A. BICUSPID AORTIC VALVE

This is the most common congenital cardiac abnormality, occurring in approximately 2% of the population. It is believed that the bicuspid valve has hemodynamic disadvantages compared with the normal tricuspid valve, leading to valvular degeneration by mechanisms that are still not fully understood. Approximately one half of all patients with bicuspid aortic valves develop at least mild aortic stenosis, usually by age 50.

B. TRICUSPID AORTIC VALVE DEGENERATION

Many patients born with normal tricuspid aortic valves eventually develop senile degeneration of the valve leaflets and leaflet calcification, thus producing valvular stenosis. Although hypercholesterolemia and diabetes have been defined as risk factors for this degeneration, these conditions account for only a small percentage of all cases. The mechanisms by which some valves degenerate and become stenotic while others remain relatively normal are unknown.

Stewart BF, Siscovick D, Lind BK et al: Clinical factors associated with calcific aortic valve disease. J Am Coll Cardiol 1997; 29:630.

Wierzbicki A, Shetty C: Aortic stenosis: An atherosclerotic disease? J Heart Valve Dis 1999;8:416.

C. CONGENITAL AORTIC STENOSIS

Fusion of the valve leaflets before birth produces congenital aortic stenosis that is occasionally detected for the first time in adulthood. In many respects, however, congenital aortic stenosis appears to differ from acquired adult aortic stenosis. The hypertrophy in congenital aortic stenosis is more exuberant, yet such patients almost never develop heart failure symptoms. The first clinical manifestation of the disease can be sudden death without the development of premonitory symptoms in about 15% of patients.

D. RHEUMATIC FEVER

Rheumatic fever still occasionally causes aortic stenosis in the United States, although this cause is more common in developing nations. Rheumatic heart disease almost never attacks the aortic valve in isolation, usually also affecting the mitral valve to some degree. Aortic stenosis in a patient with a perfectly normal mitral valve is considered to have degenerative rather than rheumatic aortic stenosis.

E. OTHER CAUSES

Systemic lupus erythematosus, severe familial hypercholesterolemia, and ochronosis have occasionally been reported to cause valvular aortic stenosis.

Clinical Findings

A. SYMPTOMS AND SIGNS

Patients with acquired aortic stenosis present with the following classic symptoms: angina, effort syncope, and congestive heart failure. Approximately 35% of patients present with angina; 15% with effort syncope; and 50% with congestive heart failure. The onset of these symptoms heralds a dramatic increase in the mortality rate for these patients if aortic valve replacement is not performed. Symptoms are therefore the guidepost for intervention, and understanding them is key to understanding and managing the disease.

1. Angina—Angina occurs in response to myocardial ischemia, which develops when left ventricular oxygen demand exceeds supply. It should be noted that although epicardial coronary artery disease may coexist with aortic stenosis, angina frequently occurs in aortic stenosis in the absence of coronary artery disease.

As noted earlier, concentric left ventricular hypertrophy develops as a compensatory response to the pressure overload of aortic stenosis. The load on individual myocardial fibers can best be described as left ventricular wall stress and defined by the Laplace equation:

$$Stress = \frac{pressure \times radius}{2 \times thickness}$$

As left ventricular pressure increases, a parallel increase in left ventricular wall thickness (concentric hypertrophy) helps to offset the pressure overload and maintain stress in the normal range. The left ventricular myocardium must produce stress in order to shorten, maintaining normal stress facilitates shortening. This compensatory mechanism is attended by negative pathophysiologic sequelae, however. Despite normal epicardial coronary arteries, the coronary blood flow is reduced; although the flow may be normal at rest, the reserve needed to offset increased oxygen demands during stress or exercise is inadequate, and thus ischemia develops. The exact mechanism by which the coronary blood flow reserve is reduced in aortic stenosis is uncertain, but low capillary density per unit of muscle is at least one operative factor.

Oxygen demand is best estimated clinically by the product of heart rate and wall stress. As noted earlier, the hypertrophy initially maintains wall stress in the normal range, and despite the pressure overload, myocardial oxygen demand is not increased. Eventually, however, the hypertrophy cannot keep pace with the pressure demands of the ventricle, and wall stress increases. This increases oxygen demand and is another factor contributing to ischemia and the symptoms of angina.

2. Effort syncope—In general, syncope results from inadequate cerebral perfusion. The syncope of aortic stenosis usually occurs during exercise. One theory for exertional syncope in aortic stenosis is that during exercise total peripheral resistance decreases, but cardiac output cannot increase as it normally does because the narrowed aortic valve restricts the output. Blood pressure is the product of peripheral resistance and cardiac output, so this imbalance causes a drop in blood pressure, leading to syncope.

Another theory is that the very high left ventricular pressure that develops during exercise triggers a reflexive vasodepressor response, leading to a fall in blood pressure. In addition, exercise can cause both ventricular and supraventricular arrhythmias, which in aortic stenosis lead to a fall in effective output and consequently a decrease in blood pressure.

3. Congestive heart failure—Both left ventricular systolic and diastolic failure occur in aortic stenosis and produce the symptoms of dyspnea on exertion as well as orthopnea and paroxysmal nocturnal dyspnea. In some patients, the attendant high left-sided filling pressure leads to pulmonary hypertension, which overloads the right ventricle and thereby produces right ventricular failure and the symptoms of edema and ascites.

Impaired diastolic left ventricular filling in aortic stenosis is primarily due to the increased wall thickness caused by concentric hypertrophy. Because the increased thickness makes the ventricle harder to fill, producing any left ventricular volume requires increased filling pressure. The increased diastolic filling pressure is referred to the left atrium and to the pulmonary veins, where pulmonary venous congestion develops, leading to increased lung water, increased lung stiffness, and dyspnea. The wall composition also changes. Collagen content increases (Figure 8–1), creating a compensatory mechanism that helps to translate the increased force generated by the myocardium into chamber contraction. Unfortunately, the increase in collagen further increases ventricular stiffness.

Systole is governed by two mechanical properties: contractility and afterload. Contractility is the ability of the myocardium to generate force; afterload is the force the ventricle must overcome to contract. Either property can impair ventricular systole, and both are operative in aortic stenosis. Although the initial concentric hypertrophy normalizes wall stress (afterload), as the disease progresses, the hypertrophy may not keep pace with the increase in pressure and wall stress increases. As stress increases, ejection fraction (EF) decreases:

$$EF = \frac{stroke\ volume}{end\ diastolic\ volume}$$

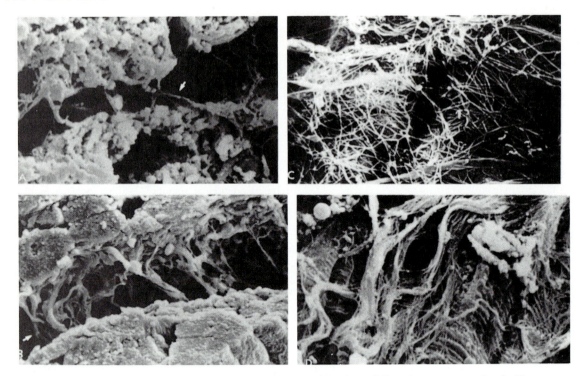

Figure 8–1. Scanning electron microscopy of normal myocardium (**A** and **C**) and pressure-overloaded hypertrophied myocardium (**B** and **D**). **B** shows denser perimysial collagen connections between in the hypertrophied myocardium (compared with **A**, **D** shows the thickened tendons in the hypertrophied myocardium (compare with normal myocardium in **C**). Adapted, with permission, from Weber KT: Cardiac interstitium in health and disease: The fibrillar collagen network. J Am Coll Cardiol 1989;13:1637.

Reduced ejection fraction is more common in men than women. Inexplicably, women tend to generate more hypertrophy, keeping wall stress low and thus maintaining normal or even supernormal ejection fraction.

Ejection fraction may also decline if contractility falls; however, the exact mechanism of reduced contractility in aortic stenosis is unclear. In the simplest sense, reduced contractility is the result of prolonged overload on the heart. Loss of contractile elements and ischemia from abnormal coronary blood flow are two of the mechanisms that have been postulated to explain the reduction.

Douglas PS, Otto CM, Mickel MC et al: Gender differences in left ventricular geometry and function in patients undergoing balloon dilation of the aortic valve for isolated aortic stenosis. Br Heart J 1995;73:548.

Julius BK, Spillmann M, Vassalli G et al: Angina pectoris in patients with aortic stenosis and normal coronary arteries. Mechanisms and pathophysiological concepts. Circulation 1997;95:892.

B. PHYSICAL EXAMINATION

1. Systolic ejection murmur—The classic murmur of aortic stenosis is a medium-pitched and often harsh systolic ejection murmur, heard best in the aortic area and radiating to the carotid arteries. In mild disease, the murmur peaks early in systole. As the disease worsens, the murmur peaks later, increases in intensity, and may be associated with a thrill palpated in the aortic area. With further progression of aortic stenosis, the murmur peaks very late in systole, it may decrease in intensity as cardiac output begins to fall, and the thrill may disappear. In advanced but still correctable disease, the murmur may become very unimpressive and be reduced to a grade II/VI or even a grade I/VI murmur, sometimes misleading the examiner into believing that severe disease is not present.

Sometimes the murmur is heard well over the aortic area, fades over the midsternum, and reappears over the apex (Gallivardin's phenomenon). The diagnostician may be misled into believing that two separate murmurs—one of aortic stenosis and one of mitral regurgitation—are present. Distinguishing between Gallivardin's phenomenon and two separate murmurs is difficult but important: The appearance of even mild mitral regurgitation in aortic stenosis is an ominous prognostic sign. If the diagnosis cannot be settled at the bedside, color-flow Doppler examination of the mitral valve will resolve the issue.

2. Carotid upstroke—Carotid upstroke in aortic stenosis is typically low in volume and delayed in reaching the peak amplitude (Figure 8–2). Palpation of this **parvus et tardus** pulse is probably the single best way to estimate the severity of aortic stenosis at the bedside. The examiner should palpate his or her own carotid artery with one hand while palpating the patient's carotid artery with the other, thus gauging the difference between normal and abnormal. A palpable shuddering sensation of the carotid pulse may also be noted. In elderly patients, increased stiffness of the carotid arteries may falsely normalize the upstroke, making it feel relatively brisk in nature. Even in this circumstance, however, the upstroke is rarely completely normal in character.

3. Second heart sound—Paradoxic splitting of the second heart sound is due to the prolonged ejection time required to expel stroke volume through the stenotic valve, which delays the closure of the aortic valve (A_2) past closure of the pulmonic valve (P_2). Although paradoxic splitting is emphasized in many texts, a more common finding is that the reduced movement of the aortic valve renders A_2 inaudible and only a soft single second sound (P_2) is heard.

4. Apical impulse—Because in aortic stenosis the left ventricle is usually concentrically hypertrophied and its volume is not increased, the point of maximum impulse is usually felt in its normal position. The apex beat, however, is abnormally forceful and sustained in nature. The left atrial contribution to left ventricular filling may be both visible and palpable; it corresponds to the fourth heart sound and is usually present in aor-

tic stenosis as a result of increased left ventricular stiffness.

5. Other findings—In far-advanced disease with congestive heart failure, a third heart sound is often heard. Pulmonary hypertension may develop, increasing the intensity of the pulmonic component of the second sound. Patients with aortic stenosis may also present initially with right ventricular failure manifested as edema and ascites.

Attenhofer Jost CH, Turina J, Mayer K et al: Echocardiography in the evaluation of systolic murmurs of unknown cause. Am J Med 2000;108:614.

Phoon CK: Estimation of pressure gradients by auscultation: An innovative physical examination technique. Am Heart J 2001;141:500.

C. DIAGNOSTIC STUDIES

1. Electrocardiography—The concentric left ventricular hypertrophy that develops in aortic stenosis is often reflected in the electrocardiogram as increased QRS voltage, left atrial abnormality, and ST and T wave abnormalities. The electrocardiogram (ECG), however, does not always demonstrate left ventricular hypertrophy even though the heart is actually hypertrophied. No ECG findings are, therefore, either sensitive or specific for aortic stenosis.

2. Chest radiography—Patients with aortic stenosis usually show a normal-sized heart in chest x-ray films. The left heart border may develop a rounded appearance consistent with concentric left ventricular hypertrophy; the aortic shadow may become enlarged because of poststenotic dilation. Occasionally, calcification of the aortic valve can be seen on the lateral view.

3. Echocardiography—Echocardiographic examination of the heart combined with Doppler investigation of the aortic valve usually can confirm the diagnosis of aortic stenosis; a technically adequate study can accurately quantify its severity. Echocardiography shows thickening of the aortic valve, reduced leaflet mobility, and concentric left ventricular hypertrophy, demon-

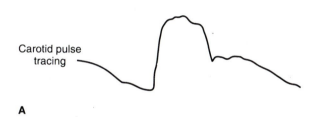

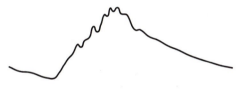

Carotid pulse tracing

A

B

Figure 8–2. **A:** A carotid pulse tracing from a normal subject. **B:** A tracing from a patient with aortic stenosis. The upstroke in **B** is quite delayed and demonstrates a shudder. Adapted, with permission, from Borow KM, Wynne J: External pulse recordings, systolic time intervals, apexcardiography, and phonocardiography. In Cohn PF, Wynne J, eds: Diagnostic Methods in Clinical Cardiology. Boston: Little, Brown, 1982.

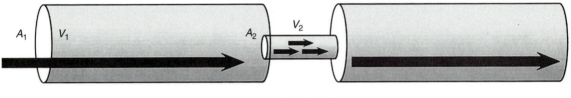

$$A_1 \times V_1 = A_2 \times V_2$$

Figure 8–3. Constant flow through a tube of different diameters. As the flow reaches the narrowed orifice A_2, velocity must increase in order for the flow to remain constant. Reprinted, with permission, from Carabello BA: Aortic stenosis. How to recognize and assess severity. Cardiol Rev 1993;1:59.

strating the presence of aortic stenosis but not quantifying its severity.

The Doppler study can be used to determine the gradient across the aortic valve and to calculate aortic valve area. Doppler quantification of aortic stenosis is based on the ability to measure blood velocity. Flow through an orifice is equal to cross-sectional orifice area times velocity. As shown in Figure 8–3, velocity must increase when a moving stream of a given flow reaches a narrowed area if the flow is to remain constant when it reaches the constriction. That is, the product of the velocity times area at the first orifice must be equal to that at the second orifice.

Measuring the area of the aortic outflow tract (A_1), the velocity of flow there (V_1), and the velocity at the stenosis (V_2), the aortic valve area (A_2) can be calculated as follows:

$$A_2 = \frac{A_1 \times V_1}{V_2}$$

The velocity of flow at the stenosis can also be used to calculate the aortic pressure gradient using the modified Bernoulli equation:

$$\text{Gradient} = 4V^2$$

Figure 8–4 shows the velocity profile from Doppler examination of a patient with aortic stenosis. The velocity of 4 m/s thus translates to a gradient of 64 mm Hg.

This technique is remarkably accurate compared with gradients measured invasively by catheter. In general, a mean gradient greater than 50 mm Hg or an aortic valve area less than 0.8 cm² indicates that the aortic stenosis is severe enough to cause the patient's symptoms. Many exceptions to this rule exist, however. Some patients remain asymptomatic despite higher gradients

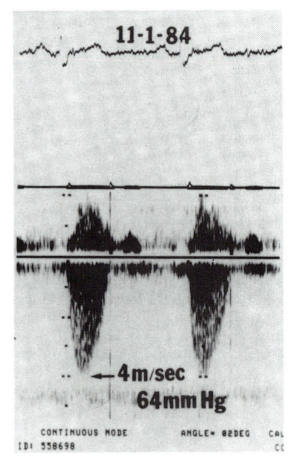

Figure 8–4. The Doppler wave form; flow across a stenotic aortic valve. Flow accelerates to 4 m/s, which translates to a gradient of 64 mm Hg. Adapted, with permission, from Assey et al: The patient with valvular heart disease. In Pepine CJ, Hill JA, Lambert CR, eds: Diagnostic and Therapeutic Cardiac Catheterization. Philadelphia: Williams & Wilkins, 1989.

and smaller valve areas, and others become symptomatic with lower gradients and larger valve areas.

4. Cardiac catheterization—Although Doppler echocardiography is an accurate means of determining the severity of aortic stenosis in most patients, other noninvasive techniques are generally not recommended. Stress testing, for example, can be dangerous, and left-ventricular hypertrophy makes cardiac perfusion imaging and the interpretation of ECGs problematic. Cardiac catheterization (whose main purpose is coronary angiography) is indicated when symptoms such as angina pectoris could be caused by coronary disease or aortic stenosis or when valve replacement surgery is planned. The presence and severity of coronary disease will influence the course of therapy, tipping the balance toward surgery when the aortic stenosis is of borderline severity.

During cardiac catheterization, cardiac output and aortic valve gradient are measured; these data are used to assess stenosis severity by calculation of aortic valve area. Great care must be used in assessing both parameters because errors in estimating the stenosis will be proportional to any measurement errors. The cardiac output is measured using the Fick principle or the indicator-dilution principle (usually thermodilution). The gradient is obtained by placing one catheter in the left ventricle (by retrograde or transseptal technique) and a second catheter in the proximal aorta on the other side of the stenotic valve. The pressure difference (gradient) is measured by recording the two pressures simultaneously. Recent studies discredit the use of a femoral artery sheath to record the downstream pressure. Left ventricular and femoral artery pressure waves occur at different times, so the tracings are aligned to compensate for this. This practice, however, may underestimate the true gradient by as much as 50%.

The cardiac output and gradient are then used to calculate the aortic valve area using the Gorlin formula:

$$AVA = \frac{CO(cm^3/min) \,/\, SEP \times HR}{44.3\sqrt{G}}$$

where AVA = aortic valve area, CO = cardiac output, G = mean aortic valve gradient, SEP = systolic ejection period (in seconds), and HR = heart rate. A valve area of less than 0.7–0.8 cm² usually indicates critical aortic stenosis, a severity of disease capable of causing symptoms, morbidity, and death. A symptomatic patient with a valve area of less than 0.8 cm² will usually require aortic valve replacement because the presence of symptoms connotes a poor prognosis and the constricted valve area suggests that the aortic stenosis is causing those symptoms. A caveat: Although the Gorlin formula is reasonably accurate in predicting the ori-

fice area in severe disease, it was validated in patients with mitral—not aortic—stenosis. When used to calculate the aortic valve area, the Gorlin formula is flow-dependent; that is, the valve area varies directly with the flow. This dependence can be the result of the increased flow physically increasing the orifice; the increased calculated area and flow can also represent a problem with the formula. In either case, the calculated area depends on the patient's cardiac output at the moment. This is not a factor in severe disease with a large transvalvular gradient for which the formula almost always correctly predicts a critically narrowed valve. In some patients with very low cardiac outputs and low transvalvular gradients, however, the formula calculates a severely narrowed aortic valve area when no severe aortic stenosis is actually present. In such cases, increasing the cardiac output by infusion of dobutamine or nitroprusside allows for recalculation of the valve area at a higher output. If the aortic valve area then exceeds 1.0 cm² or the gradient fails to increase markedly despite an increase in output, the stenosis is probably relatively mild and not the cause of the patient's symptoms or cardiac failure.

Valve resistance, which is simply the gradient divided by flow, is gaining credibility as another measure of stenosis severity. A resistance greater than 250 dynes × s × cm⁻⁵ probably indicates severe stenosis. Valve resistance (VR) is calculated using the following formula:

$$AR = \frac{Gradient \times HR \times SEP \,(in\ seconds) \times 1.33}{CO\ L/min}$$

and is expressed as dynes × s × cm⁻⁵.

The following cases are examples of patients with varying degrees of aortic stenosis (PCW = pulmonary capillary wedge):

Case 1

Symptoms: angina, dyspnea
PCW: 16 mm Hg
CO: 4.5 L/min
HR: 70 bpm
SEP: 0.33 s
G: 72 mm Hg
EF: 55%

$$AVA = \frac{4500/(0.33 \times 70)}{44.37\sqrt{2}} = 0.52\ cm^2$$

$$VR = \frac{70 \times 0.33 \times 72}{4.5} \times 1.33 = 492\ dynes \cdot s \cdot cm^{-5}$$

Both calculations indicated severe aortic stenosis; the gradient was large and the patient symptomatic. Surgery was therefore mandatory because this patient undoubtedly suffered from severe symptomatic aortic stenosis.

Case 2

Symptoms: dyspnea, orthopnea
PCW: 26 mm Hg
CO: 3.3 L/min
HR: 70 bpm
SEP: 0.28 s
G: 30 mm Hg
EF: 30%

$$AVA = \frac{3300/(0.28 \times 70)}{44.3 \sqrt{30}} = 0.70 \text{ cm}^2$$

$$VR = \frac{70 \times 0.28 \times 30}{3.3} \times 1.33 = 237 \text{ dynes} \cdot \text{s} \cdot \text{cm}^{-5}$$

In this case, the calculated aortic valve area indicated moderately severe aortic stenosis that required surgery; the valve resistance was borderline, suggesting the stenosis might be less severe. To evaluate the patient further, nitroprusside was cautiously infused and titrated. The repeat hemodynamics showed the following:

PCW: 16 mm Hg
CO: 4.5 L/min
HR: 80 bpm
SEP: 0.25 s
G: 30 mm Hg
AVA: 0.93 cm^2
VR: 177 dynes $\times$ s $\times$ cm^{-5}

Both indexes now indicated moderate—but not critical—aortic stenosis. That the disease was only moderate is further suggested by the lack of an increase in gradient when the cardiac output increased. It was also indicated by improvement in the hemodynamics with infusion of a vasodilator (which, in true aortic stenosis, could be expected to cause deterioration rather than improvement). In this case, an independent cardiomyopathy was probably responsible for the reduced ejection performance. The moderate aortic stenosis played a detrimental role but was not responsible for the patient's condition. He subsequently improved with long-term administration of an angiotensin-converting enzyme (ACE) inhibitor, a result that would not have been anticipated in severe outflow tract obstruction.

Popovic AD, Stewart WJ: Echocardiographic evaluation of valvular stenosis: The gold standard for the next millennium? Echocardiography 2001;18:59.

Rifkin RD: Physiological basis of flow dependence of Gorlin formula valve area in aortic stenosis: Analysis using an hydraulic model of pulsatile flow. J Heart Valve Dis 2000;9:740.

Treatment

The only effective therapy for severe aortic stenosis is relief of the mechanical obstruction posed by the stenotic valve. Figure 8–5 shows the natural course of aortic stenosis: Survivorship is excellent until the classic symptoms of angina, syncope, or congestive heart failure develop. At that point, survival declines sharply. Treatment includes such modalities as aortic balloon valvotomy, valve débridement, and valve replacement.

A. PHARMACOLOGIC THERAPY

There is no effective pharmacologic treatment for severe aortic stenosis, and in some instances medication may be harmful. Although digitalis and diuretics may temporarily help to improve congestive heart failure, unless the aortic valve is replaced, the heart failure will worsen and lead to death. It should also be noted that although ACE inhibitors prolong life in most cases of congestive heart failure, they are contraindicated in severe aortic stenosis. Vasodilators decrease total peripheral resistance, usually increasing cardiac output and providing a beneficial effect in other cardiac diseases. In severe aortic stenosis, however, because cardiac output across the stenotic valve cannot increase, the fall in total peripheral resistance leads to hypotension—which can be fatal. In milder disease (such as Case 2 [described earlier]) that is associated with other causes of heart failure, vasodilators can be used to treat the underlying independent cardiomyopathy. Nitrates can be used cautiously in severe disease to treat angina until surgery is performed. Beta-adrenergic blocking agents must be used with great caution or avoided entirely: They may unmask the left ventricle's dependence on adrenergic support for pressure generation and thereby cause shock or heart failure.

Although pharmacologic therapy for aortic stenosis itself may be ineffective, prophylaxis against endocarditis is mandatory. A significant pathophysiologic substrate for infective endocarditis is hemodynamic turbulence, which is indicated by the presence of a murmur. Therefore, any patient with both aortic valve disease and a murmur should receive prophylactic antibiotics prior to any bacteremia-inducing procedure, regardless of the disease's severity.

B. AORTIC BALLOON VALVULOPLASTY

This procedure involves a percutaneous catheterization in which a large-bore balloon is placed retrograde across

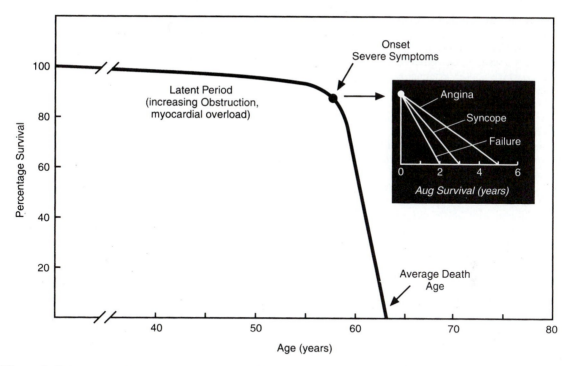

Figure 8–5. The natural history of aortic stenosis. There is little change in survival until the symptoms of angina, syncope, or heart failure develop. Then the decline is precipitous. Adapted, with permission, from Ross J Jr, Braunwald E: Circulation 1968;38(Suppl V):V-61.

the stenotic aortic valve. Inflating the balloon fractures calcium deposits in the leaflets and stretches the aortic annulus, increasing the valve area. Although the procedure is of some benefit in cases of congenital aortic stenosis, in which the leaflets are not calcified, the results in adults have been disappointing. The procedure produces no regression in left ventricular hypertrophy, the gradient is reduced acutely by only about 50%, and the valve area remains in the critical stenosis range. Six months after the procedure, 50% of the patients have completely lost even that modest benefit. The periprocedural mortality rate is 2–5%, and the ultimate mortality rate is the same as that of the natural course of the disease without intervention.

It is important that patients understand that balloon valvuloplasty is not an alternative to aortic valve replacement. Because the procedure produces only transient mild hemodynamic benefits at high risk and does not reduce the high mortality rate of untreated aortic stenosis, it should be considered only a palliative measure for patients whose other severe systemic illnesses preclude surgery. Occasionally it may provide a bridge to surgery for severely symptomatic patients who need time to recover from another illness prior to aortic valve surgery.

C. SURGICAL THERAPY

1. Aortic valve replacement—

a. **Indications for aortic valve replacement**—As noted earlier, survival in aortic stenosis drops sharply when the classic symptoms of angina, syncope, or congestive heart failure appear. Fifty percent of the patients with aortic stenosis who develop angina pectoris are dead within 5 years of its onset if aortic valve replacement is not undertaken. Half the patients developing syncope will be dead within 3 years, and 50% of the patients developing congestive heart failure will be dead within 2 years without surgical correction. The exact pathophysiologic changes that produce the onset of symptoms and begin this rapid downhill course are unknown. It is known that in some cases the stenosis can worsen relatively rapidly, going from mild to severe in a year or two. Worsening stenosis increases the pressure overload on the left ventricle, which presumably reaches a point of decompensation manifested as the onset of symptoms.

Recent studies confirm the benignity of the asymptomatic state in aortic stenosis. In asymptomatic patients with proven peak Doppler gradients equal to or greater than 50 mm Hg, the incidence of sudden death is less than 1% per year. Therefore, surgery is generally not indicated for asymptomatic patients with aortic stenosis. The surgical mortality is at least 2–3%, and even this low figure cannot be justified in the absence of symptoms. However, outcomes in asymptomatic patients vary widely. Some evidence suggests that those with severe valve calcification or rapidly increasing valvular velocity on repeated Doppler studies have a poor prognosis and perhaps should be considered for surgery despite a lack of symptoms.

It must be made clear, however, that benignity of the asymptomatic condition pertains only to adult-acquired aortic stenosis. Children in whom the disease has been present from birth respond differently, and sudden death in the absence of symptoms is common. Asymptomatic children with aortic stenosis should probably undergo surgery once a peak gradient of 75 mm Hg develops, and sooner if symptoms are present.

The mortality rate in adults rapidly increases to about 5% within 3 months of the onset of symptoms and is a remarkable 75% in 3 years if surgical correction is not undertaken. Adults with aortic stenosis should be operated on shortly after the development of symptoms. A reasonable strategy for patients with asymptomatic aortic stenosis is to obtain an initial Doppler echocardiographic study. If the mean gradient is more than 30 mm Hg, the patient should undergo a history and physical examination every 6 months— with instructions to alert the physician immediately if symptoms occur. When close questioning reveals that symptoms have developed, the Doppler echocardiographic study can be repeated to confirm that the aortic stenosis has worsened. If the patient is in the coronary-disease-prone age range, cardiac catheterization to confirm the hemodynamics and to define coronary anatomy should be performed at that time, with an eye toward aortic valve replacement in the near future.

b. Aortic valve replacement in advanced disease— Because aortic valve replacement instantaneously reduces afterload by removing or substantially reducing the pressure gradient, left ventricular performance improves immediately. Thus, patients with far-advanced disease and severe congestive heart failure may respond to aortic valve replacement with a dramatically rapid improvement following surgery. Even patients with ejection fractions of less than 20% may experience a doubling in both ejection fraction and forward output, with a reduction in filling pressures and pulmonary edema early after aortic valve replacement. Over time, left ventricular hypertrophy regresses, contractile function may improve, and ejection fraction may return completely to normal—even though it was profoundly depressed before surgery (Figure 8–6). Therefore, even when the disease is far advanced and is attended by severe congestive heart failure, it is almost never too late to perform aortic valve replacement for patients with aortic stenosis.

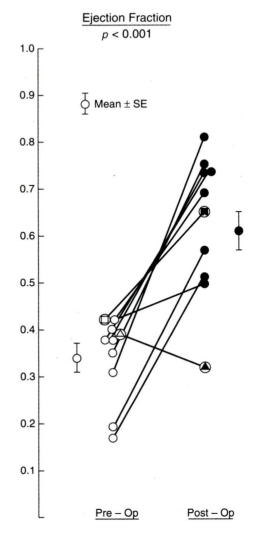

Figure 8–6. The effect of aortic valve replacement on preoperatively depressed ejection fraction. With the exception of one patient who suffered an intraoperative myocardial infarction, all patients demonstrated improved ejection fraction as afterload was reduced following surgery. Adapted, with permission, from Smith N, McAnulty JH, Rahimtoola SJ: Severe aortic stenosis with impaired left ventricular function and clinical heart failure: Results of valve replacement. Circulation 1978;58:255.

c. Contraindications to surgery—There are exceptions to this rule, however. The amount of afterload reduction that can be effected by removing the aortic valve obstruction is proportional to the gradient. In patients with a low mean transvalvular gradient, the increase in ejection fraction and cardiac output that occurs after surgery is limited because afterload reduction is limited. In fact, most patients with a low transvalvular gradient (< 30 mm Hg) and far-advanced heart failure do not improve following aortic valve replacement. It is also clear, however, that some patients do improve—even dramatically—despite a low gradient. Why some patients improve and most do not is currently unknown. Unfortunately, at this time, the outcome for the patient with a low gradient and far-advanced heart failure cannot be predicted. What is known is that such patients are at very high risk when undergoing aortic valve replacement, and such patients need to be advised of the precarious nature of the surgery if it is undertaken.

d. Effects of age—Age should not be considered a major factor when deciding if surgery should be undertaken. Although advanced age increases the risks of surgical mortality and postsurgical morbidity, it must be recognized that age is a risk factor in even apparently healthy patients without aortic stenosis. Once age is corrected for, the mortality rate following aortic valve replacement surgery for aortic stenosis approaches that of the normal population for that age range. In fact, aortic valve replacement for aortic stenosis in patients older than age 65 is one of the few conditions where cardiac surgery returns the patient to the expected longevity of the general population of that age range.

At the other end of the scale, in children with non-calcific congenital aortic stenosis, surgical commissurotomy relieves the stenosis without the need for valve replacement. This procedure, however, is ineffective in adults with calcific degenerative aortic stenosis.

e. Benefits—Replacement of the aortic valve removes or greatly reduces the pressure overload placed on the left ventricle by aortic stenosis. Left ventricular systolic pressure and afterload are significantly reduced, leading to improved ejection performance and cardiac output and reduced left ventricular filling pressure. Subsequently, the left ventricular hypertrophy regresses, most of it in the first year following surgery; full regression, however, may not occur for as long as a decade. The abnormal coronary blood flow and blood flow reserve caused by aortic stenosis also improve as the hypertrophy regresses. Although diastolic function improves as the wall thins, it may not completely return to normal because the increased collagen content (see Figure 8–1) that developed in response to the pressure overload does not regress fully. A persistently increased collagen content causes the left ventricular stiffness to be greater than normal.

f. Aortic valve replacement techniques—Aortic valve replacement can be accomplished using the pa-

tient's own pulmonic valve, a bioprosthesis, or a mechanical prosthesis. Each has its own inherent risks and benefits.

Aikawa K, Otto CM: Timing of surgery in aortic stenosis. Prog Cardiovasc Dis 2001;43:477.

Connolly HM, Oh JK, Schaff, HV et al: Severe aortic stenosis with low transvalvular gradient and severe left ventricular dysfunction: Result of aortic valve replacement in 52 patients. Circulation 2000;101:1940.

Pierri H, Nussbacher A, Decourt LV et al: Clinical predictors of prognosis in severe aortic stenosis in unoperated patients > or = 75 years of age. Am J Cardiol 2000;86:801.

Rosenhek R, Binder T, Porenta G et al: Predictors of outcome in severe, asymptomatic aortic stenosis. N Engl J Med 2000; 343:611.

Sundt TM, Bailey MS, Moon MR et al: Quality of life after aortic valve replacement at the age of > 80 years. Circulation 2000; 102:III70.

(1) Pulmonic valve transplantation (Ross procedure)—In this procedure, the patient's native pulmonic valve (autograft) is removed and sewn into the aortic position. A prosthetic valve or a pulmonic homograft is then sewn into the pulmonic position. This maneuver improves the patient's condition because the native, viable pulmonic valve with its excellent hemodynamic characteristics and durability is sewn into the high-pressure, high-stress, left-sided circuit where prostheses can fail. The bioprosthesis or homograft placed in the pulmonic position is under low pressure and low stress; it is more durable here than it would be in the aortic position.

The major disadvantage of the pulmonic autograph is the amount of surgery involved. It is a technically very demanding procedure, and, although excellent results have been reported from a few centers, it may not be applicable to every hospital's surgical program.

Oswalt JD, Dewan SJ, Mueller MC et al: Highlights of a ten-year experience with the Ross procedure. Ann Thorac Surg 2001; 71:S332.

Pessotto R, Wells WJ, Baker CJ et al: Midterm results of the Ross procedure. Ann Thorac Surg 2001;71:S336.

(2) Bioprostheses—Two general types of bioprostheses are available: heterografts and homografts. Heterografts are constructed from either porcine aortic valve leaflets or bovine pericardium (both preserved with glutaraldehyde). Heterografts have had a wide application, and much is known about their advantages and disadvantages. The major advantage of this bioprosthesis is its low thromboembolic potential. In the absence of atrial fibrillation, the risk of thromboembolism following aortic valve bioprosthetic implantation is less than 1 event per 100 patient years, and anticoagulation is not required. Atrial fibrillation substantially increases thromboembolic risk, as it does in patients with native valves. In the absence of a contraindication, anticoagulation is therefore probably ad-

visable in patients with atrial fibrillation. Anticoagulation is unnecessary in patients with normal sinus rhythm.

The major disadvantage of heterografts is their limited durability. Primary valve failure occurs in only 10% of patients 10 years following implantation of a bioprosthesis in the aortic position, but valve failure rapidly accelerates after that period; approximately 50% of valves have failed within 15 years. Calcification and degeneration of the valves leads to tears in the cusps or stenosis of the valve or flail leaflets. Degeneration is greatly accelerated in younger patients, and heterograft bioprostheses should not be used in patients younger than 35 years of age—except for young women who wish to become pregnant. Because anticoagulation with warfarin produces an unacceptable rate of fetal mortality, valve replacement with a bioprosthesis that does not require anticoagulation may be preferable. The patient must understand, however, that a second valve replacement will probably be required.

A second disadvantage to bioprosthesis is a modest obstruction to outflow and a residual pressure gradient in patients requiring implantation of small valves.

The ideal patient for heterograft bioprosthesis implantation is the elderly patient whose life expectancy is less than the durability span of the valve or the patient for whom anticoagulation poses a significant risk.

Cryopreserved homografts, which are harvested from human donors, have an excellent hemodynamic profile. They are ideal for use in patients with a small aortic root where other types of prostheses might cause a transvalvular gradient. They are also relatively resistant to bacterial endocarditis. Although homografts may be more durable than heterograft valves, long-term follow-up data on large numbers of cryopreserved homografts is currently unavailable. In addition, the use of homograft valves is limited by availability. Because many potential donors for homograft valves are also whole-heart donors, the number of available homografts is small.

(3) Mechanical valves—Compared with bioprostheses, mechanical valves, such as the bileaflet valve, have superior durability. All mechanical valves require anticoagulation, however. Thromboembolic complications possible in the absence of anticoagulation include stroke and fixation of the valve in either the open or closed position. With proper anticoagulation, these events are reduced to 1 event per 100 patient years; the risk of anticoagulant hemorrhage is approximately 0.5%/year. Anticoagulation therapy should be targeted to maintain the prothrombin time at 1.5 times control (international normalized ratio [INR] 2.5—3.5). Mechanical valves are typically implanted in younger patients for whom long-term durability is important and in whom anticoagulation can be accomplished at lower risk than in elderly patients. Although caged-ball and

tilting-disk valves were popular in the twentieth century, the bileaflet valves are most commonly employed today.

2. Aortic valve débridement—Both mechanical and ultrasonic débridement of the aortic valve to remove calcium deposits and increase leaflet mobility have met with limited success in calcific aortic stenosis. Surgical débridement usually results in significant residual stenosis that worsens in time. Ultrasonic débridement, using sound waves to pulverize the calcium deposits, dramatically reduces the aortic valve gradient and produces excellent results 6 months after surgery. Unfortunately, many patients develop aortic insufficiency shortly thereafter as the integrity of the leaflets is impaired. Most current data suggest either mechanical or ultrasonic débridement is a poor alternative to aortic valve replacement.

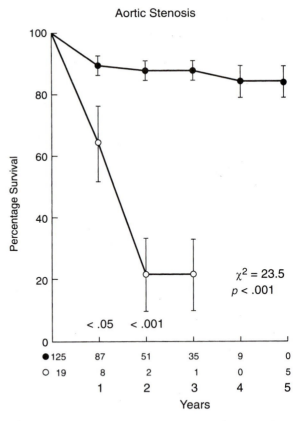

Figure 8–7. The effect of aortic valve replacement in patients with symptomatic severe aortic stenosis (solid circle) compared with the survivorship of similar patients who refused surgery (open circle). Adapted, with permission, from Schwarz F, Baumann P, Manthey J et al: The effect of aortic valve replacement on survival. Circulation 1982;66:1105.

Recently, the development of new techniques for engaging the patient with the heart-lung pump and stabilizing the heart during surgery have allowed for heart operations through limited thoracic incisions. Although results similar to conventional sternotomy have been reported for aortic valve surgery in some centers, total surgical time, pump time, and aorta cross-clamp time are significantly increased. On the other hand, patients appreciate the smaller incisions. Whether these minimally invasive approaches will replace conventional techniques is not clear at this time.

Prognosis

As noted earlier, the natural course and thus the prognosis of unoperated aortic stenosis are widely known. Once symptoms develop, aortic stenosis becomes a lethal disease with a 3-year mortality rate of 75%. Figure 8–7 compares the mortality rate of two groups of patients with symptomatic aortic stenosis: those who refused surgery, and patients who underwent it. The difference is dramatic. Overall, the 10-year survival rate following aortic valve replacement for pure aortic stenosis is 75%. The age-adjusted survivorship after surgery remains excellent even in octogenarians free of other cardiac or systemic diseases.

Asymptomatic patients generally have a good prognosis, but certain factors, such as reduced left ventricular ejection fraction, an enlarged left ventricle, and severe valve calcification, are known to reduce their survival. Also, patients with hypercholesterolemia, hy-

percalcemia, or elevated serum creatinine tend to progress more rapidly and should be followed closely. Whether progressive stenosis can be delayed or halted by altering cholesterol levels or other biologic factors is unknown.

Palta S, Pai AM, Gill KS et al: New insights into the progression of aortic stenosis: Implications for secondary prevention. Circulation 2000;101:2497.

Rossi A, Tomaino M, Golia G et al: Echocardiographic prediction of clinical outcome in medically treated patients with aortic stenosis. Am Heart J 2000;140:766.

A. COINCIDENT DISEASE

Coronary artery disease is the single most important coincident disease that affects the prognosis of aortic stenosis. Figure 8–8 shows that the prognosis for patients with aortic stenosis and coronary disease worsens almost immediately following surgery, compared with the prognosis of corrected isolated aortic stenosis. Coronary bypass surgery may improve this prognosis, but this point is controversial. What is not controversial is that even with complete revascularization the prognosis of combined aortic stenosis and coronary disease does not equal that of isolated aortic stenosis. Some experts have advocated correcting only the aortic stenosis in patients with combined disease because the addition of coronary bypass grafting has not been clearly shown to prolong survival. These results, however, were acquired before the more recent extensive use of internal mammary artery grafts, which are superior to vein grafts. Modern results may be better. Therefore,

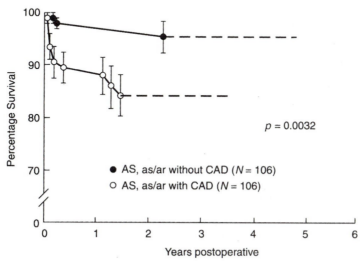

Figure 8–8. The effects of coronary disease (open circle) on survivorship of patients with aortic stenosis (AS) or aortic stenosis and regurgitation (as/ar) following surgery shown and compared with that of isolated AS or as/ar (solid circle). CAD = coronary artery disease. Adapted, with permission, from Miller DC, Stinson EB, Oyer PE et al: Surgical implications and results of combined aortic valve replacement and myocardial revascularization. Am J Cardiol 1979;43:494.

because there is no definitive answer regarding the efficacy of combined coronary bypass grafting and aortic valve replacement, grafting seems prudent when angina is one of the patient's symptoms or when left-main or three-vessel disease is present.

B. FOLLOW-UP

Implantation of a prosthetic heart valve is not curative. The severe risks of native valve aortic stenosis have instead been exchanged for the lesser risks inherent to prosthetic valves. Lifelong regular follow-up of patients with prostheses is therefore required. If anticoagulation therapy is used, periodic surveillance of the prothrombin time is needed, and alterations in dosage must be made to maintain it at 1.5 times control. The prothrombin time should be tested at least once a month and more frequently if a stable dose of warfarin and the degree of anticoagulation have not yet been obtained. Many avoidable complications of prostheses result from improper anticoagulation.

Endocarditis prophylaxis is even more important in the presence of a prosthetic valve than in the presence of an abnormal native valve. Infection of a prosthesis is often fatal, and even when the infection is cured, the valve almost always requires re-replacement. Prevention of prosthetic valve endocarditis by antibiotic administration before and after dental and other surgery is therefore imperative.

Implantation of a prosthesis makes the Doppler echocardiographic evaluation of valve function difficult. Although acoustic shadowing around the prosthesis hinders echocardiographic and Doppler interpretation, each valve has a characteristic Doppler profile that should be recorded early following surgery. If subsequent symptoms of congestive heart failure or syncope develop, another ultrasound study can be made for comparison. A significant deviation from the initial study may indicate that prosthetic stenosis or regurgitation is now present and responsible for the recurrence of the patient's symptoms. Transesophageal echocardiography usually is better able to visualize morphologic details of a prosthetic valve than transthoracic echocardiography and is indicated for suspected valve failure, thrombosis, or endocarditis. Cinefluoroscopy is also useful for assessing valve motion and diagnosing leaflet or ball-motion abnormalities. The suspicion of valve dysfunction is usually confirmed by cardiac catheterization. It should be noted, however, that when prosthetic stenosis is suspected, the gradient across the valve may be difficult to obtain invasively. Retrograde passage of the catheter across a tilting disk valve may result in catheter entrapment, a potentially fatal complication. Retrograde passage of a catheter across a bileaflet valve may damage the leaflets; this practice should be avoided. Transseptal catheterization is often the safest way to obtain a transvalvular gradient if prosthetic aortic valve stenosis is suspected.

AHA/ACC guidelines for the management of patients with valvular heart disease. A Report of the American Caollege of Cardiology/American Heart Association Task Force on Practice Guidelines (Committee on Management of Patients with Valvular Heart Disease). J Am Coll Cardiol 1998;32:1486.

Aortic Regurgitation

9

William A. Zoghbi, MD & Imran Afridi, MD

ESSENTIALS OF DIAGNOSIS

- *Following a long asymptomatic period, presentation with heart failure or angina*
- *Wide pulse pressure with associated peripheral signs*
- *Diastolic decrescendo murmur at the left sternal border*
- *Left ventricular dilation and hypertrophy with preserved function*
- *Presentation and findings dependent on the rapidity of onset of regurgitation*
- *Diagnosis confirmed and severity estimated by Doppler echocardiography or aortography*

Etiology

Normally, the integrity of the aortic orifice during diastole is maintained by an intact aortic root and firm apposition of the free margins of the three aortic valve cusps. Aortic regurgitation (AR) may therefore be caused by a variety of disorders affecting the valve cusps or the aortic root (or both) (Table 9–1). With rheumatic heart disease becoming less common, nonrheumatic causes currently account for the majority of the underlying causes of aortic insufficiency, including congenitally malformed aortic valves, infective endocarditis, and connective tissue diseases. Disorders affecting the aortic root also account for a large number of patients with AR. These conditions include cystic medial necrosis, Marfan's syndrome, aortic dissection, and inflammatory diseases. Even in the absence of any obvious pathology of the aortic valve or root, severe systemic hypertension has been reported to cause significant AR.

Pathophysiology

The presentation and findings in patients with AR depend on its severity and rapidity of onset. The hemodynamic effects of acute severe AR are entirely different from the chronic type and the two will be discussed separately.

A. CHRONIC AORTIC REGURGITATION

In response to the left ventricular volume overload associated with AR, progressive left ventricular dilation occurs. This results in a higher wall stress, which stimulates ventricular hypertrophy and which, in turn, tends to normalize wall stress. Patients with severe AR may have the largest end-diastolic volumes produced by any other heart disease and yet, their end-diastolic pressures are not uniformly elevated. In keeping with the Frank-Starling mechanism, the stroke volume is also increased. Thus despite the presence of regurgitation, a normal effective forward cardiac output can be maintained. This state persists for several years. Gradually, left ventricular diastolic properties and contractile function start to decline. The adaptive dilation and hypertrophy can no longer match the loading conditions.

Table 9–1. Causes of aortic regurgitation.

Aortic Cusp Abnormalities
Infectious: Bacterial endocarditis, rheumatic fever
Congenital: Bicuspid aortic valve, Marfan's syndrome
Inflammatory: Systemic lupus erythematosus, rheumatoid arthritis, Behçet's syndrome
Degenerative: Myxomatous (floppy) valve, calcific aortic valve
Trauma
Postaortic valvuloplasty
Diet drug valvulopathy
Aortic Root Abnormalities
Aortic root dilatation: Marfan's syndrome, syphilis, ankylosing spondylitis, relapsing polychondritis, idiopathic aortitis, annuloaortic ectasia, cystic medial necrosis, Ehlers-Danlos syndrome.
Loss of commissural support: Aortic dissection, trauma, ventricular septal defect
Increased Afterload
Systemic hypertension
Supravalvular aortic stenosis

121

The left ventricular end-diastolic pressure begins to rise and the ejection fraction drops with a decline in effective forward output and development of heart failure.

B. ACUTE AORTIC REGURGITATION

In contrast to chronic AR, when sudden severe regurgitation occurs, the left ventricle has no time to adapt. The acute ventricular volume overload therefore results in a small increase in end-diastolic volume and severe elevation of end-diastolic pressure, which is transmitted to the left atrium and pulmonary veins, culminating in acute pulmonary edema. Because the ventricular end-diastolic volume is normal, the total stroke volume is not increased and the effective forward cardiac output drops. To compensate for the low output state, sympathetic stimulation occurs, which produces tachycardia and peripheral vasoconstriction, the latter further worsening aortic regurgitation.

Clinical Findings

A. SYMPTOMS AND SIGNS

1. Chronic aortic regurgitation—Patients with chronic AR remain asymptomatic for a long time. Palpitations are common and may be due to either awareness of forceful left ventricular contractions or occurrence of premature atrial or ventricular beats. Angina may occur either from concomitant coronary disease or from a combination of low diastolic pressure and increased oxygen demand from ventricular hypertrophy. When left ventricular dysfunction supervenes, patients initially experience exertional dyspnea and fatigue. At a later stage, resting heart failure symptoms occur with orthopnea and paroxysmal nocturnal dyspnea.

On physical examination, visible cardiac pulsations are common. The area of the apical impulse is increased on palpation and is displaced caudally and laterally. The first heart sound is usually normal. The A_2 component of the second heart sound may be decreased in conditions where cusp excursion is reduced, such as with valve calcification. An S_4 is often present due to underlying hypertrophy, and an S_3 is audible when ventricular failure occurs. The characteristic auscultation of AR is a soft, high-pitched diastolic decrescendo murmur best heard in the third intercostal space along the left sternal border at end expiration, with the patient sitting and leaning forward. In the presence of aortic root disease, the murmur may be best heard to the right of the sternum. A systolic ejection murmur may be present at the aortic area due to the high flow state. Occasionally, a diastolic rumble may be heard at the apex, referred to as the Austin Flint murmur. The mechanism underlying this murmur remains unclear. A number of different causes have been proposed, the most recent being the aortic jet abutting on the left ventricular endocardium.

The systolic arterial pressure is increased due to a large stroke volume, whereas the diastolic pressure is decreased due to runoff from the aorta into both the ventricle and peripheral arteries. This is the underlying reason for a wide pulse pressure and for a variety of associated peripheral signs in chronic significant aortic regurgitation (Table 9–2). However, it must be remembered that these signs are not specific for AR and may occur in any high flow state such as occurs in anemia, thyrotoxicosis, and arteriovenous malformations. With the development of heart failure, the pulse pressure narrows and the peripheral signs of AR are attenuated.

2. Acute aortic regurgitation—In contrast to chronic AR, the majority of patients with acute severe AR are symptomatic. Initial presentation may vary depending on the underlying cause, which most commonly is aortic dissection, infective endocarditis, or trauma. In the presence of associated acute AR, patients often develop clinical manifestations of severe dyspnea, orthopnea, and weakness. The onset of symptoms is sudden, with rapid progression to hemodynamic collapse if left untreated.

In acute AR, the left ventricle has had no time to adapt to the volume overload state. The peripheral signs associated with chronic AR are therefore absent. Pulse pressure is usually normal, and hypotension may be present in severe cases. Bilateral rales are usually present on examination of the lungs and reflect underlying pulmonary edema. On precordial palpation, the apical impulse is not shifted. The first heart sound may be soft or absent due to the premature closure of the mitral valve. An S_3 is often present, but an S_4 is usually absent because there is little or no atrial contribution to

Table 9–2. Peripheral signs of aortic regurgitation.

Name of Sign	Description
Corrigan's pulse:	Rapid and forceful distension of arterial pulse with quick collapse
De-Musset's sign:	To and fro head bobbing
Muller's sign:	Visible pulsation of uvula
Quincke's sign:	Capillary pulsations seen on light compression of nail bed
Traube's sign:	Systolic and diastolic sounds (pistol shots) over the femoral artery
Durozier's sign:	Bruits heard over femoral artery on light compression by stethoscope
Hill's sign:	Popliteal cuff pressure exceeding brachial pressure by 60 mm Hg or greater

ventricular filling due to high left ventricular end-diastolic pressure. The typical diastolic murmur of AR is shortened in duration, often difficult to hear, and easily missed.

B. DIAGNOSTIC STUDIES

1. Electrocardiogram—No specific electrocardiographic abnormalities are characteristic of aortic regurgitation. Signs of left atrial enlargement, left ventricular hypertrophy, and a "strain pattern" (ST depression with T-wave inversion in lateral leads) are often seen in chronic significant AR. Arrhythmias, including ventricular ectopy and ventricular tachycardia, may occur in advanced cases with left ventricular dysfunction. In acute AR, sinus tachycardia may be the only abnormality. In cases of infective endocarditis, inflammation or abscess formation may spread to the atrioventricular node, resulting in prolongation of the PR interval or development of atrioventricular block.

2. Chest radiograph—Chest radiographic findings are not specific for AR and reflect an estimate of cardiac size and pulmonary vascular changes. In chronic significant AR, an increase in the size of the cardiac silhouette is seen. In acute AR, the cardiac size is normal; the lung fields show increased markings due to pulmonary edema. When AR is due to aortic dissection, the chest film may show an enlarged ascending aorta. If calcification of the aortic knob is present, a helpful sign of dissection is increased separation between the outer margin of the aorta and the calcific density.

3. Echocardiography and Doppler techniques—With recent technologic advances, particularly the introduction of color flow Doppler, echocardiography has become the method of choice for evaluating patients with AR. Two-dimensional echocardiography in combination with various Doppler modalities and, in selected cases, transesophageal imaging has provided a non-invasive means for not only diagnosing AR with a high sensitivity and specificity but also for assessing its etiology and severity. Furthermore, important information can be obtained on the hemodynamic impact of the regurgitant lesion, prognosis and effectiveness of therapy.

a. **Detection of aortic regurgitation**—Currently, the best noninvasive method for the detection of aortic regurgitation is Doppler echocardiography. Doppler techniques are extremely sensitive and specific in the detection of AR, manifested as a diastolic flow abnormality arising from the aortic valve, directed toward the left ventricle. Even trivial regurgitation can be detected, which commonly is not audible on physical examination. Although most cases of moderate-to-severe chronic AR have typical findings on physical examination, occasional patients with moderate lesions may be missed on examination because of the subtlety of auscultatory findings. Doppler echocardiography is also extremely valuable in patients with acute aortic regurgitation when the typical clinical findings of chronic aortic insufficiency are absent and the murmur can often be missed. Among the available Doppler techniques (including color Doppler, pulsed and continuous-wave Doppler), color Doppler echocardiography has proven to be extremely helpful in the evaluation of aortic regurgitation (Figure 9–1). Its major advantage over conventional Doppler is that it provides a spatial orientation of the regurgitant jet arising from the aortic root. A completely negative color Doppler examination in multiple planes virtually excludes the presence of aortic regurgitation. Although pulsed and continuous wave Doppler are almost equally sensitive in the detection of aortic insufficiency, eccentric aortic insufficiency jets can be missed with these techniques and are better delineated with color-flow imaging.

Echocardiographic imaging with M-mode and two-dimensional (2D) examinations cannot detect the presence of aortic insufficiency but can provide indirect clues to the presence of aortic insufficiency. These include diastolic fluttering of the anterior mitral leaflet or septum depending on the impingement of the regurgitant flow on these structures. These signs, although specific, are not sensitive for the detection of aortic insufficiency and do not relate to the severity of regurgitation.

b. **Assessment of cause**—Because 2D echocardiography can image cardiac structures, it provides valuable information on the cause of the aortic regurgitation. Structural abnormalities of the aortic valve, including calcifications or thickening, congenital deformities, vegetations, rupture, or prolapse, can be identified. Dilatation of the aortic root, calcifications, or dissection can also be evaluated. Although the majority of these pathologies can be assessed with transthoracic echocardiography, recently transesophageal echocardiography has provided high resolution images that allow for improved detection of such abnormalities, especially in technically difficult cases or in conditions such as infective endocarditis. Transesophageal echocardiography is also routinely performed when aortic pathology such as aneurysm or dissection is suspected (Figure 9–2). In patients with aortic regurgitation due to aortic pathology, precisely defining the morphology of the valve and involvement of aortic root is important in determining the surgical approach and deciding whether the valve can be preserved or requires replacement.

c. **Assessment of severity**—In addition to the detection of aortic regurgitation, Doppler echocardiography combined with 2D echocardiographic imaging has recently allowed an assessment of the severity of the lesion. Several methods have been proposed, including color Doppler assessment of regurgitant jet size, contin-

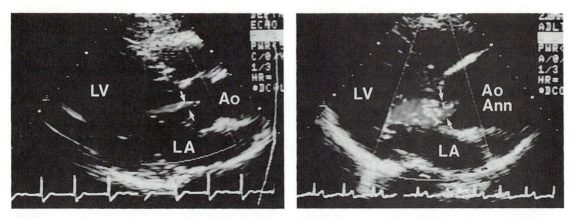

Figure 9–1. Color Doppler echocardiographic frames in diastole from the parasternal long axis view in (**A**) a patient with mild aortic regurgitation and another with (**B**) severe regurgitation. The patient with severe aortic regurgitation (**B**) has a large ascending aortic aneurysm (Ao Ann). The width of the aortic regurgitation jet in the left ventricular outflow (between arrows) provides a good estimate of the severity of aortic regurgitation by color Doppler echocardiography. Ao = aorta; AoAnn = aortic aneurysm; LA = left atrium; LV = left ventricle.

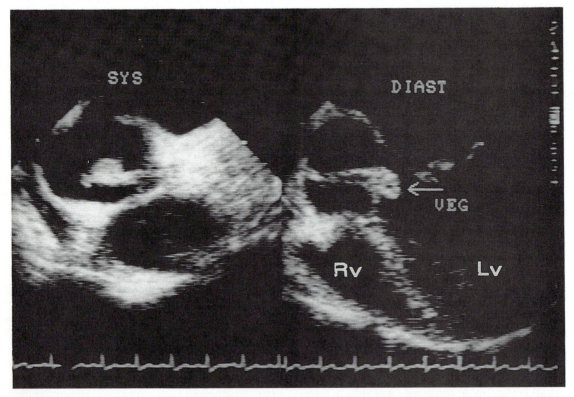

Figure 9–2. Transesophageal echocardiographic frames in systole (SYS) and diastole (DIAST), showing a vegetation attached to the aortic valve that prolapses into the left ventricular outflow tract during diastole. In this patient, transthoracic echocardiographic imaging was difficult and failed to demonstrate the large vegetation.

uous-wave Doppler using the pressure half-time method, and measurements of regurgitant fraction derived from 2D echocardiography and pulsed Doppler techniques.

With color-flow Doppler, the aortic regurgitation jet can be spatially oriented in the 2D plane arising from the aortic valve and directed toward the left ventricle. The ratio of the AR jet diameter just below the leaflets to that of the left ventricular outflow diameter has been shown to correlate well with the severity of regurgitation when compared with the angiographic standard (Table 9–3, see Figure 9–1). Similarly, a good estimation of AR severity has been found by relating the cross-sectional area of the jet at its origin to the left ventricular outflow area. Recently, measurement of the width of the AR jet at the level of the leaflets (vena contracta) has been used to quantitatively approximate AR severity. A vena contracta of > 0.6 cm is considered a sign of severe AR. On the other hand, it is important to note that the length of the AR jet does not correlate well with AR severity. This is in part because color Doppler flow mapping is also highly dependent on the velocity of regurgitation, or the driving pressure, in addition to the regurgitant volume.

Another index of AR severity that has been useful clinically is the pressure half-time derived from continuous-wave Doppler recordings of the AR jet velocity. The velocity of the regurgitant jet is related to the instantaneous pressure difference between the aorta and left ventricle in diastole by the modified Bernoulli equation: $\Delta P = 4V^2$, where ΔP is the pressure gradient in millimeters of mercury and V is the blood velocity in meters per second. The pressure half-time index is the time it takes for the initial maximal pressure gradient in diastole to fall by 50%. In patients with mild regurgitation, there is a gradual small drop in the pressure difference in diastole, whereas with severe AR, a more precipitous drop occurs (Figure 9–3). A pressure half-time greater than 500 ms is seen in mild AR, but more sig-

nificant regurgitation is usually associated with a shorter pressure half-time (see Table 9–3, Figure 9–3). The severity of aortic regurgitation using this index may be overestimated in patients who have elevated left ventricular end-diastolic pressure.

The severity of AR can also be assessed using regurgitant volume and regurgitant fraction derived from 2D and pulsed Doppler echocardiography. This method is based on the continuity equation, which states that, in the absence of regurgitation, blood flow is equal across all valves. Stroke volume at the level of a valve annulus is calculated as the product of cross-sectional area obtained by 2D echocardiography and the time velocity integral of flow recorded by pulsed Doppler. In the presence of aortic regurgitation, stroke volume at the left ventricular outflow tract is higher than that across another valve without regurgitation. Therefore, aortic regurgitant volume can be calculated as the difference between stroke volume at the left ventricular outflow and that derived at another valve site. Dividing the regurgitant volume by stroke volume across the aortic valve gives an estimate of regurgitant fraction. A regurgitant fraction of less than 20% is usually mild, whereas regurgitant fraction > 50% denotes severe aortic regurgitation (see Table 9–3). A similar approach to estimating severity of AR can be achieved using pulsed Doppler echocardiography in the proximal descending aorta. In patients with significant AR, a large reversal of flow is observed in diastole toward the aortic arch and ascending aorta. This simple method should be used routinely to qualitatively grade the severity of regurgitation and can also be used quantitatively to derive a regurgitant fraction.

Although in the majority of patients, color-flow Doppler allows a good estimation of the severity of aortic regurgitation, its accuracy depends on optimization of the color Doppler examination, including gainsettings, frame rate, and interrogation of multiple tomographic planes. The availability of other inde-

Table 9–3. Grading the severity of aortic regurgitation using Doppler techniques combined with echocardiography.

Severity of AR	Color-Flow Doppler JH/LVOH (%)	Continuous-Wave Doppler PHT (ms)	Pulsed Doppler Regurgitant Fraction (%)
Mild	<24	>500	<20
Moderate	25–45	500–349	20–35
Moderately severe	46–64	349–200	36–50
Severe	>65	<200	>50

AR = aortic regurgitation; JH/LVOH = Ratio of aortic regurgitant jet height to left ventricular outflow height in the parasternal long axis view; PHT = pressure half-time.

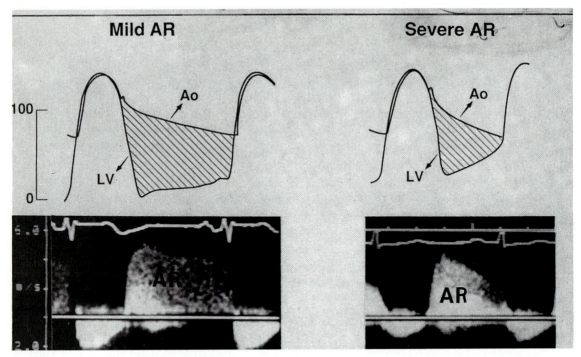

Figure 9–3. Schematic of aortic and left ventricular pressure tracings in (*left*) a patient with mild and (*right*) another with severe aortic regurgitation and corresponding examples of continuous wave Doppler recording of aortic jet velocity in such patients. In mild aortic regurgitation, a gradual small drop in the difference between aortic and ventricular pressures occurs in diastole, reflected by the small decrease in the velocity of the aortic regurgitation jet. In contrast, in severe aortic regurgitation, a more precipitous drop occurs in the pressure gradient and in the corresponding jet velocity. AR = aortic regurgitation; Ao = aorta; LV = left ventricle.

pendent Doppler indices of AR severity further allows the corroboration of color Doppler findings. This is particularly helpful in patients with eccentric AR jets, for which severity may be difficult to assess by color-flow Doppler alone. A detailed transthoracic examination usually provides all the necessary information in the vast majority of patients. When the transthoracic approach is inadequate or inconclusive, transesophageal echocardiography can be performed in this setting for the diagnosis and assessment of severity of the lesion.

Another important caveat in classifying the severity of AR is that it is in part dependent on hemodynamic status, including preload and, more importantly, afterload. Raising blood pressure may significantly increase AR severity.

d. Assessment of hemodynamic effects—The hemodynamic effects of aortic regurgitation are assessed with both echocardiographic imaging and Doppler echocardiography. Two-dimensional echocardiography provides quantitation of ventricular size and function,

in addition to the degree of left ventricular hypertrophy and ventricular mass. End-diastolic and end-systolic left ventricular dimensions and volumes as well as left ventricular ejection fraction provide important measures of the hemodynamic effects of AR and help identify patients at higher risk. In patients with acute aortic regurgitation, premature closure of the mitral valve can be demonstrated by both 2D and M-mode imaging. In these situations, diastolic mitral regurgitation can also be detected by Doppler echocardiography, reflecting the rapid rise of left ventricular pressure in diastole, exceeding that of left atrial pressure. These findings indicate severe AR. In patients with chronic AR, assessment of the ventricular and atrial filling dynamics at the mitral and pulmonary venous inflow respectively, allows for non-invasive estimation of ventricular diastolic pressure, further adding to the overall evaluation of the hemodynamic effect of AR on ventricular function. Newer modalities such as Doppler tissue imaging further enhance the accuracy of noninvasive assessment of ventricular diastolic function. Thus in patients with chronic AR, 2-D echocardiography with Doppler provides serial assessment of left ventricular volumes, hypertrophy, and function and helps assess the progression of the disease and optimum timing of surgical intervention.

4. Cardiac catheterization and angiography—Prior to the introduction of Doppler echocardiography, the evaluation of the severity of aortic insufficiency invariably required invasive testing by cardiac catheterization. With the improvement in the accuracy of noninvasive tests, routine cardiac catheterization is no longer necessary in the majority of patients. At catheterization, the detection of AR is achieved with the injection of radiopaque contrast into the aortic root and the appearance of dye in the left ventricle (Figure 9–4). In addition, aortography allows evaluation of the ascending aorta for dilatation or dissection. Some of the structural abnormalities of the aortic valve may also be identified. The severity of AR is quantitatively approximated using a grading system that takes into account the intensity of contrast dye in the left ventricle and its clearance (Table 9–4). This grading system has been helpful clinically in the assessment of AR severity. However, it is important to emphasize that, similar to other diagnostic techniques, a number of technical factors may also affect interpretation. Positioning the catheter too close to the valve may itself cause regurgitation. The volume and rapidity of contrast injection, ventricular function, and type of catheter used are important factors that may affect the interpretation of AR severity.

At catheterization, the severity of AR can also be assessed by the determination of regurgitant volume and regurgitant fraction. In the absence of regurgitation or shunts, the left ventricular stroke volume derived from contrast ventriculography is equal to right ventricular stroke volume obtained by the Fick method or thermodilution. When isolated AR is present, subtracting left ventricular from right ventricular stroke volume

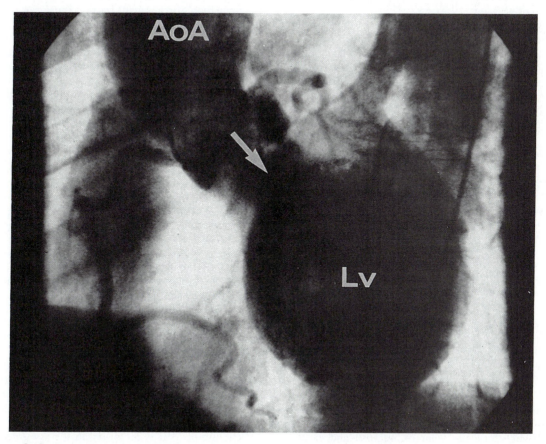

Figure 9–4. Aortic root contrast injection in the left anterior oblique projection in a patient with severe aortic regurgitation, showing significant opacification of the left ventricle. The aortography also shows an ascending aortic aneurysm. AoA = aortic aneurysm; Lv = left ventricle.

Table 9–4. Angiographic grading of the severity of aortic regurgitation.

Grade	Degree of LV Opacification	Intensity of Dye	Clearance of Dye from LV
I (mild)	Incomplete	Ao > LV	Completely cleared on each beat
II (moderate)	Complete but faint	Ao > LV	Incomplete clearance
III (moderately severe)	Complete opacification in several beats	Ao = LV	Slow
IV (severe)	Complete on first beat	Ao < LV	Slow

Ao = Aorta; LV = left ventricle.

gives the regurgitation volume. Regurgitant fraction is derived as the regurgitant volume divided by left ventricular stroke volume. In the presence of concomitant mitral regurgitation, a total regurgitant volume or fraction can only be assessed using this method. Because of inherent variability in the determination of stroke volume, a 10–15% error in these measurements is not infrequent and is similar to those obtained with Doppler echocardiography.

Cardiac catheterization provides an accurate assessment of the hemodynamic effect of aortic regurgitation. Using contrast ventriculography, preferably in biplanar projections, accurate determination of left ventricular volumes and ejection fraction can be performed. Furthermore, direct measurements of pressures in the various cardiac chambers can be recorded. In compensated chronic AR, the only abnormality that may be observed is a widened pulse pressure on the aortic pressure tracing. As decompensation occurs, left ventricular end-diastolic pressure rises. In severe, particularly acute AR, aortic and left ventricular pressures may equalize at end-diastole.

With the improvement in noninvasive testing, routine cardiac catheterization is no longer necessary in the majority of patients for the sole assessment of the lesion. Currently, cardiac catheterization is indicated in the assessment of AR severity when noninvasive testing is equivocal or discordant with the clinical presentation and, more commonly, in the assessment of coronary artery disease prior to aortic valve surgery. Preoperative coronary angiography should be performed prior to elective surgery for AR in men older than 35 years of age, premenopausal women over 35 who have risk factors for coronary artery disease, postmenopausal women, and any patients with clinical suspicion of coronary artery disease.

5. Radionuclide ventriculography—Using either first-pass or gated radionuclide ventriculography, left and right ventricular volumes, outputs, and ejection fractions can be determined noninvasively. The technique cannot be used to detect aortic insufficiency nor to assess its cause because radionuclide ventriculography allows only for the comparison of volumes or function between the two ventricles. Differences in stroke volumes can also be seen in other regurgitant lesions such as occur in mitral regurgitation or in shunts such as are present in patent ductus arteriosus. However, in patients with known aortic insufficiency, regurgitant volumes and regurgitant fractions can be calculated. A limitation of gated radionuclide ventriculography in the estimation of regurgitant fraction is its error in estimating right ventricular stroke volume due to the overlap of the right ventricle and the right atrium. Currently, radionuclide techniques are most commonly used to assess ventricular function at rest or during exercise or in serially evaluating changes in ventricular function in patients with chronic AR. The use of nuclear techniques in evaluating AR is generally reserved for patients with suboptimal echocardiographic imaging.

6. Magnetic resonance imaging—Advances in magnetic resonance imaging (MRI) have recently allowed for evaluation of patients with aortic insufficiency. At present, three basic approaches are available: spin echo imaging, gradient echo imaging (cine-MRI), and phase velocity mapping. Spin echo imaging provides an excellent approach for depicting cardiac morphology and detecting aortic root pathology. However, aortic valve visualization is poor. Using cine-MRI, aortic regurgitation is detected as a decrease in the signal intensity in the left ventricular outflow during diastole. In preliminary studies, the ratio of area of low-intensity signal to the area of the left ventricular outflow has provided an accurate estimate of AR severity. Regurgitant fractions have been determined by comparing right and left ventricular volumes and stroke volumes. Furthermore, using phase velocity mapping, flow in a region of interest can be assessed. Regurgitant fraction with this method can be derived by comparing flows in the ascending aorta and pulmonary artery.

The use of MRI is promising in the assessment of AR. It is particularly helpful in defining the severity and extent of AR. Imaging can be performed in any plane, without attenuation from lung or bone. However, this modality cannot be used in patients carrying metallic objects such as defibrillators or pacemakers. Its current drawbacks are its lack of availability and high cost. It is an alternative to echocardiography and nuclear imaging for centers with expertise in MRI.

7. Other laboratory findings—Laboratory findings depend on the underlying cause of AR. Elevated white cell count and sedimentation rate are seen in inflammatory conditions such as infection and aortitis. Abnormal antinuclear antigen and rheumatoid factor titers may be seen in patients with rheumatologic disorders. Serologic tests of syphilis may be indicated when this cause is suspected.

Nagueh SF, Middleton KJ, Kopelen HA et al: Doppler tissue imaging: A noninvasive technique for evaluation of left ventricular relaxation and estimation of filling pressures. J Am Coll Cardiol 1997;30:1527.

Nagueh SF, Koeplen HA, Zoghbi WA: Feasibility and accuracy of Doppler echocardiographic estimation of pulmonary artery occlusive pressure in the intensive care unit. Am J Cardiol 1995;75:1256.

Nagueh SF: Assessment of valvular regurgitation with Doppler echocardiography. Cardiol Clin 1998; 16:405.

Tribouilloy CM, Enriquez-Sarano M, Fett SL et al: Application of the proximal flow convergence method to calculate the effective regurgitant orifice area in aortic regurgitation. J Am Coll Cardiol 1998;32:1032.

Willett DL, Hall SA, Jessen ME et al: Assessment of aortic regurgitation by transesophageal color Doppler imaging of the vena contracta: Validation against an intraoperative aortic flow probe. J Am Coll Cardiol. 2001; 37:1450.

Treatment of Aortic Regurgitation

The treatment of AR depends on its underlying cause, severity, cardiac function, and the presence or absence of symptoms. Mild-to-moderate AR may not require any specific treatment, whereas severe acute AR due to aortic dissection is a medical and surgical emergency.

A. ACUTE AORTIC REGURGITATION

Severe acute AR carries a high mortality rate if left untreated. It requires aggressive supportive measures, a rapid assessment of cause, and institution of definitive therapy. Because early death due to left ventricular failure and hemodynamic collapse is frequent in these patients despite intensive medical therapy, prompt surgical intervention is indicated. While the patient is being prepared for surgery, pharmacologic therapy can be initiated. Vasodilator therapy with sodium nitroprusside is the treatment of choice in acute aortic regurgitation because of its afterload and preload reduction. The dose is titrated to optimize forward cardiac output and pulmonary capillary wedge pressure. Positive inotropic agents such as dobutamine can be used if the patient remains hypotensive with a low systemic cardiac output.

When acute AR is associated with hemodynamic instability, the only definitive therapy is surgical correction. The timing of surgery depends on the cause and degree of hemodynamic derangement. In infective endocarditis with severe AR, it is preferable to give 7–10 days of appropriate antibiotics prior to aortic valve replacement, provided the patient is hemodynamically stable. Indications for urgent surgery are New York Heart Association (NYHA) class III–IV congestive heart failure, systemic embolization, persistent bacteremia, fungal endocarditis, or abscess formation. When AR results from aortic dissection with disruption of commissural support, urgent surgical repair is indicated.

B. CHRONIC AORTIC REGURGITATION

1. Mild-to-moderate aortic regurgitation—Patients who have mild or moderate AR and are asymptomatic and who have normal or minimally increased cardiac size, require no therapy for the aortic regurgitation. They should be followed with clinical evaluation yearly and echocardiography at 2–3 year intervals. Antibiotic prophylaxis for endocarditis should be given to patients with structural abnormalities of the aortic valve. In patients with history of rheumatic fever, prophylaxis using either penicillin or erythromycin is indicated till the age of 25 years and 5 years after the last episode. If rheumatic carditis has already occurred, prophylaxis is recommended for life, even following valve replacement. Any occurrence of systemic hypertension should be treated because it aggravates the degree of regurgitation. Patients with AR secondary to syphilis should receive a full course of penicillin therapy. Patients with moderate aortic regurgitation should avoid isometric exercise, competitive sports, and heavy physical exertion. If such patients present with symptoms, an alternative cause for the symptoms should be considered.

2. Moderate-to-severe aortic regurgitation with symptoms and normal left ventricular function— Patients with chronic significant AR and normal left ventricular ejection fraction (LVEF) (> 50%) who have NYHA class III or IV symptoms or Canadian Cardiovascular Society class II–IV angina should undergo aortic valve replacement. Patients with NYHA class II symptoms should be evaluated on case by case basis. If the cause or severity of symptoms is unclear, an exercise test should be done. If exercise capacity is normal, treatment should be given as for asymptomatic patients as outlined in the following section. If new, even mild symptoms appear in a patient with chronic significant AR–particularly if left ventricular (LV) size is increased or the ejection fraction is on the low side of normal, then aortic valve replacement (AVR) should be considered.

Medical therapy is attempted in symptomatic patients who are awaiting surgery or are not surgical candidates due to refusal, terminal medical illness, or advanced age. The aim of therapy in these patients is primarily relief of symptoms and improvement of exercise capacity. Medical therapy includes digitalis, diuretics, and vasodilator drugs. Oral vasodilators, such as hydralazine, and angiotensin-converting enzyme inhibitors reduce afterload, allowing for greater forward cardiac output and improving exercise tolerance. Preload reduction with diuretics and nitrates is also helpful in reducing pulmonary congestion.

3. Moderate-to-severe aortic regurgitation with symptoms and abnormal left ventricular function—Symptomatic patients with mild-to-moderate LV dysfunction (LVEF = 25–50%) should undergo AVR. Treatment decision for patients with more advanced LV dysfunction (LVEF < 25% or LV end-systolic dimension > 60 mm) is difficult. The operative risk is high, and not all patients benefit from AVR. On the other hand outcome with medical therapy is poor as well. Patients with class II–III symptoms, and recent onset of LV dysfunction should be considered for surgical treatment. In patients not considered surgical candidates, aggressive medical therapy is useful in controlling symptoms. Diuretics and vasodilators are the mainstay of medical treatment. If symptoms persist, short-term inotropic support using dobutamine along with intravenous nitroprusside and diuretics may provide relief.

4. Moderate-to-severe aortic regurgitation without symptoms—The optimal timing of AVR in asymptomatic patients remains a challenging clinical decision. Clearly patients with normal LV function and good exercise capacity can live for several years without symptoms or LV dysfunction and surgery is clearly not indicated for such patients. These patients are candidates for long-term oral vasodilator therapy. It has been shown that the use of oral hydralazine in patients with AR produces a number of beneficial hemodynamic effects, including a reduction in regurgitant volume, end-diastolic and end-systolic volumes, and improvement in ejection fraction and effective cardiac output. Similar results have been shown with nifedipine and angiotensin-converting enzyme inhibitors. Vasodilator therapy has also been shown to delay onset of symptoms, occurrence of LV dysfunction and the need for aortic valve replacement.

When the evidence of LV dysfunction (ejection fraction less than 50%) is clear, despite the absence of symptoms, AVR is recommended to prevent further LV dysfunction and improve prognosis. However, once the ejection fraction is decreased, surgical risk is higher and LV dysfunction may become irreversible. The ideal time to intervene is late enough in the course of the disease to justify the surgical risk and postoperative sequelae such as anticoagulation but early enough to prevent irreversible LV contractile dysfunction. To determine the optimal time for surgery in chronic asymptomatic AR, it is important to identify preoperative variables that predict postoperative LV function. A number of parameters have been investigated in the hope of identifying the ideal predictor. Regurgitant volume or fraction are not predictors of postoperative outcome because they are significantly influenced by loading conditions. End-diastolic volume has modest correlation with surgical outcome. The cut off used varies from 150 to 250 mL/m². An end-diastolic minor dimension of greater than 70 mm has also been associated with a poor postoperative outcome. A major limitation of end-diastolic indices is their dependence on preload and thus may not reflect intrinsic myocardial contractile function. Left ventricular ejection fraction has been shown to be an important predictor of postoperative survival. An LVEF of less than 0.50 is associated with significantly reduced 3-year survival rate (64 ± 10%) compared with an LVEF greater than 0.50 (91 ± 28%). Although LVEF has high sensitivity for identifying patients with worse postoperative outcome, it is less specific. This is understandable because LVEF reflects loading conditions in addition to the inotropic state of the myocardium. Similarly, LVEF response to exercise may be modulated by multiple factors, including peripheral resistance, preload heart rate, sympathetic tone, and type of exercise. Therefore, although a decrease in EF during exercise was previously considered to predict a poor outcome in chronic AR, recent data suggest that this is a nonspecific response. However, exercise capacity by itself is an important predictor of survival in AR.

End-systolic indices are less load-dependent and have been used to predict LV function following surgery for AR. An end-systolic minor dimension > 55 mm or end-systolic volume > 60 mL/m² identifies patients with persistent LV dysfunction and a poor survival rate following AVR. Recently, a ratio of LV end-systolic dimension in millimeters and body surface area in square meters that exceeds 25 has been advocated as a marker of occult LV dysfunction. If, in addition to an increased end-systolic ventricular size, the ejection fraction is also reduced, the survival rate drops further. Even though they are preload-independent, end-systolic indices are still affected by afterload. The ratio of end-systolic pressure or wall stress to end-systolic volume has been advocated as an index of contractility, which is less dependent on loading conditions. In patients with chronic severe AR, abnormalities of the end-systolic pressure-volume relationship have been shown, despite a normal LVEF, reflecting depressed myocardial contractility. Such patients are more likely to have symptoms and a need for earlier valve replacement.

For asymptomatic patients with moderate-to-severe AR, we recommend a noninvasive evaluation of left ventricular size and function and an exercise test if functional capacity is unclear (Figure 9–5). If exercise capacity is poor or LVEF is less than 50%, surgical treatment is recommended. Those with good exercise tolerance and normal LV function should be followed at 6- to 12-month intervals. Oral vasodilators may be considered in these patients. In patients who remain asymptomatic, AVR should be considered when serial testing shows decreased exercise tolerance, progressive LV enlargement, or worsening LV function.

Bonow RO, Carbello B, de Leon AC Jr et al: ACC/AHA guidelines for the management of patients with valvular heart disease: Executive summary. A report of the American College of Cardiology/American Heart Association Task Force on Practice Guidelines (Committee on Management of Patients with Valvular Heart Disease). Circulation 1998;98:1949.

Bonow RO: Chronic aortic regurgitation. Role of medical therapy and optimal timing for surgery. Cardiol Clin 1998;16:449.

Borer JS, Hochreiter C, Herrold EM et al: Prediction of indications for valve replacement among asymptomatic or minimally symptomatic patients with chronic aortic regurgitation and normal left ventricular performance. Circulation 1998;97:525.

Prognosis

Asymptomatic patients with chronic AR have a stable course for many years. The mean rate of progression to surgery is approximately 4%/year. Symptoms are the major determinant of outcome in AR. The mortality rate for patients who develop NYHA class II–IV symptoms is over 20%/year. Even for class II patients, the mortality rate is 6%/year compared with 3% for patients in class I. In general, good results have been observed with aortic valve replacement for AR, with an average operative mortality rate of 3–4% and a 5-year survival rate of 85%. These results depend on several factors, including preoperative ventricular function, concomitant coronary artery disease, and the underlying cause of AR. Aortic valve replacement is necessary in the majority of patients. In some cases of AR secondary to loss of commissural support, aortic valve repair can be performed. In patients with excessive aortic root dilatation or aneurysm, a composite aortic graft with reimplantation of the coronary arteries is currently more frequently performed. Most patients show resolution of symptoms following surgery to correct AR. The

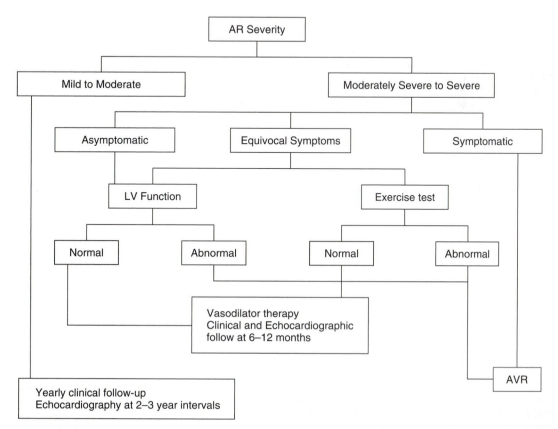

Figure 9–5. Schematic of proposed treatment of patients with chronic significant aortic regurgitation.

end-diastolic volume is reduced immediately, with some further reduction occurring over several days after surgery. The LVEF continues to improve up to 1–2 years after surgery. There is also a gradual decline in LV mass. About 20–30% of patients will have incomplete symptomatic relief and persistent LV dysfunction. These findings are associated with the presence of preoperative LV dysfunction, particularly if the duration of dysfunction is prolonged (> 18 months). Even though the outcome is less than optimal in patients with moderate LV dysfunction, with recent surgical advances, many of them still do better with surgery than with medical management. Surgery should be considered in all symptomatic patients unless LV dysfunction is very severe.

Dujardin KS, Enriquez-Sarano M, Schaff HV et al: Mortality and morbidity of aortic regurgitation in clinical practice: A long-term follow-up study. Circulation 1999;99:1851.

St John Sutton M: Predictors of long-term survival after valve replacement for chronic aortic regurgitation. Eur Heart J 2001;22:808-10.

Turina J, Milincic J, Seifert B, et al: Valve replacement in chronic aortic regurgitation. True predictors of survival after extended follow-up. Circulation. 1998;98(19 Suppl):II100.

Diet Drug Valvulopathy

Recently, observational studies have suggested a link between the diet drugs fenfluramine, dexfenfluramine, and phentermine and the appearance of valvular lesions including AR. This phenomenon was brought to light in 1997 with a report by Connolly and colleagues on a series of 24 cases of valvular lesions associated with use of these drugs. The disease affects mitral, aortic, and tricuspid valves and may involve single or multiple valves. Pathologically, the affected valves are covered with white plaques consisting of fibroblasts and an extracellular matrix, along with thickening and calcification of leaflets. The findings appear similar to carcinoid and ergot-alkaloid-induced valve disease. Since the early report, several studies have been published with conflicting data on the prevalence of this condition, ranging from less than 0.1% to over 20%. In one report the incidence of diet drug-related AR was 8%. The incidence appears related to duration of use and drug dose. Both fenfluramine and dexfenfluramine have been withdrawn from the market, but several million people have already taken these drugs for variable periods of time. Presently it is recommended that all patients who have taken any of these drugs should have a clinical examination. Those with a heart murmur, or other evidence of valvular disease should be further evaluated by echocardiography. Echocardiography should also be considered for all patients with a history of prolonged use (> 3 months) of any of these drugs at high dose. It is important to remember that a trace degree of AR may be seen in normal individuals. The presence of more than trace AR in patients with a history of diet drug use should be considered as suggestive of diet drug valvulopathy. Further care of such patients should follow standard guidelines based on the severity of regurgitation, symptoms, and LV function as described in prior sections. Endocarditis prophylaxis should be provided when needed. Serotonergic drugs should be avoided in people who have a history of fenfluramine or dexfenfluramine use.

Connolly HM, Crary JL, McGoon MD et al: Valvular heart disease associated with fenfluramine-phentermine. N Engl J Med 1997;337:581.

Jick H, Vasilakis C, Weinrauch LA et al: A population based study of appetite-suppressant drugs and the risk of cardiac valve regurgitation. N Engl J Med 1998;339:719.

Volmar KE, Hutchins GM: Aortic and mitral fenfluramine-phentermine valvulopathy in 64 patients treated with anorectic agents. Arch Pathol Lab Med 2001;125:1555.

Weissman NJ, Tighe JF Jr, Gottdiener JS et al: An assessment of heart-valve abnormalities in obese patients taking dexfenfluramine, sustained release dexfenfluramine, or placebo. N Engl J Med 1998;339:725.

Mitral Stenosis

Chad Stoltz, MD & Robert J. Bryg, MD

ESSENTIALS OF DIAGNOSIS

- *Exertional dyspnea, paroxysmal nocturnal dyspnea, orthopnea, or fatigue (later stages)*
- *Opening snap, loud S_1 (closing snap), diastolic rumbling murmur; with pulmonary hypertension, a parasternal lift with a loud P_2*
- *ECG evidence of left atrial enlargement or atrial fibrillation; right ventricular hypertrophy in later stages*
- *Chest radiographic signs of left atrial enlargement and normal left ventricular size*
- *Thickened mitral valve leaflets with restricted valve motion and reduced orifice area demonstrated on two-dimensional echocardiography*
- *An elevated transmitral pressure gradient and prolonged pressure half-time by Doppler echocardiography*

General Considerations

The normal mitral apparatus is a complex structure whose components must permit a large volume of blood to pass from the left atrium to the left ventricle. The cross-sectional area of a normal mitral valve ranges from 4 to 6 cm² in an adult and a transmitral pressure gradient develops when the valve is narrowed to <2.5 cm². Left atrial pressures begin to rise and are transmitted to the pulmonary vasculature and right side of the heart. Several congenital and acquired conditions result in impaired filling of the left ventricle and may be confused with mitral stenosis (Table 10–1).

The predominant cause of mitral stenosis in adults is rheumatic involvement of the mitral valve and approximately two-thirds of all patients with rheumatic mitral stenosis are female. However, a large proportion of patients with rheumatic valve disease—nearly 50%—have no history of rheumatic fever. Other causes

of mitral stenosis are extremely rare (Table 10–2). These figures will most likely change due to the impressive reduction of rheumatic fever in developed countries, although rheumatic fever remains a problem in developing countries and most likely reflects the reduced availability of antibiotics and the virulence of the strains of *Streptococcus.*

Acute rheumatic fever may produce a pancarditis involving the endocardium, myocardium, and pericardium. Aschoff bodies in the myocardium are very specific for a history of rheumatic carditis. Involvement of the mitral valve apparatus is the rule and may produce fusion and thickening of the commissures, cusps, and chordae tendineae. In addition, the fibrosis and calcification of the leaflets may extend to the valve ring. It is still debatable if the progression of mitral stenosis is due to a smoldering rheumatic process and recurrent infections or the constant trauma of turbulent flow produced by a deformed valve.

As the stenosis progresses, a transmitral pressure gradient develops to facilitate flow across the stenotic valve in diastole. Furthermore, the atrial contraction may augment this diastolic pressure gradient (assuming the heart is in normal sinus rhythm). Both the mitral valvular gradient (MVG) and mitral valvular flow

Table 10–1. Conditions causing left ventricular inflow obstruction.

Congenital
Valvular mitral stenosis
Subvalvular ring
Cor triatriatum
Pulmonary vein stenosis
Acquired
Valvular mitral stenosis
Atrial myxoma
Thrombus
Neoplasm
Large fungal or bacterial vegetation
Prosthetic valve dysfunction

Table 10–2. Cause of mitral valve stenosis requiring surgery (1974–1990).

Cause	Number	Percentage
Rheumatic fever	562	53.5
Rheumatic equivalents	139	13.2
Scarlet fever	111	10.6
Infective endocarditis	35	3.3
Degenerative[a]	28	2.7
Congenital[b]	13	1.2
Systemic lupus erythematosus	4	0.4
Carcinoid heart	2	0.2
Endomyocardial fibrosis	2	0.2
Rheumatoid arthritis	2	0.2
Unclassified	152	14.5

[a] Mitral annulus calcification.

[b] Lutembacher syndrome; total = 1050.

Source: Adapted, with permission, from Horstkotte D et al: Pathomorphological aspects, aetiology, and natural history of acquired mitral valve stenosis. Eur Heart J 1991;12(Suppl B):55.

(MVF) are required to assess the mitral valve area (MVA) as expressed by the Gorlin formula:

$$MVA(cm^2) = \frac{MVF}{37.7\sqrt{MVG}}$$

The mitral valvular flow is a function of cardiac output and heart rate. An increase in cardiac output or heart rate will increase the transmitral flow. As expressed by the Gorlin formula, the increased mitral valvular flow (produced by an increased cardiac output or tachycardia) elevates the mitral valvular gradient exponentially assuming the mitral valve area remains constant. The increased mitral valvular gradient produces an elevated left atrial pressure. This is an important concept for the development of symptoms.

Clinical Findings

A. Symptoms and Signs

Early in the disease, patients may be asymptomatic. However, conditions that increase cardiac output or heart rate will increase the mitral valvular gradient and left atrial pressure as described earlier. The elevated left atrial pressure is subsequently transmitted into the pulmonary circulation, leading to dyspnea, and may facilitate the early diagnosis of mitral stenosis. Common conditions that increase cardiac output or heart rate are exercise, hyperthyroidism, pregnancy, atrial fibrillation, and fever. In addition, venous return is augmented in the supine position and may produce orthopnea and paroxysmal nocturnal dyspnea in patients with moderate disease (Table 10–3).

As the disease progresses, the pulmonary artery pressure increases proportionally to the pulmonary capillary pressure. The proportional increase is termed passive pulmonary hypertension because the increased pressure produced by the right ventricle is required to drive blood across the pulmonary vascular bed into the left atrium. In some patients with severe mitral stenosis, the pulmonary artery pressure is increased disproportionally to the pulmonary capillary pressure. The disproportional increase is termed reactive pulmonary hypertension. The reactive pulmonary hypertension is secondary to pulmonary artery constriction and organic obliterative changes in the pulmonary vascular

Table 10–3. Stages of mitral stenosis.

Class	MVA (cm²)	Symptoms
1. Minimal	>2.5	None
2. Mild	1.4–2.5	Minimal dyspnea with marked exertion
3. Moderate	1.0–1.4	Dyspnea, orthopnea, paroxysmal nocturnal dyspnea, pulmonary edema
4. Severe	<1.0	Resting dyspnea; disabled (NYHA class IV); bed chair
5. Reactive pulmonary hypertension	<1.0	As in severe disease, plus fatigue, right ventricular failure.

NYHA = New York Heart Association (classification).

Source: Reprinted, with permission, from Dalen JE: Mitral stenosis. In Dalen JE, Alpert JS, eds: Valvular Heart Disease, 2nd ed. Boston: Little, Brown, 1987.

bed. These changes typically produce symptoms of right-heart failure and may not be completely reversible.

The mitral valve stenosis and atrial inflammation secondary to rheumatic fever may produce dilatation and postinflammatory changes of the left atrium. These changes predispose the patient to palpitations and atrial fibrillation. In addition, there is an increased risk of systemic embolization resulting in a stroke, myocardial infarction (coronary embolism), splenic or renal infarction, and peripheral artery occlusion. For patients in sinus rhythm, age, the presence of a left atrial thrombus, mitral valve area, and the presence of significant aortic regurgitation were positively associated with embolism. In cases of atrial fibrillation, previous embolism is positively associated with embolism; percutaneous balloon mitral commissurotomy is a negative predictor. Spontaneous echo contrast (left atrial smoky echoes) detected by transesophageal echo is associated with systemic embolism, but further studies are needed for clarification. Most emboli appear to originate from the left atrium.

Unusual conditions may occur but are extremely rare due to the altered natural history of mitral stenosis. Hoarseness (Ortner's syndrome) is an extremely rare complication and is secondary to compression of the recurrent laryngeal nerve by a massively dilated left atrium or dilated pulmonary artery. Increased pulmonary pressures and vascular congestion produce hemoptysis. Hemoptysis may present as a sudden hemorrhage (termed pulmonary apoplexy; this condition is rarely life-threatening), pink frothy sputum resulting from pulmonary edema, blood-tinged sputum associated with dyspnea or bronchitis, and pulmonary infarction due to a pulmonary embolism. Chest pain may develop and resembles angina. The chest pain is most likely the result of pulmonary hypertension and right ventricle hypertrophy and is typically relieved with correction of the mitral stenosis, although concomitant coronary artery disease should be evaluated with the development of chest pain. Endocarditis is primarily associated with mild mitral stenosis and is quite unusual with calcification in severe mitral stenosis.

B. PHYSICAL EXAMINATION

The general appearance of patients with mitral stenosis is usually unremarkable. Older studies reported mitral facies, which is characterized by pinkish-purple patches on the cheeks produced by low cardiac output, systemic vasoconstriction, and right-sided heart failure. This sign is now extremely rare. Right-sided heart failure also produces an elevated jugular venous pulse with a prominent *a* wave (assuming the heart is in normal sinus rhythm) and *v* wave (produced by tricuspid regurgitation).

The apical impulse is generally normal or decreased, representing normal left ventricular function and de-

creased left ventricular volume (Table 10–4). Palpation of the S_1 over the precordium is a pathognomonic finding and suggests that the anterior mitral valve leaflet is pliable. When the patient is in the left lateral decubitus position, a diastolic thrill may be appreciated. When pulmonary hypertension is present, a parasternal right ventricular heave develops along with a palpable P_2.

Auscultation of the heart sounds may reveal an accentuated S_1 early in the disease. Accentuation of S_1 occurs when the left ventricular pressure rises rapidly in early systole, the flexible mitral valve leaflets transgress a wide closing excursion. As the severity of mitral stenosis increases with calcification and fibrosis of the leaflets, the amplitude of S_1 subsequently diminishes. When pulmonary hypertension is present, the splitting of the second heart sound may narrow and become a single accentuated S_2. An S_3 originating from the left ventricle is absent in patients with mitral stenosis unless there is concomitant coronary artery disease, mitral regurgitation, or aortic regurgitation. An S_4, if present, originates from the right ventricle when it is hypertrophied and dilated secondary to pulmonary hypertension.

The opening snap is due to sudden tensing of the valve leaflets after they have completed their opening excursion. The vigorous opening of the leaflets is secondary to high left atrial pressures accompanied by a fall in left ventricular pressures in early diastole. The opening snap is audible (high frequency) at the apex, using the diaphragm of the stethoscope.

It is imperative to examine the patient in the left lateral decubitus position for a diastolic murmur (Figure 10–1). In addition, the murmur may be accentuated by

Table 10–4. Physical findings in mitral stenosis.

Palpation
  Point of maximal impulse (PMI) is normal or decreased
  Right ventricular heave is present if patient has pulmonary
    hypertension
  Apical diastolic thrill may be present
Auscultation
  Loud S_1
  Opening snap
  Diastolic rumble, near apex
    Middiastolic
    Presystolic
    Pandiastolic
  Variably present
    Loud P_2
    Murmur of mitral regurgitation
    Murmur of tricuspid regurgitation

Source: Reprinted, with permission, Dalen JE: Mitral stenosis. In Dalen JE, Alpert JS, eds: Valvular Heart Disease, 2nd ed. Boston: Little, Brown, 1987.

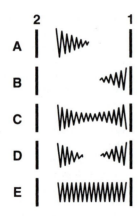

Figure 10–1. The various configurations of the diastolic murmur that may be heard in mitral stenosis. **2:** second sound; **1:** first sound. Reprinted, with permission, from Marriott HJL: Bedside Cardiac Diagnosis. Philadelphia: JB Lippincott, 1993.

having the patient exercise prior to auscultation. The murmur is described as a rumble (low frequency) and is audible at the apex, using the bell of the stethoscope. The diastolic murmur of mitral stenosis reflects the mitral valvular gradient and the duration of blood flow across the valve. In mild mitral stenosis, the early diastolic decrescendo murmur is brief and is accompanied by a presystolic murmur. The presystolic murmur is secondary to the gradient produced by the atrial contraction. However, the presystolic murmur may be produced in atrial fibrillation and is due to the narrowing of the mitral orifice produced by ventricular systole prior to S_1. A murmur of pulmonary regurgitation (Graham Steell murmur) may be present and difficult to distinguish from the murmur of mitral stenosis and aortic regurgitation (Austin Flint murmur).

Reliable indicators of the severity of mitral stenosis are the A_2–OS interval and the length (rather than intensity) of the diastolic murmur. As the severity of mitral stenosis increases, the A_2–OS interval decreases and the length of the murmur increases. The decreased interval is the result of increased left atrial pressures, producing a mitral valvular gradient at the very onset of diastole. The gradient leads to an early excursion of the valve leaflets (early OS) and continues throughout all of diastole (pandiastolic murmur). The opening snap and murmur may become inaudible when mitral stenosis is very severe and the valve leaflets are rigid.

C. Diagnostic Studies

1. Electrocardiography—Early in the disease, the electrocardiogram (ECG) typically reveals a normal sinus rhythm and is very insensitive. As the disease progresses, left atrial enlargement leads to changes in the P wave. The P wave in lead II becomes broad and notched (termed P-mitrale) along with a prominent terminal component of the P wave in lead V_1. The P wave axis migrates between +45 and –30°. Many patients subsequently develop atrial fibrillation, and the previously described findings are lost. As the pulmonary hypertension becomes severe (70–100 mm Hg), right axis deviation develops in addition to an R wave greater than the S wave in lead V_1. In pure mitral stenosis, left ventricular hypertrophy is absent.

2. Chest radiograph—Radiologic examination of the cardiac silhouette is quite advantageous. Left atrial enlargement may produce a "double-density," straightening of the left heart border, along with elevation of the left mainstem bronchus (PA view), and impingement on the esophagus due to posterior extension (lateral view). Right ventricular enlargement may occupy the retrosternal space (lateral view). The left ventricular silhouette is normal in pure mitral stenosis, and calcification of the mitral valve is difficult to see on routine chest radiograph. Radiologic examination of the lung fields reveals elevated pulmonary pressures. The pulmonary arteries are prominent, and blood flow is redistributed to the upper lobes (cephalization). Transudation of fluid into the interstitium occurs, resulting in Kerley A lines, Kerley B lines, and pulmonary edema.

3. Echocardiography—The echocardiographic examination is now the keystone of the diagnostic assessment of mitral stenosis after an appropriate history and physical, ECG, and chest radiogram. Valuable information is provided with the following three echocardiographic techniques: M-mode, two-dimensional, and Doppler.

a. M-mode— This form of echocardiography uses a relatively narrow beam of ultrasound to display valve motion and thickness. As mitral stenosis progresses, the usual M-shaped configuration of the anterior mitral leaflet is altered. The diastolic posterior motion of the anterior leaflet is reduced, producing a reduced E-F slope. In patients in sinus rhythm, the A wave, which is normally seen with an atrial contraction, may be reduced or absent. Fusion of the commissures produces a concordant motion of the anterior and posterior mitral leaflets. Although this mode of echocardiography can provide a qualitative diagnosis, it is the least reliable means of quantifying the severity of obstruction.

b. Two-dimensional echocardiography—This method provides a more complete view of the mitral valve apparatus. The parasternal long axis may reveal diastolic "doming" of the mitral valve and a "hockey stick" configuration of the anterior leaflet. Pliable leaflets with restricted mobility of the leaflet tips produce this configuration. The parasternal short axis can image the orifice of the mitral valve that demonstrates the typical "fish mouth" configuration. After visualization, the orifice is planimetered in diastole to obtain an accurate measurement of the mitral valve area. This measurement is very reliable but may be operator-dependent and prone to error. The inaccuracy is further evident after commissurotomy due to the distortion produced by commissural splitting. With the advent of percutaneous mitral balloon valvotomy (PMBV), the mitral apparatus morphology determined by two-dimensional echocardiography plays an extremely important role for selection criteria.

c. Doppler echocardiography—Doppler accurately assesses the hemodynamic effects of the mitral valve stenosis; the indicators are mitral valvular gradient, mitral valve area, and pulmonary artery pressures. The mitral valvular gradient is measured by obtaining the velocity of mitral inflow. The velocity (V) is converted to the pressure gradient between the atrium and ventricle using the modified Bernoulli equation:

$$\text{Gradient (mm Hg)} = 4(V^2)$$

The mitral valve area can be estimated using the pressure half-time method, the proximal isovelocity surface area (PISA), or the continuity of flow method. The pressure half-time is currently the most widely used technique for estimating the mitral valve area from Doppler-derived data. The pressure half-time is the time required for the peak pressure gradient between the left atrium and the left ventricle to decline to one half of its original value. Doppler velocity is converted into a pressure gradient by dividing the initial flow velocity by the square root of 2. Empirically, a pressure half-time of 220 ms correlates with a mitral valve area of 1 cm².

$$\text{MVA(cm}^2) = \frac{220}{\text{pressure half-time}}$$

As the mitral valve decreases, the pressure half-time increases. However, the pressure half-time may be inaccurate in patients with abnormalities of left atrial or left ventricular compliance, those with associated aortic regurgitation, and those with a previous mitral valvotomy. The PISA and the continuity of flow method provide more accurate estimates of mitral valve area in these circumstances.

Pulmonary artery pressures are determined using continuous wave Doppler. The velocity of tricuspid regurgitation produced by pulmonary hypertension is measured, yielding a gradient between the right atrium and right ventricle with the use of the modified Bernoulli equation described previously. The right ventricular systolic pressure is obtained by adding the estimated right atrial pressure to the gradient.

Each method has several limitations, and it is imperative to achieve cross validation. In most instances, measurements of the mitral valvular gradient, mitral valve area, and pulmonary artery pressures correlate well with one another with the use of a transthoracic echocardiogram. If correlation does not occur, a cardiac catheterization, transesophageal echocardiogram, three-dimensional echocardiogram, or exercise with simultaneous Doppler estimation of the transmitral and pulmonary pressures should be sought to clarify inconsistencies. In addition, a transesophageal echocardiogram can assess the presence or absence of left atrial thrombus in patients being considered for percutaneous mitral balloon valvotomy or cardioversion.

4. Cardiac catheterization—Direct measurements of left atrial and left ventricular pressures require a transseptal catheterization and predispose the patient to unnecessary risks. Conventional cardiac catheterization uses the pulmonary capillary wedge pressure for indirect measurement of left atrial pressures. Although the pulmonary capillary wedge accurately reflects the mean left atrial pressure, it overestimates the transmitral gradient. Presently, the cardiac catheterization has a very limited role in determining the severity of mitral stenosis due to the recent advances in echocardiography.

Binder TM, Rosenhek R, Porenta G et al: Improved assessment of mitral valve stenosis by volumetric real-time three-dimensional echocardiography. J Am Coll Cardiol 2000;36:1355.

Chiang C-W, Lo SK, Ko Ys et al: Predictors of systemic embolism in patients with mitral stenosis: A prospective study. Ann Intern Med 1998;128:885.

Faletra F, Pezzano A Jr, Fusco R et al: Measurement of mitral valve area in mitral stenosis: Four echocardiographic methods compared with direct measurement of anatomic orifices. J Am Coll Cardiol 1996;28:1190.

Haworth SG, Hall SM, Panja M et al: Peripheral pulmonary vascular and airway abnormalities in adolescents with rheumatic mitral stenosis. Int J Cardiol 1988;18:405.

Hildick-Smith DJR, Walsh JT, Shapiro LM et al: Pulmonary capillary wedge pressure in mitral stenosis accurately reflects mean left atrial pressure but overestimates transmitral gradient. Am J Cardiol 2000;85:512.

Marcus RH: The spectrum of severe rheumatic mitral valve disease in a developing country: Correlations among clinical presentation, surgical pathologic findings and hemodynamic sequelae. Ann Intern Med 1994;120:177.

Nishimura RA, Rihal CS, Tajik AJ et al: Accurate measurement of the transmitral gradient in patients with mitral stenosis: A simultaneous catheterization and Doppler echocardiography study. J Am Coll Cardiol 1994;24:152.

Olson LJ, Subramanian R, Achermann DM et al: Surgical pathology of the mitral valve: A study of 712 cases spanning 21 years. Mayo Clin Proc 1987;62:22.

Popovic AD, Thomas JD, Neskovic AN et al: Time-related trends in the preoperative evaluation of patients with valvular stenosis. Am J Cardiol 1997;80:1464.

Selzer A, Cohn KE: Natural history of mitral stenosis: A review. Circulation 1972;45:878.

Treatment

A. MEDICAL THERAPY

Primary prophylaxis consists of an early diagnosis of Group A streptococcal pharyngitis. Treatment started within 7–9 days after onset of illness may prevent rheumatic fever. Secondary prophylaxis may be individually tailored, but there are no firm guidelines. Recurrence of rheumatic fever is more common in young patients and patients who developed carditis during their initial episode. Therefore, with carditis, secondary prevention continues for 10 years or until age 25. Without carditis, secondary prevention continues for 5 years or until age 18. The prevention of repeated attacks may delay the progression of mitral stenosis.

Patients with mitral stenosis are considered to be at moderate risk for bacterial endocarditis, endocarditis prophylaxis is therefore recommended for certain procedures specified by the AHA guidelines. However, there is a recent debate concerning whether dental procedures predispose to endocarditis and whether antibiotic prophylaxis is of any value. The choice of antibiotics to treat endocarditis may be further complicated if the patient is receiving penicillin for prophylaxis against rheumatic fever. Resistance to penicillin and cephalosporins may develop in this scenario, and an alternative antibiotic should be provided for prophylaxis against endocarditis.

Medical management of mitral stenosis with normal sinus rhythm is limited. A benefit is derived from salt restriction and diuretics when there is evidence of pulmonary vascular congestion. Digitalis does not benefit patients in sinus rhythm unless an associated left ventricular dysfunction is present. Beta-blockers can significantly decrease heart rate and cardiac output. The decreased heart rate and cardiac output subsequently lead to a decrease in the transmitral gradient. Although there appears to be a physiologic advantage with the use of beta-blockers, the data are conflicting. Beta-blockers may be reserved for patients who have exertional symptoms if the symptoms occur at high heart rates. Anticoagulation is beneficial for cases with normal sinus rhythm with a prior embolic event or a left atrial dimension >55 mm Hg by echocardiography.

Medical management of mitral stenosis and atrial fibrillation can alleviate a variety of complications. Atrial fibrillation in patients with mitral stenosis is poorly tolerated due to a loss of atrial contraction and an associated rapid ventricular rate. The rate control is achieved by using a beta-blocker, calcium channel blocker, or digitalis. Electrical or chemical cardioversion should be performed with appropriate anticoagulation. Class 1A, 1C, and III agents can be used to terminate acute-onset atrial fibrillation and prevent recurrences of atrial fibrillation. Most antiarrhythmics increase the likelihood of maintaining normal sinus rhythm to approximately 50–70% of pa-

tients per year after cardioversion. Amiodarone appears to be more effective than sotalol or propafenone, although the antiarrhythmic should be tailored to the patient. In addition, a large number of patients take both digitalis and warfarin (Coumadin). The digitalis and Coumadin need to be decreased by approximately 50% due to significant drug interactions with amiodarone. Anticoagulation is necessary in patients who are unable to maintain normal sinus rhythm.

In pregnancy, the heart rate and cardiac output are increased substantially along with an increase in maternal blood volume. Nevertheless, most healthy pregnant women with mild to moderate mitral stenosis can be treated medically. Diuretics and beta-blockers appear to be safe for use in pregnancy. Quinidine or procainamide are the drugs of choice if an antiarrhythmic drug is needed to maintain normal sinus rhythm. If anticoagulation is necessary, Coumadin should be avoided and the patient should be treated appropriately with heparin.

B. PERCUTANEOUS MITRAL BALLOON VALVOTOMY

Percutaneous mitral balloon valvotomy (PMBV) was introduced by Inoue (single-balloon technique) in 1984 and involves a transseptal puncture during cardiac catheterization. The transseptal approach offers direct access to the mitral orifice, after which a single- or double-balloon commissurotomy is performed. The mechanism of action is primarily commissural splitting and fracture of calcium deposits that improve valvular function. The Inoue and double-balloon techniques produce similar long-term results.

Two newer approaches are gaining acceptance. The retrograde nontransseptal balloon mitral valvuloplasty is based on an externally steerable cardiac catheter that enters the left atrium retrograde via the left ventricle. This technique avoids the need for a transseptal puncture and dilatation of the interatrial septum. A reusable metallic valvotomy device was recently introduced and has a distinct advantage of multiple uses after sterilization, which markedly decreases the procedural cost. However, this procedure requires a transseptal route. Presently, the retrograde approach and the reusable device appear to be comparable to previous techniques and offer an alternative approach.

Balloon valvuloplasty is recommended in patients who are symptomatic, have moderate to severe mitral stenosis, have pliable leaflets, and do not have a left atrial thrombus or significant mitral regurgitation (ACC/AHA Class I recommendation). Patients who are either asymptomatic but have severe mitral stenosis or are symptomatic but have high surgical risks are considered acceptable candidates for balloon valvuloplasty (ACC/AHA Class IIa recommendation). It is not recommended in cases of mild mitral stenosis (ACC/AHA Class III recommendation). Important baseline variables include operator experience, age, New York Heart Association (NYHA) functional class, atrial fibrillation, cardiothoracic index, echocardiographic score, mean pulmonary artery pressure, and mitral regurgitation. The underlying mitral valve morphology is the most important factor in determining outcome, and echocardiographic scoring systems have been developed for assessing the morphology. The echocardiographic score developed by Abascal and colleagues in 1988 is commonly used today (Table 10–5). Patients with a score of less than 8 have a lower incidence of acute complications, decreased in-hospital cost, and a lower rate of recurrent stenosis on follow-up. Cannan and colleagues reported that the presence of commissural calcium might be a better predictor of outcome after PMBV than the Abascal echocardiographic score. The degree of commissural calcification is independent of the Abascal score and emphasizes that successful balloon valvotomy results from splitting open the fused commissures.

Cannan CR, Nishimura RA, Reeder GS et al: Echocardiographic assessment of commissural calcium: A simple predictor of outcome after percutaneous mitral balloon valvotomy. J Am Coll Cardiol 1997;29:175.

Cohen DJ, Kuntz RE, Gordon SP et al: Predictors of long-term outcome after percutaneous balloon mitral valvuloplasty. N Engl J Med 1992;327:1329.

Cribier A, Eltchaninoff H, Koning R et al: Percutaneous mechanical mitral commissurotomy with a newly designed metallic valvulotome: Immediate results of the initial experience in 153 patients. Circulation 1999;99:793.

Dajani AS, Taubert KA, Wilson W et al: Prevention of bacterial endocarditis: Recommendations by the American Heart Association. JAMA 1997;277:1794.

Eisenberg MJ, Ballal R, Heidenreich PA et al: Echocardiographic score as a predictor of in-hospital cost in patients undergoing percutaneous balloon mitral valvuloplasty. Am J Cardiol 1996; 78:790.

Falk RH: Atrial fibrillation. N Engl J Med 2001;344:1067.

Inoue K, Owaki T, Nakamura T et al: Clinical application of transvenous mitral commissurotomy by a new balloon catheter. J Thorac Cardiovasc Surg 1984;87:394.

Iung B, Garbarz E, Michaud P et al: Late results of percutaneous mitral commissurotomy in a series of 1024 patients. Analysis of late clinical deterioration: Frequency, anatomic findings, and predictive factors. Circulation 1999;99:3272.

Kang D-H, Park SW, Song JK et al: Long-term clinical and echocardiographic outcome of percutaneous mitral valvuloplasty: Randomized comparison of Inoue and double-balloon techniques. J Am Coll Cardiol 2000;35:169.

Leon MN, Harrell LC, Simosa HF et al: Comparison of immediate and long-term results of mitral balloon valvotomy with the double-balloon versus Inoue techniques. Am J Cardiol 1999; 83:1356.

Table 10–5. Echocardiographic scoring system (Massachusetts General Hospital).

Morphology	Grade	Score
Leaflet mobility	1. Highly mobile with restriction of the leaflet tips only	1
	2. Reduced mobility in midportion and base of leaflets	2
	3. Forward movement of valve leaflets in diastole mainly at the base	3
	4. No or minimal forward motion of the leaflets in diastolic	4
Valve thickness	1. Near normal (4–5 mm)	1
	2. Midleaflet thickening, marked thickening of the margins	2
	3. Thickening extends through entire leaflet (5–8 mm)	3
	4. Marked thickening of all leaflet tissue (>8–10 mm)	4
Subvalvular thickening	1. Minimal thickening of chordal structures just below the valve	1
	2. Thickening of chordae extending up to one third of chordal length	2
	3. Thickening extending to the distal third of the chordae	3
	4. Extensive thickening and shortening of all chordae extending down to the papillary muscle	4
Valvular calcification	1. A single area of increased echo brightness	1
	2. Scattered areas of brightness confined to leaflet margins	2
	3. Brightness extending into the mid-portion of leaflets	3
	4. Extensive brightness through most of the leaflet tissue	4

Meneveau N, Schiele F, Seronde MF et al: Predictors of event-free survival after percutaneous mitral commissurotomy. Heart 1998;80:359.

Roy D, Talajic M, Dorian P et al: Amiodarone to prevent recurrence of atrial fibrillation. N Engl J Med 2000;342:913.

Stefanadis C et al: Retrograde nontransseptal balloon mitral valvuloplasty: Immediate results and long-term follow-up. Circulation 1992;85:1760.

Stefanadis CI, Stratos CG, Lambrou SG et al: Retrograde nontransseptal balloon mitral valvuloplasty: Immediate results and intermediate long-term outcome in 441 cases-A multicenter experience. J Am Coll Cardiol 1998;32:1009.

Stoll BC, Ashcom TL, Johns JP et al: Effects of atenolol on rest and exercise hemodynamics in patients with mitral stenosis. Am J Cardiol 1995;75:482.

Strom BL, Abrutyn E, Berlin JA et al: Dental and cardiac risk factors for infective endocarditis: A population-based, case-control study. Ann Intern Med 1998;129:761.

Sutaria N, Northridge DB, Shaw TR et al: Significance of commissural calcification on outcome of mitral balloon valvotomy. Heart 2000;84:398.

C. Surgical Therapy

Three surgical approaches are used to treat mitral stenosis: closed commissurotomy, open commissurotomy, and mitral valve replacement. A closed commissurotomy is performed without the aid of a cardiopulmonary bypass. The surgeon enters the heart using either a transatrial or a transventricular approach. A dilator is subsequently introduced across the mitral valve without direct visualization. The lack of direct visualization is an obvious limitation, and patients are selected in a manner similar to that used for PMBV. Without cardiopulmonary bypass, the closed approach allows for a substantial reduction in cost compared with open commissurotomy and PMBV. Due to the substantial reduction of cost, closed commissurotomy is the procedure of choice in developing nations.

Open commissurotomy has several advantages over the closed procedure. Under direct visualization, the surgeon can incise commissures, débride calcium deposits, and separate fused chordae tendineae and the underlying papillary muscle. In addition, thrombi are removed from the left atrium, and many surgeons will amputate the left atrial appendage to remove a potential source of postoperative emboli. Open commissurotomy is usually preferred in patients with a left atrial thrombus or severe subvalvular and calcific disease; however, it is costly with the use of cardiopulmonary bypass.

Mitral valve replacement is primarily indicated for patients with moderate or severe mitral stenosis (MVA <1.5 cm²) and NYHA III–IV symptoms who are not considered candidates for PMBV or mitral repair. The choice of a mechanical valve versus a bioprosthetic should be individualized. A recent study suggested that there is no difference between the St. Jude and Medtronic Hall prosthesis with respect to late clinical performance or hemodynamic results. Therefore, the choice of mechanical valve should be based on the surgeon's experience and preference. Mechanical valves offer durability and a larger effective orifice area than bioprosthetics, however, mechanical valves are more thrombogenic and require continuous anticoagulation. Although there is a lower frequency of embolic complications with bioprosthetics, the rate of structural deterioration over 10 years is substantial in younger patients.

Fiore AC, Barner HB, Swartz MT et al: Mitral valve replacement: Randomized trial of St. Jude and Medtronic Hall prostheses. Ann Thorac Surg 1998;66:707.

Hammermeister K, Sethi GK, Henderson WG et al: Outcomes 15 years after valve replacement with a mechanical versus a bioprosthetic valve: Final report of the Veterans Affairs randomized trial. J Am Coll Cardiol 2000;36:1152.

Vongpatanasin W, Hillis LD, Lange RA et al: Prosthetic heart valves. N Engl J Med 1996;335:407.

Prognosis

The natural history of mitral stenosis has been profoundly influenced by the advancement of cardiovascular interventions. In most patients, rheumatic mitral stenosis is a progressive disease. In a large referral population without intervention, the mitral valve area decreased at a mean rate of 0.09 cm²/year, however, the rate of mitral valve narrowing in individual patients is variable and cannot be predicted by the initial mitral valve area, mitral valve score, or transmitral gradient, alone or in combination. The mean interval between rheumatic fever and the appearance of symptoms was 16.3 ± 5.2 years. In 84.3% of these patients death was cardiac-related and due to right-heart failure (27.7%), lung edema resistant to medical therapy (14.5%), thromboembolic (10.8%) or hemorrhagic complications (7.2%), myocardial infarction (9.3%) or infective endocarditis (3.6%); 14.5% of the patients had a sudden death. Progression from mild symptoms to severe disability is typically accelerated and the prognosis dramatically worsens (Figure 10–2).

A recent trial compared PMBV, open commissurotomy, and closed commissurotomy in 90 patients. In contrast to closed commissurotomy, PMBV and open commissurotomy produced excellent early and long-term results. The mitral valve area increased much more after PMBV (from 0.9 to 2.2 cm²) and open commissurotomy (from 0.9 to 2.2 cm²) than after closed commissurotomy (from 0.9 to 1.6 cm²). Residual mitral stenosis was 0% after PMBV or open commissurotomy and 27% after closed commissurotomy. There was no early or late mortality or thromboembolism among the three groups. At 7-year follow-up, echocardiographic MVA was greater after PMBV and open commissurotomy (1.8 cm²) than after closed commissurotomy (1.3 cm²). In addition to lower rates of restenosis, PMBV and open commissurotomy pro-

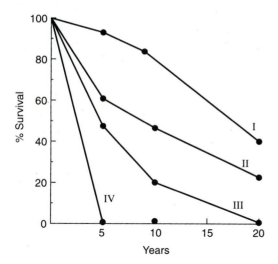

Figure 10-2. The natural history of patients with mitral stenosis for those with New York Heart Association classifications I, II, III, and IV. Reprinted, with permission, from Carabello BA: Timing of surgery in mitral and aortic stenosis. Cardiol Clin 1991;9:229.

vided lower rates of reintervention than closed commissurotomy. These results appear consistent with earlier studies. The excellent results, lower cost, and obviation of a thoracotomy and cardiopulmonary bypass advocate PMBV for all patients with favorable mitral valve morphology.

The perioperative mortality rate for mitral valve replacement is less than 5% in young healthy individuals, however, the mortality rate may exceed 20% in older patients who are in NYHA Class IV. The procedure should therefore be performed prior to the development of significant left ventricular dysfunction. Despite the increased risk of perioperative mortality, a tangible benefit is derived from mitral valve replacement (Figure 10–3).

Ben Farhat MB, Ayari M, Maatouk F et al: Percutaneous balloon versus surgical closed and open mitral commissurotomy: Seven-year follow-up results of a randomized trial. Circulation 1998;97:245.

Horstkotte D, Niehues R, Strauer BE et al: Pathomorphological aspects, aetiology and natural history of acquired mitral valve stenosis. Eur Heart J 1991;12(Supp B):55.

Reyes VP, Raju BS, Wynne J et al: Percutaneous balloon valvuloplasty compared with open surgical commissurotomy for mitral stenosis. N Engl J Med 1994;331:961.

Sagie A, Freitas N, Padial LR et al: Doppler echocardiographic assessment of long-term progression of mitral stenosis in 103 patients: Valve area and right heart disease. J Am Coll Cardiol 1996;28:472.

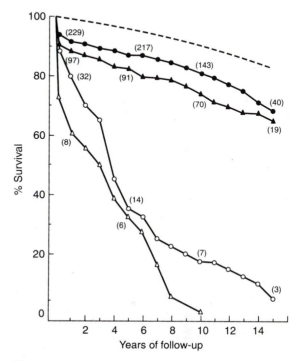

Figure 10-3. Natural history of patients with pure mitral stenosis who did not undergo surgery although it was indicated, compared with patients in whom the lesion was diagnosed invasively and who received valve replacements. The diagram also shows both the natural and the postoperative courses for patients with mitral regurgitation. Solid circle = mitral stenosis with valve replacement; solid triangle = mitral regurgitation with valve replacement; open circle = mitral stenosis, natural history; open triangle = mitral regurgitation, natural history. Reprinted, with permission, from Horstkotte D, Niehues R, Strauer BE et al: Pathomorphological aspects, aetiology, and natural history of acquired mitral valve stenosis. Eur Heart J 1991;12(Suppl B):55.

Mitral Regurgitation

11

Michael H. Crawford, MD

ESSENTIALS OF DIAGNOSIS

- *Dyspnea or orthopnea*
- *Characteristic apical systolic murmur*
- *Color-flow Doppler echocardiographic evidence of systolic regurgitation into the left atrium*

General Considerations

The mitral apparatus consists of the left ventricular walls that support the papillary muscles, the chordae tendineae, mitral leaflets, annulus, and adjacent left atrial walls. Because defects in any of these components can lead to systolic regurgitation, the list of diseases that can cause mitral regurgitation includes many types of heart disease. Anything that causes left ventricular dilatation may disrupt the alignment of the papillary muscles, impairing their function and dilating the annulus, resulting in mitral regurgitation. Myocardial infarction involving the papillary muscles or the left ventricular walls that support them can impair the function of the mitral apparatus. Mitral chordae can rupture, especially in patients with hypertension or mitral valve prolapse. The most common diseases affecting the mitral leaflets are rheumatic heart disease and the myxomatous changes of mitral valve prolapse. In addition, infectious endocarditis can destroy the mitral leaflets, and mitral annular calcification can impair the normal systolic contraction of the annulus, leading to mitral regurgitation. Finally, left atrial dilatation from any cause, can disrupt annular function and cause mitral regurgitation. Some patients have combinations of these defects, making mitral regurgitation both more likely and more severe.

For clinical purposes mitral regurgitation can be divided into two broad categories: organic and functional. The former refers to diseases that involve the valve leaflets and their immediate supporting apparatus, ie, chordae and annulus. The latter refers to diseases that affect the left ventricle and atrium, leaving the valve apparatus intact (Table 11–1). Most clinical studies involve patients with organic mitral regurgitation, so, unless otherwise specified, the following discussion focuses on organic mitral regurgitation.

Among the many causes of chronic organic mitral regurgitation, mitral valve prolapse is a unique entity in many ways. An increase in the middle connective tissue layer of the mitral valve causes an increase in leaflet size and elongated chordae. The resultant systolic prolapse of the valve into the left atrium may or may not be accompanied by regurgitation. In some patients, regurgitation depends on left ventricular volume. Large volumes tend to reduce prolapse and hence regurgitation; small volumes have the opposite effect.

Consequently, the presence or absence of regurgitation and its severity and timing in systole (the ventricle becomes progressively smaller during systole) are determined by a complex interplay of left ventricular volume, pressure, and contractile state. Patients with mitral valve prolapse are also unique because the condition can be a hereditary connective tissue disease (eg, Marfan's syndrome) or acquired (inflammation of the valve). Some patients exhibit abnormalities of connective tissue in other organs (eg, thoracic skeleton) and have demonstrable abnormalities in the autonomic

Table 11–1. Etiologic classification of mitral regurgitation.

Organic Mitral Regurgitation
  Myxomatous changes (mitral valve prolapse)
  Rheumatic heart disease
  Infectious endocarditis
  Spontaneous chordal rupture
  Collagen vascular disease
  Trauma: pentrating and nonpenetrating
Functional Mitral Regurgitation
  Coronary artery disease
  Hypertrophic cardiomyopathy
  Dilated cardiomyopathy
  Left atrial dilatation

nervous system. Thus, the clinical presentation of mitral valve prolapse varies from one that is similar to other forms of mitral regurgitation to a unique presentation that is dominated by extracardiac manifestations.

In **chronic mitral regurgitation,** the more common of the two general clinical presentations, the mitral regurgitation progressively worsens as the underlying heart disease worsens. In this situation, the heart has time to adapt to the mitral leak. The increased pressure in the left atrium during systole causes left atrial dilatation. If this is not adequate to decompress the left atrial pressure, the pulmonary arterial tone increases to protect the pulmonary capillaries from increased hydrostatic pressure, resulting in pulmonary hypertension. Because the regurgitated blood returns to the left ventricle in diastole, along with the normal atrial stroke volume, the volume load on the left ventricle results in left ventricular dilatation and eccentric hypertrophy.

Initially, the loading conditions in mitral regurgitation enhance left ventricular performance because preload is increased and afterload is normal. Preload is increased by the augmentation of left ventricular diastolic volume, which increases left ventricular systolic function via the Frank-Starling mechanism. Afterload, or the left ventricular wall tension after the aortic valve opens in systole, is not increased, despite increased left ventricular volume, because much of the increased volume is regurgitated into the left atrium in early systole before the aortic valve opens and because the continued regurgitation during systole reduces forward stroke volume and blood pressure. As the severity of mitral regurgitation increases over time, the ability of the dilated left ventricle to augment systolic function reaches its limits, left ventricular systolic function falls, and heart failure ensues.

Acute mitral regurgitation presents differently because there is insufficient time for these compensatory mechanisms to develop. Sudden rupture of the chordae tendineae, for example, may result in severe acute mitral regurgitation, which markedly increases left atrial pressure. Because the left atrium has no time to dilate, the pulmonary capillary pressure rises markedly, and pulmonary edema usually ensues. The left ventricle also does not dilate adequately to handle the tremendous volume load, and forward failure occurs because of an impaired left ventricular stroke volume. Acute mitral regurgitation (caused by the abrupt failure of a component of the mitral apparatus) can precipitate or aggravate symptoms in a patient with chronic mitral regurgitation.

Clinical Findings

A. SYMPTOMS AND SIGNS

1. Chronic mitral regurgitation—The medical history of patients with chronic mitral regurgitation may suggest its cause. Look for a possible history of acute rheumatic fever, coronary artery disease, or a cardiomyopathy. The most common symptom in patients with chronic mitral regurgitation is progressive dyspnea, beginning with dyspnea on exertion and progressing to paroxysmal nocturnal dyspnea and finally orthopnea. Patients may also complain of fatigue and other symptoms associated with congestive heart failure, such as edema. Chronic mitral regurgitation can lead to atrial fibrillation, and patients may present with palpitations or other symptoms related to this rhythm disturbance. Some patients with mitral valve prolapse may present with atypical chest pain, inappropriate sympathetic nervous system activation (eg, tachycardia, orthostatic hypotension), or even panic attacks.

2. Acute mitral regurgitation—The patient with acute mitral regurgitation is usually markedly symptomatic, with severe orthopnea or frank pulmonary edema. Although sudden pulmonary edema in itself may suggest the diagnosis, other features of the history may point to the cause of mitral apparatus failure, such as a history of acute myocardial infarction, uncontrolled hypertension, or symptoms of infectious endocarditis.

B. PHYSICAL EXAMINATION

1. Chronic mitral regurgitation—In chronic mitral regurgitation, the heart rate may be increased because of atrial fibrillation or heart failure. The carotid pulse is usually brief and of low amplitude, and blood pressure examination shows a narrow pulse pressure. These findings reflect the reduced forward stroke volume. In the presence of heart failure, the respiratory rate may be increased and rales, pleural effusion, edema, increased jugular venous pressure, or ascites may be present. Left ventricular enlargement may result in an enlarged apical impulse. The first and second heart sounds are usually normal, and the pulmonic component of the second heart sound may be increased if pulmonary hypertension is evident. A third heart sound is common because of the left ventricular volume overload, but it does not necessarily indicate heart failure. A fourth heart sound is unusual unless associated coronary artery disease or hypertension is present. The characteristic murmur of chronic mitral regurgitation is usually holosystolic and heard best at the apex, with radiation to the axilla. Occasionally, in patients with posterior leaflet defects, the direction of the regurgitant jet may be anterior, and the murmur is heard in the aortic area. With anterior leaflet defects, the direction of the mitral jet may be posterior and be transmitted to the back, where it can be heard up and down the spine. Some reports even note hearing this murmur with the stethoscope on the top of the head. In patients with mitral valve prolapse, the murmur can be crescendo and late systolic. This type of murmur, in fact, almost always represents mitral regurgitation. Often, the late systolic crescendo murmur of mitral valve prolapse is preceded by a midsystolic click from the sudden tensing of the prolapsing leaflets when the end of chordal tethering is reached. Some patients may manifest only a midsystolic click. Occasionally, mitral murmurs will be honking or musical in quality, presumably from a prolapsing leaflet that vibrates in the regurgitant stream. Some patients occasionally have other murmur configurations, whereas others with echocardiographically documented mitral regurgitation have no audible murmur, especially if the regurgitation is mild.

Because murmur configuration and radiation vary in mitral regurgitation, dynamic auscultation is of a great deal of value at the bedside for differentiating this murmur from other heart murmurs. Handgrip exercise is the favored bedside maneuver because it frequently increases the intensity of a mitral regurgitation murmur. In patients with poor grip strength, transient arterial occlusion with two blood pressure cuffs, one on each arm, is useful for producing the same effect (Table 11–2, and Chapter 1). The murmur of mitral valve prolapse behaves like that of mitral regurgitation from any cause, but it has a few unique features. Any maneuver that increases left ventricular volume will (as noted earlier) decrease the amount of mitral valve prolapse and decrease the amount of mitral regurgitation, thereby lessening the intensity of the murmur. Thus, rapid squatting will diminish the murmur of mitral valve prolapse and move the timing of the click-murmur complex later in systole (Figure 11–1). Conversely, maneuvers that decrease left ventricular volume increase the intensity

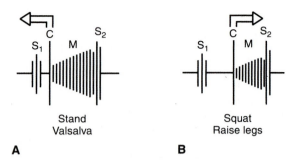

Figure 11–1. Change in the position of the click (C)-murmur (M) complex during systole and the intensity of the murmur as a result of bedside maneuvers. **A:** Maneuvers that lengthen the murmur and increase intensity. **B:** Maneuvers that shorten the murmur and reduce its intensity. Note that the position of the midsystolic click also changes with these maneuvers.

and duration of the murmur of mitral valve prolapse. Thus, standing rapidly from a squatting position will make the murmur louder and move the click-murmur complex toward early systole. Extreme left ventricular volume increases can eliminate the click-murmur and mitral regurgitation, and extreme decrease can result in a pansystolic murmur without a click. Consequently, the auscultatory findings in mitral valve prolapse vary greatly, which can make accurate clinical diagnosis difficult.

2. Acute mitral regurgitation—In acute mitral regurgitation the physical findings are different. The marked

Table 11–2. Differentiation of systolic murmurs based on changes in their intensity from physiologic maneuvers.

Maneuver	Flow	TR	AS	MR/VSD	MVP	HOCM
				Origin of Murmur		
Inspiration	– or ↑	↑	—	—	—	—
Stand	↓	—	—	—	↑	↑
Squat	↑	—	—	—	↓	↓
Valsalva's maneuver	↓	↓	↓	↓	↑	↑
Handgrip/TAO	↓	—	—	↑	↑	↓
Post-PVC	↑	—	↑	—	—	↑

AS = aortic stenosis; Flow = benign flow murmur; HOCM = hypertrophic obstructive cardiomyopathy; MR = mitral regurgitation; MVP = mitral valve prolapse; PVC = premature ventricular contraction; TAO = transient arterial occlusion; TR = tricuspid regurgitation; VSD = ventricular septal defect; ↑ = increase in murmur intensity; ↓ = decrease in murmur intensity; — = no predictable change.

increase in left atrial pressure, caused by regurgitation into a noncompliant left atrium, may raise left atrial pressure in late systole to the point that there is no longer any gradient for regurgitant flow. The murmur thus becomes an early systolic murmur rather than the holosystolic murmur characteristic of patients with chronic mitral regurgitation. In fact, when the acute mitral regurgitation is very severe, the murmur may not be audible. In mild-to-moderate acute mitral regurgitation, the murmur responds like the murmur of chronic mitral regurgitation with dynamic auscultation. More severe acute regurgitation is associated with high catecholamine tone and a lack of responsiveness to bedside maneuvers. Other characteristic features of acute mitral regurgitation include a fourth heart sound caused by vigorous atrial contraction following exaggerated expansion during ventricular systole (atrial diastole). In the presence of pulmonary hypertension, the pulmonary second sound increases, and murmurs of pulmonic and tricuspid regurgitation may be present. As mentioned earlier, acute mitral regurgitation invariably results in pulmonary edema. Consequently, the patient will have an increased respiratory rate, diffuse rales, evidence of plural effusion, increased heart rate, a narrow pulse pressure with low systolic blood pressure, and signs of acute right-heart failure, such as increased jugular venous pressure.

3. Mixed valvular disease—Patients with rheumatic valvular disease often have mixed mitral disease, which is defined as at least 2+ (on a scale of 1–4; see following section on Echocardiography) mitral regurgitation, with a mean mitral valve diastolic gradient of more than 10 mm Hg. The clinical course of mixed mitral valve disease is similar to that of mitral regurgitation, and such patients should be treated similarly. Aortic regurgitation frequently occurs with mitral regurgitation, either because of left ventricular dilatation or because the same disease process affects the aortic valve (eg, Marfan's syndrome). This places an additional volume load on the left ventricle and usually accelerates the patient's clinical deterioration.

When aortic stenosis and mitral regurgitation occur together, it is sometimes difficult to ascertain whether the same disease process (eg, rheumatic disease) involved both valves or whether the pressure load of significant aortic stenosis altered left ventricular geometry, performance, or both, resulting in functional mitral regurgitation. Diagnostic imaging studies usually resolve this issue and help direct therapy.

C. DIAGNOSTIC STUDIES

1. Electrocardiography—Patients with chronic mitral regurgitation may have evidence of left ventricular hypertrophy, left atrial abnormality, and, sometimes, right ventricular enlargement. Patients with coronary artery disease might have evidence of myocardial infarction or ischemia. Electrocardiographic (ECG) exercise testing is usually done only to confirm the patient's physical limitations, because ECG changes in the face of a left ventricular volume load are not likely to be accurate for the diagnosis of coronary artery disease. Ambulatory ECG monitoring is occasionally done in patients with palpitations to document atrial fibrillation or other intermittent rhythm disorders.

2. Chest radiograph—In cases of chronic mitral regurgitation, an enlarged left ventricle and left atrium would be expected. In severe regurgitation, right-heart enlargement and pulmonary hypertension may be evident. Patients in heart failure will show pulmonary congestion and pleural effusions. In acute mitral regurgitation, there are often signs of pulmonary congestion without enlargement of the heart.

3. Echocardiography—The color-flow Doppler identification of a systolic regurgitant jet across the mitral valve into the left atrium is diagnostic of mitral regurgitation. There are several ways of estimating the severity of mitral regurgitation by analyzing the characteristics of the regurgitant jet on color-flow Doppler. The first method is the depth of penetration of the jet into the left atrium. A penetration of 1 cm or less is considered mild; 2–3 cm, moderate; and 4 cm or more, severe. If the jet is very narrow, the actual volume of regurgitant flow may not be as great as occurs with a more voluminous flow disturbance that penetrates to the same depth. Some investigators have therefore suggested also taking the area of the jet into consideration. One problem with this assessment system, however, is that if the jet impinges on a wall of the left atrium, it appears to penetrate less and be of a smaller area than if it is free in the atrial cavity. There is thus a tendency to underestimate the severity of mitral regurgitation when the jet hits the walls. In addition, a regurgitant jet of any size occurring in a large left atrium will not appear as impressive as the same size jet in a small left atrium.

For these reasons, there has been interest in looking at the proximal isovelocity surface area maps observed where flow acceleration and convergence occur on the left ventricular side of the mitral leaflets. Fluid dynamics theory states that flow through an isovelocity surface is equal to the velocity times the surface area, which yields instantaneous regurgitant flow. This technique uses the color-flow Doppler color change inter-faces observed with accelerating velocity through the orifice to estimate isovelocity surface area. The clinician can also determine the size of the leak in the mitral valve by evaluating the jet in a cross-sectional plane at the level of the mitral valve. This method gives an estimate of the size of the hole through which the jet is originating.

Assessment of pulmonary venous flow velocity by pulsed Doppler echocardiography can also be of value in estimating the severity of mitral regurgitation. Normal pulmonary venous flow velocity is biphasic, with a predominant systolic forward velocity and a lesser diastolic forward velocity. Systolic forward velocity is reduced in patients with mitral regurgitation, and often the diastolic velocity predominates. In severe mitral regurgitation the systolic flow in the pulmonary vein signal may reverse. Unfortunately, pulmonary venous flow velocity patterns vary considerably in patients with mitral regurgitation, and the predictive value for regurgitation severity is low. Systolic flow reversal is highly specific for severe regurgitation, but sensitivity is low.. In many laboratories, all these factors are integrated to produce a composite estimate of the severity of regurgitation, usually on a scale of 1 to 4, with 4 being severe mitral regurgitation.

Doppler echocardiography can be used to quantitate regurgitant flow, which is perhaps the most accurate method for determining the severity of mitral regurgitation. The principle used is that of flow continuity. Systolic flow out the left ventricular outflow tract represents the forward flow out of the heart. This can be determined by multiplying the outflow tract area (measured on the two-dimensional echocardiographic image) times the outflow tract systolic velocity-time integral. Flow across the mitral valve in diastole represents the total flow (forward plus regurgitant flow) and can be determined by multiplying mitral annulus area times the diastolic velocity-time integral. Regurgitant flow is the difference between total and forward flow. Typically the regurgitant flow is reported as the regurgitant fraction, which is the regurgitant flow divided by the total flow. Regurgitant fractions > 60% denote severe mitral regurgitation, 40–60% is moderate, and 20–40% is mild. Unfortunately, the calculation of regurgitant flow has many possible sources of error, the largest of which is measuring the flow areas—mitral annular and outflow tract. Thus, individuals without valvular regurgitation can have regurgitant fractions of up to 20%. Also, the calculation of regurgitant flow is time-consuming and requires considerable skill. In addition, no study shows this method to be superior to semiquantitative and qualitative estimates of mitral regurgitant severity for clinical decision making. Consequently, most echocardiographic laboratories do not routinely measure regurgitant flow.

Echocardiography can be used to evaluate the anatomy of the mitral apparatus to determine where the defect lies and what its cause may be. For example, patients with rheumatic mitral valve disease have thickening of the mitral leaflets, especially at the tips, with rolled edges and regurgitation along the commissural fissure lines. Patients with mitral valve prolapse have voluminous mitral leaflets that prolapse into the left atrium in the latter part of systole. Patients with coronary artery disease have wall motion abnormalities near the papillary muscle attachments. Ruptured and flail chordae tendineae are readily detected by echocardiography, as is mitral annular calcification.

The echocardiogram is also useful for assessing the compensatory changes in the cardiovascular system resulting from mitral regurgitation. The degree of left ventricular and left atrial enlargement are related to the severity of the mitral regurgitation and its chronicity. Left ventricular systolic performance is an important determinant of prognosis in mitral regurgitation (see Prognosis). Doppler estimation of pulmonary artery pressures from pulmonic or tricuspid regurgitant jets is valuable for estimating the effect of mitral regurgitation on the pulmonary circulation. An assessment of right-heart chamber sizes and function is additional useful information. Echocardiography is also used for differentiating other conditions, such as ventricular septal defect, aortic stenosis, and hypertrophic obstructive cardiomyopathy, that might be confused on history and physical examination with mitral regurgitation.

Color-flow Doppler echocardiography can detect trivial or mild mitral regurgitation in up to half of otherwise healthy adults. The incidence increases with age and with the rigor with which the operator interrogates the valve. In the absence of anatomic abnormalities, small degrees of regurgitation are probably benign effects of aging. In most cases, mild mitral regurgitation found by echocardiography is not associated with a murmur on physical examination.

4. Radionuclide studies—Radionuclide angiography assesses regurgitant fraction by estimating right and left ventricular stroke volumes, subtracting one from the other, and dividing the difference by the left ventricular stroke volume. The result is an estimate of how much of the left ventricular stroke volume is mitral regurgitation. Unfortunately, this technique is not highly accurate, and regurgitant fractions of up to 20% can be observed in normal individuals. The estimation of left ventricular volume and ejection fraction are more useful and have prognostic implications in mitral regurgitation. Patients suspected of having coronary artery disease may be candidates for rest and exercise perfusion scanning. In patients with moderately severe to severe mitral regurgitation, however, the accuracy of perfusion scanning is questionable, and such patients might be better evaluated using coronary angiography.

5. Cardiac catheterization—Cardiac catheterization is rarely needed to diagnose mitral regurgitation, nor is it usually needed to assess the severity of the regurgitation, left ventricular size and function, or any resultant pulmonary hypertension. Coronary angiography is useful, however, for establishing artery disease as the likely cause of mitral regurgitation as well as the risk from surgical correction of mitral regurgitation from any cause.

Hemodynamic evaluation at the time of cardiac catheterization in patients with moderate-to-severe mitral regurgitation will show an increase in pulmonary artery pressures, increases in the pulmonary capillary wedge pressure (PCWP), and possibly a reduction in forward cardiac output. The PCWP tracing often displays a large v wave, which is more than 50% greater than the height of the a wave. Although much has been made of the diagnostic value of large v waves in the PCWP tracing (especially in the ICU setting) it must be remembered that any cause of left atrial pressure elevation will elevate the height of the v wave. It is only when the v wave is elevated out of proportion to the a wave that the diagnosis of mitral regurgitation is likely (> 150% of the a wave).

Left ventricular angiography can confirm the presence of mitral regurgitation, and its severity can be graded in a similar 1–4+ system, where 1+ is mild and 4+ indicates regurgitation of the angiographic dye into the pulmonary veins. This assessment method correlates well with the color-flow Doppler system. In addition, left ventricular angiography is useful for estimating left ventricular volume and ejection fraction. Cardiac catheterization can exclude the presence of other diseases, such as ventricular septal defect, hypertrophic obstructive cardiomyopathy, and aortic stenosis, that might be confused with mitral regurgitation. Certain aspects of the patient's hemodynamics, such as the presence of pulmonary hypertension, are of prognostic value in mitral regurgitation.

Enriquez-Sarano M, Dujardin KS, Tribouilloy CM et al: Determinants of pulmonary venous flow reversal in mitral regurgitation and its usefulness for determining the severity of regurgitation. Am J Cardiol 1999;83:535.

Hall SA, Brickner ME, Willet DL et al: Assessment of mitral regurgitation severity by Doppler color flow mapping of the vena contracta. Circulation 1997;95:636.

Pu M, Thomas JD, Vandervoort PM et al: Comparison of quantitative and semiquantitative methods for assessing mitral regurgitation by transesophageal endocardiography. Am J Cardiol 2001;87:66.

Simpson IA, Shiota T, Gharib M et al Current status of flow convergence for clinical applications: Is it a leaning tower of PISA? J Am Coll Cardiol 1996;27:504.

Differential Diagnosis

Because the symptoms seen in chronic mitral regurgitation are not specific for this condition, the physical examination is crucial for the differential diagnosis. The murmur of tricuspid regurgitation, for example, can occasionally be heard at the apex, especially if the right ventricle is enlarged and displaced leftward. Differentiating features include the increase in the intensity of the murmur with inspiration, the large v waves in the jugular pulse, a right ventricular lift, and a pulsatile liver. It should be noted that tricuspid regurgitation can result from pulmonary hypertension caused by mitral regurgitation, so some patients have both murmurs. In this situation, the murmur of tricuspid regurgitation is best assessed at the left or right sternal border, and those of mitral regurgitation at the apex. It may be difficult, however, to distinguish between the two murmurs in patients where both are moderately severe.

The murmur of **aortic stenosis** is often confused with mitral regurgitation, especially when the mitral regurgitant murmur is atypical or radiates to the aortic area. The murmur of aortic stenosis is usually lower in pitch than that of mitral regurgitation; it radiates to the neck and is often accompanied by an S_4 sound. In aortic stenosis the left ventricular apical impulse amplitude often increases, but not necessarily in size, as is found in patients with mitral regurgitation. On dynamic auscultation, there is no change in the murmur of aortic stenosis with handgrip exercise, but the murmur does increase in the beat following a premature ventricular contraction. Perhaps the best bedside maneuver for distinguishing between these two murmurs is the inhalation of amyl nitrite. This potent vasodilator causes the murmur of aortic stenosis to become louder and that of mitral regurgitation softer.

A **ventricular septal defect,** especially a muscular defect low in the septum, may mimic the murmur of mitral regurgitation. Because dynamic auscultation will not distinguish between these two left ventricular regurgitant murmurs, other signs must be used. The patient with ventricular septal defect usually has a large right ventricle, and a vibration (thrill) over the anterior chest may be palpable. The murmur of **hypertrophic obstructive cardiomyopathy (HOCM)** can also be confused with mitral regurgitation. The major differential features are that the murmur of HOCM increases with Valsalva's maneuver, whereas the murmur of mitral regurgitation decreases; the murmur of HOCM decreases with handgrip, and the murmur of mitral regurgitation increases. In addition, the patient with HOCM usually has a prominent fourth heart sound. However, because many patients with HOCM also have mitral regurgitation, the ability to distinguish it from mitral regurgitation is difficult in some patients.

The murmur of **mitral valve prolapse** can be difficult to distinguish from the murmur of HOCM because both murmurs change in intensity and in a similar direction with the stand and squat and Valsalva maneuvers.

In this situation, other features of each disease, such as the midsystolic click with mitral valve prolapse and the left ventricular hypertrophy evident on palpation of the chest, or the fourth heart sound in the patient with HOCM, are useful for differentiating the two conditions by physical examination. The major differential diagnosis of acute mitral regurgitation is acute **ventricular septal defect** (VSD) because both may occur in the setting of acute myocardial infarction. A palpable vibration is more common, and the right ventricle is usually more prominent with VSD, but perhaps the best differentiation is that the patient with acute VSD has much less dyspnea than does the patient with acute mitral regurgitation. The response to dynamic auscultation is the same in these two conditions.

Treatment

A. PHARMACOLOGIC THERAPY

Vasodilators are useful in acute mitral regurgitation to decrease aortic pressure and impedance, favoring forward over regurgitant flow during systole.

This decreases left ventricular size and left ventricular and atrial pressures, improves forward cardiac output, and decreases the amount of regurgitation. Studies of acute regurgitation with vasodilators, such as hydralazine, nifedipine, and nitroprusside, have demonstrated this effect in the hemodynamics laboratory and, thus, their usefulness for managing acute mitral regurgitation. Studies on the pharmacologic treatment of patients with chronic mitral regurgitation are scant, and the available data are not particularly encouraging. Because afterload is not increased in patients with well-compensated chronic mitral regurgitation, lowering it further may not improve forward flow and would more likely reduce it. Many patients experience vasodilator side effects, and if forward cardiac output is not improved, the patient's overall hemodynamic status is actually worsened. Thus, until further data are obtained there is no evidence to support vasodilator therapy for asymptomatic patients with mitral regurgitation. In mildly symptomatic patients who presumably have left ventricular dilation and dysfunction, but want to avoid surgery, vasodilators could be tried. Markedly symptomatic patients, however, are better treated surgically.

1. Digoxin—Digoxin is useful in atrial fibrillation for controlling the heart rate. Whether it is of any value for improving forward output with mitral regurgitation in patients with normal sinus rhythm is unknown. If there are other indications for using the drug, however, it is not known to be harmful to the overall hemodynamic status of patients with mitral regurgitation.

2. Oral anticoagulation—Oral anticogulation is indicated for patients in atrial fibrillation and those with concomitant mitral stenosis. Whether patients with moderate-to-severe mitral regurgitation, with large left ventricles and large left atria, who are in normal sinus rhythm and have normal left ventricular function would benefit from anticoagulants is controversial. Eccentric regurgitant jets may produce areas of stasis in the left atrium, according to color-flow Doppler studies. Furthermore, patients with moderate-to-severe mitral regurgitation are always at risk for developing atrial fibrillation. Although an argument can be made for

chronic anticoagulation in such patients, no clinical trials support this approach.

3. Antibiotic prophylaxis—All patients with mitral regurgitation require antibiotics to prevent the development of bacterial endocarditis. Patients in whom rheumatic heart disease is the likely cause of mitral regurgitation should also have rheumatic fever antibiotic prophylaxis.

B. SURGICAL TREATMENT

Patients with acute, severe, or decompensated chronic severe mitral regurgitation will need urgent surgical therapy—if it is appropriate to their general medical condition. Such patients can usually be stabilized with intravenous vasodilators, such as hydralazine or nitroprusside, and other therapies for heart failure, such as diuretics. If there is no response to pharmacologic therapy, an intraaortic balloon pump is indicated. This mechanical approach will reduce arterial and left ventricular pressure in systole, favoring forward flow rather than regurgitant and increased diastolic aortic pressure, and may improve left ventricular contractility. Most patients will stabilize on this therapy, allowing for an appropriate evaluation (eg, coronary angiography), thereby maximizing the benefits of surgery.

Patients with either acute or chronic moderately severe mitral regurgitation will eventually need surgical therapy. The issue is the appropriate timing of surgery. If the physician waits until the symptomatology is marked because of left heart failure with depressed left ventricular systolic function and severe pulmonary hypertension, the patient often does not achieve much symptomatic improvement after surgery, and left ventricular function remains depressed. On the other hand, if surgery is performed earlier, the patient may become relatively asymptomatic, with normal left ventricular function. Considerable effort has been directed at determining prognostic indicators for avoiding a poor response to surgical therapy. Prospective studies have shown that an ejection fraction of 0.60 or less and an end-systolic volume index of 50 mL/m^2 or more, or an end-diastolic dimension on echocardiography of 45 mm or more, significant pulmonary hypertension, and atrial fibrillation are all markers of a poor prognosis following surgery. Although it seems logical that surgery should therefore be performed before these indicators are obtained in a patient, even one who is asymptomatic, this decision analysis has never been tested in clinical trials (Table 11–3).

In patients with aortic and mitral regurgitation, if the mitral valve is not obviously diseased and the mitral regurgitation is mild to moderate, (1–2+), replacing the aortic valve will often diminish left ventricular size enough to reduce or eliminate the mitral regurgitation. Sometimes a mitral annular ring will be required to reduce mitral annular size. In cases where the mitral valve

Table 11–3. General indications for considering mitral valve surgery in patients with chronic severe organic mitral regurgitation.

Symptoms such as dyspnea
Left ventricular ejection fraction < 0.60
Left ventricular end-systolic dimension > 45 mm
Left ventricular end-systolic volume index > 50 mL/m²
Atrial fibrillation
Pulmonary artery systolic pressure > 50 mm Hg

leaflets and chordae are diseased or the regurgitation is severe, valve repair or replacement will be necessary—at the cost of a higher likelihood of operative mortality or postoperative morbidity. Severe aortic stenosis is often accompanied by mild-to-moderate mitral regurgitation. In this situation, the reduction in left ventricular pressure produced by aortic valve replacement usually reduces the mitral regurgitation, and further mitral surgery can be avoided.

The pulmonary hypertension that often accompanies mitral regurgitation may lead to tricuspid and pulmonic regurgitation. The latter usually resolves when the pulmonary pressure is reduced by mitral valve surgery, and pulmonary valve replacement is rarely necessary. Tricuspid regurgitation, if mild-to-moderate and associated with moderately severe pulmonary hypertension, will usually resolve after successful mitral surgery. If the tricuspid regurgitation is moderately severe but the leaflets are not diseased, a tricuspid ring may be effective; if tricuspid valve disease is present, repair or replacement will be necessary. One clinical guideline for the need for tricuspid valve repair or replacement is a mean right atrial pressure of more than 15 mm Hg; however, the decision for this is often made during surgery, after the mitral procedure has been completed.

The onset of heart failure symptoms should prompt consideration of surgical treatment. Some patients develop symptoms such as dyspnea, fatigue, and edema prior to developing the clinical and hemodynamic signs and symptoms of mitral regurgitation. The importance of other symptoms, such as a history of arrhythmias or recurrent systemic emboli, is less certain. If the hemodynamic indicators are absent, other therapies for these conditions should be attempted first, before surgery.

Other factors to be taken into account when deciding when to perform surgery are the type of operation—valve repair or replacement–and the type of prosthetic valve, should one be needed. It is now possible in many patients with mitral regurgitation to repair rather than replace the mitral valve. Patients with mitral valve prolapse, ruptured chordae tendineae, or a ruptured papillary muscle are especially likely to respond to reparative surgery, whereas patients with markedly deformed valves and fused chordae from rheumatic heart disease, patients with infective endocarditis, or patients with left ventricular disease are less likely to be helped by mitral valve repair and often require valve replacement. Repair is preferable, especially for the patient with normal sinus rhythm because there is no need for long-term anticoagulation therapy following surgery. In addition, mitral valve repair is generally associated with better preservation of left ventricular systolic function following surgery and is therefore highly advantageous for patients with a low left ventricular ejection fraction and a repairable mitral valve. Thus, if it is likely that mitral valve repair can be done, there is less reluctance about operating in asymptomatic patients that otherwise meet criteria for surgery.

If valve replacement is necessary, ventricular function can be preserved by leaving the chordae intact; chordal tethering of the papillary muscles is presumed to improve left ventricular performance. With valve replacement, the choice between a mechanical and a bioprosthetic valve may influence the timing of surgery.

In general, mechanical prosthetic valves are preferred because of their better long-term reliability. Bioprosthetic valves can be chosen when valve longevity is not an issue or when patients want to try to avoid anticoagulation therapy. The latter would apply mainly to young women with normal sinus rhythm who want to become pregnant. They will be much easier to treat without anticoagulation therapy—a feasible goal with a bioprosthetic valve. These patients must realize, however, that this valve will need to be replaced in approximately 10–15 years, as a result of deterioration. This should give these patients time for several pregnancies, if they so desire.

Generally, patients with no contraindications to anticoagulation therapy should be treated with such agents, regardless of valve type. The incidence of systemic emboli is higher with mitral than with aortic prosthetic valves (despite the lower incidence found with bioprosthetic valves); however, without anticoagulation, there is still a 1–3% per year chance of systemic emboli with a bioprosthetic valve in the mitral position. Some clinicians advocate aspirin therapy for patients with bioprosthetic valves who do not wish to use anticoagulants; this approach seems reasonable. Some data suggest the efficacy of aspirin in this situation, but whether it is as protective as warfarin therapy is unknown at present.

Prognosis

Patients with chronic mitral regurgitation have an average survival curve similar to that of patients with chronic aortic regurgitation and chronic mitral stenosis.

The cause of the chronic mitral regurgitation in individual patients influences the prognosis. In general, patients with coronary artery disease as the cause have a poor prognosis, those with the myxomatous changes of mitral valve prolapse have the best prognosis, and those with rheumatic heart disease have an intermediate prognosis, depending on the number of recurrent episodes of acute rheumatic fever. The onset of infectious endocarditis can markedly alter the prognosis. In addition, any sudden deterioration of mitral valve function that leads to acute worsening of the mitral regurgitation lessens the prognosis.

The prognosis in acute mitral regurgitation, when it is associated with acute pulmonary edema and severe symptoms, is guarded; it also depends on the cause. For example, patients with acute severe mitral regurgitation from acute myocardial infarction have a much worse prognosis than do otherwise healthy individuals who

rupture a chorda. In general, most patients with acute mitral regurgitation require immediate surgical attention, and their prognosis is not as good as that for patients with chronic mitral regurgitation.

Bonow RO, Carabello B, DeLeon AC Jr et al: ACC/AHA Guidelines for the management of patients with valvular heart disease. J Am Coll Cardiol 1998;32:1486.

Carobello BA, Crawford FA: Valvular heart disease. N Engl J Med 1997;337:32.

Enriquez-Sarano, Schaff HV, Orszulak TA M et al: Valve repair improves outcome of surgery for mitral regurgitation: A multivariate analysis. Circulation 1995;91:1022.

Hung J, Otsuji Y, Handschumacher MD et al: Mechanism of dynamic regurgitant orifice area variation in functional mitral regurgitation: Physiologic insights from the proximal flow convergence technique. J Am Coll Cardiol 1999;33:538.

Ling LH, Enriquez-Sarano M, Seward JB et al: Clinical outcome of mitral regurgitation due to flail leaflet. N Engl J Med 1996;335:1417.

Tricuspid and Pulmonic Valve Disease

12

Brian D. Hoit, MD & Michael D. Faulx, MD

TRICUSPID VALVE DISEASE

ESSENTIALS OF DIAGNOSIS

Tricuspid regurgitation
- *Prominent v wave in jugular venous pulse*
- *Systolic murmur at left lower sternal border that increases with inspiration*
- *Characteristic Doppler echocardiographic findings*

Tricuspid stenosis
- *Prominent a wave and reduced y descent in jugular venous pulse*
- *Diastolic murmur at left lower sternal border that increases with inspiration*
- *Characteristic Doppler echocardiographic findings*

General Considerations

Because valvular heart disease is an important cause of cardiovascular morbidity and mortality, clinical interest in tricuspid valve disorders has increased. Several factors account for this interest: High-resolution, noninvasive imaging techniques (primarily echocardiographic), which assess the tricuspid valve's structure and function, have been developed and validated. The frequency of tricuspid valve endocarditis has increased significantly, owing largely to an increasing population of intravenous drug abusers, patients with implanted cardiac devices or long-term central venous catheters, and, to a lesser extent, a growing number of patients with impaired host defenses. Several reparative surgical techniques with acceptable morbidity and mortality rates now exist. In addition, investigations in both animals and humans have demonstrated the influence of right-heart disease on cardiovascular performance vis-à-vis series and parallel interactions with the left ventricle.

Pathophysiology & Etiology

The tricuspid valve has three leaflets that are unequal in size (anterior > septal > posterior). The papillary muscles are not as well defined as those of the left ventricle and are subject to considerable variation in both their size and leaflet support. Like the mitral valve, the leaflets, annulus, chordae, papillary muscles, and contiguous myocardium contribute individually to normal valve function and can be altered by pathophysiologic processes (Table 12–1).

A. TRICUSPID REGURGITATION

Tricuspid regurgitation most frequently occurs with a structurally normal tricuspid valve (functional tricuspid regurgitation); a dilated right ventricle and annulus and papillary muscle dysfunction are common.

Functional tricuspid regurgitation is usually caused by disease of the left heart (eg, left ventricular [LV] dysfunction, mitral valve disease), but disease of the pulmonary vasculature (eg, primary pulmonary hypertension) or the right ventricle (eg, right ventricular infarct, arrhythmogenic right ventricular [RV] dysplasia) may be responsible.

Rheumatic tricuspid regurgitation almost always occurs in association with mitral valve involvement. Although two-thirds of patients with rheumatic mitral valve disease have pathologic evidence of tricuspid valve involvement, clinically significant tricuspid disease, which generally affects young and middle-aged women, is much less common. Rheumatic tricuspid involvement is usually mild and generally is shown clinically as pure regurgitation or mixed insufficiency and stenosis.

Tricuspid valve endocarditis, which occurs primarily in intravenous drug users and patients with chronic intravascular hardware, may complicate left-to-right shunts, burns, and immunocompromised states. The disease is typically caused by virulent pathogens that infect structurally normal valves. *Staphylococcus aureus* is the most common organism; *Pseudomonas* and *Candida* species also predominate, and polymicrobial infections are not uncommon. Fungal endocarditis should be considered when vegetations are large; occasionally,

Table 12–1. Causes of tricuspid valve disease.

Tricuspid Regurgitation	Tricuspid Stenosis
Functional (structurally normal tricuspid valve)	Rheumatic
Rheumatic	Carcinoid heart disease
Infective endocarditis	Tumors
Congenital (eg, tricuspid valve prolapse, Ebstein's anomaly)	Congenital (eg, Ebstein's anomaly)
Carcinoid heart disease	Regional cardiac tamponade
Systemic lupus erythematosus	Systemic lupus erythematosus
Catheter-induced	Whipple's disease
Trauma	Fabry's disease
Tumors	Infective endocarditis
Orthotopic heart transplantation	Endomyocardial fibrosis
Endomyocardial fibrosis	Endocardial fibroelastosis
Antiphospholipid syndrome	Methysergide therapy
	Antiphospholipid syndrome

they cause obstruction. Abscesses may involve the annulus and septum, and chordal rupture or valve perforations may cause tricuspid regurgitation.

Endocardial deposition of myofibromatous tissue leads to thickening and immobilization of the tricuspid valve in more than half of the patients.

Carcinoid tumors are a rare cause of both tricuspid and pulmonic valve disease. The vasoactive substances (principally serotonin) produced by these tumors are felt to be causal, and patients with carcinoid valvular disease have higher serum levels of serotonin and increased urinary excretion of its metabolite, 5-hydroxyindoleacetic acid (5-HIAA) than those without cardiac disease. Left-sided valve involvement is unusual due to inactivation of these vasoactive molecules by monoamine oxidase in the lungs. Tricuspid regurgitation is the most common lesion and is detected by echocardiography in virtually all patients with carcinoid tricuspid valve disease. Cardiac involvement is progressive and causes significant morbidity and mortality in such patients. Long-term survival has been reported after tricuspid valve replacement, but carcinoid plaque may deposit on the bioprosthetic leaflets.

Tricuspid valve prolapse is seen almost exclusively in patients with mitral valve prolapse and occurs in as many as 50% of cases. Isolated involvement has been confirmed, however, by both echocardiography and necropsy. Anterior leaflet prolapse is most common, followed by septal and posterior leaflet prolapse. The associated tricuspid regurgitation is usually mild. Although tricuspid valve prolapse may be a marker of generalized connective tissue disease and a poor prognostic indicator in patients with mitral valve prolapse, its clinical significance remains undefined. Like mitral valve prolapse, the precise incidence of tricuspid valve

prolapse is difficult to determine because of inconsistent clinical, echocardiographic, and angiographic definitions.

Tricuspid regurgitation is a frequent component of **Ebstein's anomaly** of the tricuspid valve because of the apical displacement of septal and posterior tricuspid leaflets. This results in atrialization of a variable portion of the right ventricle and a range of abnormalities involving the anterior leaflet and atrial septum. The downward displacement of the tricuspid valve frequently causes a tricuspid regurgitant murmur (heard best in the apical area). This uncommon congenital abnormality is associated with right-to-left intraatrial shunting, cyanosis, right ventricular dysfunction, and arrhythmias.

Tricuspid regurgitation of at least moderate severity may complicate as much as 25% of cases of **systemic lupus erythematosus;** significant tricuspid regurgitation is usually due to the pulmonary hypertension produced by lupus pulmonary disease. Libman-Sacks endocarditis that involves the tricuspid valve is far less common.

The **antiphospholipid syndrome** (antiphospholipid antibodies, vascular thrombosis, fetal loss and thrombocytopenia) has been recognized recently as a cause of valvular heart disease, including isolated tricuspid involvement. The cause of the valve disease is poorly understood, but intravalvular capillary thrombosis is felt to be a factor. Most patients present with combined tricuspid regurgitation and stenosis, and the regurgitation is typically moderate or severe. Pulmonary hypertension is usually present, and contributes to the valvular dysfunction.

Although catheter-induced tricuspid regurgitation occurs in approximately 50% of cases with catheters across the valve, the regurgitation is quantitatively small and clinically unimportant; it usually disappears when the catheter is removed. Tricuspid regurgitation can occur as a late complication of successful mitral valve replacement (MVR). In one series, Doppler-detected moderate-to-severe regurgitation occurred in two thirds of patients at a mean of over 11 years following MVR; over one third of these patients had clinically evident tricuspid regurgitation. Other causes include blunt and penetrating trauma (rupture of papillary muscles, chordal disruption or detachment, leaflet rupture, complete valve destruction), primary or secondary cardiac tumors, orthotopic heart transplantation, and endomyocardial fibrosis.

B. TRICUSPID STENOSIS

Tricuspid stenosis is an uncommon lesion that is usually rheumatic in origin and—almost exclusively—accompanies mitral stenosis. Isolated rheumatic tricuspid stenosis is rare, and subvalvular disease is usually less severe in tricuspid than in mitral stenosis. Isolated carcinoid tricuspid stenosis is also rare; tricuspid regurgitation is more frequent and often occurs with pulmonic stenosis. Right atrial myxomas and sarcomas and obstructing metastatic tumors may produce hemodynamic changes that are indistinguishable from tricuspid stenosis. Tricuspid stenosis may be congenital; it is infrequently predominant in Ebstein's anomaly. Extrinsic compression of the tricuspid valve by a loculated pericardial effusion is an uncommon cause of tricuspid stenosis. Other unusual causes include systemic lupus erythematous, Whipple's disease, Fabry's disease, antiphospholipid syndrome, infective endocarditis, and endocardial fibroelastosis; tricuspid stenosis can also occur as a sequela to methysergide therapy. It should be noted that prosthetic tricuspid valves, like all prosthetic valves, are inherently stenotic.

Bayer AS, Scheld WM: Endocarditis and intravascular infections. In: Mandell GL, Bennett JE, Dolin R (eds). Principles and Practice of Infectious Diseases, 5th ed. Philadelphia: Churchill Livingstone, 2000.

Blaustein AS, Ramanathan A: Tricuspid valve disease clinical evaluation, physiopathology, and management. Cardiol Clin 1998; 16(3):552.

Moyssakis IE, Rallidis LS, Guida GF et al: Incidence and evolution of carcinoid syndrome in the heart. J Heart Valve Dis 1997; 6:625.

Porter A, Shapira Y, Wurzel M et al: Tricuspid regurgitation late after mitral valve replacement: Clinical and echocardiographic evaluation. J Heart Valve Dis 1999;8:57.

Renzulli A, Foe DM, Carozza A et al: Surgery for tricuspid valve endocarditis: A selective approach. Heart Vessels 1999;14: 163.

Robiolio PA, Rigolin VH, Wilson JS et al: Carcinoid heart disease: Correlation of high serotonin levels with valvular abnormalities detected by cardiac catheterization and echocardiography. Circulation 1995;92:790.

Turjanski AA, Finkielman JD, Vazquez-Blanco M: Isolated tricuspid valve disease in antiphospholipid syndrome. Lupus 1999; 8:474.

Clinical Findings

A. SYMPTOMS AND SIGNS

Tricuspid valve disease can be difficult to recognize clinically. The symptoms may be overshadowed by associated illness, such as systemic lupus erythematosus, infective endocarditis, trauma, or neoplasia. The dominant presenting features may be symptoms that are usually not considered cardiac in origin: abdominal discomfort, jaundice, wasting, and inanition. In addition, patients with associated cardiovascular disease may have nonspecific symptoms (exertional dyspnea and fatigue in mitral stenosis) that obfuscate the diagnosis and deflect the suspicion of tricuspid valve disease. In patients with mitral stenosis, for example, tricuspid valve disease protects the pulmonary circulation and exertional dyspnea, pulmonary edema, and hemoptysis are less commonly reported, although a history of excessive fatigue may be elicited. Most often, however, the history is insufficient to diagnose tricuspid valve disease, and only a careful physical examination provides the necessary clues.

B. PHYSICAL EXAMINATION

1. Jugular venous pulse—Because the internal jugular veins lack effective valves, they should be inspected for an estimate of right atrial pressure (Figure 12–1 shows a normal jugular venous pulse). There are three waves (*a, c,* and *v*) and two descents, *x* and *y* (which correspond to the *a* and *v* waves, respectively). The *a* wave and the initial descent are produced by atrial contraction and relaxation, respectively. The *x* descent is interrupted by a *c* wave that is caused by isovolumetric contraction of the right ventricle and resultant bowing of the tricuspid valve toward the right atrium. The continuation of the *x* descent (sometimes called *x'* is caused by the descent of the arteriovenous (AV) ring toward the apex during right ventricular ejection. The right atrium fills and, because the tricuspid valve is closed, right atrial pressure rises, causing the *v* wave. The rapid fall in volume and pressure when the valve opens produces the *y* descent. Except for a small but variable delay, the jugular venous pulse and right atrial pressure contours are similar.

When inspecting the jugular venous pulse, the examiner should pay careful attention to the magnitude of the central venous (mean right atrial [RA]) pressure, the dominant wave (*a* or *v*), and changes in pulse contour with respiration. Tricuspid valve disease is typically associated with increased central venous pressure. In tricuspid regurgitation (Figure 12–2), a midsystolic *s* wave and prominent *y* descent occur; these findings are

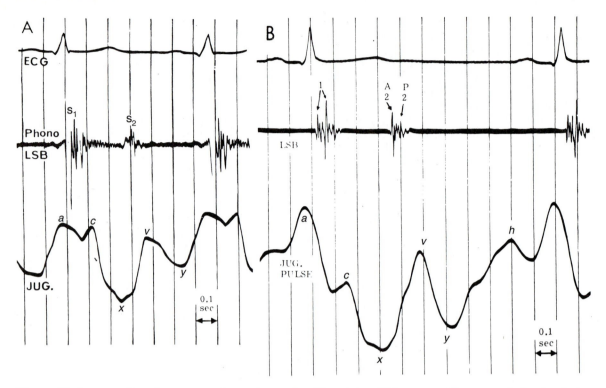

Figure 12–1. Normal jugular venous pulse tracings at fast (**A**) and slow (**B**) heart rates. The *a* wave is the dominate reflection. At slow heart rates, an *h* wave signifying the end of right ventricular filling can be seen. LSB = left sternal border. Reproduced, with permission, from Tavel ME: Clinical Phonocardiograpy and External Pulse Recoding. Yearbook Medical Publishers, 1978.

characteristically augmented during inspiration. In tricuspid stenosis (Figure 12–3), the *a* wave becomes strikingly prominent (while organized atrial activity is present) and increases with inspiration; resistance to early right ventricular diastolic filling results in a shallow *y* descent.

a. Tricuspid regurgitation—The *x* descent of the jugular venous pulse is interrupted by an early *v* wave (*c-v* wave) with a rapid *y* descent. The neck veins are distended, and the earlobes may pulsate. Because venous distention may obscure the jugular pulse contour, it is important to elevate the patient's head. Right ventricular volume overload leads to prominent pulsations over the left lower sternal border. Other characteristic, but less sensitive, findings include an enlarged, pulsatile liver and a systolic or holosystolic murmur at the left sternal border that increases with inspiration.

b. Tricuspid stenosis—In tricuspid stenosis, inspection of the jugular veins reveals a dominant *a* wave (assuming sinus rhythm) and a slow and shallow *y* descent.

2. Cardiac auscultation

a. Tricuspid regurgitation—When the right ventricle is markedly dilated, the location of the murmur may move toward the left and suggest mitral regurgitation. The auscultatory hallmark of tricuspid regurgitation is an inspiratory augmentation from increased systemic venous return and tricuspid valve flow (Figure 12–4). Under such circumstances as severe tricuspid regurgitation, markedly increased right atrial pressures, and right ventricular systolic failure, the murmur does not increase with inspiration. Although usually described as holosystolic, the timing of the murmur may be early, mid, or late systolic. The murmur may be decrescendo when tricuspid regurgitation is severe and acute and its character reflects the presence of a giant *c-v* wave; there may be a middiastolic flow rumble that resembles tricuspid stenosis. The murmur of tricuspid regurgitation is usually not accompanied by a thrill because the systolic pressure gradient across the tricuspid valve is relatively low. When the tricuspid valve is wide open in systole, there may be no murmur.

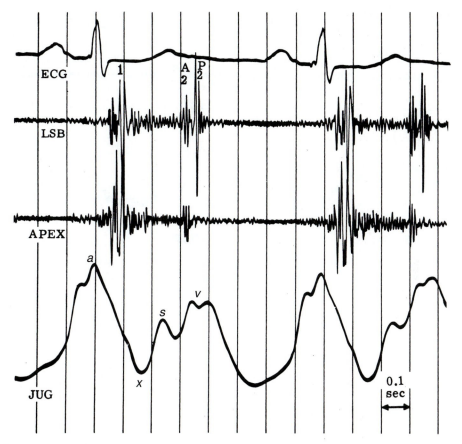

Figure 12–2. Jugular venous pulse tracing from a patient with mitral stenosis and tricuspid regurgitation secondary to pulmonary hypertension. Note the shallow *x* descent, the midsystolic *s* wave, and the respiratory increase in the *v* wave. Reproduced, with permission, from Tavel ME: Clinical Phonocardiography and External Pulse Recording. Year-book Medical Publishers, 1978.

b. Tricuspid stenosis—The tricuspid opening snap is difficult to distinguish from the mitral opening snap. Auscultatory findings may be difficult to distinguish from existing mitral stenosis. Unlike mitral stenosis, however, the diastolic rumble of tricuspid stenosis has a higher pitch, increases with inspiration, and is usually loudest at the lower left sternal border. The tricuspid stenosis murmur is often scratchy; it ends before the first heart sound and has no presystolic crescendo in patients with normal sinus rhythm. A diastolic murmur from relative tricuspid stenosis may be heard with large atrial septal defects and severe tricuspid regurgitation. In patients with normal sinus rhythm, a presystolic hepatic pulsation may be felt; this is due to reflux from atrial contraction against the stenotic valve. Unfortunately, atrial fibrillation is frequently present. Both tricuspid stenosis and regurgitation can, if chronic, lead to ascites, jaundice, wasting,

and muscle loss. Tricuspid valve disease, which is often diagnosed or suspected at the bedside, can almost always be confirmed with echocardiography.

C. DIAGNOSTIC STUDIES

The diagnostic evaluation of suspected tricuspid valve disease includes electrocardiography, plain chest film, two-dimensional and Doppler echocardiography, and cardiac catheterization. Limited experience with cine magnetic resonance imaging (MRI) suggests that, at present, the technique offers no clear advantage over Doppler echocardiography. Except for right ventricular volume and ejection fraction determinations, nuclear studies are generally not clinically useful in tricuspid valve disease. The tricuspid valve is not well visualized with computed tomography, and the ability to quantify valve regurgitation is limited.

1. Electrocardiography—P waves characteristic of right atrial enlargement with no evidence of right ven-

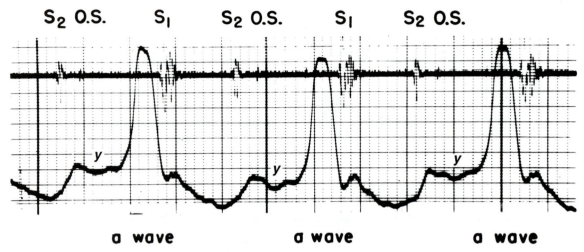

S₂ O.S.   S₁   S₂ O.S.   S₁   S₂ O.S.

a wave   a wave   a wave

Figure 12–3. Jugular venous pulse tracing and phonocardiogram from a patient with rheumatic tricuspid stenosis. Note the striking *a* waves and the shallow *y* descents. A loud S, and opening snap (O.S.) are evident on the accompanying phonocardiogram. Courtesy of NO Fowler.

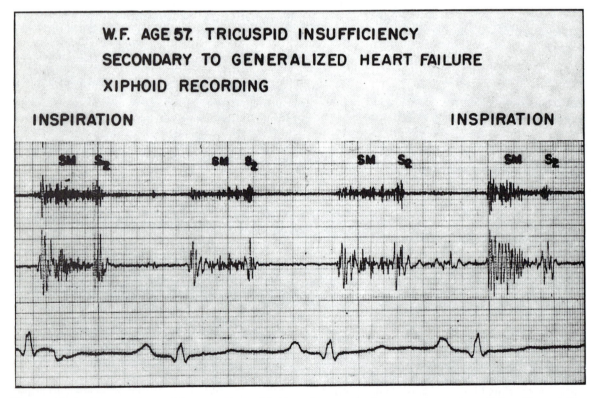

W.F. AGE 57. TRICUSPID INSUFFICIENCY
SECONDARY TO GENERALIZED HEART FAILURE
XIPHOID RECORDING

INSPIRATION   INSPIRATION

SM S₂   SM S₂   SM S₂   SM S₂

Figure 12–4. Phonocardiogram from a patient with tricuspid regurgitation secondary to heart failure. The systolic murmur increases with inspiration, seen most clearly on the lower phonocardiographic tracing. Note that the murmur does not extend to the second heart sound. Courtesy of NO Fowler.

tricular hypertrophy suggest isolated tricuspid stenosis (Figure 12–5A). Most often, however, the rhythm is an atrial fibrillation. When present, right ventricular hypertrophy indicates coexisting mitral stenosis with pulmonary hypertension. In addition, a low voltage RSR' in V_1 is frequently seen. In tricuspid regurgitation, atrial fibrillation is common; incomplete right bundle branch block and Q waves in V_1 are frequently found. Preexcitation frequently accompanies Ebstein's anomaly (Figure 12–5B).

2. Chest radiography—In tricuspid stenosis, the chest film is characterized by cardiomegaly, with a prominent right-heart border caused by right atrial enlargement, and a dilated superior vena cava and azygous vein. Pulmonary vascular markings may be notably absent. The chest film in tricuspid regurgitation shows cardiomegaly from right atrial and ventricular enlargement; pleural effusions and elevated diaphragms from ascites may be seen. In general, a dilated heart in the absence of pulmonary congestion or pulmonary hy-

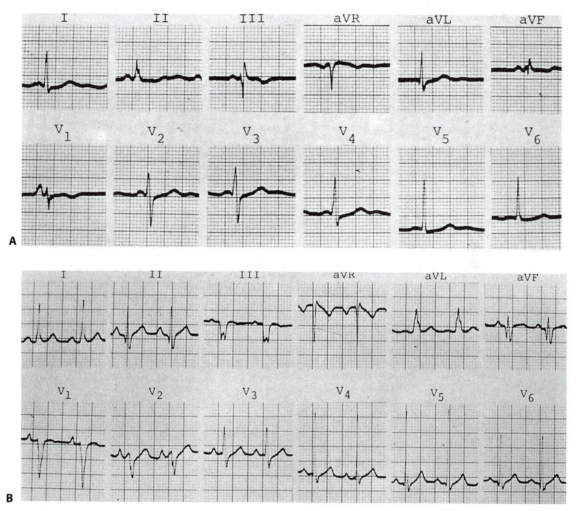

Figure 12–5. Electrocardiograms from patients with tricuspid valve disease. **A:** Mitral stenosis and isolated tricuspid stenosis. The tall initial P-wave forces in lead V, indicate right atrial enlargement. There is no electrocardiographic evidence of right ventricular hypertrophy. Reproduced, with permission, from Chou TE: Electrocardiography in Clinical Practice, 3rd ed. Philadelphia: WB Saunders, 1991. **B:** Patient with Ebstein's anomaly and preexcitation. Delta waves create a pseudoinfarct pattern. P-wave amplitude in leads II and V_2 is consistent with right atrial enlargement. Courtesy of TE Chou.

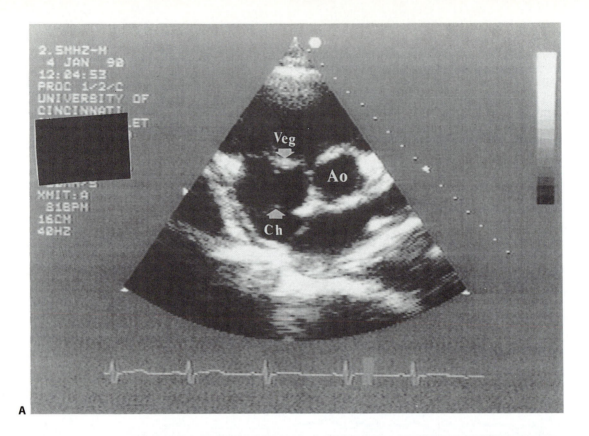

A

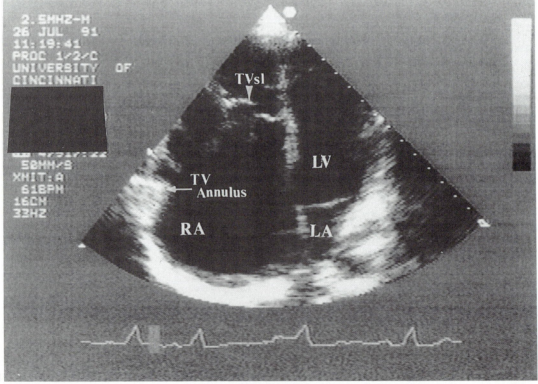

B

Figure 12–6.

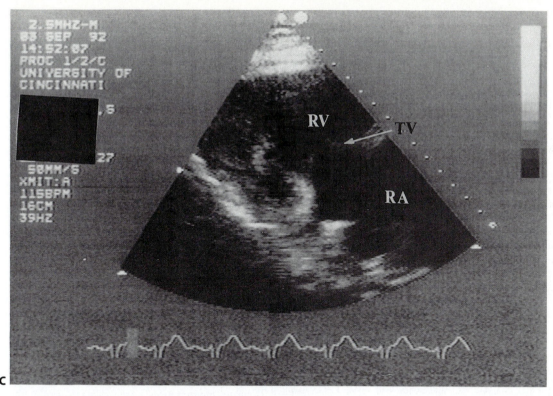

C

Figure 12–6. Two-dimensional echocardiograms illustrating abnormalities of the tricuspid valve leaflets. **A:** Infective endocarditis. Ao = aorta; Ch = Chiari network; Veg = tricuspid valve vegetation. **B:** Ebstein's anomaly. Note the displacement of the septal leaflet (TVsl) relative to the tricuspid valve annulus. LV = left ventricle; RA = right atrium. **C:** Carcinoid syndrome. Note the thickened and rigid tricuspid leaflets (*arrow*).

pertension should suggest either tricuspid valve disease or pericardial effusion. Massive right atrial enlargement suggests Ebstein's anomaly.

3. Echocardiography—Echocardiography is the most useful noninvasive diagnostic test for evaluating tricuspid valve disease. Two-dimensional and Doppler echocardiographic examinations can identify associated disease of the left ventricle and other cardiac valves (eg, mitral stenosis) and the anatomic sequelae of chronic tricuspid valve disease (eg, dilated right heart chambers), and can detect structural abnormalities of the tricuspid valve (eg, a thickened tricuspid valve with decreased mobility, compression of the tricuspid annulus, or involvement by tumor or prolapsing or displaced leaflets and vegetations; Figure 12–6). Biplane transesophageal echocardiography may be helpful when diagnostic images cannot be obtained from transthoracic views or when associated disease of the interatrial septum, atria, and mitral valve is suspected.

a. Tricuspid regurgitation—In tricuspid regurgitation, the echocardiographic findings usually show right ventricular volume overload with a dilated right ventricle, paradoxical septal motion, and diastolic flattening of the interventricular septum. Contrast or color-flow Doppler echocardiography can visualize the tricuspid regurgitant jet. Turbulence can be detected by pulsed-wave Doppler, the tricuspid valve diastolic gradient can be quantified using continuous-wave Doppler, and pulmonary arterial pressure can be estimated from the pulmonary artery acceleration time or the peak velocity of the tricuspid regurgitant jet. Two-dimensional echocardiography distinguishes between primary disease of the left heart and right ventricular disease, both of which cause functional tricuspid regurgitation and organic disease of the tricuspid valve. Contrast found in the inferior vena cava and hepatic veins following injection of agitated saline into an arm vein implies significant tricuspid regurgitation. On the other hand, a tricuspid valve annulus less then 3.4 cm in diameter during diastole virtually excludes significant tricuspid regurgitation. The temporal and spatial distribution of systolic turbulence in the right atrium, using either color-flow mapping or pulsed-wave Doppler, can be a means of estimating the severity of the regurgitation. Systolic reversal of the Doppler signal in the hepatic veins indicates significant tricuspid regurgitation. It should be recognized that Doppler-detected tricuspid regurgitation occurs commonly in normal individuals. In such cases, the Doppler signal tends not to be holosystolic, and systolic turbulence occupies only a small area of the right atrium.

b. Tricuspid stenosis—As shown in Figure 12–7, the stenotic tricuspid valve is thickened and domed and has restricted motion. The echocardiographic appearance alone may be misleading, however; many patients with two-dimensional echocardiographic findings that suggest tricuspid stenosis have normal tricuspid valve diastolic pressure gradients. Although the right atrium is usually dilated, the right ventricle is not enlarged in isolated tricuspid stenosis. The severity of the stenosis is determined with continuous-wave Doppler. Accurate peak instantaneous and mean gradients across the stenotic tricuspid valve are readily calculated using the modified **Bernoulli formula,** which relates a pressure drop (dP) to the velocity (V) across a stenosis ($dP = 4V^2$). The pressure half-time method for calculating valve orifice area, used successfully for the mitral valve, has not been validated for the tricuspid valve.

Fischer EA, Goldman EA: Simple, rapid method for quantification of tricuspid regurgitation by two-dimensional echocardiography. Am J Cardiol 1989;63:1375.

Maciel BC, Simpson IA, Valdes-Cruz LM et al: Color flow Doppler mapping studies of "physiologic" pulmonary and tricuspid regurgitation: Evidence for true regurgitation as opposed to a valve closing volume. J Am Soc Echocardiogr 1991;4:589.

Pearlman AS: Role of echocardiography in the diagnosis and evaluation of severity of mitral and tricuspid stenosis. Circulation 1991;84:I.

4. Cardiac catheterization

a. Tricuspid regurgitation—Opacification of the right atrium following injection of radiographic contrast into the right ventricle detects and estimates the severity of the regurgitation. Although right ventriculography requires a catheter across the tricuspid valve, there is no significant contrast leak into the right atrium under normal circumstances. Right atrial and ventricular pressures are elevated, and the right atrial pressure may become "ventricularized" as a result of a large c-v wave and an absent x descent (Figure 12–8A). **Kussmaul's sign** (increased RA pressure with inspiration or the absence of a normal fall in RA pressure) may be seen when the regurgitation is severe.

b. Tricuspid stenosis—In tricuspid stenosis, the mean right atrial pressure is increased; characteristically, the a wave is prominent and the y descent is slow. The hallmark of tricuspid stenosis is a diastolic gradient between the right atrium and right ventricle that increases with inspiration (Figure 12–8B). The gradients are frequently small, however; their detection is enhanced by recording right atrial and ventricular pressures simultaneously with two optimally damped catheters and

equally sensitive transducers. Because of the low gradient, calculation of the valve area is unreliable. Injection or rapid volume infusion of atropine to increase the heart rate can increase the diastolic gradient and facilitate the diagnosis.

Farb A, Burk AP, Virmani R: Anatomy and pathology of the right ventricle (including acquired tricuspid and pulmonic valve disease). Cardiol Clin 1992;10:1.

Jaffe CC, Weltin G: Echocardiography of the right side of the heart. Cardiol Clin 1992;10:41.

Kasper W, Meinertz T, Weber T et al: Incidence of tricuspid valve prolapse. Z Kardiol 1991;80:333.

Lundin L, Landelius J, Andren B et al: Transesophageal echocardiography improves the diagnostic value of cardiac ultrasound in patients with carcinoid heart disease. Br Heart J 1990; 64:190.

Ribeiro PA, Al Zaibag M, Al Kasabs S et al: Provocation and amplification of the transvalvular pressure gradient in rheumatic tricuspid stenosis. Am J Cardiol 1988;61:1307.

Stewart D, Leman RB, Kaiser J et al: Catheter-induced tricuspid regurgitation. Incidence and clinical significance. Chest 1991; 99:651.

Treatment

A. MEDICAL

Tricuspid regurgitation is well tolerated in the absence of pulmonary hypertension. When pulmonary arterial pressures increase, cardiac output falls, leading to symptoms of right-heart failure (edema, fatigue, dyspnea). Restriction of sodium and the use of potent loop diuretics decrease right atrial pressure. Medical therapy is also aimed at the cause of pulmonary hypertension, which is usually treated with positive inotropic agents or vasodilators (alone or in combination), depending on the specific cause. Treatment of associated systemic diseases is a critically important aspect of the therapeutic paradigm; it is, however, beyond the scope of this discussion. Symptomatic tricuspid stenosis is treated surgically.

B. SURGICAL

Surgery on the tricuspid valve may involve repair, reconstruction, excision, or replacement with a prosthetic valve. The decision to operate on the stenotic tricuspid valve is a straightforward one; the decision to operate on a regurgitant valve is more challenging. The surgeon must determine whether the regurgitation is functional or organic (ie, associated with a structurally normal or abnormal tricuspid valve), and if it is functional, the response of the pulmonary arterial pressure to the primary procedure should be anticipated. For example, repair may be unnecessary for functional tricuspid regurgitation if there is a high likelihood of a postoperative fall in pulmonary arterial pressure. In addition, repair of the functionally regurgitant tricuspid valve in patients with severe right ventricular dysfunction is un-

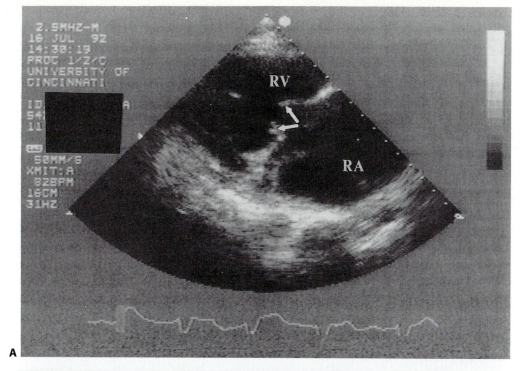

A

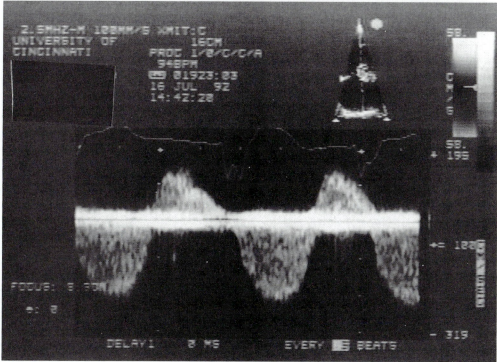

B

Figure 12–7. A: Two-dimensional echocardiogram from a patient with rheumatic tricuspid valve disease, showing a thickened and domed tricuspid valve *(arrows)*. The right atrium (RA) is considerably dilated and the right ventricle (RV) is enlarged. **B:** Continuous-wave Doppler study from the same patient confirms tricuspid stenosis and regurgitation. The high-velocity signal above the baseline during diastole represents right ventricular inflow; the signal below the baseline during systole represents tricuspid regurgitation.

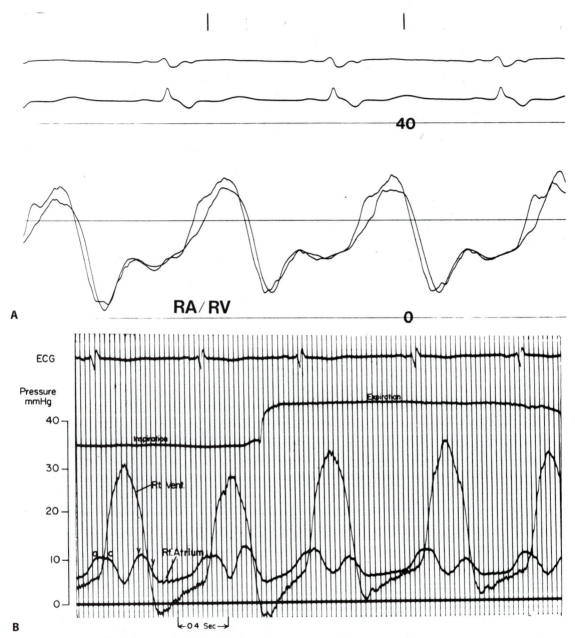

Figure 12–8. Hemodynamic recordings from patients with tricuspid valve disease. **A:** Severe tricuspid regurgitation. There is "ventricularization" of the right atrial (RA) pressures, which are indistinguishable from right ventricular (RV) pressures. **B:** Simultaneous and equally sensitive recordings of right atrial and ventricular pressures from a patient with rheumatic tricuspid stenosis. Note the RA-RV gradient throughout diastole, which increases with inspiration. Reproduced, with permission, from Fowler et al: Diagnosis of Heart Disease. New York: Springer-Verlag, 1991.

likely to improve their status. However, the response of tricuspid regurgitation to reduced pulmonary artery pressure can be difficult to predict, and as mentioned

previously, significant tricuspid regurgitation often complicates successful MVR despite reduced pulmonary artery pressures. Given the high morbidity and mortality associated with reoperation to correct tricuspid regurgitation following MVR, the presence of any degree of preoperative tricuspid regurgitation, especially organic regurgitation, warrants consideration of concurrent tricuspid valve repair.

The decision whether to repair or replace the tricuspid valve with a prosthesis depends on the suitability of valve repair, the associated surgical procedures, and the underlying disease. Thrombosis is a more frequent problem with tricuspid than with mitral prostheses. Thus, primary valve repair, when possible, is the preferred procedure. Repair of the stenotic tricuspid valve involves identifying and separating the fan chordae (the chords that support the leaflets in the area of the commissure), leaflet decalcification, and chordal or papillary muscle division.

Annuloplasty procedures correct dilatation of the tricuspid valve annulus. The dilatation, which is not symmetric, typically involves the annulus around the anterior and posterior leaflets (posterior more than anterior). The procedure involves sizing and selectively plicating the anterior and posterior annuli. Recent surgical series have shown superior results with aggressive use of tricuspid valve annuloplasty with or without valve repair.

When the tricuspid valve cannot be repaired and replacement is necessary, a porcine prosthesis is often used because of the lower risk of thrombosis, although recent changes in valve design have significantly lowered the risk of thrombosis with mechanical prostheses. Bioprosthetic valves are also more prone to late failure than mechanical prostheses. If anticoagulation is necessary for other reasons, a St. Jude prothesis is preferred by some surgeons—especially for younger patients.

The primary indications for surgery in patients with tricuspid valve endocarditis are uncontrollable infection, septic emboli, or refractory congestive heart failure. Because virulent organisms are the rule, they are not, per se, an indication for surgery. Total excision of the tricuspid valve is an attractive option in intravenous drug abusers, considering both recidivism and the threat of prosthetic valve endocarditis. As noted earlier, tricuspid regurgitation without pulmonary hypertension is well tolerated; however, 20% of these patients ultimately may require valve replacement for right-heart failure. Debridement and valve repair have been suggested as alternative procedures to valve excision.

Successful percutaneous balloon valvuloplasty has been reported for native valve tricuspid stenosis and stenotic bioprosthetic tricuspid valves. Bioprosthetic tricuspid valves tend to become obstructive and therefore do not fare as well in the long term as mechanical valves. Prosthetic valve thrombosis may be treated successfully with thrombolytic agents, however, particularly if the obstructing thrombus develops over time.

C. POSTOPERATIVE MANAGEMENT

Postoperative management is dictated largely by the surgical procedures involved. Catheters are not left across prosthetic tricuspid valves, although this does not pose a difficulty with either valve repairs or annuloplasty procedures. Cardioversion to sinus rhythm is generally not successful if preoperative atrial fibrillation was present.

Allen MD, Slachman F, Eddy AC et al: Tricuspid valve repair for tricuspid valve endocarditis: Tricuspid valve "recycling." Ann Thorac Surg 1991;51:593.

Robalino BB, Whitlow PL, Marwick T et al: Percutaneous balloon valvotomy for the treatment of isolated tricuspid stenosis. Chest 1991;100:867.

Scully HE, Armstrong CS: Tricuspid valve replacement. Fifteen years of experience with mechanical Prostheses and bioprostheses. J Thorac Cardiovasc Surg 1995;109:1035.

Shatapathy P, Aggarwal BK, Kamath SG: Tricuspid valve repair: A rational alternative. J Heart Valve Dis 2000;9:276.

Prognosis

The natural history of tricuspid valve disease is a function of the associated valvular lesions and the primary disease (eg, rheumatic fever, carcinoid syndrome, Ebstein's anomaly). Isolated lesions are rare, and their natural history is unknown.

In general, the results of tricuspid valve surgery depend on the types of valve lesions, the corrective procedures, the degree and reversibility of left and right ventricular function, and the pulmonary vascular resistance. Residual tricuspid regurgitation usually occurs when the pulmonary vascular resistance remains elevated. Many patients have small-to-moderate tricuspid valve gradients after tricuspid valve replacement; like residual tricuspid valve leaks, these are usually not clinically important.

Although most surgeons favor repair over replacement, the superiority of this approach is difficult to prove. The hemodynamics are comparable, with a greater gradient after prosthetic valve replacement and more tricuspid regurgitation following repair. Because the problem of thromboemboli is reduced, complications should be less of a problem after repair. Data suggest that long-term survival in patients may be better after repair than valve replacement, but a randomized trial has never been performed.

In a study of 109 patients undergoing aortic and mitral valve replacement and tricuspid valve repair, the 5-, 10-, and 15-year survival rates among the 79% discharged from the hospital were 70%, 42%, and 33%, respectively. Advanced age and decreased functional capacity were predictors of a poor outcome, and late mortality was due primarily to sudden death (38%) and heart failure (21%).

Mullany CJ, Gersh BJ, Orszulak TA et al: Repair of tricuspid valve insufficiency in patients undergoing double (aortic and mitral) valve replacement: Perioperative mortality and long-term (1 to 20 years) follow-up in 109 patients. J Thorac Cardiovasc Surg 1987;94:740.

PULMONIC VALVE DISEASE

 ESSENTIALS OF DIAGNOSIS

Pulmonic regurgitation
- *Diastolic murmur at the left upper sternal border that increases with inspiration*
- *Split S_2 with a loud P_2*
- *Characteristic Doppler echocardiographic findings*

Pulmonic stenosis
- *Systolic murmur at the left second intercostal space preceded by a systolic click*
- *Split S_2 with a soft P_2*
- *Characteristic echocardiographic findings*

General Considerations

The technologic advances made in the fields of noninvasive cardiac imaging, interventional cardiology, and cardiac surgery over the past few decades have had a noticeable effect on the diagnosis and management of pulmonic valve disease.

Pathophysiology & Etiology

The normal pulmonic valve is a semilunar valve with anterior, left and right leaflets. The function and texture of the valve leaflets, as well as the size of the valve annulus can be adversely affected in a variety of disease states.

A. PULMONIC REGURGITATION

Pulmonic regurgitation (PR) most commonly occurs in the setting of pulmonary hypertension. The regurgitation is caused by dilatation of the pulmonic valve ring, and any cause of pulmonary hypertension can precipitate PR. Idiopathic dilation of the pulmonary trunk and Marfan's syndrome also cause PR via a similar distortion of the valve ring. **Infective endocarditis** is the most frequently encountered cause of acquired PR, with vegetations causing dysfunction of the leaflets themselves. Although the pulmonic valve is the least likely to be seeded in endocarditis, the rising number of

intravenous drug abusers, immunocompromised hosts, and patients with subclinical pulmonic stenosis represent a growing population at risk. PR can also occur as a consequence of surgical treatment for **tetralogy of Fallot** or balloon valvuloplasty. The PR is generally mild and hemodynamically insignificant, but in rare cases it can progress to RV dilation, necessitating pulmonic valve replacement. **Rheumatic heart disease** is an infrequent cause of PR, and it invariably occurs in the setting of multiple valve disease. Other rare causes of PR include carcinoid tumors, syphilis, and catheter-related valve dysfunction. It should be noted that trivial PR is frequently encountered on routine echocardiography and is considered a normal variant.

B. PULMONIC STENOSIS

Pulmonic stenosis (PS) is a congenital disorder in over 95% of cases. Congenital PS is usually caused by a valvular lesion although subvalvular (infundibular hypertrophy) and supravalvular (rare intracardiac tumors, congenital rubella syndrome) lesions do occur. Valvular PS is most often due to fibrosis of the valve with thickening of the leaflets. The leaflets dome into the pulmonary trunk during systole, producing a narrow central aperture. Less commonly, the valve leaflets are dysplastic and rubbery with a small valve annulus. Bicuspid pulmonic valves also occur. The pathologic distinctions made earlier do have some clinical relevance, as dysplastic valves are less responsive to balloon dilatation than dome-shaped valves. **Isolated congenital PS** is the most commonly encountered congenital pulmonic valve disease in adulthood, and it typically causes valvular PS. **Tetralogy of Fallot** also causes PS with a bicuspid valve, and **Noonan's syndrome** can be associated with dysplastic PS. Other congenital syndromes associated with PS include double-outlet right ventricle, atrioventricular canal defect and univentricular atrioventricular connection.

The most common acquired form of pulmonic stenosis occurs with **carcinoid heart disease.** The proposed mechanism for carcinoid valve disease has been discussed earlier in this chapter. The whitish carcinoid plaques adhere to the valve leaflets and can cause both PS and PR. Rheumatic heart disease is a rare cause of PS and when present is generally seen with multiple valve disease. Large vegetations on an infected pulmonic valve, also rare, can cause PS.

Waller BF, Howard J, Fess S: Pathology of pulmonic valve stenosis and pure regurgitation. Clin Cardiol 1995;18:45.

Clinical Findings

A. SYMPTOMS AND SIGNS

As with tricuspid disease the symptoms of pulmonic valve disease can be subtle and overshadowed by coexisting illnesses. Patients with pulmonic regurgitation are often asymptomatic unless symptoms of pulmonary hypertension and right ventricular failure eventuate. Patients with pulmonic stenosis are also frequently asymptomatic. Symptoms can appear gradually as the pulmonic valve pressure gradient increases and include exertional dyspnea, chest pain, and fatigue.

B. Physical Examination

1. Jugular venous waveform—The presence of pulmonic stenosis is suggested by a prominent jugular venous *a* wave in the setting of a relatively normal central venous pressure.

2. Cardiac auscultation

a. Pulmonic regurgitation—The pulmonic component of S_2 is usually loud because most patients have pulmonary hypertension, and the second heart sound is often split due to prolonged right ventricular emptying. Right ventricular S_3 and S_4 gallops are sometimes heard in the left parasternal area. In the absence of pulmonary hypertension, the murmur of PR is a low-pitched, crescendo-decrescendo diastolic murmur that is best heard near the left third or fourth intercostal space. The murmur is augmented during inspiration. However, in patients with significant pulmonary hypertension the murmur assumes a different quality. The dilatation of the pulmonic valve annulus allows for a more forceful regurgitant jet, resulting in a high-pitched, decrescendo murmur that is best heard at the left parasternal border near the second or third intercostals space, the so-called **Graham Steell murmur.**

b. Pulmonic stenosis—The second heart sound is also split with PS, and this splitting is proportional to the degree of stenosis. Unlike in PR, the pulmonic component of S_2 is soft in PS, and an S_4 can frequently be appreciated over the lower left sternal border. A high-frequency systolic click can be heard near the left upper sternal border that precedes the late-peaking crescendo-decrescendo systolic murmur that typifies PS. This murmur can be associated with a thrill, and a right ventricular impulse is frequently palpable.

C. Diagnostic Studies

The diagnostic evaluation of pulmonic valve disease should include an electrocardiogram (ECG), chest film, and a transthoracic echocardiographic study with Doppler imaging. Cardiac catheterization is generally unnecessary given the high degree of agreement between echocardiographic and catheterization data in pulmonic valve disease. Indeed, the 1998 ACC/AHA Guidelines Executive Summary for the management of valvular heart disease lists cardiac catheterization as a class III (not useful, possibly harmful) intervention in the diagnosis and management of pulmonic stenosis.

1. Electrocardiography—PR and PS can both demonstrate the effects of right ventricular strain and pulmonary hypertension on surface tracings. Typical findings include right bundle branch block, right axis deviation, and right ventricular hypertrophy. Mild or moderate PS frequently presents with a normal ECG.

2. Chest radiography—Nonspecific enlargement of the right ventricle and pulmonary arteries can be seen with PR.

3. Echocardiography—In pulmonic regurgitation, the pulsed Doppler technique is used to accurately detect the presence and severity of PR. In addition, the presence of pulmonary hypertension, right ventricular hypertrophy and dilation, and coexistent valve disease can be detected. Transesophageal echocardiography has a role, however, in the evaluation of suspected pulmonic valve endocarditis.

Echocardiography determines the nature, location, and severity of the stenosis. As with PR, data regarding the status of the ventricles and other valves can also be obtained. Transesophageal studies may be useful when the location of the stenosis is unclear from the surface study.

Treatment

Pulmonic regurgitation rarely requires specific treatment. Treatment of predisposing cardiac conditions, such as pulmonary hypertension, endocarditis, or left-sided valve disease, often improves the PR. As mentioned previously, certain patients may progress to right-heart failure from PR following repair of tetralogy of Fallot. These patients may require valve replacement, often with a porcine valve or pulmonary allograft.

Pulmonic stenosis has been managed with great success by balloon valvuloplasty. Treatment is based on severity of disease: Those with mild disease (peak gradient ≤40 mm Hg) do not need treatment, but symptomatic patients with moderate disease (peak gradient 41–79 mm Hg) should receive valvuloplasty. Any patient with severe disease (peak gradient ≤80 mm Hg) should be treated. As mentioned previously patients with dysplastic valves may not respond to balloon valvuloplasty and may require valve replacement with a porcine valve or pulmonary homograft.

Prognosis

The prognosis of pulmonic valve disease per se is generally excellent. With pulmonic regurgitation one must consider the comorbidities involved (particularly pulmonary hypertension) that may influence prognosis. Patients with congenital pulmonic stenosis can expect a life expectancy comparable to that of the general population. One series that followed 85 patients for up to 10 years after balloon valvuloplasty reported that repeat balloon valvuloplasty was required in 11% of patients and surgical intervention was required in 5%.

Bonow RO, Carabello B, deLeon AC Jr et al: Guidelines for the management of patients with valvular heart disease executive summary: A report of the American College of Cardiology/ American Heart Association Task Force on Practice Guidelines (Committee on Management of Patients with Valvular Heart Disease). Circulation 1998;98:1949.

Braunwald E: Valvular Heart Disease in Heart Disease: A Textbook of Cardiovascular Medicine, 6th ed. In: Braunwald E, Zipes DP, Libby P, eds. Philadelphia, W. B. Saunders Company, 2001.

Hayes CJ, Gersony WM, Driscoll DJ et al: Second natural history of congenital heart defects: Results of treatment of patients with pulmonary valvular stenosis. Circulation 1993;87(Suppl 1):28.

Rao PS, Patana M, Buck SH et al: Results of 3 to 10 year follow up of balloon dilatation of the pulmonic valve. Heart 1998;80:591.

Shively BK: Transesophageal echocardiographic (TEE) evaluation of the aortic valve, left ventricular outflow tract, and pulmonic valve. Cardiol Clin 2000;18(4):711.

Systemic Hypertension

William F. Graettinger, MD

ESSENTIALS OF DIAGNOSIS

- *Diastolic pressure greater than 90 mm Hg, systolic pressure greater than 140 mm Hg, or both, on three separate occasions*
- *In diabetic patients, diastolic pressure greater than 80 mm Hg, systolic pressure greater than 130 mm Hg, or both, on three separate occasions*

General Considerations

Hypertension is a major modifiable risk factor for cardiovascular disease that can, if untreated, result in serious morbidity and mortality from cardiac, cerebrovascular, vascular, and renal disease. In excess of 62 million persons in the United States are estimated to have hypertension, and only slightly more than half of these individuals are aware of their diagnosis. Of those, only a third are at their therapeutic goal. The potential for death and disability is therefore quite high and represents a serious public health issue. Once the diagnosis of hypertension is made and therapy instituted, elevated blood pressure can be lowered, reducing the risk of cardiovascular disease in the vast majority of patients. Major trials in large populations have conclusively demonstrated that treating mild-to-moderate hypertension significantly decreases fatal and nonfatal stroke, coronary events, and renal failure. The wide array of antihypertensive therapy is very effective in reducing blood pressure. Despite similar blood pressure and overall mortality reductions, the reductions in incidence of stroke, coronary ischemic events, heart failure, and renal failure are not the same for all classes of antihypertensive agents. The reasons for these differences have not been totally explained and are the topic of much speculation.

A growing body of direct and inferential evidence suggests that reduction of blood pressure should not be the only goal of antihypertensive therapy. Therapy should also be directed toward controlling all of the patients' cardiovascular risk factors, including dyslipidemia, smoking, and diabetes mellitus.

MacMahon S: Blood pressure and the risk of cardiovascular disease. N Engl J Med 2000;342:50.

Pathophysiology & Etiology

Until recently, high blood pressure was synonymous with hypertension; now, however, data suggest that there is considerably more to hypertension than increased blood pressure. Several metabolic and functional abnormalities have even been observed in the children of hypertensive patients prior to blood pressure elevation that are similar to, but of a lesser magnitude than, those found in their parents. Hypertension is also associated with insulin resistance and glucose intolerance. Insulin levels are consistently higher in hypertensive patients than in normotensive controls. This condition of hyperinsulinemia is worsened by thiazide diuretics, especially in the presence of β-blocker therapy. Hyperinsulinemia produces a proliferation of vascular smooth muscle and fibrous tissue and adversely affects the serum lipid profile.

Renin and angiotensin levels are also important factors in determining both the response to therapy and the prognosis. Hypertensive patients with high renin levels have a greater incidence of myocardial infarction than do similar patients with lower levels. Normotensive young adults with a family history of hypertension have been found to have thicker left ventricular (LV) walls and alterations of LV diastolic filling in comparison with control subjects. Although not frankly abnormal, these latter two findings are similar to but less severe than those observed in hypertensive patients. Renal reserve also appears diminished in the children of hypertensive parents.

Hypertension, therefore, is a multisystem disorder with involvement of the cardiovascular, neuroendocrine, and renal systems with a strong genetic component.

A. NATURAL HISTORY

Blood pressure gradually increases throughout childhood and adolescence. The best predictor of the level of future blood pressure is the relative level of blood pressure of a child in relation to his or her peers. During childhood and adolescence, body weight is a major determinant of blood pressure, with heavier children having higher blood pressures. High blood pressure is uncommon under the age of 20; if present, it is usually associated with renal insufficiency, renal artery stenosis, or coarctation of the aorta. The initial presentation of high blood pressure usually occurs in the third to the sixth decade, and blood pressure may fluctuate significantly during the early course of the disease. The prevalence of high blood pressure increases with age and is greater in men than women. In the elderly population, this reverses, and more women than men have high blood pressure.

Everyone should be screened for the presence of high blood pressure; testing should be done routinely in the physician's office or at one of the larger community screening activities. These activities are typically targeted at those at greater risk of high blood pressure: older individuals, individuals with previously high-normal blood pressures, blacks, sedentary individuals, and those with a family history of hypertension.

Burt VL, Whelton P, Rocella EJ, et al: Prevalence of hypertension in the U. S. adult population. Results of the Third National Health and Nutrition Examination Survey, 1988–91. Hypertension 1995;25:305.

B. ETHNIC AND SOCIOECONOMIC FACTORS

Blacks have both an earlier onset and a greater prevalence of high blood pressure than do whites, Asians, and Native Americans at all ages. Over the age of 50 years, hypertension is prevalent in more than 40% of black males, compared with approximately 27% in white males. Severe high blood pressure (diastolic BP at least 115 mm Hg) is five times more common in black men than in white men and seven times more common in black women than in white women. Blacks therefore tend to have more serious complications, especially strokes, from high blood pressure. Other factors also affect the prevalence of high blood pressure. Among all ethnic groups, less-educated individuals have a greater prevalence of high blood pressure than do more highly educated individuals, especially in lower socioeconomic groups.

The level of blood pressure elevation is directly related to total cardiovascular risk, and the presence of other cardiovascular disease risk factors, especially diabetes or dyslipidemia, is synergistic with high blood pressure.

Weber MA: Cardiovascular and metabolic characteristics of hypertension. Am J Med 1991;91(Suppl 1A):4S.

Clinical Findings

Blood pressure is a continuous variable with a reasonably normal, or bell-shaped-curve, distribution across the general population. High blood pressure has been classically defined as a diastolic pressure of greater than 90 mm Hg, a systolic pressure greater than 140 mm Hg, or both. The higher the blood pressure, the greater the risk of a cardiovascular events; conversely, the lower the blood pressure, the lower the cardiovascular risk. It is important to stress that isolated systolic hypertension, a systolic pressure of greater than 140 mm Hg with a diastolic pressure of less than 90 mm Hg, is abnormal and requires attention.

The diagnosis of hypertension should not be based on measurements taken at a single office visit. Elevated readings should be confirmed at a second or third visit to establish the diagnosis, and any factors that might elevate blood pressure should be excluded. For example, the patient should refrain from smoking for at least 30 min prior to blood pressure measurement. The blood pressure should be measured, with a cuff of the appropriate size, after at least 5 min of rest in a seated or supine position. The cuff should cover approximately one third of the length of the upper arm and should completely or almost completely encircle the arm. Too small a cuff may overestimate the true blood pressure because it may only partially compress the artery, requiring a higher pressure for total occlusion. The measurements should be made twice in both arms, for a total of four measures. The average of the two measurements in the arm with the higher values is used as the baseline value of blood pressure. Systolic blood pressure is indicated by the phase 1 Korotkoff sound (onset) and diastolic pressure by phase 5, or disappearance, in adults. In children, phase 4, or muffling, has been suggested as the best indicator of diastolic pressure.

The blood pressure obtained in the physician's office, however, does not always accurately represent that experienced by the patient during routine daily living. About 20–30% of patients with mildly elevated office blood pressure may have a hyperadrenergic response to having their blood pressure measured. This hyperreactivity is called white-coat, pseudo-, or office hypertension and may be related to anxiety from merely being in the physician's office or clinic. If the blood pressure is measured in a nonthreatening situation by a friend or relative or with an automated device, the blood pressure in these individuals may be normal. Blood pressure hyperreactivity should be suspected in patients who have persistently elevated blood pressure in the office and normal pressure measurements out of the office or in patients who have hypotensive symptoms but remain hypertensive in the office despite therapy. It has not been clearly established whether the blood pressure in these individuals is truly normal or whether they have an early or different form of hypertension. Several studies have found alterations in cardiac structure and function that are somewhere between those found in normotensive subjects and those found in hypertensive patients. No large outcome studies are available.

The best way to evaluate a patient with suspected white-coat hypertension is to use an automated ambulatory blood pressure device that measures the blood pressure periodically throughout the day and night. The patient quickly becomes accustomed to the small, light-weight, portable device, and a representative series of recordings can be obtained. The accuracy of these devices allows separation of those patients with true elevations of blood pressure from those who are hyperreactors. The devices are also useful in evaluating patients with episodic hypertension and those with borderline blood pressure elevations who already have evidence of involvement of the heart, kidneys, or vasculature. Automated blood pressure monitoring can be used to evaluate the duration and effectiveness of antihypertensive medication; correlate blood pressure with damage to the heart, kidneys, or blood vessels; and determine the prognosis. Its value in routine evaluation of hypertensive patients has not been clearly established, however.

Joint National Committee: The Sixth Report of the Joint National Committee on Detection, Evaluation, and Diagnosis of High Blood Pressure (JNC VI). Arch Intern Med 1997;157:2413.

A. INITIAL EVALUATION

The initial evaluation should be focused on excluding secondary or reversible causes of hypertension and looking for the presence and severity of organ damage caused by hypertension. A reversible cause for high blood pressure is found in fewer than 5% of adult patients. Nonetheless, signs of a reversible cause should be looked for in the patient's history, the screening physical examination, blood chemistries, and urinalysis. A more exhaustive evaluation for a secondary cause is needed for patients whose blood pressure is difficult to control medically, who have malignant hypertension, or who have a sudden onset of high blood pressure.

The vast majority of patients with mild-to-moderate hypertension are asymptomatic. A careful history should be obtained, including first-degree relatives (siblings, parents, children, aunts, uncles) with high blood pressure, stroke, coronary artery disease, or diabetes; any knowledge or personal history of high blood pressure; smoking; alcohol consumption; and history of headache, sweats, palpitations, and pallor. Alcohol consumption can cause acute elevations of blood pressure; chronic consumption can cause sustained elevations. A complete evaluation of all prescription and nonprescription medications the patient is taking should be done to exclude any possible contribution to the elevation or any interaction that might limit a given drug's antihypertensive effects. In particular, the clinician should ask about use of estrogens, nonsteroidal antiinflammatory agents, and decongestants. Approximately 5% of women taking oral contraceptives have eleva-

tions of blood pressure; these usually resolve when the medication is discontinued. This side effect of oral contraceptives is more frequent in women over the age of 35 and in the presence of obesity; the use of low-dose estrogen oral contraceptives greatly reduces the incidence. Nonsteroidal antiinflammatory agents may antagonize the antihypertensive effects of antihypertensive medications, especially angiotensin-converting enzyme inhibitors (ACEI) and angiotensin receptor blockers (ARB). Any previous antihypertensive medication use should be documented as well as the blood pressure response and side effects.

B. PHYSICAL EXAMINATION

The physical findings suggestive of secondary or potentially reversible high blood pressure include abdominal or flank bruits suggestive of renovascular hypertension; absent or diminished femoral pulses suggestive of aortic coarctation; and flank or abdominal masses suggestive of polycystic renal disease or abdominal aortic aneurysm. Careful evaluation for target organ damage from hypertension should include funduscopic examination for arteriovenous nicking, arteriolar narrowing, hemorrhages, exudates, or papilledema; and cardiac examination for signs of heart failure (S_3 or a laterally displaced LV apical impulse), LV hypertrophy (S_4 or a sustained LV apical impulse). The patient should also be examined for any neurologic deficit compatible with stroke.

C. DIAGNOSTIC STUDIES

Clinical laboratory tests should be performed to screen for occult renal or cardiac disease that might contribute to the elevation of blood pressure and to assess overall cardiovascular risk. The complete blood count might demonstrate the presence of anemia, suggesting chronic renal disease. Urinalysis is a good screening tool for occult renal disease, diabetes, renal protein loss, or abnormal sediment. One should test for microalbuminuria in all hypertensive diabetics and patients with moderate to sever hypertension. Serum electrolytes; blood urea nitrogen; creatinine; fasting blood glucose; hemoglobin A_{1c}; total, high-density lipoprotein (HDL), and low-density lipoprotein (LDL) cholesterol; triglycerides; calcium; uric acid; and magnesium provide information on other potential cardiovascular risk factors and also establish a baseline for the effects of drug therapy.

1. Electrocardiography—Although not a particularly sensitive tool, an electrocardiogram should be obtained to look for left ventricular hypertrophy (LVH), which, if present, is an independent risk factor for cardiovascular morbidity and mortality. In hypertensive patients, this is a significant predictor of poor cardiovascular outcomes.

2. Echocardiography—This imaging method, which is much more sensitive for the presence of LVH, should be done in selected individuals. Although the role of echocardiography as a screening tool has not been established, it is excellent for assessing the degree of LVH and systolic functional status in hypertensive patients. Cardiac Doppler allows the assessment of diastolic filling and can suggest the presence of diastolic dysfunction, which may be associated with signs and symptoms of heart failure. Borderline hypertensive patients whose echocardiograms show LVH should probably be treated. Chest radiography is not a routine part of the screening process for the uncomplicated cases of hypertension.

D. ORGAN INVOLVEMENT

The main organs (target or end organs), which suffer the ravages of high blood pressure, are the heart, brain, kidneys, and blood vessels. High blood pressure is an independent risk factor for coronary artery disease, and cardiac involvement is responsible for the largest portion of the increase in morbidity and mortality observed in patients with high blood pressure. Up to one third of untreated patients with mild-to-moderate elevations of blood pressure have LVH. Increasing LV mass is generally associated with increasing blood pressure, although patients vary greatly in the extent of hypertrophy for any given level of blood pressure. Increased LV mass also can be present in the absence of elevated blood pressure, however, and may be related to metabolic differences in hypertensive patients. The prognosis is significantly worse when LVH is present with any amount of blood pressure elevation. Effective antihypertensive therapy will cause regression of LVH, but it is apparent that simple reduction of blood pressure is not always sufficient to cause regression. The anticipated beneficial effects of LV mass reduction with antihypertensive therapy have yet to be convincingly demonstrated.

1. Atherosclerotic complications—The most common cause of death in patients with high blood pressure are complications from atherosclerosis. These are unstable coronary syndromes characterized by angina, acute myocardial infarction, and sudden death. Large blood pressure reduction trials have shown disappointingly small decrease in the incidence of these atherosclerotic complications. When therapy is directed at reducing both blood pressure and cholesterol, the results are somewhat more encouraging—although not consistent. The addition of any of the "statins" or hydroxymethylglutaryl coenzyme A (HMG-CoA) reductase inhibitors is particularly effective in reducing acute coronary ischemic events.

2. Cardiac dysfunction—Other sequelae of long-standing high blood pressure are systolic and diastolic dysfunction. Reduced systolic function may result from myocardial ischemia, infarction, fibrosis, and or cardiomyopathy. Diastolic dysfunction results directly form

LVH and, even in the absence of systolic dysfunction, can cause symptoms of heart failure. It is estimated that 40–50% of patients admitted to hospital for heart failure have preserved systolic cardiac function. This is especially prevalent in the older (>65 years old) population. Cardiac dysrhythmias and sudden cardiac death are also more prevalent in the presence of LVH.

3. Stroke—Hypertension is the major risk factor for hemorrhagic stroke and, to a lesser extent, cerebral infarction. The level of systolic pressure is more closely related to stroke incidence than is diastolic pressure. The incidence of hemorrhagic stroke, at any raised level of systolic pressure, is significantly higher among blacks than among other groups; when stroke occurs, it also tends to be more extensive. Effective antihypertensive therapy reduces the risk of stroke to almost normotensive levels.

4. Hypertensive renal disease—Renal disease due to hypertension is characterized by nephrosclerosis with chronic renal insufficiency and ultimately renal failure. Microalbuminuria is a marker of asymptomatic renal dysfunction in hypertensive patients with renal dysfunction. The renal complications of high blood pressure can be virtually eliminated by effective antihypertensive therapy. All agents have been shown to equally effective in their renal protective effects in nondiabetic patients. The combination of hypertension and diabetes mellitus is particularly damaging to the kidneys and causes earlier onset and more rapid progression of renal insufficiency and renal failure if untreated (see section on Diabetes mellitus).

5. Aorta and peripheral blood vessels—The aorta and peripheral blood vessels are involved in the genesis of high blood pressure and in its consequences. High blood pressure is a contributing and exacerbating factor in ascending aortic dissection and contributes to abdominal aortic aneurysm by virtue of its enhancement of the atherosclerotic process. Changes in the elastic properties of the peripheral vasculature are manifest early in the course of hypertension as a decrease in arterial compliance that is related to the increase in blood pressure.

6. Eyes—The eyes suffer vascular damage as a result of untreated hypertension. The characteristic ocular findings of hypertensive retinopathy include arteriolar narrowing, arteriovenous nicking, flame hemorrhages, hard exudates, and papilledema-progressive changes related to increasing severity and duration of hypertension.

Treatment

The treatment of hypertension has evolved over the past four decades as we have accumulated knowledge of the natural history, pathophysiology, and risk factors for hypertension as well as the effects of therapy and the interactions of these factors. The goal of treating high blood pressure is to reduce blood pressure and thereby prevent or reverse end-organ damage without causing significant side effects or requiring unacceptable changes in lifestyle. We now have many classes of antihypertensive agents that effectively lower blood pressure, either alone or in conjunction with an agent from another class of drugs. Because of the potentially detrimental metabolic changes caused by some agents, their failure to reduce the incidence of myocardial infarction, and the multisystem involvement of hypertension, it is essential to choose a regimen that effectively lowers blood pressure without causing abnormalities. The following recommendations incorporate data from large long-term trials and experimental evidence from human and animal studies.

Nonpharmacologic therapy and coronary risk factor reduction should be initiated in all patients once the diagnosis of sustained hypertension is made. Individuals with mild (systolic BP, 140–159; diastolic, 90–99) or moderate (systolic, 160–179; diastolic, 100–109) hypertension can be treated with nonpharmacologic therapy for 3–6 months. If this fails to reduce blood pressure to below 140/90 mm Hg within that time, pharmacologic therapy should be initiated. If end-organ damage is already present at diagnosis, or if other major coronary risk factors such as diabetes or dyslipidemia are present, pharmacologic therapy should be initiated once the diagnosis has been made. Individuals with severe hypertension (systolic BP higher than 180; diastolic higher than 110) should have both nonpharmacologic and drug therapy initiated once the diagnosis is made.

A. NONPHARMACOLOGIC THERAPY

Nonpharmacologic therapy should be encouraged in all hypertensive patients. The approaches of proven benefit are weight reduction in obese patients, moderate aerobic exercise in sedentary patients, a reduction in alcohol consumption in all patients who drink, and a reduction of salt intake in some patients.

1. Obesity—Obesity (more than 10% over ideal weight) is associated with hypertension, diabetes, hyperlipidemia, and excess coronary mortality. In obese patients, a decrease of as much as 2 mm Hg of diastolic blood pressure can be achieved for every 3 lb of weight loss. The benefits of weight reduction start early in the course, with a loss of as little as 10–15 lb. Although all obese patients should be encouraged to lose weight, the process is usually difficult and frequently requires extensive support and sometimes a financial investment. The use of all "stimulant" type weight reduction therapies should be strictly avoided, as they tend to elevate blood pressure. The fat substitutes or avoidance therapies do not raise blood pressure but have their own side effects.

2. Exercise—Regular exercise in a previously sedentary individual may reduce diastolic blood pressure as much as 10 mm Hg. The level of exercise should be that required to raise the heart rate to 50–60% of the maximal predicted heart rate. Walking briskly for 45 min three to five times per week should suffice for most previously sedentary individuals. Increasing the amount of exercise in a previously active individual, however, seldom decreases blood pressure.

3. Alcohol consumption—Alcohol consumption causes acute increases in blood pressure and can cause sustained hypertension in a significant proportion of patients. Hypertensive patients should be encouraged to limit their alcohol consumption to 1 oz of ethanol per day, the equivalent of 2 oz of 100-proof hard liquor, 8 oz of wine, or 24 oz of beer. Even this level of alcohol consumption is associated with increased overall mortality. Alcohol decreases cardiovascular mortality and appears to decrease the onset of diabetes by improving insulin resistance. The best data for these benefits are for wine. Beer with its even higher carbohydrate load should be avoided in diabetics.

4. Sodium reduction—Reducing sodium in the diet has been shown to reduce blood pressure in most people to a modest degree. Hypertensive patients, older individuals, and blacks tend to be more salt-sensitive, and achieve larger reductions in blood pressure with salt restriction. Hypertensive patients should be encouraged to keep sodium chloride consumption to less than 4-6 g/d.

5. Stress—Stress has long been known to raise blood pressure acutely and has been implicated in the genesis of sustained hypertension, even though no clear relationship has been demonstrated. Reducing stress would seem to be a reasonable form of nonpharmacologic therapy, but no controlled studies have demonstrated significant improvement in blood pressure with stress avoidance or relaxation therapy.

Trials of Hypertension Prevention Collaborative Treatment Group: Effect of weight loss and sodium reduction intervention on blood pressure and hypertension incidence in overweight people with high normal blood pressure. Arch Intern Med 1997;157:657.

B. PHARMACOLOGIC THERAPY

The clinician is now blessed with and confused by the overwhelming number of antihypertensive medications (Table 13–1) available today. Although all of these classes of agents have been shown to be roughly equal in their ability to lower blood pressure in large population studies, they are not equally effective in all demographic groups or in preventing all complications. The initial choice for a given patient should take age, race, metabolic side effects, other cardiac risk factors, and, most importantly, concomitant diseases into considera-

Table 13-1. Common oral antihypertensive agents.

Drug	Total Daily Dose[a] (mg)	Frequency	Drug	Total Daily Dose[a] (mg)	Frequency
Adrenergic Inhibitors			**Calcium channel blockers (cont.)**		
Alpha-blockers			Verapamil	80–480	bid or tid
Doxasosin	1–16	qd	(long-acting)	120–480	qd or bid
Prazosin	1–20	bid or tid	Dihydropyridines		
Terazosin	1–20	qd	Amlodipine	2.5–10	qd
Beta-blockers			Felodipine	5–20	qd
Atenolol	25–100	qd	Isradipine	2.5–10	bid
Betaxolol	5–40	qd	Nifedipine (GITS)	30–120	qd
Bisoprolol	5–20	qd			
Metoprolol	25–200	bid	**Diuretics**		
Nadolol	20–240	bid	Thiazide-type		
Propranolol (long-acting)	60–240	qd	Bendroflumethiazide	2.5–5	qd
Timolol	20–40	qd	Benzthiazide	12.5–50	qd
Beta-blockers with ISA			Chlorthalidone	12.5–50	qd
Acebutolol	200–1200	qd	Chlorthiazide	12.5–50	qd
Carteolol	2.5–10	qd	Hydroclorthiazide	12.5–50	qd
Penbutolol	20–80	qd	Indapamide	2.5–5	qd
Pindolol	10–60	bid	Metolazone	1.25–5	qd
Alpha-beta-blockers			Methyclothiazide	2.5–5	qd
Labetalol	200–1200	qd or bid	Polythiazide	1.0–4	qd
ACE-Inhibitors			Trichlormethiazide	1.0–4	qd
Benazepril	10–40	qd/bid	Loop diuretics		
Captopril	25–50	tid	Bumetanide	0.5–5	bid
Enalapril	10–40	qd or bid	Ethacrynic acid	25–100	bid
Fosinopril	10–40	qd or bid	Furosemide	10–300	bid
Lisinopril	10–40	qd or bid	Potassium-sparing agents		
Moexipril	7.5–30	qd or bid	Amiloride	5–10	qd or bid
Perindopril	4–16	qd	Spironolactone	25–100	bid or tid
Quinapril	10–80	qd or bid	Triamterene	50–150	qd or bid
Ramipril	2.5–20	qd or bid			
Trandolapril	1–8	qd	**Centrally acting agents**		
			Clonidine	0.1–1.2	qd or bid
Angiotensin receptor blockers			Transdermal	0.1–0.3	q week
Candesartan	2–32, PO	qd	Guanabenz	4–64	bid
Eprosartan	600–800, PO	qd/bid	Methyldopa	250–2000	bid
Irbesartan	75–300, PO	qd			
Losartan	25–100, PO	qd/bid	**Peripheral vasodilators**		
Valsartan	80–320, PO	qd	Hydralazine	50–200	bid–qd
			Minoxidil	2.5–80	qd or bid
Calcium channel blockers					
Diltiazem (SR)	120–160	bid			
(CD, XR)	120–160	qd			

[a] The total daily dose should be given in divided doses at the frequency specified. The initial dose should be the smallest listed.
bid = twice a day; ISA = intrinsix sympathomimetic activity; qd = once a day; qid = 4 times a day; tid = 3 times a day.

tion. The report of the Joint National Committee on Detection, Evaluation and Treatment of High Blood Pressure recommends monotherapy with diuretics or β-blockers as initial therapy. Calcium channel blockers, angiotensin converting enzyme inhibitors (ACEI), an-giotensin receptor blockers (ARB), and α-adrenergic blocking agents are alternative first-line agents. The report does recognize special populations such as diabetics and patients with coronary disease, which need special consideration.

Joint National Committee: The Sixth Report of the Joint National Committee on Detection, Evaluation, and Diagnosis of High Blood Pressure (JNC VI): Arch Intern Med 1997;157:2413.

The traditional initial approach of monotherapy with a diuretic or β-blocker has the advantage of being both moderately effective and reasonably inexpensive. The disadvantages are that both agents may cause metabolic derangements that can adversely affect their ability to reduce coronary events and frequent side effects. A further disadvantage is that treating hypertensive patients primarily with diuretics or β-blockers fails to take ethnicity or concomitant diseases into consideration.

Table 13–2 lists the generalized response to antihypertensive therapy based on demographic groups; it is important to note that gender does not appear to affect the response. Such data can serve as a starting point in picking an initial antihypertensive agent, but they provide only an indication of the likelihood of response in an individual patient. Demographics cannot predict individual responses and therefore should not be used to exclude consideration of any class of agents in a given patient (eg, ACEI for a black patient). Because pharmaceutical agents are quite costly, the economic burden must also factor into the decision-making process. If a patient can't afford to buy his or her medications due to high cost, it is unlikely that that medication will be effective.

Concomitant diseases—Other diseases occurring along with hypertension clearly must influence the choice of initial and subsequent antihypertensive agents. In patients with diabetes, diuretics may exacerbate glucose intolerance and should be added to ACEI only if they are needed to reach target levels or to manage fluid accumulation caused by another antihypertensive agent.

Because thiazide diuretics raise plasma triglycerides and LDL cholesterol, they worsen the already present dyslipidemias prevalent in diabetics. The current recommendations are to only use low-dose diuretics, which will avoid some of the deleterious side effects but tend to be less effective when used as monotherapy. ACEIs and ARBs are extremely useful in both controlling blood pressure and slowing or preventing proteinuria and renal failure in diabetic patients.

Beta-blockers may exacerbate heart block and reactive airway disease. They may also increase plasma triglyceride levels and decrease HDL cholesterol, thereby potentially increasing atherosclerosis (see section on Beta-adrenergic blocking agents). Nonetheless, β-blockers are a good choice for patients with hypertension and angina and are recommended for all patients with known coronary artery disease. They effectively treat both conditions and can simplify patient care without sacrificing efficacy. Beta-blockers decrease mortality following myocardial infarction and should therefore not be withheld in such patients because of fears of increased atherogenesis or heart failure. Calcium channel blockers are also very effective in patients with combined hypertension and angina. ACEIs have been shown to improve survival in patients with dilated cardiomyopathy and with postmyocardial infarction systolic dysfunction.

1. Diuretics—When used as monotherapy, diuretics are effective in approximately 50% of patients and are especially effective in lowering systolic blood pressure. Several studies and meta-analyses have shown diuretic therapy to significantly decrease cardiac and stroke mortality rates. Diuretics are particularly effective antihypertensive agents in the elderly.

The adverse side effects of diuretics are urinary frequency and metabolic disturbances. They cause loss of potassium, which can precipitate cardiac dysrhythmias, renal insufficiency, and resistance to antihypertensive agents. Thiazide diuretics may induce gout in gout-prone individuals. Low doses (eg, 12.5–25 mg/day of hydrochlorothiazide) usually prevents hypokalemia and may reduce the metabolic alterations in glucose and lipids.

Table 13–2. Response by demographic group.

Group	Effective Agents	Ineffective Agents
Young white	ACEI, β-blocker	Diuretics
Older white	Calcium channel blocker, β-blocker	
Young black	Calcium channel blocker	ACEI, β-blocker
Other black	Diuretic	ACEI, β-blocker
Isolated systolic hypertension	Diuretic	ACEI

ACEI = angiotensin-converting enzyme inhibitor.

The shorter acting loop diuretics, such as furosemide, are poor antihypertensive agents and should be used for managing fluid overload. No outcome data are available for these agents in hypertension.

Spironolactone inhibits aldosterone and is a weak diuretic. It may be used in conjunction with a thiazide or loop diuretic to conserve potassium if hypokalemia occurs. Serum potassium should be monitored especially carefully when spironolactone is used with other potassium-sparing agents such as ACEI and ARBs.

2. Angiotensin-converting enzyme inhibitors— ACEI block the conversion of inactive angiotensin I to the potent vasoconstrictor substance angiotensin II. The use of this group of agents is rapidly increasing as first-line therapy, especially in the young white population, due to the low incidence of associated side effects. The success rate is 40–50% as monotherapy and when used in combination with a low-dose diuretic, β-blocker, or calcium channel blocker, ACEI are highly effective in controlling more than 80% of patients. Some of the additional benefits thought to be achieved with ACEI are related to the reduction of the potent vasoconstrictor and mitogen effects of angiotensin II on cardiac and vascular tissue. They produce no adverse effect on glucose metabolism or lipid profile and have a potent renal-protective effect in diabetic patients. ACEIs preserve renal function and avoid or delay the onset of microalbuminuria and slow or prevent the progression to proteinuria and end-stage renal disease. ACEIs work by inhibiting the renin-angiotensin-aldosterone system and may cause mild elevations of serum potassium. If supplemental potassium is concomitantly administered, life-threatening hyperkalemia may result. Renal function and potassium levels should be monitored during initiation and titration of ACEI therapy in all patients, especially those with preexisting renal insufficiency. Of special note, ACEI may cause life-threatening fetal abnormalities and should be avoided in pregnant women. A chronic nonproductive cough develops in 5–15% of patients treated with ACEI and may be bothersome enough to cause discontinuation of the agent. Recently, a rare potentially fatal side effect of angioedema has been described with ACEI use. This side effect should be aggressively treated and the patient should not be rechallenged with an ACEI.

The antihypertensive efficacy of ACEI may be attenuated by concomitant administration of nonsteroidal antiinflammatory agents (including aspirin and over-the-counter ibuprofen, naproxen, etc), which should therefore be avoided.

3. Angiotensin receptor blockers— ARBs selectively block the vascular angiotensin II (AT_1) receptors, causing vasodilation similar to the ACEI. They are as effective and very well tolerated with a side effect profile similar to that of ACEI. Angiotensin receptor blockers appear to have the same renal protective effects in diabetic patients as ACEI. No head-to-head trials of ACEI and ARBs in diabetic patients are available. Due to the much higher cost of ARBs and the proven efficacy of ACEI, diabetics should start on an ACEI, and patients intolerant of ACEI should use ARBs. The incidence of cough with ARBs is less than that observed with ACEI (< 5%) but is much higher in those patients who have already had an ACEI-associated cough. Angioedema has also been described with ARB use although it is significantly less frequent than with ACEI. If a patient has had angioedema with an agent in either of the two classes, the other class should be avoided.

4. Beta-adrenergic blocking agents— Beta-blockers are effective monotherapy in 50–60% of patients, especially those with an activated renin-angiotensin system. They lower blood pressure by decreasing both heart rate and cardiac contractility and thus cardiac output. All β-blockers are similar in antihypertensive efficacy, regardless of whether they are cardioselective (β_1-specific) or nonselective (β_1 and β_2) receptor blockers; possess intrinsic sympathomimetic activity (ISA); or are lipid-soluble. The side effect profile does differ, however, and is based on these properties. Beta$_1$-selective agents cause less bronchial constriction at lower doses but are similar to nonselective β-blockers at high doses. Agents with ISA produce less resting bradycardia than do those without. Lipid solubility determines whether the agent will cross into the brain. Lipid-soluble β-blockers, which cross the blood-brain barrier, may cause more central nervous system disturbances, including nightmares and confusion. All β-blockers depress LV systolic function, tend to reduce cardiac output, and may cause impotence. Fatigue is a frequent side effect and may limit use in young active patients. Beta-blockers also cause the alterations in lipid profile mentioned earlier; the HDL depression is less significant with cardioselective β-blockers at low doses (eg, metoprolol, 25–50 mg bid) and insignificant with the ISA β-blockers. The clinical significance of these abnormalities has not been established and the concomitant use of appropriate lipid therapy probably makes this a moot point.

5. Calcium channel blockers— Calcium channel blockers are very well tolerated and effective as monotherapy in 60–70% of patients in all demographic groups. The mechanism of antihypertensive action is vasodilatation with all such agents and a decrease in heart rate and cardiac output with the nondihydropyridines agents (verapamil and diltiazem). Because of the negative inotropic effects in all but the newest agents, calcium channel blockers should not be used in patients with cardiac failure. All calcium channel blockers are now available in formulations that can be taken once or twice daily, a regimen that greatly improves compliance. Immediate-release preparations of short-acting agents have no place in the antihypertensive armamentarium. Combinations of calcium channel blockers and a β-blocker, an ACEI, or ARB are very effective in lowering blood pressure. Concomitant use of a β-blocker and a calcium channel blocker with significant sinus and atrioventricular node-slowing properties (eg, diltiazem, verapamil) should be done with caution so as to avoid profound bradycardia or heart block. Other side effects include peripheral edema (dihydropyridines) and constipation (verapamil).

In several large meta-analyses, calcium channel blockers have been shown to be highly effective in lowering blood pressure but have a 25% excess incidence of acute myocardial infarction and heart failure. The mechanisms are as yet to be delineated. Until this is resolved, use of calcium channel blockers as monotherapy for hypertension is not encouraged.

6. Alpha-receptor blockers—Alpha-blockers act at vascular postsynaptic α-receptors to produce arterial and venous dilatation. Because the α-blockers do not reduce cardiac output, they do not adversely affect exercise tolerance. The major side effect of this group is postural hypotension, especially after the first dose, a problem that can be minimized by taking the first dose at bedtime. Alpha-blockers increase HDL cholesterol and reduce LDL cholesterol and may thereby decrease coronary risk. The LDL-cholesterol-lowering effect of doxazosin is similar in magnitude to that of 10 mg of lovastatin. It is therefore surprising that the α-blocker arm of the ALLHAT trial, a large randomized trial comparing the major antihypertensive classes, was recently stopped early due to a 25% higher incidence of major cardiac events in hypertensive patients treated primarily with α-blockers compared with diuretics. The reasons for these unexpected results are unclear. Alpha-blockers should therefore not be used as initial therapy and should be relegated to the status of add-on therapy until more data clarify the reasons for this increased risk.

ALLHAT Collaborative Research Group: Major cardiovascular events in hypertensive patients randomized to doxazosin versus chlorthalidone: The antihypertensive and lipid-lowering treatment to prevent heart attack trial (ALLHAT). JAMA 2000;283:1967-75.

7. Centrally acting agents—The group of agents with central sympatholytic action includes methyldopa, clonidine, and guanabenz. This class of drugs acts by stimulating central α_1-adrenergic receptors, which exert an inhibitory effect on peripheral sympathetic outflow and is moderately effective as monotherapy in lowering blood pressure. The predominant side effects of this class are sedation, postural hypotension, dry mouth, and fatigue. Rebound hypertension may be a significant problem if the agent is withdrawn suddenly following high-dose therapy, especially with clonidine. Gradual reduction of the dose will avoid the rebound effect. This class of agents is now used infrequently because of its significant and often limiting side effects. The transcutaneous patch formulation of clonidine, which is applied once a week, is useful in enhancing compliance in selected patients or in patients unable to take oral therapy.

8. Direct arteriolar dilators—Agents such as hydralazine and minoxidil that lower blood pressure by relaxing vascular smooth muscle do so by direct arteriolar dialtion. The resulting decrease in peripheral resistance induces a reflex tachycardia and inotropic cardiac stimulation. Because fluid retention develops almost universally, diuretics must usually be used concomitantly. Vasodilators should be avoided in patients with coronary artery disease because the reflex tachycardia may induce angina. These agents are used almost exclusively as additional agents in patients whose blood pressure is extremely difficult to control with more commonly used agents.

9. Combination therapy—Combining antihypertensive medications from different classes may be even more effective than expected from their individual responses. Many experts now recommend combination therapy to enhance efficacy and reduce side effects. This synergistic result frequently allows lower doses of each agent to be used. A low-dose thiazide diuretic, for example, will significantly augment the antihypertensive efficacy of an ACEI, an ARB, an α-blocker, a β-blocker, or a vasodilator. Beta-blockers will enhance the blood pressure-lowering effects of a vasodilator and reduce any reflex increase in heart rate. The use of lower dose combinations is highly effective and is likely to produce fewer side effects.

Pharmaceutical companies have made fixed-dose combinations of two medications in the same pill. The combinations may or may not work for a given patient, so it is recommended that blood pressure be controlled initially with appropriate doses of two or more agents and then a fixed-dose combination that approximates the effective therapy be substituted. This strategy will improve compliance.

C. Management of Complicated Hypertension

The goals of antihypertensive therapy, to lower the blood pressure to a safe level, reduce left ventricular hypertrophy, and improve other cardiovascular risk factors without adversely affecting other organ systems or risk factors, become more difficult to attain in the presence of concomitant disease of the heart, lungs, or kidneys. In tailoring antihypertensive therapy to the individual patient, it is best to simplify therapy by using medications that will improve the hypertension as well as (or at least not exacerbate) any coexisting condition (Table 13–3).

Table 13–3. Recommended initial agent in patients with concomitant disease.

Disease	Initial Agent	Alternative Agent
CAD	β-blocker	ACEI, ARB, diuretic
CHF	ACEI	β-blockers, ARB, Diuretic
CRI	β-blockers, CCB	Diuretic, clonidine
Diabetes	ACEI	β-blocker, ARB, diuretic

ACEI = angiotensin-converting enzyme inhibitor; ARB = angiotensin receptor blocker; CAD = coronary artery disease; CCB = calcium channel blocker; CHF = congestive heart failure; CRI = chronic renal insufficiency.

1. Coronary artery disease—In hypertensive patients with concomitant coronary artery disease manifested by angina, lowering blood pressure alone may improve anginal symptoms by decreasing myocardial oxygen demand. Beneficial agents include the non-ISA β-blockers, ACEI, ARBs, and calcium channel blockers. Care should be taken to avoid sudden drops in blood pressure to hypotensive levels. Patients who present with unstable angina and hypertension should receive standard therapy for unstable angina; that is, intravenous heparin and nitroglycerin, aspirin, and β-blockers. This will usually lower blood pressure to a safe level. In patients with acute myocardial infarction complicated by hypertension, β-blockers are the mainstay of therapy. Blood pressure should be reduced to < 140/90 mm Hg. Drastic reductions should be avoided because coronary perfusion pressure is directly related to mean arterial pressure; coronary vascular reserve is exhausted in the periinfarction area, and further ischemia or infarction could result. Beta-blockers have been clearly demonstrated to decrease postmyocardial infarction mortality and ischemic event rates. In several large meta-analyses, calcium channel blockers have been shown to be highly effective in lowering blood pressure but have a 25% excess incidence of acute myocardial infarction and heart failure. The mechanisms are as yet to be delineated.

2. Congestive heart failure—In patients with reduced LV systolic function (from any cause), elevated blood pressure may contribute to further signs and symptoms of heart failure. Even normal levels of blood pressure may be too high in patients with moderate-to-severe LV systolic dysfunction. The goal of therapy should be to lower systolic blood pressure as low as possible without symptoms (< 110 mm Hg and lower if tolerated). ACEIs have proved very useful in reducing blood pressure and symptoms of heart failure and improving survival rates in such patients (see Table 13–3). Diuretics augment the antihypertensive effects of ACEI and are useful additions for the hypertensive patient with or without congestive heart failure. When starting an ACEI in a patient who is already on a diuretic, the dose of the ACEI should be reduced and the diuretic should be withheld or given at a reduced dose that day to avoid hypotension. Angiotensin receptor blockers may be substituted in ACEI-intolerant patients.

Beta-blockade has been definitively shown to improve symptoms, LV systolic function, and longevity in patients with heart failure when added to ACEI or alone. Metoprolol, bisoprolol, and carvedilol are the agents that have been used in the major heart failure trials. Their use in heart failure is described elsewhere.

3. Cerebrovascular disease—Patients with symptomatic or otherwise evident cerebrovascular disease coexistent with hypertension should receive antihypertensive therapy. Such patients tend to be older and therefore respond similarly to other older patients (see Table 13–2). Acute cerebrovascular accidents are frequently accompanied by hypertension, which is sometimes severe. Rapid reduction of blood pressure in patients with acute stroke is associated with increased morbidity and mortality and should be avoided during the acute phase. In fact, unless the diastolic blood pressure is greater than 120 mm Hg, treatment should either be withheld or instituted slowly and with great caution until the patient has stabilized. Because cerebrovascular disease and coronary artery disease frequently coexist, antihypertensive therapy should be instituted judiciously in patients with stroke and evidence of ischemia or heart failure.

4. Renal insufficiency—Effective antihypertensive therapy will halt or slow the progression of renal insufficiency in most hypertensive patients (see Table 13–3). In patients with established renal insufficiency, ACEI may be very effective and improve renal function but should be used carefully, with frequent monitoring of renal function and potassium during initiation and titration of therapy. Patients with renovascular hypertension may have rapid worsening of renal function when treated with ACEI. Such patients must be monitored carefully during initiation of antihypertensive therapy for worsening of renal function or the development of hyperkalemia. Potassium supplementation or potassium-sparing diuretics should be avoided in patients with even moderate renal insufficiency. Even a modest decrease in renal function could cause serious or fatal hyperkalemia. Most patients with renal insufficiency and hypertension respond well to all types of antihypertensive therapy, however. Such patients tend to have volume-dependent hypertension and respond well to loop diuretics, although higher doses must be used as renal function deteriorates.

5. Diabetes mellitus—Diabetic patients are known for their almost universal incidence of vascular disease and increased susceptibility to cardiovascular complications. The coexistence of diabetes and hypertension markedly increases the risk of coronary artery disease, stroke, and renal failure. If dyslipidemia is also present, the risk is even greater. Hypertension should be treated aggressively in diabetic patients, using agents that are renal-protective and do not further aggravate glucose intolerance or adversely affect lipids (see Table 13–3). ACEI, β-blockers, and ARBs are extremely useful in both controlling blood pressure and preventing or slowing the onset of proteinuria and renal failure in diabetic patients. The recent Hypertension Optimal Treatment Trial (HOT) established that lowering diastolic blood pressure in diabetics to levels below 80 mm Hg decreases the risk of major cardiovascular events and mortality compared with lowering diastolic blood pressure to "normal" (< 90 mm Hg) levels. The goal for systolic blood pressure is < 130 mm Hg. Alpha-blockers, ACEI, and ARBs, which are effective in diabetic patients, are glucose- and lipid-beneficial or neutral. It is recommended that an ACEI be used as the first agent in all diabetic patients. ARBs appear to have the same renal protective effects in diabetic patients as ACEI. No head-to-head trials of ACEI and ARBs in diabetic patients are available. Due to the much higher cost of ARBs and the proven efficacy of ACEI, diabetics should start on an ACEI and ACEI-intolerant patients should use ARBs.

Hansson L, Zanchetti A, Carruthers SG, et al, for the HOT study Group: Effects of intensive blood-pressure lowering and low-dose aspirin in patients with hypertension: Principal results of the Hypertension Optimal Treatment (HOT) randomized trial. Lancet 1998;351:1755.

6. Hypertensive emergencies—Patients presenting with severe hypertension (> 220/120 mm Hg) and signs and symptoms of encephalopathy, acute myocardial ischemic syndromes, stroke, pulmonary edema, or aortic dissection should be treated emergently so as to achieve rapid reduction of their blood pressure (Table 13–4). Because of its rapid onset and short duration of therapy, which allow for smoother titration of blood pressure, intravenous sodium nitroprusside is the treatment of choice. Patients should be admitted to the intensive care unit and monitored closely during therapy. The aim is to reduce blood pressure very quickly within the first hour or two after presentation but to avoid hypotension. Patients must be monitored for thiocyanate toxicity if therapy is prolonged. A recently introduced alternative is intravenous fenoldopam, a selective dopamine-1 receptor agonist. It has a similar antihypertensive profile to nitroprusside with a rapid predictable onset of action, short half-life (9.8 min), and few side effects at effective doses. There is a linear correlation between fenoldopam infusion rate and blood pressure lowering. Its use still requires monitoring in the intensive care unit.

If aortic dissection is present, a short-acting β-blocker such as esmolol should be added to decrease shear forces in the aorta. Intravenous labetalol is highly effective and can also be used. Oral immediate-release clonidine and ACEI are effective in rapidly reducing blood pressure and can be added orally. Oral immediate-release nifedipine may cause unpredictable hypotension and should not be used.

Hypertensive urgencies defined as patients who present with severe hypertension but with minimal or no symptoms may be treated more slowly, achieving a significant reduction in blood pressure within the first 24 h. Intravenous labetalol is particularly useful in these patients.

Lip GYH, Beevers M, Beevers DG: Survival and prognosis of 315 patients with malignant-phase hypertension. J Hypertens 1995;13:915.

Prognosis

Significant reductions in blood pressure definitely reduce the incidence of stroke, renal and cardiac failure, and acute coronary syndromes. We must attempt to

Table 13–4. Antihypertensive therapy for hypertensive emergencies.

Drug	Dose	Comments
Nitroprusside	0.25–10 µg/kg/min	Treatment of choice
Fenoldopam	0.1 µg/kg/min, increased by 0.05 µg/kg/mm	Doesn't require thiocyanate monitoring
Labetalol	20–40 mg IV q10 min to 300 mg	Commonly used after surgery
Esmolol	500 µg/kg over 1 min, then 25–200 µg/kg/min	Can aggravate heart failure
Clonidine	0.1–0.2 mg PO, 0.05–0.1 mg qh until 0.8 mg	Sedation possible
Captopril	6.25–50 mg PO q 6–8 h	Excessive hypotension possible

prevent cardiac and vascular disease by taking into account all the relevant prognostic factors, not just blood pressure alone. Because coronary artery disease is the most common adverse outcome of hypertension, we must choose antihypertensive drugs not only for their blood pressure-lowering properties, but also for their effects on other critical cardiovascular, metabolic, and renal end-points. Aggressive control of all of the cardiac risk factors is essential for optimal outcomes in hypertensive patients.

Hypertrophic Cardiomyopathies

Pravin Shah, MD

ESSENTIALS OF DIAGNOSIS

- *Dyspnea*
- *Systolic ejection murmur with characteristic changes during bedside maneuvers*
- *Marked asymmetric left ventricular hypertrophy on echocardiogram*
- *Normal or hyperkinetic left ventricular systolic function*

General Considerations

The term *hypertrophic cardiomyopathy* can best be defined as a condition characterized by idiopathic or unexplained myocardial hypertrophy that is associated with small or normal ventricular cavity size, hyperdynamic ventricular function, and diastolic dysfunction. The qualifier *unexplained* is used to suggest that this condition may coexist with hypertension or aortic valve disease, although the extent and distribution of hypertrophy are disproportionate to these associated disorders. Therefore, mild-to-moderate hypertension and mild or moderate aortic valve disease cannot be implicated in massive asymmetric hypertrophy with hyperdynamic ventricular function. (The definition also requires hyperdynamic systolic function, a feature that is rarely absent even in the late stages of hypertrophic cardiomyopathy).

The condition has also been called idiopathic hypertrophic subaortic stenosis, which connotes a condition characterized by myocardial hypertrophy without underlying cause. Hypertrophic cardiomyopathy (HCM) is a more accurate term, however, in that it describes the major feature of idiopathic hypertrophy, especially in patients with no evidence of subaortic stenosis or intraventricular obstruction.

Hypertrophic cardiomyopathy can be classified as nonobstructive or obstructive, based on the presence and the location (midventricle or outflow tract) of intraventricular obstruction. Other classifications may relate to the distribution of the hypertrophy: asymmetric septal hypertrophy, disproportionate upper septal thickening, apical asymmetric hypertrophy, and the like. Such approaches are generally not fruitful except when apical hypertrophy is localized.

Pathophysiology & Etiology

The underlying cause and pathogenesis of this disease are largely unknown. The asymmetric type of HCM is commonly transmitted genetically, but sporadic cases are also recognized. An abnormal response of the myocardium to normal catecholamines has been postulated as a pathogenetic mechanism. The clinical association between HCM and pheochromocytoma, neurofibromatosis, and lentiginosis suggests a genetic disorder of neural crest tissue. More recent studies have linked familial HCM to the cardiac myosin heavy-chain genes on chromosome 14 in some—but not all—families, indicating genetic heterogeneity. The presence of different disease genes or mutations within a given gene may account for differences in the clinical expression of familial HCM.

The pathologic findings at autopsy are remarkably uniform and include massive and generally asymmetric hypertrophy. Both the atria and the ventricles are affected, with the left ventricle most commonly involved. The interventricular septum is generally far more massively hypertrophied than the free wall, a peculiar asymmetric septal hypertrophy that may provide the necessary hemodynamic conditions to cause a dynamic outflow obstruction. In this situation, the condition is referred to as hypertrophic obstructive cardiomyopathy (HOCM). Localization of such hypertrophy in the midlateral wall may result in midventricular obstruction and distribution of the hypertrophy in the right ventricular infundibulum in subpulmonic stenosis. Asymmetric localization of hypertrophy can involve virtually any segment of the left ventricle, except for the posterobasal region.

In some patients, the hypertrophy involves primarily the apical portion of the left ventricle (asymmetric apical hypertrophy) rather than the outflow tract. Such patients exhibit none of the clinical features of intraventricular obstruction.

Striking pathologic features common to most patients with left ventricular outflow obstruction include fibrous thickening of the anterior mitral leaflet and plaques in the upper interventricular septum. The thickening of the anterior mitral leaflet is thought to represent the result of frequent contact with the interventricular septum. The endocardial plaques in the septum may be the result of jet lesions distal to the obstruction. The epicardial coronary arteries are large and patent.

Microscopically, a bizarre and disorderly array of muscle fibers is a striking feature associated with increased connective tissue that interrupts and crisscrosses the muscle bundles.

At times, the hypertrophied septum assumes a peculiar catenoid shape—convex to the left in the apex-to-base plane, but concave on its left ventricular surface in the cross sections. This bizarre and characteristic shape is thought to be responsible for the adynamic nature of the septum. It is hypothesized that fiber disarray and local hypertrophy could result from isometric contraction of a catenoid septum.

A. SYSTOLIC FUNCTION

The integrity of overall systolic function is rather well preserved even in advanced cases; indeed, hypercontractility is a hallmark of the disorder. The cardiac output is generally normal or mildly increased; the ejection fraction is often supernormal. Although global function is well preserved, regional abnormalities may occur; the upper interventricular septum is often hypodynamic and shows reduced thickening during systole. The free walls are generally hyperdynamic.

Left ventricular outflow obstruction is dynamic and variable. The variability can be observed within the same cardiac cycle, from one beat to the next and from one physiologic state to another. When present, the outflow obstruction begins sometime after the onset of early uninterrupted ejection. The obstruction is caused by a sharp systolic anterior motion (SAM) of the anterior mitral leaflet, which obliterates the outflow space. The actual mechanism is not clear, although it is likely to be the result of a Venturi effect from the rapid ejection of a jet of blood through an anatomically narrowed outflow space. The degree of left ventricular outflow obstruction can be accentuated by factors that reduce preload (end-diastolic volume), diminish afterload (arterial pressure), or increase contractility or heart rate. Echocardiographic recordings have demonstrated that a sharp systolic anterior motion of the mitral valve is both accentuated and prolonged by interventions that exacerbate the outflow obstruction, and vice versa (ie, it is diminished and shortened by interventions that

reduce the outflow obstruction). Some investigators interpret intraventricular pressure gradients as not indicative of true obstruction because left ventricular emptying is normal or exaggerated and because early emptying is unimpeded. These gradients have been attributed to cavity obliteration. Echocardiographic techniques have elucidated differences between true gradients resulting from obstruction and those from cavity obliteration.

Mitral regurgitation is shown by color-flow Doppler echocardiography in more than 90% of patients with HOCM and is related to the dynamic outflow obstruction in the vast majority of them. Mitral regurgitation is more severe when a more persistent and prominent SAM accentuates outflow obstruction. The factors that decrease outflow obstruction tend to reduce the degree of mitral regurgitation.

Severe right ventricular infundibular stenosis is rare and may be either independent of or concurrent with left ventricular outflow obstruction. The mechanism of right ventricular outflow obstruction is different from that on the left side because the infundibulum is circumferentially bound by muscle. Excessive muscle contraction in this disorder results in outflow obstruction, and the factors resulting in increased contractility tend to accentuate obstruction. The tricuspid valve does not play any important role in the right-sided outflow obstruction.

B. DIASTOLIC FUNCTION

Distensibility and compliance of the hypertrophied ventricles are reduced, with resulting elevation in end-diastolic pressure without an increase in volume. The prolongation of early diastolic relaxation coupled with increased wall stiffness tends to influence the pattern of diastolic filling. Early, rapid, passive filling is notably impaired, requiring a stronger atrial contraction to deliver diastolic inflow into a relatively nondistensible left ventricle. This dependence on atrial contraction to maintain efficient flow is exemplified by a sudden drop in cardiac output when atrial fibrillation supervenes. Although this abnormality of diastolic compliance has important hemodynamic consequences (eg, elevations of left atrial and pulmonary venous pressures causing pulmonary congestion and edema), actual inflow obstruction is rare.

Clinical Findings

A. SYMPTOMS AND SIGNS

Effort dyspnea and paroxysmal nocturnal dyspnea constitute the most common symptoms (Table 14–1) and provide evidence of pulmonary congestion. Because elevations in pulmonary venous and left atrial pressures occur in the presence of a hyperdynamic, hypercontractile left ventricle, they must be attributed to increased

Table 14–1. Characteristic clinical features of hypertrophic cardiomyopathy.

Symptoms
  Dyspnea: Effort-induced, paroxysmal nocturnal, or orthopnea
  Angina: Stable or unstable
  Syncope: Generally following exertion
  Dizziness (presyncope)
  No symptoms
Signs
  Sustained bifid apical impulse
  Palpable atrial impulse (S_4)
  Brisk carotid upstroke
  Bisferious pulse with normal pulse pressure (with LVOT obstruction)
  Gallop sounds: S_4 common, S_3 uncommon
  Ejection systolic murmur along left systolic border
  Longer, higher-pitched apical systolic murmur
  Effects of Valsalva's maneuver: increased murmur intensity during peak strain phase (II) and decrease in later strain-release phase (IV)

LVOT = left ventricular outflow tract.

stiffness of the hypertrophic ventricles. In some patients, especially in those with volume overload, frank pulmonary edema may be noted.

Frank syncope and presyncope (dizziness short of loss of consciousness) are common. These symptoms may be effort-related, although not predictably so, and the frequency of the episodes is highly variable. The exact mechanism is obscure; however, it is probably related to reflex vasodilatation and hypotension induced by stretching the left ventricular baroreceptors. On the other hand, arrhythmia may play a role by producing a decrease in cardiac output.

Typical effort angina simulating symptomatic coronary artery disease is frequent, although episodes of chest pain may be prolonged and may occur spontaneously at rest. Sublingual nitroglycerin typically (but not always) fails to provide prompt relief. When the epicardial coronary arteries are large and patent, the ischemia may be due to compression of the intramyocardial coronary arteries and increased myocardial tension and muscle mass, with oxygen requirements outstripping oxygen delivery.

Palpitations may merely be the result of the patient's awareness of forcible heartbeats, especially in the left lateral decubitus position. Atrial and ventricular arrhythmias are more commonly responsible. Tachyarrhythmias are poorly tolerated and are often associated with symptoms of low output and hypotension. Isolated or short runs of ventricular and supraventricular premature depolarizations often occur without symptoms.

The physical signs also tend to vary considerably—from minimal or nonspecific to highly characteristic. The characteristic signs include evidence of left ventricular hypertrophy, obstruction of left ventricular outflow, and resistance to left ventricular inflow.

B. PHYSICAL EXAMINATION

A powerful systolic thrust of the left ventricle on palpitation indicates an increase in muscle mass; although less frequent, the characteristic bifid apex in systole is virtually diagnostic of this condition. A prominent atrial contraction imparts a strong presystolic impulse that is palpable at the apex. A trifid impulse composed of a prominent *a* wave and bifid systolic peaks is rarely palpable but can often be recorded on apex cardiogram. Such a finding is highly characteristic of this disease. S_4 is commonly observed in the presence of sinus rhythm.

A jerky arterial pulse with sharp upstroke is typical, although not diagnostic. Occasionally, a bifid pulse may be felt, especially in the carotid artery. A bifid arterial pulse in association with a normal pulse pressure is characteristic of HOCM. The pulse contour is influenced by the presence and severity of outflow obstruction. In the absence of resting obstruction, the arterial pulse is essentially normal, although with a brisk upstroke.

A systolic murmur of variable intensity is present along the left sternal border and apex. It is poorly transmitted to the aortic area and neck vessels. It is medium- or high-pitched, with onset after the S_1. The murmur resembles a long ejection murmur along the left sternal border and attains a regurgitant quality (high-pitched, blowing) toward the apex. The apical murmur may be well transmitted to the axilla. The S_2 is clearly audible, and both components are well preserved. Reverse splitting with a delayed aortic component, when present, is diagnostic of severe outflow obstruction in the absence of left bundle branch block. The signs of outflow obstruction, including intensity of the systolic murmur, are accentuated by maneuvers that augment the severity of obstruction (Table 14–2).

The blowing apical murmur of mitral regurgitation also generally varies in intensity with dynamic outflow obstruction. In a few patients, associated severe mitral valve regurgitation, independent of outflow obstruction, may be present. Its presence can be determined by raising the blood pressure with methoxamine or angiotensin, which—although relieving outflow obstruction—will not diminish the murmur's intensity if the regurgitation is unrelated to obstruction. Because these patients may be candidates for mitral valve surgery, this differentiation is clinically important.

Although a prominent atrial sound (S_4) is a common feature of a noncompliant hypertrophied left ventricle, a mitral diastolic murmur simulating mitral stenosis may occasionally lead to consideration of rheu-

Table 14–2. Effects of maneuvers on murmur intensity and obstruction severity in hypertrophic obstructive cardiomyopathy.

Maneuvers	Left Ventricular Outflow Obstruction	Severity of Mitral Regurgitation	Murmur Intensity
Upright posture	↑	↑	↑
Squatting	↓	↓	↓
Valsalva's			
Phase 2–3	↑	↑	↑
Phase 4	↓	↓	↓
Exercise	↑	↑	↑
Amyl nitrite inhalation	↑	↑	↑
Methoxamine	↓	↓	↓

↑ = increased; ↓ = decreased.

matic mitral disease. The absence of an opening snap and the presence of severe, unexplained left ventricular hypertrophy should point to a correct diagnosis.

A systolic murmur of infundibular pulmonic stenosis is often prominent at the left sternal edge. The ejection sound is absent, and the pulmonary closure sound is delayed. When infundibular obstruction accompanies left ventricular outflow obstruction, the clinical signs of the latter dominate. However, isolated right ventricular outflow obstruction may be difficult to differentiate from congenital infundibular pulmonic stenosis until evidence for unexplained left ventricular hypertrophy is demonstrable.

C. Diagnostic Studies

1. Electrocardiography—A routine 12-lead electrocardiograph (ECG) often discloses evidence of left ventricular hypertrophy with increased QRS voltage or ST-T wave changes in the lateral precordial leads (V_4–V_6). Because no signs of left ventricular hypertrophy may be present in some patients despite the massive increase in cardiac muscle mass, a normal ECG does not exclude the diagnosis of HCM. Occasionally, large, abnormal Q waves that simulate myocardial infarction are noted as a result of septal depolarization. These changes of pseudo-infarction are uncommon. Other features include a short PR interval, Wolff-Parkinson-White syndrome, left-axis deviation from left anterior hemiblock, and complete left or right bundle branch block. Atrial and ventricular premature depolarizations are common, but sometimes can be detected only with ambulatory ECG recording. Complete heart block is rare.

Deep symmetric inversion of the T waves in the precordial leads has been described with apical HCM but may also be seen in other types. These changes in a patient with chest pain are often mistaken for subendocardial infarction.

2. Chest radiograph—Posteroanterior and lateral chest x-ray films are often normal. Evidence of left ventricular enlargement may be subtle because the cavity size is not increased. Left atrial size is either normal or only slightly increased, except in a stage of advanced decompensation. Pulmonary venous engorgement may be seen, but frank pulmonary edema and signs of pulmonary arterial hypertension are infrequent.

3. Echocardiography—Echocardiography is the most important method for diagnosing HCM (Table 14–3). This technique is useful for evaluating the thickness of the interventricular septum and left ventricular posterior wall and their movements in systole; the end-diastolic and end-systolic dimensions of the left ventricular cavity along its minor axis; the left ventricular outflow size (the space between the anterior mitral leaflet and the interventricular septum); and the functional aspects of mitral and aortic valve motion. It also permits differentiation of concentric and asymmetric hypertrophy.

The presence of dynamic left ventricular outflow obstruction is diagnosed by analyzing the systolic motion of the mitral valve. Abnormal motion of the anterior mitral leaflet against the interventricular septum localizes the site of outflow obstruction in HOCM. It begins sometime after completion of early ejection and is terminated in end-systole before aortic valve closure.

The dynamic nature of the obstruction can be interpreted from variations in the extent of the systolic anterior motion with maneuvers designed to alter the obstruction. Patients without a resting obstruction usually

Table 14–3. Echocardiographic clues in diagnosis of hypertrophic cardiomyopathy.

Two-Dimensional Echocardiography
  Massive hypertrophy
  Asymmetric wall thickness
  Sparkling or granular appearance of walls
  Normal cavity size
  Dilated left atrium
  Hyperdynamic LV function (EF > 70)
  Systolic anterior motion of anterior (or posterior) mitral
    leaflet (obstructive cases)
  Thickened, elongated anterior leaflet
  Endocardiac thickening of LVOT
  Hypodynamic basal septum
Doppler Echocardiography
  Mitral regurgitation
  Mitral inflow: diastolic dysfunction pattern with impaired
    relaxation
Pulsed-Wave Doppler
  High velocities in LVOT
Color-Flow Doppler
  High velocities and turbulent flow in LVOT
Continuous-Wave Doppler
  Dagger-shaped velocity waveform in LVOT

EF = ejection fraction; LV = left ventricle; LVOT = left ventricular outflow tract.

have small and incomplete SAM, whereas those with high resting gradients tend to have a large and complete SAM that is consistently noted from one beat to the next. Systolic anterior motion has also been noted in hyperkinetic circulatory states, in aortic regurgitation, during infusion of dopamine in a patient in shock, and following mitral valve repair for myxomatous mitral valve prolapse. As a result of the dynamic midsystolic obstruction to outflow, the aortic valve cusps may show premature closure with late systolic reopening.

A combination of narrow left ventricular outflow space, thickened interventricular septum, and the typical SAM of the anterior mitral leaflet is virtually diagnostic of HOCM. When the interventricular septal wall/posterior wall thickness ratio exceeds 1.5:1.0, asymmetric hypertrophy can be diagnosed confidently. With some exceptions, patients with HCM demonstrate asymmetric septal hypertrophy. Two-dimensional echocardiography may show that the asymmetric hypertrophy involves the lateral free wall, the apex, the distal septum and, rarely, the posteroinferior wall. Additional findings include midsystolic preclosure of one or more aortic valve cusps, a hypodynamic interventricular septum with diminished systolic motion,

and reduced early diastolic slope of the anterior mitral leaflet. Two-dimensional echocardiography generally permits differentiation of SAM involving the mitral leaflet and that involving the chordae tendineae. The leaflet SAM is more characteristically associated with HOCM; the chordal motion may represent passive buckling of the chordae tendineae in a rapidly emptying left ventricle. When multiple criteria are sought, the diagnosis can be made from the echocardiographic examination alone.

Doppler echocardiography makes it possible to obtain information on flow and pressure dynamics, using pulsed- and continuous-wave modes. Pulsed-wave Doppler can localize the site of obstruction by showing high velocities in the subaortic region when the obstruction is localized in the left ventricular outflow tract; the measurement of high velocities by continuous-wave Doppler can be used to estimate the pressure drop across the subvalvular obstruction. The contour of the outflow tract velocity profile mirrors the profile of the pressure drop from the left ventricular cavity to the outflow tract and assumes a characteristic dagger shape (Figure 14–1). As ventricular ejection begins, the early velocity is in the range of 1.0–1.5 m/s, commensurate with the rapid early ejection. Subsequently, the velocity progressively increases to reach a peak in mid-to-late systole and return to baseline at the end of ejection. This profile differs sharply from that seen in fixed obstruction (eg, valvular aortic stenosis), where a smooth contour of increasing velocity is observed, even when it peaks in midsystole. The presence and severity of mitral regurgitation can also be assessed. A similar Doppler velocity contour may also be observed to evaluate right ventricular infundibular obstruction.

Doppler techniques also provide information regarding left ventricular diastolic function. The heterogenous ventricular wall relaxation is associated with flow signals that are generally directed toward the apex and suggest earlier relaxation of the apical than the basal segments. These findings are also seen in other forms of hypertrophy, however, and lack diagnostic value. The overall rate of relaxation is prolonged, resulting in a small mitral-flow, early-filling wave. The subsequent atrial contraction accounts for the major proportion of ventricular filling and results in a prominent mitral inflow *a* wave. These features of mitral inflow velocity pattern can be readily evaluated by pulsed-wave Doppler techniques and provide useful information. The pulmonary venous flow pattern detected by pulsed-wave Doppler provides supplementary information. A more forceful atrial contraction results in a more prominent retrograde flow wave into the pulmonary veins (*ar*, or *a* reversal, wave). An important limitation of these Doppler methods, however, is their dependence on loading conditions and heart rate.

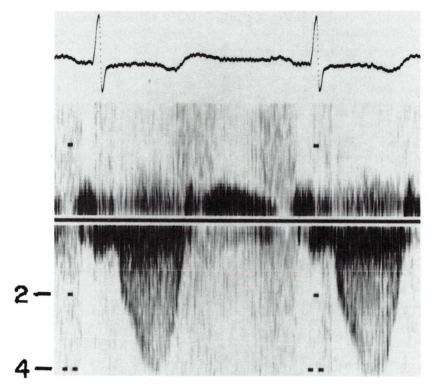

Figure 14–1. Typical dagger-shaped contour of the continuous-wave Doppler velocity obtained across the left ventricular outflow tract. The peak velocity may be used to calculate gradient across the outflow tract using a modified Bernoulli equation (Peak gradient = $4 \times V_2$). The peak gradient in this patient (with a peak velocity of 4 m/s) is 64 mm Hg.

4. Cardiac catheterization and angiography—Before the advent of echocardiography, final confirmation of the diagnosis rested on cardiac catheterization and selective cardiac angiography, specifically the demonstration of dynamic left ventricular outflow obstruction. When catheterization is necessary, special care must be taken to avoid recording an artifactual gradient caused by entrapment of the catheter. Analysis of the recorded arterial pressure and pressure gradient during a postectopic beat often provides an important clue. Typically, the arterial pulse pressure is narrower in the postectopic than in the sinus beat, in contrast to both the normal and the fixed forms of left ventricular outflow obstruction (eg, valvular aortic stenosis), when the pulse pressure is wider in the postectopic beat. Accentuation of the outflow gradient with the Valsalva maneuver, amyl nitrite inhalation, or isoproterenol infusion provides added confirmation.

Selective left ventricular cine-angiography demonstrates the characteristic anatomic and functional features of HCM. Ventricular geometry is altered, with the cavity assuming a sausage shape in the right anterior oblique projection. In a few patients, simultaneous left and right ventricular angiograms have demonstrated a massively thickened interventricular septum, especially in its midportion. Such techniques, however, are no longer routinely used because echocardiography provides a reliable, noninvasive diagnostic tool. Catheterization-angiography studies should therefore be reserved for selected patients and used on rare occasions for diagnostic confirmation.

Treatment

Both medical and surgical management are palliative (Table 14–4) since the cause of this bizarre cardiomyopathy is unknown. The major objectives of therapy include improvement of symptoms, amelioration of outflow obstruction, improvement of left ventricular compliance, suppression of arrhythmias, and the prevention and treatment of major complications such as bacterial endocarditis, thromboembolism, and sudden death.

A. MEDICAL MANAGEMENT

The cardiac drugs commonly used for symptomatic relief of dyspnea or angina in other cardiac disorders are either contraindicated or must be used with caution. Digitalis must be avoided except to treat rapid atrial fibrillation when β-adrenergic blockade and calcium channel blockers are unsuccessful or poorly tolerated. Nitrates are generally contraindicated and are often ineffective in relieving angina. Diuretics must be used with caution so as not to produce hypovolemia.

Beta-adrenergic blocking agents are used extensively. Slowing the heart rate and decreasing contractility are generally beneficial. Although exercise and β-adrenergic stimulation have been shown to ameliorate obstruction, resting gradients are reduced only in some patients with labile obstruction. Symptomatic improvement is striking in some patients and may last several years. Increasing doses are often needed, however, and other patients fail to experience sustained improvement. Although a daily dose of as high as 480 mg may be required for some patients, it is doubtful that left ventricular compliance is improved with β-adrenergic blockade. These agents have not been shown to decrease the incidence of ventricular arrhythmias or sudden death. The dose should be increased gradually and the effects monitored, especially in patients without a major component of outflow obstruction.

Calcium channel blockers (eg, verapamil, long-acting nifedipine) have provided beneficial effects, and amelioration of symptoms is frequently observed. The resting and exercise pressure gradients are reduced, and there seems to be improved compliance. The use of

Table 14–4. Management strategies in hypertrophic cardiomyopathy.

Medical Therapy
  Beta-blockers
  Calcium channel blockers
  Disopyramide
  Cautious combination of β-blockers and calcium channel
    blockers
  Judicious use of diuretics for symptom relief
  Antiarrhythmics as needed
  Antibiotic prophylaxis against endocarditis
  Anticoagulation for atrial fibrillation
Surgical Therapy
  Myectomy to relieve LVOT obstruction
  Mitral valve replacement and myectomy with severe mitral
    regurgitation unrelated to LVOT obstruction
Other Procedures
  Permanent pacemaker insertion (currently experimental)
  Appropriate AV delay to minimize LVOT gradient
  Alcohol septal ablation

AV = atrioventricular; LVOT = left ventricular outflow tract.

these agents should be carefully monitored, however. In some patients with undue hypotensive effect, severe deterioration or death may occur. Although disopyramide has been used for its negative inotropism to provide symptomatic improvement in some patients with HOCM, the frequency of side effects limits its widespread use.

In some patients with refractory symptoms, combined use of a β-blocker and a calcium channel blocker has proved successful; this regimen should be attempted under close observation, however.

Disopyramide, another negative inotropic agent, provides symptomatic improvement. Side effects include anticholinergic actions such as dry mouth and eyes, constipation, difficulty in micturition. Patients in atrial fibrillation may experience rapid ventricular rate and may require addition of β-blockers. Owing to its class IA antiarrhythmic properties, the patients should be closely monitored for proarrhythmias. Similarly, QT interval should be monitored for prolongation.

Sudden cardiac death is overwhelmingly the most common cause of demise among patients with HCM, probably from arrhythmias (their causal role has not yet been definitely established); effective antiarrhythmic agents may therefore be important. Atrial and ventricular arrhythmias are common in patients with HCM, regardless of their symptomatic or hemodynamic state. Although supraventricular tachycardias may worsen symptoms, they have not been associated with sudden death. Ventricular tachycardia and other high-grade ventricular arrhythmias have been found in at least 30% of patients monitored by 72-h ambulatory ECG recordings. Asymptomatic family members screened and found to have HCM also have a high incidence of asymptomatic ventricular arrhythmias. Although aggressive treatment of ventricular tachycardia is currently recommended, ventricular arrhythmias are generally refractory to conventional agents alone or in combination with β-adrenergic blockade. Amiodarone, a class III antiarrhythmic, has been reported (in an uncontrolled clinical trial) to prevent sudden cardiac death in this disorder, and sotalol, with its β-blocking and class III antiarrhythmic effects, may prove ideal, although systematic studies are not available.

Bacterial endocarditis is a common complication, and the use of prophylactic antibiotics at times of risk is recommended. Thromboembolism is another complication, especially in the presence of intermittent or sustained atrial fibrillation. Anticoagulation with warfarin sodium is advised in such cases, particularly if an embolic episode has been diagnosed.

B. SURGICAL MYECTOMY

Considerable experience has been reported with transaortic ventriculomyectomy in patients with HOCM. Creation of a small tunnel in the left ventricular outflow tract (by removing a small amount of muscle with a deep incision) provides postoperative relief of outflow obstruction and associated mitral regurgitation. Symptomatic improvement is often dramatic, along with reduction or abolition of the systolic murmur and other features of left ventricular outflow obstruction. Replacement of the mitral valve to relieve outflow obstruction is not indicated, unless severe independent mitral regurgitation can be demonstrated.

Surgical relief of right ventricular outflow obstruction can be carried out successfully (as it can in infundibular pulmonary stenosis). The current surgical approach to myectomy is considerably aided by intraoperative echocardiography. Multiplanar transesophageal echocardiography accurately localizes the hypertrophy and permits visualization of the resected muscle, showing the abolition of systolic anterior motion and the improvement of mitral regurgitation. The current operative risk for uncomplicated myectomy should not exceed 5%, and the obstruction should be relieved in more than 95% of cases. The surgical risk at several large centers is reported to be less than 2%.

C. Chemical Myectomy

This technique, first developed by Sigwart in 1995, uses alcohol to partially ablate the septum. During this procedure a special catheter is threaded into the septal perforator branch of the left anterior descending coronary artery to enable the injection of absolute alcohol, which produces a controlled myocardial infarction in the proximal interventricular septum. The desired end result is thinning of the upper interventricular septum and dyskinesia, thereby enlarging the left ventricular outflow tract and subsequently reducing systolic gradients. Experience at several centers has demonstrated a high level of success with hemodynamic and symptomatic improvement in most patients. The procedure-related mortality rate has been in the range of 1–2%. Additional procedure-related complications include ventricular arrhythmias, arterioventricular (AV) block often requiring permanent pacemaker implantation and large anteroseptal infarction, and coronary artery dissection. Although alcohol septal ablation is an attractive alternative to surgical myectomy, this procedure should be considered experimental and its use limited to few centers with significant experience in a sufficient number of patients. The criteria for patients who may derive most benefit are evolving, but it is clear that not all patients with outflow obstruction are suitable candidates.

D. Pacemaker Implantation

An AV sequential permanent pacemaker has been used to ameliorate obstruction of the left ventricular outflow tract. The AV delay and ventricular activation are synchronized to provide a minimum outflow tract gradient, and the pacing continues for months or years.

Long-term follow-up studies have reported substantial symptomatic and objective benefits. Further independent investigations are needed to confirm these findings. It appears that improvement with this approach, as with drugs, does not last long and may only delay rather than avoid a consideration of myectomy in symptomatic patients. This approach is therefore not recommended for general use.

E. Cardioverter Defibrillator Implantation

A subset of patients with a high risk of sudden death may benefit from implantation of a cardiac defibrillator. The risk factors for sudden death include genetic predisposition with known genotypes, sustained ventricular tachycardia or prior cardiac arrest, recurrent syncope, hypotension with exercise, and extreme hypertrophy with maximal wall thickness of 30 mm or more, particularly in adolescents and young adults.

Prognosis

The natural history of HCM is quite variable, probably because of the complexity of disease expression. In general, the earlier the onset of clinical findings, the worse the prognosis. The major problem is sudden death, which is often the first manifestation of the disease in teenagers or young adults. Sudden death rates in hospital-based populations have ranged from 2% to 6% a year; in community-based patients, the rate is probably 1%/year. Patients who survive past 35 years of age usually have a better long-term prognosis. The only factors that seem to predispose to sudden death are a history of syncope and a family history of sudden death. Although some studies have shown a link with marked wall thickness on echocardiography and nonsustained ventricular tachycardia on ambulatory ECG monitoring, these two factors have a low predictive accuracy for sudden death.

Patients who live to old age (older than 65 years) may reach the heart failure stage, characterized by a dilated, thinned left ventricle with reduced systolic function. Outflow obstruction is minimal or absent at this stage, and digoxin, vasodilators, and diuretics may be indicated to reduce congestive heart failure symptoms and signs.

Future Prospects

The genetic research on HCM has provided significant clues in the mutations in any of the ten genes of interest, each encoding proteins of the cardiac sarcomere. It promises to enable preclinical diagnosis of individuals affected by a mutant gene and characterize those likely to experience a malignant or rapidly progressive course. This could result in triage of patients with this diagnosis for selection of appropriate treatment options. A more readily available gene typical for this disorder is likely to revolutionize its management and progress.

Charron P, Dubourg O, Desnos M et al: Clinical features and prognostic implications of familial hypertrophic cardiomyopathy related to the cardiac myosin-binding protein C gene, Circulation 1998;97:2230.

Elliott PM, Poloniecki J, Dickie S et al: Sudden death in hypertrophic cardiomyopathy: Identification of high risk patients. J Am Coll Cardiol 2000;36:2212.

Elliott PM, Gimeno B, Jr, Mahon NG et al: Relation between severity of left-ventricular hypertrophy and prognosis in patients with hypertrophic cardiomyopathy. Lancet 2001;357: 420.

Faber L, Seggewiss H, Gleichmann U: Percutaneous transluminal septal myocardial ablation in hypertrophic obstructive cardiomyopathy: Results with respect to intraprocedural myocardial contrast echocardiography. Circulation 1998;98: 2415.

Fananapazir L, McAreavey D: Therapeutic options in patients with obstructive hypertrophic cardiomyopathy and severe drug-refractory symptoms. J Am Coll Cardiol 1998;31:259.

Flores-Ramirez R, Lakkis NM, Middleton KJ et al: Echocardiographic insights into the mechanisms of relief of left ventricular outflow tract obstruction after nonsurgical septal reduction therapy in patients with hypertrophic obstructive cardiomyopathy. J Am Coll Cardiol 2001;37:208.

Gietzen FH, Leuner CJ, Raute-Kreinsen U et al: Acute and long-term results after transcoronary ablation of septal hypertrophy (TASH). Catheter interventional treatment for hypertrophic obstructive cardiomyopathy. Eur Heart J 1999;20: 1342.

Heric B, Lytle BW, Miller DP et al: Surgical management of hypertrophic obstructive cardiomyopathy. Early and late results. J Thorac Cardiovasc Surg 1995;110:195.

Kizilbash AM, Heinle SK, Grayburn PA: Spontaneous variability of left ventricular outflow tract gradient in hypertrophic obstructive cardiomyopathy. Circulation 1998;97:461.

Klues HG, Roberts WC, Maron BJ: Anomalous insertion of papillary muscle directly into anterior mitral leaflet in hypertrophic cardiomyopathy. Significance in producing left ventricular outflow obstruction. Circulation 1991;84:1188.

Knight C, Kurbaan AS, Seggewiss H et al: Nonsurgical septal reduction for hypertrophic obstructive cardiomyopathy: Outcome in the first series of patients. Circulation 1997;95: 2075.

Lakkis NM, Nagueh SF, Kleiman NS et al: Echocardiography-guided ethanol septal reduction for hypertrophic obstructive cardiomyopathy. Circulation 1998;98:1750.

Lim D, Roberts R, Marian AJ: Expression profiling of cardiac genes in human hypertrophic cardiomyopathy: Insight into the pathogenesis of phenotypes. J Am Coll Cardiol 2001;38: 1175.

Maron BJ: Hypertrophic cardiomyopathy. Lancet 1997;350:127.

Maron BJ: Role of alcohol septal ablation in treatment of obstructive hypertrophic cardiomyopathy. Lancet 2000;355:425.

Maron BJ, Shen WK, Link MS et al: Efficacy of implantable cardioverter-defibrillators for the prevention of sudden death in patients with hypertrophic cardiomyopathy. N Engl J Med 2000;342:365.

Seggewiss H, Gleichmann U, Faber L et al: Percutaneous transluminal septal myocardial ablation in hypertrophic obstructive cardiomyopathy: acute results and 3-month follow-up in 25 patients. J Am Coll Cardiol 1998;31:252.

Shah PM: Controversies in hypertrophic cardiomyopathy. Curr Probl Cardiol 1986;11:567.

Shah PM, Gramiak R, Adelman AG et al: Echocardiographic assessment of the effects of surgery and propranolol on the dynamics of outflow obstruction in hypertrophic subaortic stenosis. Circulation 1972;45:516.

Shah PM, Adelman AG, Wigle ED et al: The natural (and unnatural) history of hypertrophic obstructive cardiomyopathy. Circ Res 1974;35 (Suppl):95.

Shah PM, Taylor RD, Wong M: Abnormal mitral valve coaptation in hypertrophic obstructive cardiomyopathy: Proposed role in systolic anterior motion of mitral valve. Am J Cardiol 1981;48:258.

Sigwart U: Non-surgical myocardial reduction for hypertrophic obstructive cardiomyopathy. Lancet 1995;346:211.

Yu EH, Omran AS, Wigle ED et al: Mitral regurgitation in hypertrophic obstructive cardiomyopathy: Relationship to obstruction and relief with myectomy. J Am Coll Cardiol 2000;36: 2219.

Restrictive Cardiomyopathies

15

John D. Carroll, MD & Michael H. Crawford, MD

ESSENTIALS OF DIAGNOSIS

- *Symptoms and signs of heart failure with predominant right-sided findings*
- *Normal left and right ventricular size and systolic function with dilated atria*
- *Diastolic ventricular functional abnormalities suggestive of reduced ventricular compliance*
- *Increased ventricular filling pressure (left > right) and reduced cardiac output*

General Considerations

A. DEFINITIONS AND TERMINOLOGY

1. Restrictive cardiomyopathy—The World Health Organization defines cardiomyopathies as heart muscle diseases of unknown cause and classified restrictive cardiomyopathy as having one of three forms (the others being dilated cardiomyopathy and hypertrophic cardiomyopathy). Restrictive cardiomyopathies are classified as primary (endocardial fibrosis and eosinophilic endomyocardial disease) or secondary to cardiac infiltrative diseases. Diseases with a defined cause that produce a dilated cardiomyopathy with restrictive characteristics are specifically excluded from this classification of cardiomyopathies.

For the clinician, restrictive cardiomyopathy is usually due to infiltrative diseases, such as the cardiomyopathy that occurs in systemic amyloidosis, hemochromatosis, sarcoidosis, and glycogen storage diseases (Table 15–1). These secondary cardiomyopathies are included because the cardiac involvement typically displays features of restrictive physiology that are pivotal in the diagnosis. Restrictive cardiomyopathies represent less than 1% of cases of congestive heart failure, and most of these are of the secondary form.

2. Restrictive physiology—Also known as **diastolic dysfunction** and **diastolic heart failure**, restrictive physiology requires a precise definition, even though clinical methods often yield only indirect evidence of this functional abnormality. It is characterized by elevated filling pressures and impaired ventricular filling from myocardial or endocardial abnormalities in a nondilated ventricle with no significant impairment of systolic performance. Numerous common cardiac diseases can produce the functional abnormalities of the restrictive or diastolic type, but the diseases are not classified as a restrictive cardiomyopathy.

3. Infiltrative cardiomyopathy—An alternative term applied to many of these diseases, infiltrative cardiomyopathy emphasizes that the endocardial, interstitial, or intracellular infiltration of a variety of materials (eg, extensive collagen bundles, amyloid protein) is the central histologic and pathophysiologic feature. The infiltration of material with tissue less compliant than normal myocardium and the increase in the wall thickness of the cardiac chambers reduce chamber compliance.

4. Obliterative cardiomyopathy—This term is sometimes used to describe the reduction in left ventricular

Table 15–1. Classification of restrictive cardiomyopathy.

Primary	Secondary
Idiopathic	Infiltrative disease
Familial ± skeletal myopathy	Amyloidosis
Löffler's cardiomyopathy (endocarditis parientalis fibroplastica)	Glycogen storage Hemochromatosis
Tropical endomyocardial fibrosis	Sarcoidosis
	Interstitial disease
	Radiation-induced fibrosis
	Chronic allograft rejection

chamber volume as the consequence of endocardial fibrosis and extensive mural thrombus formation.

B. Pathophysiology

1. Abnormalities in diastolic function—In restrictive cardiomyopathy abnormalities in diastolic function have several causes; the major one being a loss of ventricular chamber compliance. Fibrosis and the presence of amyloid and hemosiderin all change the intrinsic mechanical properties of the chamber wall. Furthermore, the rate and extent of myocardial relaxation and elastic recoil are reduced in restrictive cardiomyopathy, causing increased diastolic pressures, an increased rate of early diastolic filling, and a reduced rate of atrial filling. Myocardial ischemia may further compromise diastolic function. In cardiac amyloidosis particularly, the coronary arteries may be infiltrated, reducing myocardial blood supply.

2. Restrictive physiology—Restrictive physiology is best quantified by an assessment of the passive properties of the ventricles, usually of left ventricular compliance. No routine clinical methods measure chamber compliance, but a variety of tests are available to assess the consequences of altered chamber compliance. Specifically, alterations in the pattern of ventricular filling, absolute filling pressures, and pressure waveforms may be routinely determined by noninvasive and invasive techniques.

C. Etiology

1. Idiopathic restrictive cardiomyopathy—These patients have hemodynamic findings consistent with restrictive cardiomyopathy and endomyocardial biopsies that show fibrosis or variable degrees of cellular hypertrophy. The thickness of the ventricular wall need not be increased.

These patients present at an average age of 20–30 years old and are predominantly women. The clinical course is variable, with many patients being symptomatically stable for years whereas others die quickly without cardiac transplantation to treat severe heart failure.

An idiopathic restrictive cardiomyopathy has also been described in children—predominantly girls—with a mean age of 4 years. Most were dead within several years of presentation, suggesting that idiopathic restrictive cardiomyopathy in childhood has a worse prognosis than in adults.

2. Familial cardiomyopathy—Sporadic case reports describe restrictive cardiomyopathy in multiple members of families. The coexistence of a skeletal myopathy has been seen in a family with a dominantly inherited restrictive cardiomyopathy.

3. Löffler's cardiomyopathy—In 1936, Löffler described a cardiomyopathy associated with eosinophilia.

It is now established that the degree and duration of eosinophilia quantitatively relate to the extent of endomyocardial disease. Males are more commonly affected, and presentation may be as a classical restrictive cardiomyopathy. The disease has different stages and presentations; one presentation shows multiorgan involvement, evidence of a systemic inflammatory response, and thromboembolic events.

4. Tropical endocardial fibrosis—This form of restrictive cardiomyopathy is rarely seen in the industrialized societies of the West, but is quite common in subtropical and tropical regions. Although overt eosinophilia is not the rule, the gross and microscopic features of the disease resemble those of Löffler's cardiomyopathy. Overt manifestations of heart failure with ascites and edema frequently emerge in late childhood and early adulthood. The scarring process usually involves both ventricles, producing restrictive hemodynamics, although isolated right and left ventricular involvement occasionally occurs. The early stages of the disease have not been well characterized.

Management is unlike that for other causes of restrictive cardiomyopathy, and endocardiectomy may produce significant clinical improvement.

5. Amyloidosis—Cardiac amyloidosis occurs in several forms of this systemic disease; a description of each is beyond the scope of this chapter. In general, however, patients with evidence of cardiac amyloidosis should undergo an evaluation of other organ involvement, the nature of any serum gammopathy, and the nature of any plasma cell dyscrasia in the bone marrow.

Patients presenting with heart failure symptoms caused by cardiac amyloidosis are typically dead in 6 months. The severity of the restrictive hemodynamics and the independent problems of low systemic arterial pressure and renal insufficiency make treatment of these patients difficult.

6. Inborn metabolic errors—Biochemical defects, typically genetically determined, may alter a variety of metabolic pathways and lead to direct or secondary effects on cardiac function. Restrictive-cardiomyopathy-like features have been described in glycogen storage disease, Fabry's disease, Gaucher's disease, and the mucopolysaccharidoses. The result is generally an infiltrative process, although other cardiac manifestations can occur for each of these complex entities (discussion of these is beyond the scope of this chapter).

7. Hemochromatosis and hemosiderosis—These conditions can produce a restrictive cardiomyopathy. This is an unusual manifestation; most cases of cardiac involvement are associated with a dilated cardiomyopathy.

8. Sarcoidosis—Restrictive cardiomyopathy from sarcoidosis is rare. Cardiac involvement is most commonly manifested by arrhythmias and conduction abnormalities. When congestive heart failure occurs, systolic function may be reduced, and a ventricular aneurysm is occasionally produced.

9. Radiation-induced fibrosis—Radiation more often causes constrictive pericarditis, but it can produce restrictive cardiomyopathy, and the pericardial and myocardial fibrotic pictures may be combined.

10. Other causes—Other diseases have been reported (generally as case reports) with a restrictive-cardiomyopathy-type of presentation. These include pseudoxanthoma elasticum, coronary arteritis, myocardial tuberculosis, fatty infiltration of the myocardium, carnitine deficiency, neoplastic disease, and carcinoid heart disease.

Adams, Kertesz AE, Valberg LS: Clinical presentation of hemochromatosis: A changing scene. Am J Med 1991;90:445.

Falk RH, Comenzo RL, Skinner M: The systemic amyloidosis. N Engl J Med 1997; 337:898.

Kushwaha SS, Fallon JT, Fuster V: Restrictive cardiomyopathy. N Engl J Med 1997;336:267.

Lewis AB: Clinical profile and outcome of restrictive cardiomyopathy in children. Am Heart J 1992;123:1589.

Sharma OP, Maheshwari A, Thaker K: Myocardial sarcoidosis. Chest 1993;103:253.

Clinical Findings

A. SYMPTOMS AND SIGNS

The clinical presentation (Table 15–2) of most patients with restrictive cardiomyopathy is based on the hemodynamic abnormalities that produce symptoms of congestive heart failure. The symptoms are, therefore, not specific for restrictive cardiomyopathy but include dyspnea, paroxysmal nocturnal dyspnea, orthopnea, peripheral edema, ascites, and more general complaints of fatigue and weakness in everyday activities.

Anginal symptoms are not typical except in the setting of amyloidosis, where true coronary artery narrowing may be caused by vessel infiltration. Cardiac amyloidosis commonly presents as classical restrictive cardiomyopathy, although other presentations have been noted. Syncope, lightheadedness, and palpitations should suggest coexisting conduction system involvement and atrial or ventricular arrhythmias.

B. PHYSICAL EXAMINATION

Depending on the stage of the disease, the physical examination may be only slightly abnormal or may show severe congestive heart failure with extensive peripheral edema, ascites, and low cardiac output manifested by cold extremities, hypotension, and lethargy.

The arterial pressure is usually normal. Hypotension is not uncommon as the disease progresses, particularly in systemic amyloidosis, in which arterial infiltration and autonomic neuropathy may complicate the clinical picture.

Table 15–2. Characteristic findings in restrictive cardiomyopathy.

Anatomic
Nondilated left ventricle
Dilated atria
Thick chamber walls
AV valve regurgitation
Physiologic
Elevated filling pressures
Restricted filling pattern
Minimally altered systolic function
Reduced stroke volume
Clinical
Heart failure symptoms, including unexplained right heart failure
Unexplained diastolic dysfunction on Doppler echocardiography or cardiac catheterization
Arrhythmias
Conduction abnormalities
Thromboembolic events
Suspected chronic constrictive pericarditis
Cardiac abnormalities with systemic disorder known to cause restrictive cardiomyopathy

AV = atrioventricular.

The jugular venous waveform is an important aspect of the physical exam in restrictive cardiomyopathy. The absolute degree of elevation is an immediate indication of the severity of the hemodynamic impairment. The waveform also contains additional details helpful in categorizing the hemodynamic profile. The *a* wave will be absent in the presence of atrial fibrillation and a large regurgitant *v* wave will be present when tricuspid regurgitation complicates the restrictive cardiomyopathy. Rapid *x* and *y* descents should be expected in most patients with restrictive cardiomyopathy in sinus rhythm. Kussmaul's sign (lack of inspiratory decrease in pressure or increase) may be present.

The carotid pulse is often of low volume and may become very weak in the later stages of the disease characterized by a low cardiac output state.

Precordial palpitation often reveals a right ventricular heave that accompanies a moderate degree of pulmonary hypertension. Left ventricular heaves are not pronounced, and the apical impulse is usually only slightly displaced laterally.

The presence of left- and right-sided S_3 gallops is common. The intensity of the first heart sound is usually not markedly diminished, as it is with significant systolic dysfunction; an exception is a diminished S_1 intensity caused by first-degree heart block. The second heart sound often reveals an increased P_2. The splitting of the second heart sound may be increased when a right bundle branch block is present, or it may be reversed in the presence of a left bundle branch block. The S_4 gallop may be present earlier in the course of the disease and then disappear because of the development of atrial fibrillation or true atrial systolic failure (as occurs in advanced amyloidosis).

Peripheral edema and ascites are present in many cases. Hepatomegaly with a pulsatile sensation on palpation is frequently present as a result of severe tricuspid regurgitation.

C. Diagnostic Studies

The initial diagnostic studies necessary in cases of suspected restrictive cardiomyopathy include an electrocardiogram, a chest radiograph, and an echocardiogram. Based on this preliminary evaluation, further testing is often needed to more completely define the hemodynamics (with cardiac catheterization), exclude confounding coronary artery disease (using coronary arteriography), examine pericardial thickness to exclude constrictive pericarditis (with cardiac imaging), and make a tissue diagnosis (using endomyocardial biopsy).

1. Electrocardiography—Electrocardiography is used to delineate rhythm (atrial fibrillation is quite common) and assess conduction abnormalities and variations in QRS voltage and ST-T wave morphology from either hypertrophy or infiltration.

2. Chest radiograph—The chest radiograph often shows pulmonary venous congestion and pleural effusions. It also can give additional information useful in the diagnosis of sarcoidosis, neoplastic disease, scleroderma, radiation-induced disease, and other causes of restrictive cardiomyopathy.

3. Echocardiography—The central role of cardiac echocardiography in the diagnosis and management of restrictive cardiomyopathy should be emphasized. Serial echocardiographic studies are frequently useful in making the initial diagnosis and in subsequent management of this generally progressive group of diseases.

The normal-to-small-sized left ventricle with fairly well-preserved systolic performance is usually seen. Apical cavity obliteration is a feature on echocardiography that is fairly peculiar to tropical endocardial fibrosis. The dilated atria are visualized, and left atrial thrombi may be suggested by transthoracic studies and should lead to transesophageal echocardiography. Wall thickness is measured, and tissue characteristics of the myocardium are noted. Cardiac amyloidosis has unique echocardiographic features. The differential echogenicity of amyloid frequently produces a sparkling appearance of the myocardium in two-dimensional images. In addition, the relationship between electrocardiographic QRS voltage and echocardiographically determined left ventricular mass or wall thickness is characteristically altered. The reduction in QRS voltage is associated

with an increased mass due to amyloid infiltration and is easily distinguished from the reduced voltage and unaltered or reduced mass in constrictive pericarditis and from the increased voltage and increased mass in left ventricular myocardial hypertrophy.

Doppler echocardiography adds another dimension to assessing tricuspid and mitral valve regurgitation, an estimation of pulmonary artery systolic pressures, and a profile of the inflow velocities of the left and right ventricle. The mitral and tricuspid inflow velocity profile is related—but not identical—to the filling volume profile. A characteristic restrictive pattern of left ventricular filling has been described as a reduced rate of early diastolic filling with an increased atrial contribution. The diagnostic value of this approach has been severely curtailed by several factors, however. Filling velocity profiles can be normalized by elevating left atrial pressure from simple intravascular volume expansion. The inflow velocity profile is also influenced by changes in the annular dimensions of the mitral and tricuspid valves. In addition, restrictive cardiomyopathies are frequently complicated by atrial fibrillation, atrioventricular (AV) valve regurgitation, and atrial pump failure, which all independently alter the dynamics of ventricular filling. Because of these factors, a single, diagnostic restrictive filling pattern cannot be defined. However, characteristically restrictive cardiomyopathy exhibits an increased mitral Doppler inflow early velocity (E > 1.0 m/s) due to increased left atrial pressure, a decrease in the atrial inflow velocity (A < 0.5 m/s), an E/A ratio > 1.5, a reduction in mitral E deceleration time to < 125 m/s; and a reduction in isovolumic relaxation time. Pulmonary venous Doppler shows a reduction in systolic and an increase in diastolic forward velocity, as well as an increase in the atrial contraction associated backward velocity. Tricuspid E deceleration time is also reduced (< 160 ms). Hepatic vein flow velocity shows diastolic predominance and flow velocity may be reversed during inspiration.

4. Radionuclide angiography—This method can be used to assess diastolic filling characteristics. It has the advantage of quantifying volume change in the ventricle during diastole. The characteristic reduction in early diastolic filling and the rate of filling with a corresponding increase in late diastolic filling is readily determined by the multiple-gated acquisition technique. The diagnostic value of this characteristic restrictive pattern suffers from the same limitations as the Doppler technique (discussed earlier) and has an added drawback in that the sampling rate of most nuclear imaging systems may not adequately represent volume filling rates. The diagnostic image of large atria and normal-to-small-sized ventricles can be observed on radionuclide imaging, but they are better defined by echocardiography.

5. Cardiac catheterization—Many adult patients with restrictive cardiomyopathy do not need a complete cardiac catheterization; the decision depends on the quality of the noninvasive hemodynamic data, the certainty of the diagnosis, and whether the symptoms or other clinical findings suggest confounding cardiac problems such as coronary artery disease. Right- and left-heart catheterization are frequently needed to confirm the restrictive physiology and to assess the severity of the elevation of filling pressures and the reduction of cardiac output. Ventriculography may be useful in assessing the degree of mitral or tricuspid valve regurgitation. A major manifestation of a reduction in chamber compliance is elevation of filling pressures, both diastolic pressures in the ventricle and mean pressure in the atrium. The absence of elevated filling pressures in the euvolemic patient is strong evidence against a functionally important restrictive cardiomyopathy. The continued absence of elevated filling pressures after intravascular volume infusion or during exercise is definitive evidence against the presence of a restrictive cardiomyopathy. On the other hand, elevated filling pressures are so commonly found in cardiac disorders of all types that they have limited specific diagnostic value for restrictive cardiomyopathy.

The pressure waveforms recorded in the ventricles and atria may have characteristic shapes in restrictive cardiomyopathy. The right and left ventricular pressure recordings have a square-root sign (early diastolic dip followed by a plateau), and the prominent x and y descents in the right atrium produce an M or W configuration. Also, right atrial pressure usually does not change with respiration. Right ventricular systolic pressure may be elevated, but end-diastolic pressure is usually less than a third of the systolic pressure. Left ventricular end diastolic pressure is characteristically 5 mm Hg or more greater than right ventricular end diastolic pressure, but they may be nearly equal in some patients.

6. Endomyocardial biopsy—Endomyocardial biopsy is an essential test in the diagnosis of several specific diseases that lead to a restrictive cardiomyopathy, such as hemochromatosis and sarcoidosis (see Table 15–1). It is necessary to exclude these specific diseases when the final diagnosis is idiopathic restrictive cardiomyopathy. Furthermore, a negative biopsy is important information when considering thoracotomy to diagnose and surgically treat presumed constrictive pericarditis.

Endomyocardial biopsy is most commonly performed on the right ventricular aspect of the interventricular septum. The right internal jugular vein is the entry port of first choice although the femoral vein can be used, especially if the biopsy accompanies a full cardiac catheterization. Although left ventricular biopsy is not routinely done at most tertiary centers, it should be considered when selective left ventricular involvement is strongly suspected and a skilled physician is available.

The myocardial biopsy specimen is quite small, approximately 1–3 mm in diameter. Because many of the diseases in question are scattered in the wall of the septum rather than homogeneously present, at least five specimens should be taken.

7. Pericardial imaging—Computed tomography (CT), specifically fast CT, is extremely important in excluding constrictive pericarditis in many patients presumed to have restrictive cardiomyopathy. Echocardiography is frequently inadequate because the gain settings of the instrument factiously modify the true pericardial thickness. Cardiac magnetic resonance imaging is an alternative method that visualizes the pericardium as a lucent, low-intensity line bordered by opaque pericardial and subepicardial fat. Many clinicians believe magnetic resonance imaging is superior to conventional CT for defining pericardial thickness.

Differential Diagnosis

The major differential diagnosis in cases of suspected restrictive cardiomyopathy is constrictive pericarditis. Table 15–3 outlines some of the distinguishing features of each disorder. The diagnostic approach includes echocardiography, a hemodynamic profile, pericardial imaging, and endomyocardial biopsy. The Doppler echocardiographic features that distinguish between restrictive cardiomyopathy and constrictive pericarditis are shown in Table 15–4. Because hemodynamic studies cannot always correctly distinguish between these two disorders, pericardial imaging and endocardial biopsy play an important role in establishing the diagnosis in some patients.

Hurrell DG, Nishimura RA, Higano ST et al: Value of dynamic respiratory changes in left and right ventricular pressure for the diagnosis of constrictive pericarditis. Circulation 1996; 93:2007.

Katritsis D, Wilmhurst PT, Wendon JA et al: Primary restrictive cardiomyopathy: Clinical and pathologic characteristics. J Am Coll Cardiol 1991;18:1230.

Kern MJ, Aguirre FV: Hemodynamic rounds: Interpretation of cardiac pathophysiology from pressure waveform analysis. Pericardial compressive hemodynamics, Part III. Cathet Cardiovasc Diagn 1992;26:152.

Masui T, Finck S, Higgins CB: Constrictive pericarditis and restrictive cardiomyopathy: Evaluation with MR imaging. Cardiac Radiol 1992;182:369.

Oh JK, Hatle LK, Seward JB et al: Diagnostic role of Doppler echocardiography in constrictive pericarditis. J Am Coll Cardiol 1994; 23:154.

Vaitkus PT, Kussmaul WG: Constrictive pericarditis versus restrictive cardiomyopathy: A reappraisal and update of diagnostic criteria. Am Heart J 1991;122:1431.

Treatment

The therapeutic plan for treating restrictive cardiomyopathy has three directions: management of the diastolic dysfunction; treatment of rhythm, conduction

Table 15–3. Differentiating between restrictive cardiomyopathy and constrictive pericarditis.

	Restrictive Cardiomyopathy	**Constrictive Pericarditis**
At the bedside	S₃ gallop	Pericardial knock
	Increased apical impulse	Reduced apical impulse
	Regurgitant murmurs	No murmurs
Electrocardiography	Usually low voltage	Low voltage
	Atrial fibrillation common	Atrial fibrillation common
Echocardiography	Increased wall thickness	Normal-to-reduced wall thickness
Cardiac catheterization	Square root sign	Square root sign
	Increased atrial pressure with M or W configuration	Increased atrial pressure with M or W configuration
	Kussmaul's sign usually absent	Kussmaul's sign usually present
	Pulsus paradoxus occasionally present	Pulsus paradoxus occasionally present
	LV diastolic pressure usually > RV	LV and RV diastolic pressures equal
	RV systolic pressure variable	RV systolic pressure usually < 50 mm Hg
Ventriculography	Slow early diastolic LV filling	Rapid early diastolic LV filling
CT scan	Normal pericardium	Thickened pericardium

LV = left ventricular; RV = right ventricular.

system, and thromboembolic complications; and treatment of the underlying disorder, if possible.

A. DIASTOLIC DYSFUNCTION

Most patients with restrictive cardiomyopathy require diuresis to treat venous congestion in the pulmonary and systemic circulation. Unfortunately, the nature of restrictive cardiomyopathy complicates this goal in that normalization of right- and left-sided filling pres-

sures may lead to a clinically significant reduction in preload. During diuretic therapy, attention must be directed toward detecting such symptoms of excessively reduced preload and cardiac output as fatigue and light-headedness. There may be direct signs of hypotension and hypoperfusion and such laboratory evidence as rising blood urea nitrogen. In severe restrictive cardiomyopathy, a very narrow intravascular volume status may prevent overt congestion without excessively re-

Table 15–4. Differentiation of constrictive pericarditis from restrictive cardiomyopathy by Doppler echocardiography.

Parameter	Normal	Constriction	Restriction
MVE respiratory variation	< 10%	≥ 25%	None
MVEDT	> 160 ms	< 160 ms	< 160 ms
TVE respiratory variation	< 15%	> 40%	None
TVEDT	> 160 ms	< 160 ms	< 160 ms
HV velocity	Systole > diastole	Variable	Systole < diastole
HV respiratory reversal	Expiratory	More marked expiratory	Inspiratory

DT = deceleration time; HV = hepatic vein; MVE = mitral valve E wave velocity; TV = tricuspid valve.

ducing preload. No such window exists in the terminal phases of the disease. Venous congestion can also be relieved by the use of long-acting nitrates given orally or topically.

Conventional medications used to treat other heart failure states are of no proven value in restrictive cardiomyopathy. Angiotensin-converting enzyme inhibitors may be limited by a low systemic arterial pressure; they have caused complications in children with restrictive cardiomyopathy. Digitalis preparations have no proven benefit in diastolic dysfunction and may pose a risk of toxicity.

Calcium antagonists have been advocated in diastolic dysfunction found in the setting of coronary artery disease, hypertensive heart disease, and hypertrophic cardiomyopathy. Their value in restrictive cardiomyopathy is uncertain, and their use should be approached with caution because they may worsen the congestive state.

B. Cardiac Complications

1. Rhythm disturbances—

a. Atrial fibrillation—The most frequent rhythm complication in the management of restrictive cardiomyopathy is atrial fibrillation. Not only is this rhythm disturbance common in restrictive cardiomyopathy, but loss of atrial contraction may worsen diastolic dysfunction because a higher mean atrial pressure is needed to achieve an adequate preload. In addition, a rapid ventricular response in atrial fibrillation further compromises pump function. Maintenance of normal sinus rhythm is therefore a reasonable goal, and such medications as flecainide, propafenone, and amiodarone may be necessary. Atrial fibrillation cannot be successfully prevented in some patients, however.

Digoxin may also be used to control the ventricular rate if fibrillation persists, although careful attention to serum drug levels and monitoring for digitalis-induced rhythm disturbances are mandatory. In an occasional patient, especially one with restrictive cardiomyopathy from amyloidosis, atrial contractile function may be minimal. If this can be discerned by Doppler echocardiographic studies, the need to maintain normal sinus rhythm would not be as urgent as in someone in whom ventricular filling is highly dependent on atrial contraction.

b. Bradycardia—Restrictive cardiomyopathy may be complicated by advanced conduction system disease leading to complete heart block or by severe sinus node dysfunction leading to hemodynamically compromising bradycardia. Atrioventricular pacing at a reasonable rate can be achieved after pacemaker placement.

c. Ventricular arrhythmias—Ventricular arrhythmias may also complicate the course of the patient with restrictive cardiomyopathy. Management revolves around the issues of whether the arrhythmias are symptomatic, hemodynamically compromising, or sustained or whether they deteriorate into a life-threatening state. There are no special issues in managing these arrhythmias in the context of restrictive cardiomyopathy.

2. Thromboembolic complications—These complications of restrictive cardiomyopathy are similar to those of dilated cardiomyopathy. Thrombus formation in the atrial appendage or the left ventricle may occur and subsequently embolize to the central nervous system or elsewhere in the circulation. Patients with restrictive cardiomyopathy with atrial fibrillation, AV valve regurgitation, and low cardiac output are at particular risk, and prophylactic anticoagulation with warfarin should be considered. Patients with endocardial fibrosis should be particularly considered for long-term anticoagulation because of their higher thromboembolic risk and the possible progressive obliteration of the left ventricle from thrombus formation. Systemic venous thrombosis with pulmonary embolism is also a risk, especially in the bedridden, edematous patient. Heparin prophylaxis is recommended for all patients in an inpatient setting.

C. Underlying Disease

Certain treatment strategies are applied to specific causes of restrictive cardiomyopathy. Although details of these approaches are beyond the scope of this chapter, they include chemotherapy for underlying plasma cell dyscrasia in amyloidosis, treatment of underlying inflammation in sarcoidosis, treatment of underlying inflammation and hypereosinophilia in Löffler's endocardial fibrosis, and the use of iron chelation therapy in hemochromatosis.

Cardiac transplantation should be considered in patients with restrictive cardiomyopathy with intractable symptoms. This therapy is pertinent to those with idiopathic and familial restrictive cardiomyopathy and chronic allograft rejection. Although transplantation has been performed in systemic disorders such as amyloidosis, reoccurrence of the disease in the transplanted heart and the progression of disease in other organ systems argue against the use of this approach in these diseases.

The latter stage of Löffler's cardiomyopathy shows a restrictive cardiomyopathy with gross and microscopic anatomic features virtually identical to those of tropical endocardial fibrosis. Treatment of the underlying eosinophilic disorder and management of the restrictive cardiomyopathy are usually necessary. Occasionally surgical stripping of the endocardial scar (endocardiectomy) and replacement of an AV valve (if severely regurgitant) are beneficial. When endomyocardial fibrosis progresses to cause severe chamber obliteration, surgical resection should be considered.

Prognosis

As the causes of restrictive cardiomyopathy vary, so do the prognoses, depending essentially on the course of the underlying disease. Survival rates for patients with amyloidosis, for example, drop sharply within the first year, generally declining to zero within 4 years. After 10 years, patients with idiopathic restrictive cardiomyopathy have a survival rate of about 50%; those with hypertrophic cardiomyopathy, about 70%; and those with dilated cardiomyopathy, between 30% and 40%.

Hosenpand JD, DeMarco T, Frazier H et al: Progression of systemic disease and reduced long-term survival in patients with cardiac amyloidosis undergoing heart transplantation. Circulation 1991;84(Suppl 111):111.

Schneider U, Jenni R, Turina J et al: Long-term follow-up of patients with endocardial fibroelastosis effects of surgery. Heart 1998;79:362.

Surakomol S, Olson LJ, Rastagi A et al: Combined orthotopic heart and liver transplantation for genetic hemochromatosis. J Heart Lung transplant 1997;16:573.

Myocarditis

Mohammed Zaher Akkad, MD & John B. O'Connell, MD

ESSENTIALS OF DIAGNOSIS

- *New congestive heart failure with a history of an antecedent viral syndrome*
- *Elevated ESR, or cardiac markers*
- *ECG shows sinus tachycardia, nonspecific ST-T changes, atrial or ventricular arrhythmias, or conduction abnormalities*
- *Echocardiogram demonstrates chamber enlargement, wall motion abnormalities, systolic or diastolic dysfunction, or mural thrombi*
- *Endomyocardial biopsy reveals an inflammatory infiltrate with adjacent myocyte injury*

General Considerations

Myocarditis is defined simply as an inflammatory process with necrosis that involves the myocardium. In the past, the myocardial injury was believed to be a direct result of the cytotoxic effects of the relevant organisms. Even as early as 1806, however, it was thought that a persistent inflammatory process following such an infection (eg, diphtheria) of the myocardium led to progressive cardiac damage and dysfunction. When the term *myocarditis* was first introduced in 1837 as inflammation or degeneration of the heart, the diagnosis could be made only postmortem. Fortunately, endomyocardial biopsy now allows the sampling of human myocardial tissue during life and thus the accurate antemortem diagnosis of myocarditis.

Pathophysiology

The histologic hallmark of myocarditis is a focal patchy or diffuse inflammatory infiltrate with adjacent myocyte injury. The inflammation may not be restricted to the myocardium but may also involve the adjacent endocardium, pericardium, and valvular structures.

Myocarditis is most commonly initiated by viral infection (Table 16–1). Initiation of the pathophysiologic abnormalities, however, may result from a variety of insults, including drugs, toxins, hypersensitivity reactions, collagen vascular diseases, and autoimmune reactions. The most common agent associated with myocarditis in the United States and Western Europe in immunocompetent hosts is human coxsackievirus B infection. Other viruses, bacteria, rickettsiae, spirochetes, fungi, protozoans, or metazoans can also produce myocarditis; such causes are uncommon, however (see Table 16–1). Successful identification of the most common offending pathogens depends on knowledge of the geographic region's relevant endemic and epidemic infectious diseases, the inhabitants' immunization status, host immunocompetence, and the sophistication and availability of public health services.

Several mechanisms of myocardial damage have been proposed. (1) Direct injury of myocytes by the infectious agent. (2) Myocyte injury caused by a toxin such as that from *Corynebacterium diphtheriae*. (3) Myocyte injury as a result of infection-induced immune reaction or autoimmunity.

The autoimmunity hypothesis is the most widely accepted theory. It is believed that the viral infection triggers a cell-mediated immunologic response that ultimately causes myocardial injury, the myocardial injury persists despite viral clearance.

In the murine model, coxsackievirus B3 causes an infectious phase, which lasts 7–10 days, and is characterized by active viral replication. During this phase initial myocyte injury takes place, causing the release of antigenic intracellular components such as myosin into the bloodstream. Subsequently, after viral clearance, a second phase of myocyte damage will start. This phase is immune-mediated by CD8 lymphocytes and autoantibodies against various myocyte components. Antimyosin antibodies were isolated from mice that developed myocarditis following coxsackievirus B infection, as well as from patients with myocarditis. Antigenic mimicry, the cross reactivity of antibodies to both virus and myocardial proteins, occurs when an infectious agent shares an identical antigen with the normal myocyte. This mechanism is documented in animal mod-

Table 16–1. Important causes of myocarditis.

Infectious	
Viral	**Bacterial**
Coxsackie A and B	Beta-hemolytic streptococci
Influenza A and B	Corynebacterium diphtheriae
Echovirus	Neisseria meningitides
Arbovirus	Staphylococcus aureus
Cytomegalovirus	Mycoplasma pneumoniae
Human immunodeficiency virus	Salmonella typhi
Hepatitis	Mycobacterium tuberculosis
Epstein-Barr virus	Borrelia burgdorferi
Mumps	Rickettsia rickettsii
Poliomyelitis	Campylobacter jejuni
Herpes simplex	Chlamydia trachomatis
Herpes zoster	Listeria monocytogenes
Rabies	Legionella pneumophila
Rubella	Coxiella burnetii
Rebeola	
Vaccinia	
Protozoal	**Metazoal**
Trypanosoma cruzi	Echinococcus
Toxoplasma gondii	Trichinella spiralis
Fungal	
Noninfectious	
Toxic	**Hypersensitivity**
Anthracyclines	?
Catecholamines	**Autoimmune**
Interleukins	?
Alpha-2 interferon	

? = No dominant organisms.

els, and it may play a role in humans. Myocyte injury may be a direct result of CD8 lymphocyte infiltration. The local release of cytokines, such as interleukin-1, interleukin-2, interleukin-6, tumor necrosis factor (TNF), and nitric oxide may play a role in determining the T-cell reaction and the subsequent degree of au-

toimmune perpetuation. These cytokines may also cause reversible depression of myocardial contractility without causing cell death.

The popularity of the autoimmune hypothesis deemphasizes the role of the virus. Animal studies show, however, that viral proliferation itself might cause myocarditis. Some studies demonstrate the persistence of viral genomic fragments in myocardial cells of patients with active myocarditis and in some patients with dilated cardiomyopathy. Although these fragments may not be infectious, viral RNA may still serve as a persistent antigen to drive the immunologic response.

Exposure to cardiotropic viruses, presumably followed by a viral infection of the myocardium, is common. Based on the detection of serum antibodies to cardiotropic viruses, approximately 70% of the adult population has had prior exposure. Nonetheless, resultant abnormalities in cardiac function or symptomatic heart failure are unusual. The host factors predisposing to these deleterious immune responses are as yet undefined. Immunocompromised patients, such as pregnant women and patients with AIDS, are predisposed to myocarditis. The susceptibility to viral myocarditis may also be age-related, or, based on familial occurrence, genetically predetermined.

Liu PP, Mason JW: Advances in the understanding of myocarditis. Circulation. 2001;104:1076.

Mason JW: Myocarditis. Adv Intern Med 1999;44:293.

O'Connell JB et al: Inflammatory heart disease: Pathogenesis, clinical manifestations, and treatment of myocarditis. Annu Rev Med 1994;45:481.

Clinical Findings

A. SYMPTOMS AND SIGNS

Myocarditis is most commonly asymptomatic, with no evidence of left ventricular dysfunction. The clinical manifestations of myocarditis are protean, when they are present. Myocardial involvement may be overshadowed or completely masked by the constitutional symptoms of the illness or other organ dysfunction. Cardiac symptoms may result from systolic or diastolic left ventricular dysfunction or from tachyarrhythmias or bradyarrhythmias. Patients frequently present days to weeks after an acute febrile illness, particularly a flu-like syndrome. In the Myocarditis Treatment Trial, 59% of patients diagnosed with active myocarditis described an antecedent viral syndrome. Common constitutional symptoms included fever, malaise, fatigue, arthralgias, myalgias, and skin rash.

Chest discomfort is a common symptom and is typically pericardial in nature; ischemic or atypical pain may also occur. In the Myocarditis Trial, 35% of patients with myocarditis and heart failure had associated chest pain. Occasionally patients present with the syndrome of acute myocardial infarction with ischemic chest pain, electrocardiographic (ECG) abnormalities, elevated cardiac isoenzymes, or evidence of left ventricular wall motion abnormalities. Viral coronary arteritis and vasospasm have been implicated as the cause of this syndrome; the epicardial coronary arteries are usually widely patent.

The acute onset of symptoms of congestive heart failure in a young person or in a patient without known coronary artery disease often suggests the diagnosis of myocarditis. Classic symptoms of congestive heart failure, including dyspnea, fatigue, decreased exercise tolerance, palpitations, and right heart failure, may be present. This constellation of signs and symptoms may be indistinguishable from dilated cardiomyopathy. It should be noted that because the metabolic demands on the heart associated with fever or a viral illness may initiate the first episode of congestive heart failure in patients with asymptomatic left ventricular dysfunction or reduced cardiac reserve, heart failure following a viral syndrome does not necessarily imply myocarditis.

Patients may also present with other symptoms that have been described in myocarditis: dizziness, syncope, or palpitations caused by atrial and ventricular arrhythmias and conduction disturbances. Myocarditis may present as sudden death, as a result of malignant ventricular arrhythmias or complete heart block; systemic and pulmonary thromboemboli have also been noted.

Feldman AM, McNamara D: Myocarditis. N Engl J Med 2000; 19:1388.

Pisani B, Taylor DO, Mason JW: Inflammatory myocardial diseases and cardiomyopathy. Am J Med 1997;102:459.

B. Physical Examination

The findings on physical examination vary widely. The patient may appear ill because the other manifestations of a viral illness dominate the clinical picture, and myocardial involvement may become evident only later in the course of the illness. Preexisting heart disease can also obscure the findings of myocarditis on examination.

Tachycardia, hypotension, and fever are associated with myocarditis. The tachycardia may be disproportionate to the degree of fever, and the heart rate is frequently elevated both at rest and with effort. Bradycardia is seen rarely, and a narrow pulse pressure is occasionally detected. Murmurs of mitral or tricuspid regurgitation are common, but diastolic murmurs are rare. The intensity of S_1 may be decreased and the intensity of pulmonic closure increased, and S_3 and S_4 gallops may also be heard.

In more severe cases, congestive heart failure with distended neck veins, pulmonary rales, wheezes, gallops, and peripheral edema may be detected. Pleural and pericardial rubs are common in acute viral myocarditis, and a rhythm disturbance or conduction delay may be evident. Circulatory collapse and shock may occur, but these are rare.

C. Diagnostic Studies

1. Electrocardiography—Electrocardiographic abnormalities are common in patients with myocarditis even in the clinical absence of myocardial involvement. These ECG changes are often nonspecific and transient, usually appearing only in the first 2 weeks of the illness. The most common abnormality is sinus tachycardia. While the presence of ST segment and T wave changes suggest the diagnosis of myocarditis during a viral syndrome, subtle ECG changes may be caused solely by fever, hypoxia, hyperkalemia, and other metabolic abnormalities associated with the syndrome. Atrioventricular (AV) and intraventricular conduction delays are also common. Left bundle branch block occurs in approximately 20% of patients with active myocarditis. Complete AV block is not an uncommon finding and is often diagnosed after the patient presents with syncope. Heart block is usually transient but may occasionally require a temporary pacemaker. Supraventricular tachycardia is common, particularly with associated congestive heart failure or pericarditis. Ventricular ectopy may be the only clinical finding that suggests myocarditis. Other reported abnormalities include axis shifts and repolarization abnormalities.

2. Chest radiograph—The chest x-ray film may be normal, or it may demonstrate mild to moderate cardiomegaly from dilatation of the left or right ventricular cavity (or both). The cardiac silhouette may also be globular when a pericardial effusion is present, however. Evidence of venous congestion and pulmonary edema may be seen in more severe cases, and pulmonary infiltrates from concomitant pneumonia may be present.

3. Echocardiography—Two-dimensional echocardiography is a convenient and noninvasive method of evaluating chamber sizes, valvular function, and myocardial contractility. Left ventricular systolic dysfunction is commonly seen in patients with congestive heart failure. Regional wall motion abnormalities mimicking a myocardial infarction are surprisingly common; however, global hypokinesis may also occur. The left ventricular cavity may be normal in size or minimally enlarged; it may be markedly enlarged in those with fulminant disease. Mitral or tricuspid regurgitation may be present. Interestingly, an increase in wall thickness mimicking hypertrophic cardiomyopathy may be seen early in the course of the disease, presumably secondary to edematous inflammation. Mural thrombi occur in approximately 15% of cases. Echocardiography is also helpful in demonstrating abnormalities of diastolic filling that mimic restrictive cardiomyopathy and in distinguishing ventricular dilatation from pericardial effusion. Echocardiograms are commonly obtained serially to monitor the course of the illness and to evaluate therapy. Echocardiographic changes may persist, improve, or even worsen after clinical resolution of acute myocarditis

4. Radionuclide ventriculography—Radionuclide ventriculography can be used to evaluate cardiac function. This technique provides accurate estimates of chamber volumes, as well as left and right ventricular ejection fractions.

5. Myocardial imaging—Gallium-67 imaging, is a highly sensitive method for identifying active inflammation of the myocardium and pericardium. Unfortunately, the usefulness of this technique is limited by its lack of specificity.

Indium-111 monoclonal antimyosin antibody imaging has shown promise in detecting myocyte injury in patients with unexplained heart failure. This technique has sensitivity for active myocarditis of 83%, a specificity of 53%, and a positive predictive value of a normal scan of 92%. Technetium-99 pyrophosphate imaging has not been useful in humans.

Contrast media-enhanced magnetic resonance imaging using gadopentetate dimeglumine (Gd-DTPA) is a promising noninvasive tool for detecting myocardial inflammation; however low specificity remains a limiting factor.

Friedrich MG et al: contrast media-enhanced magnetic resonance imaging visualize myocardial changes in the course of viral myocarditis. Circulation 1998;97:1802.

Matsouka H, Hamad M, Honda T et al: Evaluation of acute myocarditis and pericarditis by Gd-DTPA enhanced magnetic resonance imaging. Eu Heart J 1994;15:283.

Narula I, An Khaw B, Dec GW et al: Diagnostic accuracy of antimyosin scintigraphy in suspected myocarditis. J Nucl Cardiol 1996;3:3781.

6. Cardiac catheterization—Cardiac catheterization is not routinely performed in all cases of myocarditis; however, it may help in the diagnosis when the presentation mimics myocardial infarction. Characteristic hemodynamic findings of myocarditis include an elevated left ventricular end-diastolic pressure, a depressed cardiac output, and increased ventricular volumes. Ventriculography may also confirm abnormalities seen on echocardiography or nuclear imaging. Coronary angiogram typically demonstrates normal coronary arteries.

7. Endomyocardial biopsy—Myocardial biopsy is considered the gold standard for the diagnosis of myocarditis. It is an invasive procedure, although it only involves minimal morbidity and discomfort. In the Stanford biopsy technique the bioptome is typically introduced to the right ventricular cavity. Four to six tissue fragments are obtained from the right side of the intraventricular septum. The histologic criteria for the diagnosis of myocarditis were variable among pathologists. The Dallas criteria intended for use as entry criteria in the Myocarditis Treatment Trial were developed by a group of cardiac pathologists at a meeting in Dallas, Texas. According to these criteria the diagnosis of active myocarditis is defined as an inflammatory infiltrate of the myocardium with injury to the adjacent myocytes not typical for the ischemic damage associated with coronary artery disease. The diagnosis of borderline myocarditis is made when the infiltrate is not accompanied by myocyte injury. In the Myocarditis Treatment Trial, only 214 (9%) out of 2233 patient with unexplained congestive heart failure met the criteria for active myocarditis. Many patients with negative biopsies had classical clinical presentation of myocarditis. One explanation for the low yield of endomyocardial biopsy is that the inflammation may be focal or patchy. Another reason might be that some patients have purely humoral or cytokine-mediated forms of myocarditis with little or no cellular infiltrate. Furthermore the histologic changes may be transient with rapid resolution. Thus Dallas criteria have some limitations, but they remain the most widely accepted standard for the diagnosis of myocarditis. It should be noted that endomyocardial biopsy may rule in but never rule out active myocarditis.

In recent years the role of endomyocardial biopsy has changed. It is no longer mandatory and essential in the evaluation of unexplained heart failure because the information it provides will rarely determine specific therapy. This became particularly evident after publication of the results of the Myocarditis Treatment Trial, which failed to show any benefit of the immunosuppressive therapy. It remains important to consider biopsy in some special cases of myocarditis, particularly in patients who fail to respond to conventional therapy. Some patients in this group may have giant cell myocarditis, which requires a more aggressive approach with immunosuppressive therapy and consideration for early transplantation.

The utility of endomyocardial biopsy may increase in the near future with the new focus on different markers of immunologic activation, including intracellular adhesion molecule-1 (ICAM-1), soluble FAS ligand (CD95), and human leukocyte antigen (HLA).

Aretz HT, Billingham ME, Edward WB et al: Myocarditis. A histopathologic definition and classification. Cardiovasc Pathol 1987;1:3.

O'Connell JB, Mason JW: Clinical merit of endomyocardial biopsy. Circulation 1989;79:971.

8. Other tests—An elevated erythrocyte sedimentation rate (ESR) is detected in approximately 60% of patients with active myocarditis. If elevated, the ESR may be helpful in monitoring the course of the illness and effectiveness of therapy. The accuracy of this test may be affected by coexisting hepatic congestion or hepatitis; these conditions decrease the synthesis of fibrinogen and lower the ESR.

Mild to moderate leukocytosis occurs in approximately 25% of patients, along with neutrophilia or lymphocytosis and occasionally eosinophilia, particularly in parasitic illnesses. The percentage of eosinophils may also increase in the recovery phase of myocarditis.

The creatinine phosphokinase-myocardial band (CPK-MB) fraction is elevated in approximately 6% of patients, with the degree of elevation being proportional to the degree of myocyte injury. Cardiac troponin-I (Tn I) is a sensitive and specific marker for myocyte injury. In the Myocarditis Treatment Trial elevated serum levels of Tn I were found in 34% of patients with myocarditis compared with only 11% of patient with negative biopsy results.

Measurement of serum antibody titers to various cardiotropic viruses is useful for establishing exposure to these agents. The titers may be neutralizing antibodies, complement-fixing antibodies, or hemagglutination-inhibiting antibodies. Because a fourfold rise in titer over a 4–6 week period is required to document an acute infection, serial blood samples must be obtained. It must be kept in mind that an elevated antibody titer or rise in dilution only implies infection with the offending organism. Proof of active myocarditis also requires a positive biopsy result. Cultures of throat washings, urine, and feces may help identify a viral agent. Unfortunately, viral cultures are usually negative and serologic studies are often nondiagnostic. In addition, viral recovery is usually possible only during the acute phase of the illness when active replication is occurring. Because this phase is not associated with viral injury, the diagnostic yield of culture of myocardial samples obtained by endomyocardial biopsy is minimal. Other laboratory analyses that may be useful include a Monospot test, Epstein-Barr virus titers, hepatitis serology, and urine and serum for cytomegalovirus (CMV).

The detection of viral genomic material in endomyocardial biopsies using recombinant DNA techniques is a promising diagnostic tool. Two methods are used: polymerase chain reaction (PCR) and in situ hybridization. Plus-strand RNA indicates persistent viral state, and minus-strand RNA indicates active viral replication. Unfortunately, studies have been inconsistent, with viral detection ranging between 10 and 60% of patients with dilated cardiomyopathy and myocarditis, compared with almost no viral detection in the control groups. One study showed no difference in viral detection between patients with dilated cardiomyopathy and patients with other forms of chronic heart disease like ischemic heart disease. At the present time routine viral study of endomyocardial biopsy is not recommended and remains investigational with the possibility of clinical application in the future.

Andreoletti L, Hober D, Decoene C et al: Detection of enteroviral RNA by polymerase chain reaction in endomyocardial tissue of patients with chronic cardiac diseases. J Med Virol 1996; 48:53.

Giacca M, Severini GM, Mestroni L et al: Low frequency of detection by nested polymerase chain reaction of enterovirus ribonucleic acid in endomyocardial tissue of patients with idiopathic dilated cardiomyopathy. J Am Coll Cardiol 1994;24: 1033.

Pauschinger M, Doerner A, Kuehl U et al: Enteroviral RNA replication in the myocardium of patients with left ventricular dysfunction and clinically suspected myocarditis. Circulation 1999;99:889.

Smith SC, Ladenson JH, Mason JW et al: Elevation of cardiac troponin I associated with myocarditis. Circulation 1997;95:163.

Treatment

Patients with suspected acute myocarditis should be hospitalized and monitored closely for evidence of worsening congestive heart failure, arrhythmias, conduction disturbances, or emboli. Bed rest is essential, and activities that increase cardiac workload should be strongly discouraged. In the animal model, exercise has been shown to both intensify the inflammatory process in the myocardium and increase morbidity and mortality. Activities should be restricted until clinical improvement occurs or a follow-up biopsy documents the resolution of inflammation.

Antipyretics, other than nonsteroidal antiinflammatory drugs (NSAIDs), should be given to febrile patients, and analgesics are helpful in dealing with pleuropericardial chest pain. Hypoxia, decrease in cardiac output, and tachycardia warrant the administration of supplemental oxygen. If anemia is present, correcting it may improve cardiopulmonary function. The use of tobacco and alcohol should be strongly discouraged.

Patients with congestive heart failure should be treated by restricting sodium and fluids and by administering diuretics, angiotensin-converting enzyme (ACE) inhibitors, β-blockers, and spironolactone. Patients with fulminant disease manifesting as cardiogenic shock will require more aggressive therapy with intravenous vasodilators and inotropic agents such as dobutamine or milrinone. Occasionally cases may be refractory to conservative measures and require intraaortic balloon counterpulsation or a left ventricular assist device. Recent reports have demonstrated that early aggressive approach with mechanical circulatory support might help as a "bridge to recovery." As a last resort, cardiac transplantation may be considered in patients with acute myocarditis if all other measures have failed and the patient's condition is rapidly deteriorating. Unfortunately, an increased morbidity and mortality in transplant rejection results from the activated immunologic system that the donor heart encounters.

Antiarrhythmic agents are warranted in patients with tachyarrhythmias or ventricular arrhythmias. It is best to avoid agents with strong negative inotropic effects. Occasionally amiodarone or an implantable cardioverter defibrillator may be used after all other attempts at controlling arrhythmia have failed. These measures must be used only as a last resort, however, because myocarditis frequently resolves spontaneously. Patients with symptomatic bradyarrhythmias or high-grade conduction blocks will benefit from the implantation of a pacemaker.

Anticoagulation therapy is indicated in patients with systemic or pulmonary emboli or mural thrombi detected by echocardiography or ventriculography. Patients with active myocarditis and even mild left ventricular dysfunction should probably receive anticoagulation (animal models have demonstrated a propensity toward mural thrombi). Anticoagulation may be contraindicated in patients with coexisting pericarditis.

Immunosuppressive therapy has been reported in few studies with disappointing results. The largest controlled trial to date is the Myocarditis Treatment Trial, which compared conventional therapy alone to conventional therapy plus one of two immunosuppressive combinations: the first is cyclosporine and prednisone, the second is azathioprine and prednisone. In this study significant differences in left ventricular ejection fraction (LVEF) or left ventricular diastolic diameter at 28 or 52 weeks could not be detected among the groups, largely due to unexpected spontaneous improvement in those not receiving immunosuppression therapy. No significant difference in survival occurred during the follow-up period.

Intravenous immune globulin was suggested to be useful by some reports. A recent report randomized 62 patients with recent-onset (less than 6 months of symptoms) dilated cardiomyopathy to receive intravenous immune globulin or placebo. No treatment effect was found in improving LVEF at 12 months, although both groups had a 14% increase in LVEF. Based on all available studies, immunosuppressive therapy is generally not indicated except in a few special cases.

The prognosis in giant cell myocarditis is very poor, and immunosuppressive therapy may be helpful. Another situation where immunosuppressive therapy may be indicated is myocarditis associated with underlying immune diseases like systemic lupus erythematosus (SLE). In a small percentage of myocarditis patients the disease may recur after initial resolution, in these patients immunosuppressive therapy may help in decreasing the recurrences.

A recently published study randomized 84 patients with idiopathic cardiomyopathy of more than 6 months duration to receive immunosuppressive therapy (prednisone and azathioprine) or placebo for 3 months with a 2-year follow-up. All these patients had positive HLA in their endomyocardial biopsy specimens. The author hypothesized that the presence of HLA in the myocardium will identify a population of patients with

inflammatory cardiomyopathy due to immune process. After 2 years a composite of death, heart transplantation, or hospital readmission did not differ between the study groups. The patients in the immunosuppression arm, however, showed significant improvement in LVEF at 3 months and 3 years, as well as improvement in New York Heart Association (NYHA) functional class. This study restores the interest in immunosuppressive therapy as a treatment for myocarditis; however, more work needs to be done to evaluate different immune markers that will help identify the subgroups of patients that will benefit from such treatment.

McNamara DM et al: Controlled trial of intravenous immune globulin in recent-onset dilated cardiomyopathy. Circulation 2001;103:2254.

O'Connell JB, Mason JW et al: The myocarditis treatment trial: Design, method, and patient enrollment. Eu Heart J 1995; 16,Supp O,162.

O'Connell JB, Mason JW, Herskowitz A et al: A clinical trial of immunosuppressive therapy for myocarditis: The Myocarditis Treatment Trial Investigators. N Engl J Med 1995;333:269.

Parrillo JE: Inflammatory cardiomyopathy (myocarditis). Which patients should be treated with anti-inflammatory therapy? Circulation 2001;104:4.

Parrillo JE, Cunnion RE, Epstein SE et al: A prospective randomized controlled trial of prednisone for dilated cardiomyopathy. N Engl J Med 1989;321:1061.

Wojnicz R et al: Randomized, placebo-controlled study for immunosuppressive treatment of inflammatory dilated cardiomyopathy two-year follow up results. Circulation 2001; 104:39.

Prognosis

The majority of patients with myocarditis have self-limited, asymptomatic disease without residual cardiac dysfunction. Symptomatic patients have a poorer prognosis. Patients may spontaneously recover at any point during the illness, the degree of ventricular dysfunction may stabilize, or it may progress to dilated cardiomyopathy and heart failure, especially in the face of such causes as AIDS or giant cell myocarditis. Unfortunately, a small percentage of patients will die suddenly and unexpectedly, regardless of therapy. The overall prognosis is poor. In the Myocarditis Treatment Trial, the estimated cumulative mortality rate at 5 years was about 55%. This high rate occurred despite initial improvement in ejection fraction. Progressive heart failure was the predominant cause of death. One small observational study showed that patients presenting with fulminant myocarditis have a better long-term prognosis than patients with mild acute or chronic presentations. These patients should therefore be supported aggressively with vasopressor therapy and a left ventricular assist device if necessary to give them the best chance in surviving the initial critical phase, as the likelihood of long-term recovery is high.

McCarthy RE III, Boehmer JP, Hruban RH et al: Long term outcome of fulminant myocarditis as compared with acute (nonfulminant) myocarditis. N Engl J Med 2000;342:690.

Specific Forms of Myocarditis

A. CHAGAS' DISEASE OR AMERICAN TRYPANOSOMIASIS

Chagas' disease is an endemic disease in the rural areas of Central and South America.

A few cases have been reported in the Southwestern United States among immigrants from endemic areas. It is estimated that 18–20 million people are infected with the protozoan *Trypanosoma cruzi,* the agent causing Chagas' disease; of those infected, 50,000 die each year. *Trypanosoma cruzi* is transmitted by reduviid insects (Triatominae family). The insect becomes infected when it bites an animal or human carrier. Humans acquire the trypanosomes when the insects bite them during sleep. Alternatively, the insect might deposit its feces on the skin; trypanosomes then gain access to the bloodstream by the person rubbing the abraded skin or the conjunctivae.

Approximately 1% of the people bitten by reduviid bugs will develop acute Chagas' disease. Patients may develop myocarditis in this phase; however, they usually recover within several weeks to several months. The patient may present with an erythematous, pruritic skin lesion (chagoma) at the inoculation site. Unilateral, painless, palpebral edema with local lymphadenopathy (Romaña's sign) is particularly common in children. After resolution of the acute phase, many patients enter a latent period in which they may develop a subclinical cardiomyopathy. Approximately 30% of these patients progress to chronic Chagas' disease, manifested as visceral organ enlargement (megaesophagus and megacolon) and cardiac disease, which is characterized by unrelenting congestive heart failure, malignant arrhythmias, heart block, thromboembolic phenomena, and sudden death. Cellular and humoral immune responses to *T cruzi*-altered host's cells appear to be responsible for myocardial injury. Characteristic ECG changes include right bundle branch block, with or without a left anterior fascicular block, and variable degrees of AV block. Echocardiography may demonstrate dilated ventricles, wall motion abnormalities, and specifically apical aneurysms. Active myocarditis can be demonstrated by endomyocardial biopsy using the Dallas criteria. Complement fixation test (Machado-Guerreiro test), and indirect immunofluorescent antibody assay is helpful in the diagnosis of chronic Chagas' disease.

Treatment of Chagas' disease is difficult, and primarily symptomatic. Heart failure is treated in the usual manner, and the use of anticoagulants and antiarrhythmic agents (amiodarone) may be warranted. Heart block may necessitate pacemaker placement. For life-threatening ventricular arrhythmia implantable cardioverter-defibrillator (ICD) implantation is indicated. Antiparasitic agents such as nifurtimox, benzimidazole, or itraconazole may be beneficial in both acute and untreated chronic Chagas' disease. Cardiac transplantation may be an option in some cases; however, parasitemia is a common result of immunosuppression, and nifurtimox prophylaxis should be considered.

Hagar JM, Rahimtoola SH: Chagas' heart disease. Curr Probl Cardiol 1995;20:825.

B. HUMAN IMMUNODEFICIENCY VIRUS

Infection with human immunodeficiency virus (HIV) is one of the leading causes of acquired heart diseases. The cardiac complications tend to occur late in the disease, and with lower CD4 counts. The HIV-related cardiac manifestations are likely to become more prevalent as therapy and longevity improve. Evidence of cardiac involvement is found at autopsy in more than 50% of patients dying with AIDS. There is a wide spectrum of cardiac manifestations in HIV patients, including pericardial, myocardial, and valvular involvement. Myocarditis in HIV patients is common. Causes may be a direct effect of HIV on the myocardium, or an autoimmune process induced by HIV alone or in conjunction with other viruses. About 20% of HIV-related myocarditis is caused by multiple infectious organisms, such as coxsackievirus group B, Epstein-Barr virus, cytomegalovirus, adenovirus, *Toxoplasma gondii,* and *Histoplasma capsulatum.* HIV itself is responsible for the remaining 80% of cases. HIV cardiomyopathy is probably more related to HIV than to opportunistic infections.

Clinical presentation may be asymptomatic left ventricular systolic dysfunction or congestive heart failure. Echocardiography shows increased left ventricular dimensions, and decreased function. Myocardial biopsy reveals patchy lymphocytic infiltrate, the lymphocytes consist of T cells—mostly CD8, CD2, CD3, and rarely CD4.

Prognosis in HIV cardiomyopathy is grim, and the mortality rate is high independent of CD4 count. Rapid-onset congestive heart failure carries a worse prognosis, with 50% mortality in 6–12 months. Treatment is similar to that for other forms of cardiomyopathy. Intravenous immunoglobulins have been used with some success in acute congestive heart failure and in myocarditis in HIV-infected patients.

Herskowitz A: Cardiomyopathy and other symptomatic heart diseases associated with HIV infection. Curr Opin Cardiol 1996; 11:325.

Michaels AD et al: Cardiovascular involvement in AIDS Curr Probl Cardiol 1997;22-3:109.

C. TOXOPLASMOSIS

Active myocarditis may result from acute infection by the intracellular protozoan *Toxoplasma gondii.* This form is primarily diagnosed in immunocompromised hosts, such as HIV patients, but may also occur following cardiac transplantation. The infection can be transmitted by the donor heart. Endomyocardial biopsy reveals edema, organisms within the myocytes in areas of focal myocyte necrosis, and a mixed inflammatory infiltrate containing eosinophils. Toxoplasmic cysts may also be seen, and a rise in antibody titer may be detected. The infection is usually asymptomatic, although heart failure, arrhythmias, and conduction abnormalities may occur. If detected early, pyrimethamine and sulfadiazine may be curative.

D. Cytomegalovirus

Symptomatic myocarditis caused by cytomegalovirus infection usually occurs only in immunosuppressed patients, such as those with neoplasms, HIV disease, or transplanted organs. Asymptomatic myocarditis is known to occur in the general population but is usually self-limited. Endomyocardial biopsy may demonstrate viral inclusions within myocytes, and viral DNA can be found within the myocardium. A focal lymphocytic infiltration with fibrosis is characteristic. Treatment is with intravenous ganciclovir.

E. Lyme Myocarditis

Infection with the tick-borne spirochete *Borrelia burgdorferi* causes Lyme disease, which manifests primarily with myalgias, arthralgias, headache, fever, adenopathy, and erythema chronicum migrans. Approximately 10% of infected patients will also develop symptomatic, but usually transient, cardiac involvement. Patients may present with conduction abnormalities or fluctuating degrees of AV block. Syncope secondary to complete heart block is common and may require temporary transvenous pacing. Left ventricular dysfunction is rare. Endomyocardial biopsy may reveal active myocarditis. Spirochetes have been isolated from the myocardium in some patients. It is unclear whether the myocarditis of Lyme disease is a direct result of spirochetal infection or the immunologic response to it. The course of the disease is usually benign, and complete recovery is the rule.

Treatment with penicillin or doxycycline is recommended, but it is unknown if this treatment alters the course of the cardiac disease.

F. Giant Cell Myocarditis

Giant cell myocarditis is a rare form of myocarditis characterized by multinucleated giant cells within the myocardium, particularly at the margins of necrosis. The precise cause is as yet unknown although it has been associated with several autoimmune diseases, such as ulcerative colitis, Crohn's disease, and myasthenia gravis. This form of myocarditis is rapid in onset and usually associated with fever and widespread ECG changes. Conduction abnormalities, including high-grade AV block and ventricular tachyarrhythmias, are more commonly seen in giant cell myocarditis than in viral myocarditis. The disease course is characterized by a progressive downhill trend regardless of medical therapy. Early recognition of this form of myocarditis is important, as the prognosis is far worse than viral myocarditis. It should be suspected in young patients presenting with rapidly progressive heart failure that is refractory to conventional therapy. Myocardial biopsy is usually diagnostic.

Immunosuppressive therapy with a combination of cyclosporine, azathioprine, and corticosteroids appears to be beneficial, possibly prolonging the time to transplant or death. Cardiac transplantation should be considered early despite the possibility of disease recurrence in the transplanted heart.

Cooper LT Jr, Berry GJ, Shabetai R: Idiopathic giant-cell myocarditis natural history and treatment. N Engl J Med 1997;336:1860.

G. Sarcoidosis

This systemic granulomatous disease is of unknown origin. The pathologic hallmark of this disease is noncaseating granuloma. The granuloma consists of activated helper-inducer T lymphocytes, macrophages, and multinucleated giant cells. The granulomas trigger a fibrotic response, resulting in organ damage.

The disease may be widespread or limited to a single organ. The lymphoid, pulmonary, cardiovascular, hepatobiliary, and hematologic systems are most commonly involved, with the lungs being affected in over 90% of patients. Cardiac sarcoid is more common than previously recognized and is less likely to be diagnosed antemortem than pulmonary sarcoid. Frequently, the initial presentation is sudden death. In myocardial sarcoid, portions of the myocardial wall are replaced by sarcoid granulomas. Based on the degree of myocardial involvement, the presenting signs and symptoms vary from first-degree AV block to fulminant heart failure. About 25% of deaths due to cardiac sarcoid are from heart failure, whereas sudden death accounts for about a third of the deaths. The diagnosis of cardiac sarcoid can be challenging, so evidence of other organ involvement should be sought. Chest radiograph, ECG, and echocardiography are helpful diagnostic tools. Due to the scattered nature of the granulomas, endomyocardial biopsy lacks sensitivity and seldom aids the diagnosis despite high specificity. Treatment of sarcoid has not been studied by controlled trials; however, corticosteroids can improve cardiac symptoms and reverse ECG changes in over half of the treated patients. Antiarrhythmic drugs and automatic internal defibrillator placement may be indicated to decrease the risk of sudden death.

Pericardial Diseases

17

Samer S. Kabbani, MD & Martin M. LeWinter, MD

General Considerations

A. NORMAL PERICARDIAL ANATOMY AND PHYSIOLOGY

The pericardium consists of two layers: a serous visceral layer, which is intimately adherent to the heart and epicardial fat, and a fibrous parietal layer. The pericardium encloses the greater part of the surface of the heart, the juxtacardial portions of the pulmonary and systemic veins, and the proximal segments of the great vessels. A significant portion of the left atrium, however, is not enclosed within the pericardium. The pericardium is attached by ligaments to the manubrium sterni, the xiphoid process, the vertebral column, and the central tendon of the diaphragm. The pericardium is not essential for sustaining life or health, as evidenced by continued cardiac function even if the pericardium is congenitally absent or surgically removed. The pericardium does play a role in normal cardiovascular function, however, and can be involved in a number of important disease states.

The normal functions of the pericardium include maintaining an optimal cardiac shape, promoting cardiac chamber interaction, preventing the overfilling of the heart, reducing friction between the beating heart and adjacent structures, providing a physical barrier to infection, and limiting displacement during the cardiac cycle.

B. PERICARDIAL PRESSURE

The true pressure in the normal pericardial space is a matter of some controversy. When measured with fluid-filled catheters, pericardial pressure is very similar to intrapleural pressure: from –ve 1 to –ve 2 mm Hg on average, falling to about –ve 5 mm Hg with normal inspiration. There is considerable evidence, however, that the pressure in the normal pericardial space is best considered as a contact force between visceral and parietal pericardium and therefore is more appropriately measured with flat balloons. In this case, the pericardial pressure is clearly higher than the intrapleural pressure, although its actual magnitude is a matter of conjecture. The bulk of current evidence indicates that with normal cardiac volumes, the effective pericardial pressure ranges from 0–1 mm Hg to (at most) 3–4 mm Hg.

The pericardial space between the parietal and visceral layers normally contains 15–50 mL of fluid, and the reserve volume of the pericardium is relatively small. Once this modest reserve is filled, intrapericardial pressure rises significantly with the addition of more fluid. It should be noted that with significant fluid in the pericardial space, fluid-filled catheters do provide accurate intrapericardial pressure measurements.

Pathophysiology & Etiology

A. INFECTIOUS PATHOGENS

1. Viral pericarditis—The most common clinical manifestation of viral involvement is acute pericarditis, and it seems likely that an unidentified virus underlies most cases of idiopathic pericarditis. The possibility of a viral cause is suggested when pericarditis occurs in the absence of other factors; it is supported by a more than fourfold rise in serial viral antibody titers during the initial weeks of illness. (Such measurement, however, is not a routine part of the treatment of viral pericarditis.) Frequently, a prodromal syndrome of an upper respiratory infection is present.

The viral pathogens most commonly associated with pericarditis include coxsackievirus B (most common), coxsackievirus A, echovirus 8, and human immunodeficiency virus (HIV). Although a wide range of viral agents have been implicated, no specific antiviral therapy is recommended at this time; management and outcome are described in the section on acute pericarditis.

2. Bacterial pericarditis—Bacterial infection of the pericardium can occur following thoracic surgery; as a result of a contiguous pleural, mediastinal, or pulmonary infection; as a complication of bacterial endocarditis; or as a result of systemic bacteremia. Direct extension from pneumonia or empyema with staphylococci, pneumococci, and streptococci accounts for the majority of cases. The incidence of hospital-acquired penicillin-resistant staphylococcal pericarditis after thoracic surgery has increased during the past decade. Preexisting pericardial effusions and immunosuppressed states are important predisposing factors.

Common clinical manifestations include fever, chills, night sweats, and dyspnea; pleuritic chest pain and pericardial friction rubs are present in only a minority of patients. Leukocytosis with a shift to the left is generally present, and chest radiography usually reveals an increase in the cardiac silhouette. Although electrocardiograms are frequently normal, they can show typical changes of pericarditis.

Although high intrapericardial antibiotic levels are achievable, medical therapy alone is insufficient, and prompt percutaneous or surgical drainage is essential. Cardiac tamponade may occur very rapidly with hemodynamic deterioration that can be confused with septic shock. In view of the continuing high mortality rates of 65–77%, bacterial pericarditis should be considered a medical emergency.

3. Tuberculous pericarditis—Although several decades of effective antituberculous therapy and public health measures have brought about a declining rate of tuberculous pericarditis, this condition remains a major problem in the immunocompromised host. Thus, in patients infected with HIV a common cause of symptomatic pericardial effusion is tuberculosis.

Tuberculous pericarditis usually occurs with no demonstrable pulmonary or extrapulmonary tuberculosis. Symptoms may be insidious and nonspecific. Findings are predominantly systemic, and pericardial friction rubs are found in only a few patients. Large effusions and resulting tamponade are common, and constriction occurs as a late complication. Demonstration of tubercle bacillus by stain or culture is possible in only one third to one half of the patients, and the diagnosis is often presumptively established through a history of contact or a positive purified protein derivative (PPD) skin test. High levels of adenosine deaminase, an enzyme produced by white blood cells, in pericardial fluid is a sensitive and specific test for tuberculous pericarditis. The diagnosis can often be established by culture of pericardial fluid or by noting characteristic granulomata on pericardial biopsy specimens.

Often the diagnosis of tuberculous pericarditis is made retrospectively in patients with constrictive pericarditis and a history of tuberculosis. Such cases are managed like any case of constrictive pericarditis.

Untreated tuberculous pericarditis is associated with mortality rates in excess of 80%. Management consists of triple-drug antituberculous therapy for at least 9 months. Some authorities advocate the use of corticosteroids to prevent the development of constrictive pericarditis, but data to support this approach are not conclusive. Pericardiocentesis is indicated for patients with large or compromising effusions. As much as one third of patients will require pericardial resection despite antibiotic therapy.

4. Acquired immunodeficiency syndrome—The most common pericardial abnormality encountered in acquired immune deficiency syndrome (AIDS) is asymptomatic pericardial effusion. It can be considered part of the generalized effusive process that can involve the peritoneum and pleura as well. The condition does not mandate invasive diagnostic studies or treatment because many of these effusions resolve spontaneously without specific treatment.

Symptomatic pericardial effusion with or without chest pain, friction rub, and electrocardiographic changes is often caused by a variety of opportunistic infections, and neoplasms. The most common infectious agents identified in symptomatic pericardial effusion are *Mycobacterium tuberculosis* and *Mycobacterium avium-intracellulare*. Lymphomas and Kaposi's sarcoma are the most common neoplasms associated with effusion. Pericarditis or symptomatic pericardial effusion in a patient with AIDS should therefore prompt an immediate search for infection or neoplasm. A recent study demonstrated that pericardial effusion in HIV disease usually occurs in the context of full-blown AIDS and is strongly associated with a shortened survival time independent of the CD4 count. The mortality rate at 6 months for patients with effusion was nine times greater than for subjects without effusion.

Estok L: Cardiac tamponade in a patient with AIDS: A review of pericardial disease in patients with HIV infection. Mount Sinai J Med 1998;64:312.

Heidenreich P: Pericardial effusion in AIDS: Incidence and survival. Circulation 1995;92:3229.

Fowler NO: Tuberculous pericarditis. JAMA 1991;266:99.

B. IATROGENIC CAUSES

1. Surgery-related syndromes—Several distinct pericardial syndromes may occur after heart surgery.

Cardiac tamponade may occur during in-hospital recuperation, most commonly in the first 24 h. It is identified by the hemodynamic perturbations typical of tamponade. The sudden cessation of previously brisk bleeding from drains should alert the physician to the possibility of clogged tubes. Therapy consists of prompt surgical exploration and evacuation. Cardiac tamponade is less common after the first 24 h, with fewer typical clinical manifestations, and symptoms may consist largely of nonspecific generalized complaints. Two-dimensional echocardiography establishes the presence of a significant effusion and may delineate its anatomic distribution. Pericardial effusions in this setting are often loculated and may compress only one cardiac chamber. The approach to drainage is largely dictated by the location of the effusion.

Early pericarditis, consisting of fever, chest pain, pericardial friction rubs, and typical electrocardiographic features, is common. In most cases, the syndrome resolves spontaneously, and nonsteroidal antiinflammatory agents are effective symptomatic treatment.

Postpericardiotomy syndrome is reported in as many as 30–40% of patients. This syndrome, which usually occurs during the first several postoperative weeks, consists of fever, pleuritis, and pericarditis. Diagnosis proceeds by exclusion, and treatment consists of administering nonsteroidal antiinflammatory agents; the need for steroids is rare.

Constrictive pericarditis occurs rarely as a complication for cardiac surgery. Although its incidence is estimated to occur in only 0.2–0.3% of cardiac operations, because more than 700,000 cardiac surgeries are performed in the United States annually, surgery is emerging as an important cause of constrictive pericarditis. It has been reported to occur at times ranging from 2 weeks to 21 years after the surgery. Because of the relative rarity of this complication, it has been difficult to identify specific predisposing procedural factors. In the cases of constriction reported in the literature, however, 95% have been associated with an open pericardium, which may serve as a reservoir for the collection of blood. In rare cases that occurred shortly after surgery, steroid therapy has been reported to reverse the abnormal hemodynamic findings. The mainstay of therapy, however, is still pericardiectomy.

Ling L: Constrictive pericarditis in the modern era: Evolving clinical spectrum and impact on outcome after pericardiectomy. Circulation 1999;100:1380.

2. Trauma—Traumatic hemorrhagic pericardial effusions, which can result from blunt or penetrating injuries of the chest, can also be caused by a variety of iatrogenic causes, such as cardiac catheterization, pacemaker insertion, endoscopy, and closed chest cardiac massage. The rapidity with which pericardial fluid can accumulate can quickly cause hemodynamic compromise. Hypotension in this setting should prompt both an immediate echocardiographic search for pericardial fluid and swift evacuation of any significant effusions. Delayed manifestations may include recurrent pericardial effusions and, in rare cases, constrictive pericarditis.

3. Radiation therapy—The incidence of pericardial injury from therapeutic radiation is related to dose, duration, and technical features. Pericardial damage from radiation may appear during the course of therapy or following it. The syndrome that appears during radiation therapy is acute pericarditis. The onset of clinical manifestations in the delayed form is usually within 12 months but may take many years. The clinical features of the late form range from asymptomatic pericardial effusions to acute pericarditis or constrictive pericarditis. Radiation therapy is now one of the leading causes of constrictive pericarditis. Diagnosis and management

are discussed later in the sections on pericardial effusion and constrictive pericarditis.

C. CONNECTIVE TISSUE DISORDERS

1. Rheumatoid arthritis—Pericarditis has been found postmortem in up to 50% of patients with rheumatoid arthritis. The clinical recognition of pericarditis during life, however, is far less frequent. Tamponade may occur as a complication of pericardial effusion in rheumatoid arthritis and should be treated accordingly. Patients with nodular rheumatoid arthritis are much more likely to develop pericarditis than are those without nodules, and pericarditis commonly occurs in association with arthritis and pleuritis. Symptomatic pericarditis can be treated with nonsteroidal agents. There is no evidence to support a role for steroids in preventing constrictive pericarditis; as in other conditions, the presence of constrictive pericarditis warrants pericardiectomy.

2. Systemic lupus erythematosus—Pericarditis is the most common cardiac complication of systemic lupus erythematosus (SLE) and tends to occur during periods of active disease. Clinical and electrocardiographic features tend to be typical of acute pericarditis. Although tamponade can complicate pericarditis, constrictive pericarditis is a rare complication. The pericarditis tends to subside as systemic manifestations improve in response to steroid or immunosuppressive therapy.

3. Progressive systemic sclerosis—As is true in rheumatoid arthritis, pericarditis is found at autopsy more frequently than during life. Asymptomatic pericardial effusions can be found in 40% of patients. Patients with scleroderma may present with typical symptoms of pericarditis and nonspecific electrocardiographic changes, and tamponade may occur. The prognosis is generally poor for patients with scleroderma who develop pericarditis. Pericardial involvement can also occur in association with myocardial involvement; differentiating constrictive pericarditis from restrictive cardiomyopathy may sometimes necessitate thoracotomy.

Spodick DH: Pericarditis in systemic diseases. Cardiol Clin 1990; 8:709.

D. OTHER CAUSES

1. Myocardial infarction—Clinical evidence of pericarditis can be found in 7–20% of patients within the first week after myocardial infarction, although autopsy series suggest a significantly higher incidence of clinically silent localized fibrinous pericarditis. The incidence is greater in transmural than in subendocardial infarctions. Although anticoagulant therapy does not appear to increase the incidence of pericardial effusions, it may contribute to the development of intrapericardial hemorrhage and tamponade and is therefore relatively contraindicated in the presence of pericarditis.

Thrombolytic therapy has been associated with a decreased incidence of pericarditis in placebo-controlled studies. Because these agents can also contribute to the development of tamponade, however, their use may be contraindicated when concurrent pericarditis is identified.

Dressler's syndrome (postmyocardial-infarction syndrome) occurs from 1 to 6 weeks after myocardial infarction and consists of fever, pleuropericardial pain, malaise, and evidence of pleural and pericardial effusions. The syndrome is a contraindication to anticoagulant therapy because pericardial hemorrhage can occur, increasing the likelihood of tamponade. The incidence of this syndrome has been decreasing in recent years. It is believed to have an autoimmune cause due to sensitization to myocardial cells at the time of necrosis. Antimyocardial antibodies have been demonstrated in patients with Dressler's syndrome. Management is as outlined in the section on pericarditis.

Oliva BP et al: Effect of definition on incidence of post infarction pericarditis. Is it time to redefine post infarction pericarditis? Circulation 1994;90:1537.

2. Malignancy—A variety of hematologic and solid malignancies can cause pericardial metastases that are more frequently revealed at autopsy than during life. Typically, the diagnosis of malignancy has been already established in the patient presenting with a malignant pericardial effusion, and other sites of metastatic spread are evident. On rare occasions, tamponade from the malignant effusion is the first manifestation of tumor. It is important to distinguish malignant effusions from other causes of effusion, such as radiation, infection, and uremia, because the management and prognosis of malignant and nonmalignant effusions in cancer patients differ substantially. The diagnosis is established through echocardiography and cytologic examination; the fluid will be positive in approximately 80% of malignant effusions, with the balance usually positively identified through surgical biopsy of the pericardium.

These patients may survive for a number of months after a diagnosis of malignant effusion; therapy to alleviate symptoms and prevent reaccumulation of the effusion is therefore indicated (treatment of nonmalignant effusions is discussed in the section on Pericardial Effusion). Pericardiocentesis usually provides immediate relief. Subsequent management to control the effusion may include radiation or chemotherapy for tumors, such as breast cancer, lymphoma, and leukemia, that are sensitive to these modalities. Installation of chemicals, most commonly tetracycline, into the pericardium is effective in most cases but can be associated with unpleasant side effects such as pain and fever. Surgical approaches include subxiphoid pericardiotomy or thoracotomy with either pleuropericardiotomy or pericardiectomy. The subxiphoid approach, which can frequently be carried out under local anesthetic, has the advantage of high success rates and low morbidity and mortality. Malignancies, most commonly lymphomas, can also involve the pericardium through enlargement of anterior mediastinal lymph nodes and obstruction of lymphatic drainage. Shrinking the lymph nodes by chemotherapy or radiation therapy may dramatically improve the resulting effusions.

3. Uremia—Pericardial involvement in patients with renal failure can take several forms. Many patients with chronic renal insufficiency who are asymptomatic can be found, on echocardiography, to have pericardial effusions. These effusions, which are typically small, are related more closely to the patient's volume status than other variables and usually warrant no intervention beyond clinical vigilance. The incidence of uremic pericarditis has been decreasing in recent years, a trend some observers attribute to earlier and more intensive dialysis. Uremic pericarditis typically occurs before the initiation of chronic dialysis; its development is related, in part, to the absolute levels of elevation in blood urea nitrogen (BUN) and serum creatinine levels, and it almost always responds to dialysis. Patients in this setting can present with symptoms and signs typical of acute pericarditis, or they may have few symptoms despite large pericardial effusions—with or without a pericardial rub. Although uremic pericarditis can lead to tamponade, it is more commonly associated with the slow accumulation of large, low-pressure pericardial effusions. As in any clinical setting, tamponade warrants prompt evacuation of the pericardial fluid. Echocardiography may show an effusion in the majority of patients, but the absence of an effusion in a patient with otherwise typical clinical features should not exclude the diagnosis. Classic electrocardiographic changes are present in fewer than half the patients; the abnormalities are more often nonspecific and may include atrial fibrillation. Complications from pericardiocentesis in this patient population may be more frequent than in other groups of patients with pericardial effusions.

Pericardial involvement can also occur in patients who are already undergoing dialysis. The development of dialysis-related pericardial disease is not strongly related to serum BUN or creatinine levels. Chest pain, typically pleuritic, is the most common symptom. Pericarditis in a patient undergoing dialysis presents complicated management issues. In a significant fraction of these patients, the pericarditis may have an identifiable, remediable cause that should be promptly identified. Although most patients who develop pericarditis while already undergoing dialysis respond to intensification of the dialysis regimen, a significant minority fail to improve. Clinical predictors of failure include fever of more than 102°F, evidence of heart failure, a white blood cell count higher than 15,000, a large effusion observed echocardiographically, and the use of peritoneal dialysis as a sole treatment modality. Nonsteroidal antiinflammatory agents may be tried, but a randomized, prospective study found indomethacin effective only in ameliorating fever. It did not affect the duration of chest pain and pericardial rub or the subsequent development of tamponade. These results indicate that when intensive dialysis therapy has failed to remedy the pericarditis, surgical therapy must be considered.

Rostand SG, Rutsky EA: Pericarditis in end-stage renal disease. Cardiol Clin 1990;8:701.

4. Drug-related causes—A number of pharmacologic agents have been implicated in pericardial disease. Pericarditis can occur as a feature of drug-induced SLE syndrome caused by procainamide, hydralazine, diphenylhydantoin, reserpine, methyldopa, and isoniazid. In addition to their propensity for causing myocardial inflammation, anthracycline antineoplastic agents can cause acute pericarditis. Methysergide can cause pericardial constriction as part of the syndrome of mediastinal fibrosis, and pericarditis can be part of a hypersensitivity reaction to penicillin. Minoxidil has been reported to cause pericarditis and tamponade; the mechanism is unknown.

5. Hypothyroidism—Pericardial effusion can be found in one third of patients with myxedema. The frequency of pericardial involvement is related to both the severity and duration of hypothyroidism. The accumulation of pericardial fluid in this condition appears to be a result of a combination of increased capillary permeability and retarded lymphatic drainage. Because the pericardial fluid accumulates slowly, tamponade is relatively rare. The electrocardiogram demonstrates low voltage QRS by electrocardiogram (ECG)—sometimes profoundly low. If pericardiocentesis is required before the diagnosis of hypothyroidism is made, the diagnosis can be suspected if the fluid is yellow and contains a high level of cholesterol. Pericardial disease in hypothyroidism reliably responds to thyroid hormone replacement therapy.

ACUTE PERICARDITIS

ESSENTIALS OF DIAGNOSIS

- *Central chest pain aggravated by coughing, inspiration, or recumbency*
- *Pericardial friction rub on auscultation*
- *Characteristic ECG changes*

General Considerations

Acute pericarditis is an inflammatory condition of the pericardium that can be caused by virtually any of the conditions just discussed.

Clinical Findings

A. SYMPTOMS AND SIGNS

The primary symptom of acute pericarditis is chest pain whose location, intensity, and nature are variable. The pain may be described as sharp or dull. Most often it is precordial or retrosternal in location and may be referred to the trapezius ridge, which is almost pathognomonic for pericarditis. It is characteristically aggravated by inspiration, coughing, or recumbency and lessened by sitting upright and leaning forward. Although it typically takes an hour or two to develop fully, the pain can sometimes appear remarkably abruptly. Many patients relate prodromal symptoms suggestive of a viral infection.

B. PHYSICAL EXAMINATION

Patients with pericarditis may be febrile and tachycardiac. The pericardial friction rub—the characteristic auscultatory finding—is typically scratchy and has three components corresponding to atrial contraction, ventricular systole, and early diastole. It is not unusual for only one or two components to be audible; the systolic component is most consistently present. Exercise may facilitate the identification of all three components. Because the friction rub may be evanescent, varying widely in intensity even in the course of a single day, repeated auscultation is important. Furthermore, because posture can affect the pericardial rub, auscultation with the patient in several positions, (supine, sitting, etc) is often helpful. When the intensity of the rub is modulated significantly by respiration, it is termed a pleuropericardial friction rub.

C. DIAGNOSTIC STUDIES

Evaluation of a patient with suspected pericarditis should routinely include an ECG, a chest x-ray film, a complete blood count, C-reactive protein, and erythrocyte sedimentation rate. Additional diagnostic laboratory tests should be tailored to the clinical presentation. Echocardiography is a sensitive test for detecting pericardial effusion; however, pericardial effusion can occur in the absence of pericardial inflammation.

1. Electrocardiography—Serial ECGs are valuable in diagnosing pericarditis. Four stages of ECG changes have been described (Table 17–1). In stage I, the changes accompany the onset of chest pain and consist of widespread ST-segment elevation (Figure 17–1). The ST segment is concave upward (in distinction to the elevation in myocardial infarction). ST-segment elevation is typically present in all leads except aVR and V_1, where ST-segment depression is present. The T waves are upright in the leads with ST elevation. The stage I pattern of pericarditis may be difficult to distinguish from the normal variant of early repolarization. A differentiating point that may be useful is the ST:T ratio in V_6. A T-wave apex four times (or greater) higher than the height of the ST segment is more likely to indicate early repolarization; if this ratio is less than 4, pericarditis is more likely. In addition, pericarditis causes changes in the ECG that distinguish it from early repolarization. In stage II, typically occurring several days later, the ST segments return to baseline, and the initially upright T waves flatten. In stage III, the T waves invert, and the ST segments may become depressed—changes that may persist indefinitely. Finally, in stage IV, which may occur weeks or months later, the T waves revert to normal. All four stages can be serially identified in about 50% of patients.

2. Other tests—Laboratory evidence of inflammation, such as mild leukocytosis and a modestly elevated erythrocyte sedimentation rate, is common in viral or idiopathic pericarditis. These findings are less consistent in pericarditis associated with uremia or connective tissue disorders. Cardiac enzymes may be slightly elevated when the inflammatory process involves subepicardial myocardium. Although the chest x-ray film most often reveals no abnormalities in uncomplicated pericarditis, it may occasionally show evidence of pericardial effusion (discussed in the following section). As noted earlier, although echocardiography may reveal a pericardial effusion, the absence of an effusion does not exclude the diagnosis. Gallium scans of the heart may be positive.

Treatment

The management of pericarditis associated with a specific cause is addressed primarily to that underlying cause. In the usual case of idiopathic acute pericarditis, treatment with any of the nonsteroidal antiinflammatory agents usually suppresses the clinical manifestations within 24 h—and frequently more rapidly. When these measures fail to ameliorate symptoms, steroid therapy can be initiated, with a large dose of prednisone (eg, 60 mg/day) and tapered over a week or two. If symptoms recur as the dose is lowered, the minimum dose that will suppress the illness should be maintained for 1–2 months and then tapered and discontinued.

In the majority of patients, a single course of nonsteroidal antiinflammatory therapy will effectively control the illness, and the pericarditis will resolve without sequelae. In a minority, however, a recurrence may develop over a period of weeks or months after the initial episode. The recurrences can be managed with repeated courses of nonsteroidal or steroidal antiinflammatory agents. In difficult cases of recurrent pericarditis, immunosuppressive therapy may be useful and in particular may reduce the necessity for long-term steroid therapy. Colchicine has demonstrated efficacy in the prophylaxis of recurrent pericarditis and should be considered in these patients.

In rare cases, frequent and severe recurrences despite aggressive medical therapy have prompted pericardiectomy. Unfortunately, this procedure is usually ineffective, probably because of residual pericardial tissue or a shift of the inflammatory process to the pleura. Before considering pericardiectomy, it is advisable to confirm a thickened pericardium by echocardiography or magnetic resonance imaging.

Marinella MA: Electrocardiographic manifestations and differential diagnosis of acute pericarditis. Am Fam Physician 1998;57: 699.

Adler Y et al: Colchicine treatment for recurrent pericarditis: A decade of experience. Circulation 1998;97:2183.

PERICARDIAL EFFUSION

 ESSENTIALS OF DIAGNOSIS

- *Echocardiographic demonstration of pericardial fluid*

Table 17–1. Serial electrocardiographic changes in pericarditis.

Stage	ST Segment	T Waves
I	Elevated	Upright
II	Isoelectric	Upright → flat
III	Isoelectric	Inverted
IV	Isoelectric	Upright

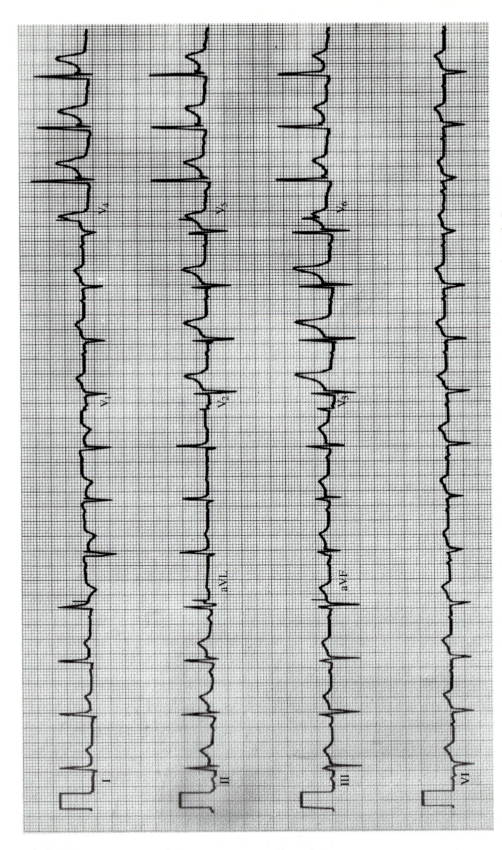

Figure 17–1. Electrocardiogram of the first stage of pericarditis demonstrating diffuse ST-segment elevation and upright T waves.

General Considerations

Pericardial effusion can develop as a result of pericarditis or an injury of any kind to the parietal pericardium. It can be encountered in the absence of pericarditis in many clinical settings, such as, uremia, cardiac trauma or chamber rupture, malignancy, AIDS, and hypothyroidism.

Clinical Findings

A. SYMPTOMS AND SIGNS

Clinical manifestations of pericardial effusion are directly related to the absolute volume of the effusion and the rapidity of accumulation. Small, incidental effusions rarely cause symptoms or complications, and patients with slowly developing pericardial effusions can accumulate large volumes of fluid without symptoms. With a slowly accumulating effusion, the pericardium can accommodate 1–2 L of fluid without a clinically significant elevation of intrapericardial pressure. Eventually, however, these large effusions are clinically manifested by compressing adjacent structures and causing dysphagia, cough, dyspnea, hiccups, hoarseness, nausea, or a sense of abdominal fullness. Rapid accumulation of even modest fluid volumes can be associated with increased intrapericardial pressures and life-threatening hemodynamic compromise.

B. PHYSICAL EXAMINATION

On examination, signs of pericardial effusion are absent in patients who have small effusions without increased pressure. Large effusions may muffle the heart sounds or cause left lower lobe lung dullness to percussion of the chest (Ewart's sign) as a result of the compression of lung parenchyma.

C. DIAGNOSTIC STUDIES

1. Electrocardiography—The ECG may be entirely normal. Large effusions can cause both reduced voltage and electrical alternans, alternating QRS voltage as a result of a swinging motion of the heart that characteristically occurs at a frequency of half the heart rate.

2. Chest radiography—An increase in the cardiac silhouette combined with clear or oligemic lung fields suggests the presence of a pericardial effusion, although the chest radiograph can appear entirely normal in the presence of a small effusion. Very rapidly accumulating fluid may result in only the subtlest of changes in the cardiac silhouette because of the restraining effect of the pericardium. With slowly accumulating fluid, the heart silhouette may assume a globular shape that has been likened to a water bottle. Radiographic differentiation of pericardial effusion and cardiac enlargement may not be possible. Occasionally, the presence of an effusion may cause increased separation of the pericardial fat-pad layers.

3. Echocardiography—Echocardiography is the fastest and most accurate means of diagnosing a pericardial effusion. The effusion appears as an echo-free space between the moving epicardium and the stationary pericardium. Although M-mode echocardiography can identify effusions as small as 20 mL, two-dimensional echocardiography has the advantage of demonstrating the full distribution of the effusion or identifying a loculated effusion. Note that quantification of the volume of effusion by echocardiography is not totally precise. Small effusions tend to be imaged only posteriorly; a posterior echo-free space, however, may reflect subepicardial fat rather than pericardial effusion. Larger effusions are distributed both anteriorly and posteriorly. On occasion, large effusions are associated with an excessive swinging motion of the heart within the fluid-filled pericardium.

Treatment

The management of a pericardial effusion is largely dictated by its size, the presence or absence of hemodynamic compromise from increased intrapericardial pressure (see next section), and the nature of the underlying disorder (discussed more specifically earlier). In most cases, a small or incidentally discovered effusion warrants no specific intervention. At the same time it should be recalled that once an effusion reaches a certain magnitude, even small additional amounts of fluid can cause a marked increase in intrapericardial pressure and rapid clinical deterioration; these patients must be monitored closely.

CARDIAC TAMPONADE

 ESSENTIALS OF DIAGNOSIS

- *Increased jugular venous pressure with an obliterated y descent*
- *Pulsus paradoxus*
- *Echocardiographic evidence of right atrial and ventricular collapse*
- *Equal diastolic pressures in all four cardiac chambers.*

General Considerations

Cardiac tamponade exists when increased intrapericardial pressure from the accumulation of fluid compromises the filling of the heart, thereby impairing cardiac output. Whether the intrapericardial pressure rises to a level that impedes filling depends on both the rapidity of accumulation and the volume of the effusion. Severe tamponade may thus ensue in the setting of a traumatic effusion where a modest volume of blood fills the pericardial space in a brief time. Conversely, in such settings as myxedema, a slowly accumulating effusion may reach a remarkably large volume without raising the intrapericardial pressure.

Clinical Findings

A. Symptoms and Signs

Patients with cardiac tamponade may complain of dyspnea and chest discomfort. In more severe cases, consciousness may be impaired, and there may be signs of reduced cardiac output; shock may also be present. The systemic arterial pressure is typically low, although it may be surprisingly well-preserved on occasion; pulse pressure is usually diminished. The patient with tamponade is typically tachycardic and tachypneic although bradycardia may ensue, especially in terminal stages.

1. Pulsus paradoxus—Pulsus paradoxus is present in most cases. (The term is actually something of a misnomer because the paradoxical pulse represents an exaggeration of the normal small decline in systolic arterial pressure that occurs during inspiration.) Pulsus paradoxus is evaluated through careful auscultation of the Korotkoff sounds as the cuff pressure is slowly released. It is measured as the difference in cuff pressure from the point at which sounds are initially heard intermittently during expiration and the point at which the sounds are audible throughout the respiratory cycle and with each ventricular systole. A pulsus paradoxus greater than 10 mm Hg is considered abnormal. In severe tamponade, the peripheral pulse reveals an obvious decrease in the stroke volume on inspiration. The presence of an abnormal pulsus paradoxus is not essential to the diagnosis of cardiac tamponade, however. It may be absent in such clinical situations as tamponade that coexists with severe atrial septal defect or aortic insufficiency. The absence of a pulsus paradoxus in these settings should not dissuade the physician from the correct diagnosis. In addition, pulsus paradoxus can be present when the inspiratory decrease in intrapleural pressure is exaggerated, such as in obstructive airway disease. Reversed pulsus paradoxus—a fall in pressure with expiration—can be seen in patients on positive pressure respirators.

2. Jugular venous pressure—This pressure is usually markedly elevated, and examination of the jugular venous pulse wave reveals obliteration of the normal *y* descent. In patients with low-pressure tamponade (see section 4, Cardiac catheterization), the venous pressure may actually be normal or only mildly elevated. Diminished heart sounds can be heard in one third of cases; a pericardial friction rub may be heard but is absent in the majority of patients. The concept of an inverse relation between the intensity of a pericardial rub (when present) and the size of the effusion cannot be used in assessing individual patients; this relationship is too variable to be reliable.

B. Diagnostic Studies

1. Electrocardiography—Electrocardiography may offer no specific diagnostic clues, although the ECG abnormalities described in pericarditis and pericardial effusion may be seen. The development of electrical alternans almost always indicates a hemodynamically significant effusion.

2. Chest radiography—Chest radiography offers no specific diagnostic signs of tamponade. As mentioned earlier, the cardiac silhouette may be remarkably normal in size in cases where a modestly sized effusion accumulates rapidly. A pericardial fat pad sign is diagnostic of pericardial effusion but does not necessarily indicate tamponade. The lung fields are frequently oligemic. Occasionally, the chest radiograph offers clues to important coexisting conditions, such as aortic dissection or malignancy.

3. Echocardiography—Echocardiography is an invaluable adjunctive tool. It confirms the presence of pericardial fluid and can provide evidence of increased intrapericardial pressure. The most useful echocardiographic sign is diastolic collapse of the right atrium and right ventricle. Though these changes are neither completely sensitive nor specific, they first occur when the pericardial pressure transiently exceeds the intracardiac chamber pressure. They can therefore be useful in identifying patients whose pericardial pressure level should be of concern. Echocardiography is extremely useful as a guide in pericardiocentesis.

4. Cardiac catheterization—In the patient with tamponade cardiac catheterization will reveal a depressed cardiac output and elevated equal or near-equal filling pressures in all four chambers. Examination of the atrial pressure waveforms reveals the loss of the normal *y* descent. The initial presentation and hemodynamic profile of tamponade may, however, be altered by a concomitant state of intravascular volume depletion, a scenario that has been called **low-pressure cardiac tamponade.** This term underscores an important feature of the pathophysiology of pericardial effusions; the hemodynamic effect is a function of both the intrapericardial pressure and the intravascular volume. Although this syndrome typically occurs in patients undergoing dialysis for chronic renal failure, it can be encountered in any setting of increased intrapericardial fluid and intravascular volume depletion. In these patients, the effusions are ordinarily insufficient to cause major hemodynamic embarrassment; they become significant when intravascular volume is depleted. The diagnosis should be considered in patients who become unusually hypotensive during dialysis. In some cases, volume expansion will result in more typical hemodynamic findings.

Treatment

Drainage of pericardial fluid is the cornerstone of therapy; reflecting the small pericardial reserve, draining even modest amounts (100–200 mL) of fluid may result in striking improvement. Drainage is most commonly achieved by subxiphoid percutaneous pericardiocentesis. Although the procedure is effective and safe, there may be complications; the most common serious complication is laceration or puncture of the heart, typically the right ventricle, because of its anterior location. Echocardiography, by confirming the presence of a sufficiently large volume of fluid in an anterior location, can decrease the risk of cardiac puncture. The presence of at least 1 cm of echo-free space anterior to the heart has been recommended as a guideline for the minimum volume of fluid that should be present before percutaneous pericardiocentesis is undertaken. In addition, the patient should be positioned in a semiupright position to allow inferior pooling of the effusion.

Several aspects of the performance of pericardiocentesis also contribute to a safe and successful outcome. The procedure is ideally carried out in the cardiac catheterization laboratory with fluoroscopic guidance and concomitant right-heart catheterization. The latter allows for hemodynamic confirmation of the diagnosis and assessment of the response to therapy. Occasionally, emergency pericardiocentesis may needed at the bedside; however, it is rare for circumstances to be so critical as to preclude confirming the diagnosis with echocardiography.

Intravenous fluids and pressors can be administered as temporizing measure until the procedure can be performed. These modalities usually will not significantly improve the clinical status, however, and should never be used in place of or allowed to interfere with prompt evacuation of the fluid.

Pericardial fluid can also be evacuated through a subxiphoid surgical pericardiotomy performed under local anesthesia; this procedure also permits pericardial biopsy in cases of suspected malignant effusion. The pericardial fluid should be sent for cultures and cytologic examination except when the tamponade is clearly traumatic. The gross appearance of the fluid is not helpful in establishing the cause, and cell counts and chemistries are also of limited value. The risks of pericardiocentesis must therefore be weighed against the

likely benefits before performing the procedure solely for diagnostic purposes. Usually a pericardial biopsy is most useful when the diagnosis is unclear.

In some cases, a single pericardiocentesis alleviates the effusion fully, but in most cases the physician should consider leaving a pericardial catheter in place for continued drainage. The catheter can be removed when the rate of drainage decreases and plans for definitive management of the pericardial disease are in place. Subsequent management is largely dictated by the specific cause of the effusion (discussed earlier).

Definitive management of pericardial fluid accumulation in some conditions may require surgical removal of the pericardium or the creation of an opening between the pericardium and left pleura. A percutaneous balloon technique for creating a pleuropericardial opening has recently been described. If tissue is not required for diagnostic purposes, this may be the preferred technique for draining a chronically recurring effusion and preventing tamponade. Pericardial windows can seal up in patients with intense inflammation, however, and pericardial stripping may be required.

Fowler NO: Cardiac tamponade: A clinical or an echocardiographic diagnosis? Circulation 1993;87:1738.

Tsang TS et al: Echocardiographically guided pericardiocentesis. Evolution and state-of-the-art technique. Mayo Clin Proc 1998;73:647.

CONSTRICTIVE PERICARDITIS

 ESSENTIALS OF DIAGNOSIS

- *Markedly elevated jugular venous pressure with accentuated x and y descents and Kussmaul's sign*
- *Pericardial knock on auscultation*
- *Magnetic resonance, computed tomography, or echocardiographic imaging showing a thickened pericardium*

General Considerations

Constrictive pericarditis can develop as the aftermath of virtually any pericardial injury or inflammation. Cardiac surgery, radiation therapy, and idiopathic causes are currently the most common. Tuberculous constriction, a leading cause in previous decades, is now rare in most of the industrialized world, but it remains significant in underdeveloped countries and may reappear in developed countries if tuberculosis continues to increase. A highly variable length of time—sometimes many years—can elapse between the initial insult and the development of constriction and its clinical manifestations.

The major physiologic perturbation of constrictive pericarditis is thickening, fibrosis, and (especially with tuberculosis) calcification of the pericardium, causing it to encase the heart in a solid, noncompliant envelope that impairs diastolic filling. In early diastole, the ventricles fill normally until the volume limit of the noncompliant pericardium is attained. At that point, diastolic filling halts abruptly. At the same time, the rigid pericardium markedly increases the intracardiac filling pressures. Because contractile function is usually normal, constrictive pericarditis can be considered an example of heart failure that is caused by diastolic dysfunction.

Clinical Findings

A. SYMPTOMS AND SIGNS

Many symptoms of constrictive pericarditis are nonspecific and are related to chronically elevated cardiac filling pressures and chronically depressed cardiac output; symptoms secondary to venous congestion are most common. Patients usually develop ascites, peripheral edema, and symptoms referable to congestion of the gastrointestinal tract and liver: dyspepsia, anorexia, and postprandial fullness. Cardiac cirrhosis may be present in extreme cases. Symptoms of left-sided congestion, such as exertional dyspnea, orthopnea, and cough, may occur but are much less frequent. The chronically low cardiac output results in fatigue and, in conjunction with the effects of visceral congestion, wasting.

B. PHYSICAL EXAMINATION

The patient may have a striking body habitus with a marked contrast between a massively swollen abdomen and edematous lower extremities and a cachectic, wasted upper torso. Ascites, hepatomegaly with prominent hepatic pulsations, and other signs of hepatic failure are common.

Patients with constrictive pericarditis have marked distention of the jugular vein; the x and y descents are prominent, typically resulting in an M or W shape of the venous waves. Kussmaul's sign—the loss of normal inspiratory decrease in the jugular venous pressure or even a frank increase with inspiration—may be present. (Kussmaul's sign may be seen in other disorders, however, including restrictive cardiomyopathy.) The arterial pulse pressure may be diminished or normal. A pulsus paradoxus is present in perhaps one third of cases.

Auscultation of the heart can reveal a characteristic early diastolic sound, the pericardial knock. The knock occurs slightly earlier in diastole than a third heart sound and has a higher acoustic frequency.

C. DIAGNOSTIC STUDIES

1. Electrocardiography—Characteristic electrocardiographic abnormalities in constrictive pericarditis are low voltage, T-wave inversions, and P mitrale or atrial fibrillation. Atrioventricular and intraventricular conduction delays or the development of Q waves are related to the extension of calcification into the myocardium and surrounding the coronary arteries.

2. Chest radiograph—The cardiac silhouette on chest radiograph can be small, normal, or enlarged. The presence of pericardial calcification is helpful in confirming the diagnosis and suggests tuberculosis as the cause. However, only a minority of patients with constriction have pericardial calcification. Conversely, a calcified pericardium does not always indicate constriction.

3. Echocardiography—Echocardiography can demonstrate pericardial thickening in most cases of constriction. As with chest radiography, however, the presence or absence of echocardiographic pericardial thickening neither establishes or excludes the diagnosis with any certainty. Pericardial imaging with echocardiography can also be misleading. Echocardiography may be useful in first raising the suspicion of constrictive pericarditis in a patient with heart failure, preserved left ventricular systolic function, and normal cardiac chamber sizes. Left ventricular function may be impaired in constriction, however, and preserved systolic function is therefore not a prerequisite for diagnosis. A variety of indices using Doppler echocardiography to assess ventricular filling in various stages of diastole have been proposed to distinguish between constrictive pericarditis and restrictive cardiomyopathy. Those that appear most useful are exaggerated respiratory variations of transmitral and hepatic vein flow and isovolumetric relaxation time. Both of these are present in constriction but absent in restrictive cardiomyopathy. It should be understood, however, that these indices have been tested in only small numbers of patients.

4. Cardiac catheterization—Cardiac catheterization can help establish the correct diagnosis. It confirms elevated—and usually virtually equal—diastolic pressures in both ventricles. The diastolic pressure waveform has been described as a square root sign, or dip and plateau: a prominent downward deflection followed by a rapid early pressure rise and plateau in the diastolic pressure. This waveform, however, is not pathognomonic for constriction; it can also be found in restrictive cardiomyopathy. Examination of the right and left atrial waveforms reveals prominent x and y descents. As with jugular venous pressures, the appearance of the atrial pressure recording has been likened to a W or an M shape. Several hemodynamic criteria are useful in distinguishing constrictive pericarditis from restrictive cardiomyopathy (Table 17–2). Although the accuracy of any one of these

Table 17–2. Hemodynamic criteria differentiating constrictive pericarditis from restrictive cardiomyopathy.

Criteria Favoring Constriction	Predictive Accuracy (%)
Difference between LVEDP and RVEDP <5 mm Hg	85
RV systolic pressure >50 mm Hg	70
RVEDP:RV systolic pressure ratio >0.33	76

LVEDP = left-ventricular end-diastolic pressure; REVDP = right ventricular end-diastolic pressure; RV = right ventricle.

criteria is far from perfect, the concordance of all three criteria favoring constriction renders the diagnosis 91% certain. Similarly, if none or only one hemodynamic criterion in favor of constriction is met, the patient has *restriction* with 94% certainty. One fourth of patients with the appropriate physiology will meet two criteria, making their chances of either diagnosis approximately equal.

5. Endomyocardial biopsy—At the time of cardiac catheterization endomyocardial biopsy can be performed to search of evidence of infiltrative cardiomyopathy. The finding of amyloidosis, sarcoidosis, or hemochromatosis precludes the need for further investigation. The finding of myocarditis, however, is not specific, and further studies may be needed.

6. Other tests—Radionuclide ventriculography may be useful in evaluating left ventricular diastolic filling. Time–activity curves can demonstrate normal filling in early diastole in constrictive pericarditis. Computed tomography (CT) and magnetic resonance imaging (MRI) are more accurate than echocardiography for direct imaging of the pericardium. Accurate measurements of pericardial thickening can be made with either technique and can be extremely helpful in both diagnosing constrictive pericarditis and distinguishing it from restrictive cardiomyopathy.

Differential Diagnosis

With the combined use of Doppler echocardiography, MRI or CT to image the pericardium, careful hemodynamic studies, and endomyocardial biopsy, it should be possible in the great majority of cases to distinguish constrictive pericarditis from restrictive cardiomyopathy. This distinction is not always possible, however, and such differentiation can sometimes be a major diagnostic challenge. Restrictive cardiomyopathy is a condition that is most commonly caused by infiltrative diseases of the myocardium such as amyloidosis, sarcoidosis, and hemochromatosis—or, in Africa, by endocardial fibroelastosis. Both constrictive pericarditis and restrictive cardiomyopathy are characterized by impaired diastolic filling of the ventricles. The two differ, however, in the degree of impairment of various phases of diastole. Unlike the rapid early diastolic filling and abrupt halt of constrictive pericarditis, ventricular filling in restrictive cardiomyopathy is impaired uniformly throughout diastole. This physiologic difference underlies many of the features that help to distinguish the two diagnoses. The correct differentiation of these two conditions is of paramount importance: Constrictive pericarditis is an eminently treatable disease; cardiac restriction of almost any cause carries a limited prognosis—despite therapy. When the distinction between constriction and restriction remains ambiguous, it may be necessary to proceed to thoracoscopy to permit direct inspection of the pericardium.

Constrictive pericarditis is sometimes virtually indistinguishable from congestive heart failure at the bedside. Disproportionate right-sided failure or ascites out of proportion to peripheral edema may be clues to the presence of constriction. Because of the relative rarity of constriction, it is often not suspected, and congestive heart failure or even noncardiac cirrhosis is diagnosed instead. Because the primary form of therapy for constriction is surgical, it is essential to be sure that the diagnosis of constriction is correct.

Treatment

Although intensive medical management may effectively control symptoms, the long-term prognosis with medical therapy alone is limited: The natural history in most cases is one of advancing severity.

Pericardiectomy is the definitive treatment for constrictive pericarditis. In most cases the procedure is straightforward, and the surgical mortality rate in recent series has ranged from 4 to 11%. Occasionally, however, the dense fibrosis and calcification extend into the epicardium, making identification of a cleavage plane impossible. The operation in this case is associated with excessive hemorrhage and an inability to relieve the compression completely. In other patients, hepatic or cardiac failure may be irreversible. The myocardium may undergo atrophy as a result of long-standing compression, and a low-cardiac-output state may persist after pericardiectomy.

In most cases patients will exhibit dramatic and sustained improvement, although full improvement may occur only after several months. When symptoms are persistent or recurrent, three possibilities need to be considered: myocardial dysfunction resulting from severe, prolonged compression; incomplete or inadequate pericardiectomy; and recurrence of the constriction. In some cases, the inflammatory and fibrotic process involves the epicardial layers and progresses after the pericardium has been removed, leading to a recurrence of constrictive physiology and symptomatology.

The combination of constrictive pericarditis and occlusive coronary artery disease is especially difficult to manage. In some cases, the coronary lesions are due to the visceral pericardial process, and stripping the pericardium may damage the coronary arteries. Bypass surgery can be extremely difficult in the presence of the dense calcium. If the coronary obstructions are not corrected, however, the increased myocardial oxygen demands of increased cardiac filling following the pericardiectomy may cause postoperative ischemia or infarction—which may severely complicate recovery from the surgery.

Mehta A et al: Constrictive pericarditis. Clin Cardiol 1999;22:334.

EFFUSIVE-CONSTRICTIVE PERICARDITIS

ESSENTIALS OF DIAGNOSIS

- *Echocardiographic demonstration of pericardial fluid*
- *Persistance of elevated intracardiac filling pressures following pericardiocentesis*

Effusive-constrictive pericarditis combines features of pericardial effusion and constrictive pericarditis. The syndrome is dynamic and may represent an intermediate stage in the development of constrictive pericarditis. The most frequent cause of effusive-constrictive pericarditis is uremia, but any cause of pericarditis can produce this condition. Echocardiography usually shows a small-to-moderate-sized effusion with strands of solid material between the visceral and parietal pericardium. Although effusive-constrictive pericarditis may be suspected on clinical grounds, the diagnosis is established through cardiac catheterization and characterization of the hemodynamics. Effusive-constrictive pericarditis can present as frank tamponade. As the effusion is drained during pericardiocentesis, elevation of intracardiac filling pressures persists and the recorded waveforms may exhibit the classic appearance of constriction.

Although pericardiocentesis may be associated with an improved cardiac output and diminished symptoms, subsequent management is essentially that for pericardial constriction. Thoracotomy with pericardiectomy is indicated to relieve the constriction in symptomatic patients.

Hancock EW: Subacute effusive constrictive pericarditis. Circulation 1971;43:1983.

Congestive Heart Failure

18

Enrique V. Carbajal, MD & Prakash C. Deedwania, MD

ESSENTIALS OF DIAGNOSIS

- *Orthopnea, paroxysmal nocturnal dyspnea, dyspnea at rest and during exertion*
- *Jugular vein distention, peripheral pitting edema, sinus tachycardia, basal rales or coarse bubbling rales throughout both lung fields, cardiomegaly, S_3 gallop sound, liver enlargement*
- *Left ventricular systolic or diastolic dysfunction*

General Considerations

Congestive heart failure (CHF) is a complex clinical syndrome characterized by dysfunction of the left, right, or both ventricles and changes in neurohumoral regulation. This syndrome is accompanied by effort intolerance, fluid retention, and shortened survival. It is often a terminal stage of heart disease, occurring after all reserve capacity and compensatory mechanisms of the myocardium and peripheral circulation have been exhausted. Initially, the syndrome was described as a state of fluid overload with congestion of the lungs caused by a failing heart. It is, however, now well recognized that in many patients the predominant symptom may be a reduction of functional capacity because of poor exercise tolerance associated with limited cardiac reserve.

Heart failure results from myocardial dysfunction that impairs the heart's ability to circulate blood at a rate sufficient to maintain the metabolic needs of peripheral tissues and various organs. It follows myocardial damage when the compensatory hemodynamic and neurohumoral mechanisms are overwhelmed or exhausted and results from the loss of a critical amount of functioning myocardium due to acute myocardial infarction (MI), prolonged cardiovascular stress (hypertension, valvular disease), toxins (eg, alcohol abuse), or infection; in some cases, there is no apparent cause (idiopathic cardiomyopathy).

Several complex interactions between myocardial and nonmyocardial compensatory events follow the initial cardiac damage, together giving rise to a clinical syndrome characterized by cardiac hypertrophy, cavitary dilatation, elevated intracardiac pressures, reduced cardiac output, and diminished functional reserve. Fundamental alterations in performance of the myocardial contractile elements ultimately result in a decline in systolic function, an increase in diastolic pressures and ventricular dimensions, and a continuous remodeling of the myocardial architecture in an attempt to compensate for the deteriorating systolic function (Table 18–1). These changes indirectly contribute to a progressively worsening clinical course. Coincident with this primary myocardial process is the activation of a number of neurohumoral (renin-angiotensin, sympathoadrenal, atrial natriuretic peptide) systems responsible for fluid retention, peripheral edema, and an increase in peripheral resistance. All these changes lead to further depression of cardiac function, reduced cardiac output, and impairment of peripheral circulation and tissue perfusion.

Heart failure is a relatively common clinical disorder, estimated to affect more than 2 million patients in the United States. About 400,000 new patients develop CHF each year. Morbidity and mortality rates are high; annually, approximately 900,000 patients require hospitalization for CHF, and up to 200,000 patients die from this condition. The average annual mortality rate is 40–50% in patients with severe (New York Heart Association [NYHA] class IV) heart failure.

Table 18–1. Sequence of events during hemodynamic adaptations in heart failure.

Increase in
Ventricular end-diastolic volume and pressure
Atrial volume and pressure
Atrial and ventricular contractility (Starling's law)
Volume and pressure in adjacent venous system
Capillary pressure and secondary transudation of fluid
Interstitial and extracellular fluid volume
Lymphatic flow from interstitial spaces

Approximately one third to one half of the deaths in patients with CHF are secondary to the progression of cardiac insufficiency and its associated conditions. The remainder of the patients with CHF die from sudden cardiac death, presumably related to electrical instability and ventricular arrhythmias, other cardiovascular conditions, as well as from noncardiovascular causes.

Data describing the natural history of CHF are limited because this condition has not been extensively studied in a prospective manner. The Framingham heart study showed that men who developed clinical symptoms of CHF had a 62% probability of dying within 5 years of the onset of symptoms. Subsequent studies in patients with dilated or congestive cardiomyopathy indicate that heart failure is a progressively deteriorating condition, with 20–40% of patients dying within 5 years after the onset of illness; other studies show that patients with advanced congestive heart failure (NYHA IV) have a 40–50% annual mortality rate.

Pathophysiology & Etiology

When an excessive workload is imposed on the heart by increased systolic blood pressure (pressure overload), increased diastolic volume (volume overload), or loss of myocardium, normal myocardial cells hypertrophy in an effort to enhance contractile force of the normal areas. The subsequent alterations in biochemistry, electrophysiology, and contractile function lead to mechanical alterations of myocardial function: The rate of contraction slows, the time to develop peak tension increases, and myocardial relaxation is delayed. Peak force development may be well preserved with enough viable myocardium and adequate time for the development of force. Thickening of the ventricular wall limits the rate of ventricular filling (diastolic dysfunction), which is worsened by increased heart rate because it shortens the duration of ventricular filling. The force of myocardial contraction is eventually reduced as cell loss and hypertrophy continue, leading to significant geometric ventricular alterations and increased volumes.

After the initial compensatory phase, the increase in intracavitary volume is usually associated with further reductions in ventricular ejection fraction (progressive systolic dysfunction) and—eventually—abnormalities in the peripheral circulation from activation of various neurohumoral compensatory mechanisms.

The ensuing CHF is characterized by a reduced contraction response to increase in volume (flattened Frank-Starling curve) and a reduced left ventricular ejection fraction (LVEF). The abnormal neurohumoral responses lead to increased systemic sympathetic tone and activation of the renin-angiotensin system. Production of angiotensin increases, causing peripheral vasoconstriction. The increase in peripheral arterial resistance limits cardiac output during exercise. The increased

levels of angiotensin II also stimulate release of aldosterone by the adrenal glands, enhancing sodium retention and thus leading to fluid retention and peripheral edema.

Myocardial (pump) failure and CHF are not necessarily closely related in time. Patients are often initially asymptomatic, with the signs and symptoms of CHF developing only after several months of myocardial failure and decreased ejection fraction. Cardiac output does not increase adequately during exercise, but it can be normal at rest during this period. Although patients may be asymptomatic or slightly symptomatic at rest, with the ejection fraction unchanged, alterations in peripheral vasculature occur with slowly rising peripheral resistance during exercise. Exercise performance slowly becomes limited because the peripheral vasculature cannot meet the increased metabolic needs of exercising skeletal muscles.

Although the precise mechanism by which hemodynamic responses and neurohumoral factors interact to cause progressive clinical deterioration in CHF is unknown, the hemodynamic and neurohumoral abnormalities that increase cardiac wall stress can lead to cell slippage, morphologic myocardial cell changes, and structural remodeling of the heart. The dilatation of the ventricular cavity and change in its shape can eventually lead to mitral regurgitation. The increase in cardiac pressures and volume may also trigger myocardial ischemia, especially in patients with underlying coronary artery disease (CAD).

The myocardial hypertrophy can enhance cardiac metabolic demands and may increase the risk of ischemia in patients with CAD. In addition, prolonged activation of neurohumoral axes may be deleterious to the heart in an independent manner: High concentrations of norepinephrine and angiotensin II can exert direct toxic effects on myocardial cells. The heightened activity of the sympathetic nervous and renin-angiotensin systems can have adverse electrophysiologic effects and may induce lethal cardiac arrhythmias—particularly in patients with electrolyte imbalances.

A. TYPES OF HEART FAILURE

1. Chronic and acute heart failure—The manifestations of heart failure depend on the rate at which the syndrome develops and whether sufficient time has elapsed for fluid to accumulate in the interstitial spaces. Generally, if the underlying cardiac abnormality develops slowly, compensatory mechanisms have time to become activated, and the patient will be able to adjust to the altered cardiac output. If the underlying condition develops rapidly or an acute precipitating factor is present, the result may be inadequate organ perfusion or acute congestion of the venous bed draining into the affected ventricle, causing sudden cardiac decompensation, with a concomitant reduction in cardiac output and an acute onset of symptoms.

In chronic heart failure, adaptive mechanisms are gradually activated and cardiac hypertrophy develops. These changes allow the patient to adjust to and tolerate a reduction in cardiac output with less difficulty. When the onset of left-heart failure is gradual, the right heart develops higher pressures in response to higher pulmonary resistance; the acute onset of similar increases in pulmonary resistance may produce acute right-heart failure. A patient with chronic heart failure may achieve compensation but then experience acute decompensation as a result of a precipitating condition (Table 18–2).

2. Left- and right-sided heart failure—Heart failure is more often limited to one side when the onset is abrupt (eg, in acute MI). The venous reservoir capacity is smaller on the left than is the systemic venous system on the right, and increased venous pressures and associated symptoms occur after a relatively smaller accumulation of fluid on the left.

Although the disease process may involve only one ventricle initially, biventricular failure usually follows, especially when the left ventricle is the site of initial damage. Both ventricles have a common interventricular septum, and biochemical changes are not confined to the stressed ventricle but involve the opposite ventricle as well. In addition, because all four cardiac chambers are enclosed in the pericardial sac, when the size of any chamber suddenly increases the opposite chambers are compressed, and the filling pressure of the normal ventricle rises (this is usually defined as ventricular interdependence). Right-sided failure often follows left-heart failure, but left-heart failure rarely follows isolated right-heart failure (eg, atrial septal defect, cor pulmonale) without a concomitant separate abnormality of the left heart (eg, CAD with ischemia or infarction). In patients with left ventricular (LV) failure, subsequent right-heart failure may relieve the respiratory symptoms (exertional dyspnea, orthopnea, nocturnal dyspnea) generally associated with left-heart failure.

3. High-output and low-output heart failure—Most cases of heart failure are associated with a low-output state that causes changes in the peripheral circulation (vasoconstriction), including cold, clammy, and pale extremities; oliguria; low pulse pressure; and an associated widened arterial-mixed venous oxygen difference. High-output heart failure, which is less common, is usually associated with a hyperkinetic circulatory state (anemia, thyrotoxicosis, pregnancy, Paget's bone disease, arteriovenous fistula). These states usually trigger heart failure when superimposed on underlying heart disease. Unlike the vasoconstriction seen in the low-output state, high-output failure is associated with vasodilatation; the patient exhibits a warm and flushed skin and a bounding pulse. The arterial-mixed venous oxygen difference is normal or decreased but usually exceeds the level encountered in patients with low-output heart failure. Although the cardiac index is usually higher than normal (>4 L/min/m^2), it is generally lower than before the onset of heart failure and is obviously insufficient to meet the increased oxygen demands.

4. Backward and forward heart failure—Increased pressure in the system draining into one or both ventricles (backward failure), inadequate cardiac output in a forward direction (forward failure), or both conditions account for the clinical manifestations of heart failure. An important tenet of the backward failure theory is the development of right-heart failure as a consequence of LV failure. The elevation of LV diastolic, left atrial, and pulmonary venous pressures causes backward transmission of pressure and leads to pulmonary hypertension that ultimately causes right ventricular failure and increasing systemic venous pressure. In addition to venous congestion of organs, backward heart failure can cause decreased cardiac output with inadequate organ perfusion (forward failure). Forward failure may account for many of the clinical manifestations of heart failure, such as mental confusion from decreased cerebral perfusion, fatigue and weakness from decreased skeletal muscle perfusion, and sodium and water retention with secondary venous congestion from decreased renal perfusion. The retention of sodium and water, in turn, augments extracellular fluid volume and ultimately leads to congestive symptoms of heart failure that are secondary to accumulation of fluid in various organs and peripheral tissues.

Table 18–2. Common precipitating factors in heart failure.

Lack of compliance (diet, drugs)
Uncontrolled hypertension
Myocardial infarction and ischemia
Cardiac arrhythmias
   Multifocal atrial tachycardia
   Atrial fibrillation, flutter
   Ventricular tachycardia
Fluid overload
Pulmonary embolism
Pulmonary infection
Systemic infection
Endocrine abnormalities
Environmental factors
Inadequate therapy
Emotional stress
Blood loss, anemia

The mechanisms that lead to both forward and backward failure operate in the majority of patients with chronic heart failure. Based on the underlying pathophysiologic process, hemodynamic abnormalities, and abruptness of disease process (eg, acute MI, acute pulmonary embolism), however, one or the other may initially be predominant. Early in the process of heart failure, cardiac output may be normal at rest. During stress, such as physical exercise and other periods of increased metabolic demand, however, the cardiac output fails to rise normally, the glomerular filtration rate declines, and the renal mechanism for salt and water retention becomes activated. Ventricular filling pressure as well as pressures in the atrium and venous system behind the affected ventricle may rise abnormally during periods of stress. This may cause transudation of fluid and symptoms of tissue congestion during exercise. In such early stages, physical rest may induce diuresis and relieve symptoms in many patients with mild heart failure; excessive and repeated strenuous physical activities will worsen the compromised hemodynamic state and cause progression of heart failure.

5. Diastolic and systolic heart failure—The symptoms and signs of heart failure can be caused by either an abnormality in systolic function that leads to a defect in the ejection of blood from the heart (systolic heart failure) or an abnormality in myocardial diastolic function that leads to a defect in ventricular filling (diastolic heart failure). Reduced LV filling caused by diastolic dysfunction leads to decreased stroke volume and associated symptoms of low cardiac output, whereas increased filling pressures lead to symptoms of pulmonary congestion. Thus, some characteristics of heart failure (eg, the inability of the left ventricle to provide adequate forward output to meet the demands of the skeletal muscles during exercise while maintaining normal filling pressures) may result primarily from diastolic dysfunction, which, in some patients, can occur with normal LV systolic function. There are no exact data on the prevalence of diastolic dysfunction leading to heart failure in the presence of normal systolic function. Several studies have shown, however, that as many as 40% of all patients with a clinical diagnosis of heart failure may have preserved LV systolic function, and many of these patients have evidence of diastolic dysfunction. Several factors can predispose to an increased risk of diastolic dysfunction in the presence of normal LV systolic function (Table 18–3).

The principal clinical manifestations of systolic failure result from inadequate forward cardiac output; the major consequences of diastolic failure relate to elevation of the ventricular filling pressure and the high venous pressure upstream to the ventricle, causing pulmonic or systemic venous congestion or both. Systolic failure is caused by the chronic contractile dysfunction

Table 18–3. Factors associated with left ventricular diastolic dysfunction.

Coronary artery disease
  Myocardial ischemia
  Scarring and hypertrophy secondary to myocardial infection
Left ventricular hypertrophy
Dilated cardiomyopathy
Volume overload
Elevated afterload
Myocardial fibrosis
Restriction to filling
  Constrictive pericarditis
  Obliterative cardiomyopathy
  Myocardial infiltrative diseases (eg, amyloidosis)

secondary to myocardial necrosis from previous infarction and by the acute depression of myocardial contractility encountered during a transient episode of myocardial ischemia. On the other hand, diastolic failure in patients with CAD is primarily due to reduced ventricular compliance and increased stiffness caused by replacement of normal, distensible myocardium with nondistensible fibrous scar tissue (eg, at the area of MI) as well as by the acute reduction in diastolic relaxation of normal myocardium during episodes of transient myocardial ischemia. Heart failure in patients with CAD is often the result of combined systolic and diastolic dysfunction.

B. Causes

The most common causes of CHF in the United States are CAD, systemic hypertension, nonischemic dilated cardiomyopathy, and valvular heart disease. Other frequent causes are myocarditis and diabetes mellitus, but there are a great many less common causes (Table 18–4). Although diabetes can predispose to CHF, the risk for CHF most commonly appears to result from some form of diabetic cardiomyopathy, particularly in insulin-dependent diabetics. Recent data suggest that the increased (twofold to tenfold) risk for CHF in diabetes patients is independent of associated CAD or hypertension and appears to be highest among women.

Many patients with heart failure have identifiable precipitating factors (see Table 18–2). The most common cause of cardiac decompensation in heart failure patients appears to be insufficient attention to the prescribed treatment regimen, eg, inadequate restriction of sodium, excessive physical activity, and noncompliance with prescribed drug therapy. Cardiac arrhythmias, including atrial or ventricular tachyarrhythmias with or without associated CAD, are common in patients with

Table 18–4. Causes of cardiac failure.

Mechanical abnormalities	**Myocardial disease** *(continued)*
Pressure overload	Metals
Aortic stenosis	Iron overload
Arterial hypertension	Primary (hemochromatosis)
Pulmonary hypertension	Secondary (chronic transfusion)
Coarctation of the aorta	Lead poisoning
Pulmonary stenosis	Cobalt poisoning
Volume overload	Acute rheumatic fever
Valvular regurgitation	Infectious
Anemia	Bacterial (staphylococcal or streptococcal infections)
Thyrotoxicosis	Viral (Coxsackie, echo, polio, and arbo; mumps and rabies;
Shunts (arteriovenous fistulas, patent ductus arteriosus,	varicella and variola; influenza, cytomegalovirus)
atrial septal and ventricular septal defect)	Parasitic (trichinosis, Chagas' disease, schistosomiasis)
Impaired ventricular filling (mitral stenosis)	Mycotic (candidiasis, histoplasmosis, toxoplasmosis)
Pericardial constriction or tamponade	Rickettsial (Q fever, typhus, scrub, psittacosis)
Ventricular dilatation/aneurysm	Connective tissue diseases
Restriction of ventricular filling	Rheumatoid arthritis
Mitral stenosis	Systemic lupus erythematosus
Constrictive pericarditis	Polyarteritis nodosa
Left ventricular hypertrophy	Scleroderma
Endomyocardial fibrosis	Dermatomyositis
Myocardial disease	Neurologic diseases
Primary	Myotonic dystrophy
Hypertrophic cardiomyopathy	Erb's limb-girdle muscular dystrophy
Restrictive cardiomyopathy	Duchenne's muscular dystrophy
Idiopathic dilated cardiomyopathy (familial, nonfamilial,	Roussy-Lévy polyneuropathy
peripartum)	Friedreich's ataxia
Secondary	Inherited diseases
Coronary artery disease	Glycogen storage disease
Myocardial infarction	Mucopolysaccharidoses
Chronic myocardial ischemia	Systemic carnitine deficiency
Silent ischemia	Hypertaurinuria
Metabolic	Fabry's disease
Alcoholic cardiomyopathy	Osteogenesis imperfecta
Nutritional	Other diseases
Thyroid disorders	Amyloid disease
Hypocalcemia	Endomyocardial fibrosis
Pheochromocytoma	Acute and chronic leukemia
Drugs	Uremic cardiomyopathy
Disopyramide/flecanaide	Henoch-Schönlein purpura
Amphetamine	Wegener's granulomatosis
Anthracyclines (doxorubicin)	Irradiation to heart
Heroin/cocaine	

heart failure and can also precipitate or intensify the signs and symptoms of CHF. Profound and inappropriate bradycardia in the presence of decreased cardiac output and atrioventricular (AV) dissociation in patients with complete AV block can also precipitate CHF because the ventricular rate is insufficient to maintain cardiac output in an already compromised heart. Acute infections, especially pneumonia, bronchitis, or other pulmonary infections, can also precipitate

heart failure. Patients with heart failure are also at increased risk of pulmonary emboli, especially when confined to bed. Other precipitating factors include physical and emotional stress, cardiac inflammation, unrelated illnesses (especially hepatorenal disorders), cardiac depressants (alcohol and other toxins), sodium-retaining drugs (nonsteroidal antiinflammatory drugs), recurrent myocardial ischemia, and progressive worsening of the underlying cardiac disorder itself.

Bonow RO, Udelson JE: Left ventricular diastolic dysfunction as a cause of congestive heart failure. Ann Intern Med 1992;117:502.

Braunwald E: The pathogenesis of heart failure: Then and now. Medicine 1991;70:68.

Grossman W: Diastolic dysfunction in congestive heart failure. N Engl J Med 1991;325:1557.

Packer M: Pathophysiology of chronic heart failure. Lancet 1992;340:88.

Clinical Findings

A. SYMPTOMS AND SIGNS

1. Shortness of breath—Dyspnea, or breathlessness (a subjective feeling of air hunger), is the earliest and most frequent symptom in CHF. Initially, dyspnea on exertion will be noted by a change in the extent of physical activity that causes shortness of breath. As heart failure worsens, the intensity of exertion required will decrease. The patient with heart failure will progressively develop paroxysmal nocturnal dyspnea, orthopnea, and eventually dyspnea at rest.

The severity of dyspnea becomes less prominent in LV failure after the patient develops right ventricular failure. In general, dyspnea is less prominent in right ventricular failure because pulmonary congestion is not present. Even patients with predominantly right ventricular failure can develop severe dyspnea when the failure advances, however. This is presumably a consequence of the reduced cardiac output and poor perfusion of respiratory muscles and associated hypoxia, leading to metabolic acidosis.

Paroxysmal nocturnal dyspnea (PND) occurs after the patient has been asleep and in the supine position for some time. Suddenly, the patient wakes up with a sensation of choking and air hunger; assuming an upright posture usually relieves the symptoms. Frequently the patient will feel better after opening a window or going outside to catch a breath of fresh air. Paroxysmal nocturnal dyspnea usually precedes orthopnea; it may be associated with bronchospasm and wheezing (cardiac asthma) and can be confused with an attack of bronchial asthma, especially in patients with prior known chronic obstructive pulmonary disease (COPD). Many patients with heart failure also have COPD; it may be difficult to distinguish between the dyspneic symptoms secondary to heart failure and those that are due to COPD (this is discussed later in more detail). Most severe episodes of PND can cause a feeling of intense suffocation and may leave the patient gasping for breath. The uncomfortable sensation may persist for 30 min or more after the patient has assumed an upright posture. Paroxysmal nocturnal dyspnea is primarily caused by mobilization of interstitial fluid (especially in patients with edema) from infrathoracic locations during recumbency. The result is increased circulating blood volume and increased pulmonary venous pressure, especially in patients with LV diastolic dysfunction.

Orthopnea is defined as dyspnea that occurs—often within a few minutes—when the patient assumes a supine position; sitting up or standing usually improves the symptoms. The most severely affected patients usually sleep upright in a chair. Orthopnea has the same cause as PND, but it represents more severe cardiac impairment.

A **dry or nonproductive cough,** rather than orthopnea, nocturnal dyspnea, or exertional dyspnea, may occasionally occur. This is due to pulmonary congestion and in patients with heart failure is usually relieved by successful treatment of the heart failure. Certain drugs used to treat heart failure can also cause cough [see section on Pharmacologic treatment, ACEI (angiotensin-converting enzyme inhibitor) safety].

2. Fatigue and weakness—Other common symptoms of heart failure include fatigue and generalized weakness, particularly in the limbs. These symptoms are secondary to low cardiac output with decreased perfusion of skeletal muscles and can occur with exertion or at rest; they may be worsened after eating because of the increased splanchnic demand for blood flow, which may stress the limited reserve. Low-output syndromes can be present, without evidence of pulmonary congestion, and limit performance during exercise testing. Extreme thirst, an often-overlooked symptom, is associated with activation of the arginine-vasopressin system and hyponatremia in patients with heart failure.

3. Nocturia and oliguria—Nocturia is a common and early symptom in heart failure. Renal filtration of sodium and water is decreased in patients with compromised LV function, in part, because of the redistribution of blood flow away from the kidneys in the upright position and during physical activity. Urine formation is enhanced in the recumbent position when renal stimulus for vasoconstriction decreases and venous return to the heart increases. Oliguria is associated with a markedly reduced cardiac output and is usually a sign of terminal heart failure; it indicates a poor prognosis.

4. Cerebral symptoms—Elderly patients with advanced heart failure may develop confusion, memory impairment, anxiety, headaches, insomnia, nightmares, and, occasionally, disorientation, delirium, and hallucinations. These cerebral symptoms are predominantly related to reduced cardiac output and poor perfusion of brain and other neurologic tissues.

5. Abdominal symptoms—Patients with heart failure may also develop gastrointestinal complaints because of hepatic congestion and edema of the abdominal wall and intraabdominal organs. Congestion of abdominal organs may be present with ascites, abdominal fullness and enlargement, easy satiety, bloating, anorexia, nausea, vomiting, constipation, and upper abdominal discomfort. The abdominal discomfort is usually described as a dull ache or heaviness that can be enhanced or reproduced by upper abdominal or hepatic palpation. This is consistent with the likely cause, the stretching of the hepatic capsule. Patients can frequently detect early reaccumulation of fluid by the recurrence of abdominal fullness before the signs become obvious. This symptom can be easily overlooked, however. Asking the patient about a recent change in waist size or a tightening of the clothing at the waist is often helpful.

B. PHYSICAL EXAMINATION

In general, patients with heart failure of recent onset appear acutely ill but well nourished. Patients with chronic heart failure, on the other hand, frequently appear malnourished, and occasionally cachectic. This appearance arises from anorexia that is secondary to hepatic and intestinal congestion or sometimes to drug therapy (digitalis) and may be, in part, caused by reasons that are unclear. Rarely, patients may experience impaired absorption of fat and, in some cases, a protein-losing enteropathy. Patients may have increased body metabolism from increased myocardial oxygen consumption, excessive work of breathing, or elevated levels of circulating catecholamines and other neurohormones. The combination of reduced caloric intake and increased energy expenditure can lead to a reduction of tissue mass and thus, in severe cases, to cachexia. In the terminal stage, a patient with advanced heart failure may resemble a patient with widespread malignancy.

Patients with LV failure may become uncomfortable if they lie flat for more than a few minutes without elevation of the head. They may appear in obvious respiratory distress following moderate activity, such as walking to the examining room from the waiting room.

Evidence of increased sympathetic activity is frequent in patients with heart failure. There may be pallor and coldness of the limbs and cyanosis of the digits because of vasoconstriction. The patient may also present with diaphoresis and abnormal distention of the superficial veins. Sinus tachycardia is often observed and usually develops in an effort to maintain the cardiac output when heart failure is decompensated or the stroke volume is significantly decreased.

Sustained periodic or cyclic respirations with regularly alternating phases of hyperpnea and apnea in a smooth crescendo-decrescendo manner (Cheyne-Stokes) can be seen in patients with heart failure. This represents an altered neurogenic control of respiration, usually from intracranial causes, but it is facilitated by a combination of pulmonary congestion, the prolonged

circulation time from lung to the brain, and decreased sensitivity of the respiratory center to hypercapnia and hypoxia. Moist rales heard initially at the lung bases result from the transudation of fluid into the alveoli that subsequently moves into the airways. In pulmonary edema, coarse bubbling rales and wheezes are heard over both lung fields and may be accompanied by frothy sputum, with or without bloodstaining. Hydrothorax (pleural effusion) is usually bilateral and can intensify the severity of dyspnea by further reducing vital capacity. Stony dullness on percussion is characteristic of pleural effusion on one or both sides. Shifting dullness can often be found with pleural effusion when the patient moves from the sitting to the lateral decubitus position. Breath sounds over the area of effusion are diminished or absent, but occasionally high-pitched bronchial sounds are present. An accompanying pleural rub usually indicates associated pulmonary infarction, infection, or inflammatory response. Hydrothorax usually is reabsorbed slowly as heart failure improves; in some cases, the pleural effusion persists for many days after the symptoms disappear.

Approximately 5 L of extracellular fluid must accumulate before peripheral edema occurs in heart failure. Pitting edema is common, with the fluid accumulating in a symmetric manner; in general, it initially involves the dependent portions of the body with higher venous pressure. This is typically noted in the feet and ankles of ambulatory patients and in the sacral area of bedridden ones. Late in the course of heart failure, edema may become massive and generalized (anasarca); it can involve the upper extremities, the thoracic and abdominal walls, and the genital area. Occasionally, with acute accumulation of edema or associated trauma, skin rupture and extravasation of fluid can occur. Chronic edema results in increased pigmentation, reddening, and induration of the skin of the lower extremities.

Cardiomegaly, with a laterally displaced, enlarged, and sustained ventricular impulse may be found on physical examination, but this is a nonspecific finding and can be absent, particularly in patients with acute heart failure. The decrease in ventricular compliance may initially become apparent by the presence of a late diastolic atrial sound (S_4 gallop). A protodiastolic sound (S_3 gallop) occurs in patients with more advanced heart failure and is caused by acute deceleration of ventricular inflow after the early filling phase. An S_3 gallop, however, can also be detected in other conditions such as mitral and tricuspid regurgitation and a left-to-right shunt. Gallop sounds are more readily audible in the presence of a rapid heart rate. The presence of a third heart sounds appears to be associated with an increased risk of death, death from pump failure, and hospitalization for heart failure. Systolic murmurs are common in heart failure and are largely secondary to mitral or tricuspid regurgitation that can result from ventricular dilatation. These murmurs frequently diminish or disappear after adequate treatment and reduction of ventricular size.

Systemic venous hypertension can be detected by abnormal distension of the jugular veins (the upper limit of the jugular venous pressure is about 4 cm above the sternal angle with the patient recumbent at a 45° angle). Although the jugular venous pressure normally declines on inspiration, it can rise in patients with right-heart failure (Kussmaul's sign). Persistent elevation of the jugular venous pressure is one of the earliest and most reliable signs of right-heart failure. The inability of the right ventricle to accept transient increases in venous return (hepatojugular reflux) is observed during transient compression (≥30 s) of the upper abdomen. Systolic pulsations of the liver may be felt in patients with tricuspid regurgitation. Liver enlargement and tenderness on palpation are marked by epigastric fullness and dullness to percussion in the right upper quadrant. These findings may persist after other signs of heart failure have disappeared because it takes longer for hepatic congestion to disappear. In some cases, the liver enlargement does not disappear because of structural changes in patients with long-standing heart failure. The presence of a elevated jugular venous pressure appears to be associated with an increased risk of death, death from pump failure, and hospitalization for heart failure.

Pulsus alternans is common in patients with CHF; when severe, it can be detected by sphygmomanometry or by palpation of peripheral pulses, particularly the femoral pulse. This sign is characterized by a regular rhythm of alternating strong and weak pulsations. Sometimes the weak beat may be so small that the aortic valve does not open and no aortic or arterial pulse is produced, resulting in total alternans and a pulse that is only half as fast as the apical beats. With total alternans, a first heart sound will occur, but no second heart sound if both the aortic and pulmonic valves fail to open. Pulsus alternans appears to be due to an alternation in the stroke volume of the left ventricle, possibly because of an incomplete recovery of myocardial cells and thus a decrease in the responsiveness of contracting cells on alternate beats. It can be persistent or paroxysmal, or it may occur only after a premature beat or with the Valsalva maneuver.

The hemodynamic response to the Valsalva maneuver has been found useful in the clinical evaluation of patients with heart failure. In this maneuver, the blood pressure cuff is inflated to just about 15 mm Hg above the systolic blood pressure before the maneuver. In a normal response, the Korotkoff sounds disappear during sustained maneuver and reappear after completion of the maneuver. An abnormal response, in which blood pressure sounds either do not disappear or are maintained throughout the maneuver, has been found

in patients with CHF. In normal patients, the decrease in blood pressure during the maneuver is associated with tachycardia, and the increase in blood pressure after release with bradycardia. No changes in heart rate are observed in CHF patients.

C. Diagnostic Studies

1. Electrocardiography—Changes in the 12-lead electrocardiogram (ECG) are generally nonspecific. Sinus tachycardia is usually present in uncompensated heart failure or in end-stage disease with a low stroke volume that requires tachycardia to maintain the cardiac output. Isolated premature ventricular beats are common, and complex ventricular arrhythmias can be detected in most patients during prolonged (24–48-h) Holter monitoring. Electrocardiographic findings suggestive of atrial and ventricular chamber enlargement may be evident. Intraventricular conduction delays are also common and include left bundle branch block as well as other, nonspecific repolarization changes.

Exercise stress testing, using a bicycle ergometer or treadmill with a progressively increasing load, can be helpful in evaluating CHF. However, the degree of LV functional impairment at rest cannot be inferred from and does not always correlate with exercise capacity measured by exercise tolerance testing. Such testing allows for close observation of the patient during graded exercise and can detect obvious difficulty in breathing at a low level of exercise or a higher workload. A more prolonged exercise assessment of heart failure patients should include monitoring the maximum oxygen consumption and anaerobic threshold (the point during exercise testing at which the respiratory quotient rises as a result of the production of excess lactate) during exercise. These measurements can be used to classify the severity of heart failure, follow the progress of the patient, and assess the efficacy of therapeutic maneuvers.

2. Chest radiograph—Cardiomegaly (cardiothoracic ratio > 50%) can be found on chest film in 87% of patients when first diagnosed with primary dilated cardiomyopathy. The lower lobes of the lung are normally better perfused than are the upper lobes; with heart failure, there is progressive vasoconstriction of vessels in the lower lobes and redistribution of the pulmonary flow to the upper lobes. Interstitial and perivascular edema develop with acute increases in pulmonary capillary wedge pressure above 20–25 mm Hg; bronchovascular markings at the bases are prominent. Interstitial edema can present as perivascular or peribronchial edema (initially in perihilar and then in peripheral zones). Kerley's lines, spindle-shaped linear opacities at the periphery of the lung bases, occur in the later stages of heart failure; pleural fluid can produce discrete interlobular-type linear opacities and subpleural fluid accumulation between the lung and adjoining pleura. The accumulation of fluid in major and minor lung fissures can be of considerable size and may be incorrectly diagnosed as a tumor mass in the lung. These "phantom tumor" shadows, however, have smooth margins and disappear with resolution of CHF. With acute increases in pulmonary capillary wedge pressures above 25 mm Hg, alveolar edema, pleural effusions, or both may occur. Chronic heart failure patients may show elevated pulmonary capillary pressures in the range of 25–35 mm Hg or more without interstitial or alveolar edema, reflecting associated increased lymphatic flow. After therapy that lowers pulmonary capillary pressure, there may be a delay of 24–48 h before improvement and clearing of pulmonary infiltrates can be seen on chest radiograph.

3. Echocardiography—The Doppler echocardiographic examination appears to be the most useful test in establishing the type of cardiomyopathy (dilated, restrictive, hypertrophic) and in evaluating the possible primary or secondary causes (valvular disease, LV aneurysm, intracardiac shunts) of heart failure.

4. Radionuclide ventriculography—This method is helpful in documenting the severity of LV systolic dysfunction and indicating whether the wall motion abnormalities are global or regional. This test is especially helpful in patients who present technical difficulties for echocardiography; it can, for example, be obtained easily even in obese patients. Comparison of right and LV stroke volumes is also helpful in establishing the severity of regurgitant lesions.

5. Cardiac catheterization—Left-heart catheterization and angiography are necessary when the presence and extent of CAD need to be determined, particularly if cardiac surgery (valve replacement, aneurysmectomy, coronary artery bypass surgery) can possibly improve ventricular dysfunction. Right-heart catheterization may be useful in evaluating and selecting patients with refractory heart failure who require customized treatment.

6. Laboratory blood tests—In severe heart failure, neurohumoral compensatory mechanisms frequently lead to hyponatremia and other significant electrolyte abnormalities, even without the use of diuretics, which (especially the thiazide type) may contribute to hyponatremia. This effect is less prominent with furosemide, the only diuretic that increases free water clearance through a mechanism that is resistant to the action of vasopressin; in fact, furosemide may be necessary to correct hyponatremia in patients with heart failure. Hypokalemia is also very common with use of diuretics, especially the long-acting thiazides. Hyperkalemia may occur in patients with very low cardiac output or renal insufficiency. It can also occur in patients who are ingesting additional potassium through salt substitutes—especially when given in addition to a potassium-sparing diuretic or angiotensin-converting-enzyme inhibitor (ACEI), such as captopril, which also blocks the release of aldosterone. Reduced renal blood flow can lead to moderate increases in the blood urea nitrogen and mild increases in sodium creatinine.

Congestion of the liver is often associated with abnormalities of liver function tests with elevated levels of liver enzyme values, particularly serum aspartic aminotransferase. A concomitant increase in serum alanine aminotransferase or other hepatocellular enzymes documents that the liver is the source of the enzyme elevation. Serum alkaline phosphatase, a hepatobiliary enzyme, may be elevated and is commonly associated with hyperbilirubinemia or even prolongation of prothrombin time as a result of decreased hepatic synthesis of clotting factors. Hyperbilirubinemia of 15–20 mg/dL and aspartic aminotransferase elevation more than ten times normal can be seen with acute hepatic congestion in patients with decompensated heart failure.

Deedwania PC: Ventricular arrhythmias in heart failure: To treat or not to treat? Cardiol Clin 1994;12(1):115.

Drazner MH, Rame JE, Stevenson LW et al: Prognostic importance of elevated jugular venous pressure and a third heart sound in patients with heart failure. N Engl J Med 2001; 345:574.

Myers J, Froelicher VF: Hemodynamic determinants of exercise capacity in chronic heart failure. Ann Intern Med 1991;115: 377.

Differential Diagnosis

Many patients with heart failure also have lung disease; the symptoms are often similar, making differentiation between cardiac and pulmonary dyspnea difficult. In the advanced stages of chronic lung disease, patients may experience orthopnea while recumbent; this position may interfere with the descent of the diaphragm or the maximal use of accessory respiratory muscles. Orthopnea can also be precipitated in patients with bronchiectasis or severe bronchitis when excessive secretions pool in the recumbent position. Although paroxysmal nocturnal dyspnea can occur in chronic lung disease, it is usually relieved by clearing the secretions—without necessarily assuming an upright position. Tachypnea associated with heart failure is characterized by rapid shallow breathing caused by the reduction in vital capacity that results when air in the lungs is replaced by blood, interstitial fluid, or both (stiff lungs syndrome). The prolonged expiratory phase seen in chronic obstructive pulmonary disease (COPD) is usually absent, however. Bronchoconstriction and wheezing from heart failure without significant pulmonary disease (cardiac asthma) is frequently associated with wet secretions (bubbly sounds, frothy sputum from bronchial congestion) and cool, dusky, and diaphoretic skin that is caused by generalized vasoconstriction.

It is important to look for both pulmonary conditions (eg, pulmonary embolism, acute bronchitis, acute asthma attack, pneumonia, pneumothorax) and precipitating causes of heart failure (eg, alteration in therapy, excessive salt and fluid intake, arrhythmias, increased physical activity, intercurrent infection, pulmonary emboli) when dyspnea suddenly worsens. Occasionally, dyspneic symptoms observed in a patient without cardiac or pulmonary illness may be related to anxiety disorders. The breathing pattern of a neurotic or anxious patient, however, is not regular, rapid, or shallow but irregular during rest or with exertion; it is usually deep and sighing. The patient may complain of lightheadedness, paresthesias, blurred vision, lump in the throat, and chest constriction—usually from hyperventilation.

Management of Heart Failure

Management of heart failure requires a treatment approach reaching into multiple areas, which includes evaluation and application of general measures, use of pharmacologic agents, and consideration of nonpharmacologic interventions.

A. GENERAL MEASURES

1. Preventive strategies—Therapeutic strategies to prevent or treat heart failure should be aimed at improving impaired ventricular function before symptoms develop. Symptomatic relief, by itself, is not an adequate treatment goal. Optimal therapy for heart failure should include the unloading of the left ventricle, reducing wall stress, lowering the myocardial oxygen demand, and lessening the degree of neurohumoral activation. Detecting and controlling hypertension, managing the metabolic abnormalities associated with diabetes, and adequately treating myocardial ischemia should be initiated before damage to the myocardium occurs.

2. Correction of precipitating factors—Some of the most important reversible causes of heart failure include endocrine abnormalities, valvular dysfunction, intracardiac shunts, and other high-output states; bradyarrhythmias or tachyarrhythmias, smoking, psychologic stress, systemic hypertension, myocardial toxins (ie, ethanol consumption), and various cardiotoxic drugs. Heart failure can also be secondary to pericardial disease, infectious or ischemic events, reversible causes of diastolic dysfunction, poor compliance with medical treatment plan, and suboptimal medical treatment. In all these situations the obvious therapeutic approach is correction of the precipitating factors and treatment of any reversible underlying cause. Because the pathophysiology of heart failure in patients with depressed LV systolic function differs from that in patients who have normal systolic function but predominant abnormalities of LV diastolic function, the therapeutic approach must be appropriate for the specific type of underlying myocardial dysfunction.

3. Changes in activity and diet—A few consistent modifications in lifestyle can help reduce both the symptoms of heart failure and the need for additional medication. In moderate-to-severe CHF, restriction of physical activities and bed rest often help improve the clinical condition temporarily. Appropriate restriction of physical activity reduces cardiac workload, improves symptoms, and allows the patient to engage in day-to-day activities. No data are available, however, to indicate that prolonged bed rest has any significant effect on the natural history of CHF. Dietary caloric restriction is particularly necessary in overweight patients because weight reduction lowers demands on the heart and can provide significant relief of symptoms.

Restricting sodium helps reduce water retention, with a concomitant reduction in cardiac work. A moderate sodium restriction (1.5–2 g/day) is usually necessary to achieve therapeutically meaningful results; however, a more stringent sodium restriction is generally not recommended.

Reducing emotional stress and providing psychologic support will also benefit patients with heart failure who must deal not only with the fear of increased mortality but also with an altered quality of life: restricted physical activities, changes in dietary habits, and chronic use of medications.

Feenstra J, Brobbee DE, Jonkman FA et al: Prevention of relapse in patients with congestive heart failure: The role of precipitating factors. Heart 1998;80:432.

B. PHARMACOLOGIC TREATMENT

Several pharmacologic agents have been used in cases of CHF due to ventricular systolic dysfunction. These include diuretics, inotropic drugs (direct and indirect), vasoactive drugs, and beta-blockers (Table 18–5).

1. Diuretics—Diuretics provide symptomatic relief of moderate-to-severe congestive symptoms. The drugs promote excretion of sodium and water and help lower plasma volume, reducing congestion in the pulmonary and systemic vascular beds and thereby improving symptoms and functional capacity. The usual goal is a ventricular filling pressure that will maintain cardiac output and relieve pulmonary congestion without causing orthostatic hypotension; the optimal pressure depends on how quickly the heart failure developed. It should be noted that overdiuresis can significantly reduce intravascular volume and cardiac output (forward cardiac failure); fluids should be given to restore optimal intravascular volume and hemodynamic parameters monitored in such cases.

Of the many diuretic agents available, oral agents are preferred in cases of mild fluid retention, whereas

Table 18–5. Pharmacologic agents used in patients with congestive heart failure.

Class	Group	Commonly Used Agent(s)
Diuretics	Thiazide diuretics	HCTZ
	Loop diuretics	Furosemide
	Potassium sparing diuretics	Spironolactone
Cardiac glycosides	Digitalis preparations	Digoxin
Inotropic drugs	Direct inotropic agents	Dobutamine
	Phosphodiesterase inhibitors	Amrinone
		Milrinone
Vasoactive drugs	Vasodilators	Hydralazine
		Isosorbide
	ACE inhibitors	Enalapril
		Captopril
		Lisinopril
		Fosinopril
		Ramipril
		Quinapril
		Benazepril
	Angiotensin receptor blockers	
		Losartan
		Candesartan
		Irbesartan
		Valsartan
Beta-blockers		Metoprolol CR/XL
		Carvedilol
Antiarrhythmic drugs		Amiodarone
		Dofetilide

ACE = angiotensin-converting enzyme; CR/XL = controlled release/extended release; HCTZ = hydrochlorothrazide.

intravenous diuretics are generally recommended for severe, progressive, or refractory heart failure. Current diuretic agents include thiazides, loop diuretics, and potassium-sparing agents.

Thiazides are organic acids that are bound to protein and work after being secreted into the lumen of the proximal convoluted portion of the renal tubule. These agents inhibit the active transport of chloride as well as the passive movement of sodium. Some thiazides (eg, metolazone) also appear to block sodium re-

absorption, producing an excretion of sodium with associated kaliuresis. Metolazone can be used with a loop diuretic in cases that appear resistant to therapy with a single agent.

Most oral thiazide agents have an onset of diuretic activity within 1 to 2 h. Both chlorothiazide and hydrochlorothiazide appear to have the shortest duration of action, usually from 6 to 12 h. In renal failure, endogenous organic acid end products may accumulate and compete with thiazide for access into the tubular lumen. Thiazides are therefore generally not effective when the glomerular filtration rate falls below 30 mL/min, as is frequently seen in severe heart failure. Metolazone appears to keep its efficacy with a glomerular filtration rate as low as 10 mL/min.

Adverse reactions associated with thiazides include hypokalemia and intravascular volume depletion with development of prerenal azotemia, hyponatremia, hypomagnesemia, and hyperglycemia. Less frequent reactions include neutropenia, thrombocytopenia, and liver dysfunction.

Loop diuretics—furosemide, bumetanide, and ethacrynic acid—exert their effect in the thick portion of the ascending loop of Henle. These drugs are generally preferred in severe CHF (NYHA classes III-IV) when the patient is unresponsive to other diuretics. For patients who do not seem to respond until a certain drug dosage has been reached, higher and less frequent doses of loop diuretics may be more effective than lower but more frequent doses. The diuretic effect of these agents is seen within 30 min and peaks in 1–2 h. A major advantage of loop diuretics is their safety and availability in intravenous form. Like the thiazides, loop diuretics are organic acids and must be secreted into the proximal tubule. They initiate diuresis by inhibiting active reabsorption of chloride in the medullary and cortical portions of the loop of Henle. Chloride is actively transported along with potassium, inhibiting the passive reabsorption of sodium.

Potassium-sparing diuretics such as spironolactone, triamterene, and amiloride act on the distal renal tubule. Active sodium reabsorption in the distal tubule and the collecting duct is accomplished in exchange for potassium and hydrogen ions. One of the mechanisms involved is mediated through the action of aldosterone and may be antagonized by spironolactone, which has competitive receptor antagonist activity (aldosterone receptor blocker). Although triamterene and amiloride directly inhibit sodium transport, their diuretic effect is similar to that of spironolactone. All these agents decrease active sodium reabsorption and potassium excretion and could potentiate hyperkalemia; this is rare when the potassium-sparing diuretic is combined with a loop diuretic. Onset of diuretic action is fairly rapid with amiloride and triamterene (2–4 h), and their effect may persist for 24 h. A more gradual onset of diuresis is exhibited with spironolactone, for which the maximum effect occurs in 3 days, which may be due in part to a progressive accumulation of drug or active metabolites. Increased diuretic activity may persist for 2–3 days after treatment with spironolactone has ended, because of the longer half-life of the active metabolites. Triamterene and amiloride are both excreted unchanged in the urine, whereas spironolactone undergoes extensive hepatic metabolism.

a. Electrolyte abnormalities—Acute diuresis with both intravenous and short-term oral agents has been associated with increases in plasma renin and aldosterone activity as well as increased plasma norepinephrine levels. Patients with heart failure are thus at risk of developing electrolyte abnormalities from neurohumoral stimulation secondary to the use of diuretic agents. Hyponatremia in advanced CHF can be caused by a combination of diuretic therapy, neurohumoral activation, and enhanced vasopressin activity.

Although it is thought that potassium-sparing diuretics used in combination with loop or thiazide diuretics may partially limit excess potassium excretion, supporting data are limited. Another concern is that use of potassium-sparing diuretics in combination with ACEI may produce hyperkalemia; here, too, no definite data are available to confirm this concern.

The excretion of magnesium appears to parallel closely that of potassium. Ongoing treatment with thiazide diuretics can lead to hypomagnesemia, which can potentially lead to life-threatening cardiac arrhythmias in patients with CHF. This problem is further magnified in patients who have concomitant hypokalemia because a combined deficiency of potassium and magnesium not only potentiates the risk of ventricular arrhythmia, but hypokalemia cannot be corrected in some cases until the magnesium levels are restored.

Diuretics used with an ACEI are usually associated with fewer adverse neurohumoral and metabolic abnormalities.

b. Electrolyte supplementation—In diuretic-induced hypokalemia associated with a metabolic alkalosis and some chloride deficiency, the preferred salt for supplementation is potassium chloride. Of the slow-release oral potassium chloride preparations frequently used in the chronic management of diuretic-induced hypokalemia, no single preparation appears to be better with regard to the ulcerogenic effects on the gastrointestinal mucosa. Potassium should be carefully administered intravenously for patients with moderate-to-severe potassium deficiency as well as those with decompensated heart failure with edema of the intestinal villi caused by inadequate absorption of potassium salts. Although the usual daily dosage for heart failure patients receiving diuretic therapy is 8–24 mEq of potassium, recent data indicate that these patients may have significantly lower potassium reserves, initially requiring 20–80 mEq daily to restore the potassium balance. The dosage should be adjusted regularly, particularly during concomitant therapy with an ACEI or a potassium-sparing diuretic.

Chronic therapy with a thiazide or loop diuretic in patients with heart failure can lead to hypomagnesemia. Some recent studies have suggested that magnesium supplementation is highly effective in controlling the complex ventricular arrhythmias that can ensue in these patients. Although the antiarrhythmic action of magnesium needs to be confirmed in large-scale clinical trials, it appears reasonable to use magnesium supplementation in patients who exhibit life-threatening ventricular arrhythmias during vigorous diuretic therapy.

c. Limitations of diuretic therapy—Although diuretics can relieve symptoms of pulmonary and systemic venous congestion, they cannot maintain most patients with heart failure in a compensated state for long periods. During the initial period of hospitalization, some patients may need larger doses of diuretics to start diuresis; doses can generally be decreased once diuresis has begun or during periods of bed rest. Somewhat larger doses may be required when the patient once again assumes routine daily activities. Patients with heart failure should be cautioned to watch for increases in weight, which can indicate retention of sodium and water. Such a weight increase should prompt the patient to seek medical help for adjustments in the diuretic dosage. This vigilance will help avoid frequent hospitalization or the need for emergency treatment, particularly in the advanced stages of heart failure. Patients with severe heart failure should also use nonsteroidal antiinflammatory agents (including aspirin) with caution because their use may interfere with diuretic action and decrease natriuresis.

d. Clinical outcomes—There is no evidence that treatment with most diuretics reduces mortality or alters the natural history of the disease. However, some recent evidence suggests a beneficial role for spironolactone in treating moderate to severe heart failure.

In the randomized Aldactone evaluation study (RALES) in patients with symptomatic heart failure, depressed LVEF), and NYHA class II–IV who were receiving ACEI and loop diuretics, compared with placebo, treatment with spironolactone (up to 25–50 mg/d) resulted in significantly reduced mortality rates for all causes, sudden death, and hospitalization. Because of these findings indicating improved clinical outcomes, the RALES trial was terminated earlier than the planned follow-up period.

Brater DC: Clinical pharmacology of loop diuretics. Drugs 1991; 42(Suppl 3):14.

Eichhorn EJ, Tandon P, DiBianco R et al: Clinical and prognostic significance of serum magnesium concentration in patients with severe chronic congestive heart failure: The PROMISE study. J Am Coll Cardiol 1993;21:634.

Kruck F: Acute and long term effects of loop diuretics in heart failure. Drugs 1991;41:60.

Pitt B, Zannad F, Remme W, et al: The effect of spironolactone on morbidity and mortality in patients with severe heart failure. The randomized Aldactone evaluation study. N Engl J Med 1999;341:709.

2. Inotropic agents—

a. Digitalis glycosides—Glycosides of digitalis, which have been used in the treatment of heart failure for more than 200 years, are the most frequently used inotropic agents and the only oral positive inotropic preparation approved for treatment of heart failure. Digitalis glycosides, of which digoxin if the agent most commonly used, relieve symptoms by improving cardiac performance through increased myocardial contractility, improved LV function, and increased cardiac output and renal perfusion. Neurohumoral modulating actions have also been reported. Several studies suggest that treatment with digitalis decreases plasma renin activity, attenuates sympathetic drive, reduces plasma norepinephrine levels, and improves baroreceptor sensitivity. These effects are seen as playing an important role in treating heart failure.

The beneficial effect of digitalis glycosides in patients with heart failure complicated by the occurrence of atrial fibrillation has been well documented and is generally well accepted by most clinicians. The results of several studies indicate that in patients with heart failure, digitalis does exert sustained beneficial hemodynamic effects accompanied by improvement in both clinical status and exercise tolerance. (Those who did not benefit from treatment with digitalis had milder degrees of heart failure or evidence of primarily diastolic dysfunction.) Because some evidence suggests that use of digitalis in suspected or confirmed MI may be associated with adverse outcome, it is appropriate to consider alternatives to treatment with digoxin for patients with MI and heart failure.

(1) Dosage and administration—Although several digitalis glycosides are available for clinical use, by far the most commonly used agent is digoxin. Although digoxin can be given intravenously or orally, the intravenous route is preferred for patients with supraventricular tachyarrhythmia and fast ventricular rate. The initial intravenous dose is 0.5 mg given slowly over 10–20 min. If necessary, additional doses (0.25 or 0.125 mg) can be given after 4 h. Younger patients generally require a total dose of about 1 mg for a full effect; smaller doses are recommended for the elderly and for patients with smaller total body mass. The initial effect is not seen until after 30 min, and the peak effect may occur at 2–3 h.

Although the therapeutic effect of oral digitalis occurs over a relatively prolonged period, it is less likely to result in overdose and toxicity. To achieve a more rapid effect orally, 1.0–1.25 mg of digoxin is given over 24 h. Preferably, a slower effect should be achieved by giving daily maintenance doses (0.125–0.25 mg). The daily requirements of digoxin may be smaller for patients with renal insufficiency because the drug is excreted primarily by the kidneys and has a half-life of 36–48 h.

The levels of digoxin may be reduced by some antibiotics and cholestyramine; however, quinidine, verapamil, and amiodarone may increase serum digoxin levels and the digoxin dosage will need to be adjusted accordingly.

(2) Digitalis toxicity—Digitalis intoxication may occur in as many as 30% of patients hospitalized for the treatment of heart failure. Common findings are nausea, vomiting, anorexia, malaise, drowsiness, headache, insomnia, altered color vision, or arrhythmia. Almost all known cardiac arrhythmias can be caused by digitalis; they are facilitated by hypokalemia, which is often associated with the concomitant use of diuretics. The most common are premature ventricular beats, junctional tachycardia, second- or third-degree heart block, and paroxysmal atrial tachycardia with block. Digoxin toxicity is usually confirmed by the reversal of symptoms or cessation of arrhythmias after withdrawal of digoxin therapy for 48 h. The severity and unpredictability of digitalis toxicity indicate that caution must be exercised while initiating treatment with digitalis glycosides as well as when continuing their use in patients with mild-to-moderate CHF.

(3) Clinical outcomes—Recent double-blind, placebo-controlled, parallel, randomized studies suggest that digoxin plays a role in the treatment of patients with stable mild-to-moderate heart failure (NYHA II-III; LVEF <0.35) who were on chronic digoxin therapy and whose disease was controlled with diuretics alone or with a combination of diuretic and an ACEI. Results of these trials revealed that patients who underwent digoxin therapy had a lower probability of developing worsening heart failure that required more diuretics, emergency room care, or hospitalization compared with patients who were not treated with digoxin. The group receiving digoxin had a significant increase in treadmill exercise time and ejection fraction compared with the group receiving placebo.

A more precise role of digoxin in patients with mild-to-moderate heart failure, depressed LVEF (≤ 0.45), and the presence of sinus rhythm was defined by the digitalis investigation group (DIG). In this study the use of digoxin, compared with placebo, was associated with a modest, nonsignificant reduction in mortality rates from all causes and death from worsened heart failure. There was also a significant reduction on the rate of hospitalization for worsened heart failure.

The data from these studies thus support a role for digoxin in patients with mild-to-moderate CHF, including patients with sinus rhythm who are being treated with diuretics or with a combination of a diuretic and an ACEI.

Garg R, Gorlin R, Smith T et al: The effect of digoxin on mortality and morbidity in patients with heart failure (DIG). N Engl J Med 1997;336:525.

Gheorghiade M, Ferguson D: Digoxin: A neurohormonal modulator in heart failure? Circulation 1991;84:2181.

Jaeschke R, Oxman AD, Guyatt GH: To what extent do congestive heart failure patients in sinus rhythm benefit from digoxin therapy? A systematic overview and meta-analysis. Am J Med 1990;88:279.

Kulick DL, Rahimtoola SH: Current role of digitalis therapy in patients with congestive heart failure. JAMA 1991;265:2995.

Tisdale JE, Gheorghiade M: Acute hemodynamic effects of digoxin alone or in combination with other vasoactive agents in patients with congestive heart failure. Am J Cardiol 1992;69:34G.

b. Sympathetic receptor agonist, quinolinone derivative, dopamine agonist, beta-1 partial agonist inotropes—Myocardial catecholamine levels are depleted in patients with advanced heart failure, probably as a result of the chronic state of increased sympathetic stimulation. Several sympathomimetic amines have been used in an effort to improve the cardiac function associated with such depletion. The clinical use of β-sympathetic receptor agonists, however, has been limited by both their adverse effects and progressive loss of efficacy as patients develop tolerance to them.

A quinolinone derivative-inotrope, a dopamine agonist, and a β_1 partial selective agonist were found, on clinical trials, to share similar clinical limitations as the sympathetic receptor agonists.

(1) Clinical outcomes—Dopamine and dobutamine are quite useful for short-term treatment of hospitalized patients with heart failure. Although intermittent intravenous dobutamine can improve hemodynamic parameters, such treatment may reduce survival—especially in patients with preexisting episodes of VT.

Limited data from a couple of studies, one being a retrospective analysis (only initial in-hospital dobutamine treatment) and another being a prospective study, both in patients with moderate to severe heart failure (NYHA III–IV) and depressed LVEF (≤ 0.25, ≤ 0.30) revealed that, compared with no-dobutamine therapy, the groups that received treatment with intravenous infusion of dobutamine while in the hospital or intravenous infusion at home (or both), experienced reduced rates of all-cause hospitalization and hospitalization for worsened heart failure during the follow-up period. However, the use of dobutamine was associated with greater rates of death from all causes, sudden death, and death due to worsened heart failure.

In another study in patients with advanced heart failure (NYHA III–IV, LVEF <0.35), who were receiving diuretics, digoxin, and an ACEI, compared with placebo treatment, the oral dopamine agonist, ibopamine, resulted in a higher mortality rate from all causes, higher risk of sudden death, and greater rate of death associated with worsened heart failure.

A subsequent evaluation of the oral quinolinone derivative inotrope, vesnarinone, in patients with symptomatic LV dysfunction (NYHA III) and LVEF ≤0.30, who were receiving conventional therapy for heart failure revealed conflicting findings. In this study, compared with placebo, high-dose vesnarinone (120 mg/day) was associated with a two to threefold increase in the risk of death during the initial period of the study. This finding prompted the discontinuation of the high-dose treatment arm. In contrast, the use of low-dose (60 mg/day) vesnarinone was associated with a significant reduction in the risk of death from all causes and a reduction in the rate of the combination events of hospitalization for heart failure and death from all causes. Also, during treatment with low-dose vesnarinone a greater proportion of patients described improved quality of life. These findings suggested a narrow therapeutic range for vesnarinone and might have instigated physician reluctance to embrace this agent for treatment of patients with CHF.

The β₁-selective partial agonist, xamoterol, was evaluated in patients with moderately severe CHF (NYHA III–IV), an LVEF <0.45, who were receiving ACEI and diuretics. Compared with placebo, xamoterol had no effect on exercise duration or on the total exertional workload achieved. A secondary analysis (secondary end points) of clinical events revealed that during treatment with xamoterol there were greater risks of death (all causes), death from worsened heart failure, and a greater risk of sudden death.

In light of these findings, intermittent dobutamine therapy with careful supervision should be restricted to patients with refractory heart failure who have failed to respond to all other therapeutic choices. The aim of such treatment should be the temporary relief of severe symptoms. Treatment with other inotropes such as the quinolinone derivative, dopamine agonist, and β₁ partial agonist inotropes appears to be associated with adverse clinical outcomes, and therefore their use seems inadvisable at this time.

Feldman A, Bristow M, Parmley W et al: Effects of vesnarinone on morbidity and mortality in patients with heart failure. N Engl J Med 1993;329:149.

Hampton JR, Veldhuisen DJ, Kleber FX et al: Randomized study of effect of ibopamine on survival in patients with advanced severe heart failure. Lancet 1997;349:971.

Oliva F, Latinie R, Politi A, et al: Intermittent 6-month low-dose dobutamine infusion in severe heart failure: DICE multicenter trial. Am Heart J 1999;138:247.

Ryden L: Xamoterol in severe heart failure. Lancet 1990;336:1.

c. **Phosphodiesterase inhibitors**—At different points in the process, phosphodiesterase inhibitors (PDI) hinder the action of cyclic adenosine monophosphate phosphodiesterase. Amrinone, milrinone, and enoximone exhibit both vasodilator and inotropic effects. Although the inotropic effects are prominent in normal hearts, the response is somewhat attenuated in the failing heart, where the myocardial levels of cyclic adenosine monophosphate are already reduced. The drugs have demonstrated a beneficial hemodynamic response during acute administration, but their long-term use is associated with a high incidence of side effects.

(1) Clinical outcomes—In two prospective studies (MMTG and PROMISE), milrinone was evaluated in patients with mild-to-moderate heart failure or in patients with moderately severe heart failure (PROMISE). In the PROMISE study, patients were in NYHA III–IV, had a LVEF ≤0.35, and were receiving digoxin, diuretics, and an ACEI. In these studies, compared with placebo, treatment with oral milrinone was associated with an increased risk of death from all causes as well as an increased risk of cardiovascular death during the follow-up period.

In a study in patients with moderate CHF (NYHA II–III) compared with placebo, the oral PDI enoximone did not improve subjective symptoms and was also associated with greater rates of death from all causes as well as cardiovascular death during follow-up.

Based on these findings, long-term treatment with PDI agents is not recommended in patients with CHF. Intravenous therapy with amrinone or milrinone could be used for patients with acute heart failure or for those with chronic heart failure when they experience acute decompensation. However, the potential adverse clinical outcome associated with the use of these drugs should be carefully considered in such patients.

Leier C: Current status of nondigitalis positive inotropic drugs. Am J Cardiol 1992;69:1206.

Packer M, Carver J, Rodenheffer R et al: Effect of milrinone on mortality in severe chronic heart failure. The prospective randomized milrinone survival evaluation (PROMISE). N Engl J Med 1991;325:1468.

Uretsky B, Jessup M, Konstam M et al: Multicenter trial of oral enoximone in patients with moderate to moderately severe congestive heart failure. Circulation 1990;82:774.

3. Vasoactive drugs—

a. **Vasodilators**—These drugs are used in the treatment of heart failure patients who remain symptomatic after administration of diuretics and digitalis; they are especially useful in patients with a dilated left ventricle, normal or increased systemic blood pressure, increased systemic vascular resistance, or valvular regurgitation. In general, these drugs are classified as venous, arterial, or mixed-vascular dilators; they have also been broadly classified as direct-acting drugs (eg, nitrates, hydralazine, minoxidil, nitroprusside) or neurohumoral antagonist drugs (eg, ACEI, α- and β-adrenoreceptor blockers, serotonin antagonists, angiotensin receptor blockers), which block the vasoconstrictive actions of neurohumoral agents and have no direct vasodilator action. Although in the past vasodilators were primarily used in managing severe CHF, they are now widely accepted for use in mild-to-moderate heart failure. Although most vasodilators produce acute beneficial hemodynamic effects, some (eg, α-blocker prazosin) have been found to be no better than treatment with placebo during large clinical trials.

(1) Venous vasodilators—Nitrates have a greater effect on venous capacitance (venodilation) than on the arterial system because of the greater degree of stimulation of cyclic guanosine monophosphate in veins than in arteries. Intravenous administration, however, may produce significant arteriolar vasodilatation. Prolonged or sustained use of nitrates can lead to pharmacologic tolerance (apparently because of the depletion of sulfhydryl groups and activation of neurohumoral axes) and offset its beneficial hemodynamic effects. Patients can develop tolerance during therapy with any nitrate preparation, whether oral, transcutaneous, or intravenous. The long-term beneficial effects of nitrates have been documented only with intermittent administration of oral preparations. Nitrate tolerance may be minimized by providing a daily nitrate-free interval of 8–12 h and by using the smallest effective dose.

Isosorbide dinitrate. Long-term administration of isosorbide has been associated with significant improvement in hemodynamic parameters, exercise capacity, and relief of symptoms in moderate-to-severe heart failure. Although isosorbide dinitrate is the only direct-acting vasodilator that produces a sustained decrease in LV filling pressure, it is also the least likely to produce activation of endogenous neurohormones. Abrupt withdrawal after long-term oral therapy may be associated with a rebound phenomenon and should be avoided.

Close monitoring of blood pressure during the initial stages of nitrate therapy is advised in patients with preexisting low systemic blood pressure, suspected normal or low central venous or LV filling pressure (eg, that secondary to overdiuresis), the presence of significant pulmonary hypertension, or a previous history of orthostatic hypotension. Patients who develop significant exertional or nocturnal dyspnea may be given sublingual nitroglycerin for acute relief of the dyspnea; this therapy causes rapid and significant pulmonary vasodilatation with pooling of blood in both the pulmonary and systemic vascular beds. Oral nitrate preparations are easy to use, provide sustained systemic venous and pulmonary vascular effects, and are well tolerated. When used alone, these agents produce only modest clinical improvement in severe heart failure, however, and are usually considered as an adjunct to therapy with other vasodilators or ACEI.

Isosorbide dinitrate (80–160 mg/day) was used in combination with hydralazine in the vasodilator heart failure trial 1 (V-HeFT) in patients with moderate CHF and LVEF < 0.45. In this study, compared with placebo, the combination of hydralazine-isosorbide was associated with a modest but significant reduction in the risk of mortality from all causes and with an improvement in the LVEF.

(2) Arterial vasodilators—Hydralazine and minoxidil are direct-acting smooth muscle relaxants that seem to dilate arterioles predominantly. During treatment with these drugs, the systemic vascular resistance decreases and the cardiac output increases both at rest and during exercise. These beneficial hemodynamic effects unfortunately do not always translate into sustained clinical benefits. When used in combination with nitrates, hydralazine and minoxidil have shown a short-term increase in cardiac output and decrease in LV filling pressure. Clinical trials, however, have not shown a significant difference in exercise tolerance between placebo and hydralazine or minoxidil in patients with heart failure.

In patients with severe heart failure, hydralazine treatment is associated with a decrease in systemic vascular resistance and with increased stroke volume and cardiac output; it has little effect on the pulmonary capillary wedge pressure or right atrial pressure. Patients who have dilated left ventricles (end-diastolic dimension ≥ 60 mm by echocardiography) appear to have a better hemodynamic and clinical response than do patients with lesser degrees of enlargement. Studies have shown marked improvement in cardiac index and stroke work with a mild but significant reduction in LV filling pressure and an improvement of prerenal azotemia in patients with ventricular enlargement; rarely did they develop significant reflex tachycardia or hypotension. In contrast, patients with smaller ventricles who are treated with hydralazine can develop clinical deterioration characterized by findings suggestive of decreased tissue perfusion: confusion, weakness, lethargy, worsening azotemia, ventricular arrhythmia, hypotension, or tachycardia. Hydralazine can produce headaches, flushing, palpitations, nausea, vomiting, myocardial ischemia, and lupus-like syndrome at the required dosage of 200–800 mg/day. The absorption of hydralazine is enhanced when it is taken with meals.

(3) Clinical outcomes—As described earlier, in the V-HeFT study in patients with moderate CHF, compared with placebo the combination of hydralazine (150–300 mg/day) and isosorbide (80–160 mg/day) resulted in an increase in the LVEF and a lower risk of death from all causes.

The combination hydralazine-isosorbide should be considered a second-line therapy to be given to patients who do not seem to tolerate other therapies, including ACEI and β-blockers.

Overall, it appears that direct-acting vasodilators have limited clinical usefulness in the management of heart failure. The lack of consistent therapeutic efficacy may be attributed to multiple factors, including suboptimal long-term hemodynamic effects, activation of endogenous neurohumoral vasoconstrictor mechanisms or the loss of direct vascular effects, the development of significant adverse effects, and poor patient compliance because of intolerance to the drugs.

Stevenson LW, Fonarow G: Vasodilators: A re-evaluation of their role in heart failure. Drugs 1992;43:15.

b. Calcium channel blockers—These drugs are arteriolar vasodilators that (compared with other arteriolar vasodilators) generally produce a smaller increase in cardiac output in response to both vasodilatation and reflex sympathetic stimulation. These agents have limited usefulness in severe CHF because of their direct negative inotropic effects, which could potentially further depress already compromised myocardial contractility. The risk of these effects appears to be proportional to the severity of the underlying disease. The depressive effects appear to be modest in mild LV dysfunction; when the dysfunction is severe, pronounced deterioration in cardiac function may occur, possibly leading to pulmonary edema and cardiogenic shock. Although all calcium channel antagonists have some negative inotropic effects, the activation of neurohumoral axes may be an additional factor contributing to attenuated hemodynamic response, lack of change in exercise capacity, peripheral edema, and clinical deterioration in patients treated with these agents.

A newer generation of dihydropyridines that appear to be more vasculoselective may prove to be safe and effective in the management of heart failure

(1) Clinical outcomes—In post hoc analyses, the use of diltiazem for treating patients with acute MI, pulmonary congestion, or evidence of depressed LV function (ejection fraction <0.40), has been associated with increased rates of morbidity and mortality. Treatment with nifedipine has also produced deterioration of right-heart function in patients with right-heart failure secondary to severe pulmonary hypertension.

Several prospective studies have evaluated the effects of calcium channel blockers on clinical outcome. One study (PRAISE) evaluated the effects of amlodipine in patients with moderate-to-severe CHF, LVEF < 0.30, and concomitant therapy with digitalis, diuretics, and ACEI. Compared with placebo, treatment with amlodipine was associated with a lower risk of mortality from all causes and nonsignificant lower risk of the combination outcome of mortality from all causes and cardiovascular death. Further analyses revealed that the subgroup with nonischemic heart failure had a significantly lower risk of mortality from all causes or the combination event of death and cardiovascular morbid-

ity. No such findings were noted in the group with ischemic heart failure.

Another study (V-HeFT III) evaluated felodipine in patients with moderate CHF, NYHA II-III, and LVEF <0.45. Compared with placebo, felodipine produced an increase in LVEF. Although treatment with felodipine was associated with lower risk of the secondary end-point of sudden death, the drug was also associated with an increased risk of other secondary end-points that included death from all causes, death with acute MI, and death from pump failure.

Mibefradil (MACH-1 study) was evaluated in more severe cases of CHF (NYHA III–IV), taking loop diuretics, and ACEI. In this study, compared with placebo, the use of mibefradil was associated with an increased risk of mortality from all causes, cardiovascular death, sudden death, and death due to worsened heart failure.

Based on the findings from the available studies, calcium channel blockers do not appear to have a role in the management of heart failure.

c. Prostacyclin analog—Epoprostenol is a prostacyclin analog with multiple properties, including the ability to reduce pulmonary vascular and peripheral vascular resistance and the ability to inhibit platelet aggregation. The drug has been associated with improved outcomes in patients with primary pulmonary hypertension. However, in CHF the drug had a rather poor record and is not recommended for treatment of CHF.

(1) Clinical outcomes—During an unblinded study (FIRST study) the effect of infusion of epoprostenol was compared with no infusion in patients with severe CHF, NYHA III–IV, depressed LVEF <0.25, who were receiving loop diuretic, digitalis, and ACEI. The use of epoprostenol was associated with a decreased risk of need for mechanical assistance for cardiac dysfunction. However, treatment with epoprostenol was associated with increased risks of mortality from all causes, worsened heart failure, and resuscitation from sudden cardiac death. Based on these findings, the trial was terminated prematurely.

4. Angiotensin-converting-enzyme inhibitors—

a. Clinical effects—In patients with heart failure, inhibition of angiotensin-converting enzyme produces a moderate increase in cardiac output (increased stroke work and cardiac index) with a concomitant significant decrease in right and left ventricular filling pressures, pulmonary and systemic vascular resistances, and mean arterial pressure, without increasing the heart rate (Table 18–6). Other beneficial effects include a reduction in the incidence of ventricular arrhythmias; decreased end-systolic and end-diastolic dimensions; and sustained improvements in symptoms, exercise duration, and quality of life. Angiotensin-converting en-

Table 18–6. Beneficial hemodynamic and neurohumoral effects of angiotensin-converting enzyme inhibitor in congestive heart failure.

Hemodynamic changes	
Central venous pressure	↓
Pulmonary capillary venous pressure	↓
Systemic vascular resistance	↓
End-diastolic LV dimension	↓
End-systolic LV dimension	↓
Stroke volume	↑
Cardiac output	↑
Cardiac index	↑
Neurohumoral activity	
Norepinephrine	↓
Vasopressin	↓
Angiotensin II	↓
Aldosterone	↓ or no change
Serum potassium	↑ or no change

LV = left ventricular.

zyme inhibitors exert their primary hemodynamic effect by inhibiting the converting enzyme responsible for the formation of angiotensin II. They may indirectly decrease the elevated levels of circulating catecholamines. Angiotensin-converting enzyme inhibitors also decrease plasma vasopressin and plasma endothelin levels, which tend to be elevated in CHF and may contribute to increased systemic vascular resistance. Because their chemical structure is similar to kininase, ACEI prevent degradation of bradykinin, thereby increasing production of nitric oxide (a vasodilator) by endothelial cells. Preliminary data indicate that ACEI may also stimulate the synthesis of vasoactive prostaglandins.

Differences among various ACEI are primarily related to pharmacokinetic and hemodynamic properties. Both enalapril and lisinopril have delayed onset of action and prolonged duration of hemodynamic effects (compared with captopril). Hypotension is delayed and prolonged and can reduce systemic perfusion, compromising both renal and cerebral functions. Because the hypotension caused by captopril is shorter in duration, it rarely compromises organ perfusion.

Captopril and lisinopril inhibit ACE directly; enalapril is the inactive ester of enalaprilic acid (the biologically active moiety responsible for ACE inhibition). Because deesterification of enalapril occurs in the liver, its pharmacokinetics may be altered in CHF with accompanying hepatic insufficiency or passive hepatic congestion. The peak hemodynamic response to captopril usually occurs within 30–90 min (Table 18–7); the peak hemodynamic response to enalapril may occur 4–5 h after administration, and that of lisinopril even later. Progressive renal failure and hyperkalemia are less prominent during treatment with captopril than with enalapril and lisinopril.

b. Short- and long-acting angiotensin-converting enzyme inhibitors—Few data are available to compare the effects of short- and a long-acting ACEI. As shown in several studies, longer-acting agents appear to have little clinical advantage over shorter-acting ones and may in fact increase the risk of adverse effects, particularly when used in large, fixed doses. Long-acting agents, however, may increase patient compliance because of their convenient once-a-day dosing.

Table 18–7. Pharmacokinetics of currently available angiotensin-converting enzyme inhibitors.

Drug	Commerical Name	ACE-binding Group	Pro-drug	Dosage (mg/d)	Peak Action (h)	Half-Life (h)	Method of Excretion
Captopril	Capoten	Sulphydryl	No	25–150	1–1.5	<2	Liver
Enalapril	Vasotec	Carboxyl	Yes	5–20	4–6	11	Renal
Lisinopril	Zestril, Prinivil	Carboxyl	No	5–40	6	12	Renal
Quinapril[a]	Accupril	Carboxyl	Yes	10–80	2–4	2	Renal
Ramipril[a]	Altace	Carboxyl	Yes	5–20	3–6	2–4	Renal and GI
Fosinopril[a]	Monopril	Phosphoryl	Yes	10–40	2–6	12[b]	Liver and renal
Benazepril[a]	Lotensin	Carboxyl	Yes	10–40	2–4	10	Renal

[a] Available but not FDA approved for heart failure.
[b] Terminal elimination.
ACE = angiotensin-converting enzyme; GI = gastrointestinal.

c. **Safety of angiotensin-converting enzyme inhibitors**—In general, most of the available ACEI are safe and well tolerated and have a similar range and incidence of adverse effects when used in recommended doses. Most adverse effects reported in controlled studies of heart failure have been mild (Table 18–8). Although these side effects are occasionally associated with significant clinical consequences, they are usually reversible with discontinuation of therapy. The most common reported adverse effects with ACEI are dizziness in up to 6% of patients, headache in approximately 5%, and fatigue in 3%. The overall discontinuation rate has been approximately 6% for ACEI, similar to rates reported for placebo in most clinical studies.

The major differences in safety appear to be the potential adverse effects of the long-acting agents on renal and cerebral function. Renal function, however, usually returns to baseline or stabilizes at a new steady state despite continued treatment with the ACEI, except in rare instances when membranous glomerulonephritis occurs. It has been suggested that captopril may be responsible for the histopathologic evidence of membranous glomerulonephritis in patients without previous renal disease who manifested proteinuria during therapy. No clear causal relationship has been established for this adverse effect, however. Based on the available data, it seems that renal complications secondary to captopril therapy occur predominantly in patients with previous renal disease and those receiving large doses (> 400 mg/day). In the majority of cases, discontinuing treatment or decreasing the dosage of the ACEI rapidly resolves the proteinuria and renal dysfunction, and this decline in renal function appears to be of little clinical significance. In major clinical trials, the incidence of discontinuation of ACEI therapy because of impairment in renal function has been low (1–3%); in some studies it was equivalent to that seen with placebo. The longer-acting ACEI, however, may be associated with a higher risk of renal dysfunction.

Some patients may be very sensitive to the hypotensive effects of ACEI, particularly patients who are initiating therapy and who are dependent on the renin-angiotensin-aldosterone system for blood pressure maintenance. This includes patients with hyponatremia or hypovolemia, those receiving high-dose diuretic therapy, and those with bilateral renal artery stenosis. The hypotension usually subsides with continued therapy and can be partly avoided by reducing the diuretic dosage for several days before initiating treatment with an ACEI. This therapy should be started under close medical supervision, and patients considered at risk for developing severe hypotension should be followed closely for the first 2 weeks of treatment. Some investigators recommend a period of brief hospitalization and close observation during the initiation of enalapril therapy until a maintenance dose is achieved.

Rare cases of neutropenia have been reported during treatment with both captopril and enalapril. Because of the presence of the active sulfhydryl group, captopril is thought to have a greater potential for bone marrow depression, which can lead to neutropenia. This adverse effect is usually seen within 3 months of therapy and in

Table 18–8. Incidence of adverse effects during treatment with angiotensin-converting enzyme inhibitors approved for congestive heart failure (in percentages).

Adverse Effect	Drug		
	Enalapril (%)	Lisinopril (%)	Captopril (%)
Fatigue	5.1	3.3	2.7
Headache	4.8	5.3	2.9
Dizziness	2.4	6.3	6.0
Diarrhea	1.6	3.2	0.5–2
Rash	1.5	1.5	4–7
Proteinuria	1.4	rare	0.6
Dry cough	1.3–10	2.9	0.5–2
Taste alterations	0.5	rare	3.1
Angioedema	0.2	rare	0.1
Neutropenia	0.06	NA	0.04

patients with evidence of renal dysfunction or collagen vascular disease; a leukocyte count is recommended every 2 weeks in high-risk patients. Taste alterations and recurrent cough have also been reported in some patients treated with ACEI; these symptoms usually subside after discontinuation of therapy or reduction in dosage.

(1) Clinical outcomes—Several ACEI have been evaluated in various degree of heart failure.

Enalapril has been compared with placebo and with the combination therapy of hydralazine and isosorbide.

In the CONSENSUS study in patients with severe heart failure and NYHA IV, compared with placebo, treatment with enalapril was associated with a greater proportion of patients with improved NYHA class. Also, enalapril was associated with a significantly lower risk of death from all causes, cardiovascular mortality, and death associated with progression of heart failure. There was a nonsignificant reduction in the risk of sudden death.

The SOLVD trial evaluated patients with cardiac dysfunction with and without symptoms of heart failure.

In the treatment arm of the SOLVD study in patients with symptoms of heart failure and LVEF ≤0.35, compared with placebo, enalapril was associated with significantly lower risk of clinical events, including death from all causes, arrhythmic death, and death associated with heart failure. In this study, there was also a nonsignificant decrease in the risk of fatal stroke and of fatal MI.

Patients with heart failure associated with acute MI also benefit from treatment with ACEI. In the SAVE study, captopril was evaluated in patients with acute MI and associated LV dysfunction (LVEF <0.40). In this study, compared with placebo, treatment with captopril was associated with lower risks for worsened heart failure, symptomatic and asymptomatic sudden death, and death from all causes. The captopril group also had a lower risk for recurrent MI and worsened heart failure.

In the AIRE study, ramipril was evaluated in patients with acute MI and moderate to severe CHF (NYHA III–IV). Compared with placebo, treatment with ramipril was associated with significant lower risk for death from all causes or for the combination event of death from all causes, worsened heart failure, reinfarction, and stroke. Evaluation of risk for separate events revealed that fewer patients receiving ramipril experienced severe resistant heart failure, reinfarction, or stroke.

High-dosage ACEI compared with low-dosage ACEI appears to be associated with only modest influence on risk of clinical outcomes. In the ATLAS study, low-dose (5 mg/day) lisinopril was compared with high-dose (35 mg/day) lisinopril. Compared with the low-dose regimen, patients in the high-dose group had a nonsignificant reduction in the risk of death from all causes. However, there was a significantly lower risk of the secondary end-points consisting of death from all causes and hospitalization for all causes. Similar findings favorable for the high-dose group were noted for other combined end-points, including death from all causes and hospitalization for cardiovascular reasons, death from all causes and hospitalization for heart failure, and acute MI and hospitalization for unstable angina.

Based on these findings, ACEI are now well established as first-line therapy for all patients with LV dysfunction and heart failure (NYHA I–IV).

d. Angiotensin-converting enzyme inhibitors and primary prevention of clinical events—The effects of enalapril and ramipril on primary prevention of clinical events have been evaluated in two large, randomized, prospective studies.

In the prevention arm of the SOLVD study enalapril was evaluated in patients with depressed LVEF ≤0.35, but without symptoms of heart failure and no prior treatment for CHF. Compared with placebo, treatment with enalapril was associated with a significantly lower risk for developing CHF. Also, treatment with enalapril was associated with a modest, nonsignificant reduction in the risk of several other outcomes including death from all causes, death from cardiovascular cause, arrhythmic death, death associated with worsened heart failure, and death from stroke. Interestingly, the risk of noncardiovascular death during treatment with enalapril increased.

In the HOPE study, ramipril was evaluated in patients without history of heart failure who were considered at future risk for developing cardiovascular events. Study patients in the HOPE trial included those with a history of CAD, stroke, peripheral arterial vascular disease, or diabetes mellitus, as well as at least one cardiovascular risk factor, including systemic hypertension, elevated low-density lipoprotein or total cholesterol levels, active smoking, or microalbuminuria.

In this study, compared with placebo, treatment with ramipril was associated with a significant reduction in the risk for the combined end-point of cardiovascular death, acute MI, or stroke. Also, the ramipril group experienced a modest but significant reduction in risk for several other outcomes, including need for myocardial revascularization, death from acute MI, death associated with stroke, and death from all causes. Patients taking ramipril also had a lower risk for developing CHF, cardiac arrest, complications from diabetes, or occurrence of new-onset diabetes mellitus.

The findings from the available studies that have evaluated ACEI provide compelling evidence to consider treatment with these drugs in patients with evidence of depressed cardiac function as well as those with normal LV function who are at high risk of subsequent cardiovascular events.

Acute infarction ramipril efficacy (AIRE) study investigators: Effect of ramipril on mortality and morbidity of survivors of acute myocardial infarction with clinical evidence of heart failure. Lancet 1993;342:821.

Cohn J, Johnson G, Ziesche S et al: A comparison of enalapril with hydralazine-isosorbide dinitrate in the treatment of chronic congestive heart failure. N Engl J Med 1991;325:303.

CONSENSUS Trial Study Group: Effects of enalapril on mortality in severe congestive heart failure: Results of the cooperative north Scandinavian enalapril survival study (CONSENSUS). N Engl J Med 1987;316:1429.

Deedwania PC: Angiotensin-converting inhibitors in congestive heart failure. Arch Intern Med 1990;150:1798.

Heart outcomes prevention evaluation study investigators: Effects of an angiotensin-converting enzyme inhibitor, ramipril, on cardiovascular events in high-risk patients. N Engl J Med 2000;342:145.

Packer M, Poole-Wilson P, Armstrong P et al: Comparative effects of low and high doses of the angiotensin-converting enzyme inhibitor, lisinopril, on morbidity and mortality in chronic heart failure. Circulation 1999;100:2312.

Pfeffer M, Braunwald E, Moye L et al: Effect of captopril on mortality and morbidity in patients with left ventricular dysfunction after myocardial infarction. Results of the survival and ventricular enlargement trial. The SAVE Investigators: N Engl J Med. 1992;327(10):669–677.

SOLVD investigators: Effect on enalapril on mortality and the development of heart failure an asymptomatic patients with reduced left ventricular ejection fractions. N Engl J Med 1992; 327:685.

SOLVD investigators: Effect on enalapril on survival in patients with reduced left ventricular ejection fractions and congestive heart failure. N Engl J Med 1991;325:293.

e. Angiotensin II receptor blockers—The angiotensin II receptor blockers (ARB) provide direct blockade of angiotensin II type-1 (AT_1) receptor activation. This action results in the effective blockade of the potentially harmful effects of angiotensin II on tissues. This action takes place regardless of angiotensin II generation by ACE-dependent pathways or ACE-independent (alternative) pathways (Figure 18–1). In addition, this effect is achieved without accumulation of bradykinin, which is considered to be responsible for some adverse reactions associated with the use of ACEI, such as persistent cough, angioedema, and significant hypotension.

Theoretically, the use of these drugs should be associated with beneficial effects on clinical outcomes similar to those seen during ACEI therapy and with fewer side effects. The ARB have produced favorable hemodynamic effects during acute and chronic administration.

(1) Clinical outcomes—Three ARBs losartan, candesartan, and valsartan have been evaluated in patients with heart failure and depressed LVEF. In these studies, each ARB has been compared with an ACEI.

The ELITE study evaluated the effect of losartan in patients with symptomatic CHF, NYHA II–IV, an LVEF ≤0.40, and no prior treatment with an ACEI. Compared with captopril, the group receiving losartan experienced a decrease in norepinephrine levels, and a lower proportion of patients developed hyperkalemia. Also, losartan was associated with a nonsignificant lower risk of the combination events of death from all causes or hospitalization for heart failure. The drug was associated with a significantly lower risk for death from all causes. During losartan therapy there were significantly fewer episodes of sudden cardiac death.

The follow-up study, ELITE II, evaluated a much larger group of patients with CHF, NYHA II–IV, LVEF ≤0.40, and most patients had no prior treatment with an ACEI. In contrast with ELITE I, in this study, compared with captopril, treatment with losartan was associated with a greater risk for adverse clinical events. Although the losartan group experienced a lower risk of outcomes such as death from worsened heart failure, noncardiovascular death, and a lower rate of hospitalizations for heart failure, treatment with losartan was associated with a nonsignificant increased risk for death from all causes, sudden death, fatal MI, stroke, and hospitalization for any reason. However, it is important to note that compared with captopril, fewer drug-related adverse reactions occurred and fewer patients discontinued receiving losartan.

In the RESOLVD study candesartan was compared with enalapril and to the combination of enalapril-candesartan in patients with CHF, NYHA II–IV, and LVEF ≤0.40 who walked a distance <500 m within 6-min. During the study, all three-treatment groups experienced a reduction in epinephrine and norepinephrine levels. Although patients receiving candesartan achieved a greater walking distance during 6 min (primary end-point) and lower levels of renin, treatment with candesartan or with the combination enalapril-candesartan was associated with a higher risk for developing renal failure and a greater risk for death from all causes, hospitalization for heart failure, hospitalization for all causes, and for the combined end-point of death from all causes and hospitalization for all causes.

The Val-HeFT study evaluated the effect of treatment with valsartan on mortality and morbidity in patients with mild-to-moderate heart failure lasting ≥3 months, LVEF <0.40, and NYHA II–IV. Compared with placebo, treatment with valsartan was associated with similar risk for death from all causes (19.3% vs 19.7%, respectively) and a significantly lower risk (32% vs 29%, P = .009, respectively) for the combined first-end point

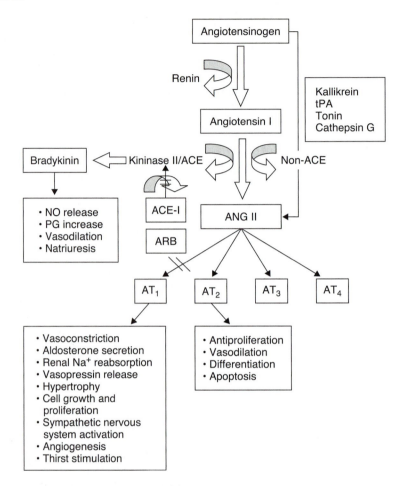

Figure 18–1. Renin-angiotensin system cascade and angiotensin II receptors. NO = nitric oxide; PG = prostaglandins; ACE = angiotensin-converting enzyme; ACE-I = angiotensin-converting enzyme inhibitor; ARB = angiotensin receptor blocker; ANG II = angiotensin II; AT_1–AT_4 = angiotensin II types 1–4.

of death, hospitalization for heart failure, resuscitated arrest, or need for intravenous inotropic or vasodilator therapy. In addition, compared with placebo, the valsartan group had a similar risk of sudden death and death due to heart failure. Treatment with valsartan also resulted in a slight but significant improvement in the relative LVEF change (3.2% vs 4.0%, P = .001, respectively), a slight but significant lower proportion of patients with worsened NYHA class (12.8% vs 10.1%, P < .001, respectively), and a slight nonsignificant lower proportion of patients with worsened NYHA class (12.8% vs 10.1%, P < .001, respectively).

Although ARB appear to be a promising class of drugs for the treatment of patients with CHF, based on the findings from the available controlled trials, results from further evaluation of these drugs in the ongoing large randomized controlled trials will be required to establish the role of ARB in treating patients with heart failure.

Cohn J, Tognoni G: A randomized trial of the angiotensin-receptor blocker valsartan in chronic heart failure. N Engl J Med 2001;345:1667.

McKelvie R, Yusuf S, Pericak D et al: Comparison of candesartan, enalapril, and their combination in congestive heart failure. The RESOLVD pilot study investigators. Circulation 1999;100:1056.

Pitt B, Poole-Wilson P, Segal R et al: Effect of losartan compared with captopril on mortality in patients with symptomatic heart failure: Randomized trial-the losartan heart failure survival study ELITE II. Lancet 2000;355:1582.

Pitt B, Segal R, Martinez F et al: Randomized trial of losartan versus captopril in patients over 65 with heart failure. Evaluation of losartan in the elderly study, ELITE. Lancet 1997;349: 747.

5. Beta-blockers—As discussed earlier, the abnormal activation of neurohumoral systems has been shown to be independently associated with higher mortality rates in patients with heart failure. The elevated circulating levels of norepinephrine indicate that a generalized activation of the adrenergic nervous system occurs as the clinical syndrome of heart failure develops. There appears to be a correlation between the extent of this activation and the limitation of functional capacity and degree of hemodynamic abnormalities. Plasma norepinephrine levels are as significant prognostically as LVEF or exercise intolerance in patients with mild-to-moderate heart failure. Although first-generation β-blocking agents (with a nonselective affinity for β_1- or β_2-receptors and no evidence of ancillary cardiovascular effects) were not well tolerated in heart failure, nonselective third-generation β-blockers with vasodilator activity (bucindolol and carvedilol) as well as the β_1-selective agent metoprolol are generally well tolerated by patients with CHF.

Several small studies have compared the effects of various β-blockers in patients with heart failure. In one study, direct comparison of carvedilol and short-acting metoprolol did not reveal significant difference on symptoms, quality of life, exercise capacity, or degree of LVEF. In another direct comparison of carvedilol and short-acting metoprolol, both drugs improved symptoms, submaximal exercise tolerance, and quality of life to a similar degree. However, compared with metoprolol, patients treated with carvedilol showed a greater increase in LVEF at rest, in LV stroke volume and in stroke work during exercise. Direct comparison of carvedilol and sustained-release metoprolol has not been performed.

a. Clinical outcomes—Clinical studies suggest that chronic β-blockade may improve hemodynamic and clinical function in patients with chronic heart failure. Patients with moderate-to-severe heart failure who received treatment with carvedilol demonstrated improvement in cardiac function and hemodynamic measurements at rest and during exercise. The beneficial effects were seen in patients with idiopathic dilated cardiomyopathy as well as in those with ischemic cardiomyopathy. More recent studies in heart failure patients treated with carvedilol demonstrated significant improvement in LVEF and invasive hemodynamic parameters, noninvasive hemodynamic variables at rest and during exercise, and the functional status of the patients.

Several recent studies have evaluated the effect of various β-blockers on clinical outcomes in patients with chronic symptomatic heart failure and depressed LVEF.

The CIBIS study evaluated bisoprolol in patients with symptoms of heart failure, LVEF <0.40, and NYHA III–IV, who were receiving "optimal" therapy with diuretics and vasodilators (ACEI preferred, hydralazine + isosorbide, digoxin, or ARB). Compared with placebo, the use of bisoprolol was associated with a nonsignificant lower risk for several events, including death from all causes, sudden death and death with documented ventricular tachycardia (VT) or ventricular fibrillation, death from heart failure, and fatal shock.

In the follow-up larger trial, the CIBIS-II study, treatment with bisoprolol was evaluated in patients with symptoms of heart failure, LVEF <0.35, and NYHA III–IV, who were receiving "optimal" therapy with diuretics and vasodilators (ACEI preferred, hydralazine + isosorbide, digoxin, or ARB). Compared with placebo, the bisoprolol group experienced a significantly lower risk for death from all causes, hospitalization for all causes, and sudden death. Also, bisoprolol therapy was associated with nonsignificant reductions in the risk of death from pump failure and the risk of fatal MI. Based on these positive findings on clinical outcomes, the CIBIS-II study was terminated earlier than the planned follow-up period. However, bisoprolol is not approved by the FDA for treatment of patients with heart failure.

In the U.S. carvedilol heart failure study (US-CarvHFSG), carvedilol was evaluated, with multiple dosage schedules, in patients with symptomatic CHF, LVEF <0.35, who were receiving ACEI and diuretic. Compared with placebo the carvedilol group experienced a significantly lower risk of secondary endpoints, including death from all causes, death from progressive heart failure, sudden death, and death associated with myocardial ischemia. Several subgroup analyses also indicated that treatment with carvedilol was associated with a reduced risk of death.

Another study (COPERNICUS) evaluated the effect of carvedilol in patients with severe heart failure (NYHA IV), LVEF <0.25, receiving diuretics, ACEI, or ARB. Compared with placebo, carvedilol was associated with a significant reduction in the risk of death from all causes and a reduction in the risk of the combined end-point of death from all causes and hospitalization for all causes.

In the CAPRICORN study, carvedilol was evaluated in stable post-MI patients with LVEF <0.40, receiving diuretic and ACEI. Similar to previous studies, compared with placebo, carvedilol was associated with significant reductions in the risk of death from all causes, cardiovascular death, and non-fatal MI. There were also nonsignificant reductions in the risk of other end-points, including death from all causes and cardiovascular hospitalization, sudden death, hospitalization for heart failure, and cardiovascular death.

Bucindolol was studied in patients with moderately severe CHF, NYHA III–IV, and LVEF ≤0.35. Compared with placebo, treatment with bucindolol resulted in improved LVEF and a reduction in plasma norepinephrine levels. However, at the conclusion of the study the bucindolol group experienced only modest nonsignificant reductions in the risk of death from all causes, sudden death, and death due to pump failure. Because of these modest, statistically nonsignificant differences, the study was terminated earlier than the planned follow-up.

Metoprolol controlled release/extended release (CR/XL) was studied in the largest β-blocker trial (MERIT-HF study) in patients with symptoms of moderate CHF, depressed LVEF, and NYHA II–IV. In this study, compared with placebo, treatment with metoprolol CR/XL was associated with significant decrease in the risk of primary and secondary clinical end-points, including death from all causes, cardiovascular mortality, sudden death, and death associated with worsening heart failure. Subsequent analyses revealed that metoprolol was associated with a significant reduced risk on several other end-points, including death from all causes or hospitalization for all causes, death or hospitalization for worsened heart failure, death or need for heart transplantation, and hospitalization for all causes.

The findings from these recent trials evaluating β-blockers in patients with varying degrees of heart failure indicate that these drugs exert a beneficial effect on LV function and improve survival as well as clinical symptoms. These findings have led to the recommendations in all guidelines for use of β-blockers in the management of heart failure (NYHA II–IV).

Beta-blocker evaluation of survival trial investigators: A trial of the beta-blocker bucindolol in patients with advanced chronic heart failure. N Engl J Med 2001;344:1659.

Bristow MR: Pathophysiologic and pharmacologic rationales for clinical management of chronic heart failure with beta-blocking agents. Am J Cardiol 1993;71:12C.

CAPRICORN investigators: Effect of carvedilol on outcome after myocardial infarction in patients with left ventricular dysfunction: The CAPRICORN randomized trial. Lancet 2001; 357:1385.

Cardiac insufficiency bisoprolol study (CIBIS): A randomized trial of beta-blockade in heart failure. Circulation 1994;90:1765.

CIBIS-II investigators and committees: The cardiac insufficiency bisoprolol study II (CIBIS-II): A randomized trial. Lancet 1999;353:9.

Eichhorn EJ: The paradox of β-adrenergic blockade for the management of congestive heart failure. Am J Med 1992;92:527.

Hjalmarson A, Goldstein S, Fagerberg B, et al: Effects of controlled-release metoprolol on total mortality, hospitalization, and well-being in patients with heart failure. JAMA 2000; 283:1295.

MERIT-HF study group: Effect of metoprolol CR/XL in chronic heart failure: Metoprolol CR/XL randomized intervention trial in congestive heart failure (MERIT-HF). Lancet 1999; 353:2001.

Metra M, Giubbini R, Nodari S et al: Differential effects of beta-blockers in patients with heart failure. Circulation 2000;102: 546.

Packer M, Bristow M, Cohn J et al: The effect of carvedilol on morbidity and mortality in patients with chronic heart failure. N Engl J Med 1996;334:1349.

Packer M, Coats A, Fowler M et al: Effect of carvedilol on survival in severe chronic heart failure. N Engl J Med 2001;344:1651.

Sanderson J, Chan S, Yip G et al: Beta-blockade in heart failure. A comparison of carvedilol with metoprolol. J Am Coll Cardiol 1999;34:1522.

6. Antiarrhythmic drugs—Patients with heart failure are at risk for sudden death presumably associated with complex ventricular arrhythmia. There has been interest in evaluating therapies targeted at reduction of this arrhythmic risk in heart failure.

The class III antiarrhythmic agents, amiodarone and dofetilide, have each been evaluated in patients with heart failure and the presence of atrial-arrhythmia or asymptomatic ventricular-arrhythmia.

Amiodarone appears to have vasodilator properties that may be of benefit in patients with heart failure. This drug is a powerful antiarrhythmic agent with little depressant effect on hemodynamic function. Available data from several studies with amiodarone show a significant increase in LVEF and improvement in exercise tolerance.

The principal focus of treatment with dofetilide was evaluation of the drug in the setting of heart failure and associated atrial fibrillation.

a. Clinical outcomes—In the GESICA study, low-dose (300 mg/day), open-label amiodarone was evaluated in patients with moderate CHF, NYHA II–IV, depressed LVEF ≤0.35, who were treated with diuretics, digoxin, and ACEI. Compared with no amiodarone, open-label amiodarone therapy was associated with statistically significant reduction in the risk of death from all causes and the combined end-point of death from all causes and hospitalization for heart failure. Also, the open-label amiodarone group experienced a lower rate of sudden death and lower risk of death associated with worsened heart failure. It is important to note, however, that in the GESICA study most patients had heart failure due to nonischemic cardiomyopathy.

In the STAT-CHF study, amiodarone was studied in patients with history of CHF; ≥ ten asymptomatic premature ventricular beats; LVEF ≤0.40; and receiving treatment with vasodilators, digoxin, and optimal diuretic therapy. Compared with placebo, treatment with amiodarone produced a greater suppression of ventricular premature beats, and a greater increase in the LVEF. However, amiodarone therapy was associated with only a nonsignificant reduction in the risk of death from all causes, sudden death, and death from pump failure.

Subgroup analyses revealed that amiodarone, did not improve survival in patients with >80% suppression of premature ventricular beats compared with patients without suppression. In addition, amiodarone also did not improve survival in patients who achieved suppression of VT episodes compared with patients without suppression of VT. Lastly, even in patients with VT at baseline, compared with placebo, amiodarone did not improve survival. However, similar to the results of the GESICA study a trend was evident toward improvement in the outcome in patients with heart failure due to nonischemic causes.

Amiodarone was also evaluated in the EMIAT study in patients with acute MI and depressed LVEF ≤0.40. In this study, compared with placebo, treatment with amiodarone resulted in no difference in death from all causes. Amiodarone was associated with small reductions in risk for arrhythmic death, and the risk for the combination end-point of death, arrhythmia, or need for resuscitation.

In the DIAMOND-CHF study, dofetilide was evaluated in patients with new or worsened moderate CHF, NYHA III–IV, and LVEF ≤0.35. In this trial, compared with placebo, treatment with dofetilide resulted in no significant difference in the end-points of death from all causes, arrhythmic death, or hospitalization for heart failure.

The findings from these studies were not encouraging and suggested that antiarrhythmic therapy needs further evaluation to help clarify the role of such therapy in patients with heart failure.

Doval H, Nul D, Grancelli H et al: Randomized trial of low-dose amiodarone in severe congestive heart failure. Lancet 1994; 344:493.

Julian D, Camm A, Frangin G et al: Randomized trial of effect of amiodarone on mortality in patients with left-ventricular dysfunction after recent myocardial infarction. Lancet 1997;349:667.

Singh S, Fletcher R, Fisher S et al: Amiodarone in patients with congestive heart failure and asymptomatic ventricular arrhythmia. N Engl J Med 1995;333:77.

Torp-Pedersen C, Moller M, Bloch-Thomsen P et al: Dofetilide in patients with congestive heart failure and left ventricular dysfunction. N Engl J Med 1999;341:857.

7. Antiischemic therapy—Coronary artery disease is the most common cause of heart failure in the United States. While most cases of heart failure associated with CAD are secondary to mechanical complications from MI (eg, pump failure, mitral regurgitation, cardiac rupture), some cases are a result of transient ventricular dysfunction related to episodes of reversible myocardial ischemia. Although not all episodes of myocardial ischemia in a given patient are associated with the development of heart failure, it seems that relatively prolonged ischemic episodes are associated

with significant abnormalities of ventricular function (diastolic dysfunction with elevated end-diastolic pressures) or mitral regurgitation from transient papillary muscle dysfunction. Conventional agents for the treatment of heart failure (eg, digitalis, ACEI, vasodilators) may prove ineffective in such cases; however, antiischemic drugs, which relieve and help prevent myocardial ischemia will effectively improve and prevent the development of symptoms of heart failure. This may help explain, in part, why β-blockers appear to be excellent drugs in patients with ischemic heart disease who suffer from recurrent episodes of angina-equivalent symptoms consistent with heart failure. These episodes may be triggered by and parallel the development of transient episodes of silent myocardial ischemia. Elderly patients frequently present with signs and symptoms of heart failure during episodes of silent myocardial ischemia. Such episodes are a common occurrence in patients with documented CAD. Simultaneous evaluation of ECG and ventricular function show that ischemic ECG changes are associated with transient depression of LVEF in some patients. Some periods of ischemia may have such a long duration that contractile function is markedly and chronically depressed (hibernating myocardium). Although irreversible myocardial damage usually does not occur in these settings, restoration of contractility may be delayed for days or weeks after the ischemia is relieved. The phenomenon of myocardial stunning is frequently observed after successful reperfusion therapy with thrombolytic agents in patients with acute MI and may also lead to transient symptoms of heart failure.

C. NONPHARMACOLOGIC TREATMENT

1. Myocardial revascularization—Heart failure associated with myocardial ischemia may be improved by myocardial revascularization.

In the 1970s, three major trials of patients with evidence of stable CAD evaluated the effects of a treatment strategy of coronary artery bypass graft surgery (CABGS) compared with no CABGS on mortality and other clinical outcomes. These trials were the VA cooperative study of surgery for coronary arterial occlusive disease (VACSS); the European coronary surgery study (ECSS); and the national heart, lung, and blood institute coronary artery surgery study (CASS).

In two of these trials (VACSS, CASS) patients with multivessel CAD and evidence of abnormal LV function were retrospectively identified as subgroups at high risk for death. The high-risk subgroups appeared to have improved clinical outcome after myocardial revascularization. In both trials a net difference in survival of 10–24% in the high-risk subgroups was observed during follow-up periods of 1–10 years. These differences were statistically significant during earlier observations and became less so during longer follow-up. In the CASS trial, compared with no-CABGS group, a similar proportion of high-risk patients developed symptoms of heart failure after CABGS (6–25% vs 5–28%, respectively) during the 1–10-year follow-up period.

Currently most clinical decisions for myocardial revascularization are based, to a great degree, on the findings from the various high-risk subgroups identified during the three major CABGS trials in patients with stable CAD. However, the findings from the post hoc analyses in patients with multivessel stable CAD and evidence of LV dysfunction have not been confirmed, as yet, in prospective, large, controlled, randomized studies.

CASS principal investigators and their associates: Coronary artery surgery study (CASS): A randomized trial of coronary artery bypass surgery. Circulation 1983;68:939.

European coronary surgery study group: Long-term results of prospective randomized study of coronary artery bypass surgery in stable angina pectoris. Lancet 1992;2:1173.

Veterans Administration coronary artery bypass surgery cooperative study group: Eleven-year survival in the veterans administration randomized trial of coronary bypass surgery for stable angina. N Engl J Med 1984;311:1333

2. Ventricular aneurysmectomy—Although patients with CAD usually experience angina in association with a LV aneurysm, heart failure may be present instead. These latter patients should be considered for surgical aneurysmectomy and myocardial revascularization. Left ventricular aneurysmectomy is usually beneficial in attenuating the symptoms of heart failure and can possibly improve survival.

3. Exercise training—Exercise is often associated with a feeling of well-being. However, there are little, if any, data to determine the effect of exercise on long-term outcomes in patients with heart failure.

The effects of exercise training were evaluated in a small study in patients with heart failure and depressed LVEF ≤0.40. In this study, patients were randomized to exercise training on a stationary bicycle over a period of 14 months or no training and then were monitored for up to 40 months. Compared with the no-training group, the training group had an improvement in LVEF as well as improvement in quality of life scores. In addition, the training group experienced a significantly lower risk of cardiac death, hospitalization for heart failure, and overall lower risk for cardiac events. Exercise training also resulted in a nonsignificant decreased risk of acute MI.

Although the findings associated with exercise training are encouraging, such results have been derived from small studies. Clearly, further evaluations from

larger ongoing studies are needed to clarify the role of exercise training on clinical outcomes in patients with heart failure.

4. Cardiac pacing—Patients with heart failure frequently have associated intraventricular conduction delay or left bundle branch block. These cardiac conduction abnormalities can trigger mechanical dyssynchrony of the ventricular contraction and adversely affect cardiac performance.

Pacing in patients with heart failure is a new concept that could lead to improved clinical outcomes. These theoretical benefits would be attained through improving the pattern of ventricular activation, reducing ventricular dyssynchrony, and optimizing synchronization between atrial and ventricular contractility. This treatment modality has been evaluated in a few uncontrolled and, more recently, some controlled trials of patients who do not require cardiac pacing due to associated bradyarrhythmias.

Uncontrolled studies in patients with heart failure who underwent cardiac pacing revealed an improvement in acute hemodynamic performance, exercise capacity, and quality of life during active pacing.

a. Clinical outcomes—Active atriobiventricular pacing was compared with inactive pacing in a crossover model after 12 weeks, in patients with heart failure, LVEF ≤0.35, NYHA II–IV, and QRS duration >120 ms, while receiving "optimal" therapy for CHF. In these patients, there was no need for cardiac pacing due to conduction problems. Compared with inactive pacing, during synchronized cardiac pacing the risks for death from all causes and death from pump failure decreased.

In another smaller study of similar format active atriobiventricular pacing was compared with inactive pacing in a crossover model after 12 weeks in patients with heart failure, LVEF ≤0.35, NYHA III, QRS duration >150 ms, and without bradyarrhythmia indication for insertion of a pacemaker. Compared with inactive pacing, during the active pacing period improvement was evident in peak oxygen consumption, distance walked during 6 min, quality of life scores, and proportion of patients with decompensation of heart failure. However, synchronized cardiac pacing was associated with an increased risk for death from all causes.

The findings from these two studies are conflicting. In addition, the periods of active therapy and follow-up were short. These factors limit the scope of conclusions that can be drawn from these limited studies. At present, further evaluation of cardiac pacing in patients with heart failure appears reasonable and will be available soon from the larger, randomized, controlled trials. Until then the use of cardiac resynchronization therapy with pacing should be only considered in very selected cases.

Cazeau S, Leclerco C, Lavergne T et al: Effect of multisite biventricular pacing in patients with heart failure and intraventricular conduction delay. N Engl J Med 2001;344:873.

Lozano I, Bocchiardo M, Achtelik M et al: Impact of biventricular pacing on mortality in a randomized crossover study of patients with heart failure and ventricular arrhythmias. PACE 2000;23(Pt. II):1711

Varmdaa C, Camm A: Pacing for heart failure. Lancet 2001;357: 1277.

5. Implantable cardiac defibrillator devices—Several studies have evaluated the effect of implantable cardiac defibrillators (ICD) on survival in patients considered at risk for complex ventricular arrhythmia and sudden death. In some studies patient eligibility criteria have included evidence of depressed cardiac function (LVEF ≤0.40). However, none of these studies have evaluated the effect of ICD on outcome in patients with clinical CHF.

a. Clinical outcomes—The Multicenter Automatic Defibrillator Implantation Trial (MADIT) evaluated the effect of ICD compared with conventional medical therapy on total mortality in patients who had suffered a Q-wave MI within 3 weeks of enrollment. Patients had experienced asymptomatic nonsustained VT 3–30 beats at > 120 bpm unrelated to acute MI, had LVEF ≤0.35, NYHA I–III, no need for revascularization <3 months. During programmed stimulation, sustained VT or ventricular fibrillation was not suppressed with procainamide or other antiarrhythmic agent. Patients received transthoracic or transvenous ICD. Conventional therapy was left at the discretion of each care provider. Antiarrhythmic drugs could be given to either group. In the MADIT study, therapy with ICD, compared with conventional medical therapy, was associated with a significantly lower risk of death from all causes (16% vs 39%, respectively, P = 0.009). Secondary analyses also revealed that treatment with ICD was associated with a nonsignificant risk for death from primary arrhythmia and nonarrhythmia death.

The MADIT study revealed improved outcome among patients with a defibrillator. However, compared with conventional therapy, a greater proportion of patients randomized to ICD received β-blockers (27% vs 5%, respectively), ACEI drugs (57% vs 51%, respectively), and digoxin (57% vs 51%, respectively). Although multivariate analyses indicated no effect of β-blockers on the primary outcome, the use of β-blockers could have certainly influenced the survival rate in patients randomized to ICD arm.

Another study, the coronary artery bypass graft patch trial (CABG-Patch), evaluated the effect of ICD, compared with no ICD, on clinical outcome in patients recovering from elective CABGS. Eligibility criteria included a LVEF <0.36 and an abnormal signal averaged ECG. In this study treatment with ICD, compared with no ICD, did not decrease risk for death from all causes (23% vs 21%, respectively) and cardiac death (16% vs 16%, respectively). In this study a similar proportion of patients on the ICD (16%) and no ICD (20%) were receiving β-blockers during the study.

A subsequent post hoc evaluation of the mode of death on the CABG-Patch study revealed that a lower proportion of ICD patients, compared with no ICD, experienced arrhythmic death (3% vs 6%, respectively). However, the treatment with ICD was associated with a greater proportion of deaths due to pump failure (7% vs 5%, respectively).

The largest study to date that has evaluated therapy with ICD is the antiarrhythmics versus implantable defibrillators study (AVID). In this study, patients were eligible for enrollment if they recovered from near-fatal ventricular fibrillation, had experienced sustained VT with syncope, or sustained VT with LVEF ≤0.40 and associated symptoms suggesting severe hemodynamic compromise due to the arrhythmia.

This study compared therapy with ICD versus antiarrhythmic drugs (mostly amiodarone). Treatment with ICD, compared with antiarrhythmic drugs, was associated with a significantly lower risk of death (16% vs 24%, respectively, $P < 0.02$). In this study, more patients in the ICD group received β-blockers (39% vs 10%, respectively). Although the proportion of patients receiving β-blockers on each group appeared to be a substantial difference, multivariate analyses indicated no apparent effect of β-blocker therapy during follow-up on the primary clinical outcome.

The Multicenter Unsustained Tachycardia Trial (MUSTT) compared the effect of programmed electrophysiologic stimulation study (PESS)-guided antiarrhythmic therapy versus no antiarrhythmic therapy on clinical outcome of cardiac arrest or arrhythmic death in patients with evidence of CAD, a LVEF ≤0.40, and asymptomatic unsustained VT (≥ three beats). Patients with sustained monomorphic VT induced by any method of stimulation and those patients with sustained polymorphic VT induce by one or two extra stimuli qualified for randomization into the study. Antiarrhythmic therapy (drugs or ICD) was not randomized.

In this study treatment with β-blockers and ACEI was encouraged. Also, nonrandomized implantation of a defibrillator device could be recommended after one or more unsuccessful antiarrhythmic drug tests.

The findings from the MUSTT study revealed that PESS-guided antiarrhythmic therapy, compared with no antiarrhythmic therapy, was associated with a nonsignificant decrease in risk (12% vs 18%, respectively) of cardiac arrest or arrhythmic death at 24 months. This risk difference (25% vs 32%, respectively, P =

0.04) became significant at 60 months follow-up. However, there was no difference between the treatment groups in regard to risk of death from all causes at 24 months (22% vs 28%, respectively), at 60 months (42% vs 48%, respectively). There was also no significant difference in the risk (34% vs 40%, respectively) of cardiac death at 5 years, or the incidence of spontaneous sustained VT (20% vs 21%, respectively).

Interestingly, during follow-up a greater proportion of patients in the PESS-guided antiarrhythmic therapy received β-blockers or antiarrhythmic drugs with β-blocker properties (63% vs 53%, respectively) and underwent nonrandomized implantation of an ICD (58% vs 3%, respectively).

Antiarrhythmics versus implantable defibrillators (AVID) investigators: A comparison of antiarrhythmic-drugs therapy with implantable defibrillators in patients resuscitated from near-fatal ventricular arrhythmias. N Engl J Med 1997;337:1576.

Bigger JT: Prophylactic use of implanted cardiac defibrillators in patients at high risk for ventricular arrhythmias after coronary-artery bypass graft surgery. N Engl J Med 1997;337:1569.

Bigger T, Whang W, Rottman J: A randomized trial of implantable cardiac defibrillator prophylaxis in patients at high risk of death after coronary artery bypass graft surgery. Circulation 1999;99:1416.

Buxton A, Lee K, Fisher J: Multicenter unsustained tachycardia trial investigators. A randomized study of the prevention of sudden death in patients with coronary artery disease. N Engl J Med 1999;341:1882.

Moss A, Hall J, Cannon D: Improved survival with an implanted defibrillator in patients with coronary disease at high risk for ventricular arrhythmia. N Engl J Med 1996;335:1933.

6. Cardiac transplantation—Patients with severe heart failure with a limited life expectancy might be considered candidates for heart transplantation (Table 18–9). The conventional criteria for consideration of heart transplantation for patients suffering from heart failure include advanced heart failure (NYHA III–IV) with objective evidence indicating severe limitation of functional ability and an estimated poor 1-month prognosis in the face of optimized or maximized medical therapy, low-output state or refractory cardiac failure requiring frequent or constant use of inotropes, cardiogenic shock or low-output hemodynamic state with reversible end-organ dysfunction requiring mechanical circulatory support, recurrence of or rapidly progressing heart failure unresponsive to optimized or maximized vasodilator and diuretic therapies. The use of ACEI, β-blockers, and spironolactone should be incorporated to the list of medications needed to optimize therapy in these patients.

Cardiac transplantation is associated with a better NYHA functional class and significantly improved hemodynamic and neurohumoral parameters. The elevated levels of norepinephrine before transplantation

Table 18–9. Criteria for cardiac transplantation.

End-stage heart disease with poor (6–12 month) prognosis and refractory to aggressive tailored medical or any other surgical treatment
NYHA functional class III or IV
Age ≤60–65 years (various programs)
Pulmonary vascular resistance <3 RU or <2.5 RU after intravenous nitroprusside
Strong self-motivation and psychosocial support
Absence of
  Malignancy
  Active infection
  Active peptic ulcerative disease
  Pulmonary infarction within 6 weeks
  Advanced insulin-dependent diabetes mellitus with end-organ damage (relative)
  Kidney or liver dysfunction beyond that expected from severe CHF
  Advanced peripheral vascular disease
  Collagen vascular diseases
  Active alcoholism or substance abuse

CHF = congestive heart failure; NYHA = New York Heart Association; RU = resistance units.

return toward baseline after the transplant, and the increased levels of norepinephrine seen at various exercise loads also tend to normalize. Patients are generally able to exercise longer and achieve a higher level of oxygen consumption during graded exercise testing after the cardiac transplant. A study evaluating pulmonary function test parameters before and after heart transplantation revealed that the forced vital capacity, forced expiratory volume in 1 second, and lung volumes improved significantly; the forced vital capacity increased in proportion to the decrease in cardiac volume after transplantation.

Not infrequently, heart failure patients might be hastily referred to undergo evaluation for possible heart transplantation. In one study the majority of patients referred for evaluation of heart transplantation were under-treated or had an absolute contraindication for transplantation. In this report, among patients with heart failure considered to be too well for heart transplantation, after stabilization with adequate treatment approximately 84% of patients were alive and well during follow-up.

a. Clinical outcomes—For several years heart transplantation has been considered a suitable treatment option in patients with advanced heart failure. Extensive clinical experience in the last 15–20 years has shown that cardiac transplantation is an effective optional therapy in advanced end-stage heart failure. In 1999, the international registry of cardiac transplantation, reported a 79% survival at 1 year with subsequent 4% mortality rate per year. However, other reports have described lower survival rates at 1 year.

The shortage of donor hearts, however, makes transplantation unavailable to most patients with end-stage heart failure, and many patients die while waiting for a donor organ. Furthermore, the stringent criteria used to select potential candidates make many patients ineligible. The qualification criteria are intended to identify the patients who are at highest risk and who may derive the greatest benefit from heart transplantation. Some patients, however, spontaneously improve while waiting for a suitable donor; this improvement has been accompanied by prolonged survival during the relatively short follow-up period. Furthermore, advances in medical and surgical therapies have been associated with improvement in clinical outcomes for patients with advanced heart failure. Compared with 10–20 years ago, these newer drug therapies have cast some uncertainty over the benefits of cardiac transplantation compared with other treatment options in advanced heart failure.

There is scarce data, if any, from prospective, randomized studies comparing the effect of aggressive medical therapy with heart transplantation on clinical outcomes in patients with severe heart failure.

Findings from a few studies in patients with heart failure suggest that the approach to treatment with heart transplant should be reevaluated in prospective, controlled clinical trials.

A couple of retrospective reports in heart failure patients who underwent heart transplantation looked into the outcomes in patients who had been on a waiting list for ≥6 months.

One report described CHF patients who underwent transplant evaluation, tailored medical therapy and, in some patients, routine transplantation. The recipient of heart transplantation was determined by time duration on the waiting list.

In this report, the actuarial survival of patients discharged on tailored therapy was 67% at 1 year without transplantation. Sudden death was the most frequent mode of death (43 of 51 deaths). The actuarial survival for posttransplantation patients was 88% at 1 year ($P = .009$) compared with medical therapy.

However, because most deaths in this study occurred within the first 6 months, the authors noted that the likelihood for survival without transplantation improved in outpatients who survived the initial 6 months. This calculation resulted in a projected subsequent survival at 1 year of 88% (similar to patients with transplantation), with or without transplantation performed at that time.

Another post hoc report described data from patients with end-stage heart failure (NYHA III IV) who had spent >6 months on a heart transplant waiting list. Patients underwent periodic clinical reevaluations after the initial assessment. Some patients did not receive heart transplantation (no-transplant group) and some patients received heart transplantation (transplant group). After ≥6 months, compared with the no-transplant group, heart transplantation was associated with similar mortality rates from all causes during a follow up of 18 months (no-transplant 18% vs transplant 24%).

A prospective observational study (German COCPIT study) in patients with heart failure who were consecutively listed for cardiac transplantation, evaluated the mortality risk while on the waiting list and the need for urgent cardiac transplantation. This study assessed clinical and prognostic profiles in order to analyze the effect of the intention-to-treat by transplantation. The a priori heart failure score was calculated and used to categorize patients into low, medium, and high risk.

Transplantation effect was reported as relative risk described as the ratio of risk of death after transplantation versus the risk of death while on the waiting list for the same period of time. A ratio <1 implied that patients benefited from transplantation. If the ratio was > 1, then survival after cardiac transplantation was not superior to survival while on the waiting list.

In this study, survival at 1 year was 71% for all patients. Survival at 1 year for the high-, medium-, and low-risk groups were 64%, 76% and 75%, respectively ($P = .02$).

The main finding from this study was the lack of survival benefit from transplantation for the group as a whole. However, heart transplantation had a beneficial effect on the high-risk group. This beneficial effect (relative risk <1) was apparent <2 weeks after transplantation but it disappeared after 8 months when the relative risk became >1. On the medium- and low-risk groups the relative risk was always >1 during follow-up, suggesting a lack of beneficial effect for heart transplantation.

A randomized trial to evaluate cardiac transplantation has been considered ethically objectionable. In addition, it has been assumed that heart transplantation will result in better quality of life and decreased mortality risk.

However, in light of recent advances in medical therapy for heart failure, findings from post hoc analyses suggesting limited benefit from heart transplantation, and the findings from the German COCPIT study indicating limited or no benefit from heart transplantation, it has been suggested that consideration should be given to a randomized trial with cardiac transplantation in patients with advanced heart failure.

Anguita M et al: Spontaneous clinical and hemodynamic improvement in patients on waiting list for heart transplantation. Chest 1992;102:96.

Deng M, Meester J, Smits J et al: Effect of receiving a heart transplant: Analysis of a national cohort entered on to a waiting list, stratified by heart failure severity. BMJ 2000;321:540.

Deng M, Smits J, Meester J et al: Heart transplantation indicated only in the most severely ill patient: Perspectives from the German heart transplant experience. Curr Opin Cardiol 2001;16:97.

Freudenberger R, Sikora J, Gottlieb S et al: Congestive heart failure. Characteristics of patients referred for cardiac transplantation: Implications for the donor organ shortage. Am Heart J 2000;140:857.

Hosenpud J, Bennett L, Keck B et al: The registry of the international society for heart and lung transplantation: Sixteenth official report: 1999. J Heart Lung Transplant 1999;18(7):611.

Hosenpud JD, Stibolt T, Atwal K et al: Abnormal pulmonary function specifically related to congestive heart failure: Comparison of patients before and after cardiac transplantation. Am J Med 1990;88:493.

Kao W, McGee D, Liao Y et al: Does heart transplantation confer additional benefit over medical therapy to patients who have waited > 6 months for heart transplantation? J Am Coll Cardiol 1994;24:1547.

Koerner M, Durand J, Lafuente J et al: Cardiac transplantation: The final therapeutic option for the treatment of heart failure. Curr Opin Cardiol 2000;15:178.

Kubo SH, Ormaza S, Francis G et al: Trends in patient selection for heart transplantation. J Am Coll Cardiol 1993;21:975.

Stevenson L, Hamilton M, Tillisch I et al: Decreasing survival benefit from cardiac transplantation for outpatients as the waiting list lengthens. J Am Coll Cardiol 1991;18:919.

7. Circulatory-assist devices—These devices can offer additional options for the treatment of patients with severe heart failure who deteriorate despite aggressive pharmacologic therapy and who may be considered candidates for heart transplantation. In general, the reasons for assisting circulation with these devices are to provide ventricular assistance and allow the heart to rest and recover its function in cases of expected recovery and to provide circulatory assistance as a bridge to cardiac transplantation in patients with extensive acute MI, acute myocarditis, or advanced end-stage heart disease or failure on whom recovery of adequate cardiac function is not expected. Several devices, which include extracorporeal membrane oxygenation, univentricular and biventricular extracorporeal nonpulsatile devices; extracorporeal and implantable pulsatile devices; the total artificial heart; and many others, are in various stages of development, and some are currently available for cardiac mechanical support. They are generally classified according to the extent of cardiac support achieved from the degree of stroke volume generated by the device and the length of support provided.

Left ventricular assist devices (LVAD) used as a bridge in patients considered for heart transplantation, provide improvement in hemodynamic status at rest and achievement of a reasonable exercise capacity.

The FDA has approved two such devices: the ThermoCardiosystems Heartmate device and the Novavcor N100 LV assist system, to be used as bridges to cardiac transplantation.

Several factors can affect the use of an LVAD: the presence of valvular heart disease (mitral stenosis or aortic regurgitation), CAD (risk of right heart dysfunction), congenital defects, and dysfunction of end organs. The presence of irreversible major neurologic deficit(s) is considered a contraindication for a LVAD as well as for cardiac transplantation.

The use of assisted circulation is associated with risk of complications as bleeding, right-sided heart failure, renal insufficiency, infection, air- and thromboembolic events, and progressive multisystem organ failure. Some of these complications, particularly infection and renal failure, carry an increased risk of death. Patients may become ineligible for heart transplantation if they develop severe complications during the period of mechanically assisted circulation.

The concept of "bridge to recovery" might become a goal for ventricular assist devices; however, several issues, particularly reliability for long-term use, need to be determined prior to wide-spread and extended use of these devices in advanced heart failure.

It is also important to keep in mind that mechanical circulatory support is expensive and can greatly tax the available resources and personnel; it should therefore be considered only in exceptional situations where reversal of the underlying condition or early transplantation is expected.

a. Clinical outcomes—Limited data are available from randomized controlled settings to help evaluate the role of LVAD in patients with heart failure.

The REMATCH study evaluated the suitability of LVAD as long-term myocardial replacement treatment in patients with severe heart failure (NYHA IV) for ≥90 days who were deemed ineligible for cardiac transplantation. In this study patients were randomized to receive a vented electric LVAD and associated medical care or to receive medical therapy aimed at optimizing organ perfusion and minimizing symptoms of CHF. Compared with optimal medical therapy, treatment with the LVAD was associated with a lower risk (89% vs 60%, $P = .001$, respectively) of death. This effect was significant (75% vs 48%, $P = .002$, respectively) at the 1-year follow-up period, but not at 2 years (92% vs 77%, $P = .09$, respectively).

Although the limited available data suggest that circulatory assist devices harbor a potential beneficial effect on clinical outcomes, further use of these devices will be closely linked to findings from large, controlled studies comparing the use of LVAD with medical therapy.

Deng M, Smits J, Meester J et al: Heart transplantation indicated only in the most severely ill patient: Perspectives from the

German heart transplant experience. Curr Opin Cardiol 2001;16:97.

Goldstein D, Mehmet O, Rose E: Implantable left ventricular assist devices. N Engl J Med 1998;339:1522.

Rose E, Gelijns A, Moskowitz A et al: Long-term use of a left ventricular assist device for end-stag heart failure. REMATCH study group. N Engl J Med 2001;345:1435.

D. TREATMENT OF ASYMPTOMATIC PATIENTS

Although it had been thought that ventricular dysfunction in the absence of overt heart failure did not warrant treatment, studies in asymptomatic patients with documented ventricular dysfunction and in patients without heart disease but considered at risk for cardiovascular events suggest that intervention in the early stages of LV dysfunction or treatment after recognition of risk may result in fewer complications and improved survival rates (Figure 18–2). Because of the use of aggressive thrombolytic therapy in acute MI, more patients now survive the acute event, many with evidence of LV systolic dysfunction. Ventricular dilatation and dysfunction occur as a function of myocardial remodeling shortly after MI. These changes in cardiac geometry and function have adverse consequences that increase the risk of complications and mortality. Early intervention with captopril is recommended to prevent LV remodeling in post-MI patients with LVEF of less than 0.35. This treatment has been associated with reduced mortality rates and a lower rate of recurrent infarctions (Figure 18–3).

Two studies have evaluated the effect of intervention with ACEI on clinical outcomes in patients with asymptomatic cardiac dysfunction and in patients considered at risk for cardiovascular events.

In the SOLVD-prevention study in patients with LV dysfunction who were asymptomatic, the use of ACEI (enalapril), compared with placebo, was associated with a nonsignificant reduction in risk for death from all causes and a significantly lower risk of developing congestive heart failure.

In the HOPE trial, patients without evidence of heart disease but who were identified at high risk for future cardiovascular events were treated with ACEI (ramipril) or with placebo. The ACEI treatment was associated with a significantly lower risk of the combined end-point of cardiovascular death, MI, or stroke. Ramipril was also associated with a lower risk for each of these outcomes separately as well as a significant decrease in the risk of developing heart failure.

The findings from these large studies in patients with newly diagnosed cardiac dysfunction or in patients considered at future risk of cardiovascular events suggest that a therapeutic strategy with preventive interventions would lead to improved clinical outcomes.

SOLVD Investigators: Effect of enalapril on mortality and the development of heart failure in asymptomatic patients with reduced left ventricular ejection fractions. N Engl J Med 1992; 327:685.

Yusuf S, Sleight P Pogue J et al: Effects of angiotensin-converting-enzyme inhibitor, ramipril, on cardiovascular events in high-risk patients. N Engl J Med 2000;342:145.

Summary

Heart failure is a complex clinical syndrome associated with adverse clinical outcome and increased likelihood of death. It can develop at various points in the natural history of a number of cardiac disorders and systemic illnesses. In general, the prognosis of patients with heart failure is closely related to the degree of ventricular dysfunction, the amount of oxygen consumption during exercise, and the extent of activation of neurohumoral axes, including the sympathetic nervous system and the renin-angiotensin-aldosterone system. Newer strategies in the treatment of heart failure are

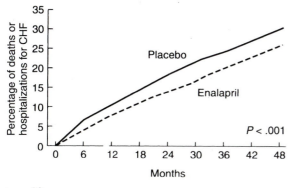

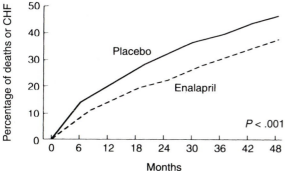

Figure 18–2. Rate of death or hospitalization for congestive heart failure (CHF), and death or development of heart failure in the Studies of Left Ventricular Dysfunction (SOLVD) prevention trial. Reprinted, with permission, from The SOLVD Investigators: Effect of enalapril on mortality and the development of heart failure in asymptomatic patients with reduced left ventricular ejection fractions. N Engl J Med 1992;327:685.

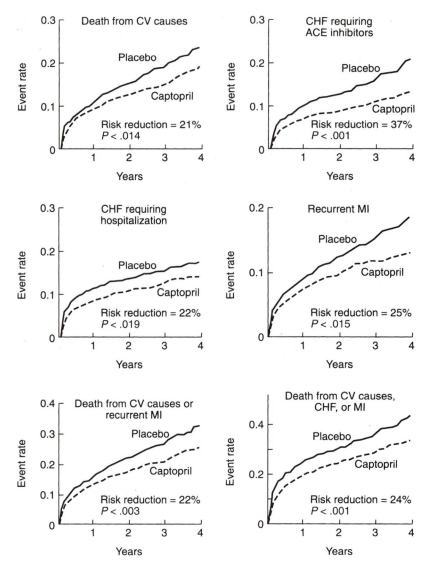

Figure 18–3. Cumulative fatal and nonfatal cardiovascular events. ACE = angiotensin-converting enzyme; CHF = congestive heart failure; CV = cardiovascular; MI = myocardial infarction. Reprinted, with permission, from Pfeffer M, Braunwald E, Moye L et al: Effect of captopril on mortality and morbidity in patients with left ventricular dysfunction after myocardial infarction. N Engl J Med 1992;327:669.

based on these and other factors that influence both the pathogenesis and prognosis of heart failure. Despite better diagnostic techniques and treatment options, however, heart failure remains a progressively deteriorating condition associated with increased morbidity and mortality.

Some clinical parameters may be useful in identifying CHF patients at an increased risk of mortality; these include: severity of LV dysfunction (measured as

ejection fraction), circulating levels of neurohormones (particularly norepinephrine), abnormalities of heart rate (fixed rapid rate), NYHA functional class, and complex atrial and ventricular tachyarrhythmias. The prognosis also appears to vary according to the cause of the underlying heart failure.

Because the prognosis of patients after they develop heart failure is quite guarded, the ideal therapeutic strategy should be directed at its prevention. This includes prompt intervention in individuals considered at risk of heart failure when evidence of impaired LV function is first detected.

Packer M: The neurohormonal hypothesis: A theory to explain the mechanism of disease progression in heart failure. J Am Coll Cardiol 1992;20:248.

Pfeffer MA, Braunwald E, Moye L et al, on behalf of the SAVE investigators: Effect of captopril on mortality and morbidity in patients with left ventricular dysfunction after myocardial infarction. N Engl J Med 1992;327:669.

Weber K, Anversa P, Armstrong P et al: Remodeling and reparation of the cardiovascular system. J Am Coll Cardiol 1992;20:3.

Supraventricular Arrhythmias

Barry M. Weinberger, DO, Roger Marinchak, MD & Peter R. Kowey, MD

INTRODUCTION

ESSENTIALS OF DIAGNOSIS

- Heart rate greater than 100 bpm
- Individual R-R interval less than 600 ms
- Rhythm supraventricular in origin

General Considerations

Supraventricular arrhythmias are rhythm disturbances localized to the atria as well as those that occur at the atrioventricular node. Much of our present knowledge arises from animal laboratory studies as well as clinical electrophysiologic evaluations. Arrhythmias occur due to a variety of mechanisms, reentry being the most common, but also including enhanced or abnormal automaticity and triggered activity. With the emergence of radiofrequency ablation and its significant success in eliminating these arrhythmias associated with a low-risk profile, there has been enormous interest in and application of this modality for patients with symptomatic arrhythmias. Pharmacologic therapy will also be reviewed (Table 19–1). This chapter will focus on supraventricular arrhythmias other than atrial fibrillation, their clinical presentation, mechanism, and therapy including radiofrequency ablation and new innovative mapping systems.

The broad category of supraventricular arrhythmias encompasses rhythm disturbances whose origins lie in the sinus node, the atrial myocardium, the atrioventricular (AV) node, and the pulmonary veins or those that perpetuate themselves by using abnormal electric circuits. Despite the variety of these arrhythmias, most are readily diagnosed through careful inspection of the electrocardiogram (ECG) or rhythm strip. This chapter deals with arrhythmias falling within the normal (60–100 bpm) and tachycardic (>100 bpm) ranges.

Bradyarrhythmias (<60 bpm) are dealt with elsewhere in this book.

Pathophysiology & Etiology

Three mechanisms account for arrhythmia genesis. **Reentrant arrhythmias,** by far the most common, sustain themselves by repetitively following a revolving pathway comprising two limbs, one that takes the impulse away from, and one that carries it back to, the site of origin. For reentry to exist an area of slow conduction must occur, and each limb must have a different refractory period (see the discussion on AV nodal reentrant tachycardia). Programmed stimulation or pacing, by inducing refractoriness in one limb of the circuit, can reliably initiate a reentrant tachycardia. Once established, pacing can terminate the tachycardia by interfering with impulse propagation in one of the limbs. The second mechanism, **automaticity,** refers to spontaneous and, often, repetitive firing from a single focus, which may either be ectopic or may originate in the sinus node. It should be noted that automaticity is an intrinsic property of all myocardial cells. This mechanism comprises two subcategories. **Enhanced automaticity** is defined as a focus that fires spontaneously and may originate in the sinus node, subsidiary pacemakers in the atrium including the Eustachian ridge, Bachmann's bundle, coronary sinus and AV valves, the AV node, His–Purkinje system, and the ventricles. The development of a junctional tachycardia resulting from the administration of a β_2-agonist, like isoproterenol, is an example of the AV junction usurping control from the sinus node. **Abnormal automaticity** is usually secondary to a disease process causing alterations in ionic flow that produces a lower (ie, more positive) resting diastolic membrane potential. Threshold potential is therefore more easily attained, thereby increasing the probability of a sustained arrhythmia.

An automatic focus may not express itself unless there is a pause or a decrease in the periodicity of the preceding predominant rhythm. Overdrive suppression by pacing, which depends on hyperpolarization of the cell membrane, does not terminate automatic rhythms because it cannot overcome the high resting potential

Table 19–1. Antiarrhythmic drugs for supraventricular arrhythmias.

Agent	Indication	Intravenous Dose	Oral Dose	Adverse Effects	Drug Interactions
Class Ia					
Quinidine	AF, AFL, AVNRT, AVRT	6–10 mg/kg over 20–30 min	200–400 mg q4–6h; q8h with long-acting preparations	Hypotension (especially IV), ventricular proarrhythmia, GI disturbance, thrombocytopenia	↑ digitalis level ↑ warfarin effect ↑ metoprolol, propranolol, propafenone levels
Procainamide	AF, AFL, AVNRT, AVRT	*Bolus:* 15 mg/kg given as 20 mg/min *Infusion:* 2–4 mg/min	50 mg/kg/day q3–4h; bid dosage with long-acting preparation	GI disturbance, hypotension, SLE, agranulocytosis, FUO hemolytic anemia, myasthenia gravis aggravation, ventricular proarrhythmia	↑ Proc level with cimetidine, quinidine & amiodarone
Class 1c					
Flecainide	AF, AFL, AT, AVNRT, AVRT	N/A	100–200 mg q12h	Ventricular proarrhythmia, CHF, GI disturbance CNS (dizziness, tremor, light-headness)	↑ digitalis level ↑ flecainide level with amiodarone, cimetidine, norpace, propranolol ↓ flecainide level with smoking
Propafenone	AF, AFL, AVNRT, AVRT	N/A	150–300 mg q8h	GI disturbance, CNS (dizziness), metallic taste, CHF, 1° AVB, IVCD, + ANA	Synergism with β-blockers
Class II (IV)					
Esmolol	Ventricular rate control for AF, AFL, ST, AT	*Bolus:* 500 µg/kg over 1–2 min *Infusion:* 50–200 µg/kg/min	N/A	CHF, AVB, bradycardia, bronchospasm	
Propranolol	Ventricular rate control for AF, AFL, ST, AT	1–5 mg at 1 mg/min	20–320 mg/day q6h, q8h, q12h or qd, depending on preparation	CHF, AVB, bradycardia, bronchospasm	
Class III					
Sotalol	AF, AFL, AVNRT, AVRT, AT	N/A	80–160 mg q12h	Dyspnea, fatigue, dizziness, CHF, bradycardia, ventricular proarrhythmia, bronchospasm	Synergism with Ca²⁺ antagonists or β-blockers

AF = atrial fibrillation; AFL = atrial flutter; ANA = antinuclear antigen; AT = atrial tachycardia; AVB = AV block; AVNRT = AV nodal reentrant tachycardia; CHF = congestive heart failure; CNS = central nervous system; FUO = fever of unknown origin; GI = gastrointestinal; IV = intravenous; IVCD = intraventricular conduction delay; LFT = liver function tests; MAT = multifocal atrial trachycardia; N/A = not applicable; NAPA = N-acetyl procainamide; SLE = systemic lupus erythematosus; ST = sinus tachycardia.

(continued)

Table 19–1. Antiarrhythmic drugs for supraventricular arrhythmias *(continued)*

Agent	Indication	Intravenous Dose	Oral Dose	Adverse Effects	Drug Interactions
Class III (continued)					
Amiodarone	AF, AFL, AVNRT, AVRT, AT	*Bolus:* 150 mg over 10 min *Infusion:* 1 mg/min × 6h, then 0.5 mg/min	100–400 mg qd	Pulmonary toxicity, CHF, tremor, bradycardia, ↑ LFTs, corneal deposits, skin discoloration, GI intolerance, hyper-/hypothyroidism	↑ digoxin levels ↑ warfarin effect ↑ quinidine, prox/NAPA, flecainide ↑ dilantin level
Ibutilide	AF, AFL	1 mg bolus over 10 min 2nd bolus, if needed, after 10-min wait	N/A	Ventricular proarrhythmia, hypotension, GI disturbance	
Dofetilide	AF, AFL	N/A	125–500 µg bid modified by algorithm	Ventricular proarrhythmia, headache, chest pain, nausea, dizziness	Contraindicated with verapamil, cimetidine, ketoconazole, trimethoprim
Class IV					
Cardizem	AF, AFL, AVNRT, AVRT, AT, MAT	*Bolus:* 0.25 mg/min over 2 min then 0.35 mg/kg in 15 min if needed *Infusion:* 5–15 mg/h	90–360 mg/day in 1–4 divided doses, depending on preparation	Hypotension, bradycardia, CHF, AVB	Synergism with β-blockers
Verapamil	AF, AFL, AVNRT, AVRT, AT, MAT	2.5–20 mg over 20 min in divided doses	40–120 mg q8h; 240–360 mg qd of long-acting preparation	Hypotension, bradycardia, CHF, AVB	Synergism with β-blockers
Class V					
Adenosine	SVT diagnosis AVNRT, AVRT, AT termination	6 mg IV rapid bolus followed by 12 mg × 2 if needed. Half dosage if administered in central line	N/A	Chest tightness, facial flushing, dyspnea, AVB	↑ activity by dipyridamole ↓ activity by theophylline
Digoxin	Ventricular rate control for AF, AFL, AT (generally not very effective in active patients)	Up to 1.0 mg bolus in divided doses followed by 0.125–0.375 mg/day	0.125–0.375 mg/ day in single dose	GI disturbance, conduction defects, atrial/ventricular arrhythmias, headache, visual disturbances	↑ *Digoxin level:* amiodarone, quinidine, verapamil, indomethacin, spironolactone, alprazolam, erythromycin, tetracycline ↓ *Digoxin level:* antacids, cholestyramine, rifampin, neomycin ↑ Risk of digitalis toxicity with potassium depleting diuretics

AF = atrial fibrillation; AFL = atrial flutter; ANA = antinuclear antigen; AT = atrial tachycardia; AVB = AV block; AVNRT = AV nodal reentrant tachycardia; AVRT = AV reciprocating tachycardia; CHF = congestive heart failure; CNS = central nervous system; FUO = fever of unknown origin; GI = gastrointestinal; IV = intravenous; IVCD = intraventricular conduction delay; LFT = liver function tests; MAT = multifocal atrial trachycardia; N/A = not applicable; NAPA = N-acetyl procainamide; SLE = systemic lupus erythematosus; ST = sinus tachycardia.

present. At best, the rhythm may be transiently suppressed. Entrance block into the abnormal tissue can also make overdrive pacing ineffective. Some of the most frequent causes of abnormal automaticity include acute myocardial infarction, electrolyte disturbance (especially hypokalemia), chronic lung disease or pulmonary infection, acute alcohol ingestion, hypoxia, and cardiac stimulants (eg, theophylline, cocaine).

In automaticity, the P waves are identical to one another but and commonly, although not always, differ from the sinus P waves. A well-defined isoelectric baseline distinguishes this rhythm from atrial flutter, and the characteristic initial warm-up period of gradual rate increase distinguishes it from reentry.

The third mechanism, **triggered arrhythmias,** depends on oscillations in the membrane potential that closely follow an action potential. In the absence of a new external electrical stimulus, these oscillations, or **after-depolarizations,** cause new action potentials to develop. Thus each new action potential results from the previous action potential. These arrhythmias can be produced by early or late after-depolarization, depending on the timing of the first after-depolarization relative to the preceding action potential (the one that spawned the triggered activity). In **early after-depolarizations,** membrane repolarization is incomplete, which allows an action potential to be initiated by a subthreshold stimulus. This type is often associated with electrolyte disturbance and may be the mechanism responsible for arrhythmogenesis related to the prolonged-QT syndrome and torsade de pointes caused by quinidine. With **delayed after-depolarization,** membrane repolarization is complete, but an abnormal intracellular calcium load causes spontaneous depolarization. The reason for the high calcium levels is unclear, but it can be related to inhibition of the sodium pump by drugs such as digoxin. In either type of arrhythmia, the process may be repetitive and lead to a sustained tachycardia.

Because reentrant, automatic, and triggered tachycardias are treated differently, it is important to be able to identify them correctly. This is discussed more fully in the section Automatic (Ectopic) Atrial Tachycardia.

General Diagnostic Approach

Rhythm interpretation is a logical process with a few simple steps that start with carefully scrutinizing the ECG tracing for P waves. Because they are frequently obscured by the larger amplitude QRS and T waves (Figure 19–1), P waves are not always readily visible. Discerning the location of the P waves requires careful scrutiny on the part of the interpreter. The optimal leads to look for P waves are II, III, aVf, and V_1. Because the diagnosis can be made or missed in this initial evaluation, its importance cannot be overemphasized.

Next, the relationship between the P waves and the QRS complexes must be examined. If there is a 1:1 relationship, do the P waves precede or follow the QRS? If there is not a 1:1 relationship, are there several P waves for each QRS (or vice versa)?

Checking the P wave in leads II, III, and aVf will show whether the atrium is being depolarized from top to bottom or from bottom to top. Each beat emanating from the sinoatrial node activates the atrium in a superior-to-inferior direction. Because the wavefront is approaching them, the inferior ECG leads record this as a positive, or upright, P wave deflection. If the atrium is depolarized in an inferior-to-superior manner, the inferior leads should inscribe a negative P wave. This would occur if an atrial premature beat (APB) were to originate from the inferior portion of the atrium or if the ventricle activates the atrium in a retrograde fashion (discussed later).

Three points regarding patient telemetry monitoring and data acquisition deserve emphasis.

- Whenever possible, a 12-lead ECG should be taken during an arrhythmia to reveal subtleties that may not be visible on a single-lead recording.
- P waves are usually best discerned in monitor leads II, III, aVf, and V_1, as mentioned earlier, but when this is not the case, different lead configurations should be tried. Monitoring with the modified chest leads (MCL; Figure 19–2), which are bipolar analogs of the standard precordial V leads, often provides good P wave identification. MCL_1 is very good for this purpose. To differentiate supraventricular tachycardia with aberrant conduction (see later discussion) from ventricular tachycardia, MCL_1, MCL_6, V_1, or V_6 is superior to a single lead II, and the two MCL leads or the two V leads used in combination are better than the usual monitoring pair of leads II and V_1.
- When P waves cannot be seen on an ECG or rhythm strip, other modalities can aid in the diagnosis.

Patients undergoing coronary artery bypass surgery often have atrial and ventricular epicardial pacing wires placed at the time of surgery. These are extended through the chest wall so that they can be connected to a temporary external pacemaker to deliver pacing therapy in the event of a rhythm disturbance. Alternatively, these wires can be attached to the channels of an ECG machine or monitor. Displaying the atrial and ventricular tracings separately solves the problem of P wave position relative to the QRS.

Tracings can also be obtained from the esophagus, which courses immediately posterior to the left atrium. A bipolar esophageal probe is advanced to the stomach or distal esophagus and then pulled back until large P waves and smaller amplitude (far-field) QRS complexes are inscribed. High-pass filter settings should be

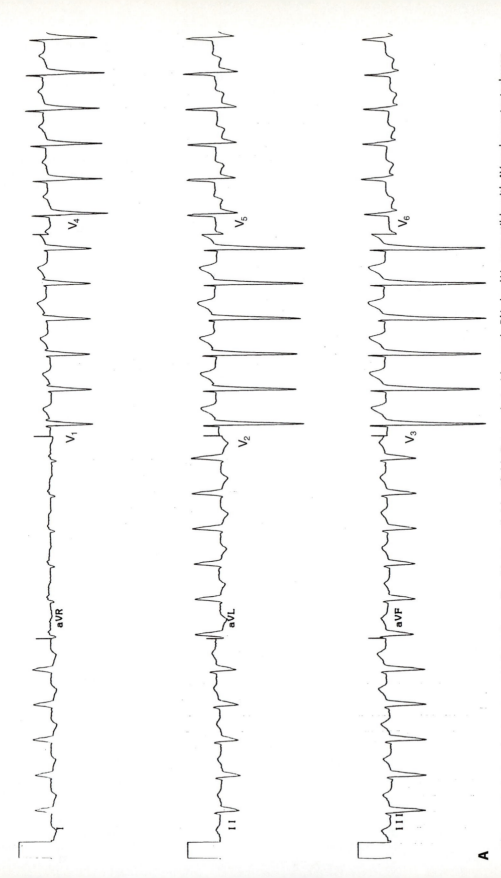

Figure 19–1. Panel A: Supraventricular tachycardia without easily identifiable P waves but with pseudo R' in lead V_1, compatible with AV node reentry tachycardia. Panel B: Postconversion tracing. Note normal QRS in lead V_1 when patient displays normal sinus rhythm.

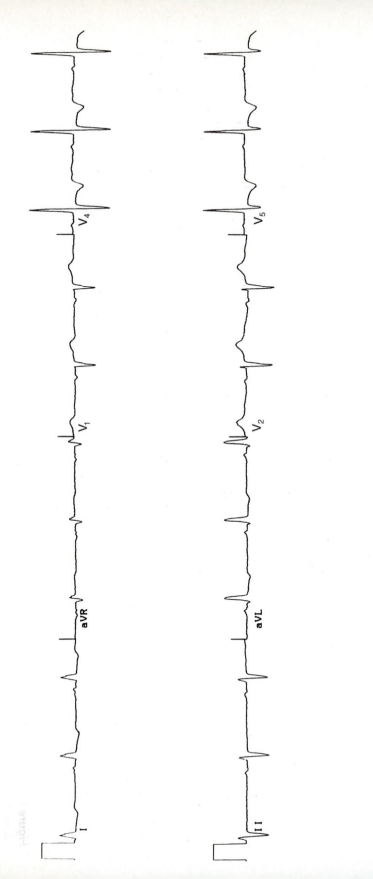
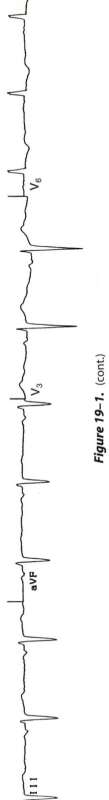

Figure 19–1. (cont.)

B

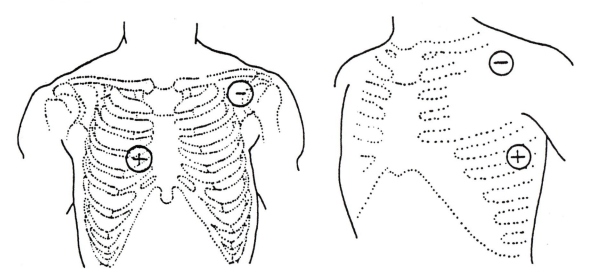

Figure 19–2. Electrode positions for obtaining the bipolar or modified precordial leads MCL$_1$ (*left*) and MCL$_6$ (*right*). Reprinted, with permission, from Drew BJ, Scheinman MM: Value of electrocardiographic leads MCL$_1$, MCL$_6$, and other selected leads in the diagnosis of wide QRS complex tachycardia. J Am Coll Cardiol 1991:18:1025.

10–20 Hz in order to exclude a low-frequency esophageal motion artifact.

Epicardial wires and esophageal recordings are especially helpful and quick ways of diagnosing atrial arrhythmias when P waves are not visible on the surface ECG and of differentiating supraventricular from ventricular tachycardia.

Electrophysiologic studies remain the definitive tool for determining arrhythmia diagnosis, mechanism, risk stratification, and treatment, however. Catheters strategically placed within various regions of the heart can yield information that is not accessible by other means.

Drew BJ, Scheinman MM: Value of electrocardiographic leads MCL$_1$, MCL$_6$ and other selected leads in the diagnosis of wide QRS complex tachycardia. J Am Coll Cardiol 1991;18:1025.

Podrid PJ, Kowey PR: Cardiac Arrhythmia, Mechanisms, Diagnosis and Management. Chapter 4.1, 2nd ed. Philadelphia: Williams and Wilkins, 2001.

Differentiation of Wide QRS Complex Tachycardia

With the exception of the AV node, the refractory period of cardiac tissue for a given beat is directly related to the interval between that beat and the preceding beat; the slower the heart rate the longer the recovery period with each beat. Furthermore, because the stability of refractoriness depends on the stability of the heart rate, a beat-to-beat change in refractoriness accompanies variability in the heart rate.

When an early supraventricular beat occurs in the midst of a regular rhythm, the tissues do not have a chance to shorten (or reset) their refractory periods; the result may be aberrant conduction (a transient functional refractoriness, or block) in one of the bundle branches. The shorter the interval between the early beat and the preceding one, the greater the probability that the early beat will be aberrant (Ashman's phenomenon). Ashman's phenomenon is also associated with the irregularity and frequent pauses of atrial fibrillation. Aberrancy may continue for a variable period before normal conduction resumes (Figure 19–3).

Aberrant conduction is often seen at the onset of any supraventricular tachycardia that uses the AV node for antegrade conduction. (This excludes tachycardias that conduct antegrade over a bypass tract.) The right bundle branch, with its longer refractory period, is more subject to block than is the left, but occasionally the left bundle becomes refractory earlier. Once the tachycardia has been established and refractory periods stabilized, this normal functional aberrancy may give way to normal conduction, with resumption of a narrow QRS.

Deciding whether a wide-complex tachycardia is supraventricular or ventricular in origin is often difficult. Only when AV dissociation or capture or fusion beats are present can a ventricular rhythm be diagnosed with certainty. The low sensitivities of these findings (20% for AV dissociation) do not provide a firm diagnosis in more than a minority of wide-complex tachycardias, however.

Classic criteria that examine V$_1$ when a right bundle branch block pattern is present, the QRS width and

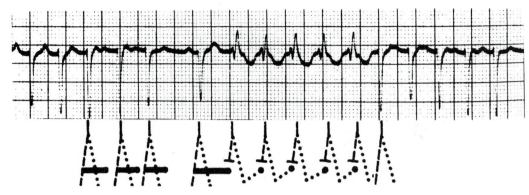

Figure 19–3. Atrial tachycardia with Wenckebach (type I) AV block, ventricular aberration from the Ashman phenomenon, and probably concealed transseptal conduction. The long pause of the atrial tachycardia is followed by five QRS complexes with right bundle branch block morphology. The right bundle branch block of the first QRS reflects the Ashman phenomenon. The aberration is perpetuated by concealed transseptal activation from the left bundle into the right bundle, with block of the anterograde conduction of the subsequent sinus impulse in the right bundle. Foreshortening of the R-R cycle, a manifestation of the Wenckebach structure, disturbs the relationship between transseptal and anterograde sinus conduction, and right bundle branch conduction is normalized. In the ladder diagram below the tracing, the solid lines represent the His bundle; the dashes, the right bundle branch; and the dots, the left bundle branch. The solid horizontal bars denote the refractory period. Neither the P waves nor the AV node is identified in the diagram. Reprinted, with permission, from Fisch C: Electrocardiography and vectorcardiography. In Braunwald E, ed: Heart Disease. A Textbook of Cardiovascular Medicine. Philadelphia: WB Saunders, 1988.

axis, the presence of positive or negative concordance across the precordium, and various combinations of QRS patterns in different leads may support a diagnosis, but they have been found lacking in diagnostic power because of their low sensitivity, low specificity, or both. A proposed algorithm separates supraventricular from ventricular tachycardia with 99% sensitivity and 97% specificity (Figure 19–4).

Brugada P, Brugada J, Mont L et al: A new approach to the differential diagnosis of a regular tachycardia with a wide QRS complex. Circulation 1991;83:1649.

SINUS TACHYCARDIA & OTHER SINUS NODE ARRHYTHMIAS

1. SINUS TACHYCARDIA

 ESSENTIALS OF DIAGNOSIS

- *Heart rate 100–160 bpm*
- *Each QRS preceded by a P wave identical to normal sinus rhythm P wave*

General Considerations

When the sinus node fires at a rate of more than 100 bpm, the rhythm is, with one exception, considered sinus tachycardia (see section on Sinus Node Reentry). The range for sinus tachycardia is 100–160 bpm; except during maximal exercise, faster rates usually imply a different mechanism. Confirming that the tachycardic P waves are identical in morphology and axis to the normal sinus rhythm P waves is essential to the diagnosis. Sinus tachycardia is usually a physiologic response, activated when the body requires a higher heart rate to meet metabolic demands or maintain blood pressure. Common causes are exercise, hypotension, hypoxemia, heart failure, sepsis, fever, hyperthyroidism, fluid depletion, and blood loss.

The heart rate achieved is proportional to the intensity of the stimulus, but the rapidity with which the heart rate increases and decreases is a function of how quickly the stimulus is applied and withdrawn. Vagal maneuvers slow the tachycardia gradually, but only while being performed; when the vagal stimulus is removed, the heart rate gradually returns to where it started. Attempting to slow the heart rate pharmacologically can be detrimental because it counteracts the compensatory mechanism provided by the tachycardia.

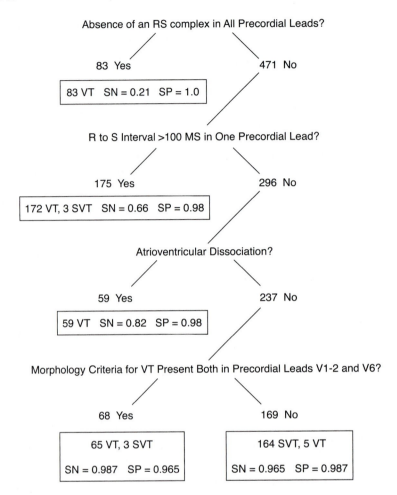

Absence of an RS complex in All Precordial Leads?

83 Yes   471 No

83 VT   SN = 0.21   SP = 1.0

R to S Interval >100 MS in One Precordial Lead?

175 Yes   296 No

172 VT, 3 SVT   SN = 0.66   SP = 0.98

Atrioventricular Dissociation?

59 Yes   237 No

59 VT   SN = 0.82   SP = 0.98

Morphology Criteria for VT Present Both in Precordial Leads V1-2 and V6?

68 Yes   169 No

65 VT, 3 SVT

SN = 0.987   SP = 0.965

164 SVT, 5 VT

SN = 0.965   SP = 0.987

Figure 19–4. Algorithm for diagnosis of a tachycardia with a widened QRS complex. When an RS complex cannot be identified in any precordial lead, the diagnosis of ventricular tachycardia (VT) is made. If an RS complex is present in one or more of the precordial leads, the longest RS interval is measured. If the RS interval is longer than 100 ms, or if atrioventricular dissociation is present, the diagnosis of VT is made. If absent, the morphology criteria for VT (see Table 19–1) are analyzed in leads V_1 and V_6. If both leads fulfill the criteria for VT, the diagnosis of VT is made. If not, the diagnosis of supraventricular tachycardia (SVT) with aberrant conduction is made. SN = sensitivity, SP = specificity. Reprinted, with permission, from Brugada P, Brugada J, Mont L et al: A new approach to the differential diagnosis of a regular tachycardia with a wide QRS complex. Circulation 1991;83:1649.

2. SINUS NODE ARRHYTHMIAS

ESSENTIALS OF DIAGNOSIS

- *Cyclic heart rate variation with respiration*
- *P-P interval variability equal to or greater than 160 ms or 10%*
- *P-wave morphology identical to normal sinus rhythm P wave*

General Considerations

A cyclic increase and decrease in heart rate normally accompanies inspiration and expiration, respectively, and the irregularity in rhythm (mediated by vagal tone) is often imperceptible. More marked degrees of rate excursion can occur, especially at slower heart rates, but these are not considered to be sinus arrhythmia unless the shortest and longest P-P interval varies by 0.16 s or more, or by 10% or more. This respiratory form of sinus arrhythmia is common in younger people. It becomes less prevalent with increasing age and in conditions associated with autonomic dysfunction, such as diabetes mellitus. Enhancement of vagal tone with agents such as digoxin and morphine may cause sinus arrhythmia. Because of its benign nature, no treatment is required.

The nonrespiratory variety of sinus arrhythmia is mostly seen in diseased hearts as a possible latent form of, or a precursor to, sick sinus syndrome. A sinus arrhythmia associated with bradycardia can develop during recovery from an acute illness or 2–3 days after an acute inferior myocardial infarction. When this arrhythmia occurs in conjunction with digoxin therapy, drug toxicity must be suspected. Treatment is directed at the underlying cause or withdrawal of the offending drug. A less common cause of this syndrome is increased intracranial pressure.

In the setting of second- or third-degree heart block or even with premature ventricular depolarizations, two consecutive sinus P waves may occur without an interposed QRS complex. If the P-P intervals that contain a QRS wave are shorter than those that do not, ventriculophasic sinus arrhythmia is said to be present. It is not known whether the early atrial depolarization following

the QRS is caused by the mechanical or vagal influences of ventricular systole on the atrium.

3. SINUS NODE REENTRY

ESSENTIALS OF DIAGNOSIS

- *Heart rate 100–160 bpm*
- *Each QRS preceded by a P wave identical to normal sinus rhythm P wave*
- *Abrupt onset and termination*

General Considerations

This uncommon rhythm accounts for less than 5% of supraventricular tachycardias. It uses the sinus node or perinodal tissue as a critical part of the reentrant circuit, producing P waves identical to those seen during normal sinus rhythm. The heart rate is similar to that seen with sinus tachycardia, falling between 100 and 160 bpm.

Longitudinal dissociation like that seen with dual AV nodal pathways may be present; this creates the conduction delay necessary to initiate the tachycardia. Unlike sinus tachycardia, sinus node reentry is initiated by an ectopic beat rather than a physiologic stimulus and possesses the characteristics typical of a reentrant circuit. It therefore begins and ends abruptly and responds to vagal maneuvers and pharmacologic interventions by terminating rather than slowing. The arrhythmia can be acutely terminated with intravenous adenosine, verapamil, or diltiazem, or via carotid massage. Chronic treatment uses β-blockers and calcium channel blockers. The largest reported series of patients treated with catheter ablation described success in all 10 patients. No complications were reported. Other smaller series described similar efficacy.

Callans DJ, Schwartzman D, Gottlieb CD et al. Insights into the electrophysiology of atrial arrhythmias gained by the catheter ablation experience: "Learning while burning, Part II." J Cardiovasc Electrophysiol 1995;6:229–243.

Sanders WE Jr, Sorrentino RA, Greenfield RA et al. Catheter ablation of sinoatrial node reentrant tachycardia. J Am Coll Cardiol 1994;23:926–934

INAPPROPRIATE SINUS TACHYCARDIA

ESSENTIALS OF DIAGNOSIS

- Heart rates greater than 100 bpm at rest or with minimal exertion
- P waves identical, or nearly identical, to sinus P waves
- Chronic duration of symptoms
- Exclusion of other causes of sinus tachycardia

General Considerations

Inappropriate sinus tachycardia is, fortunately, a rare arrhythmia with symptoms ranging from palpitations, dyspnea, chest pain, and dizziness to near syncope. Interestingly, it is most commonly found in young female health care workers. It has also been reported to occur after radiofrequency ablation of accessory pathways and after modification of the AV node, where it is a transient issue, resolving after days to months. The arrhythmia tends to be nonparoxysmal and is not associated with any underlying cardiac pathologic process. It is a diagnosis of exclusion in that other causes of sinus tachycardia must be ruled out. It is characterized by a persistently elevated heart rate with P waves identical to that seen in sinus rhythm.

The mechanism is a much-debated topic. The problem may either be due to sinus node dysfunction or alteration in the autonomic nervous system, with either excessive sympathetic tone or diminished parasympathetic tone. It appears to be due to a primary abnormality of the sinus node with elevated intrinsic heart rates and β-adrenergic hypersensitivity.

If left untreated, the arrhythmia may cause a tachycardia-induced cardiomyopathy. Therapy includes β-blockers and calcium antagonists, each sometimes requiring relatively high doses. Some studies report early success rates with catheter modification of the sinus node; however, recurrences of 20–30% have been observed. Additionally, other complications include sinus node ablation, necessitating implantation of a permanent pacemaker, and superior vena cava/right atrial junction stenosis, causing superior vena cava syndrome.

Callans DJ, Ren JF, Schwartzman D et al: Narrowing of the superior vena cava-right atrium junction during radiofrequency catheter ablation for inappropriate sinus tachycardia: Analysis with intracardiac echocardiography. J Am Coll Cardiol 1999; 33:1667–1670.

Friedman PL, Stevenson WG, Kokovic D: Autonomic dysfunction after catheter ablation. J Cardiovasc Electrophysiol 1996;7: 450–459.

Man KC, Knight B, Tse HF et al: Radiofrequency catheter ablation of inappropriate sinus tachycardia guided by activation mapping. J Am Coll Cardiol 2000 Feb;35(2):451–457.

Sergio FC, Steinberg JS: Supraventricular tachyarrhythmias involving the sinus node: Clinical and electrophysiologic characteristics. Prog Cardiovasc Dis 1998;41: 51–57.

ATRIAL FLUTTER

ESSENTIALS OF DIAGNOSIS

- Regular ventricular rate of 75–150 bpm
- Prominent neck vein pulsations of about 300/min
- Flutter waves on ECG of 250–340/min

General Considerations

Atrial flutter is usually associated with organic heart disease and is second in frequency only to atrial fibrillation in postbypass patients, with an incidence of up to 33%. It is said to be more common in males with a reported ratio of male-to-female of 4:1. With a typical atrial rate of 300 bpm (range: 250–340), atrial flutter produces a "saw-tooth" appearance (F waves). As is the case with atrial fibrillation, the ventricular rate depends on conduction through the AV node. Unlike atrial fibrillation, the ventricular impulses are transmitted at some integer fraction of the atrial rate. In rare circumstances, 1:1 conduction may occur. Fixed 2:1 or 4:1 block is the usual scenario, but variable block, with resultant ventricular rates of 75, 100, or 150 bpm, is not unusual. If flutter is suspected but F waves are not clearly visible, vagal maneuvers or pharmacologic agents can help to unmask the flutter waves by enhancing the degree of AV block.

Pathophysiology

Atrial flutter occurs in a variety of forms, the most common of which is either isthmus-dependent counterclockwise in direction, followed by the isthmus-dependent clockwise and then the atypical, nonisthmus-dependent variety. The counterclockwise flutter is recognized electrocardiographically by negative F waves in leads II, III aVf, and positive F waves in V_1. The single reentrant wavefront proceeds up the interatrial septum in a caudocranial direction, across the roof of the right atrium, down the lateral wall and across the inferior wall (Figure 19–5). Clockwise flutter, on the other hand, has positive F waves in leads II, III aVf, and negative F waves in lead V_1. The reentrant circuit in this case moves in the reverse direction. In both these types of atrial flutter, the atrial rates range between 250 and 350 bpm.

Evaluation of endocardial activation in atypical flutter demonstrates this to be a heterogeneous group of ar-

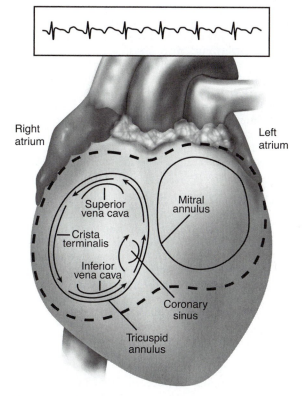

Figure 19–5. The reentry circuit of the common variety of atrial flutter (type II). The right and left atria are shown in left anterior oblique projection. The reentry circuit is confined to the right atrium and circulates in a counterclockwise direction within it (*arrows*). The shaded area between the tricuspid annulus and the inferior vena cava indicates the critical isthmus that is targeted for ablation of this type of atrial flutter. Also shown is a recording of counterclockwise atrial flutter in lead II, demonstrating the "sawtooth" pattern of flutter waves (rate, 250/min) characteristic of this type of atrial flutter. Reprinted, with permission, from Morady F: Drug therapy: Radio-frequency ablation as treatment for cardiac arrhythmias. N Engl J Med 1999;340:534–544. Copyright © 1999 Massachusetts Medical Society. All rights reserved.

rhythmias and may represent a transition between typical flutter and atrial fibrillation. Although it has not been substantiated in humans, animal studies suggest that this type of atrial flutter operates by a leading circle mechanism with a center of functional refractoriness. There is no excitable gap, making entrainment and termination by pacing impossible. The atrial rate, at 340–430 bpm, is faster than the common variety.

Whether atrial flutter is the source of peripheral embolization and stroke is an unsettled issue because most of the published studies pool their data from patients with atrial flutter and fibrillation, and most studies are retrospective in design. Additionally, many patients have bouts of both atrial fibrillation and flutter, thereby necessitating anticoagulant therapy. Nevertheless, the current recommendation is to fully anticoagulate these patients warfarin.

Clinical Findings

Symptoms attributable to atrial flutter are secondary to the ventricular response in addition to any underlying cardiac diseases. Dizziness, palpitations, angina-type chest pain, dyspnea, weakness, fatigue, and, occasionally, syncope may be the presenting symptoms. In those patients with poor left ventricular function, overt congestive heart failure may ensue.

Clinical evaluation is similar to that described for atrial fibrillation, but underlying heart disease is detected more often with atrial flutter than with fibrillation.

Treatment

A. GENERAL CONSIDERATIONS

Once the diagnosis of atrial flutter is made, assessment of the patients status will dictate whether to perform cardioversion immediately. Immediate cardioversion can be accomplished either with synchronized DC cardioversion or rapid atrial pacing to interrupt the macroreentrant circuit. For DC cardioversion, as little as 25 J may be all that is required; however, at least 50 J is recommended, and 100 J will terminate almost all episodes of atrial flutter. The major issue with this route is the need to administer an anesthetic agent.

Rapid atrial pacing is another modality, which may terminate the arrhythmia. Pacing is best performed at the high right atrium at a rate faster than the flutter rate, which allows the flutter circuit to be entered, or entrained, by the pacing impulse. If the extrinsic pacing rate exceeds the rate that can be sustained through the zone of slow conduction, the flutter wavefront can be interrupted and will no longer be present when the pacing is stopped. Pacing termination of isthmus-dependent typical atrial flutter can be achieved by several means. Although invasive, the most reliable technique is via an endocardial electrode. An alternative noninvasive method uses a swallowed transesophageal electrode. Because of the interposed tissue, a high current and long pulse width are often necessary to capture and pace the atrium reliably, which may cause significant discomfort to the patient. During bypass surgery, it is customary for surgeons to insert temporary pacing wires in both the atrial and ventricular epicardium and externalize them through the anterior chest wall. These are ideal for the pace termination of atrial flutter and can also provide a quick, noninvasive, and painless way to restore sinus rhythm. Because epicardial pacing thresholds are much higher than endocardial thresholds, a high current may be needed.

Two distinct techniques of overdrive atrial pacing are used, either fixed burst pacing or ramp pacing, beginning 10 bpm faster than the tachycardia rate. If atrial flutter does not terminate with either technique, slightly faster pacing rates should be attempted because the slower rate may only have entrained the tachycardia. Of note, overdrive pacing may precipitate atrial fibrillation, which usually terminates spontaneously after several minutes. Should the atrial fibrillation persist, however, it usually is easier to control the ventricular response when compared with atrial flutter.

Finally, rapid pharmacologic cardioversion can be considered with ibutilide, a unique intravenous class III antiarrhythmic agent. The rate of conversion with this agent is approximately 60% in patients with atrial flutter of less than 45 days duration. Cardioversion can be expected within 30 min of administration. The major complication with this agent is the development of torsades de pointes, which can occur in up to 12.5% of patients, with 1.7% requiring cardioversion for sustained polymorphic ventricular tachycardia. These occur primarily within the first hour after administration.

B. PHARMACOLOGIC THERAPY

It is difficult to assess the efficacy of antiarrhythmic drugs in suppressing recurrences of atrial flutter because studies are often contaminated with data from atrial fibrillation. Ventricular rate control and conversion and maintenance of sinus rhythm are difficult tasks to accomplish; they occur with less success than in atrial fibrillation.

Although the class Ic drugs appear to be as effective and are better tolerated than class Ia agents, the latter are still prescribed more often as initial therapy. There is, however, little data for direct comparison. When given intravenously, drugs of both classes are very effective in converting flutter to sinus rhythm. Beta-blockers alone are very effective in controlling the ventricular rate and have little or no place in conversion to sinus rhythm except in the postbypass patient. Although calcium antagonists are unable to terminate flutter, they, like β-blockers, can very effectively slow the ventricular rate. Both sotalol

and amiodarone are extremely useful in maintaining sinus rhythm. Dofetilide, also a class III antiarrhythmic agent, which blocks the rapid form of the delayed rectifier current, Ik_r, has also been found effective in converting to and maintenance of sinus rhythm. It is indicated for highly symptomatic persistent atrial fibrillation or flutter. Most studies to date have combined its rate of conversion from a mixed bag of atrial fibrillation and flutter. Its administration requires initiation in the hospital and monitored setting. Drugs that are contraindicated with its use include verapamil, ketoconazole, cimetidine, trimethoprim, prochlorperazine, megestrol and hydrochlothiazide. With regards to safety, dofetilide has a proarrhtyhmic event rate of approximately 0.9%, which is less than the 3.3% seen in patients with congestive heart failure or 2.5% in patients with previous ventricular tachycardia.

It is important that an AV nodal blocking agent be used before initiating a class I drug. If the AV node is unprotected, a type I agent could facilitate conduction of atrial flutter by improving nodal conduction or by slowing the flutter rate and paradoxically increasing the ventricular response.

C. CATHETER ABLATION AND OTHER MODALITIES

The reentrant circuit has been successfully mapped and includes an area of slow conduction bounded by the tricuspid annulus, the inferior vena cava and the os of the coronary sinus. Once it was evident that the area of slow conduction was rather contained, radiofrequency ablation was attempted in the hope of a cure for this arrhythmia. Initial reports demonstrated a success rate of 80–90%, with no inducible atrial flutter acutely. Nevertheless, early and late recurrences of 15–30% and up to 46%, respectively, were reported. Later studies demonstrated that for "success," not only was noninducibility required, but evidence of bidirectional block within the isthmus was needed. With this technique, recurrence rates of 9% are presently noted and are probably due to resumption of conduction within the isthmus. Currently, various mapping systems (electroanatomic and noncontact high resolution) are used, which may verify breakthrough areas where touchup delivery of radiofrequency energy is then used to complete the line of block. Recent data suggest advanced mapping systems aid in ablative procedures by decreasing fluoroscopic time and locating areas of breakthrough points along the flutter line Figure 19–5).

If attempts to cure flutter fail, the ventricular rate can be controlled by transcatheter ablation of the AV node or His bundle. With a long-standing flutter, there may be a subsequent improvement in left ventricular function.

Curative surgical intervention is also aimed at interrupting the zone of slow conduction.

Campbell RWF: Pharmacologic therapy of atrial flutter. J Cardiovasc Electrophysiol 1996;7:1008.

Cosio FG, Arribas F, Lopez-Gil M et al: Radiofrequency ablation of atrial flutter. J Cardiovasc Electrophysiol 1996;7:60.

Ellenbogen KA, Stambler BS, Woo MA et al: Efficacy of intravenous ibutilide for rapid termination of atrial fibrillation and atrial flutter: A dose dependent study. J Am Coll Cardiol 1996;28:130.

Falk RH, DeCara JM: Dofetilide: A new pure class III antiarrhythmic agent. Am Heart J 2000;140:697.

Kalman JM, Olgin JE, Saxon LA et al: Electrocardiographic and electrophysiologic characterization of atypical atrial flutter in man: Use of activation and entrainment mapping and implications for catheter ablation. J Cardiovasc Electrophysiol 1997; 8:121.

Schmitt H, Weber S, Tilmanns H et al: Diagnosis and ablation of atrial flutter using a high resolution, noncontact mapping system. PACE 2000;23:2057.

Shah DC, Haissaguerre M, Jais P et al: Atrial flutter: Contemporary electrophysiology and catheter ablation. PACE 1999;22:344.

Stambler BS, Wood MA, Ellenbogen KA et al: Efficacy and safety of repeated intravenous doses of ibutilide for rapid conversion of atrial flutter or fibrillation. Circulation 1996;94:1613.

Willems S, Weiss C, Ventura R et al: Catheter ablation of atrial flutter guided by electroanatomic mapping (CARTO): A randomized comparison to the conventional approach. J Cardiovasc Electrophysiol 2000;11:1223.

WANDERING ATRIAL PACEMAKER

ESSENTIALS OF DIAGNOSIS

- *Progressive cyclic alteration in P wave morphology*
- *Heart rate 60–100 bpm*

General Considerations

The presence of more than one pacemaker within the atria (which may or may not include the sinus node) causes variation in the P-P interval, P wave morphology, and the P-R interval. The heart rate remains within the normal range.

There is controversy over the cause of this rhythm. Some authorities believe that wandering atrial pacemaker and multifocal atrial tachycardia are the same rhythm artificially separated by heart rate, and that both are attributable to underlying pulmonary disease. Others believe that it is an exaggerated form of a respiratory sinus arrhythmia, with the uncovering of latent atrial and sinus node pacemakers when the primary sinus node pacemaker cycles to a slow rate with expiration.

The significance ascribed to a wandering atrial pacemaker should probably be interpreted in the setting in which it is seen. In those with lung disease, it may simply be a reflection of that process: In the elderly, it may be a forme fruste of sinus node disease or sick sinus syndrome, and in the young and athletic heart, it may represent heightened vagal tone.

The rhythm itself is benign and usually requires no intervention.

MULTIFOCAL ATRIAL TACHYCARDIA

ESSENTIALS OF DIAGNOSIS

- *Heart rates up to 150 bpm*
- *Three or more distinct P waves, in a single lead*
- *Variable P-P, P-R, and R-R intervals*

Clinical Findings

This arrhythmia, which constitutes less than 1% of all arrhythmias, is related to pulmonary disease in 60–85% of cases;, with chronic obstructive pulmonary disease (COPD) exacerbation being the most common clinical setting in which this arrhythmia is observed. It is also precipitated by respiratory failure, acute decompensated cardiac function, and infection. It has also been reported to be associated with hypokalemia, hypomagnesemia, hyponatremia, pulmonary embolism, cancer, and valvular heart disease, as well occurring in the postoperative setting. Distention of the right atrium from elevated pulmonary pressures causes multiple ectopic foci to fire, with ventricular rates not usually exceeding 150 bpm. Whether this rhythm is due to abnormal automaticity or triggered activity is uncertain, but the ability of verapamil to suppress the ectopic atrial activity by virtue of its calcium-channel-blocking properties supports the latter assumption.

Three ECG criteria must be met to diagnose multifocal atrial tachycardia (Figure 19–6):

- The presence of at least three distinct P wave morphologies recorded in the same lead
- The absence of one dominant atrial pacemaker
- Varying P-P, P-R, and R-R intervals

This rhythm is often misdiagnosed as atrial fibrillation. Although both are irregularly irregular, the former has distinct P waves with an intervening isoelectric baseline. In fact, multifocal atrial tachycardia may progress to atrial fibrillation.

Treatment

The primary treatment for multifocal atrial tachycardia should be directed at the underlying disease state.

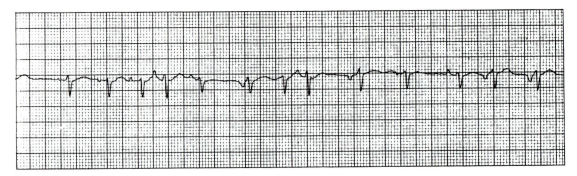

Figure 19–6. Multifocal atrial tachycardia. The presence of at least three distinct P-wave morphologies, the absence of one dominant pacemaker focus, and varying P-P, R-R, and PR intervals establish the diagnosis. Reprinted, with permission, from Goldberger A, Boldberger E: Clinical Electrocardiography. A Simplified Approach. St. Louis: Mosby Year Book, 1990.

Oral and intravenous verapamil and several formulations of intravenous β-blockers have been efficacious to varying degrees in either slowing the heart rate (without terminating the rhythm) or in converting the arrhythmia to sinus rhythm. Intravenous magnesium and potassium, even in patients with serum levels of these electrolytes within the normal range, convert a significant percentage of these patients to sinus rhythm. Digoxin is not effective in treating this condition. Moreover, treatment with digoxin may precipitate digitalis intoxication manifesting as paroxysmal atrial tachycardia (PAT) with block. Additionally, if the arrhythmia is secondary to delayed after-depolarizations, further aggravation may occur with digitalis because this drug increases delayed after-depolarizations. Medications that cause atrial irritability, such as theophylline and β-agonists, should be withdrawn whenever possible. A study of 50 patients with multifocal atrial tachycardia (MAT) demonstrated faster ventricular rates with theophylline. This may be due to theophylline's tendency to cause catecholamine-mediated delayed after-depolarizations via an increase in cyclic adenosine monophosphate (AMP).

Application of radiofrequency energy for both AV node modification and AV node ablation with subsequent implantation of a pacemaker have been reported. The numbers of patients in the studies were very small, and there are no long-term results. Nevertheless, ablation of the AV junction has been shown to reduce symptomatic MAT with improvement in quality of life, reduction in hospital admissions for recurrent symptomatic MAT, and improvement in left ventricular function.

Prognosis

Because of the severity of the precipitating underlying diseases, MAT portends a poor outcome. Mortality

during the hospitalization when the arrhythmia is first diagnosed is between 30% and 60%, with death being attributed to the disease state rather than the tachycardia itself. In one study of patients with pulmonary disease who were admitted for acute respiratory failure, the in-hospital mortality rate for those with MAT was 87%, compared with 24% for those in a different rhythm.

Tucker KJ, Law J, Rodrigues MJ: Treatment of refractory recurrent multifocal atrial tachycardia with atrioventricular junction ablation and permanent pacing. J Invasive Cardiol 1995;7: 207.

Ueng KC, Lee SH, Wu DJ et al: Radiofrequency catheter modification of atrioventricular junction in patients with COPD and medically refractory multifocal atrial tachycardia. Chest 2000; 117:52.

INTRAATRIAL REENTRANT TACHYCARDIA

 ESSENTIALS OF DIAGNOSIS

- *Heart rate of 120–240 bpm*
- *Distinct P waves that differ from sinus P waves*

General Considerations

Although similar in mechanism to atrial flutter, intraatrial reentry has a heart rate of 120–240 and distinct P waves with an interposed isoelectric baseline. The P waves differ in form from sinus P waves, which helps differentiate it from sinus node reentry tachycardia or inappropriate sinus tachycardia. This arrhythmia occurs in 6% of the population.

The substrate that makes intraatrial reentry possible is inhomogeneity of atrial conduction, refractoriness, or both. This can be confirmed by intraatrial recordings that show a stimulus-to-depolarization latency, or a delay of impulse propagation within the atrium. Unlike automatic atrial tachycardia, the reentrant form is initiated with closely coupled atrial depolarizations and does not display a warm-up phase. The arrhythmia occurs in paroxysms that are frequently sustained, responding to vagal maneuvers only 25% of the time.

In adults, the clinical setting is most often structural heart disease. In children, it often follows atrial surgery for congenital heart disease.

Treatment

Initial treatment consists of β-blockers or calcium channel blockers with negative chronotropic properties (verapamil, diltiazem) for ventricular rate control. These are often not very successful in abating symptoms, however, and more potent agents, including class IA, IC, and III antiarrhythmic preparations, may be necessary. Amiodarone achieves the goal of long-term suppression of intraatrial tachycardia twice as often as do the class I antiarrhythmic drugs. Radiofrequency catheter ablation, usually postoperative for a congenital anomaly, is directed at the area of slow conduction within the reentrant circuit and has a success rate of over 80%. Ablation of the AV node with implantation of a pacemaker is reserved for those patients who have failed attempts at curative ablation.

Dorostkar PC, Cheng JIE, Scheinman MM: Electroanatomical mapping and ablation of the substrate supporting intraatrial reentrant tachycardia after palliation for complex congenital heart disease. PACE 1998;21:1810–1819.

Feld GK: Catheter ablation for the treatment of atrial tachycardia. Prog Cardiovasc Dis 1995 Jan-Feb;37(4):205–224.

Haines DE, DiMarco JP: Sustained intraatrial reentrant tachycardia: Clinical, electrocardiographic, and electrophysiologic characteristics and long-term follow-up. J Am Coll Cardiol 1990;15:1345.

AUTOMATIC (ECTOPIC) ATRIAL TACHYCARDIA

ESSENTIALS OF DIAGNOSIS

- *Heart rate 100–180 bpm*
- *Distinct P waves that differ from sinus P waves*
- *Initiated by ectopic beat*
- *Gradual increase in heart rate during an episode*

Symptoms & Signs

Automatic, or ectopic, atrial tachycardia (the least common of the atrial tachycardias) occurs in several forms with very different presentations and prognoses. The episodes may either be brief and self-terminating or chronic and persistent, eventually leading to a tachycardia-induced cardiomyopathy if left untreated. Short nonsustained bursts of atrial tachycardia can be seen in 2–6% of young adults on Holter evaluations.

In those patients with paroxysmal sustained atrial tachycardia, there is a higher likelihood of associated organic heart disease, including coronary artery disease, valvular heart disease, congenital heart disease, and other cardiomyopathies. Frequently, patients will present with a transient automatic tachycardia the cause of which can usually be determined from the associated clinical setting. Some of the most frequent causes include acute myocardial infarction, in which case it is seen in 4–19% of patients, electrolyte disturbances (especially hypokalemia), chronic lung disease or pulmonary infection, acute alcohol ingestion, hypoxia, and use of cardiac stimulants (theophylline, cocaine). Short, unsustained bursts of paroxysmal atrial tachycardia that last only a few seconds can be seen in adults without concomitant heart disease. The heart rate is in the range of 100–180 bpm.

The form that occurs almost exclusively, and not uncommonly, in children, is a continuous tachycardia with heart rates of about 175 bpm. Symptoms are severe, and congestive heart failure frequently develops as a result of a tachycardia-induced cardiomyopathy. The arrhythmia may be transient in younger children, but when it persists in older children it should be considered permanent. Fortunately, if the tachycardia can be terminated, cardiac function returns to normal. When it appears in adults, the continuous variety manifests milder symptoms.

In all forms of PAT, the P wave morphology is unlike the sinus P waves, but it is separated by a well-defined isoelectric baseline that distinguishes this rhythm from atrial flutter.

Clinical Findings

Several features of automatic rhythms distinguish them from reentrant and triggered rhythms:

- A warm-up period of initially slower rates that speed up gradually is characteristic of automatic rhythms.

- Because they emanate from a single focus, P waves of the first and all subsequent beats of an automatic rhythm are identical. The beat that initiates a reentrant tachycardia is usually ectopic and therefore displays a different P wave from those that follow. Triggered rhythms may follow an ectopic beat or a prolongation in the sinus cycle length (long–short sequence); in either case the beats that follow have a distinct P wave morphology.

- Vagal maneuvers or pharmacologic interventions that prolong or inhibit AV nodal conduction will terminate rhythms that use the AV node as part of a reentrant circuit. They are ineffective in terminating automatic rhythms, although they may produce varying degrees of heart block.
- In contrast to reentrant and triggered rhythms, atrial extra stimulation and pacing cannot initiate automatic rhythms. Atrial overdrive pacing terminates rhythms caused by reentry, but it only temporarily suppresses automaticity.
- Direct-current cardioversion has no effect on automatic rhythms.

Treatment

A. PHARMACOLOGIC THERAPY

Automatic atrial tachycardia is more resistant to drug therapy than is any other atrial arrhythmia, but because of its low prevalence there are no controlled treatment-evaluation trials, and most data are derived from case reports. The drug with the highest long-term rate of conversion to sinus rhythm is the class III agent sotalol, with efficacy rates of 85–100% reported in some series. This is far in excess of the results seen with flecainide, the next most efficacious agent, which has a success rate of only 25%. Propafenone, also a class Ic antiarrhythmic agent, may be as effective as flecainide. Good results have also been reported with amiodarone and moricizine. Although β-blockers may slow the tachycardia heart rate, they rarely terminate the rhythm. Class Ib drugs such as mexiletine and phenytoin (Dilantin) may convert the rhythm to sinus; however, the class Ia agents, digoxin and verapamil, are uniformly ineffective in the treatment of this disorder.

B. SURGICAL THERAPY

In sharp contrast to the poor results seen with drug therapy, cure with surgery is the rule for left-sided foci; it is less certain with right-sided foci. Intraoperative mapping of the automatic focus, followed by excision or cryoablation, eliminates the arrhythmogenic substrate. It is interesting to note that gross and histologic examination of the excised tissue reveals a high incidence of focal myocarditis. When the automatic focus is found to reside in the left atrium, an alternative procedure is a left atrial isolation. The atrium is first disarticulated and then sutured back in place. Interrupting the conduit of electrical flow between the two atria confines impulses originating in the ectopic focus to

the left atrium and prevent them from reaching the AV node. With the high heart rate no longer suppressing it, the sinus node again becomes the heart's predominant pacemaker. As expected, both foci can be seen on the postoperative ECG. Catheter ablation of atrial foci has been performed with some success. With extensive experience in mapping and ablating these arrhythmias, it has been demonstrated that these arrhythmias arise from well-defined anatomic regions, including the crista terminalis, the tricuspid and mitral annuli, the right and left atrial appendage, and the region within or surrounding the pulmonary veins.

In a 1998 North American Society of Pacing and Electrophysiology registry, the success rate was found to depend on the site of origin of the tachycardia, with success rates of 80%, 72%, and 52% for right, left, and septal origins, respectively. The use of electromagnetic and noncontact mapping systems has significantly improved ablative therapy by decreasing fluoroscopic time, mapping time, and number of radiofrequency applications, thereby increasing efficacy.

Marchlinski F, Callans D. Gottlieb C et al: Magnetic electro-anatomical mapping for ablation of focal atrial tachycardias. PACE 1998;21:1621–1635.

Natale A, Breeding L, Tomassoni G et al: Ablation of right and left atrial tachycardias using a three-dimensional nonfluoroscopic mapping system. Am J Cardiol 1998;82:989–992.

Scheinman MM, Huang S: The 1998 NAPSE prospective catheter ablation registry. Pacing Clin Electrophysiol 2000;23:1020–1028.

Schmitt C, Zrenner B, Schneider M et al: Clinical experience with a novel multielectrode basket catheter in right atrial tachycardias. Circulation 1999;99:2414–2422.

Schmitt H, Weber S, Schwab JO et al: Diagnosis and ablation of focal right atrial tachycardia using a new high-resolution, non-contact mapping system. Am J Cardiol 2001;87:1017–1021.

PAROXYSMAL ATRIAL TACHYCARDIA WITH BLOCK

ESSENTIALS OF DIAGNOSIS

- *Atrial rate of 150–250 bpm*
- *AV block of 2:1*

Pathophysiology & Etiology

Although the majority of cases of PAT with block were at one time related to digoxin excess, the cause now has a stronger association with advanced organic heart disease and severe underlying pulmonary disease. Nonetheless, when PAT with block is seen, digoxin excess must be suspected. (It is still unknown whether digoxin-related PAT with block is the result of an automatic or triggered mechanism.) The atrial rate in this setting is typically 150–250 bpm. Block is usually 2:1 but may vary: It corresponds to a ventricular rate of about 100 bpm. A ventriculophasic response is often seen.

Treatment

Therapy targeted at abolishing the arrhythmia has been unrewarding, and most efforts are aimed at optimizing treatment of any underlying disorder or, when appropriate, trying to control the ventricular rate. When digoxin is implicated, treatment consists of withdrawing the drug and correcting any underlying electrolyte abnormalities, such as hypokalemia. In life-threatening cases of severe intoxication, digoxin antibodies can be administered; they are rarely needed. Dialysis is ineffective in removing digoxin from the body.

ATRIOVENTRICULAR NODAL REENTRANT TACHYCARDIA

ESSENTIALS OF DIAGNOSIS

- Heart rate 100–200 or more beats per minute
- Neck pulsations corresponding to the heart rate
- P waves not visible in 90% of cases

Pathophysiology & Etiology

The arrhythmia is more common in females. Heart rates during AV nodal reentrant tachycardia (AVNRT) usually fall in the range of 120–200 bpm, although rates up to 250 bpm have been recorded. Palpitations are almost universally reported. A feeling of diuresis, noted with other supraventricular arrhythmias, is significantly more common in AVNRT and has been correlated with elevated right atrial pressures and elevated atrial natriuretic peptide. Neck pulsations are unique to the disorder (Brugada's phenomenon) and are secondary to simultaneous contraction of the atria and ventricles against closed mitral and tricuspid valves. Dizziness and lightheadedness are common, with frank syncope occurring infrequently. Sudden death has been reported, and these patients had severe hypotension associated with the tachycardia. Although symptoms may occur at any age but rarely in childhood, the distribu-

tion of when the tachycardia and symptoms commonly appear appears to be bimodal. The initial episode may begin during the second decade of life, only to disappear and then reappear during the fourth and fifth decade of life.

Conduction from the right atrium to the ventricles is normally over a singular AV nodal pathway, with no route of reentry back into the atrium. In persons with dual AV nodal pathways, an atrial impulse may travel antegrade from the atrium over one limb of the AV node and then back to the atrium over another limb in a retrograde fashion. When only one cycle occurs, a single echo beat, in the form of a retrograde P wave, may be seen on the ECG. If this echo beat can again penetrate the AV node antegrade, the cycle can perpetuate itself, leading to AVNRT. This is the most common form of circus movement supraventricular tachycardia (SVT), accounting for almost half of all cases. It is estimated that dual AV nodal pathways exist in up to one fourth of the population, but only a fraction of these people ever manifest a tachycardia.

If each limb of the circuit had an equal ability to conduct impulses, echo beats and sustained AVNRT would be an impossibility. An atrial impulse traveling down both limbs at the same speed would cause each limb to be refractory when that impulse reached the bottom of the node, preventing the impulse in each limb from going back up the other. Instead, the limbs have varying conduction speeds (Figure 19–7A) and refractory periods. The faster conducting limb, termed the β pathway, has a longer refractory period, whereas the reverse is true for the second limb, termed the α pathway.

A premature atrial depolarization may initiate the tachycardia if it finds the fast pathway refractory; the premature impulse can then reach the ventricles through the slow pathway. The ECG manifestation of this is a P-R interval that exceeds the baseline P-R by as much as 50–300% of its value in sinus rhythm. At the same time that it enters the His–Purkinje system and the ventricles, the slow pathway impulse heads retrograde up the fast pathway, where it may block (Figure 19–7B) or continue to produce an atrial echo beat with a retrograde P wave and a short R-P interval. Right atrial mapping has shown that earliest atrial retrograde activation occurs at the anterior septum just posterior to the His bundle. If the slow pathway cannot propagate another impulse antegrade because of refractoriness, only a single atrial echo beat will occur (Figure 19–7C). If the slow pathway has recovered excitability, the circuit can again be entered. Perpetuation of this cycle will lead to a sustained episode of AVNRT (Figure 19–7D). Ventricular ectopic beats can also initiate AVNRT by the same mechanism.

Conduction up the fast pathway is usually so rapid that retrograde atrial depolarization is simultaneous or

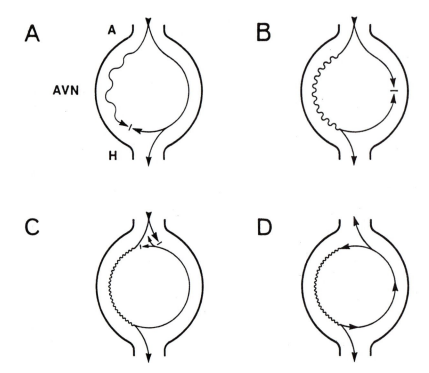

Figure 19–7. Schematic presentation of impulse propagation along with the fast (*straight line*) and slow (*wavy line*) conducting pathways. A sinus atrial impulse preferentially negotiates the His bundle via the fast pathway (**A**). Because of the longer refractoriness of the fast pathway, an atrial premature beat may block it while engaging the His bundle via the slow pathway and then penetrate the fast pathway retrograde (**B**). Depending on the recovery of tissue ahead, the returning impulse may produce a single echo beat (**C**) or sustained arrhythmia (**D**). A = atrium; AVN = atrioventricular node; H = His bundle. Reprinted, with permission, from Akhtar M: Supraventricular tachycardias. In Josephson ME, Wellens HJJ, eds: Tachycardias: Mechanisms, Diagnosis, Treatment. Philadelphia: Lea & Febiger, 1984.

almost simultaneous with antegrade ventricular activation. This causes the low-amplitude P wave to become obscured in the much higher amplitude QRS complex—and not be seen at all 50–60% of the time. In 20–30% of cases the P wave distorts the terminal portion of the QRS causing a pseudo-S wave in the inferior leads and a pseudo-R' in lead V_1, and in approximately 10% of cases the P wave distorts the initial portion of the QRS complex.

This common AVNRT is the overwhelmingly more prevalent type; it is also called **slow–fast,** referring to the antegrade and retrograde limbs taken during the tachycardia, respectively. Distinctly more unusual is the uncommon, or **fast–slow** type, seen in approximately 10% of cases. Here the slow pathway has the longer refractory period, which causes it to become blocked antegrade and then to be used as the return path to the atrium. Only 5% of the cases are of this fast–slow variety. A third variety is the so-called **slow–slow** form in which the retrograde limb causes earliest atrial activation to occur in the posterior sep-

tum, either in the vicinity of or within the coronary sinus.

One point of controversy is whether the reentrant circuit is contained within the AV node or whether some critical amount of atrial tissue is required. Nonetheless, AVNRT, once initiated, can perpetuate itself without the participation of either the atria or ventricles. If the site of dissociation from the AV node is at the level of the His–Purkinje system or ventricles, rapid and regular P waves with complete heart block and a low junctional escape rhythm are seen on the ECG.

Treatment

A. PHARMACOLOGIC THERAPY

Medical treatment of AVNRT is directed at slowing or blocking conduction in either the fast or slow pathway. Typical AV nodal blocking agents such as β-blockers, calcium channel blockers, adenosine, and digoxin are most effective on the antegrade slow pathway. The more potent class Ia antiarrhythmic drugs may be necessary to inhibit conduction in the retrograde fast pathway. Class Ic drugs, and amiodarone and sotalol (class III) affect both pathways.

Terminating an acute episode of AVNRT in the hospital setting has been made simpler with the availability of intravenous adenosine, which reaches and acts on its target within seconds of administration. With a clinical half-life on the order of 10 s, commonly reported sensations such as breathlessness, chest heaviness, and flushing disappear quickly. The routine dosage of 6 mg followed by up to two more boluses of 12 mg, should be decreased by 50% when administered via a central line. If adenosine is ineffective, intravenous verapamil can be used, but it takes longer to act. Diltiazem, given as intravenous bolus, can also be effective in aborting the tachycardia. Hypotension occurs with about a 10% incidence and is usually rapidly reversed with fluid administration. Although intravenous β-blockers, procainamide, and digoxin are other second-line choices, they can be advantageous in recurrent cases because of their slower clearance from the body.

B. Vagal Maneuvers

These maneuvers should be considered, barring any contraindications, before embarking on medical therapy. Medications may render the arrhythmia more susceptible to termination with vagal maneuvers; these should be attempted immediately after each round of drug therapy if the tachycardia persists.

C. Radiofrequency Modification in Slow–Fast AVNRT

Radiofrequency lesions delivered through a large-tipped catheter can be directed at either the fast or slow pathway; the latter is preferred.

The inferior origin of the slow pathway is variable within the triangle of Koch, but it is usually anterior and superior to (and sometimes within) the os of the coronary sinus. These anatomic landmarks and gross intracardiac electrogram patterns can be used to position the ablation catheter, or a slow pathway potential can be recorded as verification of proper catheter position. Studies have shown no significant differences between an anatomic versus electrophysiologic approach to ablation. The fast pathway is left unaltered and can still be used for transmission of sinus impulses to the ventricles. Long-term freedom from recurrent AVNRT is about 95%, and the risk of complete heart block as a result of inadvertent fast pathway damage is 0–5%.

For modification of the fast AV nodal pathway, the ablation catheter is placed across the tricuspid annulus to record the maximum His bundle electrogram and then withdrawn until the atrial-to-ventricular electrogram ratio is greater than 1 and the His electrogram

amplitude is reduced, typically to less than 0.1 mV. Radiofrequency energy is then applied and continued until the P-R interval prolongs to 50% over the baseline value. Energy delivery is discontinued if second- or third-degree heart block is seen. Using this approach, long-term success in abolishing tachycardia recurrences is equal to that of slow-pathway modification. Complete heart block with the need for permanent ventricular pacing has a reported incidence ranging from 0 to 10% (even when performed by experienced operators). When the initial approach fails, crossover to the other pathway has been shown to be 100% effective in eliminating AVNRT.

A complication that occurs in 5–15% of fast-pathway modifications is the conversion of slow–fast AVNRT to fast–slow or slow–slow reentrant tachycardia. The possible scenarios accounting for this are diagrammed in Figure 19–8. If a slow–slow tachycardia is created it may be persistent, because the prolonged conduction time in the limb carrying the impulse is always sufficient for the other limb to recover. Refractoriness is never encountered in either limb, and the tachycardia persists indefinitely. Treatment in this case is ablation of the antegrade slow pathway.

With the advent of sophisticated mapping systems, as with other arrhythmias, there has been a decrease in the procedure and in fluoroscopy time, as well as in the mean number of ablation lesions. Additionally, annotating satisfactory locations during mapping so that one can easily return to them at some later point, or marking those areas where radiofrequency energy has already been applied is also an advantageous aspect of an advanced mapping system.

A relatively new and experimental form of ablation is cryoablation, using a supercooling catheter, which can reversibly and permanently damage endocardial tissue. This novel approach, especially with regard to AVNRT and damage to the AVN region, allows for testing the acceptability of a particular site. Should heart block occur prior to irreversible tissue damage, then rewarming can be performed with no untoward effects.

D. Surgical Therapy

Although the advent of AV nodal radiofrequency catheter modification has rendered surgery almost obsolete, several operative approaches—all with good results—have been developed. The most widely used technique involves application of multiple cryoprobe lesions in Koch's triangle, in the vicinity of the exposed AV node, until P-R prolongation is seen. Although this provides evidence of fast pathway modification, the slow pathway may also become damaged to the point of being unable to participate in a tachycardia circuit. There is also a 5–10% chance of creating complete

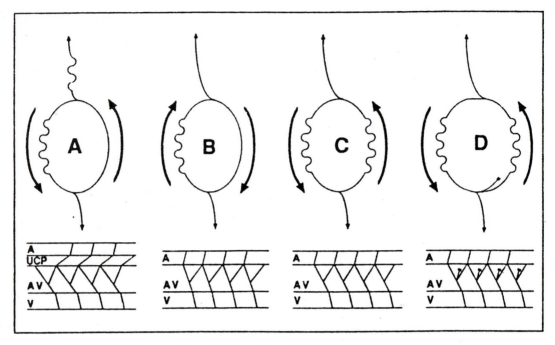

Figure 19–8. Possible mechanisms of uncommon atrioventricular nodal reentry after ablation. **A:** Continued common (up fast-down slow) tachycardia with superimposed ablation-induced upper common pathway delay. This proximal delay would prolong retrograde atrial activation time. **B:** Ablation-induced increase in fast pathway refractoriness resulting in selective retrograde fast pathway block and initiation of true uncommon (up slow-down fast) reentry. **C:** Slowing in retrograde fast pathway produced by ablative injury causes increased retrograde atrial activation time and slowing of tachycardia rate. Slower rate produces decrease in anterograde ventricular activation time. **D:** Ablation interrupts retrograde fast pathway, unmasking a second, slower retrograde pathway. A = atrium; AV = atrioventricular; V = ventricle. Reprinted, with permission, from Langberg JJ, Kim YN, Goyal R et al: Conversion of typical to atypical atrioventricular nodal reentrant tachycardia after radiofrequency catheter modification of the atrioventricular junction. Am J Cardiol 1992;69:503.

heart block, which requires implantation of a permanent pacemaker. Less often performed, but equally effective as compared with cryoablation, are incisions placed in the region of Koch's triangle.

Abe H, Nagatomo T, Kobayashi H et al: Neurohumoral and hemodynamic mechanisms of diuresis during atrioventricular nodal reentrant tachycardia. PACE 1997;20:2783–2788.

Calkins H, Yong P, Miller JM et al: Catheter ablation of accessory pathways, atrioventricular nodal reentrant tachycardia, and the atrioventricular junction: Final results of a prospective, multicenter clinical trial. The Atakr Multicenter Investigators Group. Circulation 1999 Jan 19;99(2):262–270.

Cooke PA, Wilber DJ: Radiofrequency catheter ablation of atrioventricular nodal reentry tachycardia utilizing nonfluoroscopic electroanatomical mapping. PACE 1998;21:1802–1809.

Skanes AC, Dubuc M, Klein GJ et al: Cryothermal ablation of the slow pathway for the elimination of atrioventricular nodal reentrant tachycardia. Circulation 2000 Dec 5;102(23):2856–2860.

Tebbenjohanns J, Niehaus M, Korte T et al: Noninvasive diagnosis in patients with undocumented tachycardias: Value of the adenosine test to predict AV nodal reentrant tachycardia. J Cardiovasc Electrophysiol 1999 Jul;10(7):916–923.

NONPAROXYSMAL JUNCTIONAL TACHYCARDIA (ACCELERATED AV JUNCTIONAL RHYTHM)

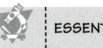

ESSENTIALS OF DIAGNOSIS

- *Heart rate 60–120 bpm*
- *Atrioventricular dissociation*
- *Gradual onset and termination*

Definition

To distinguish it from AVNRT, which presents with chronic, recurrent tachycardia episodes of sudden onset, nonparoxysmal junctional tachycardia (NPJT)is the form that is not episodic and starts almost imperceptibly. NPJT is easily differentiated from AVNRT by. a heart rate between 70 and 130 bpm, gradual onset and termination, and lack of termination with vagal maneuvers, and overdrive pacing to identify the rhythm. Although heart rates of less than 100 bpm can be seen, it is, nevertheless, a tachycardia because the rates are faster than the 40–60 bpm seen with junctional rhythm.

Pathophysiology & Etiology

A. NONPAROXYSMAL JUNCTIONAL TACHYCARDIA FROM TRIGGERED ACTIVITY

The heart rate at onset is just slightly faster than that of the rhythm preceding it, with gradual acceleration until the final rate is achieved. AV dissociation is common, occurring in 85% of cases caused by digoxin (see following discussion). With conduction to the atria intact, retrograde P waves may appear immediately before or after the QRS complex, or they may be obscured within the QRS. Discharge from the AV node is regular, but if antegrade second-degree AV block (almost always the result of digoxin excess), exit block, or atrial capture beats coexist with junctional tachycardia, the rhythm will appear irregular. Enhanced vagal tone or vagolytic agents will either slow down or speed up the arrhythmia, respectively.

Usually seen in the setting of organic heart disease, the cause of this rhythm is almost always identifiable. At one time digoxin excess accounted for up to 85% of cases of NPJT. Awareness of the drug's toxicities and the availability of other AV nodal blocking agents have diminished the incidence to about 60% of cases. Nevertheless, in those patients being treated with digoxin for atrial fibrillation, one should suspect this arrhythmia when the ECG demonstrates a regularized ventricular response. Acute inferior infarction accounts for 20% of NPJT, and this rhythm may be present in up to 10% of all infarcts in this location, with onset usually within the first 24 h, disappearing in several days. NPJT may follow open heart surgery (valve replacement more often than bypass surgery), or it can be caused by myocarditis (especially rheumatic) and, rarely, congenital heart disease. In all cases the tachycardia resolves along with the acute underlying event—or with digoxin withdrawal.

Because the rhythm rarely causes deleterious hemodynamic effects, treatment is usually not indicated. If necessary, AV sequential pacing at a rate faster than that of the NPJT may be effective by transiently suppressing the tachycardia and restoring the atrial contribution to cardiac output.

B. PERMANENT FORM OF JUNCTIONAL RECIPROCATING TACHYCARDIA

This rare cause of supraventricular tachycardia is seen almost exclusively in the infant and pediatric population, with only a handful of cases reported in adults. Permanent junctional reciprocating tachycardia (PJRT) can occur in infants and children in the perioperative period or in an idiopathic form in infants. The perioperative form is self-limiting, however, heart rates exceeding 200 bpm may cause hemodynamic collapse. The idiopathic form can be continuous and persist for years, resulting in a tachycardia-induced cardiomyopathy. As the patients mature, the heart rates decrease from approximately 200 bpm to approximately 150 bpm secondary to slowing of conduction via the retrograde limb.

P waves precede the QRS complexes and are inverted in the inferior leads. The arrhythmia is actually a variant of atrioventricular reciprocating tachycardia (see the following section) because the antegrade limb involves the AV node and the retrograde limb involves an accessory pathway with long conduction times and decremental properties, like that seen with the AV node, located most commonly in the posteroseptal region near or at the os of the coronary sinus.

Although drug therapy is frequently unhelpful in controlling this arrhythmia secondary to the prolonged conduction property of the accessory pathway, good rate control can be achieved with flecainide, propafenone, and amiodarone. Digoxin has no effect on the rate, and verapamil may accelerate it. Adults have a good response to β-blockers. Catheter-based radiofrequency ablation of the accessory pathway has a success rate greater than 95% without significant complications.

Aguinaga L, Primo J, Anguera I et al: Long-term follow-up in patients with the permanent form of junctional reciprocating tachycardia treated with radiofrequency ablation. Pacing Clin Electrophysiol 1998;21(11 Pt 1):2073–2078.

Critelli G: Recognizing and managing permanent junctional reciprocating tachycardia in the catheter ablation era. J Cardiovasc Electrophysiol 1997;8(2):226–236.

Dorostkar PC, Silka MJ, Morady F et al: Clinical course of persistent junctional reciprocating tachycardia. J Am Coll Cardiol 1999;33(2):366–375.

Yang Y, Greco C, Ciccaglioni A et al: Curative radiofrequency catheter ablation for permanent junctional reciprocating tachycardia. Pacing Clin Electrophysiol 1993;16(7 Pt 1): 1373–1379.

ATRIOVENTRICULAR RECIPROCATING TACHYCARDIA

ESSENTIALS OF DIAGNOSIS

- *Short P-R interval (<120 ms)*
- *Wide-QRS complex caused by a delta wave*
- *Supraventricular tachycardias with heart rates of 140–250 bpm*

1. BYPASS TRACTS & THE WOLFF–PARKINSON–WHITE SYNDROME

Congenital bands of tissue that can conduct impulses but lie outside the normal conduction system are called accessory pathways, or bypass tracts. These pathways are responsible for a variety of mechanistically distinct tachycardias by providing preferential conduction between different areas within the heart.

Epidemiology

Accessory pathways are quite prevalent in the general population with a 2:1 male:female predominance. The presence of a bypass tract, however, does not mean that a tachyarrhythmia is a certainty because fewer than half of those with documented bypass tracts ever sustain an arrhythmia. The actual number depends on the population studied and varies from 13% in a healthy outpatient population to 80% in the hospital setting.

Approximately 5–10% of patients with documented bypass tracts have concomitant structural heart disease. Ebstein's anomaly is the most common, accounting for 25–50% of the anomalies in this group. Of patients with Ebstein's anomaly, 8–10% have coexistent bypass tracts, mostly on the right side. The association of right-sided accessory pathways with structural heart disease is strong: 45% of patients with right-sided (and only 5% of those with left-sided) pathways display some type of heart disease. An association between mitral valve prolapse and left-sided accessory pathways has been reported, although this may simply represent two relatively common conditions that randomly coexist.

A familial tendency toward bypass tracts has been seen in some instances, with a four to tenfold increase in incidence among first-degree family members. Some investigators have postulated autosomal-dominant transmission of the trait.

Pathophysiology

A. ANATOMY

Anatomically, the atria and ventricles are in apposition, separated by an invagination known as the atrioventricular groove. Paroxysmal tachycardias mediated by accessory pathways that cross the groove and electrically link the atria and ventricles, when combined with a short P-R interval (<0.12 s), a wide QRS, and secondary repolarization abnormalities, define the Wolff–Parkinson–White syndrome. A short P-R interval and a wide QRS alone is called ventricular preexcitation.

Although the most common site of insertion is between the lateral aspect of the left atrial and ventricular myocardium, pathways can cross the atrioventricular groove anywhere in its course (except the region between the left and right fibrous trigones) to connect the left or right atrium to its respective ventricle (Figure 19–9). In noting the distribution of accessory pathways, 46–60% are located in the left free wall, 25% within the posteroseptal space, 13–21% in the right free wall and 2% in the anteroseptal space. Each location produces a distinct electrocardiographic pattern (Figure 19–10), but in the 13% of patients with two or more bypass tracts the ECG tracing can be confounding and show multiple QRS morphologies.

B. CARDIAC ELECTRICAL CONDUCTION

Unlike the AV node, whose function is to delay atrial impulses en route to the ventricles, most bypass tracts conduct rapidly and without delay, which accounts for the short P-R interval often seen in sinus rhythm in these patients.

When a sinus impulse spreads through the ventricles via the rapidly conducting His–Purkinje system, the ventricular activation time is short, and a narrow QRS is inscribed on the ECG. In contrast, impulses that reach the ventricles over a bypass tract spread through cell-to-cell conduction within the myocardium, activating the ventricles in series rather than in parallel. This much slower process is manifested as a wide QRS complex.

Sinus impulses are not restricted to using the AV node or the bypass tract only to reach the lower chambers. Instead, both may contribute to ventricular activation. This produces a QRS that is initially wide, reflecting conduction over the bypass tract, with the latter portion of the QRS appearing normal and narrow, indicating that the remainder of the ventricle has been depolarized via the normal conduction system (the AV node and His–Purkinje system). The initial slurred upstroke of the QRS, a delta wave, indicates ventricular preexcitation, which can be defined as ventricular depolarization that begins earlier than would be expected by conduction over the AV node alone.

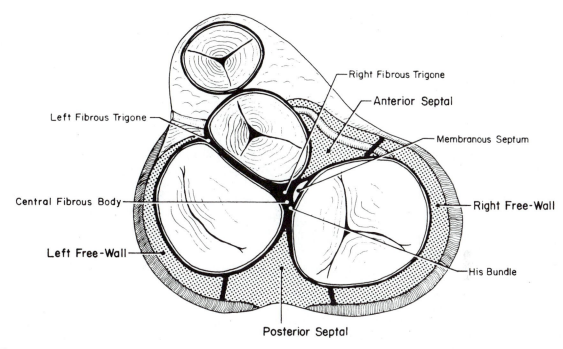

Figure 19–9. Cross-sectional diagram of the atrioventricular groove. Atrioventricular bypass tracts may cross the groove anywhere in its course except in the region bounded by the left and right fibrous trigones. Reprinted, with permission, from Cox JL, Gallagher JJ, Cain ME et al: Experience with 118 consecutive patients undergoing operation for the Wolff-Parkinson-White syndrome. J Thorac Cardiovasc Surg 1985;90:490.

The degree of preexcitation and P-R shortening depends on the proportion of ventricular activation occurring over the AV node and the bypass tract. This, in turn, is related to two factors. The first is the conduction velocity of the bypass tract relative to the AV node. The faster the bypass tract can conduct impulses to the ventricles in relation to the AV node, the earlier the ventricle will preexcite, and vice versa. The second factor is the location of the tract, and more specifically, its situation relative to the sinus node and AV node. A sinus impulse will encounter a right-sided free-wall bypass tract earlier than it will the AV node, and this favors a short P-R interval with a high degree of ventricular preexcitation (Figure 19–11A). On the other hand, a sinus beat will encounter the AV node early in its course while traveling to a pathway in the lateral left atrium, allowing ventricular activation to occur primarily by the normal conduction system. A narrow, minimally (if at all) preexcited QRS complex with a normal or near-normal P-R interval may be seen (Figure 19–11B). Changes in autonomic tone, by modifying the conduction velocity and refractoriness over both the pathway and the AV node, can produce varying degrees of preexcitation at different times in the same patient (Figure 19–11C).

If the delta wave axis of a maximally preexcited beat is discordant from the accompanying preexcited QRS axis, or if more than one preexcited QRS morphology is noted, there may be multiple bypass tracts.

C. MECHANISM

1. Atrioventricular reciprocating tachycardia—An inherent property of accessory pathways is their ability to conduct in a retrograde direction more easily than antegrade. The AV node, on the other hand, conducts more efficiently antegrade. For this reason, reentrant rhythms in this setting most commonly use the AV node to go from atrium to ventricle and the bypass tract to return to the atrium. Therefore, atrioventricular reciprocating tachycardia (AVRT) is a macroreentrant tachyarrhythmia. Orthodromic AVRT, (antegrade conduction over the AV node) accounts for 70–80% of arrhythmias in patients with atrioventricular bypass tracts, with heart rates of 140–250 bpm (Figure 19–12). Antidromic AVRT, in which the atrial impulse is carried to the ventricle over the bypass tract and reenters the atrium via retrograde conduction over the AV node, is rare, occurring in approximately 5–10% of cases. Because conduction to the ventricles during orthodromic AVRT occurs over the normal conduction

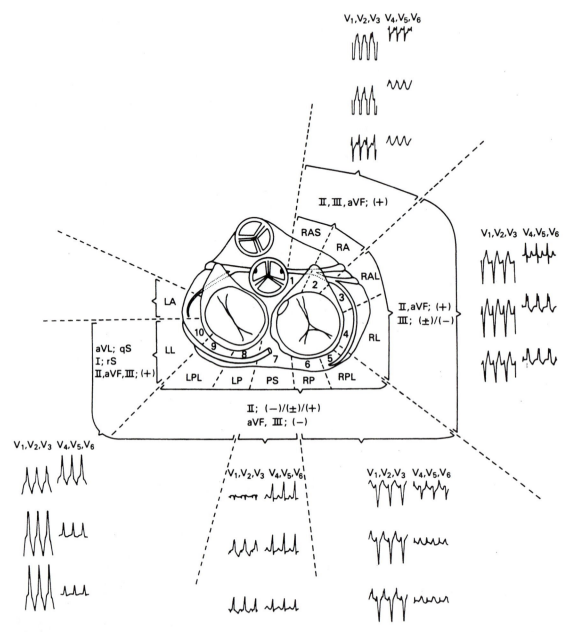

Figure 19–10. Single atrioventricular bypass-tract localization based on maximally preexcited electrocardiographic morphology. RAS/RA = right anteroseptal or right anterior accessory pathways; RAL/RL = right anterolateral or right lateral accessory pathways; RP/RPL = right posterior or right posterolateral accessory pathways; PS = posteroseptal accessory pathways; LPL/LP = left posterolateral or left posterior accessory pathways; LL = left lateral accessory pathways; + = positive delta wave; – = negative delta wave; ± = isoelectric delta wave. Reprinted, with permission, from Fananapazir L, German LD, Gallagher JJ et al: Importance of preexcited QRS morphology during induced atrial fibrillation to the diagnosis and localization of multiple accessory pathways. Circulation 1990;81:578.

system, the QRS is narrow, unless bundle branch aberrancy is present. During antidromic AVRT, the QRS is wide and maximally preexcited as a result of the complete lack of AV nodal contribution to ventricular depolarization. When two or more bypass tracts are present, each tract may act as the antegrade or retrograde limb (or both), especially with involvement of the AV node. There is a higher incidence of ventricular fibrillation in patients with multiple accessory pathways. Additionally, multiple pathways are more common in patients with antidromic supraventricular tachycardia (SVT) and in patients with Ebstein's anomaly.

Tachycardia is usually initiated by a premature atrial or ventricular beat. In orthodromic tachycardia, a premature atrial beat conducts down the AV node to depolarize the ventricle, and the bypass tract carries the impulse back to the atrium (Figure 19–13). A ventricular premature beat finding the AV node refractory

might initiate an identical tachycardia by first conducting up the bypass tract to the atrium. Antidromic tachycardia initiates in an identical fashion, but with reversal of the direction of conduction.

2. Atrial fibrillation with antegrade bypass tract conduction—Atrial fibrillation accounts for only 19–38% of arrhythmias in the population with accessory pathways, but it is potentially more lethal than the reciprocating tachycardias discussed earlier. It is more common in patients with manifest accessory pathways, ie, those with delta waves, and in pathways with a short antegrade refractory period. By virtue of their short refractory periods, bypass tracts (unlike the AV node) have the potential to conduct very rapidly to the ventricles at ventricular rates of 250–350 bpm (Figure 19–14) with the possibility of degenerating to ventricular fibrillation. A reputed marker for sudden death in

A

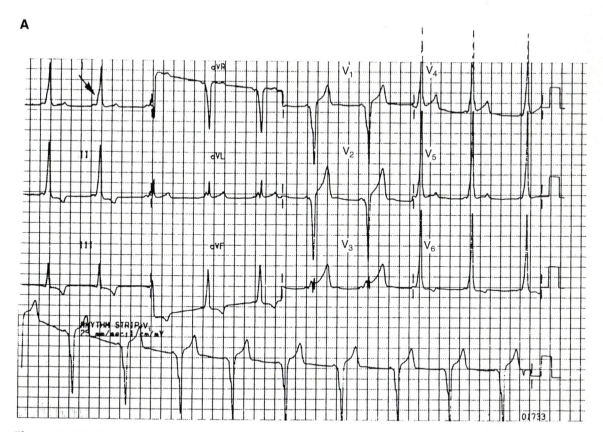

Figure 19–11. Ventricular preexcitation over a bypass tract in sinus rhythm. Note the short P-R interval. **A:** Right anterior bypass tract. The delta wave is positive in most leads (*arrow*), and negative in a VR and V_1–V_3. **B:** Left lateral bypass tract. The isoelectric delta wave in V_1 gives the appearance of a normal PR interval. Inspection of the simultaneously recorded rhythm strip leads (*lower three panels*) reveals delta wave onset to be at the end of the P wave in leads II and V_5. **C:** A short time after this tracing was obtained the patient exhibited minimal to no preexcitation. This was due to fluctuations in autonomic tone causing enhanced conduction through the AV node. *(continued)*

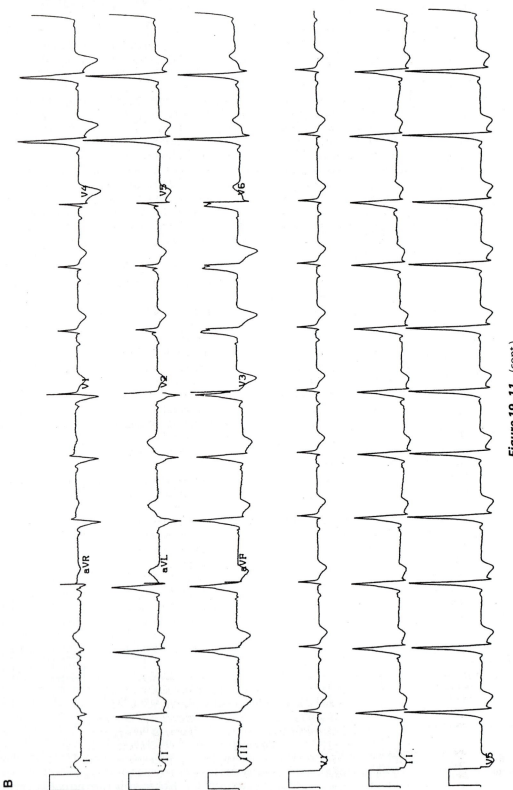

Figure 19–11. (cont.)

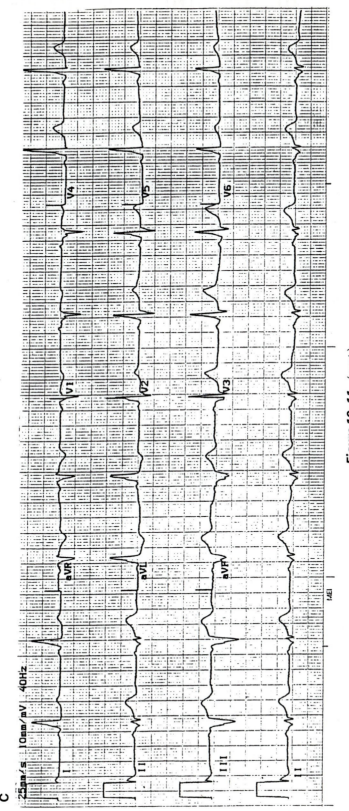

Figure 19–11. (cont.)

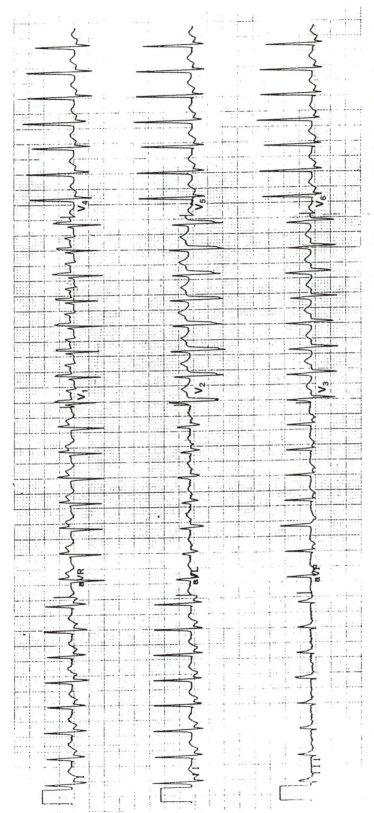

Figure 19–12. Orthodromic atrioventricular (AV) reciprocating tachycardia (O-AVRT) in a patient with a left-sided bypass tract. The circuit conducts from atria to ventricles over the AV node and from ventricles to atria retrograde over the bypass tract. This mechanism accounts for the narrow QRS and the retrograde P waves inscribed in the early portion of the T waves. Although the electrocardiogram with common AV nodal reentrant tachycardia may appear similar, a ventriculoatrial conduction time of more than 100 ms, as measured from QRS onset to P wave onset, greatly favors O-AVRT. The time in this tracing is 110 ms.

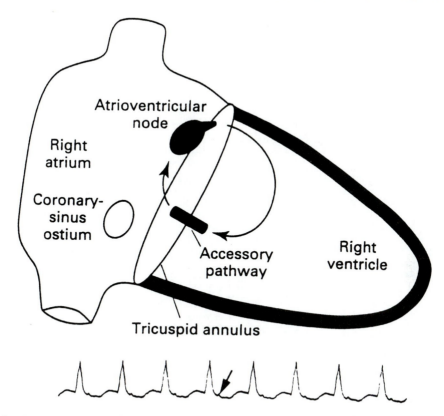

Figure 19–13. The reentry circuit of orthodromic reciprocating tachycardia. The atrioventricular (AV) node serves as the anteretrograde limb of the reentry circuit, and an accessory pathway serves as the retrograde limb. In this case the accessory pathway is located in the free wall of the right ventricle. The wave of depolarization travels from the AV node to the accessory pathway through the ventricle and from the accessory pathway to the AV node through the atrium. Because the ventricles are depolarized by the normal conduction system, the ORS are narrow unless there is a bundle branch block. Also shown is an example of orthodromic reciprocating tachycardia, at a rate of 210 per minute, recoded in lead III. A P wave is present in the left half of the RR cycle (*arrow*) because retrograde conduction through the accessory pathway is more rapid than anteretrograde conduction through the AV node. Reprinted, with permission, from Morady F: Drug therapy: Radio-frequency ablation as treatment for cardiac arrhythmias. N Engl J Med 1999;340:534. Copyright © 1999 Massachusetts Medical Society. All rights reserved.

patients with atrial fibrillation is a shortest preexcited R-R interval of ≤250 ms (corresponding to a heart rate of ≥240 bpm) between two fully preexcited beats. The finding of a short R-R interval actually has little positive predictive value, however, because sudden death in this syndrome is rare.

Atrial fibrillation is actually a very helpful diagnostic tool. Inducing it during the course of an electrophysiologic study yields two pieces of information: the shortest preexcited R-R interval, and the presence of multiple preexcited QRS complexes as a clue to multiple bypass tracts. Although more than one tract may be present, it is possible that during sinus rhythm only the tract closest to the sinus node will exhibit preexcitation on the ECG. With both atria fibrillating, distance is no

longer an issue, as all tracts have an equal opportunity to become engaged and conduct to the ventricles. Several preexcited QRS morphologies may then be seen, each representing conduction over a different accessory pathway.

During atrial fibrillation, the ECG reveals QRS complexes of varying morphologies, representing conduction to the ventricles via the AV node (normally conducted narrow complexes), the bypass tract (wide, preexcited complexes), and both (fusion beats, harboring elements of both the normally conducted and preexcited beats). Patients with AV bypass tracts have a higher incidence of atrial fibrillation than does the general population, possibly because of the degeneration of reentrant tachycardia or of microreentry within the

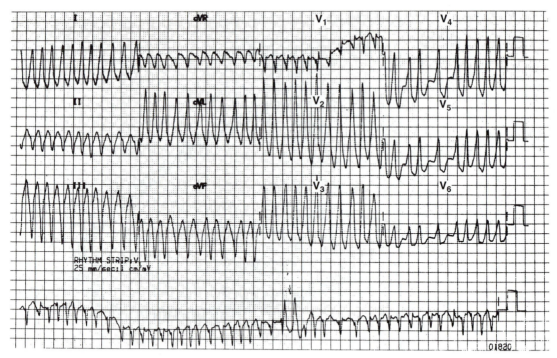

Figure 19–14. Atrial fibrillation with antegrade conduction over a left posteroseptal bypass tract. Although most beats are fully preexcited, several of the beats in the rhythm strip are narrower, indicating combined conduction over both the bypass tract and the atrioventricular node. Antidromic atrioventricular reciprocating tachycardia would have a similar appearance on 12-lead electrocardiogram, but the rhythm irregularity and the varying degrees of pre-excitation nullify this possibility. Reprinted, with permission, from Zipes DP: Specific arrhythmias: Diagnosis and treatment. In Braunwald E, ed: Heart Disease. A Textbook of Cardiovascular Medicine. Philadelphia: WB Saunders, 1988.

atrial portion of the bypass tract. Neither of these theories accounts for the fact that the site of earliest fibrillatory activity is spatially removed from the atrial insertion site of the bypass tract. If the tendency toward fibrillation is related to the presence of an accessory pathway, pathway ablation should remove the substrate and prevent recurrences.

3. Concealed bypass tracts—Between 15% and 50% of patients with no evidence of preexcitation during sinus rhythm are found to have bypass tracts that conduct in a retrograde, but not antegrade, direction. By definition, concealed bypass tracts (their presence cannot be detected by ECG) cannot display delta waves on the ECG during sinus rhythm, but they can still support an orthodromic AVRT and account for about 30% of orthodromic tachycardias.

Differentiating orthodromic AVRT from AVNRT on the ECG can be difficult. The incidence of both tachycardias being operative at different times in the same person is reported to be between 1.7% and 7%. Therefore, although the presence of a delta wave on the

nontachycardiac tracing makes it statistically unlikely that AVNRT was the documented tachycardia, it does not exclude the possibility completely.

Because of the simultaneous atrial and ventricular activation that occurs during AVNRT, the P waves formed as a result of retrograde conduction to the atrium are usually obscured within the QRS complex. Likewise, because of the short retrograde conduction time, orthodromic AVRT from septal bypass tracts may have a short R-P interval, albeit somewhat longer than with AVNRT. Usually, the P waves are located within the ST segment, ie, generally, the R-P interval is longer with AVRT than with AVNRT. Visualization of P waves following the QRS therefore favors orthodromic conduction over a nonseptal accessory pathway.

When runs of bundle branch aberrancy are interspersed with normal antegrade conduction during a tachycardia, the ventriculoatrial conduction times (VACT) should be compared. A prolongation of more than 35 ms during aberrancy indicates the presence of a bypass tract ipsilateral to the site of block. This is due to the added travel time from the contralateral bundle to the accessory pathway through the myocardium (Coumel's law). (Bundle branch block contralateral to the accessory pathway will not prolong the conduction time.) For left or right posteroseptal pathways, the VACT will prolong by less than 35 ms with ipsilateral aberrancy, if at all, because of its midline position. Although these increments are too small to be accurately measured on a 12-lead ECG being recorded at 25 mm/s, they can be easily discerned by high-speed analog and digital equipment during electrophysiologic studies.

In cases of a wide QRS tachycardia, if AV dissociation, fusion beats, or capture beats are present, the diagnosis of ventricular tachycardia is made. If these are not present and the rhythm is regular, antidromic AVRT, atrial flutter with antegrade bypass conduction, another supraventricular tachycardia with aberrant conduction, and ventricular tachycardia are possibilities. If the rhythm is associated with atrioventricular block, antidromic AVRT is excluded because participation of the ventricle is required for perpetuation of the rhythm. An irregularly irregular wide complex rhythm may represent atrial fibrillation with antegrade accessory pathway conduction.

Treatment

Because of their excellent long-term prognosis, asymptomatic patients showing delta waves on the ECG do not require treatment unless involved in a high-risk profession such as commercial pilots, police officers, firefighters, etc. Patients with occasional or rare bouts of minimal or mildly symptomatic palpitations can often be safely treated with such agents as β-blockers or calcium channel blockers. Those who experience more significant symptoms such as dizziness, presyncope, or syncope should undergo an electrophysiologic study with concomitant radiofrequency ablation. Several authorities advocate the use of exercise testing as a means of assessing sudden death risk in patients who manifest delta waves at rest. Catecholamines are known to shorten antegrade bypass-tract refractory periods. If delta waves disappear during exercise, the antegrade refractory period of the bypass tract is estimated to be longer than 300 ms. This figure has a very high negative predictive value for sudden death; however, delta waves disappear in only about 5–10% of the population, making the test difficult to apply in the majority.

A. Pharmacologic Therapy

1. Atrioventricular reciprocating tachycardia— Great care must be taken when administering drugs for antidromic AVRT. Several drugs, most notably verapamil, digoxin, and lidocaine, have the potential to accelerate antegrade conduction over the bypass tract, which may increase the rate of the tachycardia. Verapamil (only when given intravenously) does so indirectly by causing vasodilation and reflex sympathetic activation; digoxin acts directly on the accessory pathway tissue. In addition, if ventricular tachycardia is mistaken for an antidromic reciprocating rhythm (they both present with a wide QRS), and verapamil is used, its vasodilatory effect will cause severe hypotension. Because adenosine usually has no effect on accessory pathway conduction, no deleterious effect on ventricular tachycardia, and both a short time to onset and a short duration of action (5–15 s), it should be the first drug given in the acute setting. Procainamide can be used to treat both tachycardias; however, its drawbacks are potential hypotension (from vasodilation) and a long infusion time (20–40 min). With the exception of digoxin, drugs of all antiarrhythmic classes can be used for chronic therapy.

Pharmacologic treatment of recurrent orthodromic tachycardia is aimed at disabling the weaker of the two limbs of the loop, whether the bypass tract or the AV node. If β-blockers or verapamil fail to inhibit AV nodal conduction, class Ia antiarrhythmic agents can be used to target the bypass tract; class Ic and III drugs target both limbs. In the acute setting, if vagal maneuvers fail, intravenous adenosine is the drug of choice for terminating the tachycardia. If this is unsuccessful, intravenous procainamide can be used. Unless an electrophysiologic study has confirmed the absence of antegrade bypass tract conduction, digoxin and intravenous verapamil should not be used.

2. Atrial fibrillation with antegrade bypass tract conduction—Hemodynamic stability dictates the therapy here. If the patient is stable, ventricular rate control can be attempted. Because intravenous digoxin and verapamil can increase antegrade pathway conduction in this setting, their use may cause an increase in the ventricular rate, resulting in ventricular fibrillation. Except for diagnostic purposes, adenosine is of little use because of its ultrashort duration of action and its inability to terminate the underlying atrial fibrillation. Intravenous procainamide, diltiazem, or β-blockers are reasonable choices to achieve rate control. Of these, only procainamide can convert the atrial fibrillation to sinus rhythm, making it a very attractive option.

B. Radiofrequency Catheter Ablation Therapy

Patients who do not respond to or who wish to avoid drug therapy can undergo ablative therapy. The right internal jugular or femoral vein ablation approach is used for accessory pathways located on the right side of the heart. Left-sided pathways can be approached from the left ventricle with retrograde technique, or transseptally from within the left atrium using the Brockenbrough technique. Although catheter manipulation within the smooth left atrium is reportedly easier than within the muscular, trabeculated left ventricle, equal success is attained with either approach. A steerable catheter is moved around the mitral or tricuspid annulus until the site of shortest impulse transit between the atrium and ventricle is found. This mapping process localizes the bypass tract. Frequently, an impulse can be recorded directly from the bypass tract, further confirming its localization. Once isolated, radiofrequency energy delivered to the tract through the mapping catheter permanently destroys the tract and prevents further transmission of electric impulses over it.

Given its curative potential, a high success rate (95% in experienced hands, even with multiple bypass tracts), and a low complication rate, radiofrequency catheter ablation is now considered the preferred treatment for accessory pathways (Table 19–2). As with other supraventricular arrhythmias, new mapping systems have been developed that decrease fluoroscopy and procedure time as well as allowing the operator to return to specific locations if needed.

C. Surgical Ablation Therapy

Patients who have multiple pathways or pathways that are inaccessible to an ablation catheter or those patients who have a concomitant disease that requires surgery may undergo surgical division of their tract(s). The procedure involves a sternotomy, with either an epicardial or endocardial approach. Because these tracts are often several centimeters in breadth, a wide dissection along the AV groove is required for complete transection. The arrhythmia recurrence rate approaches zero following either surgical approach.

2. OTHER BYPASS TRACTS

A variety of bypass tracts other than AV tracts (Kent fibers) also exist. Lown–Ganong–Levine syndrome describes those patients with a short P-R interval, normal QRS, and recurrent SVT. Ninety percent of these cases involve accelerated AV nodal conduction, and patients may suffer from any type of rapid SVT. In a minority of patients, a bypass tract linking the atrium to the distal AV node is used as the antegrade limb, and the AV node is used as the retrograde limb of the circuit.

Atriofascicular fibers can run from the lateral right atrium to a region that sits in close proximity to the right bundle branch. The right bundle is the venue for antegrade conduction to the ventricles as well as retrograde conduction back to the atria. This bypass tract and the tachycardia it creates are unique in several regards. The tract is capable of antegrade conduction only, and it exhibits decremental conduction (longer conduction time at faster rates), as does the AV node. There is a high association with AVNRT. Because the antegrade reentrant circuit engages the right bundle branch, the QRS complex typically has a left bundle branch block pattern. Alternating long and short R-R

Table 19–2. Complications of radiofrequency ablation of accessory pathways.[a]

Complication	Prevalence (%)
Death	0.08
Nonfatal complications	
Cardiac tamponade	0.5
Atrioventricular block	0.5
Coronary artery spasm	0.2
Mild mitral regurgitation	0.2
Coronary artery thrombosis	0.1
Pericarditis	0.1
Mild aortic regurgitation	0.1
Transient neurologic deficit	0.1
Bacteremia	0.1
Femoral artery complications	
Thrombotic occlusion	0.2
Large hematoma	0.2
Atrioventricular fistula	0.1

[a] The incidence of death is based on unpublished data from the University of Oklahoma, the University of Alabama, the University of Michigan, Duke University, and the University of California, San Francisco. The incidence of nonfatal complications is based on pooled data from seven published studies.

intervals are commonly seen as a result of retrograde refractoriness of the right bundle branch. The blocked impulse may travel transseptally to engage the left bundle branch to return to the atria; the ventriculoatrial conduction time will be prolonged because of the added time it takes the wavefront to cross the septum. This allows the right bundle branch to recover retrograde conductivity by the time the next beat is delivered to it over the bypass tract, and the ventriculoatrial time is short. This cycle perpetuates itself to cause alternating short–long cycles. Tachyarrhythmias in these patients usually do not reach dangerous heart rates, and sudden death is rare. Treatment considerations are the same as for Wolff–Parkinson–White syndrome.

Podrid PJ, Kowey PR: Cardiac Arrhythmia, Mechanisms, Diagnosis and Management. Chapter 17, 2nd ed. Philadelphia: Williams and Wilkins, 2001.

Worley S: Use of a real-time three-dimensional magnetic navigation system for radiofrequency ablation of accessory pathways. PACE 1998;21:1636–1645.

Atrial Fibrillation

Melvin M. Scheinman, MD

ESSENTIALS OF DIAGNOSIS

- *Irregularly irregular rhythm*
- *Absence of P waves on the electrocardiograph*

General Considerations

Atrial fibrillation, the most common sustained clinical arrhythmia, is diagnosed by finding an irregularly irregular ventricular rhythm without discrete P waves (Figure 20–1). The QRS complex is usually narrow, but it may be wide if aberrant conduction or bundle branch block is present. Atrial fibrillation associated with the Wolff-Parkinson-White syndrome may occur with very rapid ventricular rates and may be life-threatening. This arrhythmia is diagnosed by its very rapid irregular rate associated with wide preexcited QRS complexes and requires emergency treatment (see Long-term approach).

Epidemiology

Approximately 4% of the population over age 60 years has sustained an episode of atrial fibrillation, with a particularly steep increase in prevalence after the seventh decade of life. Risk factors for development of atrial fibrillation include heart failure, hypertensive cardiovascular disease, coronary artery disease, and valvular heart disease. Moreover, both sustained and paroxys-

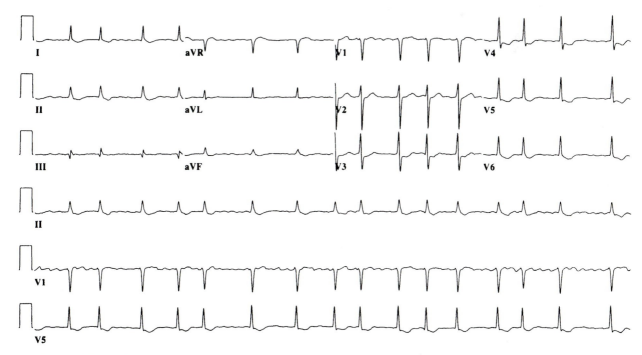

Figure 20–1. The 12-lead electrocardiogram shows the typical rapid irregular rhythm seen with atrial fibrillation.

mal atrial fibrillation have important implications for the development of a cerebrovascular accident (CVA) or other systemic emboli. It is estimated that 15–20% of CVAs in nonrheumatic patients are due to atrial fibrillation.

Clinical Findings

A. Symptoms and Signs

When called on to manage new-onset atrial fibrillation, it is important to establish the precipitating factors because the type of associated condition determines long-term prognosis. In some patients, episodes of atrial fibrillation may be initiated by caffeine, alcohol, or marijuana use. Atrial fibrillation may result from acute intercurrent ailments. For example, this arrhythmia may develop in patients with hyperthyroidism or lung disease, or after either cardiac or pulmonary surgery, especially in older patients. Atrial fibrillation is also seen in patients with acute pulmonary embolism, myocarditis, or acute myocardial infarction, particularly when the last condition is complicated by either occlusion of the right coronary artery or heart failure. When atrial fibrillation occurs in these settings, it almost always abates spontaneously if the patient recovers from the underlying problem. Hence, management usually involves administration of drugs to control the heart rate, and chronic antiarrhythmic therapy is generally not needed.

Alternatively, atrial fibrillation may occur in association with structural cardiac disease. Important associated conditions include rheumatic mitral stenosis, hypertension, hypertrophic cardiomyopathy, or chronic heart failure. In contrast to patients with acute intercurrent ailments, those with structural heart disease may expect (even with antiarrhythmic therapy) many recurrences and chronic atrial fibrillation may supervene.

Lone fibrillation is the term used to describe patients with atrial fibrillation not associated with known cardiac conditions or noncardiac precipitants. The natural history of the atrial fibrillation for those with lone atrial fibrillation is similar to that in patients with structural cardiac disease, in that episodes of atrial fibrillation are likely to recur and, eventually, the arrhythmia may become sustained.

B. Physical Examination

The initial evaluation of new-onset atrial fibrillation includes a detailed history focusing on possible precipitating factors as well as the presence of organic cardiac disease. As such, the initial evaluation includes, at a minimum, a careful physical examination, 12-lead electrocardiograph, chest radiograph, echocardiogram, and tests of thyroid function. Further testing will depend on various aspects of the history or physical examina-

tion. For example, if atrial fibrillation is usually precipitated by exercise, then an exercise treadmill test is appropriate. In the patient with frequent episodes of paroxysmal atrial fibrillation, a 24- to 48-h Holter recording may discern whether atrial fibrillation was triggered by another arrhythmia such as a premature atrial complex alone or whether the fibrillation was preceded by an episode of supraventricular tachycardia. In addition, patients with vagally mediated fibrillation will typically have episodes either after heavy meals or during sleep. These clues may help identify those patients who may respond to specific approaches (see Treatment).

Treatment

The objectives of therapy include (1) achieving rate control, (2) restoring sinus rhythm (where feasible), and (3) decreasing the risk of CVA.

A. Rate Control

If the patient presents with atrial fibrillation and a rapid rate associated with severe heart failure or cardiogenic shock, emergency direct-current cardioversion is indicated. For patients with atrial fibrillation associated with rapid rate but with stable hemodynamics, attempts to achieve acute rate control are indicated. Drugs to slow the ventricular rate in patients with atrial fibrillation (Table 20–1) include digitalis preparations, calcium channel blockers (verapamil or diltiazem), and β-blockers. If rapid rate control is desired, then calcium channel blockers and β-blockers are far more effective than digitalis, which may require many hours before rate control is achieved. In addition, a common misconception is that digitalis therapy is associated with acute conversion to sinus rhythm, but carefully controlled studies have shown that conversion to sinus rhythm is no more likely with digoxin than with placebo. As emphasized later, digitalis and intravenous calcium channel blocker therapy are contraindicated for patients presenting with Wolff-Parkinson-White syndrome and atrial fibrillation. Intravenous diltiazem has been shown to be safe and effective for patients with atrial fibrillation and a modest degree of heart failure.

In patients with a known history of congestive heart failure, use of intravenous β-blockers or calcium channel blockers may aggravate the cardiac failure. In this subset digitalis or intravenous (IV) amiodarone would be the preferred agents for rate control.

B. Chronic Antiarrhythmic Therapy and Elective Cardioversion

For patients presenting with a single, initial episode of atrial fibrillation with no significant hemodynamic problems, no specific therapy is required because repeat

Table 20–1. Intravenous pharmacologic agents for heart rate control in atrial fibrillation.

Drug	Loading Dose	Onset	Maintenance Dose	Major Side Effects
Diltiazem	0.25 mg/kg IV over 2 min	2–7 min	5–15 mg/h infusion	Hypotension, heart block, HF
Esmolol	0.5 mg/kg over 1 min	5 min	0.05–0.2 mg kg^{-1} min^{-1}	Hypotension, heart block, bradycardia, asthma, HF
Metoprolol	2.5–5 mg IV bolus over 2 min; up to 3 doses	5 min	NA	Hypotension, heart block, bradycardia, asthma, HF
Propranolol	0.15 mg/kg IV	5 min	NA	Hypotension, heart block, bradycardia, asthma, HF
Verapamil	0.075–0.15 mg/kg IV over 2 min	3–5 min	NA	Hypotension, heart block, HF
Digoxin	0.25 mg IV each 2 h, up to 1.5 mg	2 h	0.125–0.25 mg daily	Digitalis toxicity, heart block, bradycardia

HF = heart failure.

Source: Reprinted, with permission, from Fuster V, Ryden LE, Asinger RW, et al. ACC/AHA/ESC practice guidelines for the management of patients with atrial fibrillation: A report of the American College of Cardiology/American Heart Association Task Force on Practice Guidelines and the European Society of Cardiology Committee for Practice Guidelines and Policy Conference. J Am Coll Cardiol 2001; 38:266i–lxx.

episodes may not occur for many years. In contrast, patients who manifest frequent recurrences may be candidates for chronic antiarrhythmic therapy with class IA (quinidine, procainamide, and disopyramide), class IC (propafenone and flecainide), or class III (sotalol, amiodarone, and dofetilide) agents, all of which are more effective than placebo in maintaining sinus rhythm (Table 20–2).

Table 20–2. Typical doses of drugs used to maintain sinus rhythm in atrial fibrillation, listed alphabetically.

Drug	Daily Dosage	Potential Adverse Effects
Amiodarone	100–400 mg	Photosensitivity, pulmonary toxicity, polyneuropathy, GI upset, bradycardia, torsade de pointes (rare), hepatic toxicity, thyroid dysfunction
Disopyramide	400–750 mg	Torsade de pointes, HF, glaucoma, urinary retention, dry mouth
Dofetilide	500–1000 μg	Torsade de pointes
Flecainide	200–300 mg	Ventricular tachycardia, congestive HF, enhanced AV nodal conduction (conversion to atrial flutter)
Procainamide	1000–4000 mg	Torsade de pointes, lupus-like syndrome, GI symptoms
Propafenone	450–900 mg	Ventricular tachycardia, congestive HF, enhanced AV nodal conduction (conversion to atrial flutter)
Quinidine	600–1500 mg	Torsade de pointes, GI upset, enhanced AV nodal conduction
Sotalol	240–320 mg	Torsade de pointes, congestive HF, bradycardia, exacerbation of chronic obstructive or bronchospastic lung disease

AV = atrioventricular; GI = gastrointestinal; HF = heart failure.

Source: Reprinted, with permission, from Fuster V, Ryden LE, Asinger RW, et al. ACE/AHA/ESC practice guidelines for the management of patients with atrial fibrillation: A report of the American College of Cardiology/American Heart Association Task Force on Practice Guidelines and the European Society of Cardiology Committee for Practice Guidelines and Policy Conference. J Am Coll Cardiol 2001; 38:266i–lxx.

C. ANTIARRHYTHMIC DRUG THERAPY
FOR ATRIAL FIBRILLATION

For patients with lone atrial fibrillation, use of any of the antiarrhythmic drugs listed is appropriate. In general, the class IC agents (flecainide or propafenone) are the first choice in terms of efficacy and lowest incidence of side effects. It would be wise, for example, to withhold amiodarone as a first-line drug in view of the potential for adverse effects. Only two drugs have been proved safe for patients with severe congestive heart failure: dofetilide and amiodarone.

For patients with atrial fibrillation associated with coronary artery disease, consider use of sotalol as initial drug therapy. This agent has class III antiarrhythmic effects and is a potent β-blocker. Class IC drugs should not be used in patients with significant structural cardiac disease or in those with ischemic heart disease. They have, however, been found to be safe and effective for patients with hypertension and atrial fibrillation.

In addition, extra cardiac factors are very important in the choice of antiarrhythmic drugs. For example, dose adjustments are mandatory for patients with renal insufficiency. This is especially true for procainamide, sotalol, and dofetilide. Dofetilide, for example, requires hospital admission, calculation of the creatinine clearance and drug titration according to the QT corrected for heart rate as well as renal function. An algorithm for antiarrhythmic drug usage is summarized in Figure 20–2.

Even with drug therapy, recurrence rates for atrial fibrillation approach 50% per year (as opposed to recurrences with placebo therapy of 75% per year). In addition, these agents may be associated with significant side effects. For class IA drugs, these include induction of torsade de pointes, especially for those with congestive heart failure. For example, a meta-analysis compared quinidine with placebo for patients with atrial fibrillation and found that death from all causes was *higher* in the groups treated with quinidine. In addition, in the Stroke Prevention in Atrial Fibrillation (SPAF) trials, substantial numbers of patients were treated with antiarrhythmic agents; in patients with heart failure, those treated with class I drugs had significantly increased mortality rates compared with those not treated with antiarrhythmic drugs. Great care must be exercised in the use of these agents, balancing the benefits against the potential for adverse effects. General rules include avoidance of all class IA drugs or sotalol for patients with congestive heart failure and avoidance of class IC agents for patients with structural heart disease. In addition, sotalol is contraindicated for patients with severe depression of the left ventricular ejection fraction. Patients with significant sinus node or atrioventricular (AV) conduction disease may require pacemaker therapy before use of antiarrhythmic drugs because these drugs may further depress sinus node or AV conduction. The only drugs that appear to be both effective and safe for patients with heart failure and atrial fibrillation are amiodarone and dofetilide. Amiodarone is associated with a host of both cardiac (eg, severe sinus bradycardia or arrest or AV block) and noncardiac (eg, thyroid abnormalities, pulmonary fibrosis) adverse effects, but low-dose amiodarone (ie, 2 mg/day) appears to be effective and very well tolerated. Dofetilide has a narrow therapeutic window and can cause life-threatening arrhythmias; it can be used in patients with atrial fibrillation and congestive heart failure but requires an in-hospital stay for monitoring of the agent.

1. Chemical cardioversion—Recent studies have emphasized the use of drugs for acute conversion of atrial fibrillation. It has been shown that IV ibutilide or IV dofetilide (not available in the United States) are effective for conversion of approximately 35% of patients with atrial fibrillation. It should be emphasized that this drug should be used only in a monitored environment. The usual dose is 1 mg over 10 min, followed by a 10-min interlude, followed by an additional 1 mg over 10 min if necessary. Facilities with IV management, and a defibrillator should be readily available because the incidence of sustained torsade de pointes is 1–2%. Ibutilide should be avoided for patients with severe heart failure or bradycardia.

a. Other drugs for chemical cardioversion—Other drug combinations have also been found effective. For example, it has been found that use of large oral doses of either flecainide (300 mg) or propafenone (600 mg) may terminate up to 80% of episodes of atrial fibrillation within 2 h. This approach should be used only in patients who are pretreated with β-blocking drugs and in the absence of significant cardiac disease or heart failure.

b. Anticoagulant therapy—The risk of CVA in patients with nonrheumatic atrial fibrillation is 4–7% per year. Patients at particularly high risk include those over age 70 years or with hypertension, a history of heart failure, increased left atrial size, diabetes, or prior CVA. The risks of CVA are similar in patients with paroxysmal versus chronic atrial fibrillation. Numerous studies have documented the remarkable efficacy of warfarin in decreasing the risk of emboli by 45–85% in patients with nonrheumatic atrial fibrillation with a low risk of significant hemorrhage, provided the International Normalized Ratio (INR) is in the range of 2.0 to 2.5. Still controversial is the need for anticoagulant therapy in younger patients with lone atrial fibrillation because the risk of emboli is very low in this group.

The role of aspirin therapy for patients with atrial fibrillation remains controversial. In one study, 75 mg of aspirin failed to decrease the stroke risk compared with placebo (5.5%/year). In contrast, the SPAF I trials

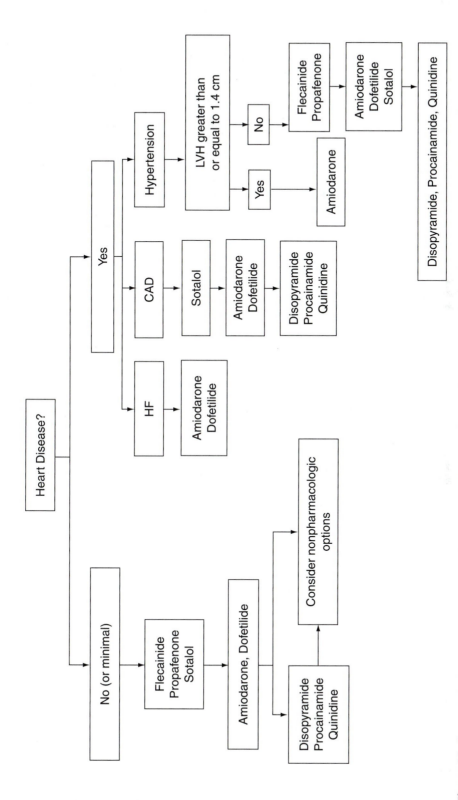

Figure 20–2. Antiarrhythmic drug therapy to maintain sinus rhythm in patients with recurrent paroxysmal or persistent atrial fibrillation. Drugs in boxes are listed alphabetically and not in order of suggested use. CAD = coronary artery disease; HF = heart failure; LVH = left ventricular hypertrophy.

showed that a higher dose of aspirin, 325 mg, appeared to be of benefit in patients under 75 years of age. In a follow-up study (SPAF II), the incidence of stroke was higher with aspirin (4.8%) compared with warfarin (3.6%). The SPAF III trials demonstrated that aspirin (325 mg/day) and fixed low-dose warfarin (1, 2, or 3 mg) were ineffective for stroke prevention. Therefore, the weight of current data favors use of warfarin with an INR of 2.0–2.5 as the best strategy to prevent systemic embolization. A number of studies involving use of antithrombin agents, clopidogrel or low-molecular-weight heparin in patients with atrial fibrillation are currently in trial stage. The advantage of these agents will be to obviate the need for blood testing of INR levels.

2. Direct current cardioversion—Direct-current cardioversion is a very effective technique for restoration of sinus rhythm. Because of the benefits of sinus rhythm in terms of improved cardiac output and decreased risk of embolic phenomena, in general, at least one attempt should be made to restore sinus rhythm. Several precautions are in order. If the patient has a history of recurrent episodes of atrial fibrillation then he or she should be pretreated with an antiarrhythmic agent because reversion to atrial fibrillation after shock therapy is very high. Use of antiarrhythmic drugs before direct-current shock, however, is inappropriate for the patient with an initial episode of well-tolerated atrial fibrillation. Unless urgent cardioversion is required because of hemodynamic decompensation, severe ischemia, or congestive heart failure, it is imperative to follow one of several options for reducing the risk of systemic embolization:

a. For patients with atrial fibrillation of less than 48 h duration it would appear to be safe to proceed with application of direct-current shock.

b. If atrial fibrillation persists for more than 48 h, then the risk of embolization increases and anticoagulants are required prior to ablation. One recommended option for patients with atrial fibrillation of more than 48 h duration is to perform transesophageal echocardiography (TEE), which is excellent for detecting clots in the left atrium or the left atrial appendage. Evidence from several studies indicates that the finding of either a clot or spontaneous echocardiographic contrast in the left atrium is associated with higher risks of systemic embolization. In the absence of such findings on TEE, systemic emboli are rare. Therefore, patients with recent-onset atrial fibrillation with no evidence of atrial clots or spontaneous contrast by TEE may undergo direct-current cardioversion after initiation of heparin therapy. A recent report from the ACUTE trial showed that treatment of patients with atrial fibrillation treated on the bases of TEE-guided therapy versus a group treated with a 3-week course of anticoagulant therapy had similar rates of thromboembolism (<1%). It must be appreciated that atrial function is depressed (atrial stunning) after cardioversion and that anticoagulant therapy is recommended for at least 1 month after cardioversion. This is true whether the duration of atrial fibrillation was either less than or greater than 48 h. For those patients with clot or dense spontaneous echocardiographic contrast with TEE, full anticoagulant therapy with an INR of 2.0–2.5 is recommended for at least 2–3 weeks before cardioversion.

c. An alternative approach is that patients with atrial fibrillation of greater than 48 h be fully anticoagulated for at least three consecutive weeks before attempting direct-current cardioversion and for about 4 weeks afterward to decrease the risk of an embolism after successful reversion to sinus rhythm. This approach tends to be less efficient than the TEE-guided approach for recent-onset atrial fibrillation but is an acceptable alternative treatment for atrial fibrillation.

Direct-current external shock is usually performed in a monitored area under supervision of an anesthesiologist. Pads are placed in an anterior-posterior orientation in order to maximize current delivered to the atrium. It is wise to check the arterial oxygen saturation, serum potassium level, digoxin, or antiarrhythmic blood drug levels before cardioversion. Direct-current shocks beginning with at least 200 J are used in an attempt to achieve sinus rhythm. Multiple shocks of lesser energy are to be avoided. If the patient fails to revert after maximal external shocks (360 J monophasic or 200 J biphasic), then successful cardioversion can almost always be achieved either by the use of a biphasic waveform defibrillator or supplemental doses of ibutilide. Ibutilide has been shown to lower the atrial defibrillation threshold. An attempt at internal cardioversion using small energy shocks delivered between the coronary sinus and the right atrium is seldom necessary because the above-described treatments are almost always effective.

3. Long-term approach—One should be especially careful to identify patients whose atrial fibrillation might be cured. Examples include patients with hyperthyroidism as well as those in whom other cardiac arrhythmias appear to trigger atrial fibrillation. For example, patients with atrial flutter or paroxysmal supraventricular tachycardia may experience atrial premature impulses that trigger atrial fibrillation. In selected patients it is possible to apply catheter ablation to cure the underlying supraventricular arrhythmia and, hence, prevent the trigger for atrial fibrillation. Therefore, in the evaluation of patients who present with atrial fibrillation, initial testing should include obtaining a thyroid-stimulating hormone assay, an echocardiogram, and a 48-h ambulatory ECG recording for those with paroxysmal atrial fibrillation. In analyses of these recordings, the clinician seeks evidence for triggering arrhythmias. In addition, one looks for vagal triggers of atrial fibrillation, such as sinus bradycardia associated with sleep or heavy meals, that initially may be treated with vagolytic antiarrhythmic agents such as disopyramide. Alternatively, if atrial fibrillation appears only with enhanced sympathetic tone, such as with exercise, a trial of β-blocker therapy is appropriate.

One important special circumstance is that of atrial fibrillation in the patient with Wolff-Parkinson-White syndrome. These patients may present with a very rapid irregular rate and wide complex tachycardia owing to conduction over the accessory pathway, Figure 20–3. After recognition of this entity appropriate acute therapy includes use of IV ibutilide or procainamide or direct-current cardioversion. It is important to remember that IV digoxin and calcium channel blockers are contraindicated. In addition, use of lidocaine, β-blockers, or adenosine is not effective and is contraindicated because they delay appropriate therapy. After the rhythm is stabilized, these patients should undergo catheter ablation of the accessory pathway.

The natural history of atrial fibrillation associated with structural cardiac disease or in patients with lone atrial fibrillation is for spontaneous recurrence of the arrhythmia. Unfortunately, no drug is universally effective, and the decision of how many drugs to try before a judgment is made to terminate antiarrhythmic drugs and focus on rate control depends on how symptomatic the patient is during atrial fibrillation. If the episodes are poorly tolerated, then multiple drug trials or even various ablative procedures may be required (see section on Nonpharmacologic Treatment of Atrial Fibrillation). On the other hand, if rate control can be readily achieved with drugs, such as digoxin, β-blockers, or calcium antagonists, that block AV nodal conduction and the patient has a good symptomatic outcome, then an acceptable alternative is to use drugs that control rate combined with chronic anticoagulant treatment. A large, randomized trial (AFFIRM) is currently underway to compare the strategy of rate control and anticoagulation versus maintaining sinus rhythm. A smaller study randomized 252 patients and compared rate versus rhythm control strategies. The groups had similar symptomatic improvements, however, exercise tolerance was improved in the rhythm-controlled group at the "expense" of more frequent hospital admissions. This relatively small study cannot be used for definitive recommendations.

D. Nonpharmacologic Treatment of Atrial Fibrillation

Because pharmacologic therapy for atrial fibrillation is not ideal, a number of nonpharmacologic treatment

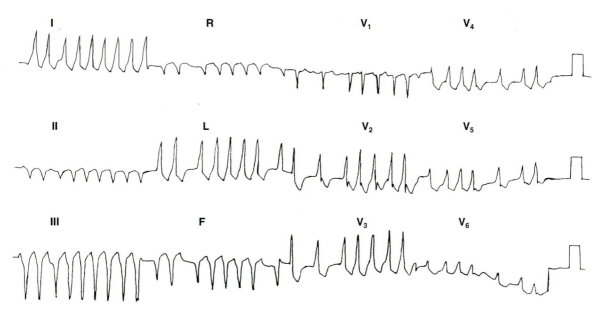

Figure 20–3. The 12-lead electrocardiogram shows a rapid irregular rhythm with broad QRS complex. This is pathognomonic of atrial fibrillation in a patient with Wolff-Parkinson-White syndrome. This arrhythmia requires urgent treatment. Acceptable therapy includes use of intravenous ibutilide or procainamide or direct-current shock.

modalities have been introduced. For atrial fibrillation that proves refractory to drug management, one time-tested approach is catheter ablation of the AV junction and permanent pacemaker insertion.

Patients with persistent tachycardia may suffer from a tachycardia-induced cardiomyopathy with left ventricular failure superimposed on their native cardiac disease. Hence, in the management of chronic atrial fibrillation, rate control is an important objective that must be achieved either via AV nodal blocking drugs or, failing these, with catheter ablative procedures. Catheter ablation of the AV junction involves insertion of an electrode catheter in the region of the His bundle with application of radiofrequency energy in order to destroy AV conduction. The chief benefit of this technique is achievement of perfect rate control without need for drugs. The drawbacks include the need for permanent pacing and a continued need for anticoagulant therapy.

It has been shown that atrial-based pacing systems will decrease the incidence of atrial fibrillation in patients with the tachycardia-bradycardia syndrome. In addition, pacing may allow for safe use of antiarrhythmic drugs. In patients with vagally mediated atrial fibrillation, atrial pacing may be effective in decreasing episodes of atrial fibrillation. Recent experimental studies have shown that either dual-site atrial pacing (ie, from coronary sinus and right atrium) or from the atrial septum in conjunction with antiarrhythmic therapy, may suppress atrial fibrillation.

An innovative approach to the management of atrial fibrillation involves use of an internal atrial defibrillator. This device has been shown to be safe and effective in conversion of atrial fibrillation in 85% of instances. The chief drawback is that although the energy required for internal defibrillation is quite low, nevertheless, internal shocks are painful and not well tolerated. Currently, atrial defibrillators are combined with ventricular defibrillators and may prove to be very helpful for patients with infrequent episodes of atrial fibrillation.

A number of surgical centers are currently using the maze procedure to try to cure atrial fibrillation. This procedure involves placing transmural lesions over both atria in such a manner that the fibrillatory impulses cannot complete a reentrant circuit. The maze procedure involves all of the risks of major open-heart surgery. This procedure should be considered for patients with atrial fibrillation who require cardiac surgery for correction of valvular diseases, coronary artery disease, or congenital heart disease.

In some patients with paroxysmal atrial fibrillation, a rapidly firing ectopic focus, often near the pulmonary veins, may cause atrial fibrillation. The current experience using catheter ablative procedures to cure atrial fibrillation has been validated by a number of studies.

It was found that attempts to ablate a specific focus within the pulmonary vein resulted in a long-term success rate of 50–60% but was associated with an unacceptable high incidence of pulmonary vein stenosis (2–8%). Currently most groups have advocated use of pulmonary vein isolation, which involves placement of a number of lesions around the ostium of the pulmonary vein in order to isolate discharges from pulmonary venous focus. Isolation procedures for at least three of the four pulmonary veins are associated with short-term success rates of 70–90% and was associated with a zero incidence of pulmonary vein stenosis. Pulmonary vein isolation is currently reserved for highly symptomatic patients with atrial fibrillation that is resistant to multiple drug trials.

Allessie MA, Konings KT, Kirchhof CJ: Mapping of atrial fibrillation. In: Olsson SB, Allessie MA, Campbell RW, eds: Atrial Fibrillation: Mechanisms and Therapeutic Strategies. Armonk, NY: Futura Pub, 1994:37.

Brand FN, Abbott RD, Kannel WB et al: Characteristics and prognosis of lone atrial fibrillation: 30-year follow-up in the Framingham Study. JAMA 1985;254:3449.

Capucci A, Lenzi T, Boriani G et al: Effectiveness of loading oral flecainide for converting recent-onset atrial fibrillation to sinus rhythm in patients without organic heart disease or with only systemic hypertension. Am J Cardiol 1992;70:69.

Cox JL, Canavan TE, Schuessler RB et al: The surgical treatment of atrial fibrillation, II: Intraoperative electrophysiologic mapping and description of the electrophysiologic basis of atrial flutter and atrial fibrillation. J Thorac Cardiovasc Surg 1991;101:406.

Fuster V, Ryden LE, Asinger RW et al: ACC/AHA.ESC guidelines for the management of patients with atrial fibrillation: A report of the American College of Cardiology/American Heart Association Task Force on Practice Guidelines and the European Society of Cardiology Committee for Practice Guidelines and Policy Conference (Committee to Develop Guidelines for the Management of Patients With Atrial Fibrillation). J Am Coll Cardiol 2001;38:1266i.

Galve E, Rius T, Ballester R et al: Intravenous amiodarone in treatment of recent-onset atrial fibrillation: Results of a randomized, controlled study. J Am Coll Cardiol 1996;27:1079.

Hart RG, Halperin JL: Atrial fibrillation and thromboembolism: a decade of progress in stroke prevention. Ann Intern Med 1999;131:688.

Hohnloser SH, Kuck KH, Lilienthal J: Rhythm or rate control in atrial fibrillation: Pharmacological Intervention in Atrial Fibrillation (PIAF): A randomised trial. Lancet 2000;356:1789.

Hohnloser SH, van de LA, Baedeker F: Efficacy and proarrhythmic hazards of pharmacologic cardioversion of atrial fibrillation: Prospective comparison of sotalol versus quinidine. J Am Coll Cardiol 1995;26:852.

Jais P, Haissaguerre M, Shah DC et al: A focal source of atrial fibrillation treated by discrete radiofrequency ablation. Circulation 1997;95:572.

Kay GN, Ellenbogen KA, Giudici M et al, for the APT Investigators: The Ablate and Pace Trial: A prospective study of catheter ablation of the AV conduction system and permanent pacemaker implantation for treatment of atrial fibrillation. J Interv Cardiol Electrophysiol 1998;2:121.

Levy S: Classification system of atrial fibrillation. Curr Opin Cardiol 2000;15:54.

Manning WJ, Silverman DI, Waksmonski CA et al: Prevalence of residual left atrial thrombi among patients with acute thromboembolism and newly recognized atrial fibrillation. Arch Intern Med 1995;155:2193.

Ricard P, Levy S, Trigano J et al: Prospective assessment of the minimum energy needed for external electrical cardioversion of atrial fibrillation. Am J Cardiol 1997;79:815.

Stambler BS, Wood MA, Ellenbogen KA: Antiarrhythmic actions of intravenous ibutilide compared with procainamide during human atrial flutter and fibrillation: Electrophysiological determinants of enhanced conversion efficacy. Circulation 1997;96:4298.

Wood MA, Brown-Mahoney C, Kay GN et al: Clinical outcomes after ablation and pacing therapy for atrial fibrillation: A meta-analysis. Circulation 2000;101:1138.

Conduction Disorders & Cardiac Pacing

21

Nora Goldschlager, MD

ESSENTIALS OF DIAGNOSIS

- *Sinus node dysfunction ("sick sinus syndrome")*

    Sinus bradycardia: Sinus rate of less than 50 bpm

    Sinoatrial exit block, type I: Progressively shorter P-P intervals, followed by failure of occurrence of a P wave

    Sinoatrial exit block, type II: Pauses in sinus rhythm that are multiples of basic sinus rate

    Sinus arrest, sinus pauses: Failure of occurrence of P waves at expected times

- *Atrioventricular block*

    First degree: Prolonged PR interval

    Second degree

    Type I: Progressive increase in P R interval, followed by failure of AV conduction and nonoccurrence of a QRS complex

    Type II: Abrupt failure of AV conduction not preceded by increasing PR intervals.

    High degree: AV conduction ratio greater than 3:1

    Complete: Independent atrial and ventricular rhythms, with failure of AV conduction despite temporal opportunity for it to occur

General Considerations

The clinical presentation of patients with conduction system disease is determined by the existence of three underlying abnormal conditions: bradycardia, inability to increase the heart rate in response to increases in metabolic needs, and inappropriately timed atrial and ventricular depolarization and contraction sequences.

Pathophysiology & Etiology

A. SINUS NODE DYSFUNCTION

Sinus node dysfunction ("sick sinus syndrome") is usually due to a degenerative process that involves the

sinus node and sinoatrial (SA) area (Table 21–1). Often, the degenerative process and associated fibrosis involve the atrioventricular (AV) node and its approaches, and the intraventricular conduction system as well as the sinus node area. As many as 25–30% of patients with sinus node dysfunction also have evidence of AV and bundle branch conduction delay or block.

Respiratory sinus arrhythmia, in which the sinus rate increases with inspiration and decreases with expiration, is not an abnormal rhythm and is most commonly seen in young healthy subjects. Nonrespiratory sinus arrhythmia, in which phasic changes in sinus rate are not due to respiration, may be accentuated by the use of vagal agents such as digitalis and morphine; its mechanism is unknown. Patients with nonrespiratory sinus arrhythmia are likely to be older and to have underlying cardiac disease, although the arrhythmia is not a marker for structural heart disease. Ventriculophasic sinus arrhythmia is an unusual rhythm that occurs when sinus rhythm and high-grade or complete AV block coexist; it is characterized by shorter P-P intervals when they enclose QRS complexes and longer P-P intervals when no QRS complexes are enclosed. The mechanism is not known with certainty but may be re-

Table 21–1. Causes of sinus node dysfunction.

Idiopathic
  Degenerative process
  Normal aging
Acute myocardial ischemia or infarction
  Right or left circumflex coronary artery occlusion
    Jarisch-Bezold reflex
Medications
  Beta-blockers
  Rate-sparing calcium channel blockers
    Diltiazem, verapamil
  Digitalis (with high prevailing vagal tone)
  Class I antiarrhythmic agents
  Class III antiarrhythmic agents (amiodarone, sotalol)
  Clonidine

lated to the effects of the mechanical ventricular systole itself: the ventricular contraction increases the blood supply to the sinus node, thereby transiently increasing its firing rate; the resulting increase in intraatrial pressure causes inhibition of the sinus rate. Ventriculophasic sinus arrhythmia is not a pathologic arrhythmia and should not be confused with premature atrial depolarizations or sinoatrial block. None of the sinus arrhythmias indicates sinus node dysfunction.

Sinus node dysfunction is present when marked sinus bradycardia, pauses in sinus rhythm (sinus arrest), SA block or a combination of these exist (Figures 21–1

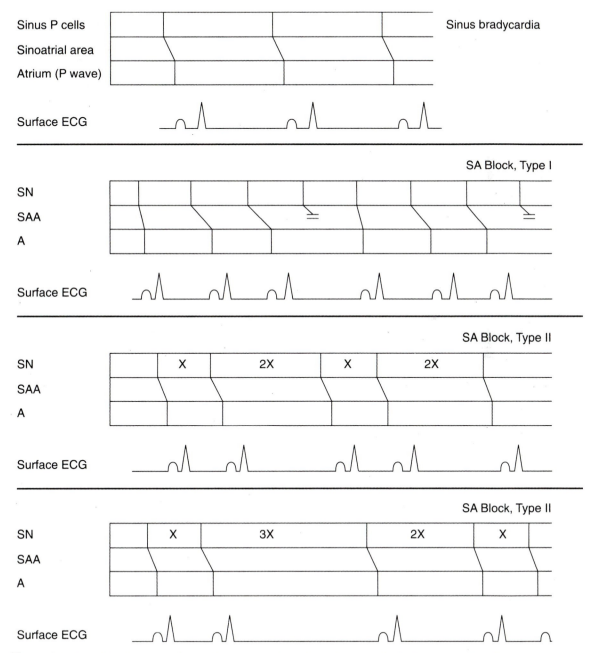

Figure 21-1. Ladder diagrams illustrating sinus bradycardia and sinoatrial block, types I and II. ECG = electrocardiogram; SA = sinoatrial; SAA = sinoatrial area; SN = sinoatrial node.

through 21–5). Some clinically normal individuals without structural heart disease can experience significant sinus bradycardia and prolonged pauses in sinus rhythm under conditions of high vagal tone such as sleep. In some subjects a trigger, such as vomiting, can be identified; in other patients, high levels of acetylcholine may be responsible. The causes in the latter case are uncertain. Vagal stimulation is also responsible for significant sinus bradyarrhythmias occurring in patients in an intensive care setting (Table 21–2), in which a trigger is often identifiable.

Sinoatrial block may take the form of progressive delay in transmission of the sinus-generated impulse through the sinoatrial node to the atrium, finally resulting in a nonconducted sinus impulse and absence of a P wave on the surface electrocardiogram (ECG) (Wenckebach, or type I second-degree exit block; see

Figures 21–1 and 21–3), or abrupt failure of transmission of the sinus impulse to the atrium (type II second-degree exit block). In type I second-degree exit block, the increment in delay in impulse transmission through the SA nodal tissue is progressively less (similar to type I AV nodal block); thus, the P-P intervals become progressively shorter until a P wave fails to occur. In type II second-degree exit block, abrupt failure of sinus impulse conduction to the atria can take the form of 2:1, 3:1 (and so on) sinoatrial block. Fixed 2:1 sinoatrial exit block cannot be distinguished from sinus bradycardia on the surface ECG.

Bradycardia-tachycardia syndrome is characterized by episodes of both bradycardias and supraventricular tachycardias (Figure 21–6). The bradycardia is due to sinus node dysfunction (sinus arrest or SA exit block)

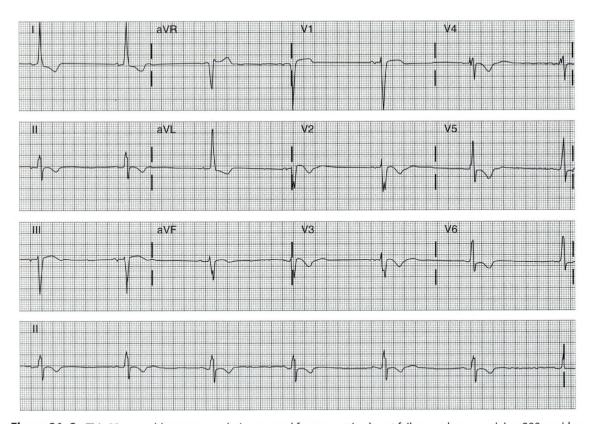

Figure 21–2. This 83-year-old woman was being treated for congestive heart failure and was receiving 200 mg/day of amiodarone for episodes of nonsustained ventricular tachycardia. She complained of profound effort fatigue but no symptoms of heart failure. Electrocardiogram reveals an atrial bradycardia at a rate of about 38/min. The P waves vary in morphology, suggesting some wandering of the atrial pacemaker. Left axis deviation, and a left intraventricular conduction delay with ST and T wave abnormalities, are present. The atrial bradycardia was presumed to be due to the amiodarone, which was discontinued, resulting in appreciable increase in a stable sinus rhythm, with amelioration of the patient's effort fatigue.

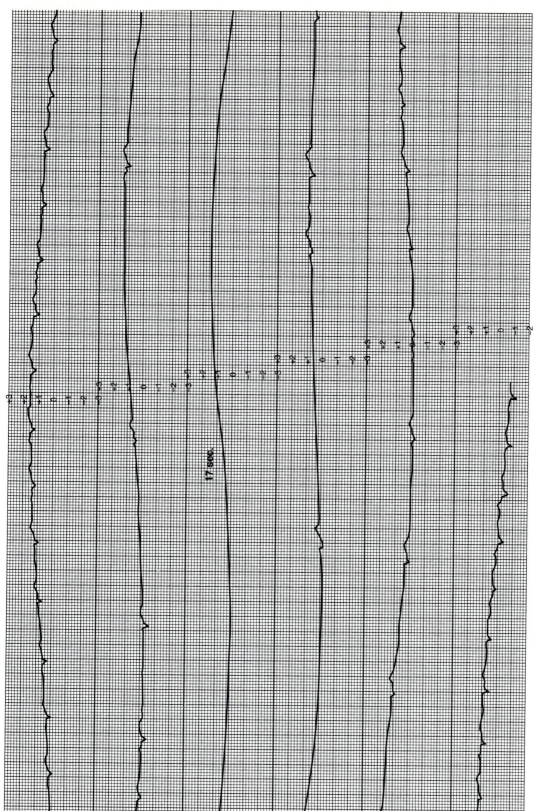

Figure 21–3. Continuous modified lead-II ambulatory electrocardiographic recording in a patient with recurrent presyncopal spells. Sinus rhythm is present in the top strip; the second strip shows marked sinus slowing, followed by a 17-s period of sinus arrest without the appearance of a QRS escape rhythm. Sinus rhythm reappears in the fourth strip, gradually increasing its rate until stable rhythm is restored in the bottom strip. The absence of an escape rhythm raises the possibility of diffuse disease of the conduction system and impulse-generating tissue.

MCL

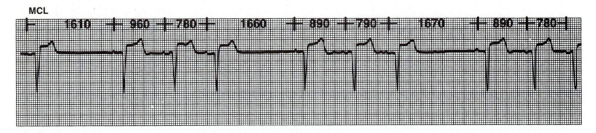

Figure 21–4. Progressive decrease in P wave cycle lengths followed by a pause in P wave rate, indicating type I second-degree sinoatrial block. The pauses in sinus rate are less than twice the preceding sinus cycle lengths, satisfying the criteria for Wenckebach periodicity. MCL = modified chest lead.

with associated junctional or ventricular escape rhythms. The supraventricular tachycardias may be atrial tachycardia, atrial flutter, atrial fibrillation or AV nodal reentry tachycardia; more than one type may occur in the same patient. Bradycardia-tachycardia syndrome represents diffuse disease of the conduction system of the heart but is not necessarily associated with structural heart disease.

Sinus bradycardia not uncommonly results from medications, particularly β-blockers, the rate-sparing calcium channel-blocking agents verapamil and diltiazem, and some commonly used antiarrhythmic agents such as sotalol and amiodarone (see Figure 21–2). If these medications are necessary to treat the patient, permanent cardiac pacing will be indicated.

The natural history of sinus node dysfunction is one of variable progression to an absence of identifiable si-nus activity, with the process taking from 10 to 30 years. The condition itself is not associated with a high risk for arrhythmic death, although the morbidity caused by a sudden onset of bradycardia can be considerable. The ultimate prognosis for patients with sinus node dysfunction depends on the presence and severity of the underlying heart disease, rather than on the bradyarrhythmias themselves.

B. ATRIOVENTRICULAR NODAL-HIS BLOCK

Like sinus node dysfunction, AV nodal-His block and bundle branch block (BBB) are often the result of sclerodegenerative processes. These processes can also involve the approaches to the AV node. Acquired AV nodal block is often due to acute ischemia and infarction (especially involving the inferior wall and right ventricle), infection, trauma, and medications (Table 21–3).

Continuous MCL₁ Rhythm Strips

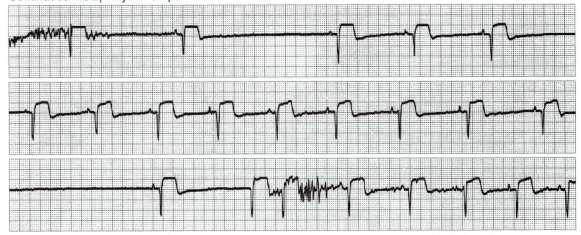

Figure 21–5. Irregular pauses in sinus rate, which occur abruptly and are not multiples of a basic sinus-cycle length. Best characterized as sinus pauses rather than sinoatrial block or sinus arrest, this rhythm indicates the existence of sinus node dysfunction. MCL₁ = modified chest lead.

Table 21–2. Conditions associated with vagally mediated bradyarrhythmias.

Highly conditioned state
Sleep
Vomiting, retching
Suctioning
Nasal intubation
Gastric intubation
Urination
Defecation
Coughing
Swallowing
Central nervous system trauma with high intracranial pressure
Isotonic exercise conditioning

Table 21–3. Causes of acquired atrioventricular nodal-His block.

Idiopathic
Degenerative process
Ischemic heart disease (inferior wall, septal area, right ventricle)
Calcific aortic and mitral valve disease
AV nodal/His ablative procedures
Medications
    Digitalis, β-blockers, calcium channel blockers (verapamil, diltiazem), sotalol, amiodarone
Infections (including aortic valve endocarditis)
Inflammatory diseases (myocarditis)
Infiltrative diseases
    Amyloidosis, neoplasm, sarcoidosis, hemochromatosis
Collagen-vascular diseases
Trauma
Aortic valve surgery

AV = atrioventricular.

The three areas of the AV node, or junction (atrionodal, central compact, and nodal-His portions) merge, without clear separation, with the His bundle. Cells of the atrionodal area have a relatively fast depolarization rate (45–60/min) and are responsive to autonomic nervous system input, whereas cells of the nodal-His region have a slower depolarization rate (about 40/min) and are generally unresponsive to autonomic influences. The site of origin of a junctional rhythm will therefore determine its rate, responsiveness to vagal and adrenergic input, and consequently the presence and severity of clinical symptoms.

Because rhythms originating in the longitudinally separated predivisional region of the His bundle can have a wide QRS complex, the QRS complex duration is an unreliable guide to the origin of a QRS rhythm.

The natural history of patients with AV block depends on the underlying cardiac condition; however, the site of the block and the resulting rhythm disturbances themselves contribute to the prognosis. First-degree AV block has little prognostic import. Chronic (ie, established) second-degree (types I and II), high-degree, and complete AV block can all be associated with adverse outcomes, including death, unless the arrhythmias are vagally mediated or are due to other reversible causes.

Clinical Findings

A. Symptoms and Signs

The symptoms resulting from conduction disorders reflect cerebral hypoperfusion, low cardiac output at rest or during exercise, and an impaired hemodynamic state. Symptoms, which are often subtle, can be episodic or chronic and can change over time. Because a patient often adapts activity levels to compensate for the impairment in heart rate response, significant symptomatology may not be evident unless the patient is closely questioned about specific activities and effort tolerance, or the clinician actually observes the patient during performance of activities of daily living such as walking or during formal treadmill exercise tests.

Syncope is the classic symptom of cerebral hypoperfusion due to bradycardia; however, symptoms of presyncope such as dizziness, lightheadedness, and confusion reflect the same pathophysiology and warrant the same aggressive approach to diagnosis and management.

It should be emphasized that patients with cerebral hypoperfusion often have impairment of memory sur-

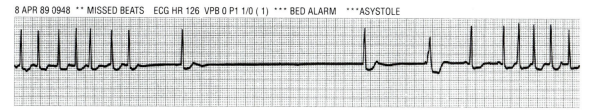

8 APR 89 0948 ** MISSED BEATS   ECG HR 126 VPB 0 P1 1/0 (1) *** BED ALARM ***ASYSTOLE

Figure 21–6. Lead II rhythm strip characteristic of bradycardia-tachycardia syndrome, recorded from a patient with palpitations and intermittent dizzy spells.

rounding the presyncopal or syncopal episodes and may therefore be unable to provide an adequate history of the events.

Patients with sinus node dysfunction or AV block, in whom the escape pacemaker is unresponsive to autonomic nervous system input, cannot increase their heart rate in response to increases in oxygen demand. They are, therefore, intolerant of effort and will report symptoms of exercise-related breathlessness, weakness, and fatigue. These symptoms, which can be disabling, are often confused with other conditions such as hypothyroidism, medication, underlying heart disease, deconditioning, or simply old age. During periods of AV block, the atria and ventricles often depolarize and contract asynchronously. Right and left atrial pressure and volume increase to variable degrees, depending on the degree to which the AV valves are open or closed at the onset of ventricular systole. The resulting atrial stretch and secretion of atrial natriuretic peptide produce reflex systemic hypotension and cerebral hypoperfusion. In addition, the increases in left atrial and pulmonary venous pressures can cause or contribute to shortness of breath and pulmonary venous congestion, including frank pulmonary edema. The mistaken diagnosis of refractory left ventricular dysfunction is not infrequently made in this situation.

Patients who have the bradycardia-tachycardia syndrome (see Figure 21–6) have symptoms referable to both the bradycardia and the tachycardia; the latter are usually perceived as uncomfortable palpitations, whereas the former cause symptoms of cerebral hypoperfusion.

More rarely, bradycardias can lead to a potentially lethal form of ventricular tachycardia known as bradycardia- or pause-dependent ventricular tachycardia (Figure 21–7). This is most often a polymorphic ventricular tachycardia and is associated with a bradycardia-related prolongation of the QT interval; symptoms in these patients can include not only palpitations, syncope, and presyncope, but also cardiac arrest.

B. Physical Examination

The physical examination of the patient with bradycardia reflects the origin of the QRS rhythm and the AV relationships to a greater degree than does the heart rate per se. Junctional or ventricular escape rhythms resulting from atrial bradycardia or AV block produce AV dyssynchrony. This results in varying degrees of atrial contribution to ventricular filling, as well as varying stroke outputs and systolic blood pressures. Because AV dyssynchrony causes changes in the positions of the mitral and tricuspid valves relative to their fully closed or open positions, the intensity of the first heart sound will vary, as will the audibility of atrial (S_4) gallop sounds and the presence and intensity of semilunar valve systolic murmur and AV valve regurgitant murmurs. Examination of the venous pulse contour in the

neck can reveal cannon *a* waves and prominent *cv* waves, which should not be confused with an elevated central venous pressure. Central venous pressure elevation is a fairly common physical finding independent of the venous pulse contour. Occasionally, especially if the *a* wave is prominent, the diagnosis of AV block can be made from the neck vein pulse contours.

The carotid pulse may vary in volume, and even upstroke velocity, in patients with AV dyssynchrony. Examination of the chest may disclose rales, which reflect increased pulmonary venous pressure and valvular regurgitation rather than systolic or diastolic ventricular dysfunction. The liver may be enlarged and may pulsate because of transmitted *a* and *cv* waves; peripheral edema may also be present if the AV dyssynchrony is chronic.

These same physical findings can also occur in patients who are being paced in the ventricle from a single-chamber ventricular pacing system and who have an atrial rhythm that is sinus because AV dyssynchrony will be present under these circumstances. In these patients, the symptoms of weakness, fatigue, and congestive heart failure, together with physical findings indicating AV dyssynchrony, constitute the pacemaker syndrome, which is treated by changing the implanted single-chamber ventricular pacing system to a dual-chambered system in which sensing of the atrial rhythm triggers a paced ventricular response to restore AV synchrony (see section on Permanent pacing).

C. Diagnostic Studies

1. Sinus node dysfunction—

a. Electrocardiography—The P waves inscribed on the surface ECG represent atrial depolarizations. Sinus node depolarization precedes atrial depolarization and is therefore not seen on the surface ECG. That P waves result from sinus-generated impulses must be inferred from their morphology and axis.

The sinus P wave has a mean frontal plane axis of +15 to +75° and is upright in leads I, II, and aVf; inverted in lead aVR; and variable in leads III and aVL. In the horizontal plane, the sinus P wave can be inverted in lead V_1 but is upright in leads V_3–V_6. Respiratory variation in the sinus P wave contour can be seen in the inferior leads and should not be confused with wandering atrial pacemaker, which is unrelated to breathing and therefore not phasic. Sinus arrhythmia is present when the P wave morphology is normal and consistent and the P-P intervals vary by more than 0.16 s. Sinoatrial block exists when some impulses generated by the sinus pacemaking cells do not exit the SA node to depolarize the atria (see Figures 21–1 and 21–4). In the absence of atrial depolarization, a P wave will not be inscribed on the surface ECG. Extreme sinus bradycardia or sinus arrest may be electrocardiographically indistinguishable from SA block. High-degree SA

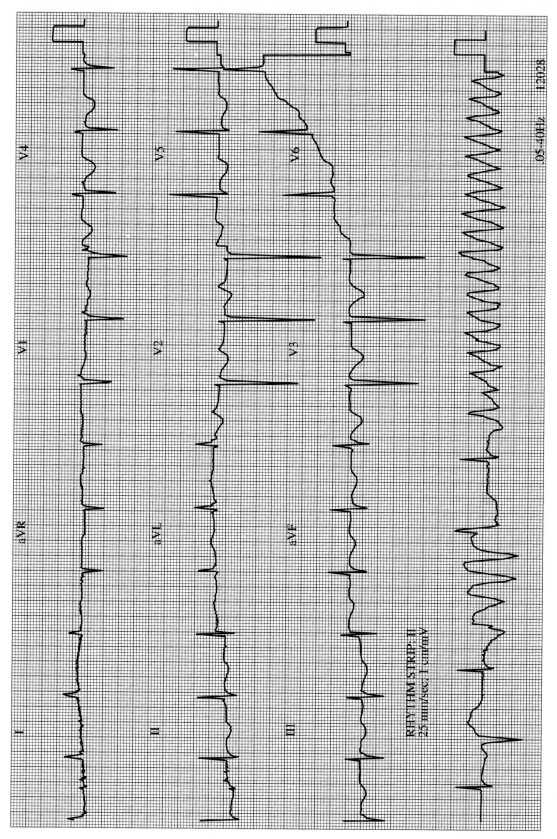

Figure 21–7. Pause-dependent ventricular tachycardia causing loss of consciousness in a patient with syncopal and presyncopal spells. Note the markedly prolonged QT interval associated with the longer RR cycle lengths.

block, in which most sinus impulses fail to exit the SA node to the atrium, is inscribed on the surface ECG as pauses in sinus rhythm. These pauses often cannot be differentiated from sinus arrest caused by failure of impulse generation. If the pauses between sinus P waves are multiples of a basic rate, however, the diagnosis of type II second-degree SA block can be made.

b. Electrophysiologic studies—Sinus node function can be evaluated in the electrophysiology laboratory by means of simultaneous surface and intracardiac electrographic recordings made during basal conditions, physiologic and pharmacologic interventions, and atrial pacing. This evaluation can be undertaken in patients with symptomatic sinus bradycardia, the bradycardia-tachycardia syndrome, or both. It can also be used in patients with recurrent syncope of unclear etiology, although the diagnostic yield is not high. Measurements include the intrinsic heart rate, the sinus node recovery time (SNRT), the sinoatrial conduction time (SACT), and the response to parasympathetic (vagal) stimulation, as assessed by carotid sinus massage.

The intrinsic heart rate (ie, the rate independent of autonomic influences) is the sinus rate during pharmacologic denervation of the sinus node using a β-blocker and atropine. The intrinsic heart rate is sometimes used to distinguish normal subjects from those with sinus node dysfunction.

Sinus node recovery time is the interval between the end of a period of pacing-induced overdrive suppression of sinus node activity and the return of sinus node function, manifested on the surface ECG by a postpacing sinus P wave. The measured SNRT depends on several factors, among them the proximity of the pacing catheter to the sinus node, the sinoatrial conduction time, the presence or absence of SA entrance block, and local neurohumoral influences. In normal subjects, atrial pacing at rates of 120–130 bpm for 15 s or more is followed by a return of sinus node activity at a reproducible interval, with the basic sinus rate generally being achieved within three postpacing beats. The usual SNRT is about 1.5 s, although considerable variation may exist, depending on the prevailing autonomic tone. The corrected sinus node recovery time can be calculated by subtracting the basic sinus rate from the sinus node recovery time; it is usually between 350 and 550 ms. In patients with sinus node dysfunction, sinus node recovery times are not reproducible and tend to be longer after more prolonged periods of pacing. Return to the basic sinus rate within three postpacing beats is inconstant and may be followed by additional (secondary) pauses in rate.

Sinoatrial conduction time reflects the time taken by a premature atrial-pacing stimulus delivered near the sinus node area to traverse the atrial tissue to reach the sinus node and prematurely depolarize it, the time to the formation of the next sinus impulse following the premature depolarization, and the return of the sinus-generated impulse through atrial tissue to the recording electrode. The SA conduction time is often prolonged in patients with clinical evidence of sinus node dysfunction other than sinus bradycardia alone.

Because the electrophysiologic tests of sinus node function are neither specific nor sensitive, they can show abnormal results in patients without sinus bradycardia and normal results in those with symptomatic sinus node disease. The test results should not, therefore, be relied on in making clinical decisions regarding either diagnosis or treatment.

Some of the problems of poor sensitivity and specificity can be overcome by recording the sinus node electrogram from an electrode catheter positioned in the vicinity of the sinus node at the junction of the superior vena cava and the right atrium. The sinus node electrogram cannot be reproducibly recorded in as many as 50% of patients, however, and both T and U waves interfere with it. Sinus node electrography can distinguish between SA exit block and sinus arrest, however, and studies have shown that most pauses in sinus rhythm are due to SA exit block. Notwithstanding these technologic advances, the diagnosis of sinus node dysfunction remains a clinical one.

c. Exercise testing—Treadmill exercise testing can be of substantial value in assessing chronotropic response ("competence") to increases in metabolic needs in patients with sinus bradycardia who are suspected of having sinus node dysfunction. The definition of chronotropic incompetence is not agreed on, but it is reasonable to designate it as consisting of either an inability to achieve a heart rate exceeding 75% of age-predicted maximum (220 − age), or 100–120/min at maximum effort. Irregular (and nonreproducible) increases, and even decreases, in sinus rate during exercise can also occur but are rare. Similarly rare are abrupt changes in rate occurring during the postexercise recovery period. Chronotropic incompetence can result from medications (see Table 21–1) and should be distinguished from intrinsic sick sinus syndrome.

The Bruce treadmill exercise protocol, which is usually used to diagnose the presence and severity of coronary artery disease, is generally inappropriate for patients with sinus node dysfunction, in whom the goal is to assess heart rate at lower workloads expected to be encountered during average daily activities. Specific protocols, such as the chronotropic assessment exercise protocol (CAEP), have therefore been developed for this purpose. In addition to documenting chronotropic incompetence, treadmill exercise testing can be used to aid in optimal programming of rate-adaptive cardiac pacemakers that are usually required in these patients.

2. Atrioventricular block—

a. Electrography and electrocardiography—The advent of intracardiac His bundle electrography has provided important information regarding normal and abnormal AV conduction in humans. The technique involves positioning a multipolar electrode catheter across the tricuspid valve in proximity to the AV nodal-His bundle to record electrical activity as it passes through these structures. Because of its location, the catheter records electrical activity at the level of the low right atrium, His bundle, and proximal right bundle branch in addition to ventricular electrical activity. The sinus node pacemaker cells normally initiate the cardiac impulse; this impulse is not registered on either the surface ECG or the His bundle electrogram. The onset of the P wave on the surface ECG signifies the beginning of atrial depolarization. Because the intracardiac electrode catheter lies at the level of the low right atrium, the early portions of atrial depolarization will not be detected by it; as the atrial depolarization wavefront passes through the region in which the catheter is located (the low right atrium), a deflection is registered (A). As the impulse traverses the His bundle another deflection is registered, representing its depolarization

(H). The His bundle deflection is followed by a ventricular deflection (V), which is registered at the time the wavefront of ventricular depolarization reaches the electrodes; this deflection often follows the onset of inscription of the QRS complex on the surface ECG.

His bundle electrography is useful in indicating the site of AV conduction delay or block. Normally, the conduction time through the AV node is 90–150 ms; the conduction time through the His-Purkinje system is 25–55 ms. In a patient with a prolonged PR interval, a prolonged A H interval signifies delayed impulse conduction within the AV node, and a prolonged HV time represents delayed impulse conduction within the His bundle or in the bundle branches. Conduction delay also occurs within the His bundle itself and is indicated by more than one His deflection ("split" His deflections).

In **first-degree AV block** (a delay in conduction between the atria and the ventricles), all atrial impulses are conducted to the ventricles; it is characterized by a prolonged PR interval that exceeds 0.2 s (Figure 21–8).

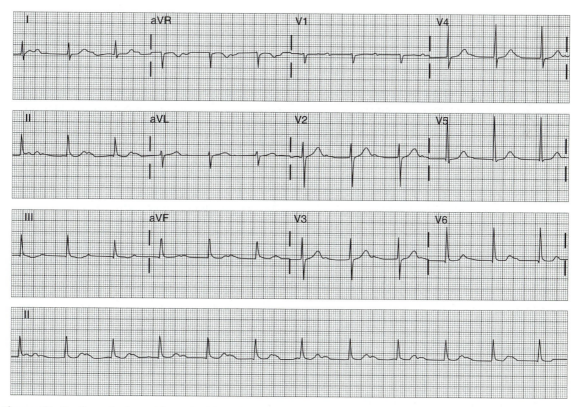

Figure 21–8. Sinus rhythm with marked first-degree atrioventricular (AV) block. All P waves are conducted to the ventricles. The PR intervals are about 0.48 s. The RP intervals are shorter than the PR intervals, which, in some patients, can cause symptoms due to suboptimal AV contraction sequences. Despite the length of the PR intervals, this conduction disturbance is generally benign; evolution to second-degree AV block can take years.

The components of the PR interval are interatrial conduction (10–50 ms), AV nodal conduction (90–150 ms), and intra-His and His-Purkinje conduction (25–55 ms). The conduction delay in first-degree AV block can thus represent prolonged interatrial, intra-AV nodal, or His-Purkinje conduction; His bundle recordings clarify the location.

In patients with a QRS complex that is narrow and normal-appearing, first-degree AV block is intra-AV nodal in more than 85% and is intra-His in under 15%. In patients with a wide QRS complex, first-degree AV block is intra-AV nodal in less than 25%, infranodal in about 45%, and at more than one site in about 33%.

In **second-degree AV block,** not all atrial impulses are conducted to the ventricles. The ratio of P waves to QRS complexes describes the AV conduction ratio. Type I (Wenckebach) second-degree AV block is present when the conduction of atrial impulses to the ventricles is progressively delayed because of AV (generally AV nodal) refractoriness, with eventual failure of conduction of an atrial impulse. The AV conduction ratio in type I second-degree AV block can be 2:1, 4:3, 8:7, and so on; this ratio is also referred to as a Wenckebach period. Because type I second-degree AV block usually occurs within the AV node, the PR interval of the first conducted P wave of the Wenckebach period is often prolonged; and because this conduction disturbance does not involve the bundle branches, the QRS complexes are expected to be narrow and normal-appearing unless preexisting bundle branch disease exists.

In a typical, or classic, **Wenckebach period,** the PR intervals progressively lengthen, the R-R intervals progressively shorten, and the R-R interval encompassing the nonconducted P wave is less than twice the preceding R-R interval. Typical Wenckebach periods are usually seen with low AV conduction ratios (3:2, 4:3, and 5:4), but as the AV conduction ratio increases (exceeding 6:5), more and more Wenckebach sequences are atypical and do not follow the rules. If the sinus rate is not constant, for example in vagal bradycardias, sequences that resemble Wenckebach conduction often occur; they should, however, not be considered type I second-degree AV block, in which the sinus rate must be constant for the diagnosis to be made.

In **type II second-degree AV block,** atrial impulses fail to be transmitted to the ventricles without progressive conduction delay prior to the conduction failure. Because prior conduction delay from the atria does not occur, the failure of antegrade conduction is often abrupt and unpredictable. In contrast to type I second-degree AV block, in which the conduction delay is usually in the AV node, the conduction delay in type II second-degree AV block can be within the bundle of His or, more commonly, distal to the bundle of His in the bundle branches. If the block is within the His

bundle, the QRS complexes will be narrow and normal-appearing or only mildly aberrant, unless preexisting bundle branch block (BBB) is present (Figure 21–9A). If the block is infra-His, the QRS complexes will show a bundle branch block pattern. In contrast to type I second-degree AV block, the PR interval of the conducted P waves is constant and often (but not always) normal (see Figure 21–9B).

Second-degree AV block with a 2:1 AV conduction ratio may represent either type I or type II AV block (Figures 21–10 and 21–11). Two consecutive PR intervals are not recorded, so the presence or absence of progressive PR prolongation cannot therefore be ascertained, and the differential diagnosis may be difficult. Certain guidelines apply: if the PR interval of the conducted P waves is prolonged and the QRS complexes are narrow and normal-appearing, type I second-degree AV block (intra-AV nodal) is probably present. If the PR interval of the conducted P waves is normal and the QRS complexes have a bundle branch block pattern, type II second-degree AV block (infra-His) is probably present. If the PR interval of the conducted P wave is prolonged and the QRS complexes have a bundle branch block pattern, or if the PR interval of the conducted P wave is normal and the QRS complexes appear normal, it may not be possible to distinguish precisely between the two types (see Figures 21–10 and 21–11), and more than one site of AV block may be present. Altering the AV conduction ratio from 2:1 to 3:2 or more by means of carotid sinus massage (to produce sinus slowing) or intravenous atropine (to enhance AV nodal conduction) will often allow identification of the nature of the AV block and thus its location (see Figure 21–9).

In **high-degree AV block** the AV conduction ratio is 3:1 or greater, and atrial impulses are occasionally conducted to the ventricles. In contrast, in complete AV block no atrial impulses are conducted to the ventricles despite temporal opportunity for this to occur, and the atria and ventricles are depolarized by their respective pacemakers, independent of each other (Figure 21–12). The atrial rate in complete AV block is almost always faster than the ventricular rate. The QRS rhythm originates distal to the site of block and may be in the AV junction, bundle of His, bundle branches, or distal Purkinje system. In high-degree and complete AV block, the QRS rhythm is an escape rhythm; the morphology of the QRS complexes and their rate will depend on their site of origin (see Figure 21–12).

If the atrial rate is not sinus, the existence of advanced or complete AV block is diagnosed by the presence of a slow ventricular rate with varying intervals between the QRS complexes, or by a slow and regular rate (Figure 21–13). Atrial fibrillation and flutter are commonly associated with advanced AV block and slow QRS rates. The rate of the ventricular rhythm, as well as the QRS-complex morphology, will depend on the site of origin of the rhythm. The regularity of the rhythm indicates that it is not being stimulated by the atrial rhythm but by an independent pacemaker originating below the level of conduction block.

In **vagotonic block,** a high degree of vagal tone, such as occurs with sympathetic withdrawal during sleep or in highly conditioned athletes, may be associated with slowing of the sinus rate; pauses in sinus rhythm; variable degrees of delay in AV conduction, manifested by (often irregular) prolongation of PR intervals; and failure of conduction of P waves, resem-

bling type I or II second-degree AV block (Table 21–4). It is important to recognize vagotonic block because it often occurs in normal individuals as well as in patients with inferior or right ventricular myocardial infarction, or any other clinical condition in which hypervagotonia is present (see Table 21–2). It not uncommonly accompanies the use of certain medications, notably β-adrenergic blocking agents, some antihypertensive drugs and, occasionally, digitalis. It can also be seen during swallowing (deglutition bradycardia), coughing (tussive bradycardia), and yawning. In the critical care setting, vagotonic bradycardia (including AV block) can

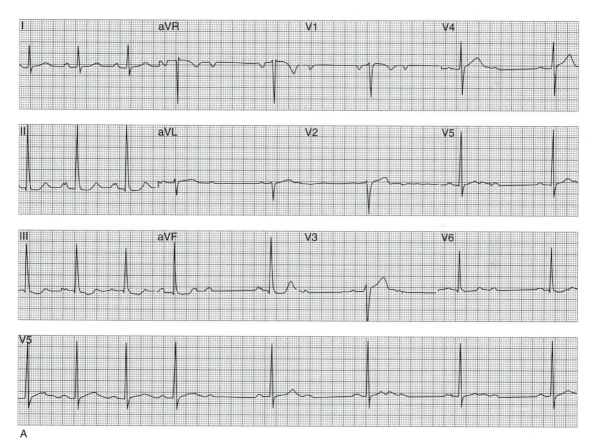

A

Figure 21–9A. This electrocardiogram was recorded in a patient with presyncopal spells who was about to undergo exercise treadmill testing. The atrial rhythm is sinus at a rate of about 68/min. The PR intervals of the conducted QRS complexes are all about 0.24 s. The QRS complexes are narrow, and nondiagnostic ST and T wave abnormalities are present. 2:1 atrioventricular (AV) conduction develops abruptly during the recording.

The prolonged PR intervals of the conducted P waves, as well as the narrow morphology of the QRS complexes (indicating absence of bundle branch system disease), could suggest that the 2:1 AV conduction represents type I second-degree (Wenckebach), which is usually AV nodal; intra-His block, however, is suggested by the absence of prolongation of the PR intervals prior to the nonconducted P waves. Changing of the AV conduction ratio from 2:1 to 3:2, 5:4, etc, would help to establish the presence of type I second-degree AV block. This could be achieved by atropine or exercise testing, during which adrenergic drive would be expected to facilitate AV conduction. *(continued)*

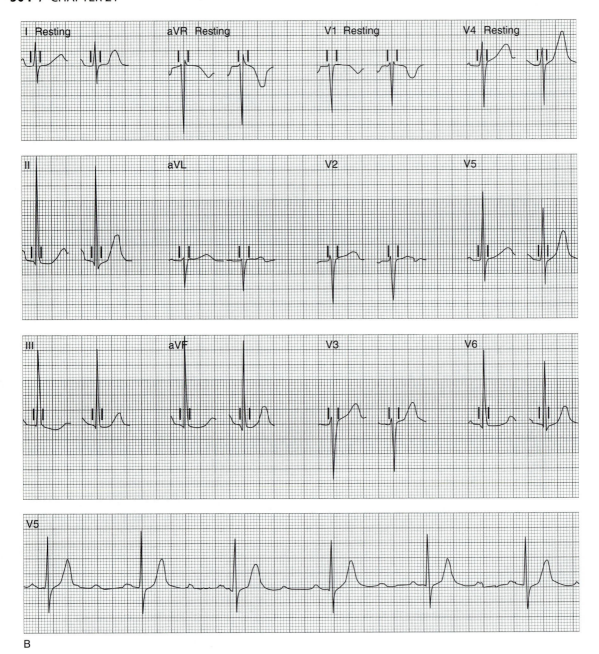

Figure 21–9B. The patient achieved stage IV of the Bruce protocol during treadmill testing. The atrial rate was 150/min. At peak effort and for the first 2 min of the postexercise recovery period, 3:1 atrioventricular (AV) block developed abruptly, and was associated with the patient's typical presyncopal symptoms. AV block developing during exercise, although decidedly rare, is always abnormal and, if the QRS complexes are narrow or normal-appearing, indicate intra-His block. Permanent cardiac pacing is required.

occur during endotracheal suctioning or esophagogastric intubation, and in patients with elevated intracranial pressure.

b. Exercise testing—Unlike the value of exercise testing in sinus node dysfunction to both document this diagnosis and evaluate chronotropic competence,

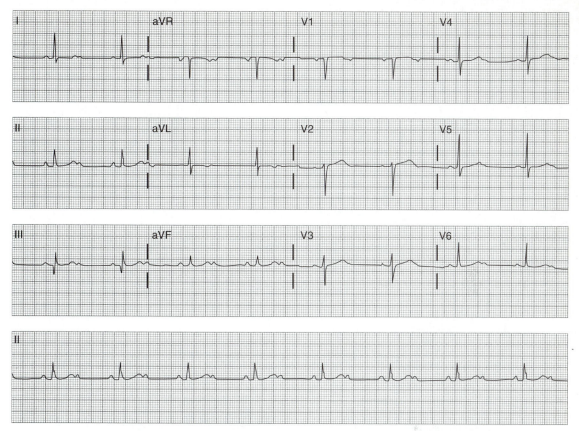

Figure 21–10. The atrial rhythm is sinus, and 2:1 atrioventricular (AV) conduction is present. The PR intervals of the conducted beats are normal at about 0.19 s. The QRS complexes are narrow and normal-appearing. The 2:1 AV conduction could represent either type I second-degree (Wenckebach) or type II second-degree AV block. When type I second-degree AV block is present, the PR intervals of the conducted complexes are often prolonged and the QRS complexes narrow and normal-appearing, whereas in type II second-degree AV block the PR intervals of the conducted complexes are generally normal and the QRS complexes broad, indicating bundle branch disease. In this tracing, the PR intervals are normal. The site of block cannot be known with certainty from this tracing, and manipulation of the AV conduction ratio by atropine or exercise, which facilitate AV conduction, might be required. Type I second-degree AV block generally does not require cardiac pacing because it is occurring within the AV node; if the block is within the His bundle (which might require electrophysiologic study to document), however, permanent cardiac pacing is indicated.

exercise testing is generally not useful in patients with AV block. The response of the AV node to vagolysis and increased sympathetic drive that occurs with exercise is enhancement of AV conduction. Thus, patients with first-degree AV block and type I second-degree AV block are expected to have shorter PR intervals during exercise; and, if type I second-degree AV block is present, to develop higher AV conduction ratios (eg, 3:2 at rest becoming 6:5 during exercise). Patients with 2:1 AV conduction in whom the site of conduction block may be uncertain can benefit from exercise testing by observing whether the AV conduction ratio increases in

a Wenckebach-like manner (eg, to 3:2 or 4:3) or decreases (eg, to 3:1 or 4:1) (see Figure 21–9). In the latter case the increase in the sinus rate finds the His-Purkinje system refractory, causing the higher degrees of block. This response is always abnormal because it indicates intra- or infra-His block, which will require permanent cardiac pacing.

Treatment

The major reversible causes of conduction system disturbances are high vagal tone and medications. High

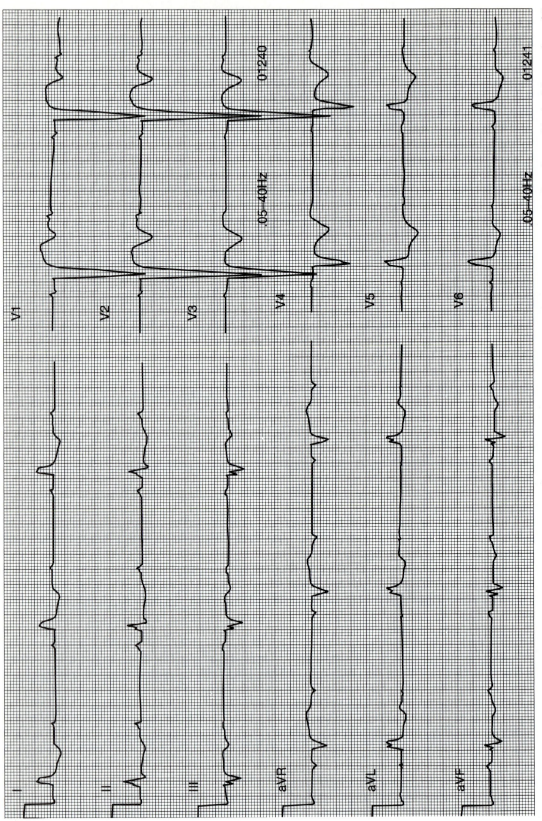

Figure 21–11. Second-degree atrioventricular block, with 2:1 conduction ratio and evidence of bundle branch disease. The first-degree block of the conducted P waves and the left bundle branch block pattern of the conducted QRS complexes make localization of the site of block difficult; electrophysiologic study may be necessary to decide whether permanent cardiac pacing is required.

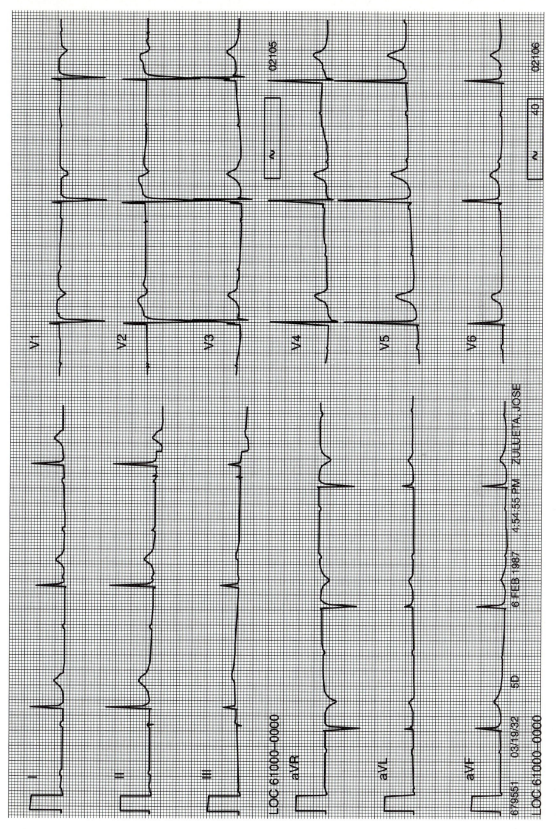

Figure 21–12. Complete atrioventricular block. The atrial and ventricular rhythms are independent of each other. The narrow, normal-appearing QRS complexes suggest that the atrioventricular block is within the bundle of His.

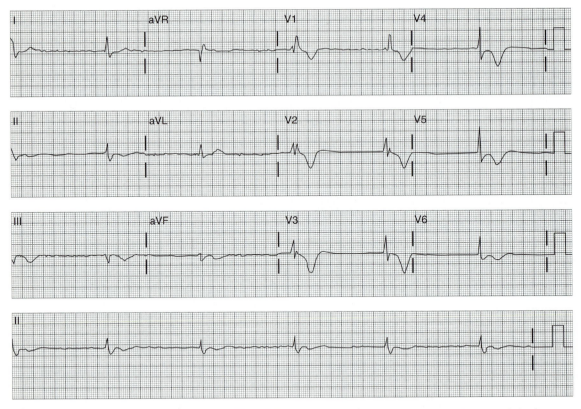

Figure 21–13. The atrial rhythm is fibrillation. The QRS rhythm is regular at a rate of about 33/min and displays a right bundle branch block pattern. The regularity of the rhythm indicates complete atrioventricular block, and the rate and morphology suggest a ventricular focus of origin. This rhythm could be due to digitalis toxicity or to the effects of calcium channel- or β-blocking agents; if offending medications cannot be discontinued, permanent cardiac pacing is indicated. This rhythm and rate are also seen in the absence of medications and after radiofrequency ablation of the AV node to treat uncontrolled ventricular rate in patients with atrial fibrillation; permanent cardiac pacing is required.

vagal tone, whether or not it is accompanied by withdrawal of sympathetic tone, can cause or contribute to both atrial and ventricular bradycardia. Vagally mediated bradycardias are usually transient and not accom-

Table 21–4. Diagnostic clues to vagally mediated atrioventricular block.

Concomitant showing of sinus rate
Changing PR intervals, often with irregularity of sinus rates
Atypical Wenckebach periods, often with inconstant PP
  intervals
Inconstant escape rates
Inconstant escape foci
Transient nature of episodes
Reversed or abolished by intravenous atropine or an increase
  in sympathetic tone

panied by symptoms of presyncope or frank syncope, and no treatment is needed. If necessary, intravenous atropine can be used to facilitate AV nodal conduction to avoid ventricular bradycardia; however, the atropine-induced increase in atrial rate can lead to a paradoxical slowing of ventricular rate as a result of more rapid stimulation of, and encroachment on, the refractory period of the AV conduction system ("time-dependent" refractoriness). Moreover, the effects of intravenous atropine are short-lived, and its chronic use is accompanied by significant side effects.

In contrast to the majority of vagally mediated bradycardias, some vasovagal episodes (hypotension with variable degrees of bradycardia or asystole) can be frequent, abrupt, unpredictable, and disabling.

These highly symptomatic episodes, also referred to as neurocardiogenic, neurovascular, or neurally mediated syncopal syndromes, can require heart rate support with oral theophylline or ephedrine. They can also require permanent dual-chamber cardiac pacing, employing special algorithms to detect an abrupt fall in heart rate and respond with tachypacing until the spontaneous heart rate increases. Intravascular volume support with fluids, support hosiery, and even mineralocorticoids is also needed. Because left ventricular baroreceptor stimulation (from vigorous systolic ventricular contraction) and its consequent reflex peripheral vasodilation play a role in this syndrome, drugs having negative inotropic effects (eg, β-blockers, verapamil, diltiazem, disopyramide) can be used in management. Alpha-agonists, such as midodrine, have also been employed. In addition, because a central effect is recognized, anticholinergic agents (eg, transdermal scopolamine and serotonin reuptake inhibitors) can be useful. Because the hypotension can exist without the bradycardia, this syndrome may not be primarily vagally mediated.

Commonly used medications that cause or contribute to bradycardia do so by enhancing vagal tone (eg, digitalis), reducing the facilitation of AV conduction that results from sympathetic tone (eg, β-blockers and antiarrhythmia agents with β-blocking properties, such as sotalol and propafenone), or direct action on SA and AV conduction tissue (eg, verapamil and diltiazem). Simple withdrawal of these medications will reverse the bradycardia, although the process may require several days. If the offending medications are necessary to treat another condition such as angina pectoris and cannot be discontinued, permanent cardiac pacing will be required (Table 21–5).

It is important to exclude AV nodal blocking medications, such as digitalis preparations, β-blockers, and some calcium channel-blocking agents, as a cause of or contributor to slow ventricular rates in atrial fibrillation and flutter; withdrawal of these drugs or reduction in dosage is associated with reversal of the AV block, and permanent cardiac pacing is usually not required. If the ventricular rhythm is slow in the absence of these agents, intrinsic AV conduction system disease is likely to be present, and permanent cardiac pacing will usually be indicated. Electrical cardioversion of the atrial arrhythmia should be undertaken with caution, if at all, in patients with slow ventricular rates in the absence of medication: because of the diffuse underlying conduction disease, postcardioversion bradycardia or even asystole can occur.

In bradycardia-tachycardia syndrome, the pauses in rhythm are often associated with symptoms of cerebral insufficiency, and cardiac pacing is required. The tachycardias are frequently associated with palpitations. Although cardiac pacing using AAIR or DDDR devices (see section on Permanent pacing) may serve to suppress the tachycardias to some degree, treatment with antiarrhythmic agents is usually required. Control of the ventricular rate is also required, but not infrequently AV

Table 21–5. Common indications for permanent cardiac pacing.

Acquired AV block
High-grade or complete
  With symptoms (including symptoms resulting from necessary medications)
  With asystole >3 s, or rate of escape pacemaker <40/min in awake patients
Second-degree
  Type I in a patient with symptoms
  Type II
Acute myocardial infarction
  With persistent second- and third-degree AV block
  With transient second- and third-degree AV block and bundle branch block
Sinus node dysfunction
With symptoms (including symptoms resulting from necessary medications)
With rates <40/min
With chronotropic incompetence
Carotid sinus hypersensitivity
With symptoms during carotid sinus massage
With asystole >3 s during carotid sinus massage in patients with recurrent syncope
In patients with unexplained syncope and a hypersensitive carotid sinus syndrome
Neurocardiogenic syndromes
With symptoms due to bradycardia, unresponsive to medications, during head-up tilt testing
With bradycardia and hypotension during head-up tilt testing in patients with refractory recurrent syncope

AV = atrioventricular.

Source: Adapted, with permission, from Gregoratos G, Cheitlin MD, Conill A et al: ACC/AHA guidelines for implantation of cardiac pacemakers and antiarrhythmia devices. A report of the American College of Cardiology, American Heart Association Task Force on Practice Guidelines (Committee on Pacemaker Implantation). J Am Coll Cardiol 1998;31:1175.

nodal blocking agents are only partially effective in achieving this control. Moreover, their use can be associated with significant side effects; radiofrequency AV node ablation, together with dual-chamber cardiac pacing, has thus emerged as a useful and cost-effective technique in the management of this rhythm disturbance. Current pacemakers used to treat the bradycardia-tachycardia syndrome employ a special algorithm to switch from a DDD or DDDR mode of operation to a VVI, VVIR, DDI, or DDIR mode on sensing an atrial tachyarrhythmia, and back again to DDD or DDDR mode when a normal atrial rate is sensed.

A. CARDIAC PACING

Temporary or permanent cardiac pacing, in which an electrical stimulus depolarizes cardiac tissue, is indicated when bradycardia causes symptoms of cerebral hypoperfusion or hemodynamic decompensation. Occasionally, patients with bradycardia-dependent ventricular tachycardia require pacing to prevent the pauses in rhythm that lead to the tachyarrhythmia (Tables 21–5 and 21–6, see Figure 21–7). Although emergency pacing can be accomplished temporarily by transcutaneous pacing systems, in all but the most critical situations stable temporary pacing is best ensured by the transvenous insertion of electrodes into the right atrium, right ventricle, or both. Permanent cardiac pacing is also usually performed through the transvenous route; in some circumstances, however, epicardial placement of electrodes via thoracotomy or a subxiphoid approach is still used.

1. Temporary pacing—

a. Transmyocardial pacing—Transmyocardial pacing involves the percutaneous placement of cardiac pacing wires into the ventricular cavity or onto the ventricular wall through a transthoracic needle. The reliability of this technique is poor, and it is a highly invasive procedure with significant potential morbidity. Transmyocardial pacing is performed only in an emergency setting, usually during cardiac arrest, when transvenous pacing cannot be accomplished rapidly or when transcutaneous pacing is unavailable or unsuccessful. The reported incidence of successful capture with transthoracic pacing varies from 5% to 90%; typically it is 21–40%.

Often, however, because of the clinical circumstances in which this type of pacing is used, electrical capture is not followed by mechanical systole. The major complications of transthoracic pacing include myocardial or coronary artery laceration, pericardial tam-

ponade, pneumothorax, and hepatic or gastric damage. Transthoracic pacing should therefore be reserved for situations of the utmost gravity where no other pacing system is feasible or available. External (transcutaneous) pacing should always be tried first, because it is probably as efficacious (if not more so) and is associated with significantly less morbidity. Transthoracic pacing should never be used in awake or stable patients.

b. Transcutaneous pacing—This method, in which electrical current is delivered to the heart through the skin via large surface electrodes, is usually reserved for standby prophylaxis in patients recognized to be at high risk for bradycardia, for example during inferior and large anterior wall acute myocardial infarctions (Table 21–7), and in some patients with suspected sinus node dysfunction who are undergoing elective cardioversion. Because of its ease of use and relative efficacy, this pacing modality has virtually eliminated the need for transmyocardial pacing in emergency situations.

The transcutaneous pacing system uses two large, low-impedance surface electrodes placed on the anterior and posterior chest walls. A long pacing stimulus output of 20–40 ms (not programmable by the operator) and current output of more than 100 mA (programmable by the operator) are often necessary to overcome the impedance offered by the chest wall, muscle and bone, and intrathoracic structures. The transcutaneous pacemaker paces the ventricle and inhibits its output when it senses spontaneous ventricular electrical activity, thus functioning in VVI (demand) mode (see section on Permanent pacing). Because the pacing pulses are 40 ms in duration and the current output is large, they create a deflection on the surface ECG recording that should not be confused with QRS com-

Table 21–6. Common uses for temporary cardiac pacing.

Therapeutic
To provide adequate heart rate in patients with symptomatic bradycardia from sinus node dysfunction or high-degree and complete AV block while awaiting definitive therapy
To terminate some supraventricular and ventricular tachycardias by overdrive suppression or entrainment (eg, atrial flutter, monomorphic ventricular tachycardia)

Prophylactic
To prevent high-degree AV block in some patients with acute myocardial infarction, and in some patients after cardiac surgery (eg, aortic valve replacement)
To prevent bradycardia-dependent ventricular tachycardia

Diagnostic
To determine the site of AV block
For evaluation for optimal type of permanent pacing system

AV = atrioventricular.

Table 21–7. Conditions considered risks for high-degree or complete atrioventricular block during acute myocardial infarction.[a]

Inferior-wall MI, especially if it involves the interventricular septum, posterior wall, and right ventricle, with first-degree AV block; second-degree AV block, type I (usually intra-AV nodal); or second-degree AV block, type II (often intra-His)
Extensive anteroseptal MI, with new bifascicular block with a normal PR interval or with first-degree AV block; second-degree AV block, type II; first-degree AV block with bifascicular block (not known to be old); or alternating bundle branch block

[a] The incidence of AV block during acute myocardial infarction has decreased considerably in the current era of fibrinolytic and direct percutaneous revascularization therapies.

AV = atrioventricular; MI = myocardial infarction.

plexes. If ventricular depolarization (capture) is occurring, the pacer output pulse will be followed by a QRS complex that is best seen on the pacemaker generator's oscilloscope and strip-chart recording. Significant distortion, or total obscuration, of the paced QRS complex can exist on the bedside rhythm monitor or surface ECG recording. Ventricular capture should always be verified by palpating the pulse. Skeletal muscle twitching occurs at a stimulus output of 30 mA, but ventricular capture does not usually occur until 35–80 mA; sedation of the awake patient is usually required to mitigate the painful muscle contractions.

Transcutaneous cardiac pacing can be effective in up to 70% of patients and has its best use in an acute emergency when pacing of short duration is required or as a bridge to permanent cardiac pacemaker implantation. The majority of pacing failures (specifically, failure to capture) occur in patients during the advanced stages of cardiopulmonary arrest. The opportunity for successful transcutaneous pacing in patients with cardiac arrest of more than 15 min duration is approximately 33–45%. Failure to capture can also occur after prolonged (hours to days) pacing and likely represents charges in impedance; repositioning of the electrodes will restore pacing capability.

c. Temporary transvenous pacing—Although transcutaneous pacing offers ease of use, rapid initiation of pacing therapy, and very low complication rates, transvenous pacing is far more stable and better tolerated if pacing is needed for longer than 20–30 min. Transvenous pacing is usually performed by placing a catheter in the right ventricle. In rare cases where temporary atrial pacing is also required, catheters can be positioned in the right atrium or in the proximal portion of the coronary sinus.

Venous access can be obtained by several approaches. The internal jugular, subclavian, and femoral veins are all potential sites for introduction of the pacing catheter into the right heart. The median basilic veins and basilic veins can also be used, but these sites are associated with a high incidence of lead dislodgement (because of arm motion) and are rarely, if ever, used today.

Prior to obtaining venous access, the existence of a bleeding diathesis or coagulopathy should be excluded or corrected if possible. If this is not possible, the femoral vein should be considered as the initial access site because it is easier to apply pressure and achieve hemostasis in this region if a complication occurs. The presence of a prosthetic tricuspid valve is a contraindication to right ventricular pacing; in this circumstance, left ventricular pacing can be performed by positioning the pacing catheter in the left ventricular veins via the coronary sinus. Other factors, such as the patient's pulmonary status, location of dialysis shunts, previous neck surgery, or radiation therapy should be taken into

account when considering the appropriate site for venous access.

Ventricular capture thresholds should be <2 mA and ideally < 1 mA (or < 1 V) in stable lead positions and should not change with coughing or deep breathing. Atrial leads are typically less stable, and capture thresholds around 2 mA (or 1 to 2 V) are acceptable. The presence of myocardial infarction, ischemia, antiarrhythmic drug therapy, hyperkalemia, and other metabolic derangements can increase capture thresholds.

Sensing thresholds can be affected by myocardial ischemia or infarction, hyperkalemia, and class I antiarrhythmic agents, leading to undersensing ("failure" to sense). Ectopic ventricular depolarizations are often undersensed because of poor signal quality. These considerations need to be borne in mind when setting the sensitivity of the pacemaker.

A daily chest radiograph and paced 12-lead ECG should be obtained and compared with prior studies to check for possible lead migration. Pacing and sensing thresholds should be checked at least daily, with any significant changes being investigated for possible lead migration, lead disconnection from the pulse generator, or change in the patient's clinical status. Battery status should be monitored by the appropriate biomedical personnel, and batteries replaced as needed. Temporary leads and access sites should be changed at least every three or four days to decrease the risk of infection and venous thrombosis.

Although temporary transvenous pacing is associated with few adverse effects, transvenous pacing does have the disadvantage of potentially serious complications. Complication rates range from 4% to 20% and include pneumothorax, hemothorax, arterial puncture, air embolism, serious bleeding, myocardial perforation, cardiac tamponade, nerve injury, thoracic duct injury, arrhythmias, infection, and thromboembolism. The risk of complications is increased if pacing is initiated in emergent situations. To minimize risk, transvenous pacing should be accomplished when the patient is relatively hemodynamically stable.

2. Permanent pacing—Because of the complexity of pacing system design, an identification code has been developed that describes the function of currently available pacemaker generators. The "mode" code consists of three primary letters. The first letter stands for the chamber in which pacing is occurring: A for atrium, V for ventricle, and D for both, or dual. The second letter stands for the chamber in which sensing of the electrical signal occurs: A, V, D, or O for neither. The third letter refers to the mode of response of the generator to the sensed signal: I for inhibited output, D for both inhibited and triggered output delivered in response to a sensed signal (eg, a paced ventricular complex delivered in response to a sensed P wave), and O for not applicable. Most currently available pacing systems incorporate one or two sensors that allow the pacing rate to increase and decrease with changes in metabolic need; sensor-based pacing systems thus adapt the pacing rate to the activities of daily living. Pacing systems with this feature add an R following the three primary letters (eg, AAIR, DDDR), indicating the existence of rate-adaptive capability. Current pacemakers have numerous functions that can be altered noninvasively by a programmer; such units are described as having multifunction programmability (Table 21–8). Several of the newer temporary pulse generators also have such features.

a. Modes of pacing—

(1) Asynchronous pacing (VOO, AOO, DOO)— In the asynchronous mode of pacemaker function no electrical signals are sensed, and the pulse generator delivers output pulses without regard to any electrical ac-

Table 21–8. Some programmable functions and parameters of cardiac pacemakers.[a]

Standby rate (base rate, low rate limit): The rate at which the patient is paced unless the spontaneous rhythm is faster

Upper rate limit: The highest rate at which the ventricles are paced 1:1 in response to the atrial rate

AV interval: The interval between the paced or sensed P wave and the delivery of the ventricular pacing stimulus

Atrial refractory period: The time after a sensed P wave or delivery of an atrial output pulse during which the atrial channel is refractory to electrical signals; the refractory period that follows a paced QRS complex, referred to as the PVARP

Ventricular refractory period: The time after a sensed QRS or ventricular output pulse during which the ventricular channel is refractory to electrical signals

Sensitivity (atrial and ventricular channels): The amplitude of the intrinsic atrial and ventricular depolarizations that are to be sensed

Energy output (atrial and ventricular channels): Volts, current and pulse duration

Modes of function: AAI, VVI, AOO, VOO, VDD, DDI, DOO, DDD, OOO

Sensor on

Sensor off

Sensor-based parameters: Time to achieve peak pacing rate; time to decline to standby rate; criteria for sensor activation

Mode switch on: Upon sensing an atrial tachyarrhythmia, a DDD(R) device will automatically switch to DDI(R) or VVI(R) mode of function, and will automatically switch back to DDD(R) mode upon sensing normal atrial rhythm

Mode switch off

---

[a] Pacemaker codes: A = atrium; D = dual; I = inhibited; V = ventricle.

PVARP = postventricular atrial refractory period.

tivity occurring spontaneously within the heart (Figure 21–14). Because the native cardiac rhythm is not sensed, competitive rhythms (paced and native depolarizations) can result. Asynchronous pacemaker generators are no longer manufactured; however, the asynchronous pacing mode can be programmed; it also occurs whenever a magnet is placed over an implanted generator to evaluate pacing function. With a magnet in place, asynchronous pacing and concomitant occurrence of the spontaneous rhythm result in iatrogenic parasystole (Figure 21–15). At the energy output of today's generators (1.5–7.5 V) repetitive ventricular or atrial rhythms are usually not observed, although this possibility exists, especially if myocardial ischemia or electrolyte imbalance is present.

(2) Single-chamber demand pacing [VVI(R), AAI(R)]—Both sensing and pacing circuits are present in these units. When a spontaneous intracardiac signal is sensed, VVI and AAI pulse generators will inhibit their output and no pacemaker stimulus artifact will appear. Electrical signals sensed by demand pacemaker generators can originate not only from the heart but also from the environment (electrocautery, cellular telephones), from the patient (muscle potentials), or from the pacing system itself (lead fracture or insulation breaks). Such sensed signals may cause inhibition of output, leading to pauses in paced rhythm; this phenomenon is termed *oversensing* (Tables 21–9 and 21–10), a problem which can generally be corrected by noninvasive programming or, in the case of lead fracture or insulation break, by replacement of the lead. Current generator design and programming capability have not only helped to reduce problems of oversensing but have also simplified their correction.

The pacing function of a demand pulse generator cannot be evaluated if the patient's spontaneous rhythm exceeds the programmed standby (base) rate of the generator. Applying a magnet over the pulse generator converts it to asynchronous mode of function, and capture (stimulation) of the atria or ventricles by the pacemaker can be confirmed, provided that the pacing stimuli fall outside the refractory period of the cardiac tissue. Conversely, if the patient's rhythm is continually paced, the sensing function of the generator cannot be evaluated. Programming the device to a lower rate may allow the emergence of a spontaneous cardiac rhythm, which should then be sensed, resulting in inhibition of pacemaker output.

(3) P-synchronous pacing systems (VDD)—These are systems in which electrodes are located in both the atrium and the ventricle. The most widely used systems employ a single lead whose tip is positioned in the right ventricular apex for ventricular sensing and pacing, and whose atrial electrodes are located on the lead, at the level of the atrium, for sensing only. When the atrial electrodes sense an electrical signal, a ventricular pacing stimulus is delivered after a programmable AV delay that corresponds roughly to the PR interval. If a spontaneous QRS complex occurs, the ventricular output is inhibited. Thus, the ventricular pacing stimulus is either triggered by a sensed atrial signal or inhibited by a native QRS event. Because atrial activity is sensed, tracking of the atrial rhythm in a 1:1 relationship occurs up to a programmed upper rate limit, allowing for changes in the ventricular paced rate to correspond to changes in sinus rate. The programmed upper rate prevents rapid ventricular paced rates should the atrial rate become too fast because this upper rate limit defines the maximum ventricular paced rate that can occur in a 1:1 relationship to atrial activity. If the atrial rate exceeds the upper rate limit, the paced ventricular rate can become irregular because of an electronic Wenckebach protection, can slow to one-half the programmed upper rate

limit, or can fall back gradually until 1:1 tracking can resume. This last feature results in disengagement of the tracking function, which causes transient AV dyssynchrony (Figure 21–16).

If no atrial activity is sensed, as occurs in sinus bradycardia, these pulse generators pace the ventricles on demand at the programmed standby rate; atrial pacing does not occur. Thus, at slow atrial rates the pacing system behaves as though it were a VVI system, and AV synchrony is lost. Although this pacing system seems ideal for patients with normal sinus rhythm and AV block, atrial bradycardia, which occurs commonly over ensuing years, either spontaneously or as a result of medications, make the VDD device ultimately suboptimal for most patients.

(4) DDD(R)—These pacing systems are capable of sensing and pacing in both the atrium and the ventricle on demand (see Figure 21–14). They therefore approach the physiology of normal AV conduction in many pa-

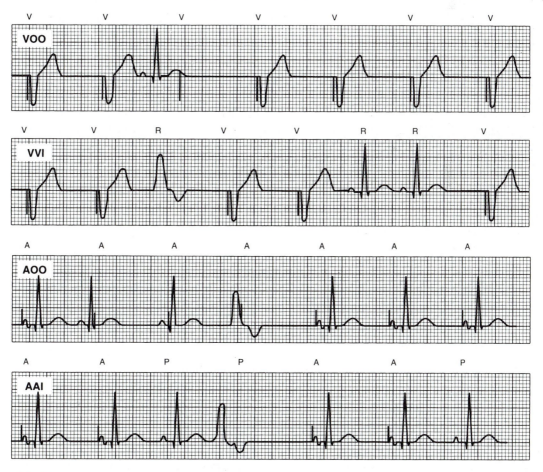

Figure 21–14. Schematic illustrations of various pacing modes. (See section on permanent pacing for explanation of symbols.) A = atrial pacing stimulus, P = spontaneous P wave, R = spontaneous QRS, V = ventricular pacing stimulus.

(continued)

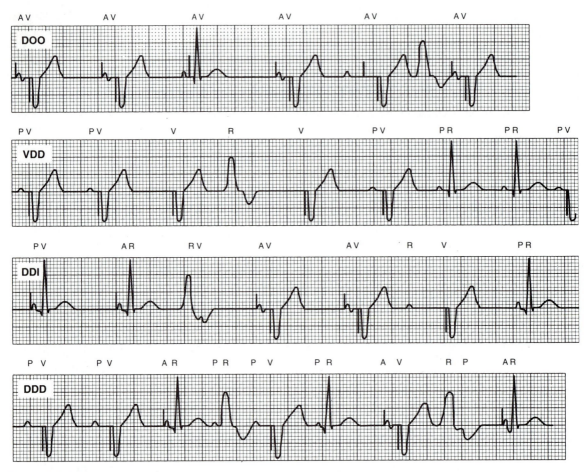

Figure 21–14. (cont.)

tients who require cardiac pacing. The ability to sense retrograde atrial depolarizations can lead to ventricular stimulus delivery and ventricular pacing in response; if the paced ventricular depolarization travels retrograde to the atrium to depolarize it, the process can become repetitive. This event creates an artificial extra-AV-nodal bypass tract, causing a pacemaker-mediated tachycardia. Specific algorithms have been designed to terminate these tachycardias and are automatic once they have been programmed.

Dual-chamber devices depend on a stable atrial rhythm for optimum function. Because of their potential for rapid paced ventricular rates, these systems should not be used with atrial rhythms such as chronic fibrillation or flutter, multifocal tachycardia, or refractory automatic tachycardia. Single-chamber VVI(R) devices should be used instead.

If the atrial tachyarrhythmias are paroxysmal, however, devices that can change automatically from dual-

to single-chamber VVI(R) function or to dual-chamber DDI(R) mode without the ability to track the atrial rate (mode switch feature) should be implanted (Figure 21–17). Studies both completed and ongoing suggest that atrial fibrillation episodes can be reduced in frequency and duration by dual-chamber pacing in these patients; progression to chronic atrial fibrillation and thromboembolism also appears to occur less commonly in these patients.

Rate-adaptive pacing systems are appropriate for patients with persistent or refractory atrial arrhythmias who are not candidates for DDD devices and for patients whose sinus node dysfunction prevents rate acceleration but who would benefit from an increase in paced atrial or ventricular rates in response to increases in metabolic demand. Sensors in current use measure muscle activity, minute ventilation, and QT interval; sensors to measure other parameters (eg, right ventricular dP/dt [rate of rise of pressure within the right ven-

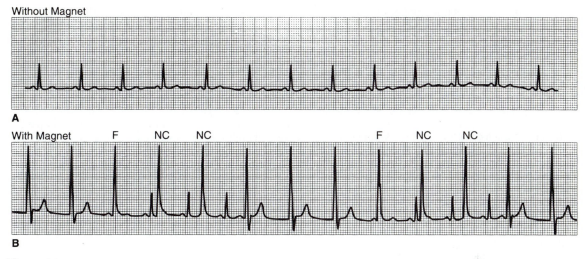

Figure 21–15. A VVI pacing system. **A:** Normal sinus rhythm is present. Sensing function is presumed to be normal because no ventricular pacing artifacts are occurring. **B:** With a magnet in place over the pulse generator, ventricular pacing stimuli are emitted asynchronously, resulting in a rhythm that competes with the sinus rhythm. The large magnitude of the pacing artifacts indicates that the lead configuration is unipolar. The large unipolar stimulus obscures the resulting QRS complex; however, because T waves are present following some of these pacing stimuli, capture is confirmed. Both sensing and pacing functions are normal. F = fusion complexes, with ventricular depolarization resulting from both sinus and paced impulses. NC = noncapture because of pacing stimuli falling in the refractory period of ventricular muscle.

tricle]) are under development. Changes within the sensor's established parameters, designed to reflect physiologic needs, result in changes in paced rates. Sensor-based pacing rates depend on the individual sensor used, however; for example, if an activity sensor is being used, the paced rate can increase in response to body vibrations that are unrelated to actual physical activity. This can cause problems in hospitalized patients, especially those in intensive care units. Several manufacturers, therefore, currently incorporate two sensors into their pacemakers to confirm the need for appropriate changes in pacing rate. For example, the activity

sensor input can be confirmed by a more physiologic sensor such as minute ventilation, resulting in a more specific and accurate response to the change in pacing rate for the particular change in metabolic need.

The type of pacing system implanted is indicated on an identification card supplied to the patient by the manufacturer; patients should carry these cards with them at all times. It is important to note, however, that such information does not guarantee the operation of a particular mode of function, rate, or any parameter that can be programmed by the patient's pacemaker physician. As pulse-generator design and function increase in

Table 21–9. Pacing system malfunctions, and clues to their recognition.

Failure to sense (undersensing)
Single-chamber systems
  ECG will show earlier-then-expected appearance of pacing-stimulus artifact.
Dual-chamber systems
  Atrial undersensing: Delivery of atrial pacing stimuli despite occurrence of spontaneous P waves; failure to track intrinsic atrial activity at the programmed AV interval
Ventricular undersensing: Delivery of ventricular pacing stimuli despite occurrence of spontaneous QRS complexes
	Oversensing
	ECG will show inappropriate inhibition of atrial or ventricular output stimuli; oversensing in the atrial channel causes earlier-than-expected ventricular pacing stimuli.
	Failure to capture
	Pacing stimuli not followed by atrial or ventricular depolarization (assuming muscle tissue is not refractory)
	Failure of output
	Absence of pacing stimulus outputs, with oversensing excluded

AV = atrioventricular; ECG = electrocardiogram.

Table 21–10. Causes of pacemaker oversensing.

Electromagnetic interference
Power transformers, power lines; welding equipment; household appliances such as razors and garage-door openers (unusual with today's pulse generators), microwave ovens operating at high power; rotating radar detectors; metal-detector gates (older generation designs); transcutaneous nerve stimulators; cardioverting and defibrillating devices (external or implanted internally); diathermy; lithotriptors; electrocautery; electrocoagulation; MRI; ionizing radiation; tasers; cellular telephones if used on the side ipsilateral to the pulse generator (some models); electronic article surveillance monitors

Physiologic intracardiac signals
R wave sensing (AAI[a] systems), T wave sensing (VVI systems), P wave sensing (VVI systems) (unusual)

Physiologic extracardiac signals
Muscle potentials (eg, diaphragm, pectoral)

Signals generated within the pacing system
Leads
Conductor-wire fracture causing a voltage transient; insulation defect
Pulse generator
Afterpotential sensing of late portions of the pacing stimulus itself (unusual); component malfunction

[a] Pacemaker codes: A = atrium; D = dual; MRI = magnetic resonance imaging; I = inhibited; V = ventricle.

complexity, it is best to assume that the pacemaker is performing normally until proved otherwise. (There are, of course, malfunctions and "pseudo" malfunctions; these are addressed in the following sections.) Similarly, ECGs in paced patients should be considered to reflect normal device function unless they are interpreted otherwise by personnel experienced in pacemaker electrocardiography.

b. Unipolar and bipolar pacing—Unipolar pacing systems have the cathode (stimulating electrode) in the heart and the anode at the generator. The distance between the cathode and anode in these systems results in the inscription of large pacing artifacts whose direction (pacing-artifact axis) in the frontal plane points toward the anode.

Bipolar pacing systems have both lead electrodes within the heart, usually 1–2 cm apart, in either or both atrium and ventricle. Either the distal (tip) electrode or the proximal (ring) electrode of the lead can serve as the cathode. Because of the small interelectrode distance, the pacing artifacts are small and their direction in the frontal plane reflects the direction of current flow (Figure 21–18).

Electrocardiograms recorded on digital rather than analog ECG machines can show marked variations in the amplitude and polarity of the pacing artifact. Because the digital equipment samples the pacing stimuli at specific time intervals and then recreates them on paper, the inscribed stimulus artifacts are not seen in real time. In some ECG leads the pacing stimuli may not be visible at all, raising the question of failure of generator output. It is important to recognize this recording artifact in patients with pacemakers so as to avoid an erroneous diagnosis of pacemaker malfunction. It is equally important to document the morphology of paced complexes so that when the pacing stimuli cannot be seen, normal pacemaker function can be assumed until accurate evaluation can be made.

Some permanent bipolar pacing systems offer lead polarity that can be programmed to unipolar; therefore, the presence of a bipolar lead on chest radiograph does not ensure bipolar lead function, and the ECG appearance of the pacing artifacts may differ from what is expected.

c. Electrocardiographic patterns of paced complexes—These patterns depend on how the myocardium is depolarized. Paced atrial complexes reflect the sequence of atrial activation initiated by the pacing impulse and thus, in part, the site of the pacing electrode(s). Because the atrial electrodes can be located in the atrial appendage or screwed into any portion of atrial tissue, paced P waves contours and axes will vary.

Pacing from the right ventricular endocardial or epicardial apical area produces paced QRS complexes having a left BBB configuration (the right ventricular myocardium is depolarized before the left), and a superior mean frontal plane axis (the apex of the heart is depolarized before the base; Figure 21–19). Paced QRS complexes usually have a duration of 0.12–0.18 s; if they are substantially longer, intrinsic myocardial disease, hyperkalemia, or antiarrhythmic drug therapy (eg, amiodarone) should be suspected.

Pacing from the right ventricular outflow tract also results in QRS complexes that have a left BBB pattern, but the mean frontal plane axis is inferiorly directed (the base of the heart is depolarized before the apex). Occasionally, pacing from the interventricular septum can result in paced QRS complexes that show an indeterminate conduction delay pattern; they can even be narrow and relatively normal-appearing. This reflects almost simultaneous activation of both the right and left sides of the interventricular septum.

Pacing from the left ventricular epicardium produces paced QRS complexes having a right BBB pattern, reflecting left ventricular myocardial activation in advance of right ventricular activation. The mean frontal-plane QRS axis will depend on the location of the epicardial electrodes relative to each other (bipolar system) or to the pulse generator serving as anode (unipolar system).

In recent years, left ventricular pacing has been accomplished from the coronary veins approached via

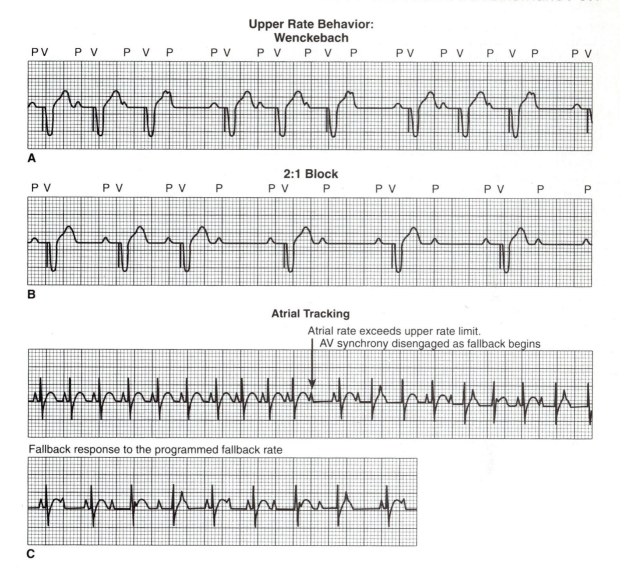

Figure 21–16. Schematic illustration of responses from pulse generators at the atrial-driven upper rate limit. The pacemaker will not allow the ventricular paced rate to exceed this programmed upper rate. Atrial rhythms that can exceed the upper rate limit include sinus tachycardia, atrial tachycardia, atrial flutter, and atrial fibrillation. The pacemaker-mediated tachycardia (see text) will also not exceed the programmed upper rate. **A:** Lengthening of the interval between the sensed P wave and the triggered ventricular-paced complex so as not to violate the upper rate limit (Wenckebach): the P wave that is not followed by a paced QRS complex falls in the refractory period of the atrial channel and is not sensed, resulting in absence (nondelivery) of the ventricular stimulus output. **B:** In 2:1 block, alternate P waves fall in the atrial refractory period and are not sensed: they are not followed by a paced ventricular event. **C:** In fallback, the ventricular paced rate gradually slows once the programmed upper rate has been achieved. During the fallback period, tracking of the atrial rate is disengaged, and AV synchrony is no longer present. The ventricular paced rate will again track the atrial rate once the latter falls below the programmed upper rate. The fallback response avoids abrupt decreases in paced ventricular rate. Pacemakers that function in a rate-adaptive mode can have their sensor-based upper rate limit exceed the above-described upper tracking limit.

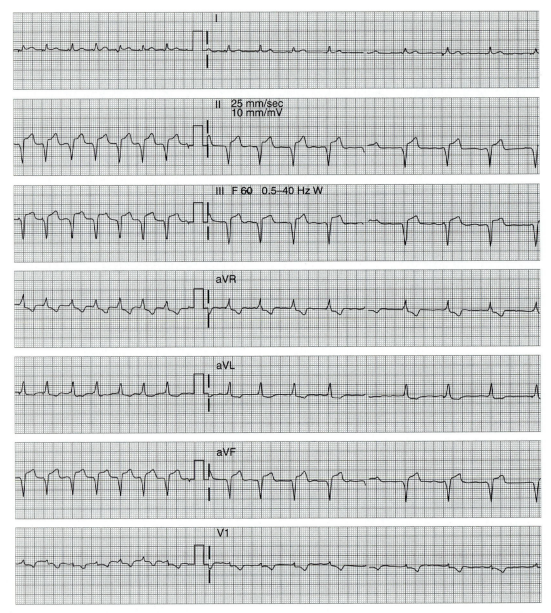

Figure 21–17. Depiction of mode-switch operation of a dual-chamber pacemaker. In the initial portion of the rhythm strip tracking of atrial fibrillation is occurring, resulting in a rapid paced ventricular rate. When the atrial tach-yarrhythmia is recognized by the algorithm in the pacemaker, automatic change of mode of function to VVIR takes place, terminating the rapid paced ventricular rate. On sensing restoration of a normal atrial rhythm, the device will automatically restore its dual-chamber mode of operation.

the coronary sinus. This technique is employed, either alone or along with simultaneous pacing from the right ventricle in patients with advanced heart failure, in order to "resynchronize" ventricular depolarization-contraction sequences; it has had its widest use in pa-tients with left BBB. The biventricular-paced QRS complexes are narrower and more normal-appearing than the patient's spontaneous QRS complexes, re-flecting the resynchronization and suggesting a benefi-cial result of this therapy. The mean frontal plane axis

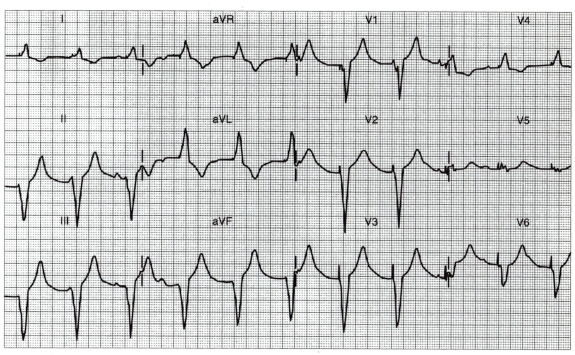

RHYTHM STRIP: II
25 mm/sec; 1 cm/mV

Figure 21–18. Bipolar VVI pacing system. All QRS complexes are paced. Note the small magnitude of the pacing artifacts. The simultaneous recordings indicate that in some leads the pacing stimuli are virtually invisible.

of the paced complexes will vary with the location of the electrodes.

Spontaneous QRS complexes occurring in patients with pacemakers often show marked T-wave inversion (Figure 21–20). Although the cause of the inversion is not understood, the ECG abnormality should not be interpreted to indicate acute or chronic myocardial disease (including ischemia and infarction).

B. PACING SYSTEM MALFUNCTIONS

System malfunctions fall into four general categories: (1) undersensing, or failure to sense; (2) oversensing, or sensing unwanted signals; (3) failure to capture and stimulate myocardial tissue; and (4) failure of output. Undersensing of cardiac electrical signals because of poor intrinsic signal quality does not represent sensing failure as such, but rather the inability to sense, or see, the suboptimal signal itself; undersensed P waves and QRS complexes are not rare. Undersensed QRS complexes tend to originate in ventricular tissue (premature ventricular depolarizations; Table 21–9 and Figure 21–21); they can occur in patients without structural heart disease and during acute myocardial infarction, or as a result of drug toxicity and electrolyte imbalance.

Undersensed P waves can be caused by changes in atrial volume, ectopic atrial rhythms, or retrograde atrial depolarizations. Failure to sense spontaneous complexes and inhibit output appropriately results in the delivery of an earlier-than-expected pacing stimulus, which can, on occasion, cause repetitive rhythms.

Occasionally, in patients with right ventricular VVI(R) or DDD(R) pacing systems, pacing artifacts occur within spontaneous QRS complexes that have a right BBB configuration. This is due to the delay in conduction in the right bundle branch: the wavefront of ventricular depolarization does not reach the lead electrode in the right ventricular apex in time to inhibit the output of the pacing stimulus. This phenomenon may also be observed in patients with inferior and right ventricular myocardial infarction and is probably due to the conduction delay resulting from ventricular scarring. Failure to sense in such cases is due to intrinsic conduction system disease rather than to a malfunctioning unit. The same principles apply to patients with left ventricular epicardial electrode(s) who have underlying left BBB and to patients with AAI(R) or DDD(R) pacing systems and right atrial electrode(s) who have an intraatrial conduction delay. The problem

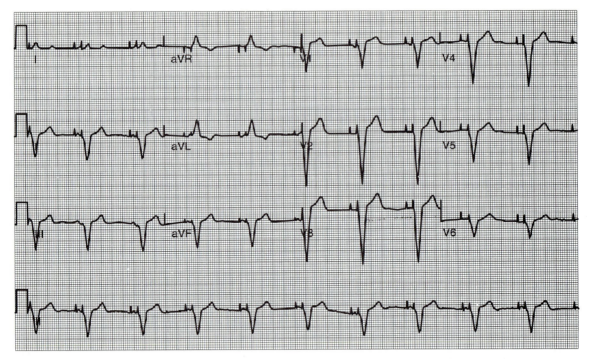

Figure 21–19. Atrioventricular pacing with ventricular pacing from the area of the right ventricular apex, yielding superiorly directed paced QRS complexes with a left BBB pattern. The paced P wave morphology and axis are similarly determined by the location of the pacing lead tip.

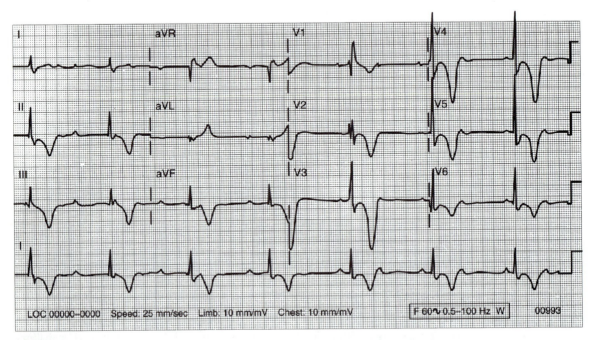

LOC 00000–0000   Speed: 25 mm/sec   Limb: 10 mm/mV   Chest: 10 mm/mV   F 60~ 0.5–100 Hz W   00993

Figure 21–20. Twelve-lead electrocardiogram in patient with a DDD pacing system, temporarily programmed to a rate of 30 bpm to permit emergence of the native rhythm. The intrinsic rhythm is sinus with complete atrioventricular block and right bundle branch block. Because no pacing artifacts are occurring, sensing function is normal in both atrium and ventricle. The deeply inverted T waves in the inferior and precordial leads represent a nonspecific abnormality commonly observed in patients with pacemakers; they do not represent myocardial injury.

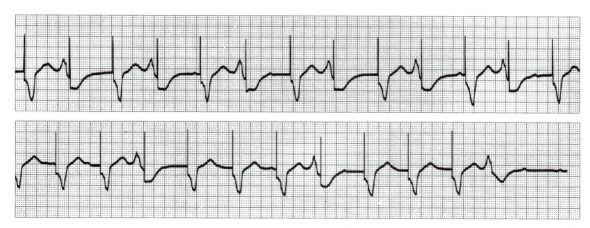

Figure 21–21. Failure to sense spontaneous ventricular complexes in a patient with a VVI pacing system. Because the signal quality of depolarization originating in ventricular tissue is often poor, this is not uncommon. Repetitive ventricular beating induced by the stimulus-on-RST complex is, however, rare in stable patients.

is managed by programming a higher sensitivity or, if necessary, by increasing the pacing rate to overdrive the native rhythm. In temporary systems, using a more sensitive setting or making the device unipolar should solve the undersensing problems.

Oversensing describes sensing of unwanted electrical signals such as T waves, myopotentials, environmental signals (eg, electrocautery; see Table 21–10). Programming the pulse generator to sense electrical signals of larger magnitude will often solve the problem. When a programmer is not available or the pulse generator cannot be identified, and therefore cannot be programmed, placing a magnet over the generator will eliminate the oversensing; definitive treatment can be undertaken at a later time. Because competitive rhythms that can cause repetitive beating can occur with the magnet in place, these patients should be in a monitored unit. In temporary units, using a less sensitive setting will achieve the desired result.

Failure to pace is present when pacing stimuli do not depolarize nonrefractory myocardium (Figure 21–22; Table 21–11). This condition may result from

poor electrode position; a subthreshold programmed output; output reduction due to battery end of life; or an increase in myocardial stimulation threshold from acute myocardial infarction, drug toxicity, electrolyte imbalance, cardiopulmonary resuscitation, or fibrosis at the pacing-catheter tip. Pacemaker noncapture can be managed by noninvasive programming of the generator's energy output; lead repositioning or implantation of a new generator (or both) may be required, depending on the underlying problem.

The difference between failure to capture when the stimulus artifact is present and a lack of stimulus output should be clearly understood. If the pacing stimulus has not been delivered (Table 21–12), capture cannot be ascertained. Applying a magnet will aid in determining the cause for the lack of stimulus output.

C. ASSESSMENT OF PACING SYSTEM FUNCTION

All patients should have a 12-lead ECG, with and without a magnet applied, to allow identification of spontaneous (where present), purely paced, and fusion P waves and QRS complexes, as well as sensing and

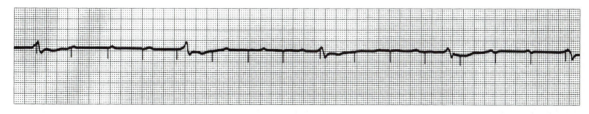

Figure 21–22. Failure to capture and sense in a patient following cardiac arrest; a temporary transvenous pacing system had been placed in the right ventricular apex. The QRS complexes are spontaneous and occur at a severely slow rate; they do not follow pacing stimuli.

Table 21–11. Causes and management of pacemaker noncapture.

Tissue refractoriness: Verify capture during temporal opportunity.
Lead dislodgement: Reposition lead, or program lead polarity.
Increase in myocardial stimulation threshold: Program higher energy output; treat underlying cause if possible.
Lead-insulation break: Repair or replace lead; unipolarize lead.
Conductor-wire fracture: Replace lead.
Inappropriately low programmed output: Program higher output.
Generator end of life: Replace generator.

---

pacing functions in both atria and ventricles. The paced rate with a magnet in place may not be the same as the programmed rate, and the mode of function with the magnet in place may differ from the programmed mode (eg, a DDD system may have a magnet mode that is VOO; Figure 21–23).

In addition, all patients should have highly penetrated posteroanterior and lateral chest radiographs; the latter may allow identification of the pacemaker's manufacturer and model number.

The number and types (unipolar, bipolar) of leads can be ascertained, as well as the positions of the lead tips and pulse generator. Lead tips lying outside the cardiac silhouette suggest the possibility of myocardial perforation. Occasionally, lead insulation degradation, wire fracture, or improper connections between the lead and generator connections can be seen. More sophisticated evaluation techniques, such as interrogation of the programmed values of the pulse generator, sensing and pacing threshold determination, and recording of intracardiac electrograms, are occasionally necessary to determine the cause of pacemaker malfunction; these evaluations are best performed by a pacemaker specialist.

Andersen HR, Nielsen JC, Thomsen PE et al: Long-term follow-up of patients from a randomised trial of atrial versus ventricular pacing for sick-sinus syndrome. Lancet 1997;350:1210.

Connolly SJ, Kerr CR, Gent M et al: Effects of physiologic versus ventricular pacing on the risk of stroke and death due to cardiovascular causes. Canadian Trial of Physiologic Pacing Investigators. N Engl J Med 2000;342:1385.

Connolly SJ, Sheldon R, Robert S et al: The North American Vasovagal Pacemaker Study (VPS): A randomized trial of permanent cardiac pacing for the prevention of vasovagal syncope. The Vasovagal Pacemaker Study Investigators. J Am Coll Cardiol 1999;33:16.

Goldschlager N, Epstein A, Friedman P et al: Environmental and drug effects on patients with pacemakers and implantable cardioverter/defibrillators: A practical guide to patient treatment. North American Society of Pacing and Electrophysiology (NASPE) Practice Guideline Committee. Arch Intern Med 2001;161:649.

Gregoratos G, Cheitin MD, Conill A et al: ACC/AHA guidelines for implantation of cardiac pacemakers and antiarrhythmia devices. A report of the American College of Cardiology/American Heart Association Task Force on Practice Guidelines (Committee on Pacemaker Implantation). J Am Coll Cardiol 1998;31:1175.

Kusumoto FM, Goldschlager N: Cardiac pacing. N Engl J Med 1996;334:89–98.

Lamas GA, Orav EJ, Stambler BS et al: Quality of life and clinical outcomes in elderly patients treated with ventricular pacing as compared with dual-chamber pacing. Pacemaker Selection in the Elderly Investigators. N Engl J Med 1998;338:1097.

Sutton R, Stack Z, Heaven D et al: Mode switching for atrial tachyarrhythmias. Am J Cardiol 1999;83(Suppl):202-D.

Wood MA, Brown-Mahoney C, Kay GN et al: Clinical outcomes after ablation and pacing therapy for atrial fibrillation. A meta-analysis. Circulation 2000;101:1138.

Table 21–12. Causes of absence of pacing stimulus output and response to magnet application.

Cause	Response to Magnet
Normal inhibition by P waves and QRS complexes	Pacing stimuli will be delivered asynchronously
Oversensing	Pacing stimuli will be delivered asynchronously
Lead fracture	Pacing stimuli may not be seen if the break in the wire is complete (current does not reach body tissues); may be seen as multiples of a basing pacing rate, or may be seen intermittently (make-break circuit); may have variable amplitude
Lead-generator disconnection or improper connection	Same as for lead fracture
Battery failure (end of life)	Pacing stimuli at slow rate, no visible pacing stimuli, noncapture, failure to sense
Battery component failure	Variable response

A. Without Magnet

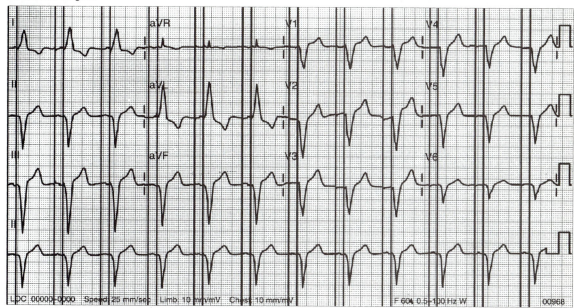

B. With Magnet

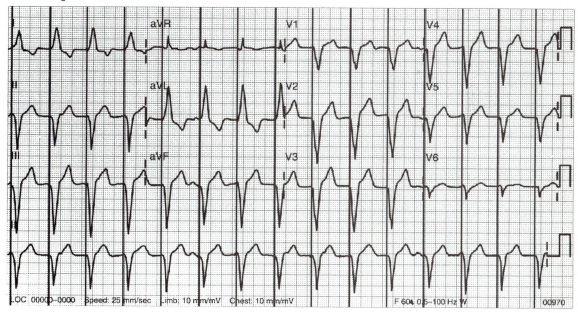

Figure 21–23. **A:** Atrioventricular sequential pacing. The large magnitude of the pacing artifacts indicate unipolar pacing in both chambers. Because atrial pacing stimuli are followed by P waves, and ventricular stimuli are followed by QRS complexes, pacing function is normal in both chambers. Sensing function cannot be evaluated because spontaneous P waves and QRS complexes are not occurring. **B:** Twelve-lead electrocardiogram, recorded with magnet in place. The mode of function is VOO (asynchronous ventricular pacing) at the factory-designated rate of about 88/min. This is normal function for this particular device.

Ventricular Tachycardia

22

Masood Akhtar, MD

ESSENTIALS OF DIAGNOSIS

- *Monomorphic ventricular tachycardia*
- *Nonsustained: Three or more consecutive QRS complexes of uniform configuration of ventricular origin at a rate of more than 100 bpm*
- *Sustained: Lasts more than 30 s; requires intervention for termination*
- *Polymorphic ventricular tachycardia: Beat-to-beat variation in QRS configuration*

General Considerations

The magnitude of ventricular tachycardia (VT), one of the most common health problems encountered in clinical practice, can best be appreciated in terms of its various clinical manifestations (Table 22–1). The most serious is its degeneration into ventricular fibrillation, producing cardiac arrest and sudden cardiac death and accounting for more than 300,000 deaths a year. The second most serious clinical presentation is syncope. Although the overall prevalence of VT-related syncope is unclear, it is estimated to be frequent because inducible VT (via electrical stimulation) is the most common arrhythmia detected in patients with unexplained syncope. A high prevalence of sudden cardiac death (more than 20% incidence within the ensuing 12 months) is noted in patients with syncope from cardiovascular causes, suggesting that undiagnosed VT

Table 22–1. Clinical manifestations of ventricular tachycardia.

Ventricular fibrillation (SCD)
Syncope, near syncope
Wide QRS tachycardia

SCD = sudden cardiac death.

may be an underlying cause of sudden death in patients with unexplained syncope. The third most significant clinical manifestation of VT is a wide QRS tachycardia that is often hemodynamically well tolerated.

A. MANAGEMENT ISSUES

1. Underdiagnosis—Ventricular tachycardia as a cause of morbidity and mortality is grossly underdiagnosed, potentially leading to mismanagement. This may be particularly true when the clinical presentation is unexplained syncope because no concomitant electrocardiographic documentation is available. In the case of cardiac arrest or sudden cardiac death (SCD) acute myocardial infarction rather than an arrhythmic problem is often assumed to be responsible. The vast majority of sudden death victims have no evidence of acute myocardial necrosis, even though the episode often occurs in patients with underlying coronary artery disease. Managing the underlying coronary artery disease with no regard to treating the concomitant VT is inadequate. Patients presenting with syncope are seldom investigated for possible ventricular tachycardia; they are more frequently thought of as having neurologic problems and therefore undergo an extensive—and usually unrewarding—neurologic workup.

2. Misdiagnosis—When hemodynamically stable VT is recorded on the surface electrocardiogram (ECG), it is often misdiagnosed as supraventricular tachycardia (SVT) with aberrant conduction. Any subsequent management is therefore directed toward SVT. Although the exact logic for this line of thinking is unclear, the main reason may be that the hemodynamic stability is associated with the broad QRS rhythm and thus the erroneous belief that the problem cannot be VT. It must be understood that approximately 80% of the patients presenting with sustained wide QRS tachycardia have VT; aberrant conduction is rare, particularly when the tachycardia is sustained for more than a few minutes. To avoid such misdiagnosis, the clinician can either use the ECG criteria that distinguish VT from SVT and aberrant conduction (discussed later in this chapter) or simply assume the presence of VT. The assumption of VT is more often correct; it is also safer because misdiagnosing VT as SVT is a riskier judgment error than vice versa.

Although VT has, in general, a life-threatening potential, not all forms of it carry such an ominous prognosis. The clinical presentation of VT depends on many factors, including rate, ventricular function, presence of concomitant coronary artery disease, the presence or absence of cardioactive drugs, and even the patient's posture at the time of onset. Hemodynamic tolerance of VT can, therefore, vary considerably in different situations; at times, it can vary in the same patient, and it is prudent not to exclude the diagnosis of VT on the basis of hemodynamic tolerance alone. It is crucial that wherever possible, a 12-lead ECG be obtained prior to intervention, particularly when the tachycardia is not associated with hemodynamic collapse.

B. DEFINITIONS

The spectrum of VT in Table 22–2 lists the two most common varieties encountered in clinical practice and their underlying causes. This classification helps approach the diagnosis in a systematic fashion and directs the physician to specific therapeutic options.

Monomorphic VT is a form of ventricular tachycardia in which the QRS complex configuration is uniform from beat to beat in all the surface ECG leads (Figure 22–1A). In **polymorphic VT,** a beat-to-beat variation occurs in the QRS complex configuration in any of the ECG leads (Figure 22–1B). These diagnoses may be difficult, however, when a single-surface ECG lead is recorded. As used in the literature, **sustained VT** is a tachycardia that lasts for 30 s or requires interven-

Table 22–2. Classification and causes of common ventricular tachycardias.

Monomorphic ventricular tachycardia
Chronic coronary artery disease
Idiopathic dilated cardiomyopathy
Right ventricular dysplasia
No structural heart disease
    Right bundle branch block configuration
    Left bundle branch block configuration
    Repetitive monomorphic VT
Other forms
Polymorphic ventricular tachycardia
Prolonged QT interval (torsade de pointes)
    Congenital
    Acquired
Normal QT interval
    Acute ischemia
    Other

tion for termination. The definition does not imply that a prolonged episode of VT lasting less than 30 s has any less clinical significance. **Nonsustained VT** is a term used to describe any three or more consecutive QRS complexes of ventricular origin with a rate of more than 100 bpm. When describing nonsustained VT, it is important to mention the number of complexes and rate in order to convey a clear picture of the event.

Once it has been determined whether the VT is monomorphic or polymorphic, the questions to be asked differ for each category. The nature of the under-

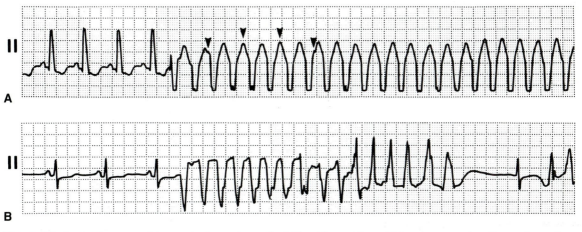

Figure 22–1. **A:** Monomorphic ventricular tachycardia (VT), with a uniform QRS appearance for all complexes. Arrowheads indicate superimposed P waves. **B:** Polymorphic VT, with a beat-to-beat variation in the QRS morphology; QT-interval prolongation follows the termination of the VT episode. Reproduced, with permission, from Akhtar M: Clinical spectrum of ventricular tachycardia. Circulation 1990;82:1561.

lying cardiac structure is crucial in monomorphic VT but not as critical for the polymorphic forms, which can occur without obvious structural heart disease. In this chapter, VT is considered sustained unless specifically stated otherwise.

MONOMORPHIC VENTRICULAR TACHYCARDIA

Diagnosis

A. MONOMORPHIC VT IN ASSOCIATION WITH CHRONIC CORONARY ARTERY DISEASE

This is the most common form encountered in clinical practice—as well as the most extensively investigated in clinical and electrophysiology laboratories. The underlying substrate is usually an area of fibrosis that provides an anatomic obstacle around which the reentrant impulse can propagate. The extent and architecture of the scar may determine the propensity to VT in a given situation. For example, a homogeneous scar with no surviving conducting tissue is less likely to cause arrhythmias than is fibrosis interspersed with streaks of healthy myocardium. In some situations, acute myocardial ischemia or infarct can produce the conditions of slow conduction and block necessary for reentry. Although nonreentrant mechanisms (eg, abnormal automaticity, triggered activity) may cause VT in these settings, reentry is the most common mechanism.

As myocardial activation spreads from the reentrant circuit, the resultant QRS morphology is determined by the direction of the activation vector. Because of the myocardial origin of this type of VT, some characteristic features are expected: (1) The initial part of the QRS complex will generally be inscribed slowly because of muscle-to-muscle propagation. (2) The resultant QRS width is often markedly increased because of this intramyocardial conduction delay. (3) Because the impulse is not activating the ventricles via the bundle branches, the QRS pattern is not likely to be typical of either the right or left bundle branch block. (4) When there is no septal scar, VT originating in the left ventricle activates the ipsilateral ventricle, followed by the interventricular septum and then the right ventricle. This causes an atypical right bundle branch block (RBBB) pattern. (5) Ventricular tachycardia that originates in the right ventricle shows a left bundle branch block (LBBB) pattern. (6) When the tachycardia originates close to a septal scar, it may show a LBBB pattern even if the reentrant circuit resides in the left ventricle.

Distinguishing ventricular tachycardia from supraventricular tachycardia with aberrant conduction is relatively easy except in patients with a regular wide QRS tachycardia from conduction over an accessory pathway (eg, Wolff-Parkinson-White syndrome). Figure 22–2 depicts, schematically, the reasons for normal and broad QRS complexes. The QRS pattern of preexcited QRS complex is difficult to distinguish from VT because in both instances the QRS starts with muscle-to-muscle conduction. Patients with ventricular preexcitation do not have myocardial fibrosis, so the QRS duration is expected to be shorter than it is in VT in association with a chronically diseased myocardium.

As noted, earlier, when VT presents as a hemodynamically stable arrhythmia, it is frequently misdiagnosed as SVT with aberrant conduction. A number of surface ECG criteria have been established to distinguish myocardial VT from aberrant conduction. If used in a systematic fashion these criteria are helpful in arriving at an accurate diagnosis. The criteria, along with their underlying electrophysiologic basis for distinction between VT and SVT with aberrant conduction appear in the following numbered sections.

1. Atrioventricular (AT) relationship—In SVT, the arrhythmia arises in the atria or AV junction and reaches the ventricles through the AV node and His-Purkinje system (HPS). Because the atrial arrhythmia is the primary event, either a 1:1 AV response or a varying degree of AV block occurs, but in either case the atrial rates equal or exceed ventricular rates. During VT, a retrograde block often leads to either AV dissociation or a varying degree of ventriculoatrial (VA) conduction ratios, but the ventricular rates equal or exceed the atrial rate. When AV dissociation can be recognized, it is the most reliable criterion for VT because SVT rarely produces such an ECG pattern. This criterion lacks sensitivity, however, because in only 25% of patients with VT can the P waves be identified on the surface ECG (see Figure 22–1). In patients with slower VT and AV dissociation, intermittent ventricular capture can result in fusion with normal complexes during the VT. This useful but rarely observed finding supports the diagnosis of VT.

2. QRS complex duration—For the reasons listed earlier, the QRS complex duration is the widest in VT and narrowest in aberrant conduction. To distinguish VT from SVT with aberrant conduction on the basis of QRS duration alone, however, some specific aspects must be considered. In the absence of cardioactive drugs and extensive myocardial fibrosis, aberrancy rarely results in a QRS duration of more than 140 ms with an RBBB pattern (Figure 22–3) or more than 160 ms with an LBBB configuration. In the presence of intramyocardial conduction delay from drugs (such as class I antiarrhythmic agents) and myocardial fibrosis, the QRS width may also exceed these values in SVT with aberrant conduction. Conversely, on a rare occasion, VT can present as a narrow QRS tachycardia (less than 120 ms) when there is near-simultaneous activation of the two ventricles, perhaps from the septum.

Narrow QRS

Wide QRS-BBB
(Aberrant conduction)

Wide QRS-Preexcitation
(Conduction via AP)

Wide QRS-VT

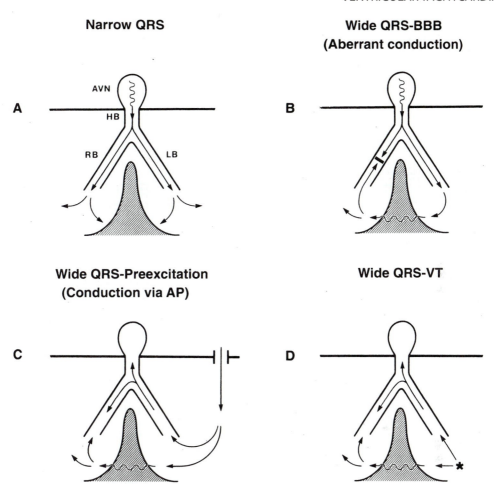

Figure 22–2. Mechanism of wide QRS. **A:** Narrow QRS from simultaneous activation of the right and left ventricles. In the three types of wide QRS shown in **B–D,** there is sequential rather than simultaneous activation of the left and right ventricle and a variable amount of muscle-to-muscle conduction. AP = accessory pathway; AVN = atrioventricular node; BBB = bundle branch block; HB = His bundle; LB = left bundle; RB = right bundle. Reproduced, with permission, from Akhtar M et al: Electrophysiological spectrum of wide QRS complex tachycardia. In Zipes DP, Jalife J, eds: Cardiac Electrophysiology. From Cell to Bedside. Philadelphia: WB Saunders, 1990.

3. Specific QRS configuration—The prevalence of LBBB versus RBBB morphology among the causes of wide QRS is comparable in both VT and SVT with aberrant conduction; it is therefore of no diagnostic value. Because of the myocardial origin of most forms of VT, however, the QRS appearance is not exactly like a typical left or right bundle branch block (see Figure 22–3). Many ECG criteria, therefore, have exploited this difference to separate VT from aberrant conduction. The typical RBBB is a triphasic complex best seen in V_1 as rsR′ or rSR′ pattern and in lead I as qRs, qRS pattern. Similarly a typical LBBB has no initial q wave in I and a small r and a rapid S wave in

V_1 such as that from onset of r to the nadir of S in V_1 measures less than 100 ms. Any deviation from these QRS morphologies should raise the suspicion of VT, particularly when a patient has a preexisting left or right bundle branch block during sinus rhythm. In this situation, a wide QRS tachycardia represent VT if there is even the slightest change in the QRS configuration. During SVT in these patients, the QRS complex should remain the same. Other morphologic features suggestive of VT are monophasic or biphasic QRS complexes in leads V_1 and V_6 and a QR complex in any of the leads. A positive QRS concordance (positive complexes V_1–V_6) is uncommon in aberrancy,

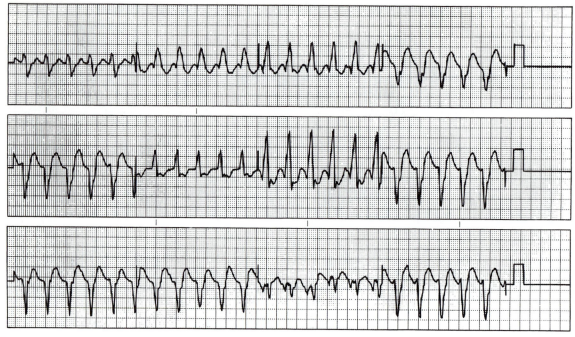

Figure 22–3. The ventricular origin of wide-QRS tachycardia is suggested here by a QRS duration of 190 ms with a right bundle branch block pattern in the absence of cardioactive drugs. The QRS appearance is not typical of right bundle branch block patterns seen in aberrancy. Atrioventricular dissociation is better appreciated in the limb leads. The electrocardiographic leads are (from top to bottom) I, II, and III and (left to right) aVR, aVL, and aVf. The last six leads are V$_1$–V$_6$ in a similar order.

but a negative QRS concordance (QS complexes V$_1$–V$_6$) can occur during aberrant conduction in a small percentage of cases.

4. QRS complex axis—The axis orientation on a 12-lead ECG ranging from normal (–30°– +90°), left (–31°– –90°) or right (+91°–+180°) has significant overlap across the causes of wide QRS complex tachycardia and is of little diagnostic value. The axis range of –91° to 180°, however, is usually not seen in aberrant conduction. The axis location of this extreme during SVT is, therefore, unlikely unless there was a nonarrhythmic reason for it, such as severe right ventricular hypertrophy or lung disease. Similarly, a combination of right axis with LBBB pattern is almost always seen in patients with VT.

After an initial documentation on the surface ECG, or when VT is suspected by virtue of underlying coronary artery disease and symptoms such as syncope, a further workup is often critical for characterization of VT. Ambulatory monitoring is of limited value because sustained VT is not commonly seen on a daily basis. In most situations, invasive electrophysiologic studies (EPS) are indicated for these patients for both diagnostic and therapeutic purposes.

B. MONOMORPHIC VT IN ASSOCIATION WITH IDIOPATHIC DILATED CARDIOMYOPATHY

Monomorphic VT associated with idiopathic dilated cardiomyopathy (IDCM) and valvular disease is indistinguishable from VT in chronic coronary artery disease in approximately 60% of patients. The underlying substrate is most probably fibrosis, providing both the anatomic obstacle and the pathway for reexcitation. Invariably, however, these patients have conduction slowing in the HPS as a part of the diffuse myocardial disease process, and the baseline ECG shows evidence of nonspecific intraventricular conduction defect. The resultant tachycardia uses the bundle branches and the bundle of His for sustained reentry. Bundle branch reentry (BBR) could manifest as either a left or right bundle branch block pattern (Figures 22–4 and 22–5). Because ventricular myocardial activation occurs via the bundle branches, a typical left or right bundle branch block configuration is generally noted. Although the prevalence of BBR is particularly high in patients with IDCM, it does occur in dilated cardiomyopathy regardless of the underlying pathology.

BBR is also fairly common in patients with aortic and mitral valve disease. Due to the close anatomic re-

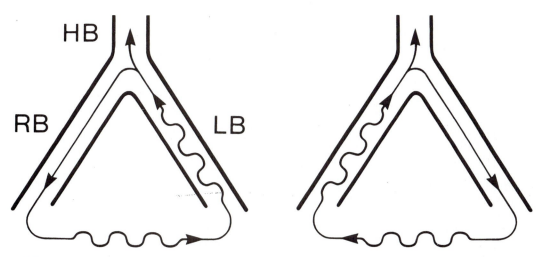

Figure 22–4. Schematic of bundle branch reentry circuit. In left bundle branch block, ventricular activation occurs via the right bundle (RB), and the impulse activates the His bundle (HB) via the left bundle (LB) to complete the circuit. A reversed impulse propagation leads to a right bundle branch block pattern.

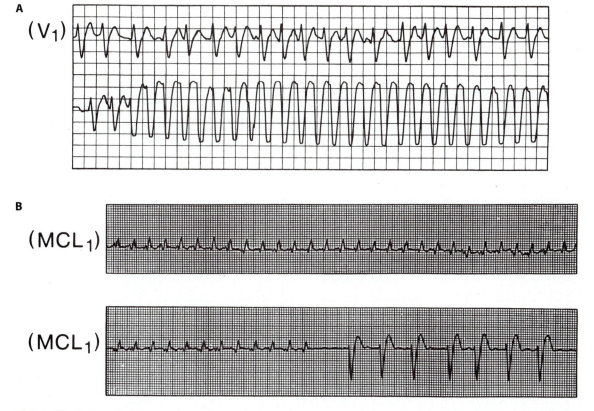

Figure 22–5. Bundle branch reentrant ventricular tachycardia with typical left (**A**) and right (**B**) bundle branch morphologies; recorded at different times in a patient with idiopathic dilated cardiomyopathy. Note the underlying intraventricular conduction defect during baseline rhythm, before onset (**A**) and after termination (**B**). Reproduced, with permission, from Akhtar M: Clinical spectrum of ventricular tachycardia. Circulation 1990;82:1561.

lationship between the proximal HPS and annuli of these valves, HPS conduction delays can occur in association with valvular disease. Frequently, sustained BBR is observed soon after valve surgery, probably related to aggregation of local substrata. In the absence of left ventricular (LV) dysfunction and coronary artery disease BBR accounted for 29% of the cases, and myocardial VT was noted in 65%. Two patients (6%) had both BBR and myocardial VT. When coronary artery disease and LV dysfunction coexisted, myocardial VT was more common.

C. MONOMORPHIC VT IN RIGHT VENTRICULAR DYSPLASIA

Because the left ventricle can be fairly normal in these patients, arrhythmic problems, primarily VT, are the main manifestations of the underlying cardiac pathology. The amount of fibrosis and fatty infiltration into the right ventricle varies, with eventual dilatation. The VT is reentrant in nature, similar to other situations with myocardial fibrosis. The QRS morphology is that of an LBBB pattern, but the axis can be right, normal, or leftward. Unless this type of VT is specifically suspected and efforts are made to elucidate right ventricular pathology, the correct diagnosis is likely to be missed. The baseline ECG often shows T wave inversion in leads V_1–V_3. This entity should be considered in patients with VT showing an LBBB morphology and left axis when there is no obvious LV pathology. Although palpitations and mild hypotension are the usual presentation, syncope and sudden cardiac death do occur in this disease.

D. MONOMORPHIC VT IN PATIENTS WITH NO STRUCTURAL HEART DISEASE

This condition is being diagnosed more frequently. When VT is seen in patients who are otherwise healthy, it is important to examine the QRS morphology as well as the axis. Depending on the site of origin (eg, left versus right ventricle), the tachycardia may have a different response to therapeutic agents.

1. Monomorphic VT with a right bundle branch configuration—The origin of this tachycardia is in the inferoapical region of the left ventricle. The axis orientation is leftward unless the tachycardia originates elsewhere; a normal-to-rightward axis can be seen occasionally. A somewhat rapid initial inscription of the QRS in this ventricular tachycardia suggests a possible origin in the peripheral Purkinje network. Both reentry and triggered activity have been suggested as underlying mechanisms. Because this VT responds to intravenous verapamil it is often referred to as verapamil-sensitive VT (Figure 22–6). The usual presentation is

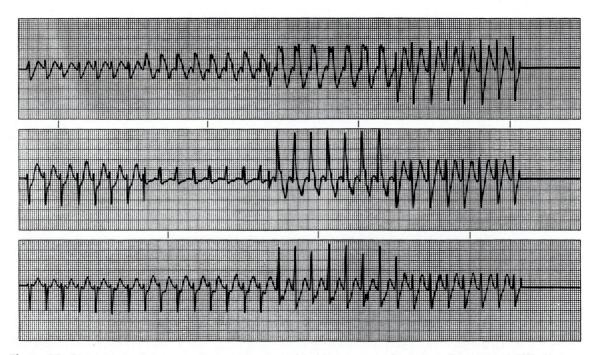

Figure 22–6. Twelve-lead electrocardiogram showing typical appearance of a verapamil-sensitive ventricular tachycardia with no associated structural cardiac abnormality. Reproduced, with permission, from Akhtar M: Clinical spectrum of ventricular tachycardia. Circulation 1990;82:1561.

palpitation. Presyncope and syncope are sometimes noted, but sudden cardiac death is rare.

2. Monomorphic VT with a left bundle branch block configuration—Several somewhat different types of VT may present with this QRS morphology in patients who have no obvious structural cardiac abnormality (Figure 22–7). The axis is typically rightward and sometimes normal. In some patients, the tachycardia is provoked by exercise and isoproterenol infusion, suggesting that catecholamines triggered after depolarization may be the underlying mechanism. Because of easy induction, however, reentry is suggested in other cases. In some situations intravenous adenosine will terminate the VT, and triggered activity dependent on cyclic adenosine monophosphate (AMP) may be the mechanism. Even though the underlying mechanisms of VT with an LBBB configuration may be diverse, it seems to be a clinically identifiable entity. It is unclear at present whether subtle myocardial abnormalities exist in this population that are not detectable with the routine diagnostic workup. Sudden cardiac death is rare, but syncope and presyncope as a clinical presentation are fairly common.

3. Repetitive monomorphic VT—This condition is also seen in patients with no structural heart disease. Unlike the aforementioned varieties, it is characterized by repeated brief runs of VT. Its precise mechanisms and underlying substrate are poorly understood because these patients seldom have an in-depth evaluation. The clinical presentation is rather benign in the vast majority of cases; these patients are either asymptomatic or have a feeling of palpitations. Asymptomatic patients often come to medical attention because of irregularity of the pulse or ECG recording for unrelated reasons.

E. OTHER FORMS

Aside from repetitive monomorphic VT, the ventricular tachycardias described earlier are sustained forms. In rare situations, sustained VT can also occur in other clinical settings, and any type of sustained tachycardia may present in a nonsustained form as well. When the nonsustained VT is symptomatic, it should be managed like the sustained variety. Asymptomatic nonsustained VT, however, particularly with brief runs (fewer than 10 beats) and a slower rate (less than 150/min) generally does not require treatment unless associated with poor LV function (left ventricular ejection fraction [LVEF] ≤0.35).

Diagnostic Studies

Patients with sustained ventricular tachycardia that is either documented via ECG or suspected from symptoms such as syncope or presyncope should undergo further studies. These can confirm the diagnosis of wide QRS tachycardia, determine whether VT is the cause of unexplained symptoms, identify the underlying substrate, and determine the direction of therapy.

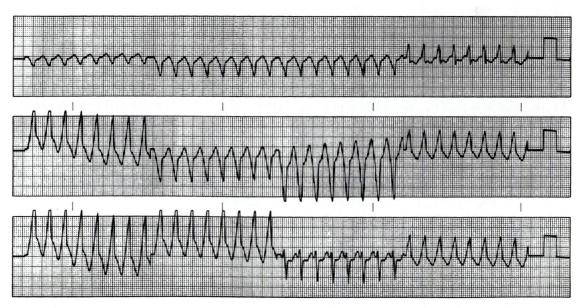

Figure 22–7. In this electrocardiogram, the appearance of the left bundle branch block pattern and right-axis deviation is typical of ventricular tachycardia in the absence of structural heart disease, originating in the left ventricular outflow tract. Reproduced, with permission, from Akhtar M: Clinical spectrum of ventricular tachycardia. Circulation 1990;82:1561.

In most patients with documented sustained VT the critical components of the workup include assessment of the nature and extent of any underlying heart disease and an electrophysiologic evaluation. A noninvasive cardiovascular workup includes ambulatory monitoring to detect heart rate variability or a daily fluctuation of arrhythmia; exercise testing to detect coronary artery disease or provoke catecholamine-sensitive VT; and an echocardiographic examination to uncover structural heart disease. Cardiac catheterization is strongly recommended for patients suspected of coronary artery disease.

Although a 12-lead ECG is usually adequate to make an accurate diagnosis of VT (versus SVT), the precise nature may not be clear in many patients unless electrophysiologic studies are performed.

When VT is suspected but not documented, its induction in the laboratory is critical to the decision to undertake any therapeutic approach. By inducing or replicating VT in the laboratory, its rate, morphology, origin, hemodynamic tolerance, and response to intravenous drugs can be evaluated.

Serial drug testing can be carried out using oral antiarrhythmic agents and EPS. Complete suppression of VT inducibility is considered a desirable endpoint. Significant slowing of the VT rate is also associated with a lower incidence of cardiac arrest. The lack of a response to antiarrhythmic drugs with EPS quickly establishes a high-risk group needing such nonpharmacologic treatments as surgery, catheter ablation, or implantation of a cardioverter-defibrillator. Because the newer generation of implantable cardioverter-defibrillators (ICDs) has the option of tiered therapy, in which overdrive-pacing termination of VT is attempted first, it is helpful to determine the feasibility of terminating VT by pacing.

Catheter ablation using radiofrequency or electrical energy is an effective form of treatment in patients with BBR, VT in association with a structurally normal heart and, in some cases, VT in association with prior myocardial infarction. Thorough electrophysiologic testing is crucial for a successful outcome in these cases.

Many patients with VT have extensive cardiac pathology, including abnormalities of sinus node function and AV conduction. These abnormalities can be further aggravated with the administration of antiarrhythmic drugs. EPS can frequently identify the nature and determine both the extent of these abnormalities and the need for additional therapeutic interventions (eg, permanent pacing for bradycardia).

Aside from arrhythmia assessment and cardiac substrate identification, the role of further tests in this population is dictated by the initial findings. When reversible abnormalities, such as myocardial ischemia, are detected, every attempt should be made to correct them. Paying separate attention to arrhythmias is critical because monomorphic VT is unlikely to be controlled without addressing specific VT management.

Management of Monomorphic Ventricular Tachycardia

Because monomorphic VT is most commonly due to underlying myocardial fibrosis, the pharmacologic treatment outlined here primarily relates to this substrate. The same approach can be used in other situations, but it may not be as applicable.

A. ACUTE TERMINATION

The method of VT termination in the acute settings depends on the hemodynamic tolerance of the tachycardia. When the patient loses consciousness or has severe hypotension, a synchronized DC cardioversion (200–300 J) should be attempted. Sedation prior to cardioversion is advised in patients who are awake. With hemodynamically well tolerated VT, there is ample time to gather complete information, including a 12-lead ECG, before initiating therapy. Although a bolus of lidocaine (2–3 mg/kg) is often used initially, its efficacy in chronic VT is not proven; VT in association with acute myocardial infarction may respond to lidocaine, however. Intravenous procainamide (10–15 mg/kg) at a rate of 50–100 mg/min is more effective. In some situations, intravenous amiodarone may be necessary. If administration of any of these agents results in the termination of VT, it is customary and frequently desirable to initiate a continuous infusion of the effective agent. Intravenous calcium channel blockers such as verapamil should not be administered unless you are certain about the supraventricular nature of a sustained wide QRS tachycardia (SVT with aberrant conduction). The only type of VT that responds to verapamil is uncommon. When VT is triggered or aggravated by exercise, intravenous β-blockers may be tried as the initial therapy unless there are contraindications to their use. If there is any uncertainty regarding the safety of β-blockers in patients with VT, it is somewhat safer to use agents with a short half-life, such as esmolol.

When pharmacologic intervention fails, overdrive termination can be tried. It does require insertion of a pacing catheter but can be quite useful in patients with frequent recurrent VT. Cardioversion is necessary in many situations, particularly if a prolonged VT episode is undesirable, such as in the setting of ischemic heart disease. It should also be emphasized that careful attention should be paid to other factors contributing to ventricular arrhythmogenesis, such as acidosis, hypoxia, electrolyte abnormalities, and the use of drugs. If such factors are involved, pharmacologic treatment alone may fail to control the VT.

B. PREVENTION

Although acute termination of VT is relatively straightforward in most situations, the prevention of recurrences is often a challenge. The empiric use of antiarrhythmic drugs is not encouraged because of potential harm to the patient—as well as their unproven efficacy. Because VT represents a potentially life-threatening arrhythmia, establishing an effective form of therapy is desirable before the patient is discharged–especially for patients who present with VT-related syncope or cardiac arrest. In most situations, the therapy must be individualized, which requires understanding the type of VT, any underlying heart disease, LVEF, and the clinical presentation.

1. Pharmacologic therapy—For monomorphic VT in association with chronic coronary artery disease or any other type of fibrosis, a variety of therapeutic options are now available. These include antiarrhythmic drugs, VT focal ablative therapy, and ICDs. Among the antiarrhythmic drugs, class I agents (Table 22–3) have moderate efficacy; quinidine and procainamide (class Ia) have been used extensively. In recent years, however, their use has progressively declined because of both excessive patient intolerance and lack of efficacy. Class Ib drugs such as mexiletine are weak antiarrhythmic agents when used alone, but they seem more useful in combination with Ia drugs. Class Ic drugs have moderate efficacy but a significant proarrhythmic potential. At present, class III agents (amiodarone, sotalol, etc) are the most promising antiarrhythmic agents for control of VT and ventricular fibrillation (VF). After a loading dose of 1200–1800 mg/day for 1–2 weeks, amiodarone can be used in a maintenance dose of 200–400 mg/day. The usual daily dose of sotalol is 240–480 mg/day. It should be pointed out that in high-risk patients with coronary artery disease and reduced LV function, amiodarone has not been shown to decrease mortality rates as compared with placebo. When using class I drugs or sotalol, it is important to have some objective means of documenting VT control, such as serial Holter monitors or EPS. The latter may be the only option when VT does not recur as frequently as it does in most patients with VT and VF. Exercise-induced VT generally responds well to β-

blockers, and serial exercise stress tests can be used to judge drug efficacy. Because other forms of VT in patients with coronary artery disease may respond to β-blockers, they are frequently used alone or in combination with other antiarrhythmic drugs when the patient can tolerate them.

Regardless of the method used, a failure of drug response is usually an indication for nonpharmacologic treatment, which can produce excellent results.

2. Nonpharmacologic therapy—

a. Implantable cardioverter-defibrillators—These devices clearly provide the most effective form of therapy for preventing sudden cardiac death in patients with VT. In our experience, the outcome of these high-risk patients over 5 years is better with an ICD than with any form of drug therapy. The ICD does not prevent VT from occurring, however; it is designed only to terminate the tachycardia or fibrillation. Most episodes of VT can now be terminated with overdrive pacing; this form of therapy is usually not perceptible to the patient. There are relatively few contraindications to ICD treatment; these include incessant VT and VF secondary to reversible causes such as antiarrhythmic drugs, electrolyte abnormalities, and acute ischemia.

Several recent publications representing the results of randomized trials have shown superiority of ICDs compared with conventional drug therapy or no therapy. In the multicenter amiodarone versus defibrillator trial (MADIT) prior myocardial infarction patients with spontaneous nonsustained VT resistant to IV procainamide were randomized to ICD or conventional drug therapy. A significant mortality rate reduction ($P < 0.009$) in the ICD limb necessitated premature termination of the trial (Figure 22–8). The MUSTT (multicenter unsustained tachycardia trial) had a somewhat similar population and again demonstrated better outcomes with ICD. Another large randomized trial,

Table 22–3. Antiarrhythmic drugs.

Class	Drug
Ia	Quinidine, procainamide, disopyramide
Ib	Mexilentine, lidocaine
Ic	Flecainide, propafenone, others (ethmozine)
II	Beta-blockers
III	Amiodarone, sotalol, bepridil
IV	Calcium channel blockers

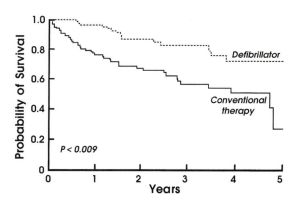

Figure 22–8. Probability of survival over 5 years in MADIT patients randomized to a defibrillator versus conventional therapy.

amiodarone versus ICD (AVID) showed ICD efficacy that was greater than the amiodarone limb in patients with prior VT/VF (Figure 22–9). The MADIT and MUSTT are considered primary prevention trials because prior to study entry the population did not have life-threatening symptomatic VT/VF. AVID, on the other hand included patients with prior symptomatic VT/VF. Several more trials in patients with VT/VF are ongoing, and the results should be available in the near future.

b. Surgical ablation—In patients with coronary artery disease and prior myocardial infarction, the VT often originates close to the infarct, thus providing the opportunity for surgical destruction of the VT site of origin. It should be considered in patients undergoing coronary artery bypass surgery who have a ventricular aneurysm or infarction and mappable VT. In patients with a LVEF of at least 0.25, this type of surgery can be carried out with relatively low risk and a cure rate of approximately 75%.

c. Catheter-based ablation—With its lower success rate, catheter-based ablation plays a limited role in patients with myocardial VT. It is almost always curative, however, for sustained VT from BBR from any cause seen in patients with dilated cardiomyopathy. This method of treatment has also proven its value in patients with VT who have no obvious structural heart disease. Catheter-based ablation techniques using radiofrequency as an energy source have already established their value in the management of SVT and are likely to play a greater role in VT as well.

POLYMORPHIC VENTRICULAR TACHYCARDIA

Recognition of polymorphic VTs and their distinction from the monomorphic variety represent the crucial

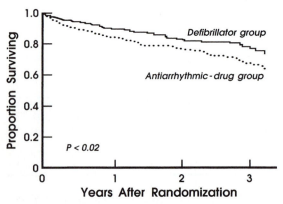

Figure 22–9. Proportion of AVID patients surviving 3 years after randomization to a defibrillator versus antiarrhythmic drug therapy.

first step toward appropriate management. These tachycardias tend to be rapid; they generally produce symptoms of hypotension and can readily degenerate into ventricular fibrillation. At least two types can be recognized that must be distinguished by the presence or absence of prolonged myocardial recovery.

A. POLYMORPHIC VT IN THE SETTING OF PROLONGED QT INTERVAL

This condition is often referred to as torsade de pointes. It can be congenital or acquired. Although the precipitating factor can differ between the two varieties, both show a prolonged QT (QTc) interval and slow, prominent, or unusual-looking T waves.

1. Congenital prolonged QT interval syndrome— This syndrome occurs with or without associated deafness. It is mainly characterized by episodes of torsade de pointes that are often triggered by adrenergic stimulation, which can be brought about by physical exertion or mental or emotional stress. The clinical presentation includes light-headed spells, near syncope, syncope and, in some cases, cardiac arrest. There are no obvious associated cardiac abnormalities. The QT interval prolongation may be subtle and can be unmasked by long pauses or adrenergic stimuli such as exercise. Exercise testing and the administration of epinephrine to trigger torsade de pointes have also sometimes been used. It is now clear that congenital long QT syndrome has a genetic basis. At least six genetic mutations at different loci have been identified. QT_1 and QT_2 are K^+ channel abnormalities, but QT_3 is a Na^+ channel mutation. Undoubtedly a clear picture regarding the basis for arrhythmia management will emerge in years to come. The electrophysiologic mechanism may be early after-depolarization for initiation and reentry for sustenance.

The mainstay of treatment is β-blockade, and up to 5 mg/kg/day of propranolol may be necessary in some situations. Because cardiac slowing can also be arrhythmogenic, permanent pacing is often performed. Clearly, drugs that prolong the QT interval must be avoided. Left stellate sympathectomy has been carried out with variable success in difficult cases. In individuals with recurrent syncope or cardiac arrest, ICDs remain a viable option to prevent sudden cardiac death.

2. Acquired prolonged QT interval—A variety of pharmacologic agents and metabolic factors can trigger this type of polymorphic VT (a partial list is given in Table 22–4). The main electrocardiographic abnormality is that of prolonged QT interval and often an unusual appearance of the T wave, frequently referred to as the slow wave (Figure 22–10). The QT interval prolongation may not always be striking at the normal rates but should show a measurable increase after a pause, for example, following a premature beat. Even

Table 22–4. Causes of acquired prolonged QT interval.

Pharmacologic agents
   Quinidine, procainamide, disopyramide, amiodarone, sotalol, bepridil
   Erythromycin, chloroquine, amantadine, and pentamidine
   Tricyclic antidepressants, phenothiazines
   Liquid-protein diets
   Organophosphorous insecticide poisons
   Antihistamines such as astemizole, terfenadine
Electrolyte abnormalities
   Hypokalemia, hypomagnesemia, hypocalcemia

---

excessive slowing of the heart rate will often make a subtle QT interval prolongation more obvious.

The offending agents ordinarily cause some prolongation of myocardial recovery. In vulnerable individuals, however, excessive QT prolongation may occur in association with the emergence of torsade de pointes. This type of arrhythmogenic vulnerability is not always easy to predict. Once it is manifested by any individual, however, extreme caution must be exercised because a recurrence is likely if challenged with the same triggers. The underlying mechanism of this form also appears to be early after-depolarization. The latter can be triggered in animal models by slow heart rates, hypokalemia, and quinidine. It is likely that each of these makes an independent contribution and that a combination of the three could be particularly arrhythmogenic. This, in part, might explain the emergence of torsade de pointes in individuals who have been stable for a long time on the agents listed in Table 22–4. It is conceivable that the presence of hypokalemia or bradycardia, despite stable drug levels, may precipitate such an occurrence. The actual list of potentially offending agents may be quite long because many pharmacologic agents have not been tested for such adverse side effects as prolongation of the QT interval, and only the widely known culprits are listed in the table.

The key to managing torsade de pointes related to acquired prolonged QT interval is recognizing it. Frequently these patients have underlying monomorphic VT that is being treated with antiarrhythmic agents. The emergence of torsade de pointes in this setting may not be interpreted correctly as a side effect of the medication but as a lack of sufficient control that requires more aggressive but similar therapy. When the proper diagnosis is made, the treatment is withdrawal of the offending agent and replacement of electrolytes. A routine workup should include a thorough history regarding drugs, diuretics, and alcohol. The prompt replacement of magnesium, potassium, and calcium is critical. Because hemodynamic stability is necessary to excrete the offending pharmacologic agent, the immediate suppression of torsade de pointes is desirable and can be accomplished with overdrive pacing. Further administration of agents known to cause prolonged my-

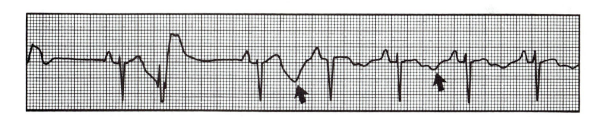

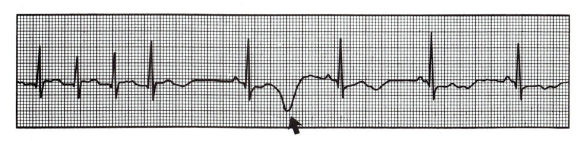

Figure 22–10. Prolonged QT interval with slow wave. The T wave has an unusual appearance, and both the QT-interval prolongation and T-wave morphologic abnormality are more pronounced after the pause. The slow wave is indicated by the arrows. Reproduced, with permission, from Jackman WM et al: The long QT syndromes: A critical review, new clinical observations and a unifying hypothesis. Prog Cardiovasc Dis 1988;31:115.

ocardial recovery must be avoided. Once the precise precipitating event is found, torsade de pointes can be prevented. When it is related to pauses and bradycardia, pacemaker support may be needed.

B. POLYMORPHIC VT WITH A NORMAL QT INTERVAL

It is not uncommon to see short episodes of polymorphic VT without any QT interval prolongation. Sustained forms of such arrhythmias can lead to ventricular fibrillation. The true nature of this problem can be readily appreciated by observation of the QT interval prior to the tachycardia and, more reliably, following the pause that ensues after termination of VT. If no QT prolongation is noted, the following possibilities must be entertained.

Acute ischemia should be suspected with polymorphic VT in the presence of a normal QT interval. Although the exact prevalence of this type of VT is unknown, it is probably more common than realized. The VT tends to be rapid and has a tendency to degenerate into ventricular fibrillation (Figure 22–11). Acute ischemia must be excluded in all patients presenting with polymorphic VT in association with normal QT interval. The acute ischemia might be related to underlying coronary stenosis or coronary artery spasm brought about by a variety of factors. Prompt diagnosis and therapy are critical for preventing VT-related sudden cardiac death in these patients. The workup includes coronary arteriography and an assessment for coronary artery spasm. The traditional diagnostic criteria—history of chest pain or obvious ST abnormalities—may not be present prior to the episode. A high index of suspicion is likely to lead to a correct diagnosis. This type of VT can seldom be induced in the laboratory, and the electrophysiologic mechanism for it remains unclear. The treatment, in essence, is directed toward eliminating myocardial ischemia; it might include myocardial revascularization or antiischemic drugs such as β-blockers or calcium channel blockers.

Polymorphic VT with normal QT interval can also occur in patients without substrates for myocardial ischemia but with chronic fibrosis or hypertrophy; sometimes, it can occur with no obvious pathology. It is prudent to exclude all the previously mentioned correctable causes before a diagnosis of this idiopathic variety is made. In some cases, the polymorphic VT may be inducible, suggesting a reentrant nature. Although such an arrhythmia can occur in patients with healed myocardial infarction, it is also sometimes seen in patients with hypertrophic and congestive cardiomyopathy. This type of polymorphic VT does not provide a reliable endpoint for drug testing or VT surgery. Antiarrhythmic drugs, particularly amiodarone, may be useful as are ICDs in preventing sudden cardiac death in this population.

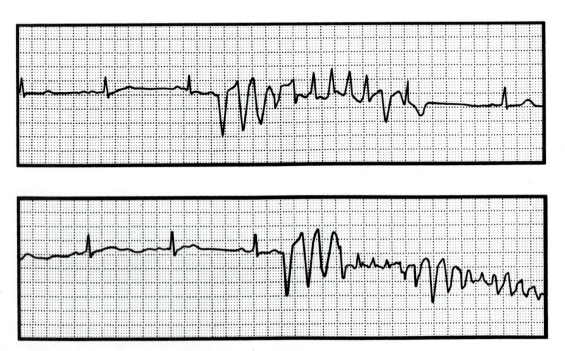

Figure 22–11. Polymorphic ventricular tachycardia and normal QT interval in a patient with severe three-vessel disease. **A:** Several nonsustained polymorphic VT episodes. **B:** Degeneration to VF, requiring DC cardioversion.

Prognosis

Ventricular tachycardia as a warning sign for sudden cardiac death differs vastly in various clinical situations. The initial presentation and the LVEF are, perhaps, the most important determinants. Recurrent cardiac arrest or sudden cardiac death is more likely in patients who have had a previous similar presentation, and syncope resulting from VT also carries a poor prognosis. On the other hand, sudden cardiac death in the event of VT recurrence is less likely in patients with hemodynamically well tolerated VT. Reduced LV function and VT carry a worse prognosis than does either alone.

Akhtar M: Clinical spectrum of ventricular tachycardia. Circulation 1990;82:1561.

Antiarrhythmics versus Implantable Defibrillators (AVID) Investigators: A comparison of antiarrhythmic drug therapy with implantable defibrillators in patients resuscitated from near-fatal ventricular arrhythmias. N Engl J Med 1997;337:1576.

Buxton AE, Lee KL, DiCarlo L et al, for the Multicenter Unsustained Tachycardia Trial Investigators (MUSTT): Electrophysiologic testing to identify patients with coronary artery disease who are at risk for sudden death. N Engl J Med 2000:342:1937.

Cairns JA, Connolly SJ, Roberts R et al: Randomized trial of outcome after myocardial infarction in patients with frequent or repetitive ventricular premature depolarisations: CAMIAT. Lancet 1997;349:675. (Erratum, Lancet 1997;349:1776.)

CAST Investigators: Preliminary report: Effect of encainide and flecainide on mortality in a randomized trial of arrhythmia suppression after myocardial infarction. N Engl J Med 1990; 321:393.

Dhein S, Muller A, Gerwin R et al: Comparative study on the proarrhythmic effects of some antiarrhythmic agents. Circulation 1993;87:617.

Gomes JA, Winter SL, Ip J et al: Identification of patients with high risk of arrhythmic mortality: Role of ambulatory monitoring, signal-averaged ECG, and heart rate variability. Cardiol Clin 1993;11:55.

Grogin HR, Scheinman M: Evaluation and management of patients with polymorphic ventricular tachycardia. Cardiol Clin 1993;11:39.

Julian DG, Camm AJ, Frangin G et al: Randomized trial of effect of amiodarone on morality in patients with left-ventricular dysfunction after recent myocardial infarction: EMIAT. Lancet 1997;349:667. (Errata, Lancet 1997;349:1180,1776.)

Klein LS, Shih HJ, Hackett FK et al: Radiofrequency catheter ablation of ventricular tachycardia in patients without structural heart disease. Circulation 1992;85:1666.

Mason J: A comparison of electrophysiologic testing with Holter monitoring to predict antiarrhythmic drug efficacy for ventricular tachyarrhythmias. N Engl J Med, 1993;329:445.

Morady F, Harvey M, Kalbfleisch SJ et al: Radiofrequency catheter ablation of ventricular tachycardia in patients with coronary artery disease. Circulation 1993;87:363.

Moss AJ, Hall WJ, Connom DS et al: Improved survival with implanted defibrillator in patients with coronary artery disease at high risk for ventricular arrhythmia. N Engl J Med, 1996; 335:1933.

Narasimhan C, Jazayari MR, Sra J et al: Ventricular tachycardia in valvular heart disease-facilitation of sustained bundle-branch reentry by valve surgery. Circulation 1997;96:4307.

Sra JS, Jazayari MR, Dhala A et al: Neurocardiogenic syncope: Diagnosis, mechanisms, and treatment. Cardiol Clin 1993;11: 183.

Sra JS, Anderson AJ, Sheikh SH et al: Unexplained syncope evaluated by electrophysiologic studies and head-up tilt test. Ann Intern Med 1991;114:1013.

Syncope

Christopher S. Cadman, MD

ESSENTIALS OF DIAGNOSIS

- *Sudden, unexpected and transient loss of consciousness and postural tone*
- *Spontaneous and full recovery*

General Considerations

Syncope can be defined as a sudden, transient loss of consciousness and postural tone that fully resolves spontaneously without specific intervention (eg, CPR, electrical or chemical cardioversion). The common pathophysiologic mechanism responsible for the majority of syncopal spells is a transient reduction in cerebral blood flow and cerebral hypoperfusion. Reduced cerebral blood flow from cardiovascular and neurocardiogenic causes accounts for most cases in which a diagnosis can be made. Even when cerebral blood flow is normal, a reduced delivery of such essential cerebral nutrients as oxygen and sugar can occasionally cause altered consciousness.

Syncope is a common condition experienced by 5–20% of adults by age 75. It is responsible for 3% of hospital admissions and 6% of emergency room visits. Physicians are frequently consulted to evaluate this symptom and—more commonly—presyncope, dizziness or lightheadedness, which may have a similar pathogenesis.

Syncope has many causes (Table 23–1), the majority of which have a benign prognosis. Because cardiac causes are associated with greater morbidity and mortality, early recognition of structural heart disease or other cardiogenic causes is important in order to prevent sudden death or injury.

Pathophysiology & Etiology

A. CARDIAC CAUSES

1. Obstruction to blood flow—Any structural lesion of the left or right side of the heart can critically reduce

the cerebral blood flow. Exertional symptoms are common with obstructive lesions because cardiac output

Table 23–1. Major causes of syncope.

Cardiac
  Obstruction to blood flow
    Valvular stenosis
    Hypertrophic cardiomyopathy
    Prosthetic valve dysfunction
    Atrial myxoma
    Congenital heart disease
    Pericardial tamponade
    Pulmonary hypertension
    Pulmonary emboli
    Pump failure (myocardial infarction or ischemia)
  Arrhythmias (decreased cardiac output)
    Bradyarrhythmias
      Sinus bradycardia
      Sick sinus syndrome
      Atrioventricular block (Stokes-Adams attacks)
      Pacemaker malfunction
      Drug-induced bradyarrhythmia
    Tachyarrhythmias
      Ventricular tachycardia
      Supraventricular tachycardia
      Torsade de pointes
Neurocardiogenic
  Vasovagal
  Vasodepressor
  Carotid sinus hypersensitivity
  Situational (tussis, micturition, defecation, deglutition)
Other Causes
  Seizures
  Drugs
  Hypoglycemia
  Hypoxia
  Hypovolemia
  Cerebral vascular insufficiency
  Extracranial vascular disease
  Orthostatic hypotension
  Neuralgia
  Psychogenesis
  Hyperventilation

does not rise normally with exercise and cerebral perfusion is not maintained. Obstruction to left ventricular outflow occurs with aortic valve stenosis, mitral stenosis, left atrial myxoma, prosthetic aortic or mitral valve dysfunction, and hypertrophic cardiomyopathy. The ventricular arrhythmias that can occur with valvular heart disease may be responsible for both exertional and nonexertional syncope as well as sudden death.

Lesions that obstruct flow through the right side of the heart include right atrial myxoma, pulmonary stenosis, tricuspid stenosis, pulmonary hypertension, and pulmonary emboli. Limitations to right ventricular outflow diminish the cardiac output and the ability to increase the output with exertion. Exertional syncope is common with severe pulmonary hypertension and severe pulmonic stenosis.

Patients with congenital heart disease, such as tetralogy of Fallot, septal defect, or patent ductus arteriosus, can experience syncope caused by obstruction to flow and hypoxia. These patients frequently have left-to-right shunts that can suddenly reverse with exertion, lessening arterial oxygenation and resulting in hypoxia and syncope.

Nonexertional syncope can be the result of pulmonary emboli (hypoxia and obstruction of right ventricular outflow) and aortic dissection with pericardial tamponade, which impedes right ventricular filling and decreases cardiac output.

2. Electrical disturbances—

a. Bradyarrhythmias and atrioventricular block—Both bradyarrhythmias and tachyarrhythmias can cause transient decreased cardiac output with resultant cerebral hypoperfusion. Bradycardias result in symptoms when the rate is so slow that the compensatory increase in stroke volume is inadequate to maintain blood pressure. Periods of ventricular asystole as short as 5 s can cause syncope (from the ensuing cerebral hypoperfusion). Mechanisms of symptomatic ventricular bradycardia and asystole include sinus node disease (sinus exit block, sick sinus syndrome, marked sinus bradycardia, or sinus arrest) and second- or third-degree atrioventricular (AV) block. Syncope from Mobitz II second-degree AV block with paroxysms of several consecutive P waves that fail to conduct to the ventricle is classically termed a **Stokes-Adams** attack. Medications can also cause syncope, and any patient with syncope from bradycardia must be thoroughly questioned regarding medications. Calcium channel blockers, digoxin, β-blockers (including optical formulations), sympatholytics, primary antiarrhythmics, and other medications can all decrease heart rate and increase AV block—enough to cause symptoms in susceptible patients.

Pacemaker malfunction is another possible cause. If a pacemaker was previously implanted for sinus node disease or high-degree AV block and the patient has a recurrence of syncope, there may be a pacemaker system problem, such as battery failure or lead fracture.

b. Tachyarrhythmias—Transient decreased cardiac output during ventricular or supraventricular tachycardias results when the ventricular rate is fast enough to decrease diastole significantly and thus decrease ventricular filling (preload). Concomitant peripheral vasodepression with resultant hypotension may also play a role in the pathophysiology of syncope with supraventricular arrhythmias.

Ventricular tachycardia occurs most frequently in patients with organic heart disease, particularly coronary artery disease with previous myocardial infarction. Ventricular tachycardia is an important and ominous cause of syncope because ventricular tachycardia usually precedes ventricular fibrillation, resulting in sudden cardiac death. Symptoms and prognosis are related to the degree of underlying myocardial dysfunction, and the rate and duration of the arrhythmia.

Supraventricular arrhythmias are more likely to cause palpitations and presyncope than true syncope. Although they occur often in young patients with structurally normal hearts, they are also prevalent in structurally abnormal hearts. As with ventricular arrhythmias, the severity of the symptoms is related to the ventricular rate of the arrhythmia and the degree of underlying myocardial dysfunction. Mechanisms associated with syncope include atrial arrhythmias (fibrillation, flutter, tachycardia) with rapid ventricular response, AV nodal reentrant tachycardia, and supraventricular arrhythmias associated with accessory pathways.

Torsade de pointes is a rapid polymorphic ventricular arrhythmia classically known to cause syncope in association with quinidine (*quinidine syncope*). Because this arrhythmia can also cause sudden cardiac death, it is very important to understand the reversible conditions that can precipitate it. Most cases of torsade are associated with acquired long-QT syndromes that can occur with several drugs (class IA and III antiarrhythmics, erythromycin, certain antihistamines, and tricyclic antidepressants), electrolyte abnormalities (hypomagnesemia, hypokalemia, hypocalcemia), myocardial ischemia, and central nervous system disorders. Rarely, long QT syndrome occurs congenitally, in hereditary forms of prolongation of the QT interval (with or without associated deafness).

B. NEUROCARDIOGENIC CAUSES

1. Vasovagal syncope—This is the most common mechanism of syncope in young, otherwise healthy individuals, constituting approximately 60% of cases. The underlying mechanism is a paradoxical autonomic reflex resulting in profound hypotension (vasodepression) that is often associated with bradycardia (vasovagal). It has received more attention in the literature in the last decade than any other mechanism listed in Table 23–1. The underlying pathophysiology of vasovagal syncope has been elucidated with the aid of tilt-table testing (see the section on Noninvasive Studies). This technique provides a controlled means of reproducing vasovagal syncope and serves as a means to guide medical therapy. Before the development of tilt-table testing, the diagnosis of vasovagal syncope was largely a matter of exclusion.

Despite extensive study by numerous investigators, several controversies still remain regarding the underlying pathophysiology of vasovagal syncope. When one stands, a significant amount of venous pooling occurs, which can shift from 300 to 800 mL of blood away from the central circulation. To counteract this gravitational effect, baroreceptors in the carotid sinus, aortic arch, and left ventricle sense decreased stretch (low pressure) and send afferent neural messages to the vasomotor center in the brainstem's medulla, which in turn sends efferent stimuli to increase peripheral sympathetic and cardiac tone (vasoconstriction and increased heart rate and contractility) and decrease vagal tone. This is the normal neural reflex arc that maintains cerebral arterial pressure and prevents hypotension or syncope with orthostatic changes.

It is believed that this reflex arc goes awry in susceptible individuals, resulting in a mixed response of vasodepression (hypotension) and cardiac inhibition (bradycardia). This symptomatic reflex arc, commonly known as a vasovagal episode, can occur as pure vasodepression or, rarely, pure cardiac inhibition; the classic mixed response is most common, with hypotension often preceding the bradycardia.

Vasovagal syncope is often, but not always, preceded by predisposing factors such as fear, pain, injury, fatigue, prolonged standing, or such medical procedures as venipuncture. During the initial phase, it is believed that blood pressure and heart rate increase in response to circulating catecholamine increase, sympathetic nerve stimulation, and vagal withdrawal. This is abruptly followed by hypotension, bradycardia, and syncope caused by inhibition of sympathetic vasoconstrictor and cardiac stimulatory activity and increases in vagal tone.

Although the exact pathophysiology is not understood, two conditions are thought to bring on the para-

doxical reflex in susceptible individuals: reduced left ventricular filling (an empty ventricle) from decreased venous return; and increased left ventricular pressure from increased contractility caused by cardiac stimulation from circulating catecholamines. A vigorously contracting empty ventricle is thought to paradoxically increase left ventricular pressures (mimicking hypertension), which are sensed by left ventricular stretch receptors (C fibers). This afferent neural arc to the nucleus tractus solitarius in the medulla results in an efferent arc that paradoxically decreases sympathetic and increases vagal tone, causing hypotension and bradycardia, respectively. Because both the sinus node and AV node are richly innervated with autonomic nerves, bradycardia can be caused by both vagal depression of sinus node automaticity and decreased AV nodal conduction with AV block. Assuming a supine posture provides spontaneous resolution because the gravitational effects on cerebral blood flow are immediately neutralized. Figure 23–1 shows a two-lead ambulatory recording of a classic vasovagal episode in a patient with previously undiagnosed syncope.

Vasovagal syncope is usually considered a benign form that can often be treated with patient education and avoidance of the precipitant. Some individuals, however, have frequent severe spells that result in injuries and, rarely, sudden death. Several therapies (discussed later) are available for patients who require intervention.

2. Carotid sinus hypersensitivity—The carotid sinus has baroreceptors located in the internal carotid artery just above the bifurcation of the common carotid artery. These are sensitive to stretch and pressure and give rise to afferent impulses to the vasomotor center in the medulla. In susceptible individuals, particularly the elderly, activation of this reflex results in vagal efferent stimulation, which causes marked bradycardia or AV block (the cardioinhibitory response) with vasodepression (from efferent sympathetic inhibition). In contrast to vasovagal syncope, the cardioinhibitory response is usually dominant. Syncope from carotid sinus hypersensitivity usually is suggested by historical factors: precipitation with turning the head, shaving the neck, or wearing a tight shirt collar. Spontaneous attacks can also occur. Full consciousness is usually regained in less

---

Figure 23–1. Consecutive two-lead rhythm strips recorded from a patient wearing an ambulatory monitor during a vasovagal near-syncope spell, illustrating the classic response. **A:** In his diary, the patient indicates that he is possibly passing out. Because heart rate and rhythm are normal, the symptom is due to initial hypotension from vasodepression. **B:** As the episode proceeds, sinus bradycardia develops from vagal cardiac inhibition. **C:** Later still sinus rhythm is completely suppressed, resulting in a junctional escape rhythm; *open arrow* shows first junctional beat. **D:** Vagal inhibitory effect on the AV node is also shown because a sinus beat did not conduct to the ventricle *(solid arrow)*. **E:** Complete resolution to normal sinus rhythm, correlated with spontaneous full recovery.

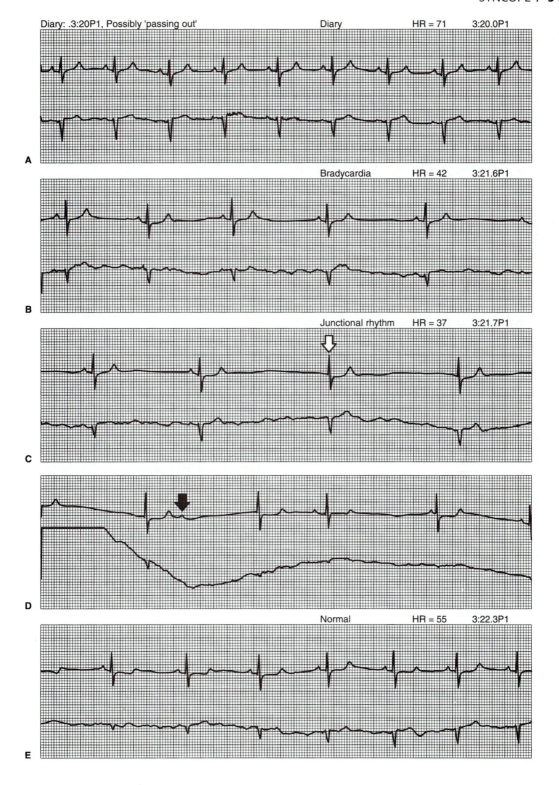

Diary: .3:20P1, Possibly 'passing out'   Diary   HR = 71   3:20.0P1

A

Bradycardia   HR = 42   3:21.6P1

B

Junctional rhythm   HR = 37   3:21.7P1

C

D

Normal   HR = 55   3:22.3P1

E

than a minute after attaining a supine position. Carotid sinus massage (CSM) can be used to diagnose this condition in suspected individuals; hypersensitivity is generally defined as cardiac asystole of 3 s or more or a decline in systolic blood pressure of at least 50 mm Hg.

3. Situational—The pathophysiologic mechanisms of syncope associated with micturition, defecation, coughing, and swallowing are not precisely elucidated. It is suggested that the vagal-sympathetic autonomic reflex (hypotension and bradycardia) is involved, with afferent neural stimulation coming from the involved viscera. The Valsalva maneuver (used during micturition, defecation, and coughing) is thought to contribute to hypotension by decreasing venous return, which decreases cardiac output.

In micturition syncope, which classically occurs on waking, a combination of physiologic changes that occur during sleep (eg, sudden decompression of the bladder, decreased heart rate and blood pressure) may contribute to syncope. Tussive syncope classically occurs in middle-aged men who drink alcohol, smoke, have chronic lung disease, and experience paroxysms of severe cough; it is thought to be largely due to decreased venous return caused by the Valsalva-like action of coughing. Deglutition syncope is believed to be entirely due to dysfunction of the afferent-efferent reflex arc and is associated with structural abnormalities of the esophagus (eg, diverticula, diffuse esophageal spasm, achalasia, stricture) and heart (acute rheumatic carditis, myocardial infarction).

C. ORTHOSTATIC HYPOTENSION

Volume depletion, medications, and autonomic dysfunction (primary and secondary) can all lead to cerebral hypoperfusion and syncope. Primary chronic autonomic dysfunction is associated with Shy-Drager syndrome, Parkinson's disease, and other rare dysautonomias. Secondary autonomic dysfunction with syncope has been described with diabetes mellitus, anemia, amyloidosis, multiple sclerosis, and HIV infection. Medications that commonly cause orthostatic hypotension include diuretics, antihypertensives (angiotensin-converting enzyme [ACE] inhibitors, β-blockers, calcium channel blockers), and ethanol.

Essential to the diagnosis of orthostatic hypotension is evaluation of postural changes in blood pressure. Normal reflex mechanisms maintain blood pressure on standing (see discussion of neurocardiogenic syncope). The inability to maintain cerebral flow when standing or sitting upright, with resultant hypotension, dizziness, or syncope, is called orthostatic hypotension. Quantitatively, it has been defined as a 20 mm Hg or greater decline in systolic pressure or a 10 mm Hg or greater decline in diastolic pressure on assuming an upright position. Because this finding is frequent and asymptomatic in the elderly, the clinical diagnosis of

syncope from orthostatic hypotension requires the presence of symptoms with blood pressure changes.

D. PSYCHIATRIC DISORDERS

Syncope has been well described in patients with several psychiatric disorders, including anxiety disorder with panic attacks, major depression, somatization, and substance abuse. Unfortunately, these patients may also present with pseudo or fictitious syncope. Syncopal episodes with these disorders are often associated with hyperventilation.

E. NEURALGIA

Both glossopharyngeal and trigeminal neuralgia can precipitate syncopal spells through paradoxical neural reflexes. Glossopharyngeal neuralgia is characterized by severe unilateral pain in the oropharynx or ear precipitated by swallowing, chewing, or coughing. Syncope is thought to occur through an afferent reflex arc involving the glossopharyngeal nerve, with resultant efferent vagal stimulation that causes a cardioinhibitory response (bradycardia or asystole). Trigeminal neuralgia involves a reflex arc as well, with paroxysmal facial pain episodes precipitating vasodepressor, cardioinhibitory, or mixed responses.

F. SYNCOPE OF UNKNOWN CAUSE

No cause of syncope may be found in as many as 34% of patients according to several studies reported in the 1980s. However, over the past decade with the increased use of tilt-table testing (see section on Head-up tilt-table testing), some investigators estimate that between 50 and 66% of cases of unknown cause may be neurally mediated.

Clinical Findings

A. HISTORY AND PHYSICAL EXAMINATION

According to several prospective studies, the initial clinical evaluation establishes the cause of syncope or suggests the necessary diagnostic test in up to 85% of the patients in whom a diagnosis will eventually be made. A detailed history and physical examination are therefore essential parts of the initial clinical evaluation. A detailed history can potentially reduce the number of undiagnosed cases (approximately 50% in several series). Relevant historical information includes all details leading up to the event, precipitating factors (micturition, cough, exertion), premonitory symptoms (aura), onset (sudden or slow), associated symptoms (palpitations, chest pain, headache), activity (at rest or with exercise), position (standing, sitting, changing position), and details about the episode (injury, incontinence, rapid recovery versus postictal state) and the frequency and severity of the events. The history should include factors suggestive of cardiac or other systemic illnesses, such as a family history of cardiac illness, arrhythmias, syncope, sudden death, or pacemaker implantation. Because up to 9% of syncope is caused by the use of medications and recreational drugs, information regarding their use, prescribed dosages, and the amount actually taken is very important. All witnesses to the event (family, friends, bystanders) should be thoroughly interviewed because they can often supply details that the patient cannot. These witnesses may be able to provide information about the patient's complaints just prior to the event and observations during both the event (eg, pulse rate and rhythm, color, presence of spontaneous breathing, seizures, or seizure-like activity) and recovery. Electrocardiographic recordings made by paramedics at the scene or recorded en route to the hospital and in the emergency room may provide important clues.

All patients need a complete cardiac, peripheral vascular, and neurologic examination, including an assessment of positional blood pressure and heart rate. Cardiac murmurs may be suggestive of structural heart disease, such as valvular stenosis. Differential blood pressure and pulse intensity may suggest aortic dissection or subclavian steal syndrome. Focal neurologic findings may point to seizure, stroke, or transient ischemic attack. The development of similar symptoms with upright posture and a corresponding decrease in blood pressure implicates orthostatic hypotension.

Several bedside maneuvers can be used to provoke syncope or presyncopal symptoms in appropriate patients. Arm flexion and extension may be used to provoke symptoms of subclavian steal syndrome; neck flexion and extension may elicit the symptoms of vertebrobasilar insufficiency. Open-mouthed hyperventilation for 1–3 min may elicit symptoms described in the history. Carotid sinus massage (when not contraindicated by presence of bruits or known carotid arteriosclerotic disease) can be performed at the bedside with electrocardiographic (ECG) and blood pressure monitoring. Although the technique is not standardized, carotid massage is usually performed with the patient in the supine position, with 5 s of firm massage of each carotid body. Note that simultaneous bilateral massage is never done. A positive test is defined as at least 3 s of asystole with hypotension or reproduction of symptoms. Because of the high false-positive rate for carotid sinus massage in the elderly, the diagnosis of carotid sinus hypersensitivity should only be considered if clinical events are associated with activities that press or stretch the carotid sinus.

Toxicology screens and medication levels may provide useful information, however, and should be ordered if suggested by the patient's or the witness's history. Figure 23–2 outlines a suggested diagnostic approach.

B. Noninvasive Studies

1. Twelve-lead electrocardiogram—A 12-lead ECG should be part of the routine clinical evaluation of syncope. A normal 12-lead ECG generally portends a good prognosis, with a very low incidence of either cardiogenic causes or diagnostic findings during invasive electrophysiologic testing. Unfortunately, the initial ECG rarely establishes arrhythmia as the cause unless complete heart block, ventricular tachycardia, or another abnormality is present at the time of the tracing. Given the unpredictably episodic nature of syncopal spells and the fact that most patients recover completely from them prior to the ECG, it is rare that the 12-lead ECG is diagnostic. More often, certain findings will suggest the possibility of a specific diagnosis. For example, Q waves suggestive of previous myocardial infarction correlate with abnormal electrophysiologic studies and the presence of inducible ventricular arrhythmias. Delta waves suggestive of Wolff-Parkinson-White syndrome make supraventricular tachycardia a very likely diagnosis. A long QT interval suggests torsade de pointes, and bifascicular block correlates with abnormal electrophysiologic findings, including high-degree AV block and inducible ventricular arrhythmias.

The most common abnormalities found in patients presenting with syncope are bifascicular block, prior myocardial infarction, left ventricular hypertrophy, sinus bradycardia, and first-degree, or Wenckebach AV block. Although these findings are all nonspecific, they may suggest a cardiac cause. The ECG or rhythm strips recorded by paramedics, the emergency department, or hospital ward lead to a specific diagnosis in about 11% of presenting patients. The most common diagnoses include ventricular tachycardia and bradyarrhythmias caused by sinus node dysfunction or high-degree AV block.

2. Echocardiography—Although no studies specifically evaluate the utility of echocardiography in syncope, it is often the first test performed after a 12-lead ECG. In patients with suspected underlying heart disease, abnormal ECG, or suspected arrhythmias, the echocardiogram is a valuable diagnostic tool. Echocardiography may diagnose the likely cause of syncope (aortic stenosis, hypertrophic heart disease); but, more commonly, it is useful in directing further evaluation. Because morbidity and mortality with syncope are directly related to the presence and severity of structural heart disease, the echocardiogram can aid the physician in assessing the patient's prognosis and the necessity for further invasive evaluation. Unsuspected findings on echocardiography are reported in 5–10% of unselected patients with syncope. Although this is similar to the ECG, the cost of the study limits it to persons with suspected underlying heart disease.

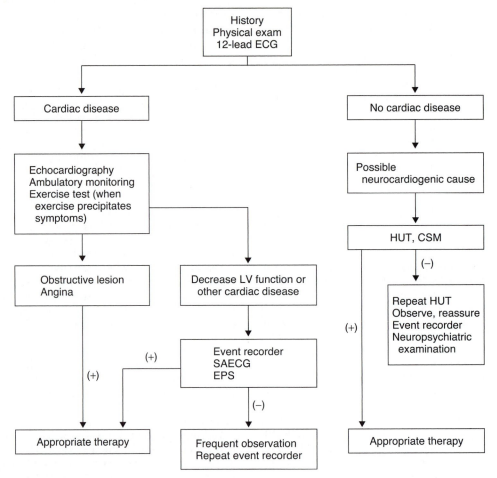

Figure 23–2. Diagnostic approach to syncope. CSM = carotid sinus massage; ECG = electrocardiogram; EPS = electrophysiology; HUT = head-up tilt-table testing; LV = left ventricular; SAECG = signal-average ECG.

3. Ambulatory monitoring—Prolonged electrocardiographic monitoring can be useful for documenting transient brady- or tachyarrhythmias. The most common method used is Holter ambulatory recording. Typically, two surface ECG leads are recorded for a period of 24 to 48 h. Although the optimal duration of monitoring is unknown, several studies suggest that the longer recordings are no more likely to establish a diagnosis. Holter recording can be particularly helpful in diagnosing bradyarrhythmias, such as significant sinus pauses and transient high-degree AV block. When interpreting Holter recordings, one must recognize that several abnormalities can occur in healthy, asymptomatic patients, and correlation with symptoms is often essential. Premature atrial and ventricular contractions, brief and paroxysmal atrial tachycardia, episodic AV Wenckebach block, sinus bradycardia, sinus pauses of up to 3 s especially when asleep, and nonsustained ventricular tachycardia can all be seen in normal, asymptomatic patients. Sinus pauses of longer than 3 s, Mobitz II AV block, complete heart block, and frequent nonsustained ventricular tachycardia are far less prevalent.

Because the correlation of symptoms with an arrhythmia in patients with syncope provides the most valuable information, it is essential for the patient to keep an accurate diary of symptoms and activity during the recorded interval. Ambulatory monitoring is often useful in excluding arrhythmia mechanisms of syncope when patients experience syncope or presyncope without associated arrhythmias. Conversely, ambulatory monitoring may reveal significant conduction abnormalities or arrhythmias when the patient is asymptomatic. Frequent sinus pause of ≥3 s with associated atrial fibrillation indicates significant sinoatrial dysfunction. Asymptomatic Mobitz II AV block suggests distal conduction disease, with the possibility of prolonged AV block resulting in Stokes-Adams attacks. Nonsustained ventricular tachycardia in patients with significant left ventricular dysfunction (ejection fraction <40%) correlates with a risk of sudden death from sustained ventricular arrhythmias and warrants further electrophysiologic evaluation (see section on Invasive Electrophysiology Studies).

A significant limitation of Holter ambulatory recording is how infrequently patients experience either syncope or associated symptoms. The results of studies suggest that Holter monitoring captures the heart rhythm during spontaneous syncope in only 4–10% of patients. For this reason, external ambulatory loop recorders have been used extensively for the evaluation of syncope. These devices record a single ECG lead continuously and can be worn by a patient for weeks to months. When activated by the patient or an observer, a rhythm strip is saved that includes several minutes surrounding the syncopal or presyncopal episode (Figure 23–3). The rhythm strip is produced using transtelephonic equipment for added convenience for the patient and physician. Loop recorders are useful for evaluating patients with episodic syncope, presyncope, or dizziness, with or without associated palpitations. They are particularly helpful in the evaluations of the structurally normal heart.

A recent advancement in ambulatory monitoring is the implantable loop recorder (ILR). Although similar to the external loop recorder described earlier, the ILR is implanted under the skin and can be programmed to record episodes of bradycardia or tachycardia automatically. In a recent study of 60 patients with unexplained syncope, ILR was compared to "conventional" testing (external loop recorder, tilt-table testing, and electrophysiology testing). Prolonged monitoring with the ILR resulted in a diagnosis in 55% versus 19% of patients. Bradycardia was the most common cause in 40% of patients. Some investigators now recommend earlier implantation of the ILR rather than reserving it for patients who have exhausted all other diagnostic strategies, including external loop recorders.

4. Exercise stress testing—Exercise stress testing (EST) may be useful in patients presenting with exertional symptoms. Exertional hypotension may occur as a result of underlying structural heart disease, chronotropic incompetence, or severe conduction disease resulting in AV block with increased atrial rates. Supraventricular and ventricular arrhythmias may be provoked with exercise. Hypotension and bradycardia at the termination of exercise can be diagnostic of reflexive vasomotor instability. Although the diagnostic yield is less than that with ambulatory monitoring, EST can useful in selected patients.

5. Head-up tilt-table testing—Gravitational shifts in blood volume have long been recognized as a stimulus to neurocardiogenic syncope (also known as vasomotor, vasovagal, neurally mediated, or neurocardiogenic syncope). The use of the tilt table as a provocative maneuver in the diagnosis of unexplained syncope is increasing exponentially, although there is currently a great deal of controversy regarding the most sensitive and specific protocol (there is no consensus for a standardized protocol). One approach is to strap the supine, fasting patient to a specially designed table. The patient is monitored for 10 min in the horizontal position, using noninvasive brachial or finger blood pressure, O_2 saturation, continuous ECG, and if somatization disorder is suspected, EEG (true syncope can be differentiated from malingering). The patient is then tilted 60–80° for up to 45 min; in children and adolescents, positive tests tend to occur sooner, and a period of 30 min is sufficient. The tilt produces a shift in blood volume distribution away from the central circulation and thorax to dependent peripheral vessels. This causes a decrease in central venous pressure, ventricular filling, stroke volume, and mean arterial blood pressure. Normally, activation of the baroreceptor-vasomotor reflex (described above) and renin-angiotensin system and release of catecholamines results in maintenance of blood

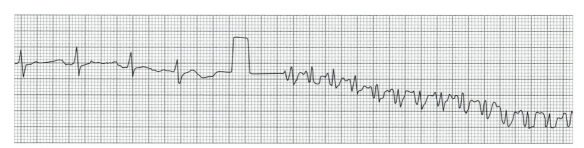

Figure 23–3. Event recorder monitor strip received from a patient with a prior history of syncope, recurrent presyncope, and structural heart disease. The patient underwent an electrophysiology study and was found to have inducible monomorphic ventricular tachycardia that was treated with an implantable cardioverter-defibrillator.

pressure through increased heart rate and vasoconstriction. Monitoring of a normal passive tilt would show a small decrease in systolic blood pressure, with an increase in diastolic blood pressure, mean arterial pressure, and heart rate. All of these are considered normal adjustments to gravitational stress.

The test is considered positive if syncope or presyncope occurs with hypotension, with or without bradycardia. The patient is then quickly placed in the horizontal position, where normal compensatory mechanisms restore blood pressure and consciousness. The test is considered negative if symptoms and hemodynamic abnormalities fail to occur by 45 min of tilt. The tilt can be repeated with a provocative agent, such as the β-agonist isoproterenol, in selected patients (discussed later).

As previously discussed, susceptible patients develop various degrees of hypotension and bradycardia secondary to a paradoxical reflex that increases vagal tone and decreases sympathetic tone. Both hypotension and bradycardia are present (a mixed response) in most patients. Hypotension usually predominates, however, and tends to occur before bradycardia (as shown in Figure 23–1). Hypotension that occurs alone, without bradycardia, is considered a purely vasodepressor response. Rarely, a patient may have a purely cardioinhibitory response (asystole).

The test has been shown to be 80–90% reproducible and specific, with a low false-positive rate (<10%) in asymptomatic individuals. It is becoming the procedure of choice, recommended before electrophysiologic testing when the ECG and ambulatory monitoring are normal, when no structural heart disease is present, and when the history is compatible with a vasovagal episode. Several controversial areas remain to be investigated, however. There is no standardized protocol regarding the optimal tilt angle and length, invasive or noninvasive monitoring, fasting or nonfasting patients, hydrated as opposed to nonhydrated patients, the best means of securing the patient to the table, and the lab environment. Also debated are the use of such provocative agents as isoproterenol, epinephrine, edrophonium, nitrates, or adenosine triphosphate if the baseline tilt is negative, and the use of tilt-table testing to guide chronic medical or pacemaker therapy. Sensitivity and specificity are also difficult to measure because no gold standard exists for the diagnosis of syncope.

With regard to testing with a provocative agent, administration of 1–5 μg/min of intravenous isoproterenol, with subsequent retilt after a negative baseline tilt, provides the most clinical experience to date. A 1 μg/min intravenous drip of isoproterenol is started with the patient in the horizontal position, gradually increasing the rate, in 1 μg/min increments, to 5 μg/min or until a 20% increase in heart rate over baseline is seen. The patient is then retilted for 10 min and similar endpoints are monitored. Although most investigators believe this is a useful maneuver to diagnose syncope of unknown origin, some investigators question its usefulness because of a higher rate of false-positive tilts using isoproterenol in normal, asymptomatic subjects. Therefore, although isoproterenol has been clearly shown to increase sensitivity in detecting neurocardiogenic syncope, it does so at the cost of decreased specificity.

6. Signal-average electrocardiogram—Low-amplitude signals (late potentials) can be recorded from the body surface using signal averaging and filtering techniques. These high-frequency, low-amplitude components of the terminal QRS have been correlated in some studies with a high incidence of inducible ventricular arrhythmias at electrophysiology study (EPS) in patients with prior myocardial infarction. However, no studies of the usefulness of signal-average electrocardiogram (SAECG) have been done in unselected patients.

Studies using SAECG to identify patients at risk for ventricular arrhythmias as a cause of their syncope have reported a sensitivity ranging from 73 to 89% and a specificity ranging from 89 to 100% compared with inducibility of ventricular tachycardia at EPS. The utility of SAECG is its negative predictive value—the absence of a late potential is strongly predictive of an inability to induce ventricular tachycardia at EPS. Unfortunately, SAECG has many limitations. It has no role in the evaluation of sinoatrial or AV nodal dysfunction. Using the most common techniques, SAECG cannot accurately be used in patients with marked intraventricular conduction delay or bundle branch block, including patients with pacemakers. Although SAECG may be useful in patients with coronary artery disease but preserved left ventricular systolic function, its role in the evaluation of patients with syncope of unknown cause remains controversial. In addition, it is limited to the evaluation of ventricular arrhythmias and is often bypassed in favor of invasive EPS testing. For these reasons, the SAECG is currently used less frequently in the evaluation of syncope.

7. Other testing—Routine laboratory tests (blood counts and chemistries) rarely reveal useful diagnostic information. Unless specifically suggested by the history and physical examination, it is not recommended in the evaluation of syncope. Likewise, electroencephalography (EEG), CT, or MRI studies are of little use in patients whose history is not suggestive of a neurologic cause. These tests should be considered only in those patients whose neurologic history and physical examination are suggestive of seizure or other neurologic pathology. Although routinely performed, the utility of transcranial Doppler ultrasonography in patients with syncope is unclear. Transient ischemic attacks rarely result in syncope without other associated symptoms. In patients with bruits on physical examination, ultrasonography is reasonable and may be useful in leading to a diagnosis.

C. INVASIVE ELECTROPHYSIOLOGY STUDIES

An invasive electrophysiology study is an invasive procedure using multielectrode catheters inserted percutaneously and guided under fluoroscopy to specific cardiac locations. Electrode recording and pacing protocols are then performed to assess the patient's conduction system, including sinoatrial and AV nodal function and the distal conduction system (His-Purkinje). In addition, supraventricular and ventricular arrhythmias may be induced and their mechanisms determined in susceptible patients. In selected patients, ablation of the arrhythmic substrate with radiofrequency energy can be performed, curing the patient of the condition.

Because patients are generally supine and sedated during EPS, one significant limitation is the inability to definitely correlate induction of arrhythmias with syncope; however, a rapid tachycardia associated with a significant decrease in systolic blood pressure generally supports the clinical importance of inducible arrhythmias. Induction of certain arrhythmias, such as atrial fibrillation, atrial flutter, polymorphic ventricular tachycardia, and ventricular fibrillation, can be a nonspecific finding. Asymptomatic patients with normal hearts can have all these induced with aggressive stimulation protocols.

According to the ACC/AHA Guidelines for Clinical Intracardiac Electrophysiological and Catheter Ablation Procedures, EPS is indicated in persons at risk for or with manifestations of cardiac disease with syncope that remains unexplained after appropriate evaluation. In addition, EPS is reasonable in patients with recurrent unexplained syncope without structural heart disease and a negative head-up tilt test. In patients with no structural heart disease, normal ECG, normal ambulatory monitoring, and recurrent syncope not associated with injury, EPS is usually not diagnostic. EPS is not indicated in patients with a known cause of syncope for whom treatment will not be guided by electrophysiology testing.

The most significant finding at EPS is the induction of ventricular tachyarrhythmias. In addition, the induction of supraventricular tachycardias with associated hypotension is considered a "positive" study. Other significant findings include a prolonged corrected sinus node recovery time longer than 1000 ms, prolongation of the His-to-ventricle activation interval greater than 100 ms (normally 35–55 ms), or induction of infra-Hisian conduction block during rapid atrial pacing. These three findings are associated with significant bradyarrhythmias. Unfortunately, the diagnostic sensitivity of EPS for bradyarrhythmias is low, and further

ambulatory monitoring is often necessary after a nondiagnostic EPS.

Due to variations in patient populations, study protocols, and diagnostic definitions in published studies, it is difficult to assess the utility of EPS in the diagnosing of syncope of unknown origin. In general, the mean proportion of negative or nondiagnostic findings has been 60%. When the test is suggestive of a diagnosis, the mean proportion of positive findings has been 35% ventricular tachycardia, 35% conduction system disease, 20% supraventricular tachycardia, and 10% other abnormalities, such as carotid sinus hypersensitivity.

Interpreting the success of therapy guided by EPS is also difficult. Published studies have been based on relatively short follow-up (1–3 years) for a condition that is inherently sporadic. Noncompliance of patients, side effects of therapy, or an incorrect initial diagnosis add to the difficulty in interpreting reoccurrence.

The AVID (antiarrhythmics versus implantable defibrillators) study was designed to compare initial treatment with an implantable cardioverter-defibrillator (ICD) to antiarrhythmic drug in patients with documented ventricular fibrillation or tachycardia with hypotension. Although not enrolled in the trial, patients with structural heart disease experiencing out-of-hospital unexplained syncope and an inducible and symptomatic ventricular arrhythmia during EPS were also included in the registry. The AVID trial was stopped prematurely because of the marked benefit of the ICD over amiodarone or sotalol. Of 5989 patients screened, 4595 were registered and 1016 were randomized. In the registry group, the mortality rate for patients with cardiac arrest was 17% (238 deaths out of 1399 patients), and with unexplained syncope and positive EPS it was 12.3% (48 deaths out of 390 patients). Because these patients appear to be at high risk for sudden death, most electrophysiologists now recommend EPS for patients with structural heart disease (ejection fraction <40%) and unexplained syncope; moreover, an ICD is indicated if significant ventricular arrhythmias are induced.

Differential Diagnosis

A. SEIZURE

True seizures are rarely established as the cause of a syncopal event, although they are frequently considered. A history of loss of bowel or bladder tone, witnessed convulsions, a preceding aura, and slow recovery with prolonged postictal state strongly suggest seizure. Syncope occurs frequently without a preceding aura or loss of sphincter tone and characteristically has a rapid spontaneous recovery without postictal state.

Some factors blur the distinction between these two entities: Convulsions may occur with syncope (from cerebral anoxia or ischemia), the episode may be unwitnessed, the patient may not be able to recall associated symptoms, and the patient may have temporal lobe epilepsy, in which loss of consciousness is not associated with tonic-clonic movements. Temporal lobe epilepsy can also cause arrhythmias. Electroencephalography is indicated when the history cannot provide a clear distinction between syncope and seizure.

B. Metabolic Disorders and Hypoxia

Any condition that starves the cerebrum of essential nutrients (electrolytes, oxygen, glucose) or markedly changes pH can cause somnolence or coma. These conditions are not usually associated with spontaneous recovery (ie, without intervention); they tend to be longer lasting, and treatment is directed at the underlying abnormality. Hypoglycemia in outpatient diabetics, resulting from excessive insulin injection, can cause somnolence with a normal pulse and blood pressure; it is rapidly correctable with glucose.

C. Cerebral Vascular Insufficiency and Extracranial Vascular Disease

Although altered states of consciousness are known to occur with cerebral vascular events, true syncope is an uncommon presentation. Diseases of the intracranial and extracranial vessels can cause strokes and transient ischemic attacks, rarely syncope. Focal neurologic defects found during the physical examination are clues to the presence of cerebral vascular insufficiency, and differential peripheral arterial pressures or bruits suggest extracranial arterial disease. The extracranial arteries most commonly involved are the vertebrobasilar (occlusion), carotids (occlusion, emboli), aortic arch (dissection), and subclavian artery (stenosis), which may produce the subclavian steal syndrome.

D. Psychiatric Disorders with Hyperventilation and Pseudoseizure

Psychiatric illnesses are an important cause of syncope, especially in younger patients with multiple episodes and no organic heart disease. Depression, anxiety attacks, somatization disorder, panic disorder, and substance abuse (eg, alcohol, cocaine, sedatives) have all been associated with syncopal spells. In addition, patients may present with pseudoseizure that may or may not be associated with true seizure disorder.

Hyperventilation may cause syncope by producing hypocapnia and metabolic alkalosis, both of which stimulate cerebral arterial chemoreceptors to produce cerebral arterial vasoconstriction and decrease blood flow. Hyperventilation is frequently associated with such psychiatric illnesses as anxiety, depression, and panic attacks, but it can also occur sporadically in patients without psychiatric disease. A history of rapid breathing and perioral numbness is suggestive. A monitored hyperventilation maneuver that reproduces the patient's symptoms helps to confirm the diagnosis.

Treatment

Medical therapy is primarily targeted toward tachyarrhythmias, but pacemakers are generally used for bradyarrhythmias. In some situations, however, both are needed. For example, in sick sinus syndrome, a pacemaker is needed to prevent sinus bradycardia and pauses, and antiarrhythmic medications are needed to prevent the tachycardia (paroxysmal atrial fibrillation and flutter). Moreover, antiarrhythmic drugs can exacerbate bradycardia in some patients and necessitate implantation of a pacemaker to prevent medication-induced bradycardia and syncope.

A. Pharmacologic

Supraventricular arrhythmias can be treated with an assortment of antiarrhythmic medications (sodium channel blockers, β-blockers, potassium channel blockers, calcium channel blockers) with a wide range in therapeutic efficacy. Inherent in the medical treatment of arrhythmias, unfortunately, is a consistently high rate of side effects and the occurrence of proarrhythmia, worsening the arrhythmia or creating new arrhythmias such as quinidine-induced torsade de pointes. Sustained ventricular arrhythmias can be suppressed with antiarrhythmic drugs; however, recent studies favor their use only in combination with an ICD in the majority of patients.

Coronary artery, valvular, and other structural heart disease can usually be handled medically. If the disease has reached the point of causing syncope, however, it is usually severe enough to warrant surgical intervention or, in selected cases of coronary disease, percutaneous transluminal angioplasty.

Neurocardiogenic and situational syncope can be treated in a number of ways (Table 23–2). Education and avoidance of known precipitants are a first step. Alpha-agonists such as ephedrine, midodrine, or etilefrine can be used to enhance vasoconstriction and counteract the vasodilation portion of the reflex arc. Beta-blockers (eg, metoprolol, pindolol) have been used effectively; they are thought to work by decreasing ionotropy and preventing the afferent loop of the paradoxical reflex arc. Propantheline and scopolamine have been used for their anticholinergic effects against the vagal efferent loop of the reflex. The sodium channel blocker disopyramide has been used successfully, although its mechanism of action against neurocardiogenic syncope is poorly understood. Theophylline, an adenosine antagonist, has also been used successfully (adenosine is thought to be a mediator of vasodepression in the reflex arc). Some success has been reported using the antidepressants (serotonin reuptake inhibitors) fluoxetine and

Table 23–2. Medical treatment of neurocardiogenic syncope.

Class	Drug	Dosage Range
Alpha-agonists	Ephedrine	24 mg, bid–qid
	Etilefrine	15–30 mg/day
	Midodrine	2.5 mg, bid–tid, up to 40 mg/day
Beta-blockers	Metoprolol	25–100 mg, bid
	Pindolol	5–30 mg, bid
Anticholinergics	Propantheline	7.5–15 mg, tid
	Scopolamine patch	1.5 mg over 3 days
Sodium channel blocker	Disopyramide CR	150–300 mg, bid[a]
Adenosine antagonist	Theophylline	200–450 mg, bid[a]
Serotonin antagonist	Sertraline	50–200 mg/day
Antidepressant	Fluoxetine	20–80 mg/day
Mineralocorticoid	Fludrocortisone	0.1 mg/day

[a] Dose can be guided by serum levels.
CR = controlled release.

sertraline. Although the mechanism of action is not fully understood, serotonin is believed to play a central role in the development of vasovagal syncope. Volume expansion with liberalization of salt and water intake, administration of the mineralocorticoid fludrocortisone, and the use of thigh-high elastic stockings are effective because they can augment venous return.

None of these therapies has been shown to have any particular therapeutic advantage over the others, although most investigators consider β-blockers the first choice. The specific therapy chosen should be based on the patient's age, lifestyle, and medication side effects. Each can be given an empiric trial until an effective agent is found, or a repeat tilt-table test response can be used as a guide to chronic therapy.

When drug-induced syncope is suspected, the offending agent should be discontinued and the patient followed closely for recurrence. In the case of documented or suspected torsade de pointes, the underlying drug; electrolyte abnormality; or thyroid, neurologic, or cardiac cause must be sought and corrected. Intravenous magnesium, lidocaine, or isoproterenol or temporary ventricular pacing can be used to stabilize a patient with torsade while the underlying problem is corrected.

B. Nonpharmacologic Therapies

Implantable devices, such as the ICD and pacemakers, surgical procedures, and catheter ablation have all been used to treat syncope in appropriate patients. Besides causing syncope, ventricular tachycardia has the potential to degenerate to ventricular fibrillation. Many electrophysiologists consider syncope with ventricular tachycardia to be aborted sudden cardiac death. For this reason, patients with structural heart disease, documented ventricular tachycardia, and associated syncope are best managed with an ICD; moreover, patients with structural heart disease, syncope of unknown origin, and inducible ventricular arrhythmias during EPS are also most commonly managed with an ICD. The device continuously monitors the patient's heart rate and can apply a DC shock to convert the patient from ventricular fibrillation or tachycardia to sinus rhythm. ICDs have been found to reduce the likelihood of mortality in appropriate patients when compared with antiarrhythmic drugs. Although an ICD does not always prevent syncope, it effectively prevents sudden cardiac death. In addition, and ICD can terminate some ventricular tachycardias with rapid ventricular antitachycardia pacing (ATP). This therapy is painless and often unnoticed by the patient.

Ventricular tachycardia with associated ventricular aneurysm has also been successfully treated with open heart surgical ablation. With the development of nonthoracotomy ICD implantation, surgical ablation has become less common. In addition, nonsurgical catheter ablation techniques have been developed that allow for the treatment of some selected patients in the electrophysiology laboratory. In the great majority of patients, surgical or catheter ablation is used to reduce frequent appropriate ICD shocks and does not replace ICD therapy.

Single- and dual-chamber pacemakers are very effective in reducing symptomatic recurrences and preventing sudden death in patients with syncope caused by bradyarrhythmias from sinus node dysfunction, sick sinus syndrome with brady- and tachyarrhythmias, high-degree AV block, and carotid sinus hypersensitivity. Pacemaker therapy has been shown to have little role in treating neurocardiogenic syncope, largely because vasodepression is often the dominant component of the reflex and is not corrected by pacing. Pacemaker implantation may occasionally be appropriate for these patients if temporary pacing shows that the symptoms can be minimized (converting syncope to dizziness only) or if the episodes are purely cardioinhibitory. It may also be considered if multiple medications have been ineffective in severely diseased patients with mixed (vasodepressive and cardioinhibitory) episodes and the desired goal is to convert syncopal to presyncopal spells by abolishing the cardioinhibitory component.

Surgery can be performed to correct congenital heart disease, severe valvular disease, severe coronary disease, hypertrophic cardiomyopathy, and atrial myxoma, and heart transplantation can be performed in patients with severe end-stage muscle dysfunction.

In the past decade, electrophysiologic percutaneous catheter techniques using radiofrequency energy as an ablative source have been more than 95% effective in curing patients with supraventricular arrhythmias from AV nodal reentry or accessory pathways. Although successful ablation of atrial tachycardias, atrial flutter, some ventricular tachycardias, and even atrial fibrillation can be performed in selected patients, recurrence is not uncommon. In the case of atrial fibrillation with an uncontrollably rapid and symptomatic ventricular response, creation of complete heart block with catheter ablation and implantation of an activity-modulated ventricular pacemaker can effectively ameliorate symptoms.

Prognosis

The studies to date suggest that mortality rates in patients presenting with syncope are strongly correlated with the presence or absence of underlying structural heart disease. Dividing syncope patients into three groups is helpful for assessing their prognosis. In patients with cardiac causes of syncope, mortality is high at 1 year, ranging from 18 to 33%. In patients with noncardiac causes of syncope, 1-year mortality is much lower and ranges from 0 to 12%. Patients in whom syncope remains of unknown origin (despite an appropriate directed workup) do fairly well with a 6% 1-year

mortality rate. The incidence of sudden death in the cardiac patients is also much higher than in the other two groups. Recurrence rates in all three groups are similar: up to 15% per year. Recurrences do not predict an increase in mortality, although they are associated with increased morbidity (eg, fractures, soft tissue injury).

Recurrent syncope of unknown origin remains a difficult management problem. Patients with multiple atraumatic episodes and structurally normal hearts are more likely to have psychiatric illness or neurocardiogenic syncope and less likely to have electrophysiologic abnormalities at EPS. Memory-loop event recorders (to rule out brady- and tachyarrhythmias), tilt-table testing, and neuropsychiatric evaluation are probably the best means of evaluating these patients further. Patients with syncope of unknown origin and no structural heart disease have an excellent prognosis. They need to be reassured, but close follow-up and episodic reevaluation are also recommended. Intensive follow-up and reevaluation are needed for the patient with underlying heart disease and syncope of unknown origin. Such patients are not rare, and therapy should be directed at likely causes (such as EPS-induced sustained ventricular tachycardia). Empiric therapy (such as antiarrhythmic medication to suppress ventricular ectopy) is not without significant risk, however, and cannot be recommended as a general approach.

Ammirati F, Colivicchi F, Santini M: Permanent cardiac pacing versus medical treatment for the prevention of recurrent vasovagal syncope. Circulation 2001;104:52.

Anderson JL, Halstrom AP, Epstein AE et al: Design and results of the antiarrhythmics vs implantable defibrillators (AVID) registry. Circulation 1999;99:1692.

Bachinsky WB, Linzer M, Weld L et al: Usefulness of clinical characteristics in predicting the outcome of electrophysiologic studies in unexplained syncope. Am J Cardiol 1992;69:1044.

Bass EB, Curtiss EI, Arena VC et al: The duration of Holter monitoring in patients with syncope. Is 24 hours enough? Arch Intern Med 1990;150:1073.

Benditt DG, Remole S, Bailin S et al: Tilt-table testing for evaluation of neurally mediated (cardioneurogenic) syncope: Rationale and proposed protocols. PACE 1991;14:1528.

Brignole M, Menozzi C, Gianfranchi L et al: A controlled trial of acute and long-term medical therapy in tilt-induced neurally mediated syncope. Am J Cardiol 1992;70:339.

Cadman CS: Medical therapy of neurocardiogenic syncope. Cardiol Clinics 2001;19:203.

Chen XC, Chen MY, Remole S et al: Reproducibility of head-up tilt-table testing for eliciting susceptibility to neurally mediated syncope in patients without structural heart disease. Am J Cardiol 1992;69:755.

Crawford MH, Berstein SJ, Deedwania PC et al: ACC/AHA guidelines for ambulatory electrocardiography: Executive summary and recommendations. Circulation 1999;100:886.

Davis TL, Freemon FR: Electroencephalography should not be routine in the evaluation of syncope in adults. Arch Intern Med 1990;150:2027.

Fitzpatrick A, Theodorakis G, Vardas P et al: Methodology of head-up tilt testing in patients with unexplained syncope. J Am Coll Cardiol 1991;17:125.

Grubb BP, Gerard G, Rousch K et al: Differentiation of convulsive syncope and epilepsy with head-up tilt testing. Ann Intern Med 1991;115:871.

Grubb BP, Temesy-Armos P, Moore J et al: Head-upright tilt-table testing in evaluation and management of the malignant vaso-vagal syndrome. Am J Cardiol 1992;69:904.

Kapoor WN: Diagnostic evaluation of syncope. Am J Med 1991; 90:91.

Kapoor WN: Evaluation and management of syncope. JAMA 1992; 268:2553.

Kapoor WN: Syncope. N Engl J Med 2000;343:1856.

Krahn AD, Klein GJ, Yee R et al: Randomized assessment of syncope trial: Conventional diagnostic testing versus a prolonged monitoring strategy. Circulation 2001;104:46.

Kushner JA, Kou WH, Kadish AH et al: Natural history of patients with unexplained syncope and nondiagnostic electrophysiologic study. J Am Coll Cardiol 1989;14:391.

Linzer M, Prichett EL, Pontinen M et al: Incremental diagnostic yield of loop electrocardiographic recorders in unexplained syncope. Am J Cardiol 1990;66:214.

Linzer M, Caria I, Pontinen M et al: Medically unexplained syncope: Relationship to psychiatric illness. Am J Med 1992; 92(Suppl 1A):18S.

Linzer M, Yang EH, Estes NA 3rd et al: Diagnosing syncope part 1: Value of history, physical examination, and electrocardiography. Ann Intern Med 1997;126:989.

Linzer M, Yang EH, Estes NA 3rd et al: Diagnosing syncope part 2: Unexplained syncope. Ann Intern Med 1997;127:76.

Middlekauff H, Stevenson WG, Saxon LA et al: Prognosis after syncope: Impact of left ventricular function. Am Heart J 1993; 125:121.

Olshansky B: Is syncope the same thing as sudden death except that you wake up? J Cardiovasc Electrophysiol 1997;8:1098.

Olshansky B: Syncope: Overview and approach to management. In Grubb B, Olshansky B, eds: Syncope: Mechanisms and Management. Armonk NY: Futura Publishing Company, 1998:15.

Sheldon R, Splawinski J, Killin S: Reproducibility of isoproterenol tilt-table tests in patients with syncope. Am J Cardiol 1992; 69:1300.

Sra JS, Jazayeri MR, Avitall B et al: Comparison of cardiac pacing with drug therapy in the treatment of neurocardiogenic (vasovagal) syncope with bradycardia and asystole. N Engl J Med 1993;328:1085.

Sra JS, Anderson AJ, Sheikh SH et al: Unexplained syncope evaluated by electrophysiologic studies and head-up tilt testing. Ann Intern Med 1991;114:1013.

Sra JS, Murthy JS, Jazayeri MR et al: Use of intravenous esmolol to predict efficacy of oral beta-adrenergic blocker therapy in patients with neurocardiogenic syncope. J Am Coll Cardiol 1992;19:402.

Zimetbaum PJ, Josephson ME: The evolving role of ambulatory arrhythmia monitoring in general clinical practice. Ann Intern Med 1999;130;848.

Zipes DP, DiMarco JP, Gillette PC et al: Guidelines for clinical intracardiac electrophysiological and catheter ablation procedures. A report of the American College of Cardiology/American Heart Association Task Force on Practice Guidelines (Committee on Clinical Intracardiac Electrophysiologic and Catheter Ablation Procedures), developed in collaboration with the North American Society of Pacing and Electrophysiology. J Am Coll Cardiol 1995;26:555.

Sudden Cardiac Death

24

John P. DiMarco, MD, PhD

ESSENTIALS OF DIAGNOSIS

- *Unexpected death occurring within an hour of onset of symptoms*
- *Primary electrical mechanisms include ventricular fibrillation, ventricular tachycardia, asystole, and pulseless electrical activity*

General Considerations

Each year in the United States, more than 300,000 individuals die suddenly from some form of cardiovascular disease. Because of the many advances made during the past 30 years in our ability to identify and modify the risk factors associated with sudden death, to resuscitate victims of cardiac arrest, and to prescribe specific antiarrhythmic therapy to prevent recurrences, age-adjusted sudden death mortality rates have declined dramatically. However, the number of elderly individuals in the population has increased, and the total number of sudden cardiac deaths has remained relatively stable.

In a simplistic sense, any death can be considered sudden. For general clinical purposes, however, the term **sudden cardiac death** is usually reserved for those deaths in which the patient had stable cardiac function until the terminal event, with death occurring within a short time (often defined as less than 1 h) of the onset of symptoms. A further subclassification of sudden death uses the term, *instantaneous death*—namely, death with immediate collapse without preceding symptoms. Instantaneous death is usually assumed to be due to primary arrhythmia, but other catastrophic events, such as a massive pulmonary embolism, the rupture of an aortic aneurysm, or a stroke, can also cause instantaneous death. It is also important to note that not all arrhythmic deaths are sudden. For example, a patient who is resuscitated from a cardiac arrest may die days or weeks later from complications of the arrest. This death would be due to an arrhyth-

mia but would not meet a standard definition for sudden death.

Effective evaluation and treatment of patients at risk for cardiac arrest and sudden death require an understanding of the responsible pathophysiologic mechanisms, the strategies proposed for primary prevention, the techniques and results of resuscitation, and the treatment modalities for secondary prevention in survivors of an initial episode.

Pathophysiology & Etiology

A number of different electrophysiologic mechanisms may be responsible for sudden cardiac death. When ambulatory electrocardiographic (ECG) recordings from the time of an out-of-hospital cardiac arrest are examined, ventricular fibrillation and rapid ventricular tachycardia are the most commonly documented arrhythmias. Bradyarrhythmias, including atrioventricular block, asystole, or electromechanical dissociation, can also be observed. The prevalence of these latter arrhythmias increases among sudden death victims with very advanced underlying heart disease and in patients whose sudden death is precipitated by an acute catastrophe, such as a pulmonary embolism, an acute myocardial infarction, rupture of a major vessel, or a major neurologic insult. The focus of this chapter will be primarily those sudden deaths for which an arrhythmia was the primary cause.

A. CORONARY ARTERY DISEASE

Although sudden death occurs in all forms of heart disease, in the United States and Europe, coronary artery disease is the most common cardiac diagnosis seen in sudden death victims (Table 24–1). Several mechanisms can produce potentially fatal arrhythmias among patients with coronary artery disease, and it is often difficult to define the precise factors that underlie a given episode. At one extreme is the patient with a previously normal ventricle who has an acute occlusion of a major epicardial coronary artery and then develops ventricular fibrillation during the first minutes of an acute infarction. This patient represents an example of pure ischemic injury without associated prior scar. At the

Table 24–1. Cardiac conditions associated with sudden death.

Diseases of the coronary arteries
  Atherosclerotic
    Acute ischemia or infarction
    Prior myocardial infarction
  Congenital coronary anomalies
  Others
    Spasm, arteritis, dissection, etc.
Diseases of the aorta
  Marfan's syndrome, aortic aneurysm
Diseases of the myocardium
  Hypertrophic cardiomyopathy
  Dilated cardiomyopathy
  Valvular heart disease
  Arrhythmogenic right ventricular cardiomyopathy
  Congenital heart disease
  Infiltrative cardiomyopathy
  Primary pulmonary hypertension
  Myocarditis
Primary electrophysiologic disorders
  Long-QT syndrome
    Acquired and congenital
  Preexcitation syndromes
  Brugada's syndrome
  Catecholaminergic polymorphic ventricular tachycardia
  Congenital AV block
Other
  Drug ingestion, commotio cordis, electrolyte disorders, diet related, etc.

---

other end of the spectrum is the patient with a history of a single-vessel occlusion and an old myocardial infarction, in whom postinfarction scarring has provided the anatomic substrate for a rapid reentrant ventricular tachycardia that results in hemodynamic collapse and sudden death. Acute ischemia need not be involved. For the majority of victims with coronary artery disease, the immediate causation for sudden death lies between these extremes; they have both multivessel disease and myocardial scarring from one or more prior infarctions. As treatment of acute myocardial infarction has become more aggressive during the past 10–15 years, the nature of the typical scar that results from a myocardial infarction has also changed. Dense scar tissue with aneurysm formation, the classic substrate associated with uniform morphology ventricular tachycardia, is now less frequently seen. After pharmacologic or mechanical reperfusion—the current standards of therapy, the area of infarcted myocardium shows patchy fibrosis, and in such areas disorganized arrhythmias predominate. In patients with this complex substrate, sudden death is thought to result from a complex interaction between some triggering event, such as ischemia, auto-

nomic nervous system dysfunction, electrolyte imbalance, or drug toxicity, and the unstable electrophysiologic milieu created by prior infarction.

Autopsy and clinical studies have highlighted this complexity. Coronary artery thrombi or plaque rupture may be detected in up to 50% of sudden death victims, but only about 25% of patients resuscitated from an out-of-hospital cardiac arrest will develop new Q wave myocardial infarctions. Although persistent repolarization abnormalities and enzymatic evidence of necrosis may be noted in another 25% of patients, these changes are not specific for a new infarction and may be caused by prolonged hypotension during an arrest from any cause. Angiographic studies in cardiac arrest survivors have shown that a high proportion of subjects have long, diffusely irregular, and ulcerated coronary lesions similar to those seen in patients with unstable angina. If patients who are resuscitated from an out-of-hospital cardiac arrest undergo urgent catheterization, a high proportion will show a recent or acute coronary artery occlusion. Chest discomfort preceding an arrest is also difficult to interpret. Chest pain can occur during any significant tachycardia and may be either a consequence or a cause of an arrhythmia. Sudden death is more common among patients with evidence for silent ischemia on ambulatory ECG recordings, but in the relatively small number of sudden death victims with recordings at the time of arrest, ischemic changes have been only occasionally noted. Therapy directed at ischemia does reduce the incidence of sudden death. Aggressive surgical revascularization has been shown to decrease late sudden death mortality. In the Coronary Artery Bypass Graft (CABG-Patch) trial, no survival benefit over control was seen in the patients who received an implantable cardioverter defibrillator at the time of their revascularization surgery. Based on this confusing overall picture, it is prudent in any individual with coronary disease to consider ischemia as an important, potentially reversible contributor to sudden death, even if its precise role cannot be defined. In previously asymptomatic individuals, coronary artery disease may still be the cause of sudden death. Significant coronary artery disease may be asymptomatic or unrecognized, and the general population contains a large number of such individuals. Up to 50% of all sudden cardiac deaths due to coronary artery disease may occur in individuals not previously known to have the condition.

Other diseases of the coronary arteries are rare causes of sudden death. An anomalous origin of a coronary artery may give rise to either myocardial scarring with late ventricular tachycardia or to arrhythmias mediated by acute intermittent ischemia. Similar mechanisms affecting patients with coronary artery spasm, embolism, trauma, dissections, or arteritis may lead to sudden death.

B. Hypertrophic Cardiomyopathy

Sudden death is a well-recognized complication of non-ischemic cardiomyopathies. In hypertrophic cardiomyopathy, sudden death tends to occur in young adults who often have had no prior cardiac symptoms. There appears to be an excess of events during vigorous exercise. Teenagers or young adults in some kindreds with familial hypertrophic cardiomyopathy have a higher incidence of sudden death than do older members. In other families, an early event is uncommon, and sudden death usually occurs only after signs or symptoms of heart failure have developed.

Several clinical risk factors for sudden death in patients with hypertrophic cardiomyopathy have been determined. These include a family history of sudden death, recurrent, unexplained syncope, nonsustained ventricular tachycardia during ambulatory monitoring, and severe left ventricular hypertrophy. The genetics of hypertrophic cardiomyopathy are under intense study. Some mutations (eg, those in troponin T) may be associated with a high risk for sudden death even in the absence of marked left ventricular hypertrophy. It is hoped that, at some point, specific genetic patterns can be characterized as either high or low risk, but at present, family history is still the most valuable indicator. Polymorphic ventricular tachycardia or ventricular fibrillation, rather than monomorphic ventricular tachycardia with an intramyocardial circuit, is thought to be the initial arrhythmia at the time of cardiac arrest in patients with hypertrophic cardiomyopathy. Due to the severe hypertrophy and conduction system disease seen in patients with this disease, sustained ventricular tachycardia due to reentry in the His-Purkinje system may occur and result in hemodynamic collapse with sudden death. Patients with hypertrophic cardiomyopathy are also at risk for sudden death due to atrioventricular block and supraventricular arrhythmias because any change in rhythm that produces significant ischemia in the hypertrophied ventricular wall may degenerate to a fatal arrhythmia.

C. Idiopathic Dilated Cardiomyopathy

Nonischemic dilated cardiomyopathy is the primary cardiac diagnosis in about 10% of resuscitated cardiac arrest victims. Sudden death accounts for about half of all deaths in patients with this diagnosis. In contrast to the situation in some forms of hypertrophic cardiomyopathy, sudden death tends to occur relatively late in the course of dilated cardiomyopathy, after hemodynamic symptoms have been present for some time. A variety of arrhythmias have been implicated in patients with this condition; both monomorphic and polymorphic ventricular tachycardias are seen in patients with nonischemic dilated cardiomyopathies. When a monomorphic ventricular tachycardia, particularly one with a left bundle branch block morphology, is seen in a pa-

tient with a baseline intraventricular conduction delay, a specific form of ventricular tachycardia involving macroreentry using the His-Purkinje system should be suspected. In patients with this arrhythmia, catheter ablation of one of the bundle branches may be curative. If His-Purkinje reentrant tachycardia is not detected, electrophysiologic testing is of limited value in patients with dilated cardiomyopathy in determining the cause of a cardiac arrest. Even in patients with well-documented clinical episodes of ventricular tachycardia or fibrillation, similar arrhythmias frequently cannot be induced with programmed stimulation during an electrophysiologic study. In patients with cardiomyopathies and very advanced heart failure, bradyarrhythmias, rather than tachyarrhythmias, may account for up to 50% of cardiac arrests.

D. Other Cardiac Diseases

In **valvular heart disease,** sudden death can occur in several ways. Sudden death is usually related to exertion in young adults with congenital aortic stenoses. Although the responsible mechanism is uncertain, sudden changes in either ventricular filling or aortic obstruction with a secondary arrhythmia are suspected. In the acquired forms of valvular heart disease, sudden death is usually a late occurrence seen in patients with advanced heart failure and ventricular hypertrophy. Although symptomatic atrial and ventricular arrhythmias are common in patients with mitral valve prolapse, truly life-threatening arrhythmias are extraordinarily rare, except in the presence of some complicating condition, such as a long-QT syndrome, electrolyte imbalance, or drug toxicity. In pulmonary hypertension, sudden death may occur from hemodynamic causes, bradyarrhythmias, or tachyarrhythmias.

Arrhythmogenic right ventricular cardiomyopathy is a regional myopathy with primarily right ventricular involvement. Several pathologic patterns may be seen. In one, gross right ventricular dilatation and dysfunction may be present, but symptoms of heart failure are absent or mild. In localized areas where the myocardium has been replaced by fat and fibrous tissue, dysplasia can be seen. These patients usually present with a ventricular tachycardia with an ECG pattern that resembles left bundle branch block. Some patients with arrhythmias due to a predominantly right ventricular myopathy, however, have a more fulminant course, with both progressive heart failure and life-threatening arrhythmias. Arrhythmogenic right ventricular cardiomyopathy can occur in both familial and sporadic forms.

In most forms of **congenital heart disease,** sudden arrhythmic death in the absence of severe heart failure, ventricular hypertrophy, or hypoxemia is uncommon. In patients who have undergone a successful surgical repair of Fallot's tetralogy, however, late arrhythmias may develop in the region of the right ventriculotomy or on either side of the septal repair.

E. Patients Without Structural Heart Disease

Several electrophysiologic abnormalities can produce sudden death without associated major structural heart disease. **Supraventricular arrhythmias,** if associated with very rapid ventricular rates, can cause hemodynamic collapse and degenerate to ventricular fibrillation. Atrial fibrillation with rapid conduction over an accessory pathway in a patient with **Wolff-Parkinson-White syndrome** is the supraventricular arrhythmia most frequently associated with sudden death, but other supraventricular arrhythmias have also occasionally been implicated. Although sudden death due to a ventricular preexcitation syndrome is rare, it may be the first clinical manifestation of the condition. **Bradyarrhythmias** may also be associated with sudden death. In **congenital complete heart block,** the escape pacemaker may deteriorate over time, with ventricular arrhythmias appearing as the patient's bradycardia becomes more and more inappropriate. Most previously healthy adults who develop a bradycardia as a result of sinus node dysfunction or heart block will have some functioning escape pacemaker that can, at least briefly, support vital organs. Therefore, sudden death is uncommon with these arrhythmias in the absence of severe ventricular dysfunction, another complicating disease, electrolyte imbalance, or drug toxicity.

The **congenital long-QT syndrome** is a family of disorders characterized by prolongation of cardiac repolarization with a prolonged QT interval on the scalar ECG and a tendency to develop polymorphic ventricular tachycardia that may degenerate to ventricular fibrillation. The basic defect in these syndromes is a mutation in a gene coding an ion channel protein (Table 24–2). The dysfunctional channel results in a prolonged repolarization phase of the ventricular action potential, which promotes polymorphic ventricular tachycardia triggered by oscillations in the action potential called early after depolarizations. Electrolyte imbalance, bradycardia or pauses, sudden sympathetic stimulation, and drug effects all may further prolong repolarization in individuals with these mutations and precipitate acute episodes. It is important to recognize patients with the long-QT syndrome because standard antiarrhythmic drugs may worsen their condition.

The **Brugada syndrome** is another familial condition associated with sudden death. These individuals have a incomplete or complete right bundle branch block on their ECG with ST segment elevation in V_1 and V_2. These patients will manifest spontaneous episodes of polymorphic ventricular tachycardia and ventricular fibrillation, often during sleep. Similar arrhythmias are usually also inducible at electrophysiologic study. The syndrome has been linked to a mutation in the sodium channel gene with a decrease in the inward sodium current during the plateau phase of the action potential. The unusual ECG manifestations are believed to be due to more pronounced ion channel dysfunction in the right ventricular epicardium.

Some patients without structural heart disease who have been resuscitated from an episode of cardiac arrest exhibit none of the previously detailed characteristics. Although changes in the autonomic nervous system's influence on the heart have been postulated as being responsible for a fatal arrhythmia in some individuals with the familial syndrome of **catecholaminergic poly-**

Table 24–2. Genetic syndromes associated with sudden death.

Syndrome	Gene	Current or Protein Affected
Long-QT		
LQT1	KvLQT1	I_{Ks}
LQT2	HERG	I_{Kr}
LQT3	SCN5A	I_{Na}
LQT4	?	?
LQT5	KCNE1 (minK)	I_{Ks}
LQT6	KCNE1 (MiRP1)	I_{Ks}
Brugada	SCN5A, others	I_{Na}, others
Arrhythmogenic right ventricular cardiomyopathy	Several	Ryanodine receptor, others
Hypertrophic cardiomyopathy	Several	Myosin light and heavy chains, troponins, others

morphic ventricular tachycardia, the full scope of the problem remains poorly defined. Usually, electrophysiologic studies and Holter monitoring are either normal or reveal only polymorphic arrhythmias that may be poorly reproducible.

Although these syndromes that are caused by a single gene mutation account for only a small proportion of sudden deaths in the population, it seems likely that single nucleotide polymorphisms in these and other genes may result to a genetic predisposition to sudden death when they exist in combination with various forms of heart disease or unusual physiologic stress.

All ventricular arrhythmias in patients with structurally normal hearts do not carry a risk for sudden death. Sudden death is very rare in individuals with structurally normal hearts who initially present with a well-tolerated **monomorphic ventricular tachycardia,** even when the tachycardia is sustained. The two most common forms of sustained monomorphic ventricular tachycardia in patients with structurally normal hearts arise either from the right ventricular outflow tract with a left bundle branch block pattern and an inferior axis or from the inferior septal region with a right bundle branch block and left axis pattern. Both these forms of ventricular tachycardia are usually hemodynamically well tolerated and rarely result in hemodynamic collapse.

A recently recognized syndrome of sudden death in young individuals with structurally normal hearts has been named **commotio cordis.** Victims develop ventricular fibrillation after receiving a sharp blow to the chest, often while engaged in sports. In animal models, it has been shown that a critically timed and placed chest impact during a vulnerable portion of the T wave can initiate ventricular fibrillation. It is assumed that a similar mechanism is responsible for the human syndrome.

F. Drug-Induced Arrhythmias

Drug toxicity can also result in sudden death. A variety of medications can affect cardiac electrophysiology and lead to fatal arrhythmias. Even when prescribed for atrial fibrillation or supraventricular tachycardia, all antiarrhythmic drugs may be associated with a proarrhythmic response in the ventricle. The pattern of proarrhythmia that is seen depends on the electrophysiologic action of the drug involved. Class 1a drugs (quinidine, procainamide, and disopyramide) can result in both monomorphic ventricular tachycardia and polymorphic ventricular tachycardia with a long-QT interval (torsades de pointes). The characteristic drug-induced arrhythmia seen with class 1c agents (flecainide and propafenone) is an incessant ventricular tachycardia with a very wide QRS complex. Atrial proarrhythmia (eg, atrial flutter with 1:1 conduction) and worsened arrhythmias during ischemia are also

seen with class 1c drugs. Among the class III drugs, sotalol and dofetilide have been associated with torsades de pointes; amiodarone rarely causes it. Incessant ventricular tachycardia and bradycardias may, however, complicate therapy with amiodarone.

A large number of noncardiac drugs can also cause potentially life-threatening arrhythmias—usually because they have secondary effects to block the delayed component of the inward-rectifying potassium channel, I_{Kr}, which is important for repolarization. On several occasions, both cardiac and noncardiac drugs with secondary actions on ion channels have been withdrawn from market release because of their tendency to produce arrhythmias in susceptible individuals under certain conditions. The phenothiazines, bepridil, cisapride, the nonsedating antihistamines, terfenadine and astemizole; erythromycin, pentamidine, several fluoroquinolones, azole antifungals, and several antipsychotic agents have been shown to prolong QT intervals in vitro and produce arrhythmias. Clinical reports of sudden deaths during therapy with some of these agents have appeared. Cocaine use has been associated with unexpected sudden death, with both primary and ischemically mediated arrhythmias suspected as the cause. Other drugs that are abused can also cause arrhythmias. Alcohol is frequently implicated in sudden death, with both respiratory depression and alcohol-induced arrhythmias probably responsible. Overuse of inhalers containing sympathomimetic amines has been implicated as a precipitant of fatal arrhythmias in patients with asthma. Some herbal medications contain compounds that may cause arrhythmias in susceptible individuals or in overdose situations. Patients with severe electrolyte disturbances and abnormal dietary histories (eg, anorexia nervosa and liquid protein diets, etc) are also susceptible to potentially fatal ventricular arrhythmias.

Management of Cardiac Arrest: Initial Resuscitation

The introduction of transthoracic defibrillation 40 years ago sparked the development of community-based programs to resuscitate victims of out-of-hospital cardiac arrest. A successful system involves both an educated lay public that can provide at least basic cardiopulmonary resuscitation (CPR) and an organized structure to provide advanced life support in the field. Because the time period for delivering effective therapy to the victim of a cardiac arrest is very short, even the best community programs will have survival-to-hospital discharge rates of only 20–30%. Several factors have been identified with a favorable outcome. Probably the most important is the time from arrest to restoration of an organized cardiac rhythm. If an effective rhythm is not restored within 4–8 min, survival with preserved higher neurologic function becomes unlikely. Bystander CPR extends this window for survival, but by only a few minutes.

Because early defibrillation is the key to survival, community programs to speed defibrillation have been widely introduced but with variable success. Initial efforts involved emergency medical technicians trained in both basic and advanced cardiac life support who responded to the emergency call. The success of these programs was limited by the ability of these trained responders to reach the victim within the first critical minutes after the arrest. The extensive training required to achieve competency in advanced cardiac life support limited the implementation of these programs.

Public access to automatic external defibrillators (AEDs) offers the potential to improve survival further for out-of-hospital cardiac arrest victims. When an AED is connected to an unconscious individual by electrode pads placed on the chest, a microprocessor within the device analyzes the patient's rhythm. Ventricular fibrillation and rapid ventricular tachycardia are accurately identifiable as "shockable" rhythms, and the AED instructs the rescuer to push a button to deliver a shock. AEDs were first successfully introduced for use by emergency medical technicians, fire fighters, and police officers. Recent studies have shown benefit with AED use by security officers in casinos and by airline and airport employees. AEDs designed for home use by minimally trained lay family members are now commercially available, and a "wearable" vest AED that does not require a rescuer for activation has recently been introduced.

A discussion of the techniques for basic and advanced cardiac life support are beyond the scope of this chapter. For patients with ventricular tachycardia or fibrillation, early cardioversion or defibrillation is the key to survival. For patients with asystole or pulseless electrical activity, the prospects for survival are dismal unless some reversible cause can be identified and immediately corrected.

Management of Cardiac Arrest Survivors: In-Hospital Phase

Even in communities that have effective programs for prehospital cardiac care, only a minority of cardiac arrest patients will survive to hospital admission. Optimal management for these survivors of an episode of cardiac arrest requires a systematic approach. First, potential complications of the resuscitation must be identified and treatment instituted. Next, the probable cause, including reversible precipitating events, the nature and severity of any underlying heart disease, and the arrhythmia probably responsible for the episode, should be determined. Finally, therapy can be selected and its potential for success evaluated.

A. Complications of Resuscitation

Only a minority of cardiac arrest victims who receive early defibrillation will be alert and oriented with full recovery of function at the time of hospital admission. Most patients will have pulmonary, cardiac, or neurologic complications resulting from the period of arrest or the resuscitation itself. Pulmonary complications are usually due either to aspiration of gastric contents or to mechanical injury to the thoracic cage during closed-chest compressions. The chest wall should be carefully inspected, palpated, and stabilized, if necessary. In extreme cases, bony thoracic fractures may result in a flail chest, or hepatic or splenic lacerations may occur. Chest radiography may be helpful in detecting aspiration, but repeated examinations may be necessary to document the delayed appearance of infiltrates. If a central line has been placed, the chest radiograph is also useful to confirm catheter position and to exclude a pneumothorax. Mechanical ventilation is often required in the early period after admission to allow adequate oxygenation and pulmonary cleansing; this may require the use of muscle relaxants and sedation.

Cardiac arrest produces a period of global cardiac ischemia, frequently resulting in a period of cardiac stunning defined as a reversible depression in cardiac systolic function. This has two important implications. First, inotropic or even mechanical (eg, intraaortic counterpulsation) support may be necessary to maintain vital organ perfusion during the early phase after resuscitation. Second, any acute assessment of ventricular function may overestimate the amount of permanent dysfunction. Thus, a low ejection fraction measured in the first several days after arrest should not be a reason to discontinue support. ECG and enzymatic data obtained after an arrest are often difficult to interpret. It is usually wise to reserve a definite diagnosis of an acute infarction as the primary event for those patients with chest pain preceding collapse and documented ST segment elevation or new Q waves. Without a documented new infarction, it may be hoped that the patient's cardiac function will eventually recover to its status before the arrest, but this may take several weeks. Even if transient ischemia were the immediate trigger for the arrest, full recovery of function may occur if the culprit vessel has regained patency. Arrhythmias are frequently seen during the immediate period after resuscitation. They may be similar to the disturbance that originally produced the arrest, or they may be new rhythm disturbances caused by poor hemodynamic function and multiorgan failure. No single therapy will be predictably effective against these arrhythmias, and antiarrhythmic agents, β-adrenergic blockers, positive inotropic agents, and other measures to improve hemodynamic function must be tried. Recent studies using intravenous amiodarone prior to hospital admission have demonstrated improvements in rates of return of spontaneous circulation and survival-to-hospital admission but no clear benefit in survival-to-hospital discharge.

Neurologic damage occurs quickly during a cardiac arrest. Unless defibrillation with restoration of spontaneous circulation was almost immediate, patients will be unconscious when admitted to the hospital, and an accurate evaluation of the potential for functional recovery is often difficult in this early stage. Brain stem reflexes may be preserved, but their presence does not necessarily predict a favorable outcome. Generalized or focal seizure activity, decerebrate or decorticate posturing, and involuntary respiratory efforts may make mechanical ventilation difficult, and neuromuscular blocking agents, anticonvulsants, and sedation are often required, further hampering any ability to make an accurate neurologic assessment. In the absence of some severe concomitant disease, it is usually wise to withhold any decisions concerning withdrawal of support for at least 24 h. After that time, attempts should be made to withdraw sedatives and neuromuscular blockers. The prognosis is good for patients who regain consciousness within 72 h of arrest, and many of them will recover completely with no or minimal long-term neurologic impairment. If coma persists longer than 72 h, few patients survive. Those who do will often have persistent severe motor and cognitive deficits. Decisions about prolonged artificial support of these latter patients are often difficult and require that a variety of medical, ethical, and social factors be taken into consideration.

B. Diagnostic Studies

1. Noninvasive Evaluation for Structural Heart Disease—Once the patient has recovered to the point that long-term survival seems likely, efforts should be made to define fully the type and extent of underlying cardiac disease.

a. Electrocardiography—Although the ECG usually provides the first information available, the initial ECG after defibrillation may be misleading. Transient ST-segment elevation in leads with prior Q waves is common; it should not be interpreted as indicating a new infarction as the primary cause of the arrest. Only if ST elevation has been documented during normal rhythm before the arrest, or if new Q waves appear, should a definite diagnosis of an acute infarction be made. This distinction is critical because the prognosis associated with resuscitated ventricular fibrillation precipitated by a new acute infarction is not significantly different from that associated with an infarct of similar size without arrest. More commonly, the ECG will show such evidence of chronic disease, including old Q waves, conduction defects, or hypertrophy. ST segment and T-wave abnormalities appear in virtually all patients following resuscitation and are of limited signifi-

cance. The ECG may also be useful in the diagnosis of congenital and acquired long-QT syndromes, the Brugada syndrome, preexcitation syndromes, cardiomyopathies, and congenital heart disease.

b. Echocardiography—Echocardiography performed in the coronary care unit can provide a noninvasive assessment of cardiac function and anatomy shortly after resuscitation. An early, two-dimensional echocardiogram can provide valuable information about chamber size, valvular abnormalities, and ventricular function. Serial studies are often helpful in documenting recovery of function after an initial period of stunning.

c. Other noninvasive tests—Other noninvasive tests may also be appropriate in some cases. Magnetic resonance imaging is particularly valuable in patients with arrhythmogenic right ventricular cardiomyopathy. Positron emission tomography, magnetic resonance imaging, and isotope perfusion scans may be useful for assessing viability in regions of poor ventricular function. Preserved viability may influence decisions concerning the appropriateness of any attempts at revascularization. Signal-averaged electrocardiography is of limited value in a patient who has already had a cardiac arrest. Although an abnormal study increases the probability that a monomorphic ventricular tachycardia caused the arrest and will be inducible at electrophysiologic study, the values found in cardiac arrest survivors are often within normal limits. In-hospital monitoring may identify spontaneous arrhythmias that require suppression.

2. Invasive evaluation for structural heart disease—Cardiac catheterization provides the most complete assessment of the structure, function, and blood supply of the heart, and it should be performed for virtually all survivors of cardiac arrest. Coronary artery disease is found in about 80% of cardiac arrest victims in the United States and Europe. In coronary disease, unanticipated cardiac arrest occurs primarily in three clinical settings: acute infarction; transient ischemia, usually in the presence of prior infarction or severe multivessel disease; and with chronic arrhythmias in patients with prior healed infarctions. In the first two settings, polymorphic ventricular tachycardia or ventricular fibrillation are the arrhythmias observed, whereas both monomorphic and polymorphic arrhythmias can occur in the cases of prior healed infarction.

The prognosis of a patient who survives a cardiac arrest in the acute phase of a myocardial infarction is determined by the total amount of ventricular damage, the severity of residual ischemia, and the completeness of recovery from any noncardiac complications of the arrest. Treatment of these patients should be similar to that for other infarct survivors, and special steps to define and control a specific arrhythmia are not required. The role of ischemia in cardiac arrest patients without new Q wave infarction is controversial. As noted earlier, long, ulcerated coronary artery lesions are often seen on coronary angiograms in cardiac arrest survivors and at autopsy in those with sudden death. If these lesions are seen in patients with totally normal ventricular function, ischemia from these lesions alone may be responsible for the arrest. Correcting the ischemia through revascularization is the most appropriate—and sometimes the only required—therapy. More commonly, both a potential for ischemia and a fixed scar will be evident, and a complex interaction between the two will be responsible for the event.

Other procedures may be indicated when no coronary artery, valvular, or myocardial disease is detected during routine catheterization. Ventricular biopsy may be helpful if an acute myocarditis or amyloidosis is suspected. A diagnosis of sarcoid heart disease may be confirmed by biopsy in about 50% of patients with the condition.

3. Diagnosis of arrhythmias—A variety of arrhythmias can cause cardiac arrest and sudden death. Supraventricular arrhythmias with rapid ventricular rates and primary bradyarrhythmias are infrequent causes of cardiac arrest. However, it is important to identify patients with these arrhythmias because they will require a different approach to therapy. Ventricular tachycardia and ventricular fibrillation are the most common causes of out-of-hospital cardiac arrest, and the evaluation and treatment of these arrhythmias will be the focus of the rest of this chapter.

a. Noninvasive evaluation—The role of noninvasive testing in patients with a cardiac arrest is limited because a history of cardiac arrest has already placed them in a high-risk group. Noninvasive tests, however, are often used to assess risk for future events in patients with known cardiac disease. Signal-averaged electrocardiography detects subtle delays in intraventricular conduction that may predispose a patient to sustained ventricular tachycardia. ECG signals are filtered and then averaged to eliminate random noise, allowing amplification of small voltage signals in the terminal portion of the QRS. These voltages are considered abnormal and are called **late potentials** when the total filtered QRS duration exceeds a certain threshold (usually between 113 and 120 ms), when the root mean square voltage in the terminal QRS is lower than 20 μV, or when the duration of the signal below 40 μV is prolonged (*greater than* 38 ms). The presence of late potentials is a risk factor for death after myocardial infarction; they are present in most coronary disease patients and patients with arrhythmogenic right ventricular dysplasia with recurrent sustained monomorphic ventricular tachycardia. Late potentials are present less reliably in cardiac arrest survivors, and their absence in these patients has no diagnostic value.

Exercise testing may be useful in some cases of exercise-induced ventricular tachycardia or in some patients with cardiac arrest to determine the presence of inducible ischemia. Abnormal prolongation of the QT interval in patients with the long-QT syndrome and the appearance of arrhythmias in patients with congenital heart block may also be useful markers of future risk. In most cases, however, exercise testing is used to provide information about the potential for ischemia, rather than to diagnose the mechanism of arrhythmia or to guide therapy.

Ambulatory ECG monitoring is rarely useful in cardiac arrest survivors, but the presence of frequent and complex ventricular premature beats and abnormal heart rate variability are risk factors for sudden death during follow-up in patients with many forms of heart disease. In population studies, frequent or complex ventricular ectopy is associated with an increased risk of both sudden and nonsudden cardiac death. Unfortunately, the prognostic value of ambulatory ECG monitoring data in any individual patient is limited by poor day-to-day reproducibility of the data. The use of antiarrhythmic drug therapy guided by suppression of ventricular ectopic activity has not been shown to improve survival.

b. Invasive evaluation—Invasive evaluation involves a baseline electrophysiologic study that uses programmed electrical stimulation to initiate and characterize the patient's arrhythmia. Early, observational studies indicated that this technique could be used to assess the effects of antiarrhythmic drugs. Three hypotheses were the basis for this approach: (1) that most ventricular arrhythmias are due to reentry over well-established electrophysiologic pathways; (2) that systematic programmed ventricular stimulation could artificially recreate the conditions necessary for reentry to occur; and (3) that changes in the response during repeat stimulation during therapy would correlate with subsequent clinical events. Unfortunately, when examined in controlled trials, serial electrophysiologic testing has not been demonstrated to be sufficiently accurate to serve as a predictor of long-term outcome. The ability to identify initially an effective drug is limited, and the failure rate of drug therapy selected by the technique is unacceptably high. Therefore, electrophysiologic studies now play a secondary role in the diagnosis and treatment of cardiac arrest survivors. The primary value of these studies will be to identify those patients with associated supraventricular arrhythmias or abnormal atrioventricular conduction who will require a specific treatment. A few types of ventricular tachycardia can potentially be eliminated by catheter ablation, and electrophysiologic studies should be performed if reentry in the His-Purkinje system or a right ventricular outflow tract tachycardia is suspected. Electrophysiologic studies are useful for characterizing the effects of drug therapy on tachycardias. Drug therapy may change the rate of many ventricular tachycardias and can affect defibrillation thresholds. Data obtained from electrophysiologic studies during drug therapy can be used to guide programming of implantable cardioverter defibrillators (ICDs).

Treatment of Cardiac Arrest Survivors

Treating the cardiac arrest survivor requires a comprehensive strategy that must consider both aggressive and appropriate management of the underlying cardiac disease process as well as specific antiarrhythmic therapy.

A. ANTIARRHYTHMIC DRUG THERAPY

The role of antiarrhythmic drugs in the treatment of cardiac arrest survivors has changed substantially in the last 15 years. This change in strategy has been based on the results of randomized clinical trials for the primary and secondary prevention of sudden death. These trials have shown that therapy with class I antiarrhythmic drugs does not improve, and may worsen, survival when used for primary prevention in patients after myocardial infarction. When used in patients with a history of sustained ventricular tachycardia or ventricular fibrillation, class I drugs are inferior to sotalol and amiodarone. The latter drugs have, in turn, been shown to be less effective for improving survival than is therapy with an ICD.

Antiarrhythmic drugs, however, are still of value in individual patients. Unstable arrhythmias are common in the immediate period after resuscitation. Intravenous amiodarone and β-blockers are the most effective treatments in this setting. Many patients with an ICD, in the absence of drug therapy, would have frequent episodes of sustained or nonsustained ventricular tachycardia that would trigger ICD therapy. Sotalol, a class III agent with β-adrenergic blocking activity, has been shown in a randomized trial to decrease the need for ICD therapy. Amiodarone and β-adrenergic blockers are also thought to have a similar effect on the frequency of ICD therapy, but these agents have not been studied in a similar, randomized trial. The usual dose range for sotalol is 120–160 mg bid. Sotalol is cleared by the kidney, and the dose should be adjusted in patients with renal insufficiency. *d, l*-Sotalol is a potent β-adrenergic blocker, and bradycardia may limit therapy. Sotalol may also lower defibrillation threshold. Amiodarone is usually administered with a loading dose of 5–10 g in the first 1–2 weeks of therapy, followed by a daily dose of 200-300 mg daily. Common adverse reactions during amiodarone therapy include thyroid dysfunction, photosensitivity and skin discoloration, neuromuscular complaints, and abnormal liver function tests. Amiodarone-induced pulmonary toxicity can be life-threatening if unrecognized and occurs in approximately 1–2% of patients in the first year of therapy and in 0.5% of patients per year thereafter. Some patients will not be candidates for or not desire ICD therapy. In those cases, sotalol or amiodarone would be the drugs of choice. The role of new antiarrhythmic drugs, including dofetilide and azimilide in patients with ventricular arrhythmias, remains undefined.

B. REVASCULARIZATION

Revascularization may play an important role in the care of both survivors of cardiac arrest and patients at risk for sudden death. In patients with ischemic heart disease and chronic stable angina, coronary revascularization decreases sudden death rates, with the greatest benefits being observed in patients with multivessel disease and depressed left ventricular function. Among cardiac arrest survivors, revascularization is indicated in patients with evidence of active ischemia or extensive areas of hibernating, dysfunctional but viable, myocardium. If no significant prior scarring is evident, revascularization alone may provide effective therapy for selected patients. In the presence of prior scar, however, revascularization alone may not be effective at preventing future arrhythmias. Cardiac transplantation plays an important role in patients with both arrhythmias and intractable ischemia or severe heart failure and in patients whose arrhythmias cannot be controlled with any less drastic form of therapy.

C. SURGICAL OR CATHETER ABLATION

Direct surgical or catheter approaches designed to eliminate or ablate the myocardial areas where the reentry circuit responsible for ventricular tachycardia arises, have been developed. Both approaches involve induction of tachycardia using programmed stimulation, mapping to determine critical portions of the tachycardia circuit, and either resection or ablation at the sites identified. Map-guided surgical resection procedures are no longer commonly performed due to the substantial likelihood of mortality associated with these procedures. Although catheter ablation has been successfully used in patients with sustained ventricular tachycardia, the highest success rates have been in patients with well-tolerated tachycardias or no structural heart disease. At present, the most frequent use of catheter ablation in cardiac arrest patients is as an adjunct treatment to lessen the frequency of arrhythmias in patients who also have ICDs. New ablation approaches designed to isolate large areas of arrhythmogenic myocardium are now being studied and may be effective in some patients with rapid and unstable arrhythmias.

Catheter ablation of an accessory atrioventricular connection will be curative in patients with cardiac arrest in association with atrial arrhythmias. In patients with ventricular tachycardia caused by macroreentry in the His-Purkinje system, ablation of the right bundle will eliminate further episodes.

D. IMPLANTABLE CARDIOVERTER DEFIBRILLATORS

The first implantable automatic defibrillator was implanted for clinical use in 1980. Primitive by today's standards, the early devices clearly demonstrated the validity of the concept that a totally implanted device could be used to terminate automatically life-threatening arrhythmias. Advances in defibrillator technology have extended the applications of these devices, and ICD therapy is now considered the primary therapeutic option for cardiac arrest survivors.

An ICD has two basic components: the ICD generator and the lead system for pacing and shock delivery to which it is connected. An ICD generator contains sensing circuits, memory storage, capacitors, voltage enhancers, a telemetry module, and a control microprocessor. Advances in miniaturization and complexity in all of these components have permitted a tremendous reduction in size of the generator itself despite increased functionality. The original implantable defibrillator was designed to recognize the disorganized electrical activity characteristic of ventricular fibrillation only. The ability to recognize ventricular tachycardia was added shortly thereafter. Subsequent generations of devices have added extensive programming options, antitachycardia pacing, single- and dual-chamber rate-responsive pacing for bradycardia, biphasic defibrillation waveforms, enhanced arrhythmia detection features, and innovations in lead systems. The original systems required a thoracotomy to place epicardial patches, and, as a result, the implant procedure itself was associated with substantial morbidity and mortality rates. After transvenous leads were developed that allowed successful defibrillation and the generator

size was reduced, subcutaneous implants in the pectoral region became standard. Current systems can be implanted by electrophysiologists using local anesthesia in a cardiac laboratory.

From the point of their introduction, there was little doubt that ICDs were very effective for terminating episodes of ventricular tachycardia and ventricular fibrillation. Initially, they were implanted chiefly in patients who did not respond to antiarrhythmic drug therapy as assessed by repeat ECG monitoring or electrophysiologic testing. As the limitations of antiarrhythmic drugs became more apparent, ICDs began to be used as the first treatment option. Three large randomized trials have compared ICD therapy to antiarrhythmic therapy in survivors of cardiac arrest or hemodynamically unstable ventricular tachycardia (Table 24–3). In the Antiarrhythmics versus Implantable Defibrillator (AVID) study, 1016 patients were randomly assigned to either drug therapy (amiodarone or, rarely, sotalol) or an ICD. Survival analysis showed a decrease in total mortality rates of 39%, 27%, and 31% at follow-up points of 1, 2, and 3 years, respectively. The Cardiac Arrest Study Hamburg (CASH) randomly assigned 346 cardiac arrest survivors to either an ICD or drug therapy with one of three agents: amiodarone, metoprolol, or propafenone. The propafenone arm was terminated early due to an excessive mortality rate among those patients. At 2-year follow-up, the mortality rate was 37% lower in the ICD group than in the combined metoprolol and amiodarone group. In the Canadian Implantable Defibrillator Study (CIDS), 650 patients with cardiac arrest, sustained ventricular tachycardia, or inducible ventricular tachycardia with unexplained syncope were treated with either an ICD or amiodarone. The mortality rate at 2-year follow-up was 19.7% lower in the ICD group. These three studies

Table 24–3. Implantable cardioverter defibrillator trials.

| Trial | Follow-Up (years) | Total Mortality | | Overall Risk Reduction in ICD Group (%) |
		Drug or Control Group (%)	ICD Group (%)	
AVID	2	25.3	18.4	27
CASH	2	19.6	12.1	37
CIDS	3	30.0	25.0	20
MADIT I	4	44	22	54
CABG-Patch	4	24	27	−7

AVID = Antiarrhythmics Versus Implantable Defibrillator; CABG-Patch = Coronary Artery Bypass Graft; CASH = Cardiac Arrest Study Hamburg; CIDS = Canadian Implantable Defibrillator Study; ICD = implantable cardioverter defibrillator; MADIT I = Multicenter Automatic Implantable Defibrillator Trial.

provide convincing evidence that an ICD should be a primary option in a cardiac arrest survivor. ICD therapy results in the greatest probability of benefit in those at the highest risk for repeat events (ie, those with lower ejection fractions). In fact, a meta-analysis of data from AVID, CIDS, and CASH failed to show improved survival with ICD therapy if the patient's left ventricular ejection fraction was above 0.35.

ICD therapy has a number of limitations, however. An ICD terminates arrhythmias by using either anti-tachycardia pacing or direct current shocks. The latter produce significant discomfort, and patients who receive multiple shocks report significant negative effects on their quality of life. Although an ICD may be programmed to employ various pacing strategies that may decrease arrhythmia frequency, these steps are not always effective, and antiarrhythmic drugs are often required as adjunctive therapy. Sotalol, amiodarone, and β-adrenergic blockers are the agents most commonly used in patients with an ICD. Disease progression often limits the usefulness of an ICD. In AVID, CIDS, and CASH, the mortality benefit of ICD therapy was virtually gone after 6 years of follow-up. Hardware deterioration, although rarely life-threatening, continues to be a problem and may lead to a need for multiple invasive procedures. Finally, ICD therapy is very costly. Estimates of added cost over drug therapy per quality of life year saved in the AVID and CIDS populations exceeded $100,000.

Identification of Patients at Risk

Even in communities with the most advanced systems for emergency response and out-of-hospital resuscitation, only a minority of patients are resuscitated and survive to hospital discharge without significant residual deficits. In many areas, it is logistically impossible to rescue more than a minor fraction of cardiac arrest victims. It is, therefore, important to be able to identify patients at high risk for sudden death and to determine what specific interventions would be effective in this population.

A. Risk-Assessment Studies

The most comprehensive assessments of factors that predict risk for future sudden death have been undertaken in populations of patients with recent myocardial infarction. In general, an adverse prognosis has been associated with laboratory or clinical findings of residual ischemia, ventricular dysfunction, and electrical instability. A number of findings have been identified as markers for chronic electrical instability. The presence of frequent or complex ventricular premature beats (VPBs) is a risk factor for sudden death after myocardial infarction. An increase in risk can be identified in patients with as few as 3–6 VPBs per hour on a 24-h ambulatory recording. Poor day-to-day reproducibility in both the frequency and patterns of spontaneous ventricular arrhythmias limits the value of this finding in individual patients. Other findings during ambulatory monitoring may be useful. A decrease in the normally observed variability in R-R intervals during ambulatory ECG monitoring is a marker for heightened adrenergic tone and an increased risk of sudden death. The signal-averaged ECG is used to detect abnormal delays of ventricular activation that would be indistinguishable from noise in a routine ECG. These late potentials (discussed earlier) are frequently seen in patients with sustained monomorphic ventricular tachycardia and are predictors of mortality in patients after myocardial infarction. Microvolt alternation in T-wave amplitude during exercise is another finding thought to be a marker of increased risk.

The usefulness of risk assessment in populations other than postmyocardial infarction patients is not well established. Signs and symptoms of heart failure, clinical evidence for increased adrenergic tone, and spontaneous arrhythmias appear to correlate with an adverse prognosis, but there are no firm values for the relative risk associated with specific findings for patients with nonischemic heart disease.

B. Primary Prevention of Sudden Death

Primary prevention of sudden death remains an elusive goal. Although many risk factors have been identified, it has been difficult to show in clinical trials that therapy directed at any single risk factor is effective. Beta-adrenergic blocking agents, cholesterol-lowering drugs, and angiotensin-converting enzyme (ACE) inhibitors have been shown to decrease both sudden and nonsudden deaths in patients with heart failure or after myocardial infarction, but these agents are not thought to treat arrhythmias in a specific fashion. Clinical trials have shown that class I antiarrhythmic drugs did not decrease sudden death mortality rates. In fact, the most definitive study—the Cardiac Arrhythmia Suppression Trial (CAST)—showed a higher mortality rate among patients who were randomized to drug therapy after it was shown that their spontaneous VPBs could be suppressed. Several studies using empirically prescribed amiodarone have reported improved survival after myocardial infarction, but the largest, placebo-controlled studies—the European and Canadian amiodarone myocardial infarction trials (EMIAT and CAMIAT)—have shown the benefit to be small, if any. Dofetilide and azimilide have been tested in patients after myocardial infarction, and dofetilide in patients with chronic heart failure. Treatment with these two drugs showed no change in mortality rates. Studies of biventricular pacing in patients with heart failure and intraventricular conduction defects are now ongoing.

Several randomized trials have indicated that ICD therapy may be of benefit. In the Multicenter Automatic Implantable Defibrillator Trial (MADIT), patients with a prior myocardial infarction, an ejection fraction (35%, and documented nonsustained ventricular tachycardia underwent electrophysiologic study. Those with inducible ventricular tachycardia that was not suppressed by intravenous procainamide were then randomly assigned to either ICD therapy or "conventional" therapy, that is, the investigator selected the drug therapy. The ICD group showed a highly significant decrease in mortality rates. The Multicenter Unsustained Tachycardia Trial (MUSTT) tested whether an electrophysiologic study was an effective predictor of risk and whether therapy guided by serial electrophysiologic studies among those with inducible ventricular tachycardia would improve survival. Patients with an inducible arrhythmia that was not specifically treated had a higher 2-year mortality likelihood than did those without an inducible arrhythmia. However, both groups had a substantial mortality rate, and although the difference between them was statistically significant, the electrophysiologic study did not clearly distinguish high- and low-risk groups. In the treatment portion of MUSTT, guided antiarrhythmic therapy did improve outcome, but all benefit was in the subgroup of treated patients who received an ICD. Amiodarone and sotalol were only rarely used in MUSTT, so this trial largely confirmed the adverse potential of class I antiarrhythmic drugs. A number of other studies involving drug therapy or ICD therapy in high-risk populations are now at or near completion. One of these—the Sudden Cardiac Death in Heart Failure Trial (SCD-HeFT)—enrolled 2500 patients with heart failure and low ejection fractions and randomly assigned them to placebo, amiodarone, or an ICD. Hopefully, the results of these studies will further clarify the role of ICD therapy in patients with heart failure treated with an aggressive regimen. The MADIT II trial enrolled coronary artery disease patients with an ejection fraction ≤ 0.30 and randomly assigned them to either ICD therapy or "conventional" antiarrhythmic therapy. Patients were not required to have either spontaneous nonsustained or inducible sustained ventricular tachycardia. In MADIT II, the ICD group had a 30% reduction in overall mortality. Additional trials are still in progress.

Other, novel approaches are also under investigation. AEDs suitable for home use by lay, family members are now being marketed. An external, wearable vest AED is now approved for use. Issues concerning the cost-effectiveness and efficient use of these strategies remain to be addressed in clinical trials.

Amiodarone Trials Meta-analysis Investigators: Effect of prophylactic amiodarone on mortality after myocardial infarction and in congestive heart failure: Meta-analysis of individual data from 6500 patients in randomized trials. Lancet 1997;350: 1417.

Antiarrhythmics versus Implantable Defibrillators (AVID) Investigators: A comparison of antiarrhythmic drug therapy with implantable defibrillators in patients resuscitated from near-fatal ventricular arrhythmias. N Engl J Med 1997;337:1576.

Bigger JT Jr: Prophylactic use of implanted cardiac defibrillators in patients at high risk for ventricular arrhythmias after coronary artery bypass graft surgery. N Engl J Med 1997;337: 1569.

Buxton AE, Lee KL, Fisher JD et al: A randomized study of the prevention of sudden death in patients with coronary artery disease. N Engl J Med 1999;341:1882.

Buxton AE, Lee KL, DiCarlo L et al: Electrophysiologic testing to identify patients with coronary artery disease who are at risk for sudden death. N Engl J Med 2000;342:1937.

Connolly SJ, Gent M, Robert S et al: Canadian Implantable Defibrillator Study (CIDS): A randomized trial of the implantable defibrillator against amiodarone. Circulation 2000;101:1297.

Eisenberg MS, Mengert TJ: Cardiac resuscitation. N Engl J Med 2001;344:1304.

Hohnloser SH, Klingenheben T, Zabel M et al: Prevalence, characteristics, and prognostic value during long-term follow-up of nonsustained ventricular tachycardia after myocardial infarction in the thrombolytic era. J Am Coll Cardiol 1999;33: 1895.

Kuck KH, Cappato R, Siebels J et al: Randomized comparison of antiarrhythmic drug therapy with implantable defibrillators in patients resuscitated from cardiac arrest: The Cardiac Arrest Study Hamburg (CASH). Circulation 2000;102:748.

Maron BJ, Shen WK, Link MS et al: Efficacy of implantable cardioverter-defibrillators for the prevention of sudden death in patients with hypertrophic cardiomyopathy. N Engl J Med 2000;342:365.

Moss AJ, Hall WJ, Cannom DS et al: Improved survival with an implanted defibrillator in patients with coronary disease at high risk for ventricular arrhythmia. N Engl J Med 1996; 335:1933.

Moss AJ, Zareba W, Hall WJ et al: Prophylactic implantation of a defibrillator in patients with myocardial infarction and reduced ejection fraction. N Engl J Med 2002;346:877.

Myerburg RM: Sudden cardiac death: Exploring the limits of our knowledge. J Cardiovasc Electrophysiol 2001;12:369.

Naccarelli GV, Wollbrette DL, Dell'Orfano JT et al: A decade of clinical trials in postmyocardial infarction, congestive heart failure, and sustained ventricular tachyarrhythmia patients: From CAST to AVID and beyond. J Cardiovasc Electrophysiol 1998;9:864.

Pacifico A, Hohnloser SH, Williams JH et al: Prevention of implantable-defibrillator shocks by treatment with sotalol. N Engl J Med 1999;340:1855.

Prior SG, Barhanin J, Hauer RN et al: Genetic and molecular basis of cardiac arrhythmias: Impact on clinical management. Circulation 1999;99:518.

Priori SG, Aliot E, Blomstrom-Lundqvist C et al: Task Force on Sudden Death of the European Society of Cardiology. Eur Heart J 2001;22:1374.

Sra J, Dahla A, Blanck Z et al: Sudden cardiac death. Curr Probl Cardiol 1999;24:461.

Takata TS, Page RL, Joglar JA: Automated external defibrillators: technical considerations and clinical promise. Ann Intern Med 2001;135:990.

de Vreede-Swagemakers JJ, Gorgels AP, Dubois-Arbouw WI et al: Out-of-hospital cardiac arrest in the 1990s: A population-based study in the Maastricht area on incidence, characteristics, and survival. J Am Coll Cardiol 1997;30:1500.

Zipes DP, Wellens HJ: Sudden cardiac death. Circulation 1998;98:2334.

Pulmonary Embolic Disease

Samuel Z. Goldhaber, MD

ESSENTIALS OF DIAGNOSIS

- *Otherwise unexplained dyspnea, tachypnea, or chest pain*
- *Clinical, ECG, or echocardiographic evidence of acute cor pulmonale*
- *Elevated plasma D-dimer ELISA*
- *Positive spiral chest CT scan with contrast*
- *High-probability ventilation-perfusion lung scan or high-probability perfusion lung scan with a normal chest radiograph*
- *Positive venous ultrasound of the legs with a convincing clinical history and suggestive lung scan*
- *Diagnostic contrast pulmonary angiogram*

General Considerations

The term venous thromboembolism (VTE) encompasses both pulmonary embolism (PE) and deep venous thrombosis (DVT) and accounts for more than 250,000 hospitalizations per year in the United States. Venous thromboembolism constitutes one of the most common causes of cardiovascular and cardiopulmonary illnesses in Western civilization. Pulmonary embolism causes or contributes to at least 50,000 deaths per year in the United States, a rate that has probably remained constant for the past three decades. For those who survive PE, further disability includes the potential development of chronic pulmonary hypertension or chronic venous insufficiency. Survivors worry whether family members are predisposed to PE. They may also wonder whether they themselves harbor an occult carcinoma. Most emotionally devastating is the psychologic burden of a potential recurrent PE after discontinuation of anticoagulation.

Etiology

"Primary" PE occurs in the absence of surgery or trauma. Patients with this condition often have an underlying hypercoagulable state, though we may not be able to identify a specific thrombophilic condition. A common scenario is a clinically silent tendency toward thrombosis, which is precipitated by a stressor such as prolonged immobilization, oral contraceptives, pregnancy, or hormone replacement therapy. Recently, there has been an increased appreciation of the risks of VTE among patients with medical illnesses, including cancer (which itself may be associated with a hypercoagulable state), congestive heart failure, and chronic obstructive pulmonary disease.

The prevalence of "secondary" PE is high among patients undergoing certain types of surgery, especially orthopedic surgery of the hip and knee, gynecologic cancer surgery, major trauma, and craniotomy for brain tumor. Pulmonary embolism in these patients may occur as late as a month after discharge from the hospital.

A. THROMBOPHILIA

Principal thrombophilic risk factors for VTE are listed in Table 25–1. The two most common genetic mutations that predispose to VTE are the factor V Leiden and the prothrombin gene. Both are autosomal-dominant. Whether factor V Leiden predisposes to recurrent VTE after anticoagulation is discontinued remains controversial. The prothrombin gene mutation is associ-

Table 25–1. Thrombophilic risk factors for venous thromboembolism.

Common
Factor V Leiden
Prothrombin gene mutation
Anticardiolipin antibodies (including lupus anticoagulant) as a feature of the antiphospholipid antibody syndrome
Hyperhomocysteinemia (usually due to folate deficiency)
Uncommon
Antithrombin III deficiency
Protein C deficiency
Protein S deficiency
Mutations of cystathionine β-synthase or methylene tetrahydrofolate reductase (MTHFR)
High concentrations of Factors VIII or XI (or both)

ated with an increased risk of recurrent VTE after discontinuation of anticoagulation, especially in patients who have coinherited the factor V Leiden mutation.

Elevated levels of homocysteine are usually easily treated with folate. The presence of anticardiolipin antibodies suggests the need for prolonged and intensive anticoagulation.

Screening for deficiencies of antithrombin III, protein C, and protein S is a low-yield strategy that produces positive findings in fewer than 5% of patients. Heparin decreases the antithrombin III level, whereas warfarin, pregnancy, and oral contraceptives decrease the protein C and S levels, thereby resulting in potentially spurious diagnoses of these hypercoagulable states.

B. WOMEN'S HEALTH

Pulmonary embolism poses a special threat for women because VTE is associated with the use of oral contraceptives, pregnancy, and hormone replacement therapy.

One third of pregnancy-related VTE occurs postpartum. The risk of DVT is present throughout pregnancy and increases during the third trimester. Of all antepartum DVT, about one fifth occur during the first trimester, one third during the second trimester, and almost half during the third trimester. After delivery, two of the most important risk factors for VTE are increased maternal age and cesarean section. Emergency cesarean section increases the VTE risk by about 50% compared with elective cesarean section.

Thrombophilia increases the risk of VTE during pregnancy and puerperium. Among women with a history of VTE during pregnancy or puerperium in one study, the prevalence of factor V Leiden was 44% and the prevalence of the prothrombin gene mutation was 17%. Compared with controls, the Leiden mutation increased the risk of VTE ninefold, and the prothrombin gene mutation increased the risk by a factor of 15. The combination of the Leiden and prothrombin gene mutations increased the VTE risk to more than 100 times that seen in the controls. Irrespective of factor V Leiden, pregnancy itself causes hypercoagulability because it induces a relative state of activated protein C resistance.

The traditional teaching was that hormone replacement therapy (HRT) did not predispose to VTE. In 1996, this assumption was shattered when three separate large data sets implicated HRT as doubling, tripling, or even quadrupling the risk of VTE. As with oral contraceptives, the risk of VTE peaks during the first year of HRT.

Daly E, Vessey MP, Hawkins MM et al: Risk of venous thromboembolism in users of hormone replacement therapy. Lancet 1996;348:977–980.

Gerhardt A, Scharf RE, Beckmann MW et al: Prothrombin and factor V mutations in women with a history of thrombosis during pregnancy and the puerperium. N Engl J Med 2000; 342:374–380.

Grodstein F, Stampfer MJ, Goldhaber SZ et al: Prospective study of exogenous hormones and risk of pulmonary embolism in women. Lancet 1996;348:983–987.

Jick H, Derby LE, Myers MW et al: Risk of hospital admission for idiopathic venous thromboembolism among users of postmenopausal oestrogens. Lancet 1996;348:981–983.

Miles JS, Miletich JP, Goldhaber SZ et al: G20210A Mutation in the prothrombin gene and the risk of recurrent venous thromboembolism. JACC 2001;37:1–4.

Nguyen A: Prothrombin G20210A polymorphism and thrombophilia. Mayo Clin Proc 2000;75:595–604.

Price DT, Ridker PM: Factor V Leiden mutation and the risks for thromboembolic disease: A clinical perspective. Ann Intern Med 1997;127:895–903.

Ridker PM, Miletich JP, Stampfer MJ et al: Factor V Leiden and risks of recurrent idiopathic venous thromboembolism. Circulation 1995;92:2800–2802.

Simioni P, Prandoni P, Lensing AWA et al: The risk of recurrent venous thromboembolism in patients with an Arg[506] (r) Gln mutation in the gene for factor V (factor V Leiden). N Engl J Med 1997;336:399–403.

Wicki J, Perrier A, Perneger TV et al: Predicting adverse outcome in patients with acute pulmonary embolism: A risk score. Thromb Haemost 2000;84:548.

Clinical Findings

Pulmonary embolism is often difficult to diagnose. Despite the availability of lung scanning, chest computed tomographic (CT) scanning, and pulmonary angiography, many emboli are not discovered until postmortem examination. Appreciation of the clinical settings that make patients susceptible to PE and maintenance of a high degree of clinical suspicion are, therefore, of paramount importance.

A. SYMPTOMS AND SIGNS

The most common symptoms or signs of PE are nonspecific: dyspnea, tachypnea, chest pain, or tachycardia. Patients with life-threatening PE are apt to have a painless presentation with dyspnea, syncope, or cyanosis. Pulmonary embolism should be suspected in hypotensive patients who have evidence of, or predisposing factors for, venous thrombosis and clinical findings of acute cor pulmonale (acute right ventricular failure), such as distended neck veins, an S_3 gallop, a right ventricular heave, tachycardia, or tachypnea.

Patients who present with severe chest pain or with hemoptysis usually have anatomically small PE near the periphery of the lung. This is where innervation is greatest and where pulmonary infarction is most likely to occur from a dearth of collateral bronchial circulation.

1. Clinical scoring systems—Traditionally, the clinical likelihood of PE has been estimated subjectively by "gestalt" as low, moderate, or high. More recently, quantitative clinical scoring systems have been devised. This new approach provides standardization and objectivity. If widely used, clinical scoring systems will improve communication among members of the health care team when they are considering the diagnosis of PE.

The Ottawa Scoring System has a maximum of 12.5 points (Table 25–2). The greatest emphasis is placed on the presence of signs or symptoms of DVT (3 points) and whether an alternative diagnosis is unlikely (3 points). If the score exceeds 4 points, the overall likelihood of PE being confirmed with imaging tests is 41%. However, if the score is 4 points or less, the likelihood of PE is only 8%. Although this scoring system has the advantage of simplicity and rapidity, it offers a somewhat subjective approach with regard to the important, heavily weighted category of "alternative diagnosis unlikely." The Geneva Scoring System is more objective but also more complex (Table 25–3).

B. DIAGNOSTIC STUDIES

1. Nonimaging studies—

a. Electrocardiography—Electrocardiography (ECG) may show evidence of acute cor pulmonale, manifested by a new $S_1 Q_3 T_3$ pattern, new incomplete right bundle branch block, or right ventricular ischemia.

b. Arterial blood gases—Neither measurement of room air arterial blood gases (Figure 25–1) nor calculation of the alveolar-arterial oxygen gradient (Figure 25–2) is useful in excluding the diagnosis of PE.

Table 25–2. Ottawa scoring system.

Signs or Symptoms	Points
Clinical signs and symptoms of DVT (minimum of leg swelling and pain with palpation of the deep veins)	3.0
An alternative diagnosis is less likely than PE	3.0
Heart rate greater than 100 bpm	1.5
Immobilization or surgery in the previous 4 weeks	1.5
Previous DVT or PE	1.5
Hemoptysis	1.0
Malignancy (on treatment, treated in the last 6 months or palliative)	1.0

DVT = deep vein thrombosis; PE = pulmonary embolism.

Source: Reprinted, with permission, from: Wells PS, Anderson DR, Rodger M, et al: Derivation of a simple clinical model to categorize patients probability of pulmonary embolism: Increasing the models utility with the SimpliRED D-dimer. Thromb Haemost 2000;83:416–420.

Among patients suspected of PE, neither test helped to differentiate patients with a confirmed PE at angiography from those with a normal pulmonary angiogram. Therefore, arterial blood gases should not be obtained as a screening test for suspected PE.

c. Plasma D-dimer enzyme-linked immunosorbent assay—Endogenous fibrinolysis, though ineffective in preventing PE, almost always causes the release of D-dimers from fibrin clot in the presence of established PE. Therefore, elevated levels of the D-dimer enzyme-linked immunosorbent assay (ELISA) serve as a highly sensitive screening test for patients suspected of PE. However, such results are not specific and are elevated in many other conditions, such as myocardial infarction, pneumonia, cancer, sepsis, or the postoperative state. Normal D-dimer ELISA levels have a high negative predictive value in patients suspected of acute PE. Among patients with a normal D-dimer level, the likelihood of no PE is approximately 95%. The combination of low clinical suspicion, ideally quantified with a validated scoring system, and a normal D-dimer ELISA, makes PE exceedingly unlikely.

d. Troponin levels—Screening for troponins is now the standard blood test for cardiac injury, and it is obtained routinely when acute myocardial infarction or unstable angina is suspected. Circulating troponin indicates irreversible myocardial cell damage and is much more sensitive than creatine kinase or its myocardial muscle isoenzyme. Cardiac markers of injury should not be used, however, as a primary diagnostic test for acute PE. Nevertheless, elevation of cardiac troponin has recently been recognized as an adverse prognostic factor in patients with acute PE. Elevated levels are associated with a markedly increased mortality rate and requirement for inotropic support and mechanical ventilation. Troponin elevation also correlates with ECG evidence of right ventricular dysfunction. This suggests that release of troponin from the myocardium during PE may result from acute right ventricular microinfarction due to pressure overload, impaired coronary artery blood flow, or hypoxemia caused by the PE.

2. Imaging studies—

a. Chest radiography—Chest radiography can help exclude diseases such as lobar pneumonia, pneumothorax, or cardiogenic pulmonary edema, which can have clinical presentations that mimic acute PE. However, patients with these disorders can also have concomitant PE.

b. Lung scanning—This study has served as the principal diagnostic imaging test for PE but is now with increasing frequency being superseded by chest CT scanning. Lung scanning is most useful when unequivocally normal or when highly suggestive of PE (Figure 25–3). Neither intermediate nor low-probability scans (in the presence of high clinical suspicion) ex-

Table 25–3. Geneva diagnostic scoring system-multivariate predictors of pulmonary emboism and development of the clinical score.

Variable	Logistic Regression Coefficients	Adjusted Odds Ratio (95% CI)	*p*	Point Score
Age, years				
60–79	0.6	1.9 (1.3–2.7)	.002	+1
≥80	1.0	2.8 (1.8–4.4)	<.001	+2
Previous PE or DVT	1.1	3.0 (2.1–4.4)	<.001	+2
Recent surgery	1.5	4.6 (2.6–8.3)	<.001	+3
Pulse rate >100/min	0.5	1.6 (1.1–2.2)	.008	+1
$Paco_2$ mm Hg				
<36 mm Hg	1.1	2.9 (1.9–4.4)	<.001	+2
36–40 mm Hg	0.6	1.9 (1.1–3.2)	.02	+1
Pao_2 mm Hg				
<50	2.0	7.2 (3.2–15.8)	<.001	+4
50–59	1.4	3.9 (2.2–6.8)	<.001	+3
60–72	1.0	2.6 (1.6–4.2)	<.001	+2
73–82	0.6	1.8 (1.1–2.9)	.03	+1
Chest radiograph				
Platelike atelectasis	0.7	1.9 (1.3–2.9)	.001	+1
Elevation of hemidiaphragm	0.5	1.6 (1.1–2.4)	.02	+1

Source: Adapted, with permission, from: Wicki J, Perneger TV, Junod AF, et al: Assessing clinical probability of pulmonary embolism in the emergency ward: A simple score. Arch Intern Med 2001;161:92–97.

clude PE. For example, with the combination of a low-probability scan and high clinical suspicion for PE, the likelihood of PE is 40%. When lung scanning is performed, the ventilation scan is being used less frequently than previously because its contribution to the diagnostic decision is only marginally better than the combination of a perfusion scan and chest radiograph.

c. Chest computed tomographic scanning—The chest CT is diagnostic of PE when an intraluminal pulmonary arterial filling defect is surrounded by contrast material. Computed tomographic scanning has two major advantages over lung scanning: (1) direct visualization of thrombus, and (2) establishing alternative diagnoses on CT images of the lung parenchyma that are not evident on chest film.

Conventional chest CT scanning relies on imaging a series of consecutive sections of the chest. With the introduction of spiral chest CT scanning, patients can

now be scanned continually. As patients are advanced through the spiral CT scanner, the x-ray source and single-row detector array rotate around them. These scans are performed during a single breath-hold, thereby eliminating respiratory motion artifact that previously limited thoracic imaging. Overlap data from adjacent slices are acquired, thus reducing the possibility of missed pathology. Scans are performed in less than 30 s; excellent vascular opacification of the pulmonary arteries with contrast agent can usually be achieved (Figure 25–4). However, the major limitation has been failure to detect PEs beyond third-order pulmonary arterial branches.

Further innovations occurred with the introduction of multirow detector CT scanners, which are replacing single-row detectors. This newer technology permits four slices to be acquired simultaneously during each rotation of the x-ray source. Resolution is improved from

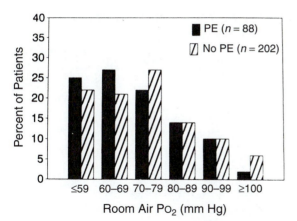

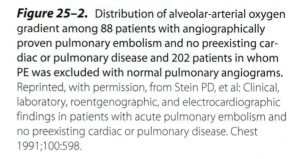

Figure 25–1. Distribution of partial pressure of oxygen in arterial blood (Po_2) while breathing room air. The group included 88 patients with angiographically proven pulmonary embolism and no preexisting cardiac or pulmonary disease and 202 patients in whom PE was excluded with normal pulmonary angiograms. Reprinted, with permission, from Stein PD, et al: Clinical, laboratory, roentgenographic, and electrocardiographic findings in patients with acute pulmonary embolism and no preexisting cardiac or pulmonary disease. Chest 1991;100:598.

Figure 25–2. Distribution of alveolar-arterial oxygen gradient among 88 patients with angiographically proven pulmonary embolism and no preexisting cardiac or pulmonary disease and 202 patients in whom PE was excluded with normal pulmonary angiograms. Reprinted, with permission, from Stein PD, et al: Clinical, laboratory, roentgenographic, and electrocardiographic findings in patients with acute pulmonary embolism and no preexisting cardiac or pulmonary disease. Chest 1991;100:598.

5 mm to 1.25 mm. Subsegmental vessels can generally be well visualized with multirow detector scanners. Compared with conventional spiral CT, the sensitivity of multirow detector scanners for the diagnosis of acute PE increases from about 70% to more than 90%. Fewer motion artifacts occur because the gantry rotates around

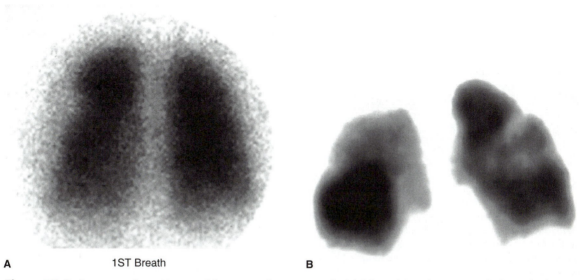

A   1ST Breath   **B**

Figure 25–3. Lung scan for a 63-year-old woman who presented with idiopathic pulmonary embolism. The lung scan showed **A:** normal ventilation and **B:** multiple segmental perfusion defects, indicating a ventilator perfusion mismatch and high probability of pulmonary embolism.

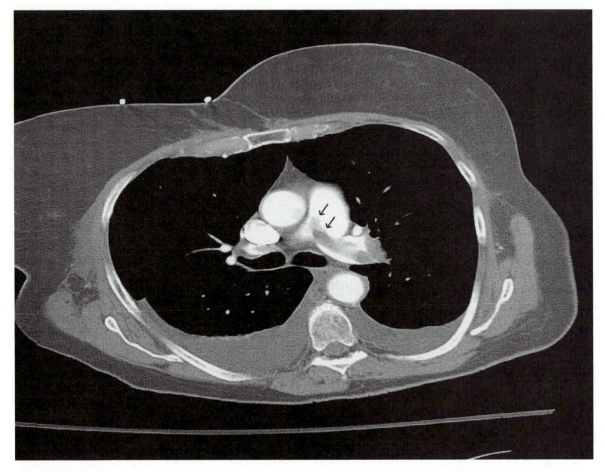

Figure 25–4. Spiral computed tomography scan of massive bilateral pulmonary arterial filling defects *(arrows)* in the main pulmonary arteries of a 72-year-old woman who suffered acute pulmonary embolism after general surgery.

the patient in less than 1 s; the total examination time can be eight times faster than with single-row detector systems. With these newer scanners, the combination of shorter scan times, narrow collimation, and narrow reconstruction intervals greatly enhances accuracy.

d. Venous ultrasonography—In combination with color Doppler imaging, venous ultrasonography is known as duplex sonography and is the principal diagnostic imaging test for suspected acute DVT. Sonographic evaluation employs compression ultrasound along the full length of the femoral, popliteal, and calf veins. The transducer is held transverse to the vein and, normally, the vein collapses with gentle manual compression. The compressed vein appears as if it is winking. The main criterion for diagnosing DVT is lack of compression of a deep vein. This diagnosis can be confirmed by direct visualization of thrombus on ultrasound or by abnormal venous flow on Doppler exami-

nation (eg, loss of physiologic respiratory variation or loss of the expected augmentation of blood flow during calf compression).

Among symptomatic patients, duplex sonography is very accurate, with high sensitivity and specificity. Its sensitivity decreases when assessing asymptomatic patients. Major limitations include an inability to image directly pelvic vein thrombosis and difficulty diagnosing an acute DVT superimposed upon a chronic one. Magnetic resonance imaging may be useful under these circumstances.

Importantly, many PE patients do not have evidence of leg DVT, probably because the thrombus has already embolized to the pulmonary arteries. Therefore, if the clinical suspicion of PE is high, patients without imaging evidence of DVT have not necessarily been ruled out for PE.

e. Echocardiography—Echocardiography should not be used routinely to diagnose suspected PE because the majority of PE patients have normal echocardiograms. However, the echocardiogram, like the troponin level, is an excellent tool for risk stratification and prognostication. Echocardiography is useful diagnostically when the differential diagnosis includes pericardial tamponade, right ventricular infarction, and dissection of the aorta, as well as PE.

Imaging a normal left ventricle in the presence of a dilated, hypokinetic right ventricle strongly suggests the diagnosis of PE (Figure 25–5). Echocardiographic findings in PE patients are listed in Table 25–4. Despite moderate or severe right ventricular free-wall hypokinesis, PE patients with abnormal echocardiograms often have relatively normal contraction and sparing of the right ventricular apex. This finding has become widely known as McConnell's sign and helps to distinguish between right ventricular dysfunction due to PE and dysfunction due to other conditions such as primary pulmonary hypertension.

The pulmonary arterial systolic pressure can be estimated by measuring the peak velocity of the tricuspid regurgitant jet obtained with Doppler echocardiography. The gradient across the tricuspid valve can be estimated by using the modified Bernoulli equation, $P = 4V^2$, where V is the peak velocity of the regurgitant jet, and P represents the peak pressure difference between the right atrium and right ventricle. The estimated right atrial pressure is added to the gradient to obtain an estimate of pulmonary arterial systolic pressure.

Transesophageal echocardiography for suspected PE is best reserved for critically ill patients. Transesophageal echocardiography diagnoses PE by direct visualization of thrombus, assesses its extent, and provides guidance regarding its surgical accessibility. Transesophageal echocardiography may also have a valuable role in detecting unexplained sudden cardiac arrest and pulseless electrical activity due to acute PE. Pulmonary embolism represented 5% of those who presented with cardiac arrest in a series of 1246 patients in Vienna. Of those with PE, 63% presented with pulseless electrical activity. Therefore, occult PE should be considered when patients present with pulseless electrical activity.

f. Pulmonary angiography—This imaging method is rapidly becoming a lost art and is being undertaken primarily for therapeutic interventions (such as suction catheter embolectomy) rather than to solve diagnostic dilemmas. Most diagnostic questions can be resolved with the new generation chest CT scanners, which provide resolution to subsegmental branches. A constant intraluminal filling defect seen in more than one projection is the most reliable angiographic diagnostic feature for PE.

This procedure can almost always be accomplished safely. Selective angiography should be performed, with the equivocal portion of the perfusion lung scan or chest CT scan serving as a road map. To avoid damaging the intima of the pulmonary artery, soft, flexible

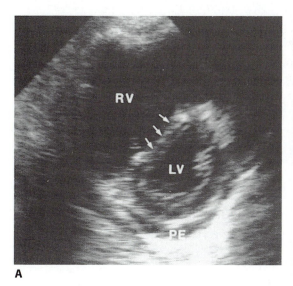 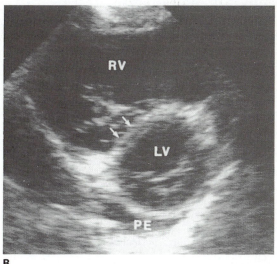

A   **B**

Figure 25–5. Parasternal short-axis views of the right ventricle (RV) and left ventricle (LV) in **A:** diastole and **B:** systole. Diastolic and systolic bowing of the interventricular septum *(arrows)* into the left ventricle is evident, which is compatible with right ventricular volume and pressure overloads, respectively. The right ventricle is appreciably dilatated and markedly hypokinetic, with little change in apparent right ventricular area from diastole to systole. PE = small pericardial effusion. Reprinted, with permission, from Come PC: Echocardiographic evaluation of pulmonary embolism and its response to therapeutic interventions. Chest 1992;101[Suppl]:151S.

Table 25–4. Abnormal echocardiographic findings in pulmonary embolism.

Abnormal Finding	Description
Right ventricular dilatation and hypokinesis	Associated with leftward septal shift; the ratio of the RVEDA to LVEDA exceeds the upper limit of normal (0.6). Associated with right atrial enlargement and tricuspid regurgitation.
Septal flattening and paradoxical septal motion	Right ventricular contraction continues even after the left ventricle starts relaxing at end-systole; therefore, the interventricular septum bulges toward the left ventricle.
Diastolic left ventricular impairment with a small difference between left ventricular area during diastole and systole, indicative of low cardiac output	Due to septal displacement and reduced left ventricular distensibility during diastole; consequently, Doppler mitral flow exhibits a prominent A wave, much higher than the E wave, with an increased contribution of atrial contraction to left ventricular filling.
Direct visualization of PE	Only if PE is large and centrally located; much more easily visualized on transesophageal than on transthoracic echocardiography.
Pulmonary arterial hypertension detected by Doppler flow velocity in the right ventricular outflow tract	Shortened acceleration time, with peak velocity occurring close to the onset of ejection. Biphasic ejection curve, with midsystolic reduction in velocity.
Right ventricular hypertrophy	With mildly increased right ventricular thickness (often about 6 mm, with 4 mm as upper limit of normal); clear visualization of right ventricular muscle trabeculations.
Patent foramen ovale	When right atrial pressure exceeds left atrial presure, the foramen ovale may open and cause worsening hypoxemia or stroke.

LVEDA = left ventricular end-diastolic area; PE = pulmonary embolism; RVEDA = right ventricular end-diastolic area.

catheters with side holes should be used, rather than stiff catheters with end holes. Low-osmolar contrast agents minimize the transient hypotension, heat, and coughing that often occur with conventional radioactive contrast agents.

3. Integrated diagnostic approach—I favor an integrated diagnostic approach for cases of suspected PE (Figure 25–6). The diagnostic work-up should begin by quantifying the clinical suspicion with a precise clinical scoring algorithm. If the patient has no obvious acute comorbid illnesses, such as acute myocardial infarction, metastatic cancer, sepsis, or recent surgery, then a plasma D-dimer level should be obtained. If the D-dimer ELISA is normal, then the diagnosis of PE is almost always excluded. To pursue the diagnosis of PE with imaging tests, chest CT scanning is the single most useful exam, but a normal lung scan is also very reliable. If a diagnostic dilemma persists because of an equivocal chest CT scan, then venous ultrasonography of the legs can be undertaken. If the ultrasound is negative and the clinical suspicion remains very high, then pulmonary angiography is indicated.

Giannitsis E, Muller-Bardorff M, Kurowski V et al: Independent prognostic value of cardiac troponin T in patients with confirmed pulmonary embolism. Circulation 2000;102:211–217.

Kürkciyan I, Meron G, Sterz F et al: Pulmonary embolism as cause of cardiac arrest: Presentation and outcome. Arch Intern Med 2000;160:1529–1535.

McConnell MV, Solomon SD, Rayan ME et al: Regional right ventricular dysfunction detected by echocardiography in acute pulmonary embolism. Am J Cardiol 1996;78:469–473.

Meyer T, Binder L, Hruska N et al: Cardiac troponin I elevation in acute pulmonary embolism is associated with right ventricular dysfunction. J Am Coll Cardiol 2000;36:1632–1636.

Pattynama PMT, Kuiper JW: Second-generation, subsecond multislice computed-tomography: Advancing the role of helical CT pulmonary angiography in suspected pulmonary embolism. Semin Vasc Med 2001;1:195–203.

Wells PS, Anderson DR, Rodger M et al: Derivation of a simple clinical model to categorize patients probability of pulmonary embolism: Increasing the models utility with the SimpliRED D-dimer. Thromb Haemost 2000;83:416–420.

Wicki J, Perneger TV, Junod AF et al: Assessing clinical probability of pulmonary embolism in the emergency ward: A simple score. Arch Intern Med 2001;161:92–97.

Management

A. Risk Stratification

Not all PEs are created equal. The most important concept in PE management is that acute PE spans a wide range of risk, from small asymptomatic emboli to massive thromboembolism with catastrophic cardiovascular

Brigham and Women's Hospital Integrated Approach

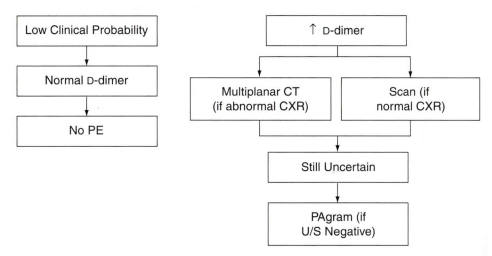

Figure 25–6. Strategy for diagnosing pulmonary embolism. CT = computed tomographic scan; CXR = chest x-ray film; PAgram = pulmonary angiogram; PE = pulmonary embolism; U/S = ultrasound.

collapse and death due to right ventricular failure. Therapy must be geared to patient risk. Low-risk patients will do well with anticoagulation alone, whereas high-risk patients will require thrombolysis or embolectomy in addition to anticoagulation.

Investigators in Geneva have developed a clinical risk score to predict adverse outcomes after PE (Tables 25–5 and 25–6). The maximum number of points, based on clinical parameters, is 8. Those patients scoring 5 or more points had a more than 50% likelihood of a major adverse clinical event, such as recurrent thromboembolism, major bleeding, or death. Other nonimaging markers of poor prognosis include hypoxemia despite oxygen, physical examination evidence (accentuated pulmonic component of the second heart sound or left parasternal heave, or distended neck veins) of pulmonary hypertension or right ventricular strain, or an elevated troponin level.

The most important imaging test for risk stratification is echocardiographic assessment of right ventricular function. In a cohort of 209 consecutive PE patients, 65 (31%) presented with the combination of normal systemic arterial pressure and echocardiographic evidence of right ventricular dysfunction. Of this group, 6 (10%) developed cardiogenic shock within 24 h of diagnosis and 3 (5%) died during the initial hospitalization. Conversely, none of the 97 normotensive patients with normal right ventricular function on echocardiography died from PE.

Pulmonary hypertension, as estimated by Doppler echocardiography, that persists for more than 5 weeks after the diagnosis of PE is associated with an adverse long-term prognosis. In a study of 78 PE patients followed prospectively, those who had persistent pulmonary hypertension and right ventricular dysfunction were nine times more likely to die during the ensuing 5 years than those whose pulmonary arterial pressures and right ventricular function had normalized.

Table 25–5. Geneva point score to assess pulmonary embolism prognosis.

Variable	Point Score
Cancer	+2
Heart failure	+1
Prior DVT	+1
Hypotension	+2
Hypoxemia	+1
DVT on ultrasound	+1

DVT = deep vein thrombosis.

Source: Reprinted, with permission, from: Wicki J, Perrier A, Perneger TV, et al: Predicting adverse outcome in patients with acute pulmonary embolism: A risk score. Thromb Haemost 2000;84:548–552.

B. TREATMENT

1. Unfractionated and low-molecular-weight heparins—Unfractionated heparin and low-molecular-weight heparins are used for 5–7 days in the initial

Table 25–6. Geneva adverse outcome score.

Number of Points	Number of Patients	Cumulative %	Percent of Patients with Adverse Outcome (*n*)
0	52	19.4	0 (0)
1	79	48.9	2.5 (2)
2	49	67.2	4.1 (2)
3	56	88.1	17.8 (10)
4	22	96.3	27.3 (6)
5	7	98.9	57.1 (4)
6	3	100	1 00 (3)

Source: Reprinted with permission from: Wicki J, Perrier A, Perneger TV, et al: Predicting adverse outcome in patients with acute pulmonary embolism: A risk score. Thromb Haemost 2000;84:548–552.

treatment of PE and are continued until a therapeutic effect has been achieved with oral anticoagulants such as warfarin. Although unfractionated heparin has served as the standard foundation of PE treatment for more than 40 years, this anticoagulant has important limitations. Its variable protein binding leads to an often unpredictable dose response and makes it a drug that is difficult to administer properly in everyday clinical practice. Subtherapeutic levels of heparin increase the risk of recurrent PE; excessive levels of heparin increase the risk of major bleeding.

Unfractionated heparin for PE treatment is usually ordered as an intravenous bolus followed by a continuous intravenous infusion. The required dose is unpredictable and must be adjusted according to the activated partial thromboplastin time, which is not well standardized among different hospital laboratories. In general, the target partial thromboplastin time is 60–80 s. Heparin can be dosed by weight-based nomograms,

but none of the nomograms provides a consistent dose response. An alternative approach is to initiate administration of unfractionated heparin in an arbitrary dosing regimen of 5000–10,000 U as a bolus, followed by 1250 U/h. At Brigham and Women's Hospital in Boston, we have implemented a weight-based nomogram for using unfractionated heparin to treat PE or DVT and have incorporated it into our computerized order entry system (Table 25–7).

Low-molecular-weight heparins have revolutionized the initial management of venous thromboembolism (Table 25-8). They have a much more predictable dose response than unfractionated heparin and can usually be administered on the basis of weight alone, without any blood testing to modify the dose. The only exceptions occur in cases of renal insufficiency and massive obesity, for which we have developed a weight-based nomogram at Brigham and Women's Hospital (Table 25–9). Low-molecular-weight heparins appear to be

Table 25–7. Unfractionated heparin weight-based nomogram for acute venous thromboembolism.

PTT	Repeat Bolus	Stop Infusion (min)	Rate Change	Repeat PTT (h)
<35	70 units/kg[a]	0	Increase 3 units/kg/h	6
35–59	35 units/kg[b]	0	Increase 2 units/kg/h	6
60–80 target	0	0	No change	6
81–100	0	0	Decrease 2 units/kg/h	6
>100	0	60	Decrease 3 units/kg/h	6

[a] Maximum bolus 10,000 units.

[b] Maximum bolus 5000 units.

PTT = activated partial thromboplastin time; measured in seconds.

Table 25–8. Comparison of unfractionated heparin versus low-molecular-weight heparin.

Characteristic	UFH	LMWH
Molecular weight (average in daltons)	15,000	5,000
Ratio of anti-Xa to anti-IIa (thrombin) activity	1	>1
Metabolism	Hepatic	Renal
Bioavailability	Fair	Excellent
Frequency of subcutaneous administration	X2–X3/day	X1–X2/day
Frequency of heparin-induced thrombocytopenia	1–2%	0.1–0.2%
Osteoporosis after prolonged exposure	Rare	Very rare
Laboratory assay of anticoagulant effect	Activated partial thromboplastin time	Anti-Xa level
Reversal of anticoagulant effect	Protamine	Protamine
Spinal or epidural anesthesia	OK	Heed the FDA warning

safer than unfractionated heparin because osteopenia and heparin-induced thrombocytopenia occur far less often than with unfractionated heparin.

In the United States, two low-molecular-weight heparins are approved for treatment of patients who present with symptomatic DVT, with or without (asymptomatic) PE: enoxaparin and tinzaparin (Table 25–10).

2. Treatment for deep vein thrombosis—The use of low-molecular-weight heparins to treat DVT has dramatically converted the therapy of this illness from a 5- to 6-day hospitalization to primarily outpatient or overnight in-hospital management. The FDA-approved outpatient therapy for DVT with the low-molecular weight-heparin, enoxaparin 1 mg/kg bid, is based on the landmark randomized trial of Levine and colleagues.

These Canadian investigators assigned patients either to enoxaparin 1 mg/kg bid, often with no hospitalization or with an overnight admission, versus a conventional 5- to 7-day intravenous regimen of unfractionated heparin as a "bridge" to warfarin. They found no significant differences in such adverse outcomes as recurrent venous thromboembolism or major bleeding. However, those patients randomly assigned to enoxaparin had an average hospital length of stay of 1 day compared with patients treated with unfractionated heparin whose average hospital stay was 6 days. Based on a separate inpatient trial of DVT treatment, the FDA also approved enoxaparin in the once daily dose of 1.5 mg/kg.

By converting uncomplicated DVT to an outpatient illness or one that merely requires overnight admission, hospital beds can be set aside for the care of more

Table 25–9. Low-molecular-weight heparin weight-based nomogram for enoxaparin in the presence of renal insufficiency or marked obesity.

Renal Insufficiency Creatinine Clearance (mL/min)	Enoxaparin Dose	Anti-Xa Monitoring (Heparin Level)*
>70	1 mg/kg q12h	None
35–69	0.75 mg/kg q12h	3–6 h after the third injection
<35	1 mg/kg q24h	3–6 h after the third injection
Obese Weight	**Enoxaparin Dose**	**Anti-Xa Monitoring (Heparin Level)***
<100 kg	1 mg/kg q12h	None
100–130 kg	1 mg/kg q12h	3–6 h after the first injection
>130 kg	130 mg q12h	3–6 h after the first injection

*Therapeutic level is 0.5–1.0 units/ml.

Table 25–10. FDA-approved low-molecular-weight heparins for the initial treatment of DVT (with or without asymptomatic PE).

Enoxaparin 1 mg/kg twice daily
Enoxaparin 1.5 mg/kg once daily
Tinzaparin 175 U/kg once daily

acutely ill patients. With the establishment of a hospital-based outpatient treatment program, even diverse inner-city patients with DVT can be cared for with a low incidence of adverse events. This approach requires the infrastructure of a centralized anticoagulation service, usually staffed by a nurse or pharmacist who is supervised by a physician.

In a meta-analysis of randomized DVT treatment trials comparing low-molecular-weight heparins with unfractionated heparin, low-molecular-weight heparins were found to be more effective and safer. Their use resulted in fewer recurrent thromboemboli, less bleeding, less thrombocytopenia, and an improved quality of life and patient satisfaction. The strategy of using low-molecular-weight heparins was also more cost-effective.

3. Pulmonary embolism treatment—In an inpatient trial, patients who presented with symptomatic PE but who did not require thrombolytic therapy were randomized to subcutaneous injection of once daily tinzaparin 175 U/kg versus continuous intravenous unfractionated heparin as a bridge to oral anticoagulation. Both groups of patients were hospitalized for an average of 1 week. Those receiving once daily tinzaparin had no significant difference in outcome compared with those receiving continuous intravenous unfractionated heparin. The FDA has not approved any low-molecular-weight heparin for patients presenting primarily with symptomatic PE.

a. Warfarin—Although warfarin is the standard oral anticoagulant used in the United States, it is limited by a narrow therapeutic index. Too little anticoagulant effect leads to thromboembolism, and excessive anticoagulation leads to bleeding. The drug is plagued by a long list of interactions with other drugs that either decrease or increase warfarin's anticoagulant effect. The consumption of vitamin K-containing foods such as green leafy vegetables decreases the anticoagulant effect, whereas the ingestion of alcohol increases the likelihood of hemorrhage.

Warfarin dosing is adjusted according to a standardized prothrombin time by using the International Normalized Ratio (INR). For PE and DVT, the target INR is ordinarily between 2.0 and 3.0.

Recently, several advances facilitated optimal warfarin dosing. First, it has become evident that aceta-

minophen in high doses makes an unintended increase in the INR more likely. Second, we now initiate warfarin in a dose of about 5 mg once daily for an ordinary sized adult, rather than initiating much higher loading doses. Third, we are now aware that 2–3% of patients have a genetic mutation that results in slow metabolism of warfarin. We therefore test the INR after several doses of warfarin, rather than waiting for 5 days after initiation of therapy. Finally, for patients who require lifelong anticoagulation, we consider prescribing point-of-care INR testing machines used at home. Patients obtain a drop of their own blood by finger stick puncture. We then train them to self-adjust their warfarin doses, based on the results of the INR.

b. Reversal of warfarin—When the INR exceeds 5.0 in the absence of clinical bleeding, we hold further warfarin doses and administer oral vitamin K, usually in a dose of 2.5 mg. We prefer to administer vitamin K orally, but we give it subcutaneously for those patients whose gastrointestinal absorption is uncertain. This strategy replaces the previous classic teaching in which patients were prescribed 10 mg of subcutaneous vitamin K, often for three consecutive days. This approach, now abandoned, effectively reversed warfarin but created resistance to resumption of anticoagulation for at least the ensuing week.

Occasionally, patients will require immediate reversal of excessive anticoagulation. This can be accomplished by the emergency administration of fresh frozen plasma, usually two units. However, to ensure continued reversal, vitamin K should be administered concomitantly.

c. Optimal duration of anticoagulation—The optimal duration of anticoagulation for patients with acute PE remains extremely controversial, especially for patients with idiopathic PE that occurs without relation to cancer, surgery, or trauma. Schulman and coworkers found that 6 months of oral anticoagulation after PE halved the recurrence rate over the ensuing 2 years, compared with a strategy of 6 weeks of anticoagulation. Consequently, 6 months of anticoagulation is the usual duration of therapy under these circumstances. However, in a provocative study by Kearon and colleagues, patients with venous thromboembolism were randomized to 3 months or to 2 years of anticoagulation. The trial was stopped early because of the markedly lower rate of recurrence in the group receiving prolonged anticoagulation. With an average follow-up period of 10 months, there were 17 recurrences among those on the 3-month regimen compared with one event among those receiving long-term anticoagulation.

A more recent randomized trial of 736 DVT patients found that shortened duration of anticoagulation appeared effective and safe in patients who had no predisposing risk factors for recurrence. After 1 year of follow-up, it seemed that patients with isolated calf DVT could be treated with 6 weeks rather than 3 months of anticoagulation. Patients with proximal DVT were effectively treated with 3 months rather than 6 months of anticoagulation.

However, prolonged anticoagulation may simply forestall but not prevent a recurrent thrombosis. Furthermore, the increased bleeding with prolonged anticoagulation may negate any potential benefit of fewer recurrences. In the Warfarin Optimal Duration Italian Trial (WODIT) by Agnelli and colleagues, 267 patients with idiopathic proximal DVT were randomized to either 3 or 12 months of anticoagulation. They were followed clinically for at least 2 years. The mortality and recurrence rates were the same in both groups. The average time to recurrence was 11 months among patients who received 3 months of anticoagulation, compared with 16 months in the group that received 12 months of anticoagulation. Importantly, 3% of patients receiving 12 months of anticoagulation had major nonfatal bleeding during the fourth through twelfth month of therapy. Thus, in WODIT, extending the 3-month course of anticoagulation to 1 year was not associated with long-term net clinical benefit.

It is possible that a lower intensity of anticoagulation therapy, after the initial phase of full-dose warfarin, might reduce bleeding complications associated with a long-term regimen and yet maintain a low frequency of recurrent events. To test this hypothesis, the NIH-sponsored Prevention of Recurrent Venous Thromboembolism (PREVENT) Trial is evaluating the efficacy of prolonged treatment with low-intensity warfarin to prevent recurrent events. Patients with a history of documented idiopathic venous thrombosis who have completed a standard course of anticoagulation are being enrolled in an ongoing randomized, double-blind, placebo-controlled trial comparing low-intensity anticoagulation and a target INR of 1.5 to 2.0, to usual care without anticoagulants. Trial end-points include recurrent VTE, major bleeding, and death from all causes. So far, more than 500 patients have been enrolled in this NIH-sponsored trial. Follow-up will take place for at least 4 years. For additional information and potential enrollment of patients, please contact me at sgoldhaber@partners.org.

In summary, despite the high rate of recurrent venous thrombosis after discontinuation of anticoagulation, there are currently insufficient data to recommend indefinite warfarin therapy following an initial acute PE. Clinical trials are under way to test the strategy of prolonged anticoagulation, particularly with less than standard intensity of anticoagulation. The hope is that this approach will reduce both recurrent events and hemorrhagic risk associated with long-term anticoagulation. Further research will be required to identify those

patients prospectively who are at highest risk of recurrence after discontinuation of anticoagulation.

d. Thrombolysis—PE thrombolysis remains a debatable indication because large clinical trials using survival as an end-point have not been carried out. A definitive clinical trial is long overdue. Nevertheless, successful thrombolysis usually reverses right heart failure rapidly and safely, thereby preventing a downhill spiral of cardiogenic shock. Thrombolysis may also prevent chronic pulmonary hypertension over the long term and thus improve exercise tolerance and quality of life. It is certain that thrombolysis should be considered only for those patients at high risk of an adverse clinical outcome with anticoagulation alone. Although no precise indications currently exist in the absence of massive PE with cardiogenic shock, the clinician should be wary of conservative management in the presence of risk factors for a poor prognosis (Table 25–11).

For patients with massive PE and cardiogenic shock, thrombolysis can be life-saving. In a small clinical trial, patients with hypotension and heart failure due to PE were randomized to thrombolysis (streptokinase 1,500,000 U administered over 1 h) plus anticoagulation versus anticoagulation alone. The trial was stopped after the first 8 of a planned 40 patients were enrolled, because all 4 patients allocated to the anticoagulation alone group died; in contrast, the 4 patients who received thrombolysis all survived. Of the four patients who died, three underwent postmortem examination and had right ventricular myocardial infarction (without significant coronary arterial obstruction) in addition to massive PE. Thus, this small trial, consisting of only eight patients, is the sole investigation

Table 25–11. Pulmonary embolism patients at high risk (in the absence of systemic arterial hypotension and cardiogenic shock).

Physical findings of right ventricular dysfunction (eg, distended neck veins, accentuated P_2, tricuspid regurgitation murmur)

Electrocardiographic manifestations of right ventricular strain (eg, new right bundle branch block, new T wave inversion in leads V_1–V_4)

Right ventricular dilatation and dyskinesis on echocardiogram

Patent foramen ovale

Free-floating right-heart thrombi

Doppler echocardiographic pulmonary arterial systolic pressure >50 mm Hg

Elevated troponin level

Age >70 years

Cancer

Congestive heart failure

Chronic obstructive pulmonary disease

demonstrating that thrombolysis reduces the likelihood of mortality from PE; the presumed mechanism is rapid reversal of the right heart failure that is causing cardiogenic shock.

We tested the hypothesis that among hemodynamically stable PE patients, recombinant tissue-type plasminogen activator (rt-PA) followed by anticoagulation accelerates the improvement of right ventricular function and pulmonary perfusion more rapidly than anticoagulation alone. In this multicenter controlled trial, 101 patients were randomized: 46 to rt-PA 100 mg/2h followed by heparin and 55 to heparin alone.

No clinical episodes of recurrent PE occurred among rt-PA patients, but there five (two fatal and three nonfatal) clinically suspected recurrent PEs occurred within 14 days in patients randomized to heparin alone ($P = .06$). All five presented initially with right ventricular hypokinesis on echocardiogram, despite normal systemic arterial pressure at baseline. Thus, echocardiography helps identify a subgroup of PE patients with impending right ventricular failure who appear to be at high risk of adverse clinical outcomes if treated with heparin alone.

Right ventricular wall motion was assessed qualitatively, and the right ventricular end-diastolic area from the apical four-chamber view was planimetered on serial echocardiograms at baseline, 3 h, and 24 h. At baseline, slightly more than half of the patients with PE had entirely normal right ventricular function. Qualitative assessment of right ventricular wall motion at baseline versus 24 h later demonstrated that 39% of the rt-PA patients improved and 2.4% worsened, compared with 17% improvement and 17% worsening among those who received heparin alone ($P = .005$). Quantitative assessment showed that rt-PA patients had a significant decrease in the right ventricular end-diastolic area, indicating improved right ventricular function, during the 24 h after randomization, compared with none among those allocated to heparin alone ($P = .01$).

With respect to complications, one patient who was randomized to heparin suffered a fatal recurrent PE and during resuscitation was given rt-PA off protocol, which resulted in a nonfatal intracranial bleed. She had fallen on her head when she initially presented with syncope and should have been excluded from the trial. Three rt-PA patients received blood transfusions: two for augmentation of hematocrit and one for groin puncture site bleeding. One patient on the heparin alone protocol received a blood transfusion for augmentation of hematocrit. A second patient on the same protocol had a more than 10-point decrement in hematocrit, which was ascribed to rectal bleeding.

Recently, Nass and colleagues showed quantitatively that most patients who receive thrombolytic therapy for PE achieve recovery of regional as well as global right ventricular function. At baseline, right ventricular areas were significantly larger than normal at end-diastole and at end-systole. Diastolic and systolic right ventricular areas decreased after thrombolysis. The area of the right ventricle most severely affected (and most improved after therapy) was the mid-right ventricular free wall.

e. Embolectomy—Patients at high risk for an adverse outcome with anticoagulation alone should be considered for embolectomy if they have contraindications to thrombolytic therapy. Embolectomy can be performed as a catheter-based procedure in the interventional laboratory or in the operating room. Catheter embolectomy has a very limited application because it cannot successfully remove large amounts of thrombus, due to limitations in available catheter devices.

Surgical embolectomy for acute PE is an entirely different operation from embolectomy for chronic thromboembolic pulmonary hypertension. Embolectomy for acute PE should be considered for patients who would otherwise receive thrombolytic therapy but who have contraindications to this treatment modality. The operation is best performed on a warm beating heart with continuous transesophageal echocardiographic monitoring, after performing a median sternotomy and placing the patient on cardiopulmonary bypass. The embolus should be removed under direct visualization, never "blindly." With experience, all lobar and most segmental pulmonary artery branches can be visualized. It is crucial to refer high-risk PE patients as soon as their prognosis with anticoagulation has been established. Taking a "watch and wait" approach and delaying referring until the onset of cardiogenic shock requiring pressors yields poor results. At Brigham and Women's Hospital, we have formed an interdisciplinary clinical team to evaluate and refer patients for open surgical embolectomy. Within the past 2 years, we have performed 29 emergency embolectomies, with a survival rate of 89%.

To manage severe chronic pulmonary thromboembolic hypertension due to prior PE, a separate and more technically challenging operation can be performed, a pulmonary thromboendarterectomy. Patients requiring this surgery may be virtually bedridden with breathlessness caused by high pulmonary arterial pressures. If successful, this operation can reduce and possibly cure pulmonary hypertension. This surgery requires dissecting the old thrombus, which has turned whitish and hardened, from the walls of the pulmonary arteries. Complications include pulmonary arterial perforation and hemorrhage; pulmonary steal syndrome, in which blood rushes from previously well-perfused lung tissue to newly perfused tissue; and reperfusion pulmonary edema. For patients who are not candidates for pulmonary thromboendarterectomy, balloon pulmonary angioplasty can be considered.

f. Inferior vena caval filters—There are two indications for placing an inferior vena caval filter for patients with acute PE: (1) major bleeding requiring transfusion or any intracranial hemorrhage, (2) recurrent PE despite prolonged intensive anticoagulation. Though filters reduce the frequency of PE, they do not halt the thrombotic process and are associated with a doubling of the rate of DVT.

g. Adjunctive measures—Occasionally, PE patients will develop respiratory failure and will require ventilatory assistance. Such patients, along with the rare patient who requires pulmonary artery catheterization to determine optimal fluid management, need to be placed in an intensive care unit. The vast majority of patients with acute PE, however, can be cared for in an intermediate care or step-down unit. Most will benefit from supplemental oxygen. Narcotics usually do not relieve the chest discomfort that they may be experiencing. Nonsteroidal antiinflammatory agents are often effective, and combining them with anticoagulation usually does not pose an undue risk of bleeding complications.

Pulmonary embolism patients with concomitant DVT of the leg should wear below-knee graduated compression stockings (ideally 30–40 mm Hg or, if not tolerated, 20–30 mm Hg) to provide leg support while ambulating. The stockings help prevent distention of the vein wall and may mitigate the syndrome of chronic venous insufficiency—most often characterized by leg swelling and discomfort—that the majority of DVT patients experience.

Although PE can be as devastating emotionally and physically as myocardial infarction, the burden on individual patients may be even greater because the general public does not have as good an understanding of PE, particularly in terms of the potential incomplete recovery from it and long-term disability it engenders. Young patients with PE repeatedly voice a common theme. Although they appear healthy, they have actually suffered a life-threatening illness. Because of their youth and healthy appearance, however, they may find family and friends unable to empathize with their fears and feelings about the illness.

Virtually all patients with PE will wonder why they were stricken with the illness and whether they harbor an underlying coagulopathy (or "bad" gene) that predisposed them. When anticoagulation is discontinued after an adequate course of therapy, patients are often fearful of recurrent PE. Physicians can ease the emotional burden of PE by taking the time to discuss the implications of the illness with the patient and family. By encouraging patients to express their underlying concerns, we can begin to address the psychosocial burden that usually accompanies the physical illness.

Agnelli G, Prandoni P, Santamaria MG et al: Three months versus one year of oral anticoagulant therapy for idiopathic deep venous thrombosis. Warfarin Optimal Duration Italian Trial Investigators. N Engl J Med 2001;345:165.

Aklog L, Williams CS, Byrne JG et al: Acute pulmonary embolectomy: A contemporary approach. Circulation 2002;105:1416.

Decousus H, Leizorovicz A, Parent F et al: A clinical trial of vena caval filters in the prevention of pulmonary embolism in patients with proximal deep-vein thrombosis. Prevention du Risque d'Embolie Pulmonaire par Interruption Cave Study Group. N Engl J Med 1998;338:409.

Fedullo PF, Auger WR, Kerr KM et al: Chronic thromboembolic pulmonary hypertension. N Engl J Med 2001;345:1465.

Feinstein JA, Goldhaber SZ, Lock JE et al: Balloon pulmonary angioplasty for treatment of chronic thromboembolic pulmonary hypertension. Circulation 2001;103:10.

Goldhaber SZ, Haire WD, Feldstein ML et al: Alteplase versus heparin in acute pulmonary embolism: Randomised trial assessing right-ventricular function and pulmonary perfusion. Lancet 1993;341:507.

Gould MK, Dembitzer AD, Doyle RL et al: Low-molecular-weight heparins compared with unfractionated heparin for treatment of acute deep venous thrombosis. A meta-analysis of randomized, controlled trials. Ann Intern Med 1999;130:800.

Grifoni S, Olivotto I, Cecchini P et al: Short-term clinical outcome of patients with acute pulmonary embolism, normal blood pressure, and echocardiographic right ventricular dysfunction. Circulation 2000;101:2817.

Jerjes-Sanchez C, Ramirez-Rivera A, de Lourdes GM et al: Streptokinase and heparin versus heparin alone in massive pulmonary embolism: A randomized controlled trial. J Thromb Thrombolysis 1995;2:227.

Kearon C, Gent M, Hirsh J et al: A comparison of three months of anticoagulation with extended anticoagulation for a first episode of idiopathic venous thromboembolism. N Engl J Med 1999;340:901.

Levine M, Gent M, Hirsh J et al: A comparison of low-molecular-weight heparin administered primarily at home with unfractionated heparin administered in the hospital for proximal deep-vein thrombosis. N Engl J Med 1996;334:677.

Merli G, Spiro TE, Olsson CG et al: Subcutaneous enoxaparin once or twice daily compared with intravenous unfractionated heparin for treatment of venous thromboembolic disease. Ann Intern Med 2001;134:191.

Nass N, McConnell MV, Goldhaber SZ et al: Recovery of regional right ventricular function after thrombolysis for pulmonary embolism. Am J Cardiol 1999;83:804,A10.

Pinede L, Ninet J, Duhaut P et al: Comparison of 3 and 6 months of oral anticoagulant therapy after a first episode of proximal deep vein thrombosis or pulmonary embolism and comparison of 6 and 12 weeks of therapy after isolated calf deep vein thrombosis. Circulation 2001;103:2453.

Ribeiro A, Lindmarker P, Johnsson H et al: Pulmonary embolism: One-year follow-up with echocardiography Doppler and five-year survival analysis. Circulation 1999;99:1325.

Schulman S, Rhedin AS, Lindmarker P et al: A comparison of six weeks with six months of oral anticoagulant therapy after a first episode of venous thromboembolism. Duration of Anticoagulation Trial Study Group. N Engl J Med 1995;332:1661.

Simonneau G, Sors H, Charbonnier B et al: A comparison of low-molecular-weight heparin with unfractionated heparin for acute pulmonary embolism. The THESEE Study Group. Tinzaparine ou Heparine Standard: Evaluations dans l'Embolie Pulmonaire. N Engl J Med 1997;337:663.

C. PREVENTION

Pulmonary embolism is easier and less expensive to prevent than to diagnose or treat; therefore, virtually all hospitalized patients should receive prophylaxis against VTE. Unfortunately, such prophylaxis is underutilized, even for high-risk patients. Furthermore, prophylaxis, even when instituted, may not be effective. Nonetheless, prevention programs should be es-

tablished at all hospitals to ensure that adequate measures are implemented. Nurses and physicians must collaborate to achieve this goal by instituting protocols that are both streamlined and standardized. In addition, quality assurance personnel should adopt a proactive stance to encourage the development of such programs.

The preventive measures should be based on an assessment of the patient's level of risk for PE and whether the optimal strategy will be nonpharmacologic, pharmacologic, or combined modalities. Because the risk of PE continues after discharge from the hospi-

Table 25–12. FDA-approved low-molecular weight regimens for orthopedic and general surgery prophylaxis.

Indication	Drug and Dose	Duration	Timing of Initial Dose
Hip replacement ("USA-style") with enoxaparin	Enoxaparin 30 mg q12h or 40 mg q24h	≤14 days	12–24 h postoperatively, providing that hemostasis has been achieved
Hip replacement ("European-style") with enoxaparin	Enoxaparin 40 mg q24h	≤14 days	12h ± 3 h preoperatively
Hip replacement with dalteparin (option #1)	Dalteparin 2500 units preoperatively and first dose postoperatively, followed by 5000 units q24h	≤14 days	First dose within 2 h preoperatively; second dose at least 6 h after the first dose, usually on the evening of the day of surgery; omit second dose on the day of surgery if surgery is done in the evening
Hip replacement with dalteparin (option #2)	Dalteparin 5000 units q24h	≤14 days	First dose on the preoperative evening; second dose on the evening of the day of surgery (unless surgery is done in the evening)
Extended hip prophylaxis	Enoxaparin 40 mg q24h	An additional 3 weeks after initial hip replacement prophylaxis	After the initial hip replacement prophylaxis regimen has been completed
General surgery with enoxaparin	Enoxaparin 40 mg q24h	≤12 days	2 h preoperatively
General surgery with dalteparin (moderate risk for venous thromboembolism)	Dalteparin 2500 units q24h	5–10 days	1–2 h preoperatively
General surgery with dalteparin (high risk for venous thromboembolism: option # 1)	Dalteparin 5000 units q24h	5–10 days	Preoperative evening
General surgery with dalteparin (high risk for venous thromboembolism: option #2)	Dalteparin 2500 units preoperatively and first dose postoperatively, followed by 5000 units q24h	5–10 days	First dose 1–2 h preoperatively; second dose 12 h later

tal, prophylaxis should be continued at home among those patients at moderate or high risk for VTE.

1. Nonpharmacologic prevention—The most commonly used nonpharmacologic measures are graduated compression stockings (GCS) and intermittent pneumatic compression (IPC) devices ("boots"). Vascular compression with either stockings or boots is effective among surgical patients, because it counters the otherwise-unopposed perioperative venodilation that appears causally related to postoperative venous thrombosis. Even among low-risk general surgery patients, GCS can substantially reduce the frequency of venous thrombosis and should therefore be considered first-line prophylaxis against PE in all hospitalized patients, except those with peripheral arterial occlusive disease whose condition may be worsened by vascular compression.

Intermittent pneumatic compression boots, which provide intermittent inflation of air-filled cuffs, prevent venous stasis in the legs; they also appear to stimulate the endogenous fibrinolytic system. Because it appears that GCS and IPC work through somewhat different—although complementary—mechanisms, these modalities can be used in combination in patients at moderate or high risk of venous thrombosis.

2. Pharmacologic prevention—Drugs can be used instead of or in addition to nonpharmacologic prophylaxis (Table 25-12). The most comprehensive randomized, controlled trial of low-dose heparin as prophylaxis against fatal postoperative PE was the 1975 International Multicentre Trial involving 4121 patients. Treatment consisted of 5000 units of heparin administered subcutaneously, 2 h preoperatively and every 8 h thereafter for 7 days. Eligible patients were over age 40 and were scheduled to undergo elective major surgery. Of the autopsied patients, 16 in the control group versus only 2 in the heparin group died of PE. Although more wound hematomas occurred in the heparin-treated patients, there was no increase in the number of deaths from hemorrhage.

A meta-analysis of data from 78 randomized controlled trials involving almost 16,000 patients confirmed the International Multicentre Trial results: Heparin-treated patients had a 40% reduction in nonfatal PE and a 64% reduction in fatal PE. The heparin-treated patients also had about one third as many DVTs as the control patients, regardless of the type of surgery. Although excessive bleeding was more likely to occur among patients assigned to heparin therapy—especially those who underwent urologic procedures—the absolute excess in bleeding was only about 2%. There was no significant difference in fatal hemorrhage between the heparin and control groups.

3. Future directions—In the future protocol-driven prophylaxis will be used for all hospitalized patients, especially for medical patients hospitalized in intensive care units. The emphasis on preventive strategies will also increase at the time of hospital discharge or transfer to a skilled nursing facility or rehabilitation hospital. Orders to prescribe these prophylactic measures will be prompted by computerized order entry.

Collins R, Scrimgeour A, Yusuf S et al: Reduction in fatal pulmonary embolism and venous thrombosis by perioperative administration of subcutaneous heparin. Overview of results of randomized trials in general, orthopedic, and urologic surgery. N Engl J Med 1988;318:1162–1173.

Prevention of fatal postoperative pulmonary embolism by low doses of heparin. An international multicentre trial. Lancet 1975;2:45–51.

Pulmonary Hypertension

Robert A. Taylor, MD

ESSENTIALS OF DIAGNOSIS

- *Right ventricular lift*
- *Increased intensity of the pulmonic component of the second heart sound*
- *Elevated jugular a waves*
- *Electrocardiographic evidence of right ventricular hypertrophy*
- *Elevated pulmonary artery pressures by Doppler echocardiography or cardiac catheterization*

General Considerations

Pulmonary hypertension is a pathologic state in which the systolic pressure in the pulmonary artery is consistently elevated above normal at rest or with exertion. Elevation of the pressures of the usually low-pressure pulmonary vascular bed is often accompanied by increased vascular resistance and diminished cardiac output. In essence, pulmonary hypertension is the result of a reduction in the caliber of the pulmonary vessels, an increase in pulmonary blood flow, or both. The normal values for peak systolic pulmonary artery pressure are in the range of 20–30 mm Hg, with diastolic pressures of 6–10 mm Hg, and a mean of 12–16 mm Hg. Pulmonary artery pressure is determined using Ohm's law by flow (cardiac output) and resistance (pulmonary vascular), typically described in dynes×sec×cm^{-5}. Pulmonary vascular resistance reflects such variables as the cross-sectional area of the vessels and the total surface area of the pulmonary vascular bed. Several disease processes may alter the cross-sectional area of the pulmonary vasculature and ultimately may lead to pulmonary hypertension.

Pathophysiology & Etiology

The specific causes of pulmonary hypertension can be categorized according to the underlying process that produces the elevation of pulmonary artery pressures (Table 26–1). Conditions producing disease intrinsic to the pulmonary arteries, such as the vasculitides, constitute a substantial proportion of the disorders that cause pulmonary hypertension. Also in this category is primary pulmonary hypertension. This rare disease affects women twice as often as men, has no clear cause, and may represent a final common pathway for various disease processes.

Perhaps the largest group of causative disorders includes those diseases that affect the pulmonary parenchyma directly, such as chronic obstructive pulmonary disease and pulmonary fibrotic processes. Fortunately, the parenchymal disorder and its concomitant symptoms usually bring the patient to medical care relatively early and raise the suspicion of secondary pulmonary hypertension. These same conditions, however, often make bedside and noninvasive assessment of elevated pulmonary artery pressures more difficult. Many factors lead to the elevation of the pulmonary artery pressures in these disorders. One key factor is the hypoxia and hypercapnia produced by ventilation and perfusion mismatch caused by obstruction and loss of vascular elements in the pulmonary vascular bed. Hypoxemia in particular has been shown to stimulate vasoconstriction and decrease vasodilator responses. Chronic changes in the histologic architecture as well as hyperviscosity from erythrocytosis also contribute to pulmonary hypertension in these patients.

Diseases leading to left atrial and pulmonary venous hypertension also commonly result in pulmonary hypertension. Lesions of the left heart, such as aortic and mitral valvular disease, the cardiomyopathies, and coronary artery disease can lead to elevation of the left-sided pressures. Left atrial hypertension is transmitted to the pulmonary vessels and right cardiac chambers. The pulmonary artery pressure must elevate to allow forward blood flow across the pulmonary vascular bed. Rare diseases such as cor triatriatum and left atrial myxomas, which produce outflow obstruction of the left atrium, also increase left atrial pressures and with time can lead to pulmonary hypertension. Relief of the obstruction, just as with surgical repair of mitral and aortic valvular disease, may reverse the pulmonary vascular lesions and

Table 26–1. Causes of pulmonary hypertension.

Conditions directly affecting the pulmonary arteries
Primary pulmonary hypertension
Toxin-induced (ie, anorexic agents)
Vasculitides
  Granulomatoses, collagen-vascular disorders, arteritis
Hepatic cirrhosis/portal disease
Congenital heart disease (eg, Eisenmenger syndrome [ASD, VSD, PDA])
Infection
  Human immunodeficiency virus
Conditions affecting the pulmonary parenchyma
Chronic obstructive lung disease
Infiltrative/granulomatous diseases
  Sarcoidosis, pneumoconiosis, radiation, fibrosis, neoplasm, pneumonia, collagen-vascular diseases
Cystic fibrosis
Upper airway obstruction
High-altitude disease
Arteriovenous fistulas within the lung
Restrictive lung diseases
Conditions affecting the thoracic cage and neuromuscular system
Obesity-hypoventilation/sleep apnea
Pharyngeal-tracheal obstruction
Kyphoscoliosis
Pleural fibrosis
Neuromuscular disorders
  Myasthenia gravis, poliomyelitis, central respiratory disorders
Conditions causing left atrial/or pulmonary venous hypertension
Elevated left ventricular diastolic pressure
  Systolic failure, diastolic dysfunction, constrictive pericarditis
Aortic valve disease
Mitral valve disease
Cor triatriatum
Left atrial masses
  Myxoma or neoplasm, thrombus
Fibrosing mediastinitis
Congenital pulmonary vein stenosis
Anomalous pulmonary venous connection
Pulmonary venoocclusive disease
Nonvasculitis conditions that result in pulmonary artery obstruction
Acute and chronic thromboembolism
Hemoglobinopathies (eg, sickle cell disease)
Primary or metastatic malignancies
Peripheral pulmonic stenosis
Congenital pulmonary hypoplasia

---

decrease pulmonary hypertension over time. Pulmonary venous disease resulting from mediastinal fibrosis, inflammation, or neoplasm are often more difficult to treat.

Congenital cardiac abnormalities are an infrequent but more clinically obvious group of conditions that result in pulmonary hypertension. The end result of these lesions may be Eisenmenger's syndrome (see Chapter 27), in which patients with congenital heart disease and severe pulmonary hypertension have reversal of their left-to-right cardiac shunt. Conditions that cause this syndrome include atrial septal defect, ventricular septal defect, and patent ductus arteriosus. Initially, pulmonary artery pressures are elevated due to high pulmonary artery blood flow caused by left-to-right shunting. Over time, pathologic changes occur in the pulmonary vasculature, which decrease the cross-sectional area of the pulmonary arterial bed. This results in increased pulmonary vascular resistance and worsening pulmonary hypertension.

Disorders of the thoracic cage, such as kyphoscoliosis, and neuromuscular abnormalities, represent a small group of causes of pulmonary hypertension. Similar to pulmonary parenchymal diseases, pulmonary artery pressures are elevated by pulmonary vasoconstriction stimulated by chronic hypoxia. These syndromes, however, generate hypoxia by hypoventilation. Other diseases in this group include obstructive sleep apnea, which may prove very difficult to diagnose, and pleural fibrosis.

Thromboembolism and sickle cell anemia, which are hemoglobinopathic-thrombotic disorders, ultimately result in mechanical obstruction of the lumen of the pulmonary vasculature but do not result from intrinsic vascular abnormalities per se, although some secondary vascular injury does occur.

In general, the different categories (intrinsic vascular disease, parenchymal disease, thromboembolic, etc) lead to injury of the vascular endothelium. Once initiated, pathophysiologic alterations in the vascular wall occur that decrease vascular reactivity; increase thrombosis; and stimulate the proliferation of smooth muscle cells, fibroblasts, and inflammatory cells. Over time, these histologic changes perpetuate the increases in pulmonary artery pressures by decreasing vascular dilation, increasing vasoconstriction, and promoting in situ thrombus formation.

Certain historical features may help direct the search for an underlying cause. Prior use of anorectic agents, intravenous drugs, or crack cocaine may point to the cause. A history of deep venous thrombosis or a family history of a thrombotic disorder such as protein C deficiency increases the suspicion for thromboembolic pulmonary hypertension. More than half of the patients presenting with thromboembolic pulmonary hypertension have had a prior diagnosed deep venous thrombosis. Associated involvement of the kidney, skin, or joints may point toward a collagen vascular disorder.

Aberhaim L, Moride Y, Brenot F et al: Appetite-suppressant drugs and the risk of pulmonary hypertension. N Engl J Med 1996;335:609.

Alpert MA: Obesity cardiomyopathy: Pathophysiology and evolution of the clinical syndrome. Am J Med Sci 2001;321:225.

Moraes DL, Colucci WS, Givertz MM: Secondary pulmonary hypertension in chronic heart failure: The role of the endothelium in pathophysiology and management. Circulation 2000;102:1718.

Shimoda LA, Sham JS, Sylvester JT: Altered pulmonary vasoreactivity in the chronically hypoxic lung. Physiol Res 2000:49:549.

Clinical Findings

A. SYMPTOMS AND SIGNS

One of the major problems in pulmonary hypertension is the failure to make the diagnosis early. This is frequently difficult because the symptoms may be unreliable, subtle, and often vary from patient to patient. Many times, the symptoms occur only after pulmonary artery pressures are three to five times normal values. The most common symptoms in pulmonary hypertension tend to be nonspecific. Early symptoms include exertional dyspnea, syncope, and varying types of chest pain—musculoskeletal, pleuritic, and anginal. Although the presence of pulmonary parenchymal disease may raise the clinician's index of suspicion for pulmonary hypertension, new or more prominent nonspecific symptoms may be attributed to progression of the underlying parenchymal process rather than to new or worsened pulmonary hypertension. For this reason, pulmonary hypertension often goes unrecognized for months or years. In one study of patients referred to surgery for chronic thromboembolic pulmonary hypertension, the mean time from the onset of the symptoms to surgery was 4.5 years. Later in the course, symptoms of right-sided fluid overload such as peripheral edema, abdominal distension from ascites, and fatigue occur as a consequence of a failing right ventricle.

B. PHYSICAL EXAMINATION

The physical findings of pulmonary hypertension can be subtle. A careful examination, however, provides important clues into the presence of pulmonary hypertension. It may also suggest an underlying cause and estimate the severity of the disease. An increase in the intensity of the pulmonic component of the second heart sound is not always present. An early systolic click may be heard as a consequence of the interruption of pulmonic valve opening. A midsystolic flow murmur across the pulmonic valve can usually be appreciated. In dramatic cases, it may be possible to feel the tap of a pressure-overloaded right ventricle along the left sternal border as well as a palpable P_2 in the second intercostal space. Other findings, such as tricuspid and pulmonic regurgitation, elevated jugular venous pressure, ascites,

hepatojugular reflux, hepatomegaly, pulsatile liver, and peripheral edema, are variable manifestations of right-sided cardiac failure. The severity of these findings usually correlates with the degree of pulmonary hypertension.

The murmur of tricuspid regurgitation is not always easy to hear, despite the presence of moderate or severe regurgitation. In addition, because of high pressure in the right atrium, respiratory variation of the tricuspid regurgitation murmur, as classically described, may be absent, causing the murmur to be mistakenly identified as mitral regurgitation. Unlike most mitral regurgitation murmurs, however, the murmur of tricuspid regurgitation is usually not audible in the axilla.

Findings of pulmonary parenchymal disease or the diastolic murmurs of mitral stenosis, if present, should direct the search for an underlying cause once pulmonary hypertension is considered. Cyanosis and clubbing usually point toward congenital cardiac conditions in the absence of findings of parenchymal disease. A systolic or continuous murmur in the lung fields is unique to thromboembolic pulmonary hypertension or congenital pulmonary artery branch stenosis. Arthritis, rash, or other skin changes (ie, sclerodactyly) may suggest underlying rheumatologic disorders.

C. DIAGNOSTIC STUDIES

1. Electrocardiography—The electrocardiogram (ECG) often shows abnormalities that suggest right ventricular hypertrophy (Table 26–2). These include right-axis deviation, prominent anterior forces, and inverted T waves in the precordium. It is not uncommon for computer-interpreted ECGs to be read as suggesting anterior ischemia instead of the strain pattern of right ventricular hypertrophy. Incomplete or complete right bundle branch block and right atrial abnormalities are also common. As with the chest radiograph, these ECG findings occur more frequently in patients with severe, chronic pulmonary hypertension; the ECG may be entirely normal in patients with moderate pul-

Table 26–2. Electrocardiographic criteria for right ventricular hypertrophy.

1	Frontal-plane right-axis deviation >90°
2	R–S amplitude in precordial lead V_1 >1.0
3	R-wave amplitude in precordial lead V_1 ≥7 mm
4	S-wave amplitude in precordial lead V_1 <2 mm
5	qR pattern present in precordial lead V_1
6	R-wave amplitude in precordial lead V_1 plus S-wave amplitude in precordial leads V_5 or V_6 >10.5 mm
7	R–S amplitude in precordial leads V_5 or V_6 ≤1.0
8	S-wave amplitude in precordial lead V_5 ≥7 mm
9	R-wave amplitude in precordial lead V_5 <5 mm

monary hypertension even of fairly long duration. The ECG findings can reverse early after reduction of pulmonary artery pressures (Figure 26–1).

2. Chest radiography—A chest radiograph can be helpful in raising the suspicion of pulmonary hypertension (Figure 26–2). Unfortunately, radiographic findings, such as prominent proximal pulmonary artery vessels with distal pruning as seen in primary pulmonary hypertension, are frequently not present until late in the course of the disease. This is also true for filling of the retrosternal space by the right ventricle on the lateral projection. The presence of pulmonary venous congestion, left atrial enlargement, and a large cardiac silhouette should direct the search for a left-sided disorder. Hyperinflation suggests chronic obstructive pulmonary disease, whereas kyphosis or scoliosis may reflect conditions producing restrictive lung disease. It is important to recognize that although abnormalities on the chest radiographs may be helpful to the

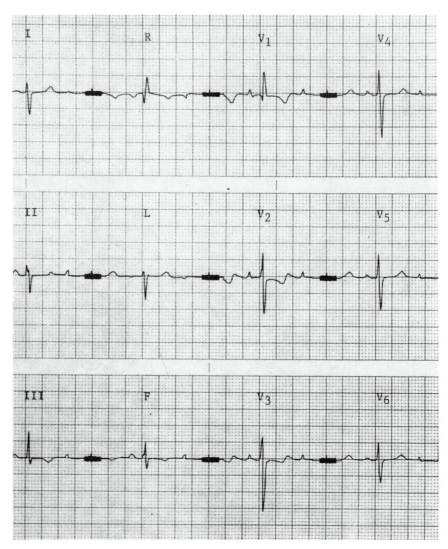

Figure 26–1. **A:** Electrocardiogram from a patient with severe, chronic thromboembolic pulmonary hypertension (mean pulmonary artery pressure of 65 mm Hg) with eight of nine electrocardiographic criteria for right ventricular hypertrophy (See Table 26–2). **B:** Same patient 36 days after pulmonary thromboendarterectomy that normalized pulmonary artery pressures. the ECG is essentially normal; no criteria for right ventricular hypertrophy are present.

(continued)

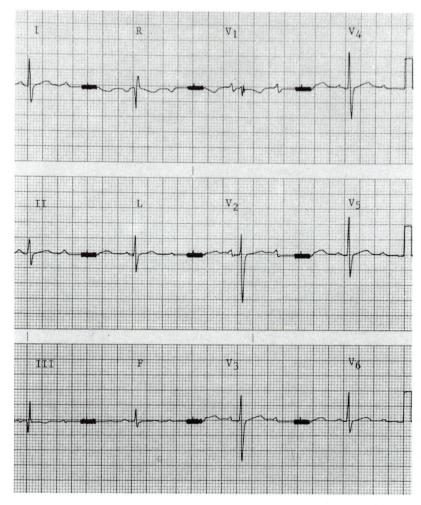

Figure 26–1. (cont.)

diagnosis, the frequency of normal chest films in pulmonary hypertension is high, even in the setting of long-standing disease.

3. Pulmonary function tests—Pulmonary function tests may be entirely normal in patients with disease intrinsic to the pulmonary vasculature or may show characteristic patterns of obstructive or restrictive disorders. (A complete discussion of these abnormalities is beyond the scope of this chapter.) Obviously, the evaluation of patients with pulmonary hypertension requires the use of pulmonary function tests when parenchymal, obstructive airway, restrictive, or neuromuscular disorders are considered.

4. Radionuclide lung scans—The ventilation-perfusion scan can be invaluable in establishing the underlying cause of pulmonary hypertension. The perfusion scan is diagnostic in thromboembolic pulmonary hy-

pertension, demonstrating one or more segmental defects mismatched by the ventilation scan. In primary pulmonary hypertension, the scan is often normal or shows mottled, subsegmental defects (Figure 26–3). Other conditions that cause pulmonary hypertension may have normal scans or show perfusion defects matched by ventilation defects that point toward airway or parenchymal disease. Because surgical correction may be curative in patients with pulmonary hypertension due to thromboembolic disease, a perfusion lung scan should be part of the diagnostic evaluation in all patients with pulmonary hypertension of unknown cause.

5. Echocardiography—Two-dimensional (2-D) and Doppler echocardiographic studies to establish right-sided cardiac hemodynamics are extremely helpful, not only during the initial diagnostic evaluation but also af-

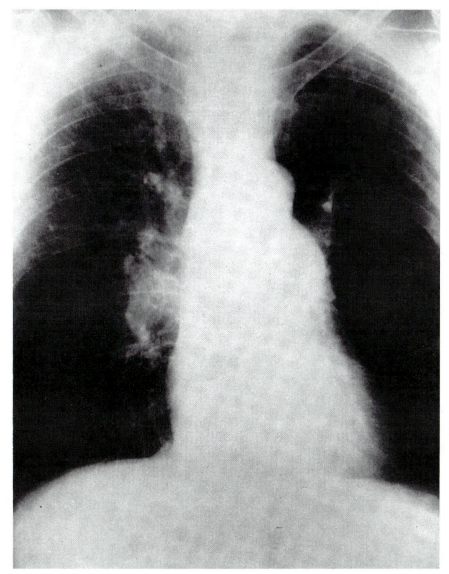

Figure 26–2. Posteroanterior chest x-ray of a patient with pulmonary hypertension. Note the dilated proximal pulmonary arteries with a relative lack of pulmonary vasculature in the periphery. No cardiomegaly is noted in the PA projection.

ter therapy to lower pulmonary artery pressures has been initiated. The echocardiogram may show flattening of the septum (**D**-shaped septum) in both diastole and systole. If the flattening is seen only during diastole, the cause may be a volume overload with no accompanying pulmonary hypertension. This is commonly seen when the right ventricular contraction appears normal or even hyperdynamic. Pulmonary hypertension that causes a pure right ventricular pressure overload results in concavity of the interventricular sep-

tum toward the left ventricle with a dilated, hypertrophied, and hypocontractile right ventricle (Figure 26–4). The left ventricle is often small and demonstrates normal systolic function but abnormal transmitral filling characteristics. Ratios of early-to-late peak velocities are reversed, and deceleration of early filling is slowed. These changes are linked to the abnormality of the interventricular septum and are reversible with interventions that lower pulmonary artery pressure. Similarly, the right ventricular dysfunction and right-

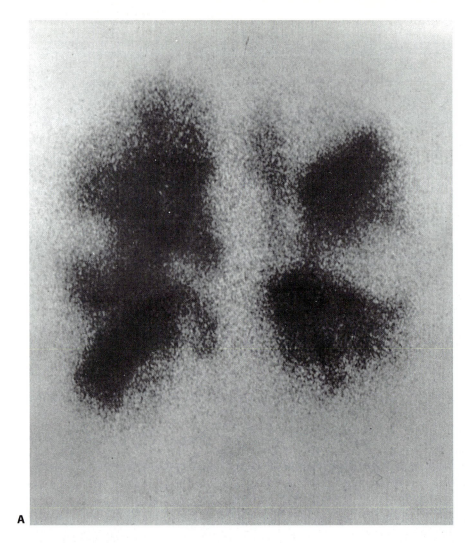

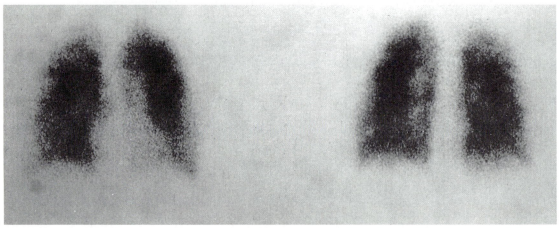

Figure 26–3. **A:** Perfusion lung scan from a patient with thromboembolic pulmonary hypertension, demonstrating multiple segmental defects in both lungs. **B:** Perfusion lung scan from a patient with primary pulmonary hypertension, demonstrating only a slight mottled appearance.

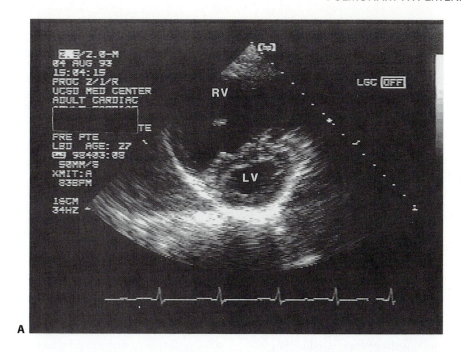

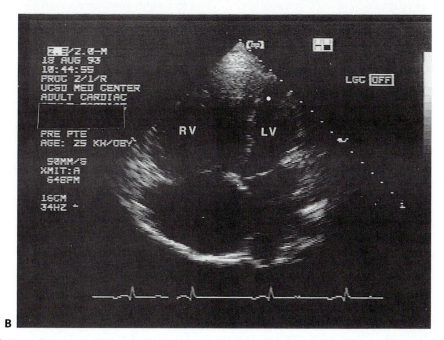

Figure 26–4. Two-dimensional echocardiographic images from the parasternal short axis (**A**) and the apical four-chamber views (**B**) in a patient with severe pulmonary hypertension. Note the flattened interventricular septum, the strikingly dilated right ventricle (RV), and the compressed left ventricle (LV).

sided chamber dilatation, which is commonly found in pulmonary hypertension, return to normal early after reduction of pulmonary artery pressures in patients with thromboembolic pulmonary hypertension.

Two-dimensional and Doppler echocardiography are also essential tools for the evaluation of the underlying cause of the elevated pulmonary artery pressures. Left-sided cardiac abnormalities such as left ventricular dysfunction and mitral valvular disease can be excluded. The existence of intracardiac shunts (ie, atrial septal defect [ASD] or ventricular septal defect [VSD]) can also be detected.

Color-flow Doppler evaluation of tricuspid regurgitation jet often suggests significant regurgitation in the absence of significant auscultatory findings. This is particularly common in patients with intrinsic airspace disease in which the increased intrathoracic volume (barrel chest) diminishes all cardiac sounds. Continuous-wave Doppler of the tricuspid regurgitant jet can be extremely helpful for noninvasively estimating the pulmonary artery systolic pressure and can be used to follow changes in pulmonary artery pressure after surgery for thromboembolic pulmonary hypertension (Figure 26–5) or to evaluate response to medical therapy. Other acceptable, although less accurate, methods for estimating right-sided pressures involve determining the preejection period and the systolic acceleration time of the right ventricle outflow-tract flow. The preejection period spans the time from the electrocardiographic QRS to the onset of systolic flow across the pulmonic valve. The acceleration time (from valve opening to the peak of the velocity waveform) should be obtained at 100-mm/s paper speed and is inversely related to pulmonary artery pressure and somewhat less so to pulmonary vascular resistance. Continuous-wave Doppler of the pulmonic insufficiency waveform estimates pulmonary artery diastolic pressure. The end-diastolic velocity of the pulmonic insufficiency waveform, when added to an estimate of right atrial pressure (equivalent to right ventricular diastolic pressure) correlates well with pulmonary artery diastolic pressure. Midsystolic notching (or diminished flow) of the pulmonary Doppler flow also suggests pulmonary hypertension. Other Doppler velocity techniques have been used with varying success to estimate right-sided cardiac hemodynamics in pulmonary hypertension.

M-mode Doppler of the pulmonic valve leaflets may demonstrate midsystolic notching and an absent *a* wave, qualitatively suggesting pulmonary hypertension. This technique, however, does not allow for the quantitative measurement of pulmonary pressures.

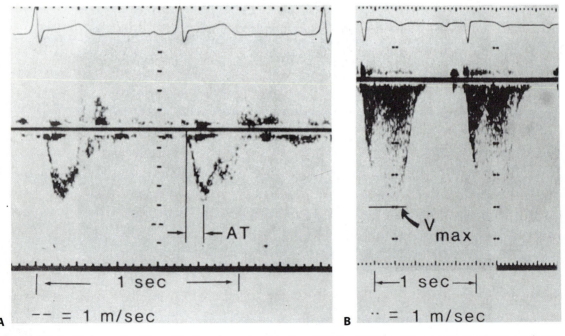

Figure 26–5. Right ventricular outflow-tract acceleration time (AT) in ms (**A**) and tricuspid regurgitation velocity waveform, showing a maximum velocity (V_{max}) of 4 m/s (**B**). Reprinted, with permission, from Chow LC et al: Doppler assessment of changes in right-sided cardiac hemodynamics after pulmonary thromboendarterectomy. Am J Cardiol 1988;61:1092.

Imaging of the pulmonary arteries with 2D echocardiography has had limited success. Transthoracic echocardiography can establish that proximal vessels are dilated and, in a minority of patients, identify very proximal thrombi. Transesophageal imaging of the pulmonary arteries is superior to the transthoracic approach but still remains limited primarily to the main, right, and left pulmonary artery branches and the origins of the lobar vessels. Echocardiographic identification of thrombotic material or tumor is possible, but it is inferior to other imaging modalities described later.

6. Angiography and cardiac catheterization—Cardiac catheterization, specifically right-sided catheterization, is crucial in establishing the diagnosis in many cases of pulmonary hypertension. Right-heart catheterization documents pulmonary artery pressure and allows measurement of pulmonary vascular resistance. In some acutely ill patients with pulmonary artery pressures equal to systemic arterial pressures, the procedure is performed with an increased risk. Adequate oxygenation and avoidance of vasovagal reactions (eg, from pain) reduce the risk to these patients undergoing right-sided heart catheterization. Although cardiac catheterization is necessary for the accurate measurement of shunts in congenital heart disease, the anatomic abnormality can frequently be established with thoracic and transesophageal echocardiography. Abnormalities of the left heart, such as aortic and mitral stenosis, regurgitation, cor triatriatum, or left ventricular dysfunction, elevate the pulmonary artery wedge pressure, pointing to a left-sided cause for the pulmonary hypertension.

Pulmonary angiography is confirmatory in the diagnosis of primary pulmonary hypertension and diagnostic in thromboembolic disease of the major pulmonary arteries. Levophase angiography can make the diagnosis of pulmonary venous disease, including venoocclusive disease or extrinsic compression of the pulmonary veins (eg, in fibrosing mediastinitis; Figure 26–6). Although posing a risk in patients with acute pulmonary embolism and even moderate levels of pulmonary hypertension, selective pulmonary angiography is considered safe in patients with severe, chronic pulmonary hyper-

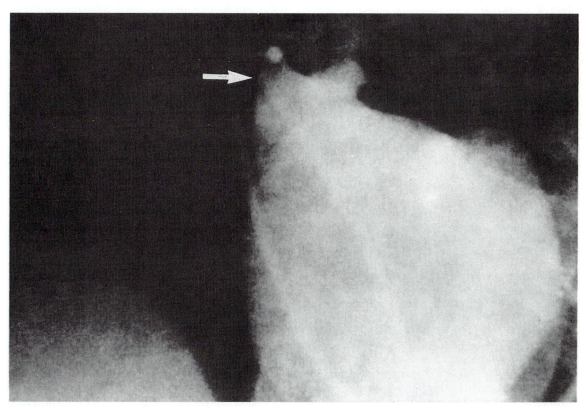

Figure 26–6. A retrograde left atrial angiogram from a patient with fibrosing mediastinitis. The tip of the catheter is placed at the mouth of a right pulmonary vein (*arrow*) with good opacification of the left atrium but no retrograde filling of the totally occluded pulmonary vein.

tension from a thromboembolic cause. Characteristic abnormalities on the pulmonary angiogram, including webs, abrupt cutoffs, and poststenotic dilatation, have been found in patients with chronic thromboembolic disease. However, chronic emboli may organize, causing angiography to underestimate the extent of the occlusive vascular disease.

During catheterization, the response of the pulmonary artery pressures and pulmonary vascular resistance to vasodilators such as nitroprusside, prostacyclin, or nitric oxide should be tested. Improvement of greater than 20% with these therapies suggests reversible increases in the vascular bed pressures, which implies a better response to therapy and improved overall prognosis.

Cockrill BA, Kacmarek RM, Fifer MA et al: Comparison of the effects of nitric oxide, nitroprusside, and nifedipine on hemodynamics and right ventricular contractility in patients with chronic pulmonary hypertension. Chest 2001;119:128.

7. Computed tomography and magnetic resonance imaging—Computed tomography (CT) and magnetic resonance imaging (MRI) of the chest can provide useful information in parenchymal disorders and several other conditions that cause pulmonary hypertension. The CT scan of the mediastinum demonstrates characteristic findings in patients with fibrosing mediastinitis caused by histoplasmosis, in which large, calcified lymph nodes can block or compress pulmonary arteries and veins. Similarly, MRI may show disease within the mediastinum, flow abnormalities, and or tumor within the pulmonary arteries. Electron-beam and spiral CT and MRI provide an accurate definition of right-heart chamber dimensions and volumes. Additionally, these imaging modalities can evaluate for thromboembolic disease with similar accuracy to pulmonary angiography.

Fleischmann D, Scholten C, Klepetko W et al. Three-dimensional visualization of pulmonary thromboemboli in chronic thromboembolic pulmonary hypertension with multiple detector-row spiral computed tomography. Circulation 2001; 103:2993.

8. Pulmonary angioscopy and intravascular ultrasonography—Advances in fiberoptics and the miniaturization of ultrasound transducers have allowed for the development of intravascular angioscopy and ultrasonography, which can be used in the pulmonary arteries. Both technologies are particularly useful in identifying thrombus in major vessels, and angioscopy permits the differentiation between acute and chronic thrombus. This capability has important implications for treating thromboembolic pulmonary hypertension because the success of thromboendarterectomy rests in part on selecting patients with anatomically accessible thrombotic disease.

9. Lung biopsy—A lung biopsy is infrequently required to confirm the cause of pulmonary hypertension. A biopsy can identify injected particulate matter from pulverized tablets in intravenous drug addicts with pulmonary hypertension and other pulmonary vascular disorders. In general, however, these disorders are systemic, and biopsy of other organs may be enough to confirm the diagnosis. Pulmonary hypertension is reversible when the pulmonary vessel demonstrates only medial hypertrophy and when vasoconstriction is present. If histologic abnormalities, including necrotizing arteritis and plexiform lesions, are present, pulmonary hypertension is generally irreversible.

10. Other diagnostic tests—Because the list of causes for pulmonary hypertension is so extensive, other specific tests, such as hemoglobin electrophoresis or serologic analysis, may be needed to confirm a diagnosis. In such cases, the history and physical examination will direct the clinician toward the appropriate tests.

Treatment of Secondary Pulmonary Hypertension

Pulmonary hypertension that is due to known causes is, of course, best managed by directing therapy at the underlying disease process. In some cases, such as mitral stenosis, surgery or balloon valvuloplasty may completely eliminate the left atrial pressure elevation driving the pulmonary hypertension. In many other conditions, however, the chronic effects on the pulmonary vasculature are irreversible, and correcting the problem may still leave residual pulmonary hypertension. More often, the underlying cause cannot be either effectively treated or reversed to an extent that will allow reversal of the pulmonary hypertension. Chronic obstructive lung disease or interstitial disease may be stabilized, for example, but even maximal therapy will not reverse the pulmonary hypertension.

In cases of congenital heart disease, heart or heart-lung transplantation or surgical correction of the congenital abnormality combined with either single- or double-lung transplantation is now performed with some frequency. It is important to remember, however, that in Eisenmenger's syndrome, the pulmonary hypertension has become irreversible, and correction of the congenital defect alone will be of no value and will most likely prove fatal. Therefore, either single- or double-lung transplantation must accompany the repair of the congenital defect.

Some conditions that affect the pulmonary parenchyma may be partially or completely reversed. For example, vascular diseases and fibrotic conditions may be amenable to treatment with corticosteroids or chemotactic agents. In addition, parenchymal disorders with significant hypoxia may be effectively treated with chronic administration of supplemental oxygen; the direct vasodilator effect of which reduces pulmonary artery pressures. Patients with hypoxia caused by a significant right-to-left shunt may, however, derive no symptomatic benefit from the supplemental oxygen.

It appears that most of the agents used for pulmonary vasodilation in primary pulmonary hypertension (see section on Vasodilators) have not been found to be particularly effective in patients with pulmonary parenchymal disease and secondary pulmonary hypertension. This is probably due to the relative lack of vascular reactivity, especially once hypoxia is treated with supplemental oxygen. Other isolated forms of secondary pulmonary hypertension may respond, however.

In conditions that affect the thoracic cage and neuromuscular system, the pulmonary hypertension can be relieved completely with treatment with supplemental oxygen and or positive airway pressure (continuous positive airway pressure [CPAP] or bilevel positive airway pressure [BiPAP]). Obstructive sleep apnea can also be treated with positive airway pressure. Additionally, weight loss may have a dramatic clinical effect in patients with obstructive sleep apnea. Severe cases of pharyngeal or tracheal obstruction that cause obstructive sleep patterns can be surgically corrected, producing a pronounced reduction in pulmonary hypertension over time.

Several of the conditions causing left atrial and pulmonary venous hypertension can be treated surgically. Revascularization to improve left ventricular systolic and diastolic function, and aortic and mitral valve disease therapy can reverse pulmonary hypertension. The same is true for the surgical repair of cor triatriatum, pericardiectomy for constrictive pericarditis, surgical resection of obstructing left atrial myxomas or neoplasms, and rarely surgical treatment of fibrosing mediastinitis. This last condition, almost always caused by histoplasmosis, is generally beyond medical therapy with antifungal agents by the time it is diagnosed. Unfortunately, the surgery for fibrosing mediastinitis is extremely tedious and technically difficult, with significant failure rates to reduce the pulmonary hypertension; mortality rates are also high. The conditions unrelated to vasculitis that result in pulmonary artery obstruction can sometimes be surgically treated. In cases of primary or metastatic malignancies, appropriate chemotherapeutic agents and or radiation may be needed as an adjunct to surgical resection.

The most well established treatment for secondary pulmonary hypertension is in the group of patients presenting with chronic thromboembolic pulmonary hypertension. These patients, if carefully selected for organized, proximal pulmonary artery thrombi, can undergo thromboendarterectomy (Figure 26–7) and achieve near normalization of pulmonary artery pressures (Figure 26–8). More recent studies report a 30-day mortality rate of 8.7%, which is significantly improved from mortality rates of 22% in the early days of this surgery. New York Heart Association functional class and exercise capacity are improved dramatically at the time of discharge and at the 1-year follow-up.

Successful reversal of pulmonary hypertension is accompanied by remarkable changes in cardiac size and function as documented by 2-D and Doppler echocardiography. Within the first month after surgery, normal left ventricular diastolic function returns and right-sided cardiac-chamber sizes and pressures diminish. Normalization of pulmonary artery pressures continues, and at the 1-year follow-up, patients have been found to have further decreased pulmonary artery pressures and increased cardiac output. It is clear that after reversal of pulmonary hypertension, the right ventricle, despite being massively dilated with severely depressed function, can return to normal size and function. This reversal of right-sided cardiac abnormalities is particularly relevant when considering the use of single- and double-lung transplantation in other conditions that cause severe, chronic pulmonary hypertension. The results have encouraged the use of isolated lung transplantation rather than combination heart-lung transplantation, thereby increasing the availability of donor organs.

McKane CL: Pulmonary thromboendarterectomy: An advance in the treatment of chronic thromboembolic pulmonary hypertension. Heart Lung 1998;27:293.

Menzel T, Wagner S, Kramm T et al: Pathophysiology of impaired right and left ventricular function in chronic embolic pulmonary hypertension: Changes after pulmonary thromboendarterectomy. Chest 2000;118:897.

Treatment of Primary Pulmonary Hypertension

A. CARDIAC GLYCOSIDES

The value of agents such as digoxin to improve right-heart hemodynamics, although commonly used, is not established in the treatment of primary pulmonary hypertension. The risk of toxicity may outweigh any potential benefit, particularly in patients with hypoxia and those in whom diuretic therapy for edema might result in hypokalemia.

B. SUPPLEMENTAL OXYGEN

As noted earlier, pulmonary parenchymal disorders that result in hypoxia require the use of oxygen. Although low-flow oxygen may—or may not—be beneficial for patients with primary pulmonary hypertension, some patients will desaturate with activity and thus benefit from supplemental oxygen. Patients with severe right-

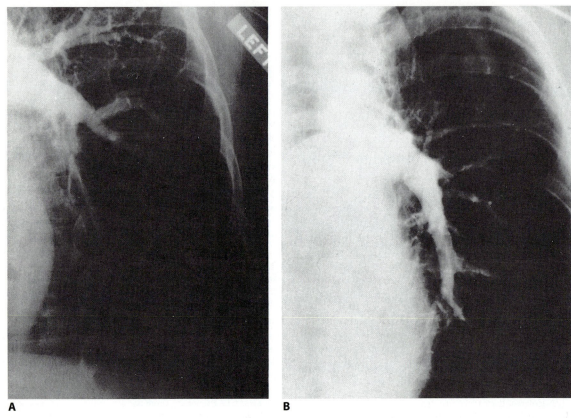

A   B

Figure 26–7. Left pulmonary artery angiogram from a patient with thromboembolic pulmonary hypertension before (**A**) and after (**B**) pulmonary thromboendarterectomy. Note the opacification of the lower lobe vessel, which was not seen preoperatively.

sided cardiac failure and hypoxia at rest should receive supplemental oxygen continuously.

C. DIURETICS

Patients with right ventricular failure caused by severe pulmonary hypertension frequently develop peripheral edema and hepatic congestion, both of which may be substantially improved by the use of diuretics. Care should be taken not to decrease right ventricular preload excessively because of the right ventricle's reliance on adequate preload for filling. Overaggressive diuresis can, in these cases, prove catastrophic. Close scrutiny of electrolyte balance is important, especially in patients with associated hypoxia, to decrease the risk of sudden cardiac death.

D. ANTICOAGULANTS

Based on small clinical trials, many clinicians recommend chronic anticoagulant therapy with warfarin in patients with primary pulmonary hypertension. It is also recommended in some patients with secondary pulmonary hypertension. Such therapy is clearly indicated for those patients with pulmonary thromboembolic disease in whom life-long anticoagulation must be maintained. These patients may additionally have inferior vena cava filters placed to prevent further lower-extremity thrombi from entering the lung vasculature. Some studies suggest that the use of anticoagulant therapy in patients with primary pulmonary hypertension may improve survival rates, compared with those who were not treated with anticoagulants. In some patients, a sedentary state, diminished cardiac output, and peripheral venous insufficiency may present a milieu that predisposes to deep venous thrombosis. Because pulmonary embolism could be catastrophic in such patients with pulmonary hypertension from any cause, the judicious use of anticoagulant therapy is recommended for patients with chronic pulmonary hyperten-

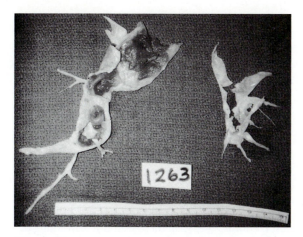

Figure 26–8. Well-organized thrombus surgically removed from subsegmental pulmonary arteries of a patient with thromboembolic pulmonary hypertension.

sion—regardless of its cause. Additionally, the endothelial injury of primary pulmonary hypertension predisposes the pulmonary arterioles to in situ thrombosis.

E. Vasodilators

The most effective oral vasodilators are the calcium channel blockers. Unfortunately, no agents are selective as pulmonary vasodilators, and systemic vasodilators—which may produce pulmonary vasodilation—must be chosen with care. The goal of therapy is to reduce pulmonary artery pressure and right ventricular afterload, allowing for improved right ventricular hemodynamics and an increase in overall cardiac output. This must be accomplished without producing symptomatic systemic hypotension. Approximately 25% of patients treated with agents such as nifedipine (30–240 mg/day) or diltiazem (120–900 mg/day) will have a sustained reduction in pulmonary artery pressure. In some cases, right ventricular hypertrophy has regressed in these patients. In others, however, vasodilators cause an increase in cardiac output without a significant drop in pulmonary artery pressure. Functional capacity may improve in these patients, but the long-term benefits with respect to survival are unknown. A small percentage of patients receiving vasodilators will have neither a reduction in pulmonary artery pressure nor an increase in cardiac output, but instead will suffer from reduced systemic arterial pressure. These patients should not receive vasodilator therapy because survival is not improved and the precipitation of right-to-left shunting is increased.

Tests with prostacyclin have been found useful in determining which patients respond to oral agents (eg, nifedipine, diltiazem). Other agents such as acetylcholine,

inhaled nitric oxide, and adenosine are useful as short-acting agents to determine vasoreactivity at the time of right-sided heart catheterization. Unfortunately, no clinical or hemodynamic variables accurately predict the response to vasodilators.

Once a patient is determined to have an appropriate vasodilator response to a titratable agent, therapy with a longer acting oral agent can be started. These agents should be started slowly and titrated to a maximal hemodynamic effect without causing such significant adverse effects as systemic hypotension, bradycardia, or atrioventricular block. Calcium antagonists such as verapamil, which have a more pronounced negative inotropic effect, should probably be avoided. Other vasodilators, such as nitrates, or direct-acting agents, such as hydralazine, have been of limited value because of their peripheral dilator effects. In addition, angiotensin-converting enzyme inhibitors have not been found to be particularly useful for treating pulmonary hypertension.

Regardless of which drug is chosen, it is important not to undertake vasodilator therapy in an uncontrolled setting because the consequences can be fatal. Often central venous catheters are placed to measure cardiac output, pulmonary artery pressures, and vascular resistance, whereas the medications are titrated in dose over time.

F. Prostacyclin

Patients with pulmonary hypertension can best be treated with a short-acting titratable vasodilator such as intravenous prostacyclin (PGI_2), administered during right-sided cardiac catheterization. This agent (given in 2–20 mg/kg/min doses) is valuable because of its 3–5 min half-life and the rapidity with which it can be studied. Long-term continuous intravenous infusion of prostacyclin has been shown to decrease pulmonary artery pressures and resistance in some patients with primary pulmonary hypertension. Improvements in symptoms as well as exercise tolerance and long-term survival have also been demonstrated (4-year survival approaching 75%). Prostacyclin can be delivered through a portable infusion pump connected to a central catheter inserted into a jugular or subclavian vein. The main difficulties with this approach have been complications related to infection, thrombosis at the catheter site, and pump malfunction. Inhaled and subcutaneous preparations are now becoming available. To date, prostacyclin has become the most effective therapy for intrinsic pulmonary vascular disease.

Galie N, Ussia G, Passarelli P et al: Role of pharmacologic tests in the treatment of primary pulmonary hypertension. Am J Cardiol 1995:75:55A.

Hoeper MM, Schwarze M, Ehlerding S et al: Long-term treatment of primary pulmonary hypertension with aerosolized iloprost, a prostacyclin analogue. N Engl J Med. 2000;342;1866.

McLaughlin VV, Genthner DE, Panella MM et al: Reduction in pulmonary vascular resistance with long-term epoprostenol (prostacyclin) therapy in primary pulmonary hypertension. N Engl J Med 1998;338:273.

Rich S, Kaufmann E, Levy PS: The effect of high doses of calcium-channel blockers on survival in primary pulmonary hypertension. N Engl J Med 1992;327:76.

Shapiro SM, Oudiz RJ, Cao T, et al: Primary pulmonary hypertension: Improved survival with continuous intravenous epoprostenol infusion. J Am Coll Cardiol 1997;30:343.

G. TRANSPLANTATION

Experience with combined heart-lung or single- or double-lung transplantation is growing. Initially, it was believed that because of the right ventricular failure found in many patients with pulmonary hypertension, combined heart-lung transplantation would be necessary. As noted earlier, however, in patients with severe right ventricular dysfunction undergoing pulmonary thromboendarterectomy, the right ventricle was able to function normally after reduction of afterload. Results with lung transplantation alone have been very gratifying. One-year actuarial survival rates after lung transplantation for end-stage pulmonary hypertension are now reported at 91%. Five-year survival rates are approximately 50%. Obviously, such surgery must be selected for patients with underlying disease processes that will not cause secondary pulmonary hypertension in the transplanted organ.

H. OTHER FORMS OF THERAPY

In some patients with pulmonary hypertension who have a patent foramen ovale, it has been suggested that survival is extended because of the right-to-left shunt, which allows for unloading of the right atrium. Overall right-heart hemodynamics and right ventricular perfusion are improved. Because of these findings, blade or balloon atrial septostomy as a palliative measure has been advocated for some patients awaiting transplantation.

Rich S, Dodin E, McLaughlin VV: Usefulness of atrial septostomy as a treatment for primary pulmonary hypertension and guidelines for its application. Am J Cardiol 1997;80:369–371.

Prognosis

The underlying cause of the pulmonary hypertension is the key determinant to the prognosis and natural history of the disease. When the underlying source (eg, mitral valve disease) can be treated effectively, the pulmonary hypertension may reverse with an accompanying substantial improvement in survival. For example, patients with chronic thromboembolic disease who undergo successful pulmonary thromboendarterectomy may expect to return to a normal lifestyle with normal anticipated survival rates. In contrast, those cases left untreated may result in death in the first decade after diagnosis. The prognosis varies from individual to individual depending on the duration of time between onset and diagnosis and the extent of pressure elevation. The degree of preserved vascular reactivity is also an extremely important factor.

When pulmonary hypertension cannot be corrected, the underlying cause appears to influence survival. Patients with congenital heart disease leading to Eisenmenger's syndrome have a 6-month actuarial survival rate of 89%; those with emphysema, 81%; those with cystic fibrosis, 74%; and those with interstitial lung disease, 38%.

Survival in cases of primary pulmonary hypertension depends on several factors and is difficult to predict. The usual causes of death are right ventricular failure in about two thirds of patients, followed by sudden death (7%) and pneumonia (7%). Overall survival may range up to 10 years or more, and a few case reports tell of survival beyond two decades, with rare instances of spontaneous reversal of pulmonary hypertension.

Some hemodynamic parameters give clues to the prognosis of the patient with primary pulmonary hypertension. According to the Patient Registry for the Characterization of Primary Pulmonary Hypertension, patients with a mean pulmonary arterial pressure of 85 mm Hg or more have a median survival of 12 months, and those with a mean pulmonary artery pressure less than 55 mm Hg, have a median survival of 48 months. Right atrial pressure and cardiac index are also predictors of survival. Patients with a cardiac index less than 2 L/min/m² have a median survival of only 17 months. Low mixed venous oxygen saturations also predict decreased survival.

Clinical features, such as the functional classification of the patient, are important factors in determining prognosis. Survival for patients with New York Heart Association classes I and II was approximately 59 months (median); for patients in classes III and IV, it ranged between 6 and 30 months. Because symptoms of right-heart failure are a late development and a consequence of right ventricular dysfunction, their presence may suggest both a more severe course and a later stage in the disease. Presence of right-heart failure predicts early mortality. Hemodynamic variables, as noted earlier, in concert with symptomatic classification can provide a general predictive score for patient survival.

Archibald CJ, Auger WR, Fedullo PF: Outcome after pulmonary thromboendarterectomy. Semin Thorac Cardiovasc Surg. 1999; 11:164.

Bennett LE, Keck BM, Daily OP et al: Worldwide thoracic organ transplantation: A report from the UNOS/ISHLT International Registry for Thoracic Organ Transplantation. Clin Transpl 2000:31.

D'Alonzo GG et al: Survival in patients with primary pulmonary hypertension: Results from a natural perspective registry. Ann Intern Med 1991;115:343.

Congenital Heart Disease in Adults   27

Nikola Tede, MD & Elyse Foster, MD

General Considerations

Over the past three decades the number of patients surviving with congenital heart disease, both in the United States and worldwide, has increased significantly. Over 85% of infants born with cardiovascular anomalies now can expect to reach adulthood. Reduced mortality rates can be attributed to improved diagnostic abilities, enhanced surgical techniques, and advances in intensive care. For the first time the number of adults with congenital heart disease nearly equals the number of children with the disorder.

The increase in the number of adults with congenital heart disease requires that the physician who must manage the care of these patients have improved knowledge of simple and complex anatomy and physiology. Although actual numbers are difficult to assess, it has been estimated that more than 750,000 adults in the United States alone currently have congenital heart disease and that the number of patients reaching adulthood with treated congenital heart disease will increase by approximately 9000 per year.

These patients fall into several broad categories: those surviving into adulthood without surgical intervention, those surviving with curative surgical or nonsurgical intervention (catheter-based stenting, coiling, or device occlusion), and those surviving with palliative surgical or nonsurgical intervention. The patients who are today making the transition into the adult congenital heart disease population have different hemodynamic and cardiac problems from those of previous decades. Surgical techniques have evolved, intervention occurs earlier and is often definitive rather than palliative, and a greater number of patients with complex single-ventricle physiology and various modifications of cavopulmonary anastomoses (Glenn shunt, Fontan procedure) will reach adulthood.

Although many patients are referred by pediatric cardiologists, others may present for the first time in adulthood. Examples of cardiac pathology that may not be readily apparent in childhood include secundum atrial septal defects (ASD), coarctation of the aorta, Ebstein's anomaly of the tricuspid valve, congenitally corrected transposition (ventricular inversion),

and coronary artery anomalies. Endocarditis remains an ongoing concern in many adult congenital cardiac patients and varies considerably in relative risk from one lesion to another; it is also dependent on whether the patient has been surgically treated. The risk of endocarditis and the need for prophylaxis are summarized in Table 27–1.

Morris CD, Reller MD, Menashe VD: Thirty-year incidence of infective endocarditis after surgery for congenital heart defect. JAMA 1998;279(8):599.

Perloff JK, Warnes CA: Challenges posed by adults with repaired congenital heart disease. Circulation 2001;103:2637.

Thirty-second Bethesda Conference: Care of the adult with congenital heart disease. JACC 2001;37:1161.

Wren C, O'Sullivan JJ: Future demand for follow-up of adult survivors of congenital heart disease. Heart 2001;85:438.

ACYANOTIC CONGENITAL HEART DISEASE

The most common acyanotic congenital heart defects include abnormalities of the heart valves and great vessels, ventricular or atrial communications with left-to-right shunting, and such lesions as partial anomalous pulmonary veins and anomalous coronary arteries.

CONGENITAL AORTIC VALVULAR DISEASE

 ESSENTIALS OF DIAGNOSIS

- *History of murmur since infancy, coarctation repair, or endocarditis*
- *Early systolic ejection click, harsh crescendo-decrescendo systolic, or early decrescendo diastolic murmur*
- *Left ventricular hypertrophy*
- *Abnormal bicuspid or dysplastic aortic valve with stenosis or regurgitation on Doppler echocardiography*

Table 27–1. Congenital heart disease in adults.

Defect	M:F	Associated Defects	Risk of Endocarditis	Prophylaxis
Acyanotic				
Bicuspid AV	4:1	Coarctation	High	Yes
Valvar PS	1:1	VSD (see TOF), Noonan's syndrome	Low (mild PS), intermediate (severe PS)	No Yes
ASD secundum	1:2	Mitral valve prolapse	Low	No
ASD primum AV canal		Bridging AV valve leaflets, trisomy 21	Intermediate (with MR)	Yes
VSD	1:1	PS (see TOF), AR	Intermed-high (unoperated or w/AR) Low (operated without AR)	Yes No
PDA	1:2–3	Coexists with many complex syndromes	Low (ligated), Intermediate (patent)	No Yes
Coarctation	2:1	Bicuspid AV	Low (operated[a]), intermediate (without treatment)	No Yes
C-TGV	M > F	VSD, infundibular PS	Low (isolated C-TGV)	No
Ebstein's anomaly	1:1	ASD PFO	Low-intermediate	Yes
Coronary AV fistulae	1:1		Intermediate	Yes
Cyanotic				
TOF	1.5:1	RAA, ASD	Intermediate	Yes
Eisenmenger's syndrome	M < F	VSD, ASD, PDA	Low	Yes
Tricuspid atresia	1:1[b]	Pulmonary atresia, ASD, VSD	?	Yes
Pulmonary atresia/ Intract septum	1:1		?	Yes
D-TGV	2–4:1	ASD, PFO, PDA, VSD, PS, RAA	Intermediate	Yes
Postoperative				
Fontan			Variable	Depends on associated defects
Glenn			Variable	Depends on associated defects
Blalock-Taussig			High	Yes
RV-PA conduit			High	Yes

[a] Unless there is associated bicuspid AV.

[b] In TA with transposition, M > F.

AR = aortic regurgitation; ASD = atrial septal defect; AV = aortic valve; C-TGV = congenitally corrected transposition of the great vessels; MR = mitral regurgitation; PA = pulmonary artery; PDA = patent ductus arteriosus; PFO = patent foramen ovale; PS = pulmonic stenosis; Pul Atr = pulmonary atresia; RAA = right-sided aortic arch; RV = right ventricle; TOF = tetralogy of Fallot; VSD = ventricular septal defect.

General Considerations

Congenital aortic stenosis is the most common anomaly encountered in the adult population and constitutes approximately 7% of all forms of congenital heart disease. The term **bicuspid aortic valve** is actually a misnomer; a raphe caused by commissural fusion of two leaflets usually exists. The valve is often dysplastic, with thickening and rolling of the leaflets. The predominant pathophysiology results from a mildly obstructed non-laminar (disturbed) flow across the abnormal valve. A left ventricle-to-aorta pressure gradient of variable severity occurs, setting the stage for the inevitable deterioration of the valve with long-term calcium deposition and progressive stenosis or regurgitation. In a study of young adults with aortic stenosis who presented for surgery between the ages of 21 and 38, diastolic murmurs were audible in 75%, and calcification was found at surgery in 75%. The valve is also at risk for endocarditis, which can lead to early destruction and regurgitation.

Clinical Findings

A. Symptoms and Signs

The individual with congenital aortic stenosis is usually asymptomatic unless hemodynamically significant stenosis or regurgitation is present. Routine physical examination reveals a normal carotid pulse contour and left ventricular (LV) impulse, a normal S_2, an early systolic click or sound, and an early-peaking systolic murmur. Identifying these patients in the asymptomatic stage is important. They must be educated on the need to protect the valves with endocarditis prophylaxis and good dental hygiene. Refraining from high-level isometric exercise should also be encouraged for preservation of valve function. The presence of a diastolic murmur of aortic regurgitation in a patient with a febrile illness should alert the clinician to the possibility of endocarditis and prompt the performance of appropriate diagnostic tests (eg, blood cultures, echocardiogram).

Congenital aortic stenosis is progressive; once a patient develops evidence of hemodynamically significant valvular disease, generally in the fifth or sixth decade of life, the symptoms and signs are identical to those of a patient with acquired aortic valvular disease. The patient presents with the classic triad of symptoms: dyspnea, chest pain, and exertional syncope. When stenosis predominates, the carotid upstroke is delayed and diminished in volume, the systolic click is no longer present, S_2 is single, and the systolic murmur is crescendo-decrescendo, peaking in late systole. The murmur of aortic regurgitation is often present.

B. Diagnostic Studies

1. Electrocardiography and chest radiography— The major electrocardiographic (ECG) findings include left ventricular hypertrophy (LVH) with high QRS voltage, left-axis deviation, and repolarization changes; left atrial enlargement may also be present. The chest radiographic findings are nonspecific. With predominant valvular aortic stenosis, the cardiothoracic ratio may be normal, but LV enlargement and calcification may be evident in the region of the aortic valve on the lateral film. A dilated ascending aorta or a prominent aortic knob may be seen. The cardiac silhouette is enlarged in patients with predominant aortic regurgitation. Pulmonary vasculature may be prominent in the presence of congestive heart failure (CHF).

2. Echocardiography—In the child and younger adult, the abnormally thickened leaflets of the congenitally abnormal valve are readily seen, and the bicuspid valve with its ovoid appearance in systole is apparent (Figure 27–1). On M-mode echocardiography, the point of closure may be eccentric. Heavy calcification often obscures the original valve morphology in the older individual with stenosis. The peak systolic gradient in severe aortic stenosis is usually greater than 64 mm Hg (peak velocity >4 m/s by continuous-wave Doppler). Aortic valve area can be accurately calculated by the continuity equation. Severe or critical aortic stenosis is defined as a valve area of less than 0.8 cm² or 0.5 cm²/m². The left ventricle shows concentric hypertrophy with thick walls and normal cavity dimensions, and the LV ejection fraction is usually normal. In cases with reduced ejection fraction, however, the peak gradient across the aortic valve is generally lower.

In hemodynamically significant aortic regurgitation, the high-velocity diastolic color-flow jet is broad at its site of origin below the aortic valve. Spectral Doppler imaging demonstrates a dense diastolic velocity signal with a short pressure half-time (<400 ms), and diastolic flow reversal can be recorded in the descending aorta. The left ventricle shows eccentric hypertrophy with normal LV wall thickness and a dilated cavity.

Transesophageal echocardiography (TEE) has proven to be of great value in patients with poor precordial windows. This technique allows the valve leaflets with the commissural fusion and asymmetric sinuses of Valsalva to be well visualized. Systolic doming of the leaflets can be easily seen in the long axis view of the LV outflow tract, which also allows measurements to be taken of the aortic valve annulus, sinuses of Valsalva, sinotubular ridge, and ascending aorta.

3. Cardiac catheterization—Indications for cardiac catheterization in congenital aortic valve disease have changed significantly because most of the diagnostic

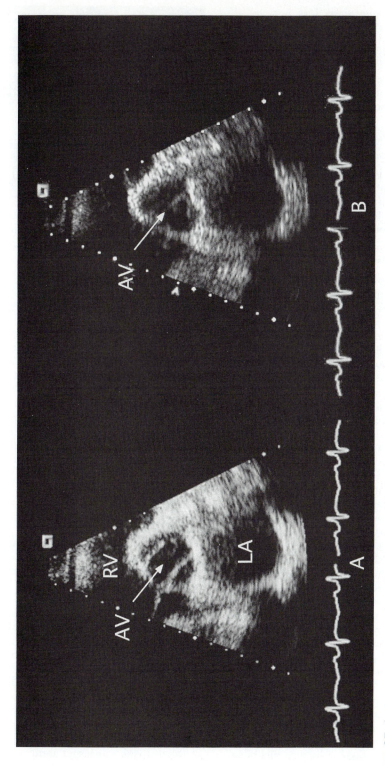

Figure 27–1. Transesophageal echocardiographic views of a patient with bicuspid aortic valve. **A:** Systolic frame showing two leaflets of the aortic valve (AV) with an ovoid opening (*arrow*). **B:** Diastolic frame showing the single line of coaptation (*arrow*). LA = left atrium, RV = right ventricle.

data are now available noninvasively. It is, however, almost always indicated in the following situations:

- Symptoms and signs suggesting that stenosis is more severe than indicated by Doppler findings
- Any individual older than 40 years of age, with cardiovascular risk factors or an abnormal myocardial perfusion study, to rule out coronary artery disease

When Doppler information is adequate, the procedure can often be limited to coronary arteriography.

4. Magnetic resonance imaging—Serial imaging with magnetic resonance imaging permits accurate and reproducible follow-up of aortic dilatation and is accepted as the standard of care for follow-up of repaired coarctation, a frequent association with a bicuspid aortic valve.

Differential Diagnosis

A fibrous membrane may characterize discrete subaortic stenosis, which is more frequently encountered in adults, or by a tubular fibromuscular channel that usually presents in childhood. Aortic regurgitation, commonly associated with this anomaly (in approximately 60% of cases), increases in frequency with age. It is attributed to the high-velocity jet, which causes direct trauma to the aortic leaflets, resulting in leaflet thickening, or interference of leaflet closure by the membrane may occur. The aortic valve appearance and the severity and mechanism of aortic regurgitation must be carefully assessed.

Recurrent stenosis caused by regrowth following surgical resection of the fibromuscular ridge is sometimes encountered in the adolescent or adult. Discrete subaortic stenosis and congenital valvular aortic stenosis must also be distinguished from dynamic LV outflow-tract obstruction caused by hypertrophic obstructive cardiomyopathy (see Chapter 14).

When aortic regurgitation is the predominant lesion and ascending aorta dilatation is present, the condition must be distinguished from Marfan's syndrome. This latter condition is characterized by dilatation of the aortic root at the level of the sinuses of Valsalva (Figure 27–2). The aortic valve leaflets are not thickened, and regurgitation is caused by failure of leaflet coaptation caused by the root dilatation. With valvular stenosis, the aorta narrows toward normal at the sinotubular junction, and the descending thoracic aorta is spared. In some patients with a bicuspid aortic valve an underlying abnormality of the medial layer of the aorta above the valve predisposes to the dilatation of the aortic root, which may progress to aneurysm formation or rupture. All components of the vessel wall, smooth muscle, elastic fibers, collagen, and ground substance can be affected and should be recognized as a potential risk in the surgical patient.

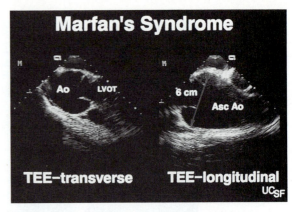

Figure 27–2. Transesophageal echocardiographic views of the ascending aorta (Asc Ao) measuring 8 cm in a patient with Marfan's syndrome. LVOT = left ventricular outflow tract.

Prognosis & Treatment

The natural history of aortic stenosis presenting in childhood depends largely on the severity of the stenosis at the time of diagnosis. During a 25-year follow-up period, approximately one third of the children (with a peak systolic gradient of less than 50 mm Hg) who were treated medically required surgery, in contrast to 80% of those with an intermediate gradient (50–79 mm Hg). Of those treated surgically for a gradient of more than 79 mm Hg, approximately one fourth required reoperation; reoperation was more common in those treated with initial valvotomy (30%) than aortic valve replacement (5%). The overall 25-year survival rate is approximately 85%; sudden death accounts for approximately one half of the cardiac-related deaths.

Once the patient develops symptoms of aortic stenosis, the prognosis without valve replacement is poor; the 5-year mortality rate is approximately 90%. Although percutaneous valvuloplasty has been successful in children and adolescents, the results in adults (even those with congenitally abnormal valves), have been disappointing. Therefore, surgery with aortic valve replacement, rather than percutaneous valvuloplasty, is generally mandated. Surgery is indicated in the symptomatic patient with a valve area of less than 0.8 cm^2 (or <0.5 cm^2/m^2). It should be considered in the asymptomatic patient with critical stenosis when the patient requires cardiac surgery (eg, coronary artery bypass surgery) for another lesion or prior to noncardiac surgery under general anesthesia.

Patients with a bicuspid aortic valve and concomitant annuloaortic ectasia may show a more rapid progression of aortic regurgitation and require surgical intervention earlier than those patients with pure aortic stenosis.

An ideal substitute for replacing the aortic valve does not exist. Homografts and bioprosthetic valves can develop rapid calcific degeneration, causing valve dysfunction, particularly in the younger cohort of patients. Mechanical valves, although extremely durable, require anticoagulation to decrease the complication of thromboembolism. The risks associated with long-term anticoagulation have made surgical options to avoid the use of mechanical valves desirable alternatives. The Ross procedure (in which the autologous pulmonary valve replaces the aortic valve, and an aortic or pulmonary homograft replaces the pulmonary valve) has been increasingly performed for a variety of LV outflow tract diseases, including aortic insufficiency and valvar aortic stenosis with or without other forms of obstruction (subaortic stenosis, supravalvar stenosis, arch hypoplasia, etc). Although the Ross procedure is more complex than simple aortic valve replacement, it can be carried out with a low mortality rate in selected patients. The pulmonary valve autograft advantages include freedom from anticoagulation and the absence of compromise from host reactions and autograft growth, making it an attractive option for aortic valve replacement in infants and children. It is recognized, however, that the pulmonary homograft will require replacement for degenerative disease and size restriction in children. In adults who are confronting surgery for a stenotic aortic valve in the fifth or sixth decade of life, the Ross procedure has shown to be an acceptable alternative to the usual mechanical or bioprosthetic valve. These patients also benefit from the absence of anticoagulation, and growing data show good longevity of the homograft in the pulmonary position. Contraindications to a Ross would include advanced three-vessel coronary artery disease, poor LV function, a severely calcified aortic root, or pulmonary valve pathology.

Gerosa G, McKay R, Ross DN: Replacement of the aortic valve or root with a pulmonary autograft in children. Ann Thorac Surg 1991;51(3):424.

Keane JF, Driscoll DJ, Gersong WM et al: Second natural history study of congenital heart defects: Results of treatment of patients with aortic valvular stenosis. Circulation 1993; 87(Suppl 1):16.

Knott-Craig CJ, Elkins RC, Santangelo KL et al: Aortic valve replacement: Comparison of late survival between autografts and homografts. Ann Thorac Surg 2000;69:1327.

Lambert V, Obreja D, Losay J et al: Long-term results after valvotomy for congenital aortic valvar stenosis in children. Cardiol Young 2000;10(6):590.

Masani N: Transesophageal echocardiography in adult congenital disease. Heart 2001;86(Suppl II):ii30.

Niwa K, Perloff JK, Bhuta SM et al: Structural abnormalities of great arterial walls in congenital heart disease: Light and electron microscopic analyses. Circulation 2001;103(3):393.

PULMONARY VALVE STENOSIS

 ESSENTIALS OF DIAGNOSIS

- *History of murmur since infancy*
- *Systolic ejection click and an early systolic murmur in the second left intercostal space with transmission to the back. S_2 may split widely*
- *Right ventricular hypertrophy on electrocardiograph*
- *Dilatation of main and left pulmonary arteries on chest radiograph*
- *Right ventricular hypertrophy, systolic doming of the pulmonary valve, and a transpulmonic gradient by Doppler echocardiography*

General Considerations

Pulmonary valve, or pulmonic stenosis, is the second most common form of congenital heart disease in the adult. Although many cases are so mild as to require no treatment, it often coexists with other congenital cardiac abnormalities (ASD, ventricular septal defect [VSD], patent ductus arteriosus, or tetralogy of Fallot [TOF]). It is characterized by a conical or dome-shaped pliant valve with a narrow outlet at its apex. Right ventricular (RV) outflow is obstructed depending on the size of the orifice, and RV stroke volume may not rise appropriately during exercise. In response to the pressure overload, the right ventricle hypertrophies, with an increase in wall thickness. This compensatory hypertrophy can involve the infundibulum and potentially lead to reversible dynamic subpulmonic stenosis once the valvular stenosis is relieved (see section on Pulmonary Valve Stenosis). If the stenosis remains untreated, RV failure may ensue. It is important to differentiate pulmonary valve stenosis from stenoses of the peripheral pulmonary arteries and primary infundibular stenosis (often associated with ventricular septal defect; see the section on tetralogy of Fallot). Pulmonary stenosis from a thickened, dysplastic valve is seen in patients with Noonan's syndrome (a nonchromosomal malformation syndrome with autosomal-dominant inheritance).

Clinical Findings

A. SYMPTOMS AND SIGNS

The patient with pulmonic stenosis (PS) usually presents with exercise intolerance in the form of exertional fatigue, dyspnea, chest pain, or syncope. Right ventricular failure with systemic venous congestion occurs late in the course of the disease. If the foramen ovale is patent or a concomitant ASD exists, shunting of blood from the right atrium to the left may occur, causing cyanosis and clubbing. The volume overload of pregnancy may precipitate failure in patients with severe PS, although mild and even moderate stenosis are usually well tolerated.

In significant PS, the physical examination demonstrates a parasternal RV heave, a delayed and diminished or absent P_2, and a late-peaking crescendo-decrescendo murmur. If the valve is pliable, an ejection click precedes the murmur. This pulmonic ejection sound, best heard in the second left intercostal space, is the only right-sided event that decreases in intensity during inspiration and increases during expiration. As the stenosis becomes more severe, the systolic murmur will peak later in systole and the ejection click moves closer to the first heart sound, eventually becoming superimposed on it. The jugular venous pulse shows a prominent *a* wave, as a result of the diminished RV compliance, but jugular venous pressure is increased only in the late stages when RV failure occurs. Similarly, there may be an RV S_4 gal-

lop early in the course of the disease and a right-sided S_3 in the later stages.

B. DIAGNOSTIC STUDIES

1. Electrocardiography and chest radiograph—The ECG demonstrates evidence of right ventricular hypertrophy (RVH) with right-axis deviation, prominent R waves in the right precordial leads, and deep S waves in the left precordial leads (Figure 27–3). There may also be evidence of P-pulmonale with peaked inferior (II, III, aVF) P waves.

The chest radiograph shows a normal cardiac silhouette in mild-to-moderate PS but may become enlarged in severe stenosis when right-heart failure occurs. The main and left pulmonary arteries are dilated because of poststenotic dilatation. Dilatation may be seen even in cases of mild PS and may be related to intrinsic abnormalities of the pulmonary artery (idiopathic pulmonary artery dilatation).

2. Echocardiography—The poor near-field resolution of transthoracic echocardiography (TTE) often limits definition of pulmonary valve morphology in the adult

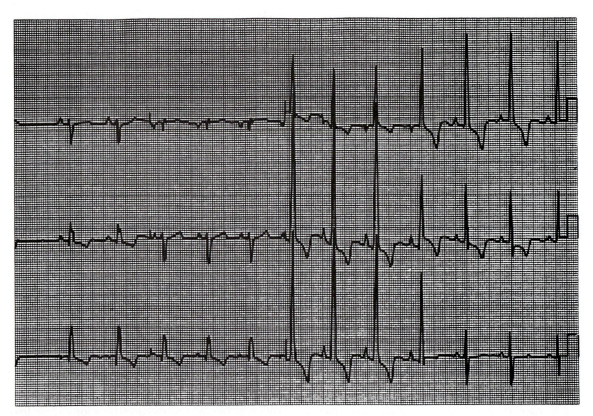

Figure 27–3. Electrocardiograph in congenital pulmonic stenosis with severe right ventricular hypertrophy and marked right-axis deviation.

patient. When visualized in the parasternal short-axis view, the valve may appear thickened (rarely calcified) and usually manifests systolic doming. In the absence of right heart failure, the RV dimension is normal or only mildly increased, but the RV wall thickness is increased (more than 5 mm). In severe cases, the septum may be deviated toward the left ventricle from the pressure overload of the right ventricle. The right atrium and ventricle dilate late in the course of the disease. Contrast echocardiography should be performed in all patients with pulmonary valve stenosis to exclude an ASD or a patent foramen ovale.

Color-flow Doppler imaging demonstrates high-velocity flow within the pulmonary artery and is helpful in excluding a ventricular septal defect or a patent ductus arteriosus. Continuous-wave Doppler demonstrates a high-velocity jet across the RV outflow tract (Figure 27–4B). This signal is best obtained from the parasternal short-axis view where flow is axial to the Doppler beam. Unfortunately, because of the lack of range resolution, continuous-wave Doppler cannot localize the level of the obstruction. The morphology of the valve by echocardiography and pulsed-wave Doppler mapping may provide localizing information, but additional diagnostic procedures are often necessary.

Transesophageal echocardiography, provides excellent definition of the RV outflow tract and pulmonary valve in the basal longitudinal views and allows for good visualization of the atrial septum. As a result, noninvasive methods may now be adequate for establishing the diagnosis, even in adults.

3. Cardiac catheterization—In most patients cardiac catheterization is therapeutic as well as diagnostic because percutaneous balloon valvuloplasty has virtually replaced surgery for treatment of pulmonary valve stenosis (see below). During right-heart catheterization, the level of the stenosis can be confirmed by pressure monitoring during pullback from the pulmonary artery. In valvular stenosis, there is a rise in peak systolic pressure as the catheter exits the pulmonary artery into the infundibulum. In contrast, when the stenosis is in the infundibulum, the systolic pressure increases when the catheter is pulled into the body of the right ventricle. As mentioned earlier, in PS, secondary hypertrophy may result in some degree of infundibular stenosis, and a pressure differential may be demonstrated at both levels on pullback (Figure 27–5). If the level of obstruction is still uncertain, cine-angiography may show the hypertrophied infundibulum or, alternatively, the domed and thickened pulmonary valve. Of course, both levels of obstruction may coexist.

Unlike aortic valve stenosis, the valve area is not calculated from the Doppler or invasive hemodynamic data, and the gradient alone is used to determine the severity of the obstruction and guide therapy.

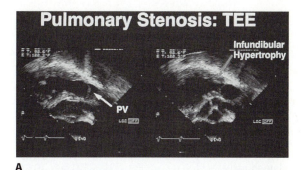

Figure 27–4. **A:** Transesophageal echocardiographic views of a pregnant woman with severe pulmonary valve (PV) stenosis. The left image demonstrates the doming pulmonary valve in systole. The right frame illustrates the severe infundibular hypertrophy. **B:** Continuous-wave Doppler recording from the same patient demonstrated a peak velocity of 6 m/s corresponding to a peak transvalvular gradient of 144 mm Hg.

Prognosis & Treatment

In severe untreated pulmonary valve stenosis, the average life expectancy is approximately 30 years. The natural history of medically treated mild (gradient <50 mm Hg) or moderate (gradient 50-79 mm Hg) PS and surgically treated severe (gradient >80 mm Hg) PS is excellent with a 25-year survival rate of 95%. Surgical valvotomy via a pulmonary artery incision has been extremely effective in long-term relief of pulmonary valve obstruction. Although approximately 50% of patients have mild-to-moderate regurgitation following surgery, it is seldom of hemodynamic significance, and reoperation is rarely necessary.

In children treated conservatively for PS, the likelihood of eventually requiring surgery is dependent on the initial gradient: less than 25 mm Hg, 5%;

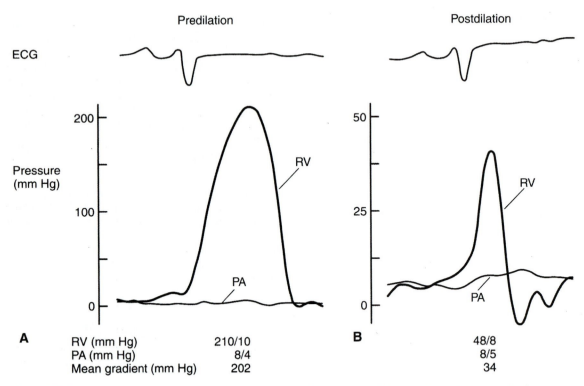

Figure 27–5. Hemodynamic tracings in pulmonic stenosis. **A:** Predilation: Mean gradient of 202 mm Hg between right ventricle (RV) and pulmonary artery (PA). **B:** Postdilation: Residual gradient of 34 mm Hg between RV infundibulum and pulmonary artery. Reprinted, with permission, from McGregor J, Ports TA: Catheter balloon valvuloplasty. In Parmley WW, Chattergee KD, eds: Philadelphia: Lippincott, 1993.

25-49 mm Hg, 20%; and 50-79 mm Hg, 76%. In the adult, the indication for treatment of pulmonary valve stenosis is a peak systolic gradient in excess of 50 mm Hg. When the gradient is between 40 and 50 mm Hg, the decision to treat is based on the presence of symptoms, the age of the patient, and the degree of RVH (by echocardiography or electrocardiography [ECG]). Echo- cardiography, pre and post exercise may be an important technique to assess RV function in the presence of an increased gradient.

As mentioned above, most patients (including adults) with pulmonary valve stenosis are currently treated with percutaneous balloon valvuloplasty. The Registry of the Valvuloplasty and Angioplasty of Congenital Anomalies has listed 35 patients over the age of 20, among them a 76-year-old man. No significant complications occurred in adult patients, and the gradient was reduced from approximately 70 to 30 mm Hg, with about 50% of the residual gradient caused by infundibular hypertrophy. Ongoing assessment of these patients indicate sustained long-term relief of the pul-

monary valve gradient with progressive infundibular remodeling causing further reduction in the outflow tract gradient over time. Recent technical improvements leading to the development of low profile balloon have decreased the risk of pulmonary regurgitation after dilatation. Based on these results, percutaneous balloon valvuloplasty appears to be the treatment of choice in adults with pulmonary valve stenosis.

Brickner ME, Hills LD, Lange RA: Congenital heart disease in adults. N Engl J Med 2000;342(4):256.

Chen CR et al: Percutaneous balloon valvuloplasty for pulmonic stenosis in adolescents and adults. N Engl J Med 1996; 335(22):1688.

Perloff JK: Physical Examination of the Heart and Circulation, 3rd ed. Philadelphia: WB Saunders, 2000.

Sadr-Ameli MA et al: Late results of balloon pulmonary valvuloplasty in adults. Am J Cardiol 1998;82:398.

Teupe CH et al: Late (five to nine years) follow-up after balloon dilation of valvar pulmonary stenosis in adults. Am J Cardiol 1997;80:240.

ATRIAL SEPTAL DEFECT

ESSENTIALS OF DIAGNOSIS

- *A widely fixed and split S_2 and a mid systolic murmur are characteristic. If the shunt is large a mid-diastolic rumble of relative tricuspid stenosis may be audible at the lower left sternal border*
- *Incomplete RIGHT BUNDLE BRANCH BLOCK with vertical QRS axis (ostium secundum ASD) and superior axis (ostium primum ASD) on ECG*
- *Prominent pulmonary arteries and right ventricular enlargement (decreased retrosternal air space) on chest radiograph. Increased pulmonary vascular markings*
- *Right ventricular dilatation, increased pulmonary artery flow velocity, and left-to-right atrial shunt by Doppler echocardiography*
- *O_2 step-up within the right atrium; right-sided catheter can pass into the left atrium across the defect*

General Considerations

Atrial septal defects make up 10% of congenital heart disease cases in newborns and are regularly encountered as new diagnoses in adults. The defects vary in size from the smallest fenestrated ASD (a few millimeters) to the largest defect—the complete absence of the atrial septum, or common atrium. The most common atrial communication is a patent foramen ovale (PFO) that is anatomically and physiologically not classified as an ASD.

Classification of ASDs is according to location (Figure 27–6): ostium secundum in the region of the fossa ovalis, ostium primum in the lower portion of the atrial septum (actually part of an atrioventricular (AV) canal defect, discussed below), sinus venosus in the upper part of the septum near the entrance of the superior vena cava or at the entrance of the inferior vena cava, and unroofed coronary sinus (communication between the coronary sinus and left atrium). Important associated abnormalities include anomalous drainage of the right upper pulmonary vein into the superior vena cava associated with a superior sinus venosus ASD, a persistent left superior vena cava with secundum or primum ASDs, and a cleft anterior mitral leaflet and mitral regurgitation associated with an ostium primum ASD. Ostium primum ASD is a common cardiac anomaly in

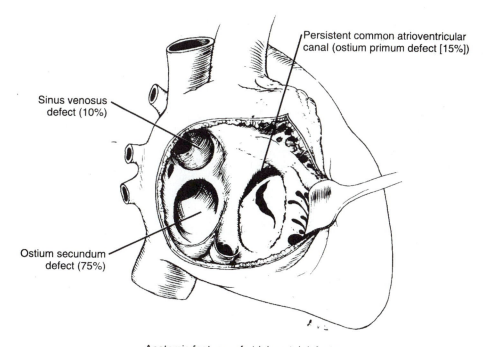

Anatomic features of atrial septal defects.

Figure 27–6. Anatomic location of atrial septal defects. Adapted from Cheitlin M, Sokolow M, McIlroy M: Congenital heart disease. In Clinical Cardiology. Norwalk, CT: Appleton & Lange, 1993.

trisomy 21 (Down syndrome) and is part of the spectrum of AV septal "canal" defects (discussed later).

The pathophysiologic consequences of an ASD depend on the quantity of blood shunted from the systemic to pulmonary circulation. The size of the shunt is in turn dependent on the size of the defect and the relative compliance of the right and left ventricles. Little or no shunting occurs immediately after birth because of the high pulmonary vascular resistance (PVR), but as resistance falls, the more compliant right ventricle receives the shunted blood mainly in diastole, when all four chambers are in communication. In the compensated patient with ASD, pulmonary resistance is usually low. The older adult with the LV diastolic abnormalities of hypertension, coronary artery disease, and aging may experience increased left-to-right shunting and, consequently, right heart failure. Atrial arrhythmias, especially atrial fibrillation, are common over the age of 50.

Clinical Findings

A. SYMPTOMS AND SIGNS

The young adult with an uncorrected ASD and normal PA pressures is usually asymptomatic, with normal or minimally diminished exercise tolerance. After the age of 30, however, exertional dyspnea and atypical chest pain increase in frequency. As mentioned earlier, the frequency of atrial arrhythmias increases with age and occurs in a high percentage of patients over the age of 50 who have not been treated surgically. Signs and symptoms of RV failure may occur because of pulmonary hypertension or as a result of long-standing volume overload.

Important findings of the physical examination in an uncomplicated ASD include a prominent RV impulse along the lower-left sternal border, a palpable pulmonary artery, a systolic ejection murmur that does not vary in intensity with respiration, and the almost pathognomonic fixed split second heart sound. There may be an associated right-sided diastolic flow rumble and S_3 gallop from increased flow across the tricuspid valve. The patient with ostium primum ASD usually has a holosystolic murmur of mitral regurgitation. If pulmonary hypertension is present, P_2 is increased and a high-pitched murmur of pulmonary regurgitation (Graham Steele murmur) may be audible. Signs of RV failure with elevated jugular venous pressure and venous congestion may be apparent in the later stages of this disease.

B. DIAGNOSTIC STUDIES

1. Electrocardiography and chest radiograph—The ECG shows an incomplete right bundle branch block (RBBB) in 90% of cases (Figure 27–7). In ostium secundum and sinus venosus ASDs, the QRS axis is vertical or rightward. In the patient with ostium primum ASD, the axis is superior and leftward. Abnormal sinus node function in patients with sinus venosus ASD often results in an ectopic atrial rhythm with a superior P-wave axis.

The chest radiograph shows prominent main and branch pulmonary arteries with a small aortic knob and RV enlargement. The right atrium may appear enlarged. In the absence of pulmonary hypertension, the lung markings are increased as a result of increased pulmonary blood flow.

2. Echocardiography—The findings on TTE include right-heart enlargement and increased pulmonary artery flow. Color-flow Doppler often can identify the interatrial flow, especially in the subcostal four-chamber view. An intravenous saline contrast injection should be used in all patients with these findings to exclude an unsuspected ASD. In the presence of an ASD, a negative contrast effect can be seen in the right atrium as the unopacified left atrial blood is shunted from left to right. A small degree of bidirectional shunting nearly always is present and microbubbles can be seen in the left atrium as a result of right-to-left shunting. The shunting across a patent foramen ovale is purely right to left and occurs only during transient (eg, Valsalva maneuver, coughing) or persistent elevations in right atrial pressure.

Pulmonary artery pressure can be estimated from the peak velocity of the tricuspid regurgitant jet. Echocardiographic measurements may be used to determine shunt flow, eliminating the need for an invasive assessment. In adults, however, the TTE is somewhat limited in quantifying the magnitude of shunts and the size of the defect and in locating sinus venosus defects or anomalous pulmonary veins. As noted earlier, TEE has been found to be more accurate in determining the size and location of atrial communications (Figure 27–8). Biplanar and multiplanar transesophageal views are particularly useful in identifying sinus venosus type ASD (Figure 27–9).

3. Cardiac catheterization—In some younger individuals with unequivocally large defects on noninvasive imaging, cardiac catheterization may be avoidable. In others, however, invasive studies may be necessary to accurately quantitate the shunt, measure PVR, and exclude coronary artery disease. Right-heart catheterization with repeated blood sampling for oxygen saturation demonstrates an O_2 step-up (ie, an increase in saturation) from the vena cava to the right atrium. In general, the higher the pulmonary arterial oxygen saturation, the greater the shunt, with a value greater than 90% suggesting a large shunt. The ratio of pulmonary to systemic flow can be calculated by the following formula:

$$\frac{Q_P}{Q_S} = \frac{S_{AO_2} - M_{VO_2}}{P_{VO_2} - P_{AO_2}}$$

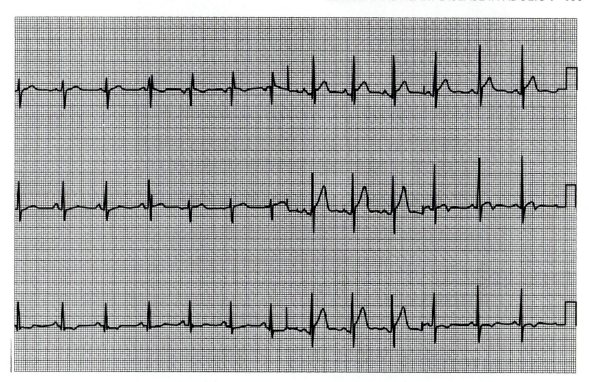

Figure 27–7. Electrocardiograph in atrial septal defect with right-axis deviation, incomplete right bundle branch block and right ventricular hypertrophy.

Where SAO_2, MVO_2, PVO_2 and PAO_2 are systemic arterial, mixed venous, pulmonary venous, and pulmonary arterial blood oxygen saturations, respectively.

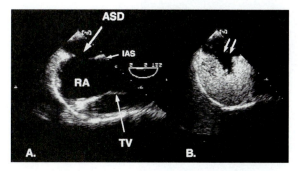

Figure 27–8. Transesophageal echocardiogram of a patient with an ostium secundum atrial septal defect (ASD). **A:** The image clearly demonstrates the position of the ASD in the midportion of the interatrial septum (IAS). **B:** The image is obtained after intravenous injection of agitated saline, which opacifies the right atrium (RA). The negative contrast effect produced by the unopacified left atrial blood entering the RA is clearly demonstrated (*double arrow*). TV = tricuspid valve.

A pulmonary vascular resistance that is more than 70% of the systemic vascular resistance suggests significant pulmonary vascular disease, and surgery is best avoided.

Prognosis & Treatment

Although patients with an uncorrected ostium secundum ASD generally survive into adulthood, their life expectancy is not normal—only about 50% survive beyond age 40. The mortality rate after the age of 40 is about 6% per year. Small ASDs (a pulmonary-to-systemic-flow ratio of less than 1.5–2:1) may cause problems only in the advanced years, when hypertension and coronary artery disease cause reduced LV compliance, resulting in increased left-to-right shunting, atrial arrhythmias, and potential biventricular failure. In addition, intrinsic abnormalities in LV diastolic function may develop in patients with ASDs unrelated to acquired heart disease. Only 5–10% of patients with large shunts (>2:1) develop severe pulmonary hypertension during young adulthood. Although most adults with ASDs have mild-to-moderate pulmonary hypertension, the late development of severe pulmonary hypertension in older adults appears to be quite rare. Pregnancy, in the absence of pulmonary hypertension,

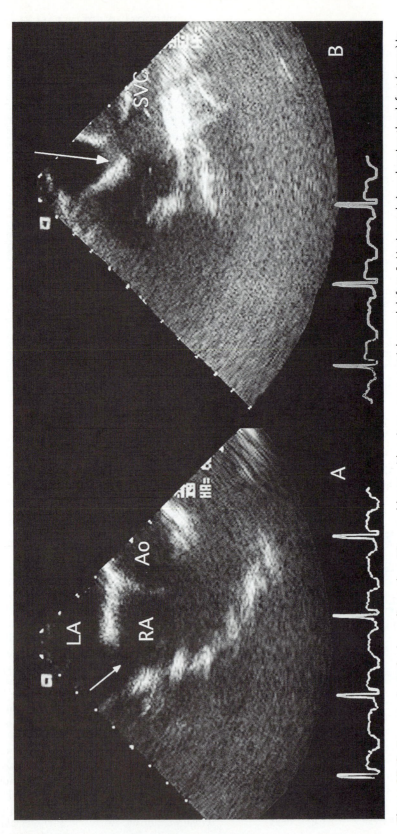

Figure 27–9. Transesophageal echocardiography a 50-year-old man with a sinus venosus atrial septal defect. **A:** Horizontal view showing the defect (*arrow*) in the superior portion of the interatrial septum. **B:** The defect (*arrow*) is clearly demonstrated in this longitudinal plane view. Ao = aorta, LA = left atrium, RA = right atrium, SVC = superior vena cava.

is usually uncomplicated. Another potential complication of ASD (including even the smallest patent foramen ovale) in the adult patient is paradoxical embolization. Endocarditis is rare in patients with ASD, and prophylaxis is not routinely recommended unless associated lesions with higher risk exist.

The natural history of sinus venosus ASDs is similar to that of ostium secundum, although many of these patients have associated partial anomalous pulmonary venous drainage. Adults with an ostium primum ASD are less commonly encountered and may have additional complications resulting from mitral regurgitation caused by the cleft leaflet (see the discussion on AV canal defects, later in this chapter).

Ostium secundum ASDs have been surgically repaired for more than 40 years. No late cardiac deaths occurred in those who had early surgical repair of ASDs (before the age of 18) among patients in a large registry. The Mayo Clinic experience with 123 patients who underwent surgery between 1956 and 1960 (a follow-up of approximately 30 years) included patients older than 24, with elevated pulmonary systolic pressure (>40 mm Hg), at the time of surgery. The poorest survival rate was in patients older than 41 at the time of operation (40%, versus 59% survival in younger patients), and late complications included heart failure, atrial arrhythmias, and stroke.

Despite the poorer surgical results in adults older than 40, surgery is probably superior to medical therapy and is recommended in patients with predominant left-to-right shunts (Qp:Qs >1.5:2:1) and PVR less than 10 units/m². Although mortality rates increase when the resistance exceeds this level, surgery can be performed safely in many patients with PVR between 10 and 15 units/m². Surgery will improve functional class and eliminate the risk of paradoxical embolization, but closure does not reduce the incidence of atrial arrhythmias. Device closure has now become standard of care for adolescents and adults with appropriately selected ostium secundum defects. In patients with patent foramen ovale who have suffered embolic phenomena, device closure is also becoming a standard intervention although evidence from a randomized controlled trial is lacking.

Berger F, Vogel M: Comparison of results and complications of surgical and Amplatzer device closure of atrial septal defects. J Thorac Cardiovasc Surg 1999;118:674.

Gatzoulis MA, Freeman MA, Siu SC et al: Atrial arrhythmia after surgical closure of atrial septal defect in adults. N Engl J Med 1999;340:839.

Hung J, Landzberg MJ, Jenkinskj et al: Closure of patent foramen ovale for paradoxical emboli: Intermediate term risk of recurrent neurological events following transcatheter device placement. J Am Coll Cardiol 2000;35:1311.

Konstantinides S, Geibel A, Olschewski M et al: A comparison of surgical and medical therapy for atrial septal defects in adults. N Engl J Med 1995;333:469.

VENTRICULAR SEPTAL DEFECTS

 ## ESSENTIALS OF DIAGNOSIS

- *History of murmur appearing shortly after birth*
- *Holosystolic murmur at left sternal border radiating rightward*
- *Left atrial and left ventricular or biventricular enlargement*
- *High-velocity color-flow Doppler jet across ventricular septal defect*
- *Increased pulmonary-flow velocities*

General Considerations

Because of the tendency for many VSDs to close spontaneously (see later discussion) and the tendency of larger defects to appear in early childhood as CHF, it is relatively uncommon to encounter adults with previously undiagnosed VSDs of hemodynamic consequence. Ventricular septal defects in adults are usually either small and hemodynamically insignificant or large and associated with Eisenmenger's syndrome. The importance of identifying the former is that they pose an ongoing risk for endocarditis and the potential complication of progressive aortic regurgitation. Eisenmenger's syndrome is discussed later in this chapter.

Classifications of VSDs can be based on anatomic location or physiology. The anatomic classification includes defects of both the membranous and muscular portions of the ventricular septum (Figure 27–10). Membranous VSDs can be subdivided into supracristal (also known as doubly committed subarterial), perimembranous (the inlet portion of the membranous septum), and malalignment (found in TOF with an overriding aorta) defects. The muscular VSDs, often multiple, may be located in the inlet or outlet regions or within the trabecular portion of the septum. Classifying VSDs physiologically is based on the size of the defect as well as the relative vascular resistances within the systemic and pulmonary circulation. A high-pressure gradient exists across a small restrictive VSD, with normal or mildly elevated PA pressure and predominant left-to-right shunting. A large nonrestrictive VSD permits equalization of RV and LV pressures with obligatory pulmonary hypertension (in the absence of RV outflow-tract obstruction) and bidirectional shunting. The smallest VSD (maladie de Roger) is characterized by a hemodynamically insignificant shunt, a loud murmur, and an intermediate-to-high risk for endocarditis.

In the infant, left-to-right shunting occurs only when pulmonary vascular resistance falls below sys-

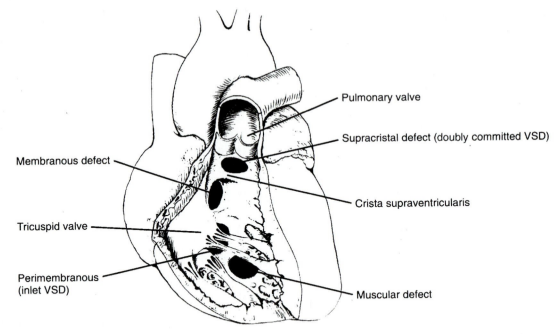

Figure 27–10. Anatomic location of ventricular septal defects. Adapted, with permission, from Cheitlin M, Sokolow M, McIlroy M: Congenital heart disease. In Clinical Cardiology. Norwalk, CT: Appleton & Lange, 1993.

temic vascular resistance, and the murmur usually becomes audible in the first month of life. With a large nonrestrictive defect, PVR may not fall; if the defect is not surgically closed by age 2, irreversible pulmonary hypertension may ensue. The volume overload caused by a large restrictive VSD may cause CHF in the first 6 months of life. Approximately 40% of VSDs close spontaneously by age 3, and a smaller percentage close before age 10. Generally, the smaller defects are more likely to close, but even in infants with heart failure, 7% will experience spontaneous closure.

Three late complications of VSD are worth mentioning. Tricuspid regurgitation may rarely result when the septal leaflet of the tricuspid valve is deformed by the ventricular septal aneurysm that causes spontaneous closure of a perimembranous VSD. Aortic regurgitation is common in patients with doubly committed subarterial VSDs (supracristal, or outlet, VSDs), as a result of herniation of the right aortic sinus into the defect; it also occurs in those with perimembranous VSDs. Infundibular PS from hypertrophy of the RV outflow tract can develop with formation of a double-chambered RV and right-to-left shunting, if the degree of stenosis becomes significant.

Clinical Findings

A. Symptoms and Signs

The young adult with an uncorrected VSD and normal PA pressures is usually asymptomatic, with normal or minimally diminished exercise tolerance. Like those with defects of the atrial septum, patients with VSDs develop exertional dyspnea after the age of 30 when the shunt ratio exceeds 2–3:1. Individuals with smaller shunts rarely report symptoms. The most disabled group with pulmonary hypertension and cyanosis (Eisenmenger's physiology, or syndrome) will be discussed later.

Physical findings depend on the size of the VSD. The patient with uncomplicated VSD is acyanotic, and the LV apical impulse is displaced laterally and may be hyperdynamic. A holosystolic murmur occurs, often associated with a systolic thrill, heard best in the fourth or fifth intercostal space along the left sternal border, with radiation to the right parasternal region. Because of the increased flow across the mitral valve, an S_3 gallop and a diastolic rumble may be present. Additional signs of tricuspid insufficiency (prominent jugular venous v wave and systolic murmur) or aortic valve regurgitation (diastolic blowing murmur, increased arterial pulses) will be present in patients with these complications.

B. Diagnostic Studies

1. Electrocardiography and chest radiography—In the presence of a large shunt, the ECG is suggestive of LVH or biventricular hypertrophy, with biphasic QRS complexes in the transitional precordial leads. Evidence of left or right atrial enlargement is present in only about 25% of patients.

Cardiac enlargement with an increased cardiac silhouette is evident on chest radiograph only in the presence of a large left-to-right shunt. In the absence of pulmonary hypertension, there is evidence of pulmonary vascular engorgement with a plethora of the peripheral vasculature as well as enlargement of the proximal vessels. Left atrial enlargement may be evident on the lateral chest radiograph.

It is important to remember that in most adults with a small VSD (<1.5–2:1 shunt), both the ECG and radiograph are normal, even in the presence of a loud murmur. On the other hand, the presence of pulmonary hypertension alters the ECG and radiograph findings.

2. Echocardiography—Two-dimensional and Doppler echocardiography can usually define the location and often the size of a VSD, although accurate Doppler shunt quantitation may not be possible in the adult. There is evidence of left atrial and ventricular dilatation. The right-heart chamber dimensions are usually normal, although the main pulmonary artery may appear dilated. The presence of RVH usually signifies pulmonary hypertension or associated PS (with right-to-

left shunting and cyanosis). Usually only the largest defects, often located in the membranous septum, can actually be visualized echocardiographically (Figure 27–11). The aneurysmal pouch of a ventricular septal aneurysm may be seen in the parasternal short-axis view just below the aortic valve in the inlet portion of the septum near the septal leaflet of the tricuspid valve. Saline contrast administration shows a negative contrast effect within the RV, and a small degree of bidirectional shunting is usually present, with microbubbles appearing in the left ventricle.

Color-flow Doppler imaging demonstrates a high-velocity (aliased) systolic jet across the ventricular septum into the right ventricle. The location of the jet provides the best guide to the location of the defect. In the parasternal short-axis view, the jet from a membranous VSD may be seen in the region of the tricuspid valve (perimembranous) or toward the pulmonary artery (doubly committed subarterial, or supracristal). Muscular VSD jets are best seen in the apical or subcostal four-chamber views (Figure 27–12).

In continuous-wave Doppler, the peak velocity of the jet across the ventricular septum provides the peak systolic LV-RV gradient (using the modified

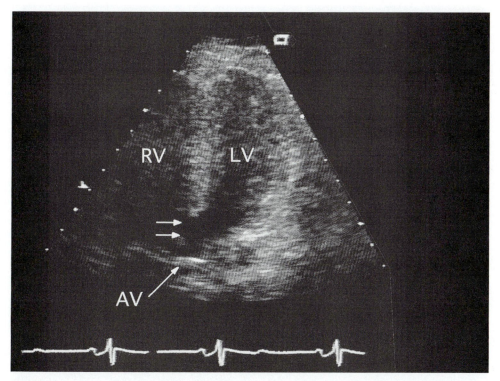

Figure 27–11. Transthoracic echocardiogram of a 40-year-old woman with a large membranous ventricular septal defect (*double arrow*). The right ventricle (RV) was enlarged because of pulmonary hypertension. AV = aortic valve; LV = left ventricle.

Bernoulli equation). Subtracting this gradient from the systolic blood pressure gives the peak RV systolic pressure. In the absence of a pressure gradient across the RV outflow tract—including the pulmonary valve (which should be carefully sought)—the RV systolic pressure is equivalent to the pulmonary artery (PA) systolic pressure. Additional Doppler evidence of the left-to-right shunt is found in the increased PA flow velocity.

In the postrepair patient, the VSD patch may or may not be apparent, depending on the size of the original defect. Once endothelialized, the patch does not cause acoustic shadowing (or distal echo blockout). Color-flow Doppler may demonstrate patch leaks at the peripheral suture lines of the patch in a small percentage of patients. Spontaneous closure of a VSD involving juxtaposed tricuspid valve tissue may cause significant tricuspid regurgitation. Varying degrees of aortic regurgitation may be present and are most often associated with membranous VSDs.

3. Cardiac catheterization—Although the diagnosis is often made noninvasively, the decision to close a VSD rests on accurate measurements of the shunt ratio and the level of pulmonary vascular resistance. Catheterization is therefore often necessary for therapeutic decision making.

Right-heart catheterization with sequential measurements of oxygen saturation reveals a step-up within the body of the right ventricle. As with an ASD, the higher the RV oxygen saturation, the greater the degree of shunting. For the calculation of Qp:Qs, the same formula is used as for ASD. Pulmonary artery pressures and vascular resistance should be measured and a gradient across the RV outflow tract, including the infundibulum and the pulmonary valve, must be excluded. Left ventriculography in the cranial left anterior oblique projection will reveal the location of the defect as contrast enters the right ventricle.

Prognosis & Treatment

As previously mentioned, adults with uncorrected VSDs are uncommonly encountered. In a series of 67 patients with an uncorrected VSD, the overall 10-year survival rate after initial presentation was 76%. Survival was adversely affected by functional class greater than New York Heart Association I, cardiomegaly, and ele-

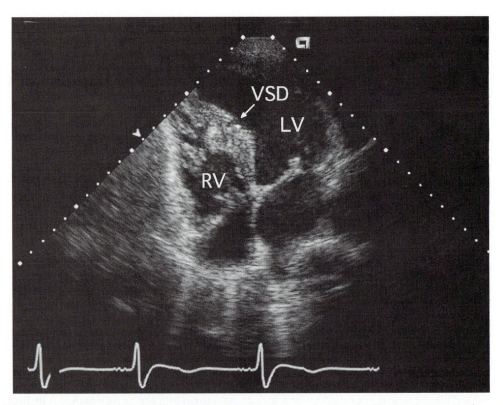

Figure 27–12. Transthoracic echocardiogram of a 45-year-old woman with a small muscular ventricular septal defect (VSD). LV = left ventricle; RV = right ventricle.

vated PA pressure (>50 mm Hg). As in patients with ASD, surgery is generally recommended when the magnitude of the systemic-to-pulmonary-shunt ratio exceeds 2:1. Other indications for surgery may include recurrent endocarditis and progressive aortic regurgitation.

Surgery for closure of VSDs has been available for more than 40 years, and long-term follow-up data are available. Surgery prior to age 2—even in infants with a large VSD, high pulmonary blood flow, and preoperative pulmonary hypertension—almost always prevents the development of pulmonary vascular obstructive disease. In patients operated on in the 1960s and 1970s, there is an approximately 20% incidence of residual left-to-right shunt and a persistent risk of endocarditis. Ventricular arrhythmias and RBBB are more common with a repair performed via right ventriculotomy (eg, muscular or subarterial VSD); when possible, the right atrium is the preferred approach. The risk of sudden death and complete heart block is low. Most patients who have VSDs repaired in childhood survive to lead normal adult lives.

Device closure, particularly for defects located in the muscular septum may eventually be a reasonable alternative to surgery, however these are not yet widely available.

Kidd L, Driscoll DJ, Gersong WM et al: Second natural history study of congenital heart defects: Results of treatment of patients with ventricular septal defects. Circulation 1993;87 (Suppl I):I-38.

Moodie DS: Adult congenital heart disease. Curr Opin Cardiol 1994;9:137.

Neumayer U, Stone S, Somerville J: Small ventricular septal defects in adults. Eur Heart J 1998;19:1573.

PATENT DUCTUS ARTERIOSUS

 ESSENTIALS OF DIAGNOSIS

- *Continuous machinery-like murmur, loudest below the left clavicle*
- *Left ventricular hypertrophy*
- *Pulmonary plethora, left atrial and ventricular enlargement; in older adults, calcification of the ductus on chest radiograph*
- *Left atrial and ventricular dilatation with normal right-heart chambers on echocardiography*
- *Continuous high-velocity color Doppler jet with retrograde flow along lateral wall of main pulmonary artery near left branch*

General Considerations

The patent ductus arteriosus (PDA) is a remnant of the normal fetal circulation. In the fetal circulation, superior vena cava blood enters the right atrium and characteristically is directed across the tricuspid valve into the right ventricle. It is then delivered into the systemic circulation via the ductus arteriosus, which connects the left pulmonary artery to the descending aorta just distal to the insertion of the left subclavian artery (Figure 27–13). In the normal full-term newborn, the ductus closes within the first 10–15 h following birth. If the ductus fails to close after birth when pulmonary vascular resistance falls, the direction of blood flow within the ductus reverses, producing a left-to-right shunt. Patients with nonrestrictive PDA (large left-to-right shunts) usually develop congestive heart failure within the first year of life. As with ventricular septal defect, it is relatively unusual—but by no means rare—to encounter an adult with uncorrected PDA.

An anatomic variant of the PDA is the aortopulmonary window (See Figure 27–13), which is usually a relatively large communication between the ascending aorta and the main pulmonary artery. The pathophysiology is similar to that of the PDA and is dependent on the size of the shunt and the level of PVR. The degree of pulmonary hypertension depends on the directly transmitted aortic pressure, which in turn depends on the size of the channel and the amount of pulmonary blood flow. If LV failure occurs, pulmonary venous hypertension may contribute further to the pulmonary hypertension. In the minority of patients, pulmonary vascular resistance rises above systemic vascular resistance and the shunt reverses. Because the site of the PDA is distal to the left subclavian, the head and neck vessels continue to receive oxygenated blood—but the descending aorta receives the desaturated blood, with the development of differential cyanosis.

When present in isolation, the PDA may lead to heart failure from pulmonary overcirculation. In conjunction with other defects, however, it may represent the sole pulmonary (eg, pulmonary atresia with intact ventricular septum) or systemic (eg, aortic atresia) blood supply, and survival may depend on persistent patency.

Clinical Findings

A. SYMPTOMS AND SIGNS

The mothers of patients with PDA may have a history of maternal rubella, and the patient may have had a murmur since infancy. If CHF has not developed by age 10, the majority of patients will be asymptomatic as adults. A few patients develop CHF in their 20s and 30s, however, and present with exertional dyspnea, chest pain, and palpitations.

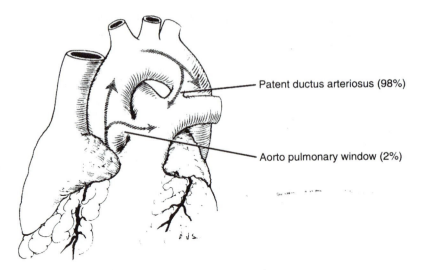

Figure 27–13. Anatomic locations of patent ductus arteriosus and aortopulmonary window. Adapted, with permission, from Cheitlin M, Sokolow M, McIlroy M: Congenital heart disease. In Clinical Cardiology. Norwalk, CT: Appleton & Lange, 1993.

The patient is almost always acyanotic; but when cyanosis and clubbing are present the upper extremities are usually spared. Thus, the lower extremities and sometimes the left hand may show clubbing and cyanosis, but the right hand and head are always pink. The pulse pressure may be widened, and the pulses are collapsing. The LV impulse is hyperdynamic and often laterally displaced. The classic murmur of the uncomplicated PDA is best heard below the left clavicle and gradually builds to its peak in late systole; it is continuous through the second heart sound and wanes in diastole. There may be a pause in late diastole or early systole. With a significant LV volume overload caused by a large shunt, an S_3 gallop and a diastolic murmur of relative mitral stenosis (similar to that of the large VSD) may be present. The murmur varies as pulmonary vascular resistance increases and shunting reverses, first with a decrease in the diastolic component and then a decrease in the systolic component. Finally, the murmur is silent and the physical findings are consistent with pulmonary hypertension (see Eisenmenger's Syndrome).

B. DIAGNOSTIC STUDIES

1. Electrocardiography and chest radiograph—The ECG is normal when the shunt is small; it shows left atrial and ventricular hypertrophy in the presence of a large shunt. When pulmonary hypertension is present and the shunt is predominantly right to left, the ECG may show P-pulmonale, right-axis deviation, and evidence of RVH.

The chest radiograph is also normal in the presence of a small shunt. With a significant shunt, LV prominence is evident with an enlarged cardiac silhouette and pulmonary vascular plethora. In the presence of pulmonary hypertension pruning of the peripheral pulmonary vessels is present, with prominence of the central pulmonary arteries. The ductus may be calcified in the older adult.

2. Echocardiography—The two-dimensional echocardiogram shows left atrial and ventricular enlargement, but imaging of the ductus itself is usually difficult in the adult. Color-flow Doppler imaging is diagnostic and reveals continuous high-velocity flow within the main pulmonary artery near the left branch. Flow is predominantly retrograde within the pulmonary artery and can be detected by continuous-wave Doppler. In an aortopulmonary window, continuous color-flow is detected, but it is most often antegrade, which distinguishes it from the flow through a PDA. Pulmonary artery pressure can be estimated from the almost ubiquitous tricuspid regurgitant jet.

3. Cardiac catheterization—Right-heart catheterization is performed to measure the PA pressure, pulmonary vascular resistance, and the flow ratio (Qp:Qs). The O_2 step-up is at the level of the pulmonary artery, and when the ductus is large enough, the descending aorta can be entered from the pulmonary artery. The ductus can also be visualized during aortography in the left lateral position. Because echocardiography is noninvasive and diagnostic, cardiac catheterization may become exclusively therapeutic in the future. Techniques for coil occlusion are well established and currently represent the treatment of choice for simple PDAs in many institutions.

Prognosis & Treatment

Patients who survive into adulthood with a large uncorrected PDA generally develop CHF or pulmonary hypertension (with right-to-left shunting and differential cyanosis) by about age 30. Most adults with PDA and normal or only mildly elevated PVR (<4 units) are either asymptomatic or mildly impaired and can undergo surgical ligation or percutaneous closure with good results. In the group with severely elevated PVR (>10 units/m²), survival is poor. Approximately 15% of patients older than 40 years of age may have calcification or aneurysmal dilatation of the ductus, which can complicate surgery. Surgical ligation or percutaneous coil or device occlusion of a PDA can be performed with low morbidity and mortality and is recommended—independent of the size of the shunt—because of the high risk of endocarditis in uncorrected cases. Division of an isolated restrictive PDA in childhood can be curative of congenital heart disease. If repaired after childhood, the morbidity and mortality rates depend on the degree of pulmonary hypertension, LV volume overload, and calcification of the ductus. Unless persistent shunting is present following a surgical ligation, endocarditis prophylaxis is not recommended after the sixth postoperative month.

Harrison DA, Benson LN, Lazzam C et al: Percutaneous catheter closure of the persistently patent ductus arteriosus in the adult. Am J Cardiol 1996;77:1094.

Takenaka K, Sakamoto T, Shiota T et al: Diagnosis of patent ductus arteriosus in adults by biplane transesophageal color Doppler flow mapping. Am J Cardiol 1991;68:691.

COARCTATION OF THE AORTA

ESSENTIALS OF DIAGNOSIS

- *Elevated systolic blood pressure in the upper extremities (always in right arm); normal or diminished systolic blood pressure in lower extremities (and often left arm); radial-femoral pulse delay.*
- *Left ventricular hypertrophy, LV prominence, "3" sign, rib-notching on chest radiograph*
- *Visualization of the coarctation by imaging*
- *Distal aortic pressure drop by Doppler echocardiography or catheterization*

General Considerations

Coarctation of the thoracic aorta predominates in males and is often associated with a congenitally abnormal aortic valve. The most common location is distal to the origin of the left subclavian artery (postductal; Figure 27–14), but the narrowing may also be proximal (preductal). Infrequently, the origin of the right subclavian is distal to the left, causing reduced pressures in the right upper extremity. There is considerable variability in the degree and extent of narrowing, ranging from a localized shelf to a long tubular narrowing. Multiple discrete sites are rarely encountered. Coarctation of the abdominal aortic is less common than that of the thoracic aorta; it is found equally in males and females and presents with symptoms of claudication. Additional coexisting problems may include congenital mitral valve disease and aneurysms of the circle of Willis. Collateral circulation to the distal aorta develops mainly via the subclavian and intercostal arteries, in addition to the vertebral and anterior spinal arteries.

Aortic coarctation is usually diagnosed during childhood in the asymptomatic phase by routine examination of blood pressure and femoral pulse palpation. In cases of severe obstruction, the infant may present with CHF. Symptoms may arise in the adult during the 20s and 30s, and evidence of coarctation should always be sought in patients of this age group presenting with hypertension. Early detection and repair are highly desirable because repair forestalls the associated accelerated development of coronary artery disease.

Clinical Findings

A. SYMPTOMS AND SIGNS

The adult with uncorrected coarctation is usually asymptomatic. When symptoms occur, they are nonspecific: exertional dyspnea, headache, epistaxis, and leg fatigue. Congestive heart failure can occur in the adult with long-standing hypertension secondary to coarctation. Additional significant complications, usually occurring between the ages of 15 and 40, include aortic rupture or dissection of the proximal thoracic aorta or an aneurysm distal to the coarctation, infective endocarditis on an associated bicuspid aortic valve or endarteritis at the site of coarctation, and cerebrovascular accidents, which are most often due to rupture of an aneurysm of the circle of Willis.

The systolic blood pressure is elevated in the right arm and often the left arm, with reduced systolic blood pressures in the lower extremities. Diastolic blood pressures are not usually affected. Simultaneous palpation of the brachial and femoral pulses reveals delayed arrival of the femoral pulse. Adult patients with highly developed collateral circulation may no longer exhibit these signs, however. The jugular venous pulse is nor-

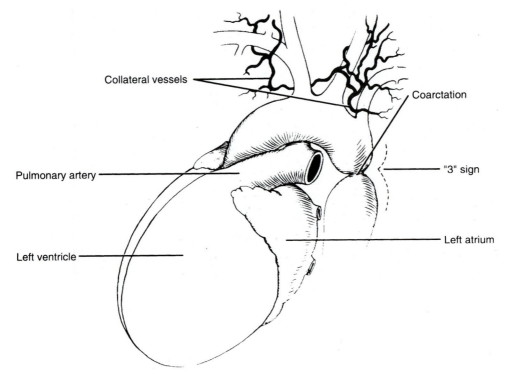

Figure 27–14. Anatomic features of aortic coarctation. Reproduced, with permission, from Cheitlin M, Sokolow M, McIlroy M: Congenital heart disease. In Clinical Cardiology. Norwalk, CT: Appleton & Lange, 1993.

mal, the carotid upstroke is usually brisk, and the aorta may be palpable in the suprasternal notch. Cardiac examination reveals a nondisplaced, but forceful, LV impulse. The first heart sound is normal, and the aortic component of the second heart sound may be accentuated. A late systolic murmur is present (as a result of the coarctation) that is best heard between the scapulae to the left of the spine. The murmur caused by collateral flow through the intercostal and internal mammary arteries is longer, but it is not necessarily continuous. An ejection check and systolic murmur as well as a blowing diastolic murmur of aortic regurgitation may be associated with a bicuspid aortic valve.

B. DIAGNOSTIC STUDIES

1. Electrocardiography and chest radiograph—The ECG is nonspecific, with LVH and, in the later stages, left atrial enlargement. As in other patients with long-standing hypertension, atrial fibrillation may occur.

   On the other hand, the radiograph finding of rib notching is highly specific, although it is not 100% sensitive even in adults. Notching is present on the bottom of the rib where the intercostal arteries are located. In preductal coarctation (ie, proximal to the left subclavian), the rib notching is present only on the right side,

and, in abdominal coarctation, it is limited to the lower ribs. Another classic radiograph finding is the "3" sign, with the dilatated left subclavian artery forming the upper curvature and the dilatated distal aorta forming the lower. There may be radiologic evidence of LV and atrial enlargement.

2. Echocardiography—It is extremely difficult to visualize the actual site of the coarctation in the adult patient with precordial two-dimensional echocardiography. Color-flow Doppler identification of flow acceleration in the descending aorta from the suprasternal notch, however, can often identify obstruction even when images are suboptimal. The peak systolic velocity can be used to estimate the gradient, but the presence of persistent antegrade flow in diastole (Figure 27–15A) and decreased acceleration time beyond the coarctation provide additional confirmation of hemodynamic significance. Further localization of the coarctation is now possible with imaging of the descending aorta in the longitudinal plane during multiplanar transesophageal echocardiography. The anatomy of the aortic valve should be carefully defined, and careful Doppler interrogation for evidence of stenosis or insufficiency is essential.

3. Magnetic resonance angiography—Magnetic resonance angiography can localize and define the extent

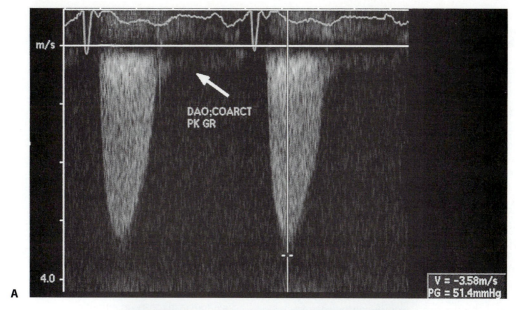

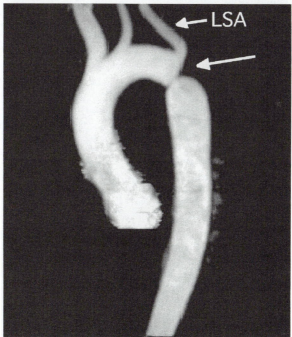

Figure 27–15. **A:** Continuous-wave Doppler from transthoracic echocardiogram in a patient with coarctation of the descending aorta (DAO). There was a peak gradient (PK GR) of 51.4 mm Hg with runoff in diastole (*arrow*). **B:** Three-dimensional reconstruction of a magnetic resonance angiogram of the thoracic aorta demonstrates a discrete coarctation (*lower arrow*) in the typical location after the take-off of the left subclavian artery (LSA).

of narrowing with a high degree of accuracy (Figure 27–15B). Aneurysmal dilatation is visible, and postoperative evaluation is possible.

4. Cardiac catheterization—Aortography is necessary only when the diagnosis is not adequately confirmed clinically or the anatomy cannot be fully defined noninvasively. Premature coronary disease is common, and if it is clinically suspected, coronary arteriography should be performed. Balloon dilatation with or without stent placement across native and recurrent coarctation has been attempted in cases of discrete narrowing (see later discussion).

Prognosis & Treatment

The importance of identifying coarctation in adults lies in the tendency toward LVH and CHF, premature coronary artery disease, and cerebral hemorrhage. In an autopsy series of uncorrected coarctation, 50% of patients had died by about age 30 and 90% by age 60. Proximal aortic rupture and cerebral hemorrhage often occur before the age of 30, and the incidence of CHF continues to increase after the age of 40.

Surgery for correcting coarctation presents a considerable challenge in patients over the age of 15 years because of often-huge intercostal aneurysms and atheromatous changes in the aorta near the shelf. It should be noted that surgical repair even in childhood is often only palliative, and these patients require continued surveillance, particularly in the presence of associated cardiac lesions or preoperative systemic hypertension. Hypertension persists in approximately one third of patients operated on after the age of 14. The major determinants of long-term survival following repair of aortic coarctation are the presence of associated lesions and the age at operation. The postsurgery cardiac mortality rate after age 20 is approximately 5% in patients with isolated coarctation. Causes of late cardiovascular deaths (in order of frequency) include coronary artery disease, sudden death, aortic regurgitation and heart failure, hypertension and heart failure, and cerebrovascular accidents. Approximately 10% of patients require subsequent cardiovascular surgery, the majority for aortic valve replacement. The incidence of recurrent coarctation requiring surgery or percutaneous intervention varies significantly depending on surgical technique and can be 16–60%.

The surgical methods of repair have undergone considerable evolution since their initial introduction in the late 1950s. In part this is due to the considerable morphologic variability which has precluded using a single method for correction. The removal of the abnormal coarctation tissue as occurs in an end-to-end anastomosis is most desirable, but depending on other factors a subclavian flap repair or an interposition graft may be necessary. Less reliance is placed on the patch angioplasty because long-term studies have shown late aneurysm formation due to thinning of the posterior wall. It is now almost universally accepted that recoarctation can be managed by percutaneous transluminal balloon angioplasty, with or without stent implantation. Angioplasty is not generally indicated in uncomplicated native coarctation.

Amato JJ, Douglas WI, James T et al: Coarctation of the aorta. In Williams WG, ed: Seminars in Thoracic and Cardiovascular Surgery. Pediatric Cardiac Surgery Annual 2000. Philadelphia: WB Saunders, 2000.

Kaemmerer H, Oelert F, Bahlman J et al: Arterial hypertension in adults after surgical treatment of aortic coarctation. Thorac Cardiovasc Surg 1998;46:121.

Yetman A, Nykanen D, McCrindle BW et al: Balloon angioplasty of recurrent coarctation: A 12-year review. J Am Coll Cardiol 1997;30:811.

EBSTEIN'S ANOMALY

ESSENTIALS OF DIAGNOSIS

- *History of dyspnea, atypical chest pain, or intermittent cyanosis*
- *Palpitations associated with supraventricular arrhythmias and preexcitation syndrome*
- *Right parasternal lift, widely split S_1, systolic clicks, and systolic murmur of tricuspid regurgitation (without inspiratory accentuation)*
- *Right atrial enlargement, right ventricular conduction defect of right bundle branch block type, posteriorly directed delta waves with accessory pathway by ECG. Frequent first-degree AV block*
- *Normal or reduced pulmonary vascularity without pulmonary artery enlargement, right atrial enlargement, normal left-sided cardiac silhouette on chest radiograph*
- *Apical displacement of septal tricuspid valve leaflet; variable degrees of tricuspid regurgitation originating from apical portion of right ventricle; and enlarged right atrium on echocardiography*

General Considerations

Ebstein's anomaly is characterized by deformity of the tricuspid valve with apical displacement of the septal and posterior leaflets (Figure 27–16) and their adhesion to the RV wall. The anterior leaflet is elongated and has been described as sail-like. Tricuspid regurgitation arises from the apically displaced site of leaflet coaptation with considerable variability in the extent of tricuspid leaflet displacement and the degree of tricuspid regurgitation. The portion of the right ventricle proximal to the leaflets is atrialized (thinned), and if the remaining right ventricle is diminutive in size, pump function may be inadequate. Cyanosis may be present as a result of right-to-left shunting across an ASD or patent foramen ovale in the presence of significant tricuspid regurgitation or elevated right atrial pressures. Atrial septal defect is the most common associated anomaly.

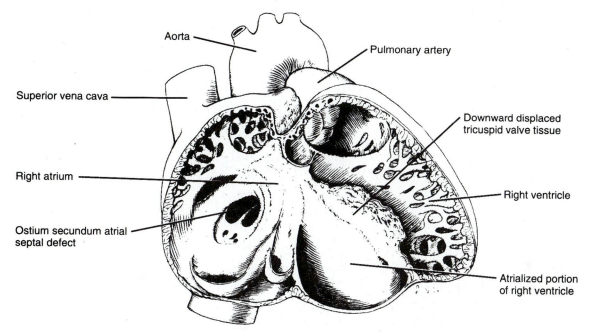

Figure 27–16. Anatomy of Ebstein's anomaly. Redrawn from The CIBA Collection of Medical Illustrations, Volume 5, HEART. Reproduced, courtesy of CIBA-GEIGY Limited, Basle (Switzerland). All rights reserved.

Tremendous variability in morphologic and clinical presentation occurs in patients with Ebstein's anomaly. In severe cases, the patient may present during infancy with CHF. At the opposite end of the spectrum, an adult with only mild tricuspid valve displacement may be asymptomatic or symptomatic only because of supraventricular tachyarrhythmias. The latter are an important feature of Ebstein's anomaly, as a result of its association with preexcitation in 25–30% of patients. The accessory pathway is usually posteroseptal or posterolateral in location.

Clinical Findings

A. SYMPTOMS AND SIGNS

Cyanosis may be the most important clinical feature in early life, but in older patients long-standing RV volume overload and right atrial distension results in congestive failure and dysrhythmias, including the Wolff-Parkinson-White syndrome are frequent. These patients may present with dyspnea, arrhythmias, decreased exercise tolerance and intermittent or exercise-induced cyanosis (with associated right-to-left shunting across an ASD or patent foramen ovale).

Physical examination reveals right parasternal lift, widely split S_1, systolic clicks (from delayed tricuspid valve closure, the "sail" sounds), and the systolic murmur of tricuspid regurgitation. The latter does not usually increase in intensity during inspiration, because the noncompliant RV cannot accept an increase in venous return. On the other hand, the RA is compliant, and systemic venous congestion is uncommon; the jugular venous pulse is therefore usually normal. S_3 and S_4 gallops may be present as may an early diastolic snap from the opening of the elongated anterior leaflet.

B. DIAGNOSTIC STUDIES

1. Electrocardiography and chest radiograph—The ECG shows evidence of right atrial enlargement and a RV conduction defect of the RBBB type. The PR interval may be prolonged, except in the presence of an accessory pathway. In 25–30% of patients, ECG findings are consistent with Wolff-Parkinson-White syndrome; the PR interval is short, and delta waves from a posterolateral or posteroseptal bundle of Kent are evident (Figure 27–17). Atrial fibrillation may be present in older patients.

The chest radiograph shows normal or reduced pulmonary vascularity without pulmonary artery enlargement; it also shows cardiac enlargement to the right of the sternum caused by right atrial enlargement. The left ventricle and atrium are normal in size.

2. Echocardiography—The classical M-mode description of this anomaly included increased excursion of the anterior tricuspid valve leaflet and delayed tricuspid valve closure (> 40ms) following mitral valve closure. Two-dimensional and Doppler echocardiography are diagnostic in most adults. The four-chamber apical and

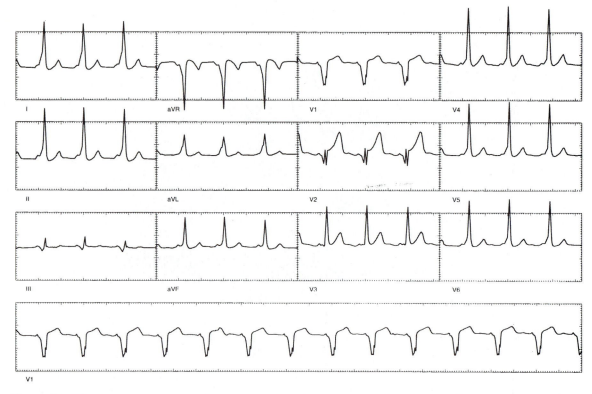

Figure 27–17. Electrocardiogram in Ebstein's anomaly with associated Wolf-Parkinson-White syndrome.

subcostal views provide most of the necessary information. The right atrium is enlarged and the right ventricle is usually small, consisting of the atrialized portion and the remaining pumping chamber. The septal leaflet of the tricuspid valve is apically displaced, and color-flow Doppler imaging shows the regurgitant jet arising from the apical point of coaptation (Figure 27–18). The degree of tricuspid regurgitation can be estimated from the extent of RA filling by color-flow and from the density of the continuous-wave Doppler signal. The PA systolic pressure estimated from the continuous-wave tricuspid regurgitation jet is nearly always normal.

Although color-flow imaging may reveal a patent foramen ovale or an ASD, it is mandatory to perform a saline contrast examination to reliably exclude these sources of right-to-left shunting. When precordial echocardiography is inadequate, TEE can be used to exclude associated lesions of the atrial septum.

3. Cardiac catheterization—During right-heart catheterization, simultaneous recordings of a RV electrogram and an RA pressure tracing are obtained with a catheter in the atrialized portion of the right ventricle. This finding is considered pathognomonic of Ebstein's anomaly, but catheterization is now rarely necessary for diagnosis.

Prognosis & Treatment

The chance of surviving to age 50 is about 50%, with survival dependent on the degree of the anatomic and physiologic abnormalities. As mentioned, 25–30% of patients have supraventricular arrhythmias, many associated with accessory pathways that are now amenable to catheter ablation. Although tricuspid annuloplasty and tricuspid valve reconstruction, with creation of a monocuspid valve, are often possible, tricuspid valve replacement may be required in some patients. Improvement in exercise tolerance following tricuspid valve replacement or repair has been observed, especially in patients with associated ASD. In other patients, a Fontan-like procedure (see Palliative surgical procedures) may be the only suitable choice. In patients who are symptomatic predominantly on the basis of exercise-induced cyanosis, device closure of the interarterial septal defect may be adequate treatment.

Celermajer DS, Bull C, Till JA et al: Ebstein's anomaly: Presentation and outcome from fetus to adult. J Am Coll Cardiol 1994; 23:170.

DiRusso GB, Gaynor JW: Ebstein's Anomaly: Indications for repair and surgical technique. In Spray TL, ed: Seminars in Thoracic and Cardiovascular Surgery. Pediatric Cardiac Surgery Annual 1999. Philadelphia: WB Saunders, 1999.

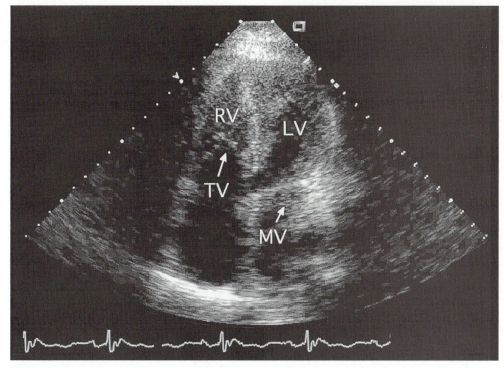

Figure 27–18. Transesophageal echocardiogram in a 50-year-old woman with Ebstein's anomaly. This four-chamber view shows the apically displaced tricuspid valve (TV) in relation to the normal mitral valve (MV). LV = left ventricle; RV = right ventricle.

CONGENITALLY CORRECTED TRANSPOSITION OF THE GREAT ARTERIES

ESSENTIALS OF DIAGNOSIS

- *Prominent left parasternal impulse, soft S_1, accentuated A_2, soft or inaudible P_2*
- *PR prolongation, variable degrees of AV block, Q waves in right precordial leads with absence in left precordial leads on ECG*
- *Absence of left-sided aortic knob on chest radiograph*
- *Rightward and posterior pulmonary artery with leftward and anterior aorta, apical displacement of right-sided AV valve, coarsely trabeculated left-sided systemic ventricle with moderator band (the morphologic right ventricle) on cardiac imaging*

General Considerations

In congenitally corrected transposition of the great arteries (C-TGA), the visceroatrial relationship is normal with the right atrium to the right of the left atrium (Figure 27–19). The systemic venous blood drains into the right atrium, through a bileaflet (mitral) valve into a morphologic left ventricle pumping into a posterior and rightward pulmonary artery. The pulmonary venous blood drains into the left atrium, through a trileaflet tricuspid valve into a morphologic right ventricle pumping into an anterior and leftward aorta. This occurs because of atrial-ventricular discordance (ventricular inversion) causes the right ventricle to be located to the left of the left ventricle with the left ventricle located to the right of the right ventricle. The great arteries are transposed, with the aorta arising from the right ventricle and the pulmonary artery rising from the left ventricle. The result is functional correction, in that oxygenated blood comes into the left atrium, goes to the anatomic right ventricle, and then flows out of the aorta. The patient is acyanotic and is usually asymptomatic in the absence of associated lesions.

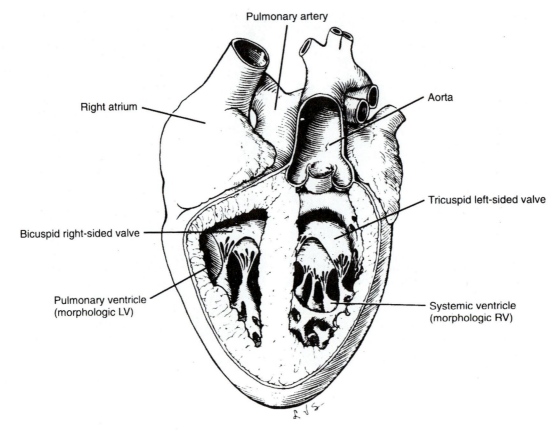

Figure 27–19. Anatomy of congenitally corrected transposition of the great vessels. LV = left ventricle; RV = right ventricle. Redrawn from The CIBA Collection of Medical Illustrations, Volume 5, HEART. Reproduced, courtesy of CIBA-GEIGY Limited, Basle (Switzerland). All rights reserved.

The most common complications are complete heart block (occurring with an incidence of approximately 2% per year) and other associated anomalies, most commonly ventricular septal defect, subvalvular PS, and abnormalities of the systemic AV valve. Coronary anomalies are uncommon, and the coronary circulation is usually concordant; that is, a right coronary artery supplies the right ventricle. Eventually, the systemic ventricle (a massively hypertrophied right ventricle) is subject to pump failure, even in cases of isolated C-TGA. The relative degree of PS and the size of the VSD determine whether cyanosis is present. In the absence of PS, the patient with a large VSD may develop CHF from the volume overload of the systemic ventricle and is at risk for pulmonary vascular disease.

Clinical Findings

A. Symptoms and Signs

The majority of patients with isolated C-TGA are asymptomatic in childhood and young adulthood. The highly prevalent complication of complete heart block may present with syncope, sudden death or, less dramatically, with exercise intolerance. More often, the clinical picture is dominated by associated lesions.

Exertional dyspnea and easy fatigability may develop with systemic AV valve regurgitation. Pulmonary venous congestion from pump failure of the anatomic right ventricle may occur in middle age.

The physical examination depends largely on the associated anomalies. The left parasternal impulse is prominent as a result of the hypertrophied systemic ventricle. In the presence of a prolonged PR interval, S_1 is diminished in intensity. The proximity of the aorta to the chest wall causes an accentuated A_2; conversely, the posterior displacement of the pulmonary valve causes a soft or inaudible P_2. Systolic thrills occur in the presence of PS, with and without VSD. If PS is present, the murmur is best heart in the third left intercostal space, radiating to the right. The murmur of a VSD is usually typical, but the murmur of left-sided AV valve regurgitation radiates to the left sternal border in C-TGA.

B. Diagnostic Studies

1. Electrocardiography and chest radiograph—The electrocardiographic and radiologic findings of C-TGA are dominated by its associated lesions. The ECG shows variable degrees of AV block, from simple PR prolongation to complete heart block. The absence of Q waves in I, V_5 and V_6 or the presence of Q waves in V_4r or V_1 is characteristic of the condition. This pattern results because the ventricular septal depolarization proceeds from the embryonic left ventricle to right ventricle (Figure 27–20). The typical chest radiograph finding in isolated C-TGA is a straight, left upper cardiac border, formed by the ascending aorta and loss of the pulmonary trunk contour.

2. Echocardiography—The anatomic features of isolated C-TGA are usually apparent by TTE, even in adults. Transesophageal echocardiography may be useful in defining the anatomy of associated lesions such as infundibular obstruction and the severity of left-sided AV valve regurgitation. In the basal parasternal short-axis view, the aortic valve is anterior and usually to the left of the pulmonic valve. Because the two great arteries arise in parallel, there is a "figure-eight" appearance, rather than the usual arrangement of the pulmonary artery in long axis surrounding the aortic valve. On careful inspection, the coronary arteries can be identified as

they emerge from the aortic root. In the long axis view (obtained from a more vertical and leftward scan) the aorta arises from the posterior ventricle and is not in fibrous continuity with the AV valve. The heavily trabeculated and hypertrophied right ventricle with its moderator band is posterior and to the left and the smoothly trabeculated left ventricle is anterior and to the right (Figure 27–21). The systemic AV (anatomically a tricuspid) valve has three leaflets and septal attachments, is apically displaced, and may show variable degrees of regurgitation. In contrast, the subpulmonary AV (anatomically a mitral) valve has two leaflets and no septal attachments.

It is essential to identify associated lesions because these are the primary determinants of survival, specifically a VSD and infundibular pulmonary valve stenosis. Doppler echocardiography should be used to determine the pulmonary valve gradient and to estimate the degree of pulmonary hypertension. Left-sided Ebstein's anomaly may coexist, with the systemic AV valve leaflets displaced apically. Furthermore, morphologic abnormalities of the tricuspid valve are frequently found in patients with C-TGA. Autopsy studies of patients with this lesion have documented tricuspid valve abnormalities in >90% of cases, most commonly an Ebstein-like anomaly with short, thickened chordae tendineae. Clinically significant tricuspid regurgitation

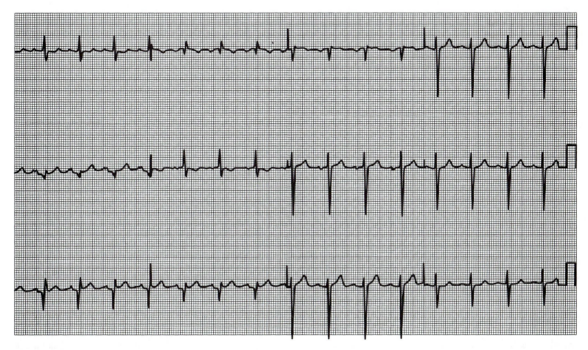

Figure 27–20. Electrocardiograph in congenitally corrected transposition of the great vessels with associated pulmonic stenosis and ventricular septal defect.

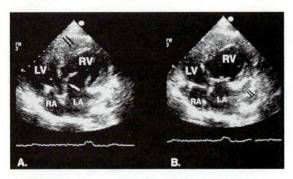

Figure 27–21. Apical transthoracic echocardiographic views in a patient with congenitally corrected transposition of the great vessels. **A:** The moderator band is clearly visualized (*double arrow*) in the left-sided morphologic right ventricle (RV). **B:** The narrow based atrial appendage (*double arrow*) clearly identifies this as a left atrium. The right ventricle (RV) is spherically dilated, reflecting the pressure overload of this chamber. The left ventricle (LV) is small and compressed. RA = right atrium. The left-sided atrioventricular (AV) valve is a morphologic tricuspid valve and the right-sided AV valve is a morphologic mitral valve.

has been reported in 20% to 50% of patients with C-TGA.

3. Cardiac catheterization—When noninvasive data are diagnostically conclusive, the role of cardiac catheterization is for preoperative evaluation in patients with surgically remediable lesions. The pulmonary artery may be difficult to enter; fluoroscopically, the venous catheter is noted to enter a posterior and rightward vessel. The pulmonary vascular resistance must be measured to rule out irreversible pulmonary vascular disease in patients with VSD. Although angiography can indicate the abnormally positioned great arteries, it is important only for identification of anomalous coronary arteries, which are infrequently encountered.

Prognosis & Treatment

Survival in congenitally corrected transposition of the great arteries is usually determined by other, associated lesions, but even in its isolated form, survival may not be normal. The natural history and postoperative outcome of patients with C-TGA and the commonly associated lesion of VSD and PS are known to be less satisfactory than those of patients with normal AV connections and similar intracardiac lesions. The propensity for AV conduction abnormalities, for tricuspid valve dysfunction, and the much-debated capability of the right ventricle to function adequately in the systemic circulation may all affect survival.

A constant feature of C-TGA is the development of complete heart block, estimated to occur at a rate of about 2% per year. AV conduction abnormalities of varying degrees are seen in nearly 75% of patients with this anomaly; many will require permanent pacemaker insertion. Periodic surveillance for the development of high-degree AV block is important: sudden death may be the first manifestation of this complication. However, it is the morphologic abnormalities of the tricuspid valve resulting in severe valvular dysfunction/regurgitation which have been shown to be the most critical determinant for survival. The systemic right ventricle in C-TGA appears to be less tolerant than an anatomic left ventricle of similar degrees of valvular incompetence, and there is an acceleration of the usual vicious cycle. The right ventricle's inability to cope with significant tricuspid regurgitation leads to decreased contractility and annular dilation that in turn exacerbates the degree of regurgitation. Theoretically, the anatomic right ventricle is subject to progressive pump failure from the obligatory pressure overload of the systemic circulation, potentially hastened by systemic hypertension, coronary artery disease, and volume overload from a regurgitant AV valve. Because the circulation is functionally corrected, the indications for surgery are those of the associated lesion requiring surgery (eg, VSD with a Qp:Qs of 2:1, VSD with PS causing cyanosis). Repair or replacement of the tricuspid valve is often indicated, however 10-year survival after surgical intervention is low. A "double switch" operation has been proposed for patients whose tricuspid valves are severely insufficient. An atrial switch combined with an arterial switch (see the section on Transposition of the Great Arteries) in the absence of LV outflow obstruction or with a **Rastelli** procedure (right ventricle to pulmonary artery conduit) has been successfully performed. After surgery, the left ventricle and mitral valve are restored to systemic circulation. Improvement in tricuspid valve function in a low-pressure right ventricle has been documented after these operations. This procedure carries significant risk, and late complications relating to the atrial switch component (baffle obstruction, sick sinus syndrome) are of additional concern. Heart transplantation remains the final option for patients with C-TGA, intractable tricuspid regurgitation and RV failure.

Connelly MS, Liu PP, Williams WG et al: Congenitally corrected transposition of the great arteries in the adult. Functional status and complications. J Am Coll Cardiol 1996;27:1238.

Graham TP Jr, Bernard YD, Mellen BG et al: Long-term outcome in congenitally corrected transposition of the great arteries: A multi-instrumental study. J Am Coll Cardiol 2001;36:255.

Prieto LR, Hordof AJ, Secic M et al: Progressive tricuspid valve disease in patients with congenitally corrected transposition of the great arteries. Circulation 1998;98:997.

Yeh T, Connelly MA, Coles JG et al: Atrioventricular discordance: Result of repair in 127 patients. J Thorac Cardiovasc Surg 1999;117(6):1190.

OTHER ACYANOTIC CONGENITAL DEFECTS

Partial anomalous pulmonary venous return usually involves abnormal drainage of the right upper pulmonary vein into the superior vena cava and is often associated with sinus venosus ASD. Other sites of drainage include the coronary sinus and the inferior vena cava (scimitar syndrome). The need for surgical correction depends on the size of the shunt, which in turn depends on the number of pulmonary veins draining into the pulmonary circulation.

Atrioventricular septal ("canal") defects (also known as **endocardial cushion defects**—a term out of favor with many anatomists) are particularly common in children born with trisomy 21. These defects include an ostium primum ASD, a membranous VSD, and a mitral valve malformation, consisting of a cleft in the anterior leaflet or anterior and posterior bridging leaflets (Figure 27–22). Irreversible pulmonary vascular disease with shunt reversal may lead to cyanosis (see section on Eisenmenger's Syndrome) and is extremely common in the adult who has had no attempt at repair. Residual mitral regurgitation is often encountered following repair. Even when the valve is competent in the early postoperative period, late regurgitation occurs in a small percentage of patients.

Coronary artery anomalies are rarely seen as an isolated defect in the adult patient. They are found in approximately 1% of patients undergoing coronary arteriography and in approximately 0.3% of autopsies. The most common anomaly is the left main coronary artery arising from the pulmonary trunk. This may present in infancy as cardiomyopathy and CHF from myocardial ischemia and systolic dysfunction. A small minority of patients may develop sufficient myocardial collaterals from the right coronary artery to allow survival into adulthood. Physical examination may reveal a continuous murmur, and clinical assessment may be remarkable for angina pectoris, myocardial infarction, dyspnea, syncope, and sudden death. Treatments include surgical closure of the left main artery with possible bypass to the left anterior descending artery, or, primary reanastomosis of the anomalous artery from the pulmonary artery to the aorta or the subclavian artery. There are many anatomic variations of the less severe coronary anomalies. When the left coronary artery arises from the right or noncoronary cusp and passes between the aorta and pulmonary artery, however, the patient is at increased risk for ischemia and sudden death. This diagnosis should be considered in young patients with exertional chest pain. Transesophageal echocardiography may visualize anomalous coronary ostia. Although MRA may be diagnostic in the future,

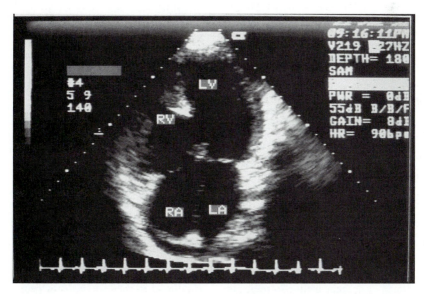

Figure 27–22. Apical four-chamber view from a transthoracic echocardiogram in a patient with atrioventricular septal defect and Down syndrome. The crux of the heart is missing, and a large ostium primum atrial septal defect and large ventricular septal defect are evident. LA = left atrium; LV = left ventricle; RA = right atrium; RV = right ventricle.

coronary angiography is currently the diagnostic gold standard.

Coronary arteriovenous fistulas are more likely to permit survival to adulthood. Large fistulas draining into the right side of the circulation may be associated with a sizable shunt and can rarely present with CHF in infancy. Coronary steal may occur, leading to myocardial ischemia. In the adult, there may be a history of exertional dyspnea or chest pain and a continuous murmur on physical examination. TTE detects the dilated fistulous coronary artery in approximately 50% of patients. Abnormal continuous jets within the cardiac chambers (RV is most common) or in the pulmonary artery seen in color-flow Doppler should suggest this diagnosis. Cardiac catheterization showing the dilated coronary artery and fistulous communication confirm the diagnosis.

Congenital **sinus of Valsalva aneurysms** have the potential for catastrophic rupture with development of acute severe aortic regurgitation or pericardial tamponade. Although the perforation may be subacute with mild regurgitation, it nonetheless poses an ongoing risk for endocarditis. Echocardiography, with a transesophageal approach if necessary, is diagnostic. Surgical repair with a pericardial patch is indicated when rupture is present.

Hoffman J: Congenital anomalies of the coronary vessels and the aortic root. In Emmanoulidies GC, Allen HD, Riemenschneider TA, Gutgesell HP, eds: Heart Disease in Infants, Children and Adolescents: Including the Fetus and Young Adult. Philadelphia: Williams & Wilkins, 1995.

Taylor AJ, Virmani R: Coronary artery anomalies in adults: Which are high risk? ACC Curr J Rev 2001;10(5):92.

Taylor AM, Thorne SA, Rubens MB et al: Coronary Artery Imaging in Grown Up Congenital Heart Disease. Complementary role of magnetic resonance and x-ray coronary angiography. Circulation 2000;101:1670.

CYANOTIC CONGENITAL HEART DISEASE

Patients with cyanotic congenital heart disease have arterial oxygen desaturation resulting from the shunting of systemic venous blood to the arterial circulation, or from cardiac anatomy, which mandates mixing of systemic and pulmonary venous return. The shunting can occur at the level of the atrium (ASD), the ventricle (VSD), or the great vessels (PDA or aortopulmonary window). If a right-to-left shunt is present, it implies a right-sided obstruction distal to that level, or the presence of pulmonary vascular obstructive disease causing reversal of flow through a previous left-to-right shunting lesion. Thus, right-to-left shunting through an ASD (or patent foramen ovale) may be due to tricuspid atresia, tricuspid stenosis, severe PS, or atresia with an intact ventricular septum or pulmonary vascular disease. Also, in Ebstein's anomaly (sometimes classified with acyanotic heart disease) with severe tricuspid re-

gurgitation and an associated ASD or patent foramen ovale, right-to-left shunting is due to the increased right atrial pressure. Right-to-left shunting at the ventricular level (through a VSD) may be due to RV outflow obstruction created by pulmonary valvular or infundibular stenosis (TOF) or increased pulmonary vascular resistance (Eisenmenger's syndrome). Right-to-left shunting across a patent ductus is almost always due to pulmonary vascular disease.

In d-transposition of the great arteries (D-TGA), the aorta arises from the right ventricle carrying desaturated blood to the body and the pulmonary artery arises from the left ventricle carrying oxygenated blood to the lungs. The result of D-TGA is complete separation of the pulmonary and systemic circulations. Infants with this condition have severe cyanosis. Survival depends on saturated blood entering the systemic circulation via an intracardiac (ASD or VSD) or interarterial (PDA) communication.

In patients with a single ventricle (double-inlet ventricle), both AV valves are connected to a main, single ventricular chamber. One great artery arises from the main chamber, the other arises from a rudimentary chamber. Because almost complete mixing of the systemic and pulmonary venous return takes place in the single ventricle, the systemic arterial saturation is primarily determined by the amount of pulmonary blood flow. Cyanosis of varying degrees is present from birth.

Untreated cyanotic heart disease carries an extremely high mortality rate in the infant and child; therefore, most patients reaching adulthood have had reparative or palliative surgery. Those who reach adulthood without surgery are usually those with TOF or irreversible pulmonary vascular disease (eg, Eisenmenger's syndrome) from underlying complex congenital cardiac lesions. The importance of recognizing cyanotic heart disease in the adult lies not only in the potential for possible surgical or nonsurgical intervention but also for appropriate management of the extracardiac manifestations of long-standing cyanosis. The systemic complications of cyanotic heart disease include the development of secondary erythrocytosis, an associated bleeding diathesis, thrombocytopenia and hyperuricemia secondary to increased red cell turnover. Urolithiasis and urate nephropathy rarely occur, but gout is common. Neurologic abnormalities include infectious, hemorrhagic, and hypoxic disorders. Counseling of the young adult with reference to contraception, pregnancy, and exercise is especially important in this group of patients.

Palliative surgical procedures for complex cyanotic congenital heart disease performed during infancy or childhood in the early years of pediatric cardiothoracic surgery, were associated with unique physical findings and specific complications. These procedures, such as aortopulmonary anastomoses (Waterston, Potts, Blalock-Taussig) and atrial switches (Senning and Mustard), are still commonly encountered in adult patients. They are associate with unique physical findings and specific complications. Most of these procedures are no longer performed in children as surgical techniques, which optimize physiology and reduce complications, have evolved over the years.

Brickner EM, Hillis DL, Lange RA: Medical Progress: Congenital heart disease in adults. N Engl J Med 2000;342(5):334.

Foster E, Graham TP Jr, Driscoll DJ et al: Task Force 2: Special health care needs of adults with congenital heart disease. J Am Coll Cardiol 2001;37:76.

Perloff JK, Child JS: Cyanotic congenital heart disease: A multisystem disorder. In: Perloff JK, Child JS, eds: Congenital Heart Disease in Adults, 2nd ed. Philadelphia: WB Saunders, 1998.

TETRALOGY OF FALLOT

 ## ESSENTIALS OF DIAGNOSIS

- *History of exercise intolerance and squatting during childhood*
- *Central cyanosis, mildly prominent right ventricular impulse, murmur of pulmonic stenosis (with sufficient pulmonary blood flow) and absent P_2*
- *Mild right ventricular hypertrophy; occasionally left ventricular hypertrophy*
- *Chest radiograph shows classic boot-shaped heart (coeur en sabot) in severe cases without left-to-right shunt; left ventricular enlargement and post-stenotic pulmonary artery dilatation in milder cases; right-sided aortic arch in approximately 25% of patients*
- *Echocardiogram shows right ventricular hypertrophy, overriding aorta, large perimembranous ventricular septal defect, and obstruction of the right ventricular outflow tract (subvalvular, valvular, supravalvular, or in the pulmonary arterial branches)*
- *Gradient across pulmonary outflow tract, normal pulmonary artery pressures, equalization of right and left ventricular pressures*
- *Possibly anomalous branches of right coronary artery crossing right ventricular outflow tract on coronary angiography*

General Considerations

Tetralogy of Fallot is the most common form of cyanotic congenital heart disease. Without surgical intervention, most patients die in childhood; however, occasionally an acyanotic patient with only mild-to-moderate

PS and minimal right-to-left shunting is encountered (pink TOF). Although it is called a tetralogy, only the membranous nonrestrictive VSD and PS contribute to the pathophysiology of this disorder (Figure 27–23). The severity of PS determines the RV systolic pressure and thus the degree of right-to-left shunting. The PS can be valvular or, more commonly, infundibular with an obstructing muscular band in the RV outflow tract. The other two components of the tetralogy include the aortic override and the secondary RVH. Both cyanotic and acyanotic patients are at high risk for endocarditis, much like patients with complicated VSD.

Common associated anomalies include ASD (15%; the pentalogy of Fallot), right-sided aortic arch (25%), and anomalous coronary distribution (about 10%). It is important to identify the origin of the left anterior descending artery from the right coronary cusp preoperatively because the artery courses over the RV infundibulum, a potential incision site for the repair. Tetralogy of Fallot is a form of conotruncal malformation that may occur in conjunction with DiGeorge syndrome. Routine screening for the chromosome 22q11.2 deletion is now recommended to appropriately guide management and identify those patients whose offspring will be at increased risk for congenital heart disease.

Clinical Findings

A. SYMPTOMS AND SIGNS

The patient with tetralogy was typically a blue baby, cyanotic at birth. There is usually a history of exercise intolerance and squatting during childhood. Characteristic "tet spells," which are typified by episodic faintness and worsening cyanosis, are believed to be due to infundibular spasm and are generally diminished or absent by adulthood. Worsening cyanosis also occurs during exercise because of the associated systemic vasodilation and increased right-to-left shunt.

In severe cases of PS or atresia, the patient may have had life-saving surgical palliation with an aortopulmonary shunt. In the past, total repairs were not attempted until school age, but they are now being performed in infancy in many centers.

Physical examination reveals cyanosis and, less frequently, clubbing. The precordium is generally quiet, although a mild RV heave may be present. The intensity and duration of the pulmonic flow murmur vary with the degree of PS; P_2 is usually absent. In cases of pulmonary atresia with VSD (an extreme form of TOF), a continuous murmur over the back may be audible due to aortopulmonary collaterals. Patients who have had a "classic" Blalock-Taussig shunt, anastomosis of the subclavian to the side of the pulmonary artery, will have an absent pulse in the ipsilateral arm and a continuous murmur as long as the shunt is patent and functioning properly. A "modified" Blalock-Taussig

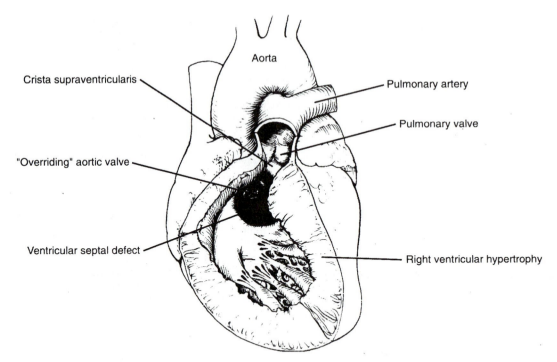

Figure 27–23. Anatomy of tetralogy of Fallot. Adapted, with permission, from Cheitlin M, Sokolow M, McIlroy M: Congenital heart disease. In Clinical Cardiology. Norwalk, CT: Appleton & Lange, 1993.

shunt, interposing a small Gore-Tex tube between the subclavian artery and the pulmonary artery, preserves the brachial pulse and is easily occluded at the time of intracardiac repair. In patients who have had intracardiac repair, a low-pitched pulmonary regurgitation murmur is commonly audible. When the murmur occurs only in early diastole, it suggests clinically important residual regurgitation.

B. DIAGNOSTIC STUDIES

1. Electrocardiography and chest radiograph—The electrocardiographic findings depend on the severity of the PS and the relative degree of shunting. If PS is severe, RVH is usually evident. If the PS is mild and the shunt is predominantly left to right, LVH may be evident. P waves are usually normal. Following intracardiac repair with infundibular resection, RBBB and varying forms of heart block are common. Postoperative atrial and ventricular arrhythmias are well-recognized complications.

The radiographic findings also depend on the underlying individual pathophysiology. The typical boot-shaped *coeur en sabot* is seen when PS is severe and the left ventricle is small. In these cases, pulmonary blood flow is reduced. Poststenotic pulmonary artery dilatation and a right-sided aortic arch may be visible on chest radiograph.

2. Echocardiography—Transthoracic two-dimensional and Doppler echocardiography demonstrates the features of this defect in its native and repaired state. The typical findings in patients with unrepaired TOF include severe RVH and a thickened, malformed pulmonary valve with poststenotic dilation. Alternatively, the level of stenosis may be primarily infundibular, with marked hypertrophic narrowing of the RV outflow tract. (Figure 27–24) Systolic color-flow aliasing and a continuous-wave Doppler gradient are detectable across the RV outflow tract or pulmonic valve. Two-dimensional imaging reveals a perimembranous VSD with evidence of right-to-left shunting by color-flow imaging; the peak velocity of the VSD jet seen by spectral Doppler is usually low. The aortic root is variably enlarged and overrides the VSD. Aortic insufficiency, usually mild, may be present. Multiplanar TEE is particularly suited to define the anatomy of the RV outflow tract and the pulmonary valve when precordial imaging is difficult. In pulmonary atresia with VSD (previously called truncus arteriosus, type IV), aortopulmonary collaterals arising from the descending aorta can also be imaged by TEE.

Complications of TOF repair that can be detected noninvasively by echocardiography include residual outflow obstruction, severe pulmonary valve regurgitation, RV outflow-tract aneurysms, and VSD patch leak.

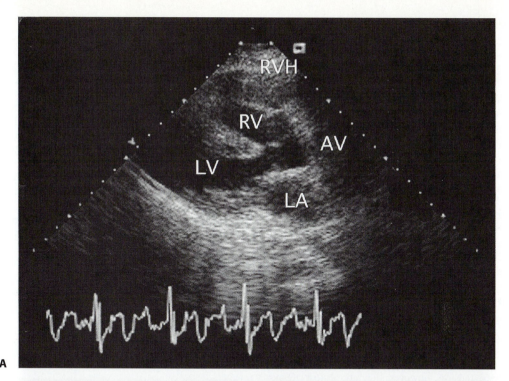

A

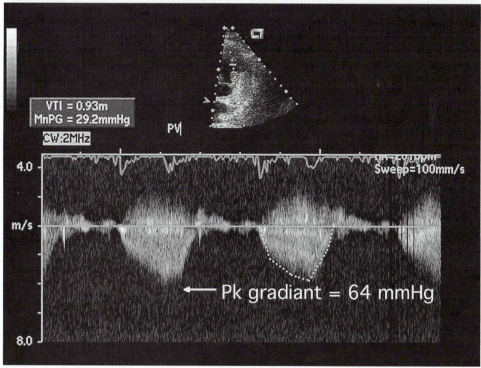

B

Figure 27–24. Transthoracic echocardiogram in patient with tetralogy of Fallot. **A:** The parasternal long axis view shows the VSD, overriding aorta. AV = aortic valve; LA = left atrium; LV = left ventricle; RVH = right ventricular hypertrophy; RV = right ventricle. **B:** Continuous-wave Doppler signal across the right ventricular outflow tract shows a high-velocity, late-peaking jet. This demonstrates severe outflow tract obstruction. The late peak suggests a component of dynamic obstruction due to the hypertrophied infundibulum.

In rare cases, an anomalous left anterior descending artery that was severed during surgery results in a LV apical aneurysm.

3. Cardiac catheterization—Cardiac catheterization reveals a gradient across the pulmonary outflow tract, usually normal PA pressures, and equalization of RV and LV pressures. Angiography may better define the anatomy of the RV outflow tract and the size of the VSD (this information is now usually available noninvasively). Coronary arteriography may demonstrate anomalous origins of the left coronary artery.

4. Other laboratory findings—Arterial saturation is variably reduced, and secondary erythrocytosis is present in the adult who has had no reparative surgery. In those with adequate surgical repair, arterial saturation should be normal.

Prognosis & Treatment

Only 11% of individuals born with this lesion survive without palliative surgery beyond the age of 20, and only 3% survive beyond the age of 40. Because the PS protects TOF patients from the development of pulmonary hypertension, however, they are almost always surgical candidates as adults. Medically, it is important to avoid systemic vasodilator therapy in the patient whose TOF is uncorrected because a reduction in arterial blood pressure can increase right-to-left shunting. Endocarditis is common in unrepaired TOF.

Total intracardiac repair with closure of the VSD and correction of the pulmonary or infundibular stenosis is indicated in the cyanotic patient to reduce symptoms and forestall complications attributable to cyanosis. The infundibulum is incised and resected to alleviate obstruction, with patching of the RV outflow tract or pulmonary annulus when necessary. This is considered one of the most successful operations in congenital heart disease surgical treatment. The indications for surgery in the occasional acyanotic patient with TOF are similar to those of a patient with VSD. Important considerations prior to surgery include the presence of anomalies in the pulmonary and coronary arteries (approximately 15% and 35%, respectively). In pulmonary atresia with VSD, which can be considered the extreme form of TOF, survival depends on the presence of well-developed bronchopulmonary or systemic-to-pulmonary collaterals. In the rare adult presenting with this lesion, surgical repair is either more complicated, requiring multiple procedures, or it is not feasible.

In patients who undergo intracardiac repair for TOF, potentially significant postoperative anatomic sequelae are possible, including residual outflow obstruction, pulmonary valve regurgitation, RV aneurysms, and VSD patch leak. Pulmonary regurgitation may develop as a consequence of surgical repair of the RV outflow tract (transannular patch). Although even substantial regurgitation can be tolerated for long periods, enlargement of the right ventricle eventually occurs, with resultant RV dysfunction, and repair or replacement of the pulmonary valve may be required.

A recent large retrospective study looking at risk stratification for arrhythmia and sudden death in these patients underscores the importance of vigilant assessment of electrocardiographic parameters (QRS duration), and hemodynamic characteristics (pulmonary regurgitation/obstruction) with timely intervention as a means of modifying the risk for sudden cardiac death in these patients. It is hoped that two current trends in surgery will reduce the incidence of arrhythmias. The first is avoidance of RV outflow tract incisions by either a transatrial or transpulmonary approach. Secondly, earlier surgical intervention may allow less time for the development of ventricular fibrosis.

Maeda J, Yamamishi H, Matsuoka R et al: Frequent association of 22q11.2 deletion with tetralogy of Fallot. Am J Med Genet 2000;92(4):269.

Owen AR, Gatzoulis MA: Tetralogy of Fallot: Late outcome after repair and surgical implications. In Williams WG, ed: Seminars in Thoracic and Cardiovascular Surgery. Pediatric Cardiac Surgery Annual 2000. Philadelphia: WB Saunders, 2000.

Therrien J, Siu SC, Harris L et al: Impact of pulmonary valve replacement on arrhythmia propensity late after repair of tetralogy of Fallot. Circulation 2001;103:2489.

EISENMENGER'S SYNDROME

 ESSENTIALS OF DIAGNOSIS

- *History of murmur or cyanosis in infancy, symptoms of dyspnea and exercise intolerance since childhood*
- *Hemoptysis, chest pain, and syncope in the adult*
- *Clubbing, cyanosis, and prominent P_2*
- *Compensatory erythrocytosis, iron deficiency, and hyperuricemia*
- *Right ventricular hypertrophy; large central pulmonary arteries with peripheral pruning on chest radiograph*
- *Severe right ventricular hypertrophy and right atrial enlargement, elevated pulmonary artery pressures, pulmonary insufficiency*
- *Detection of bidirectional shunt*

General Considerations

Three related, but not identical, clinical terms bear the name of Eisenmenger. The development of pulmonary hypertension in the presence of increased pulmonary blood flow is called the **Eisenmenger's reaction.** **Eisenmenger's syndrome** is a general term applied to pulmonary hypertension and shunt reversal in the presence of a congenital defect, including VSD, ostium primum ASD, AV canal defect, aortopulmonary window, or PDA. **Eisenmenger's complex,** as originally described, is the association of a VSD with pulmonary hypertension and shunt reversal. Patients usually develop pulmonary hypertension before puberty. Occasionally, however, patients with ostium secundum ASDs frequently develop Eisenmenger's reaction and acquire pulmonary vascular disease after puberty.

In approximately 10% of patients with nonrestrictive VSDs, the PA pressure does not fall normally in the neonatal period. Therefore, a large left-to-right shunt and CHF are not present. If the VSD goes undetected and the problem is not repaired before the infant reaches the age of 1 year, irreversible pulmonary vascular disease may result. The same is true for the other lesions associated with Eisenmenger's syndrome. In patients with ostium secundum ASD, pulmonary vascular resistance almost always falls to normal levels in the neonatal period, and the development of irreversible pulmonary hypertension is far less common.

Hemoptysis in Eisenmenger's syndrome may occasionally be due to bronchitis or pneumonia. Pulmonary infarction, a potentially fatal complication, and pulmonary arteriolar rupture must be excluded. Pregnancy is accompanied by an unacceptably high rate of maternal and fetal mortality and is virtually contraindicated in patients with Eisenmenger's syndrome.

Clinical Findings

A. SYMPTOMS AND SIGNS

Patients usually have a history of murmur or cyanosis during infancy. Exertional dyspnea is the most commonly encountered symptom. Chest pain, hemoptysis, and presyncope are less common. Transient bacteremias can result in brain abscess as a result of right-to-left shunting and entry of bacteria into the cerebral circulation without the normal filtering through the pulmonary circulation.

Physical examination reveals cyanosis (differential when the cause is PDA); cardiovascular examination is most remarkable for findings associated with pulmonary hypertension. The LV impulse is not displaced and an RV parasternal heave is present. The jugular venous pressure may be elevated in the presence of RV failure and the *a* wave may be prominent. The first heart sound is normal, and P_2 is markedly accentuated. A systolic murmur of tricuspid regurgitation may be present, and a high-pitched diastolic murmur of pulmonary regurgitation (Graham Steele murmur) is com-

mon. In the presence of RV failure, hepatomegaly, ascites, and peripheral edema may be present.

B. DIAGNOSTIC STUDIES

1. Electrocardiography and chest radiograph—The ECG shows evidence of RA enlargement and RVH with a rightward axis (Figure 27–25A). The presence of a leftward or superior axis suggests an ostium primum ASD or AV canal defect as the underlying cause (Figure 27–25B). Chest radiograph findings include RV enlargement with filling-in of the retrosternal air space, prominent proximal pulmonary arteries with pulmonary oligemia, and pruning of the peripheral pulmonary vessels.

2. Echocardiography—Severe RVH and right atrial enlargement is evident (Figure 27–26A). Right ventricular function may be normal until the late stages of the disease, at which time the right atrium enlarges. The left ventricle appears small and underfilled; the septum deviates toward the left ventricle. The level of shunt can be determined by two-dimensional imaging, aided by color-flow Doppler and saline contrast injection (Figure 27–26B). When a VSD is present, the flow velocity across the defect is low because of pressure equalization between the two ventricles. On the other hand, the tricuspid regurgitant velocity is increased and can be used to estimate the peak RV systolic pressure (Figure 27–26C). Pulmonary insufficiency with a high-velocity regurgitant jet is a frequent finding. Other valvular lesions are uncommon except in ostium primum ASD or AV canal defects, when mitral regurgitation is invariably present.

Eisenmenger's syndrome can usually be differentiated from primary pulmonary hypertension noninvasively by TTE, although shunting across a patent foramen ovale may mimic an ASD with Eisenmenger's syndrome. In these cases, further investigation with TEE or cardiac catheterization is indicated.

3. Cardiac catheterization—The pathognomonic hemodynamic findings are elevated PA pressure, increased pulmonary vascular resistance, and right-to-left shunting. The degree of residual left-to-right shunt should be measured. Oxygen should be administered during catheterization to determine whether pulmonary vascular reactivity persists. If pulmonary vascular resistance falls during O_2 or NO (nitric oxide) administration, increased left-to-right shunting can be measured. In this case, the patient may be a candidate for surgical repair.

4. Other laboratory findings—The arterial oxygen saturation by pulse oximetry or arterial blood gas measurements is markedly decreased. The hematocrit is elevated, with an overall increase in red cell mass. Iron deficiency is common, particularly after injudicious phlebotomies. Hyperuricemia caused by increased red cell turnover may be present.

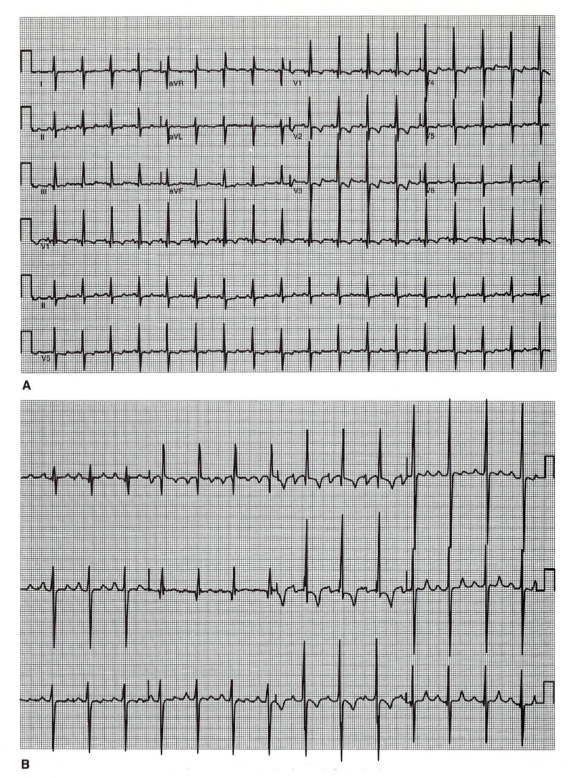

Figure 27–25. **A:** Electrocardiograph in Eisenmenger's syndrome from ostium secundum atrial septal defect with right ventricular hypertrophy and right-axis deviation. **B:** Electrocardiograph in Eisenmenger's syndrome and atrio-ventricular canal defect with right ventricular hypertrophy and left anterior hemiblock.

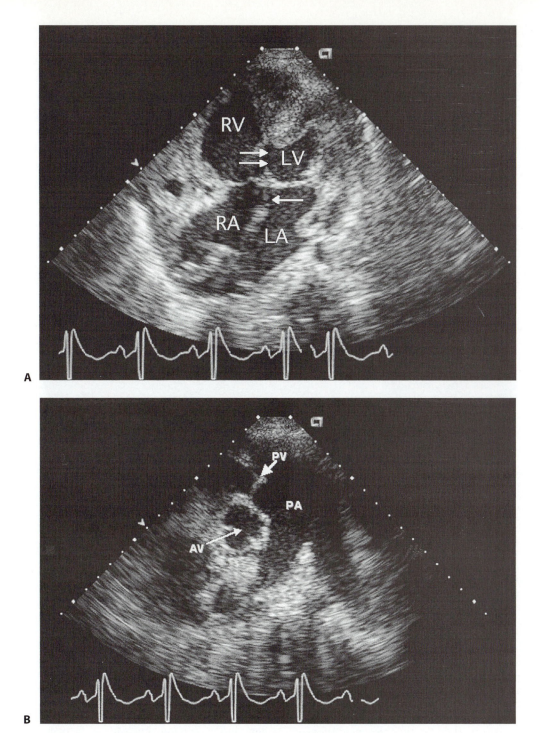

Figure 27–26. **A:** Transthoracic echocardiogram in a 32-year-old woman with Down syndrome. She has Eisenmenger's syndrome due to an atrioventricular septal defect. Four-chamber view shows hypertrophied right ventricular (RV) wall, ventricular septal defect (*double white arrow*), and ostium primum atrial septal defect (*single white arrow*). **B:** Parasternal short-axis view showing markedly dilated pulmonary artery (PA). AV = aortic valve. PV = pulmonary valve. **C:** Subcostal view after intravenous injection of agitated saline. The right atrium (RA) and right ventricle (RV) are opacified and there is rapid appearance of contrast in the left atrium (LA) and ventricle (LV) (*double black arrow*). A moderate pericardial effusion (PE) is also noted.   (continued)

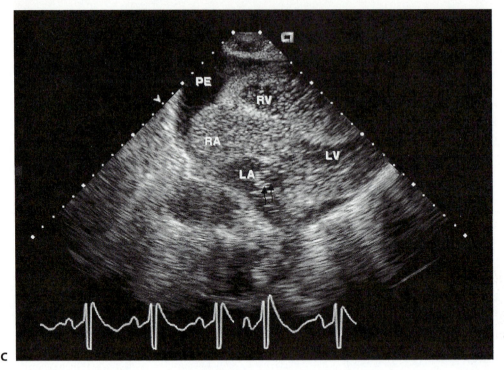

Figure 27–26. (cont.)

Prognosis & Treatment

Life expectancy is markedly shortened in patients with Eisenmenger's syndrome; however, meticulous medical management can result in improved longevity in adults with this and other forms of cyanotic heart disease. The causes of death include pulmonary infarction with uncontrollable hemoptysis, arrhythmias with sudden death, progressive RV failure, and brain abscess.

Surgical repair is contraindicated when the pulmonary vascular disease is fixed; that is, pulmonary resistance does not fall in response to O_2 or NO inhalation. In these patients, closure of the VSD (or other defects) increases the work of the right ventricle, with a resultant excessively high mortality rate. Heart-lung transplantation, offers hope for the adolescent and young adult with Eisenmenger's syndrome, but the results support only guarded optimism. In addition, some centers are looking at the feasibility of intracardiac repair in children after treatment with intravenous prostaglandin to decrease the pulmonary vascular resistance.

Careful medical management of the complications of cyanotic congenital heart disease is crucial in these patients. Hematologic disorders in adults with cyanotic congenital heart disease, including adult Eisenmenger's syndrome, can significantly influence morbidity and mortality rates. Patients with secondary erythrocytosis have been classified as either **compensated** or **decompensated.** Patients with compensated erythrocytosis are in equilibrium with stable hematocrits, no evidence of iron depletion, and few (if any) symptoms of hyperviscosity. Even with hematocrits above 70%, they do not appear to be at increased risk for cerebrovascular accidents and do not require phlebotomy. Patients with decompensated erythrocytosis have increased hematocrits (>65%) with symptoms. Because iron deficiency and dehydration may mimic hyperviscosity, these conditions should be excluded and, if present, treated before phlebotomy is undertaken. Generally, phlebotomy is not recommended for patients with hematocrits of less than 65%. A bleeding diathesis is also associated with cyanotic heart disease; it is usually mild and requires no specific therapy except for the avoidance of heparin and aspirin. Because severe life-threatening bleeding can occur during surgical procedures, preoperative phlebotomy to attain a hematocrit just below 65% is recommended. Gout can be treated with conventional therapy, taking care to avoid the antiplatelet properties of antiinflammatory agents.

Counseling regarding contraception is crucial in these patients, and pregnancy should be avoided if at all possible (see later discussion).

Hopkins WE: Severe pulmonary hypertension in congenital heart disease: A review of Eisenmenger syndrome. Curr Opin Cardiol 1995;10:517.

Perloff JK, Child JS: Cyanotic congenital heart disease: A multisystem disorder. In Perloff JK, Child JS, eds: Congenital Heart Disease in Adults, 2nd ed. Philadelphia: WB Saunders, 1998.

Rosenzweig EB, Kerstein D, Barst RJ: Long-term prostacyclin for pulmonary hypertension with associated congenital heart defects. Circulation 1999;99:1858.

TRANSPOSITION OF THE GREAT ARTERIES

ESSENTIALS OF DIAGNOSIS

- *History of cyanosis that worsens shortly after birth at the time of ductal closure*
- *Prominent right ventricular impulse, palpable and delayed A$_2$; murmurs from associated defects (eg, VSD, PS)*
- *Chest radiograph shows narrowing at base of heart in region of great vessels; prominent pulmonary vascularity unless pulmonary vascular resistance is increased*
- *Right atrial enlargement, right ventricular hypertrophy; occasionally biventricular hypertrophy (with an associated ventricular septal defect)*
- *Great arteries discordant with anterior and rightward aorta arising from the right ventricle and leftward and posterior pulmonary artery arising from the left ventricle. Atria and ventricles usually in normal position with severe right ventricular hypertrophy*

General Considerations

The key to the pathophysiology of transposition of the great arteries (D-TGA) is that the pulmonary and systemic circulations exist in parallel rather than in the normal series relationship (Figure 27–27). Survival after birth therefore depends on mixing saturated and desaturated blood via a PDA or an ASD or VSD. If an ASD or VSD does not coexist with D-TGA, an atrial communication must be created (usually percutaneously via an atrial balloon septostomy [the Rashkind procedure]) to permit survival in the newborn once the ductus closes. Prostaglandin E$_1$ may be given to restore or maintain patency of the ductus arteriosus; however, this does not always provide adequate mixing. When a VSD is present, the physiologic consequences depend largely on whether associated PS

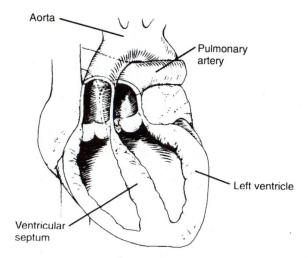

Figure 27–27. Anatomy of transposition of the great vessels. Reproduced, with permission, from Cheitlin M, Sokolow M, McIlroy M: Congenital heart disease. In Clinical Cardiology. Norwalk, CT: Appleton & Lange, 1993.

is present. In the absence of PS, there is a risk of developing pulmonary vascular disease because of the increased pulmonary blood flow; in the presence of PS, an aortopulmonary shunt may be necessary to increase pulmonary blood flow.

Clinical Findings

A. SYMPTOMS AND SIGNS

Males predominate (3:1) in this condition. There is a history of cyanosis at birth that worsens shortly thereafter when the ductus closes. In the infant with a large VSD, heart failure can occur with lesser degrees of cyanosis. In addition to profound central cyanosis, physical examination reveals a prominent RV impulse, a palpable and delayed A$_2$, and murmurs caused by associated defects (eg, VSD, PS). The findings usually associated with a large patent ductus arteriosus (see previous discussion of PDA) may be absent. The physical examination is often nondiagnostic and may actually provide more information about associated anomalies than about the presence of transposition.

B. DIAGNOSTIC STUDIES

1. Electrocardiography and chest radiograph—The ECG usually demonstrates right atrial enlargement, a rightward QRS axis, and RVH. In the presence of a VSD, biventricular hypertrophy may be evident. The chest radiograph shows narrowing at the base of the heart in the region of the great vessels. In the newborn, prior to surgery, pulmonary vascularity is prominent unless the pulmonary vascular resistance is increased by the associated pulmonary vascular disease. The right ventricle and right atrium are prominent.

2. Echocardiography—The atria and ventricles are usually in the normal position with severe RVH. The great vessels are discordant with the anterior and rightward aorta arising from RV, and leftward and posterior PA arising from the LV. In the newborn, complete examination, using combined two-dimensional and color-flow Doppler imaging should confirm or exclude the presence of an associated ASD, VSD, or PS. Virtually all surviving adults have had palliative surgical procedures, most often an atrial-switch (Mustard or Senning) operation. In these patients, baffle obstruction and leaks can be detected by color-flow Doppler and contrast echocardiography. Late obstruction of the superior vena cava can be detected by contrast echocardiography with agitated saline injected into an arm vein, opacifying the inferior vena cava. Arterial switch procedures may show regurgitation of the neoaorta or stenosis of the neopulmonary valve. Magnetic resonance imaging may also be helpful in determining the anatomy of the vena cava and pulmonary veins.

3. Cardiac catheterization—Invasive studies confirm the noninvasive diagnosis and the presence of associated defects. In the newborn, catheterization with a percutaneous atrial balloon septostomy is therapeutic and usually life-saving as well as diagnostic. The administration of intravenous prostaglandin E_1 to maintain ductal patency may preclude the need for an atrial septostomy if the oxygen saturations are adequate. In the adult with associated VSD, cardiac catheterization may be indicated to determine pulmonary vascular resistance or the severity of PS.

Prognosis & Treatment

Without treatment, isolated D-TGA carries a mortality rate of greater than 90% in the first year of life. Infants with an ASD, a VSD, or a large PDA have higher O_2 saturations and better survival rates, but early surgery is indicated to prevent the development of irreversible pulmonary vascular disease.

Definitive repair of this defect was first undertaken in the early 1960s. The atrial switch operation (Mustard or Senning) redirects the pulmonary and systemic venous return at the atrial level. The atrial septum is excised, and using either a pericardial or prosthetic baffle, the systemic venous return is directed across the mitral valve into the left ventricle and the pulmonary venous return flows across the tricuspid valve into the right ventricle. The postoperative physiology after an atrial switch procedure is similar to that of patients with C-TGA, in that the right ventricle continues to supply the systemic circulation. Many of these patients have survived to lead productive lives; however, they are potentially faced with significant late postoperative complications, including sick sinus syndrome, atrial and ventricular tachyarrhythmias, baffle obstruction and leaks (approximately 15%), and systemic ventricular dysfunction (10–15%). The late (30-year) mortality rate is approximately 20%. The majority of deaths are sudden, and the presence of atrial flutter is a precursor to sudden death, probably the result of rapid 1:1 conduction, leading to ventricular fibrillation. On the other hand, the loss of sinus rhythm (at a constant rate of 2.4% per year) does not predict death, although many patients do require a pacemaker.

Repair since the early 1980s has favored the arterial switch procedure pioneered by Jatene. This repair reestablishes the left ventricle as the systemic ventricle, and has ameliorated many of such long-term complications of the atrial switch as arrhythmias, RV dysfunction, baffle stenosis, and tricuspid regurgitation.

Follow-up of patients after arterial switch procedures has recently become available. The late mortality rate is low, and good LV function and sinus rhythm have been maintained. Postoperative aortic regurgitation and the potential for development of coronary artery ostial stenosis and late supravalvular narrowing at the anastomotic sites are of concern but will require ongoing assessment.

Kiriavainen M, Happmen JM, Louhimo I: Late results of Senning operation. J Thorac Cardiovasc Surg 1999;117:488.

Losay J, Touchot A, Serraf A et al: Late outcome after arterial switch operation for transposition of the great arteries. Circulation 2001;104(12 Suppl I):I-121.

Von Bernuth G: Twenty-five years after the first arterial switch: Mid-term results. Thorac Cardiovasc Surg 2000;48(4):228.

Wilson NJ, et al: Long-term outcome after the Mustard repair for simple transposition of the great arteries. J Am Coll Cardiol 1998;32:758.

TRICUSPID ATRESIA

 ESSENTIALS OF DIAGNOSIS

- *History of either cyanosis (70%) or congestive heart failure (30%)*
- *Cyanotic patient with absent right ventricular impulse and prominent left ventricular impulse*
- *Oligemic lung fields, right atrial and left ventricular prominence without RV enlargement in retrosternal airspace on chest radiograph*
- *Evidence of left ventricular hypertrophy, absent or atretic tricuspid valve, atrial septal defect, small right ventricle*

General Considerations

Atresia of the tricuspid valve cannot be viewed as a single congenital anomaly. In these patients the tricuspid valve is absent, the right ventricle is hypoplastic, and the inflow portion of the right ventricle is absent. Although an atrial communication is invariably present, the additional associated anomalies determine the ultimate pathophysiology and clinical presentation (Figure 27–28). Tricuspid atresia is usually classified according to the presence or absence of pulmonary stenosis and of transposition of the aorta and pulmonary artery. The great arteries are normally related in about 70% of the cases and are transposed in 30%. Pulmonary blood flow is supplied by either a PDA or aortopulmonary collaterals. Palliative surgery in this group is aimed at increasing pulmonary blood flow by a systemic venous or an arterial-to-pulmonary-artery shunt (see Palliative surgical procedures). In the 30% of patients born with tricuspid atresia and associated transposition of the great vessels, a VSD is usually present and no pulmonary obstruction is evident. These infants present with CHF; pulmonary banding in the first year of life may prevent the development of irreversible pulmonary vascular disease and allow a later intracardiac repair to be performed.

Almost all adults with tricuspid atresia have had previous surgery, and their clinical condition at presentation depends on their underlying anatomy as well as the adequacy of the palliative procedure.

Mair DD, Puga FJ, Danielson GK: The Fontan procedure for tricuspid atresia: Early and late results of a 25-year experience with 216 patients. J Am Coll Cardiol 2001;37:933.

Clinical Findings

A. SYMPTOMS AND SIGNS

A history of cyanosis predominates in patients with normally related great arteries, restrictive VSD, or PS or atresia. Patients with associated transposition of the great vessels and nonrestrictive VSD, usually have a history of CHF from LV volume overload.

Physical examination is highly variable, but the absence of a RV impulse with a prominent LV impulse in a cyanotic patient suggests tricuspid atresia. The second heart sound is often single. A continuous murmur may be present as a result of aortopulmonary collaterals or a Blalock-Taussig shunt.

B. DIAGNOSTIC STUDIES

1. Electrocardiography and chest radiograph—The ECG reveals RA enlargement and LVH. In the adult,

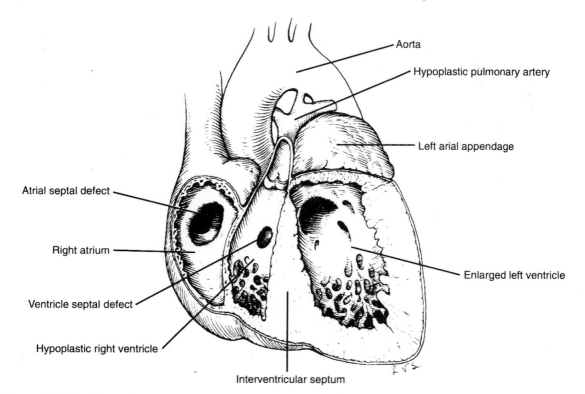

Figure 27–28. Tricuspid atresia. Reproduced, with permission, from Cheitlin M, Sokolow M, McIlroy M: Congenital heart disease. In Clinical Cardiology. Norwalk, CT: Appleton & Lange, 1993.

the chest radiograph usually shows oligemic lung fields and RA and LV prominence without RV enlargement in the retrosternal airspace.

2. Echocardiography and magnetic resonance imaging—Constant echocardiographic features include an absent or atretic imperforate tricuspid valve, ASD, and a small right ventricle. More variable features include the size of the right ventricle, the presence and size of a VSD, the presence of pulmonary atresia or stenosis, and relationship of the great vessels (normal or transposed). Doppler examination can estimate the degree of PS and the gradient across the VSD. When PS is not present, the estimated RV systolic pressure reflects the PA systolic pressure. Color-flow Doppler imaging is helpful in confirming the pattern of flow and the site of the VSD (Figure 27–29). Magnetic resonance imaging can also be helpful in defining the anatomy.

3. Cardiac catheterization—Cardiac catheterization is used to determine operability by measuring pulmonary vascular resistance and the size of the pulmonary arteries. The right ventricle cannot be entered through the right atrium, and the pulmonary artery (in the absence of atresia) must be entered from the left ventricle through the VSD. Catheterization can also be used to assess the patency of palliative shunts.

PULMONARY ATRESIA WITH INTACT VENTRICULAR SEPTUM

 ESSENTIALS OF DIAGNOSIS

- *History of cyanosis at birth, worsening at the time of ductal closure*
- *Single S_2; continuous murmur is rare*
- *Prominent left ventricular forces*
- *Oligemic lung fields, enlarged cardiac silhouette on chest radiograph*
- *Atrial septal defect, small right ventricle, absent pulmonary valve. In adults, a palliative shunt or right-ventricle-to-pulmonary-artery conduit*

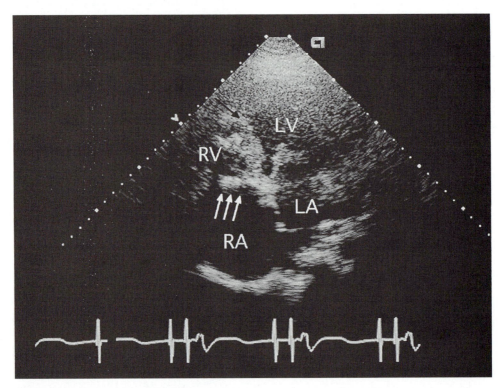

Figure 27–29. Transthoracic echocardiogram in a 30-year-old woman with tricuspid atresia. This four-chamber view demonstrates the plate-like imperforate tricuspid annulus *(three white arrows)*. The right atrium (RA) is markedly dilated, and the right ventricle (RV) is hypoplastic. A ventricular septal defect *(black arrow)* is noted. LA = left atrium, LV = left ventricle.

General Considerations

Pulmonary atresia with intact ventricular septum is rarely encountered in the adult population with congenital heart disease. The pulmonary valve is absent or imperforate, and blood flow is entirely through a PDA in the newborn. As in tricuspid atresia, an atrial communication exists through which the left atrium receives all of the systemic and pulmonary venous return. The volume-overloaded left ventricle pumps the total blood flow into the aorta and, in most cases, all the pulmonary blood flow is received retrograde via the ductus. When the ductus closes, cyanosis may worsen acutely, and pulmonary blood flow must be restored by a palliative shunt. The right ventricle may be diminutive, normal, or increased in size, and the tricuspid valve is, respectively, atretic, normal, or severely regurgitant. The high pressure in the right ventricle is decompressed through dilated coronary circulation (ie, coronary sinusoids) into the left or right coronary artery. The presence of the sinusoids directly relates to RV pressure and inversely to the amount of tricuspid regurgitation. These factors largely determine the clinical and echocardiographic findings.

Clinical Findings

Patients have a history of cyanosis at birth that worsens shortly afterward, at the time of ductal closure. The physical examination is variable, and the findings depend on the size of the right ventricle and the presence of tricuspid regurgitation. The chest radiograph may reveal oligemic lung fields and an enlarged cardiac silhouette, caused by the enlargement of the left ventricle. The main pulmonary artery segment is concave. The echocardiogram most commonly shows an ASD; a hypertrophied RV wall with a small cavity; a patent but small tricuspid valve; and a thickened, immobile, atretic pulmonary valve with no Doppler evidence of blood flow through it. The ductus arteriosus is seen running vertically from the aortic arch to the pulmonary artery (ie, vertical ductus). In adults, a palliative shunt (see section on Tricuspid Atresia) or a right-ventricle-to-pulmonary-artery conduit (the Rastelli procedure) is almost always present. Cardiac catheterization reveals systemic or supersystemic RV pressures, and the catheter cannot be passed from the right ventricle to the pulmonic artery. Angiography of the right ventricle fails to opacify the pulmonary arteries, and contrast may fill the sinusoidal vessels that often communicate with the coronary arteries.

Prognosis & Treatment

Three categories of surgical intervention exist for infants with pulmonary atresia with intact ventricular septum. The intervention selected depends on the size of the right ventricle and the presence or absence of coronary sinusoids or coronary artery anomalies. When the right ventricle is of adequate size for anticipated future growth, a connection is established between the right ventricle and main pulmonary artery to prepare for a two-ventricle repair. A systemic-to-pulmonary-artery shunt is performed at the same time. Generally, a right-ventricle-to-pulmonary-artery conduit (with or without a valve) can be placed in the older child. Problems from valvular obstruction or degeneration and conduit obstruction caused by pseudo-intimal thickening can be detected by Doppler echocardiography. A two-ventricle repair is not possible in the subset of these patients with severely hypoplastic right ventricles. Therefore a systemic-to-pulmonary-artery shunt without the connection to the right ventricle is performed, with anticipation of a Fontan procedure at a later date. Patients who have a rudimentary right ventricle and sinusoidal channels serving as the major source of coronary circulation, with perfusion by desaturated blood, represent a special problem. Decompression of the right ventricle by connection with the pulmonary artery may result in a reversal of coronary flow into the right ventricle, thereby producing myocardial ischemia. If coronary anomalies are identified by an aortogram, the sinusoids are left alone, and a systemic-to-pulmonary-artery shunt is performed in anticipation of a future Fontan-type operation. Overall, the prognosis in pulmonary atresia is limited, and although palliative surgery improves longevity, these patients require careful surveillance for complications of the surgery in addition to the underlying cyanotic heart disease.

OTHER CYANOTIC CONGENITAL HEART DEFECTS

It is increasingly common to encounter adults with complex forms of cyanotic congenital heart disease that have had some sort of palliative surgery. In addition to the conditions already discussed, there are many variants of the single-ventricular and double-outlet-ventricular anomalies. Most common among these are the **double-inlet left ventricle, double-outlet right ventricle,** and **hypoplastic left heart.** The anatomic features of the dominant ventricle that identify it as a right or left ventricle on echocardiography include the trabeculae (coarse in a right ventricle, smooth in a left ventricle), the presence of the moderator band (right ventricle), and the presence of septal attachments of the AV valve (right ventricle). Sometimes a rudimentary second ventricle occurs. In the absence of pulmonary or infundibular stenosis, pulmonary vascular disease is prevalent; subaortic stenosis and AV valve regurgitation are also common. Survival into adulthood is more likely in patients with PS.

The defect in **truncus arteriosus** arises from a failure of the single truncus in the embryo to divide into pulmonary and aortic vessels; and the pulmonary artery, aorta, and coronary arteries arise from a single main trunk. Although the anatomy of this lesion varies, a VSD is always present. The single semilunar valve, often with more than three cusps, is usually incompetent. The left ventricle is faced with not only the volume overload of both pulmonary and systemic circulations but also that caused by truncal valve regurgitation. The mortality rate in the first year of life from CHF is high. Pulmonary branch stenosis and increased pulmonary vascular resistance may improve prognosis by decreasing the likelihood of CHF. Treatment consists of closure of the VSD, surgical separation of the pulmonary arteries from the truncus, and placement of a valved conduit to connect them to the right ventricle. Late sequelae include progressive truncal valve regurgitation, progressive pulmonary vascular disease, and the need for conduit revision because of patient growth and valve degeneration.

In **total anomalous pulmonary veins,** the pulmonary venous flow enters the right atrium either directly or by one of many possible connections including the coronary sinus, superior vena cava, inferior vena cava, portal vein, hepatic vein, and ductus venosus. There is an atrial communication, and the degree of cyanosis depends on the size of the ASD and the pulmonary vascular resistance. If left untreated, most (80%) die within the first year of life. The subdiaphragmatic anomalous veins are more likely to be associated with pulmonary venous obstruction. Surgical correction consists of connecting the common pulmonary venous channel to the left atrium. Obstruction may recur following surgery in those patients who originally presented with obstruction; in others, the postoperative course is usually uncomplicated.

Palliative Surgical Procedures

In cyanotic congenital heart disease associated with diminished pulmonary blood flow, palliative procedures have been aimed at increasing pulmonary blood flow by directly or indirectly shunting blood from the systemic veins or systemic circulation. These procedures have continued to evolve.

The **Fontan procedure** (with its many modifications), the final common pathway for single ventricle repair, precludes the need for a right ventricle by rerouting the venous return from the superior and inferior vena cava directly to the pulmonary circulation, thus separating the systemic and pulmonary venous return. This operation was originally used in patients with tricuspid atresia but currently is the palliative procedure of choice for a variety of congenital heart defects, including hypoplastic left heart syndrome and morphologic single ventricle. The Fontan procedure has also been shown to be an effective palliation for selected adults with single-ventricle physiology when the pulmonary bed has been protected by congenital or palliative (ie, pulmonary band) stenosis. The Fontan procedure performed in adulthood carries a relatively low perioperative risk and leads to relief of cyanosis and improved functional class. However, arrhythmias, protein-losing enteropathy, and progressive ventricular dysfunction remain ongoing concerns. The extracardiac Fontan procedure (direct cavopulmonary anastomosis) may decrease the incidence of arrhythmias. The modified, or bidirectional, **Glenn procedure** (superior vena cava to confluent PA) can be used as a staging procedure for a future Fontan procedure or as a palliative shunt that can increase pulmonary blood flow when a Fontan is contraindicated because of high PA pressures or poor ventricular function. Because RA distension does not occur, atrial arrhythmias may be less common.

In cyanotic patients with inadequate pulmonary blood flow (eg, TOF, pulmonary and tricuspid atresia), early surgical **systemic-to-pulmonary shunts** are lifesaving procedures. The **Waterston** (ascending-aorta-to-pulmonary-artery) and **Potts** (descending-aorta-to-pulmonary-artery) shunts have been abandoned because of the high frequency of pulmonary hypertension, stenosis distal to the shunt sites, and considerable difficulty with surgical take down, but adult patients with these types of shunts are still encountered. Pulmonary artery pressure can be estimated noninvasively using the brachial artery systolic cuff pressure and continuous-wave Doppler echocardiography to measure the gradient between aorta and PA across the shunt. The classic **Blalock-Taussig shunt** (subclavian artery anastomosed to the PA) has a much lower risk of pulmonary vascular disease, with preferential blood flow into one lung (usually the left). Even when pulmonary vascular disease develops in the ipsilateral lung, the other lung is usually protected and late intracardiac repair may be possible. Because the subclavian artery is diverted, the ipsilateral arm is pulseless. The modified Blalock-Taussig shunt (now more commonly performed) uses a synthetic conduit and maintains perfusion to the arm. These shunts can become obstructed with recurrence of cyanosis, loss of the continuous murmur on physical examination, and decreased flow on Doppler echocardiography.

In the **Rastelli procedure,** extracardiac conduits from the right ventricle to the PA may be used in pulmonary atresia and C-TGA with PS, truncus arteriosus, and double-outlet right ventricle with PS. They can be synthetic (heterograft) or cadaveric (homograft) and may or may not contain valves. Problems are caused by valvular obstruction or degeneration and obstruction of shunts, baffles, and conduits. Continued clinical and noninvasive follow-up is essential in this group of patients.

Some further considerations are necessary when dealing with patients with congenital heart disease. Congestive heart failure and arrhythmias may occur as part of the natural history of the congenital defect or as a result of acquired heart disease. In managing CHF in these patients, diuretics must be used judiciously to avoid dehydration, especially in cyanotic patients, who may also be more susceptible to digoxin toxicity. In addition, the benefit of digoxin is unproven in right-heart failure associated with pulmonary vascular disease. Arrhythmias, including atrial flutter and fibrillation, are precursors to sudden death. Empiric treatment with antiarrhythmic agents should be avoided, and consultation with an electrophysiologist experienced in the care of these individuals is advised.

As many young adults with congenital heart disease have entered or are about to enter their reproductive years, genetic counseling and issues regarding pregnancy are important. The risk of congenital heart defects increases to 5–10% (higher in specific disorders) in their offspring; fetal echocardiography is becoming routine when the parent or previous offspring is affected. Maternal and fetal mortality rates vary with functional class: in NYHA class I, they are 0% and 0.4%, respectively; in NYHA class IV, the rates are 30% and 6.8%, respectively. Although pulmonary edema occurs less commonly than in patients with acquired heart disease, it may be useful to assess ventricular function noninvasively in the early months of pregnancy. Because Eisenmenger's syndrome is associated with the greatest maternal mortality rate, at approximately 50%, patients with severe pulmonary vascular disease (including primary pulmonary hypertension) should be advised against pregnancy. Women with acyanotic congenital heart disease can have successful pregnancies, however. Prophylaxis during vaginal delivery is generally recommended for those at high risk for endocarditis (see Table 27–1). General recommendations regarding exercise should be individualized to the patient following a complete clinical and noninvasive evaluation. Exercise testing and Holter monitoring should be included in this evaluation to detect significant asymptomatic arrhythmias.

It is important not to ignore the presence of acquired heart disease in adults with congenital heart disease. Acquired and congenital heart lesions may interact in unexpected ways, for example, the association of rheumatic mitral stenosis causing increased shunting across an ASD in Lutembacher's syndrome. Impaired diastolic function from hypertension or coronary artery disease in a patient with an ASD may also increase the magnitude of the left-to-right shunt. Similarly, increased systemic vascular resistance from hypertension in a patient with a VSD may worsen the shunt. The clinician must exclude coronary artery disease as a cause of chest pain in adults with congenital aortic stenosis and pulmonary hypertension. In addition, the progression of atherosclerotic coronary disease may be accelerated in association with aortic coarctation.

Ammash NM, Warnes CA: Survival into adulthood of patients with unoperated single ventricle. Am J Cardiol 1996;77:542.

Gates RN, Laks H, Drinkwater DC Jr et al: Fontan procedure in adults. Ann Thorac Surg 1997;63:1085.

Drinkwater DC, Laks H, Perloff JK: Operation and Reoperation. In Perloff JK, Child JS, eds: Congenital Heart Disease in Adults, 2nd ed. Philadelphia: WB Saunders, 1998.

Gatzoulis MA, Munk MD, Williams WG et al: Definitive palliation with cavopulmonary or aortopulmonary shunts for adults with single ventricle physiology. Heart 2000;83:51.

Chronic Anticoagulation for Cardiac Conditions

28

Richard W. Asinger, MD & Richard D. Taylor, MD

General Considerations

Intracardiac thrombi, which complicate many types of heart disease, are important because of their potential to embolize. Those in the left atrium and ventricle may embolize to the systemic circulation and are a significant cause of stroke.

The aim of antithrombotic therapy is to safely lower the rate of thromboembolism in various types of heart disease, using such methods as risk stratification and the safest effective intensity of anticoagulation. Effective primary or secondary prevention is possible with short- and long-term anticoagulation.

A. ACUTE ANTICOAGULATION

Acute anticoagulation can be a temporary bridge to chronic anticoagulation in selected clinical settings. Acute anticoagulation can be achieved with either unfractionated heparin or low-molecular-weight heparin.

1. Unfractionated heparin—Unfractionated heparin is a glycosaminoglycan that acts as an anticoagulant through an interaction with antithrombin III that accelerates antithrombin III's ability to inactivate coagulation enzymes, in particular thrombin. Unfractionated heparin may be given intravenously or subcutaneously, and its anticoagulant effect is immediate. The anticoagulant effect of unfractionated heparin can be monitored by the activated partial thromboplastin time and activated clotting time. Importantly, the anticoagulant effect of unfractionated heparin can be reversed quickly with protamine. Although it is primarily used intravenously in the hospital setting, it can also be used for chronic anticoagulation. Major disadvantages of long-term anticoagulation with subcutaneous unfractionated heparin · include heparin-induced thrombocytopenia and osteoporosis.

2. Low-molecular-weight heparin—Low-molecular-weight heparins are derived from standard heparin through a chemical or enzymatic depolymerization process. Their molecular size is approximately one third of heparin and they exhibit reduced protein and cellular binding compared with unfractionated heparin,

leading to a more predictable dose response. They are clinically effective when given subcutaneously, but their anticoagulant effect cannot be easily measured or immediately reversed. They play a major role in prevention and treatment of deep vein thrombosis following surgical procedures and are also effective in acute coronary syndromes. They are also used as a bridge to chronic anticoagulation in a variety of other clinical settings although evidence for efficacy in this circumstance is less robust. Their decreased protein and cellular binding probably explain the lower incidence for heparin-induced thrombocytopenia and osteoporosis and makes them more attractive than unfractionated heparin for long-term outpatient use.

B. LONG-TERM ORAL ANTICOAGULATION

This therapeutic method is aimed at safely reducing thromboembolism. In North America, this is almost exclusively accomplished with warfarin, which interferes with the synthesis of vitamin-K-dependent clotting factors. The reduction of these factors is determined by the Quick prothrombin time test. The time required for thrombin formation (prothrombin time) is expressed as the ratio of the tested plasma to an average prothrombin time for normal plasma; this ratio is referred to as the PTR. Thromboplastin reagents vary in their sensitivity to depletion of vitamin K clotting factors. A single batch of human brain thromboplastin has been designated the first international standard preparation by the World Health Organization. The calibration system adopted to standardize PTRs to this thromboplastin is referred to as the International Normalized Ratio (INR). It is based on the assumption that a linear relationship exists between the logarithms of prothrombin times determined by the standard reference thromboplastin and those used in the clinical laboratory. The International Sensitivity Index (ISI) is defined as the slope of this relationship determined by linear regression. The INR equals the PTR raised to the ISI power of the thromboplastin used (INR = PTR^{ISI}). The ISIs of commercially available thromboplastins used in North America varied in the past, and an INR calculation must have been made in order to compare the PTRs determined by various thromboplastins. This can be done with a nomogram (Figure 28–1).

As long as thromboplastins with variable ISIs are used clinically to determine the prothrombin time, the INR is theoretically safer than the PTR for monitoring long-term oral anticoagulants. Much of the concern over varying sensitivities of thromboplastins has been obviated recently with the change to commercial thromboplastins with an ISI of 1.0.

The intensity level of anticoagulation recommended for most clinical indications is an INR of 2.0–3.0. For patients with mechanical prosthetic valves and those who have experienced thromboembolism while on lower intensities of anticoagulation, a higher intensity (an INR of 2.5–3.5) is recommended. If thromboem-

bolism still occurs with an appropriate level of anticoagulation, 80–160 mg/day of aspirin, clopidogrel 75 mg/day, or dipyridamole 200 mg in divided doses daily may be added.

Pathophysiology & Etiology

A. PATHOGENESIS OF INTRACARDIAC THROMBUS

In the nineteenth century, Virchow theorized that stasis of intracavitary blood, endocardial injury, and a hypercoagulable state were necessary for intracardiac thrombosis. In the normally functioning heart, stasis and thrombosis do not occur, but a high incidence of thrombosis is noted in cardiac chambers that are enlarged or have low flow. Left atrial thrombi complicate mitral stenosis and atrial fibrillation; left ventricular

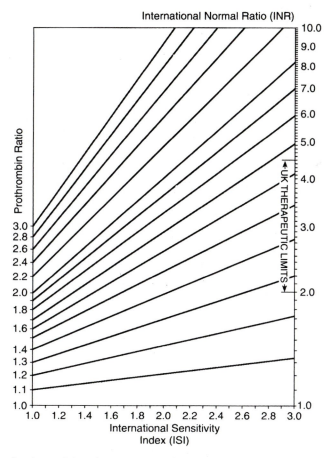

Figure 28-1. Nomogram for determining the International Normalized Ratio (INR), given the patient's prothrombin ratio and the International Sensitivity Index (ISI) of the thromboplastin used over a range from 1.0 to 3.0 United Kingdom (UK) therapeutic reference, INR of 2.0–4.5 indicated on right margin. Modified, with permission, from Hirsh J, Dalen JE, Deykin D et al: Oral anticoagulants: Mechanism of action, clinical effectiveness, and optimal therapeutic range, Chest 1992;102:316S.

thrombi can occur with acute myocardial infarction, left ventricular aneurysm, and dilated cardiomyopathy. In these clinical settings, there is generalized or localized low flow in either the left atrium or left ventricle.

Acute myocardial infarction causes stasis of intracardiac blood (secondary to the dysfunction of part of the left ventricle) in the setting of a hypercoagulable state, and left ventricular thrombosis is common particularly if reperfusion therapy is not given or is not effective. These thrombi usually develop at the apex of the left ventricle 2–7 days after anterior infarction; they rarely develop with inferior infarction (Table 28–1). Because the left anterior descending coronary artery usually supplies the apex, apical stasis occurs with anterior infarction. The apex is the portion of the left ventricle farthest from the inflow and outflow areas—the areas with the highest blood flow velocities. Severe apical wall motion abnormalities, such as akinesia, dyskinesia, and aneurysm, precede thrombus formation in acute infarction. Endocardial injury that occurs during acute infarction may also contribute to thrombosis.

Myocardial necrosis including the endocardium may occur with infarction and contribute to thrombus development. Endocardial abnormalities may also be present in other clinical settings such as atrial fibrillation in which elevated von Willebrand factor is noted in the left atrium. The introduction of a foreign mate-rial, such as a prosthetic valve (discussed in the section on Prosthetic Heart Valves), into the heart can provide the nidus for thrombus formation. An inflammatory process that involves the myocardium, secondary to myocarditis or noninfectious endocarditis, may also be responsible for thrombus formation, particularly when there is a coexistent hypercoagulable state. Reduced ventricular function can also contribute to thrombosis with myocarditis. Eosinophils presumably cause the endothelial injury with Löffler's endocarditis that leads to thrombus formation.

The final prerequisite for intracardiac thrombosis is a hypercoagulable state, and activation of the coagulation system can be found in conditions associated with intracardiac thrombi, including acute myocardial infarction and atrial fibrillation. Rare cases have been reported in which, even with normal wall motion and presumably normal blood flow, intracardiac thrombi develop because of a hypercoagulable state. Platelets may also play an active role in the formation of intracardiac thrombi and are activated in such clinical situations as acute infarction and atrial fibrillation.

Although all three of Virchow's prerequisites are operative in specific settings, most clinical data indicate an complex interaction exists with stasis the most frequent—or perhaps the most easily demonstrated—factor leading to intracardiac thrombosis.

Table 28–1. Incidence of left ventricular thrombus following transmural myocardial infarction.

Study	Total Number of Patients	Anterior Infarction			Inferior Infarcion		
		Patients (#)	LVT (#)	LVT (%)	Patients (#)	LVT (#)	LVT (%)
Asinger, 1981	70	35	12	34	35	0	0
Friedman, 1982	52	21	8	38	13	2	15
Johannessen, 1984	90	53	15	28	28	0	0
Visser, 1984	96	65	21	32	31	1	3
Weinreich, 1984	261	130	44	34	131	2	2
Gueret, 1986	90	46	21	46	44	0	0
Nihoyannopoulus, 1989	87	53	21	40	34	0	0
Keren, 1990	198	124	38	31	74	0	0
Total	944	527	180	34	390	5	1

LVT = left ventricular thrombus.

Source: Data from Asinger RW et al: Incidence of left ventricular thrombosis after acute myocardial infarction. N Engl J Med 1981;305:297. Friedman MJ et al: Clinical correlations in patients with acute myocardial infarction and left ventricular thrombosis detected by two-dimensional echocardiography. Am J Med 1982;72:894.

B. Embolization of Thrombi

With the exception of prosthetic valve thrombosis, intracardiac thrombi rarely cause clinical manifestations independent of embolization. It has even been proposed that the left ventricular thrombi that complicate acute myocardial infarction are beneficial because they may prevent rupture of the left ventricular free wall by reducing wall stress in the area of acute infarction.

Unlike Virchow's triad of prerequisites for the development of intracardiac thrombus, prerequisites for embolization of existing thrombi have not been defined. Theoretically, the reversal of any member of the triad could result in embolization of an existing intracardiac thrombus. Because myocardial dysfunction causes stasis of blood and leads to thrombus formation, recovery of function may eliminate stasis and promote embolization. This could explain why left ventricular thrombi usually develop within the first week following infarction but embolization occurs 5–21 days following infarction. Improving myocardial function at the margins of a thrombus could theoretically change its shape from mural to protruding and lead to embolization. A protruding thrombus provides a greater surface area to circulating blood and may account for the reported high frequency of embolization.

Recovery of mechanical function of the left atrium has also been implicated in embolization of left atrial thrombi. The fibrillating left atrium is enlarged and has low flow, including its appendage, where thrombosis may occur. Restoration of normal sinus rhythm (spontaneously or following pharmacologic or electrical cardioversion) restores mechanical systole to the atrium and may cause systemic embolization. It is also important to remember that the return of effective mechanical function of the atrium after successful cardioversion may require several weeks. Stasis may occur during this period of stunning, allowing thrombi to develop. With the return of mechanical function, these thrombi may be expelled from the left atrium or its appendage resulting in systemic embolization and may explain reports of patients with no left atrial or appendage thrombus on transesophageal echocardiography (TEE) who experience systemic embolization several days after cardioversion from atrial fibrillation to normal sinus rhythm if they are not therapeutically anticoagulated.

The role of endocardial healing following acute myocardial infarction may play a role in embolization of a thrombus. Lysis at the endothelial contact of the thrombus may lead to embolization.

Endogenous thrombolysis may cause embolization of an existing thrombus. As previously noted, protruding and—especially—mobile thrombi are associated with embolization. The mechanism of thrombus protrusion and mobility may involve spontaneous thrombolysis independently or in combination with improving segmental or global chamber function. Thrombolytic drugs, in doses used for acute myocardial infarction, have been given to patients with recently developed left ventricular thrombi; serial echocardiography showed rapid and dramatic changes in the shape of thrombi. Over a period of hours, some thrombi become protruding and mobile, with clinical systemic embolization occasionally occurring. Low-dose urokinase administered over a longer period, however, is reported to lyse recently formed thrombi successfully, without clinical evidence of systemic embolization.

Gueret P et al: Effects of full-dose heparin anticoagulation on the development of left ventricular thrombosis in acute transmural myocardial infarction. J Am Coll Cardiol 1986;8:419.

Johannessen KA, Nordrehaug JE, Gerhard L: Left ventricular thrombosis and cerebrovascular accident in myocardial infarction. Br Heart J 1984;51:553.

Keren A et al: Natural history of left ventricular thrombi: Their appearance and resolution in the post-hospitalization period of acute myocardial infarction. J Am Coll Cardiol 1990;15:790.

Nihoyannopoulos P et al: The natural history of left ventricular thrombosis in myocardial infarction: A rationale in support of masterly inactivity. J Am Coll Cardiol 1989;14:903.

Visser CA et al: Long-term follow-up of left ventricular thrombosis after acute myocardial infarction: A two-dimensional echocardiographic study in 96 patients. Chest 1984;84:532.

Weinreich DJ, Burke JF, Pauletto FJ: Left ventricular mural thrombi complicating acute myocardial infarction: Long-term follow-up with serial echocardiography. Ann Intern Med 1984;100:789.

Diagnostic Studies

Prior to the advent of accurate imaging techniques, most knowledge of intracardiac thrombi was derived from postmortem studies. Echocardiography is an accurate, noninvasive technique for detecting intracardiac thrombi during life; it surpasses routine contrast radiographic techniques. Transthoracic echocardiography is sensitive and specific for detecting left ventricular thrombi, but TEE is required to reliably detect left atrial thrombi.

The use of serial echocardiography has greatly enhanced our knowledge of the natural history of intracardiac thrombosis associated with acute myocardial infarction. The precise onset of the pathophysiologic thrombotic process can be accurately defined with acute myocardial infarction, allowing serial study of thrombus development. Meticulously performed Doppler studies of blood flow within the left ventricle of patients who develop thrombosis show that apical patterns of low flow precede thrombosis. Because these high-risk factors, anterior infarction and severe apical wall motion abnormality, are present and can be detected prior to thrombus development, it is possible to initiate prophylactic treatment with anticoagulants and decrease the development of thrombus and, presumably, subsequent systemic emboli.

Spontaneous echo contrast ("smoke") detected in a cardiac chamber represents low flow and early rouleaux formation and is frequently associated with thrombus. Patients with spontaneous echo contrast in the left atrium accompanying rheumatic mitral stenosis, a prosthetic mitral valve, or nonvalvular atrial fibrillation have a high incidence of left atrial thrombi and thromboembolism.

Indium-111-labeled platelets can also be used to detect left ventricular thrombi. This radionuclide imaging technique allows determination of thrombotic activity at the thrombus-blood interface and has predictive value for subsequent systemic embolism. It also allows evaluation of the effectiveness of antithrombotic treatment. High-speed contrast, computed tomography and magnetic resonance imaging can also be used to reliably detect intracardiac thrombus, especially in the left ventricle. These three techniques, however, require specialized equipment not readily available, are expensive, and used infrequently.

Bussey HI, Force RN, Bianco TM et al: Reliance on prothrombin time ratios causes significant errors in anticoagulant therapy. Arch Intern Med 1992;152:278

Cerebral Embolism Task Force: Cardiogenic brain embolism: The second report of the Cerebral Embolism Task Force. Arch Neurol 1989;46:727.

Delemarre BJ, Visser CA, Bot H et al: Prediction of apical thrombus formation in acute myocardial infarction based on left ventricular spatial flow pattern. J Am Coll Cardiol 1990; 15:355.

Hirsh J, Dalen J, Anderson DR et al: Oral anticoagulants: Mechanism of action, clinical effectiveness, and optimal therapeutic range. Chest 2001;119:8S.

Hirsh J, Warkentin TE, Shaughnessy SG et al: Heparin and low molecular weight heparin: Mechanisms of action, pharmacokinetics, dosing, monitoring, efficacy, and safety. Chest 2001; 119:64S.

Keren A, Goldberg S, Gottlieb S et al: Natural history of left ventricular thrombi: Their appearance and resolution in the post-hospitalization period of acute myocardial infarction. J Am Coll Cardiol 1990;15:790.

Manning WJ, Leeman DE, Gotch PJ et al: Pulsed Doppler evaluation of atrial mechanical function after electrical cardioversion of atrial fibrillation. J Am Coll Cardiol 1989;13:617.

Maze SS, Kotler MN, Parry WR: Flow characteristics in the dilated left ventricle with thrombus: Qualitative and quantitative Doppler analysis. J Am Coll Cardiol 1989;13:873.

Tsai LM, Chaen JH, Fang CJ et al: Clinical implications of left atrial spontaneous echo contrast in nonrheumatic atrial fibrillation. Am J Cardiol 1992;70:327.

Vecchio C, Chiarella F, Lupi G et al: Left ventricular thrombus in anterior acute myocardial infarction after thrombolysis: A GISSI-2 connected study. Circulation 1991;84:512.

Virchow R: Phlogose und thrombose in gefassystem. In: Gesammelter Abhandlungen zur wissenschaftlichen Medicin. Meidinger 1856:458-636.

Treatment of Conditions That Require Chronic Anticoagulation

A. Prosthetic Heart Valves

The purpose of replacing diseased native heart valves is primarily to improve hemodynamics and hence functional status and long-term survival. The first prosthetic valves were mechanical, and although the hemodynamic status improved following implantation, thromboembolic complications occurred and caused such disastrous complications as stroke. Initially it was unclear whether thromboembolism was caused by the introduction of a foreign body into the circulation or by the underlying pathology. Thromboembolic risk continues well after endothelialization of the sewing ring has occurred, suggesting that the mechanical prosthesis or underlying cardiac abnormality is the cause. Whatever the mechanism, it is apparent that these complications can be reduced with anticoagulation.

Because a mechanical prosthesis necessitates lifelong anticoagulation, it is important to evaluate patients for hemorrhagic risk prior to valve surgery. For women of child-bearing age, an important consideration is the type of valve (mechanical or biologic) to be implanted because of the risks of anticoagulation with pregnancy (this is discussed later in this chapter).

When using anticoagulation to reduce the thromboembolic complications associated with prosthetic valves, however, it is important to recognize that no antithrombotic regimen guarantees a thromboembolus-free course or a hemorrhage-free valve implant.

1. Mechanical valves—Such valves include ball-cage, unileaflet tilting-disk, and bileaflet tilting-disk prostheses. Although flow characteristics vary, all prosthetic valves are foreign material (the sewing ring and the mechanical portions of the prosthesis) placed in the central circulation, providing a potential nidus for thrombus formation. The underlying pathologic processes, as well as atrial fibrillation and decreased systolic performance of the left ventricle, are also important risk factors for postimplant thromboembolism.

The thromboembolic rate of patients with mechanical valves treated with moderate or high-intensity anticoagulation is similar; the hemorrhagic rate is, however, much higher for those on high-intensity anticoagulation (Table 28–2).

All studies of mechanical valves indicate that a certain thromboembolic rate continues despite anticoagulation. In a direct comparison of anticoagulation with warfarin versus antithrombotic treatment with dipyridamole, warfarin had a significantly lower thromboembolic rate. Agents that interfere with platelet function in addition to anticoagulation, however, could conceivably lower the thromboembolic rate even more. A reduction in cardiovascular mortality rates has been re-

Table 28–2. Anticoagulation intensity for artificial cardiac valves and incidence of thromboembolic and other events.

	Events per 100 Patient-Years	
Mechanical Valves		
Saour JN		
Anticoagulation intensity	PTr 1.5; INR 2.65 $n = 122$	PTr 2.5; INR 9 $n = 125$
Thromboembolic events	4.0	3.7
Bleeding episodes	6.2	12.1
Altman R		
Anticoagulation intensity	INR 2.0–2.99 $n = 51$	INR 3.0–4.5 $n = 48$
Thromboembolic events	1.9	4.9
Bleeding episodes	3.8	24.7
Biologic Valves		
Turpie AGG		
Anticoagulation intensity	INR 2.0–2.25 $n = 102$	INR 2.5–4.0 $n = 108$
Major thromboembolic events	2.0	1.9
Minor thromboembolic events	10.8	10.2
Hemorrhagic complications	5.9	13.9

Note: Both moderate- and high-intensity groups also received aspirin (330 mg) and dipyridamole (75 mg) twice daily.

Source: Data from Saour JN et al: Trial of different intensities of anticoagulation in patients with prosthetic heart valves. N Engl J Med 1990;322:428.

ported on patients with mechanical valves treated with warfarin and aspirin compared with those receiving warfarin alone.

Currently, warfarin alone is an acceptable anticoagulant for patients with mechanical valves (INR 2.5–3.5); the addition of aspirin (80–160 mg/day), clopidogrel (75 mg/day), or dipyridamole (200 mg/day in divided doses) is optional. Patients who have had thromboembolic events on standard anticoagulation therapy should also receive aspirin in low doses (80–160 mg/day), clopidogrel (75 mg/day), or dipyridamole (200 mg/day in divided doses).

2. Biologic valves—Despite the advantages of biologic valves in terms of central flow and less-thrombogenic valve material, thromboembolic complications do occur, particularly in the early postoperative period. The presumed mechanism in this setting is thrombus formation on the sewing ring. A randomized trial of two intensities of anticoagulation following bioprosthetic valve replacement showed similar rates of thromboembolism but fewer hemorrhagic complications for low-intensity anticoagulation (see Table 28–2). Therefore, low-intensity therapeutic anticoagulation (INR of 2.0–3.0) for the first 3 months following the biologic valve implant is recommended. After that period, anticoagulation for bioprosthetic cardiac valves is generally considered optional—except for patients at high risk for thromboembolism, where continued low-intensity anticoagulation (INR 2.0–3.0) is recommended. High-risk features include previous thromboembolism, atrial fibrillation, congestive heart failure, and an enlarged left atrium. For patients without these risk factors, the use of aspirin alone is an option, but reports of its efficacy are based on limited data.

B. ATRIAL FIBRILLATION

Atrial fibrillation is the most commonly encountered arrhythmia in clinical practice and complicates many types of heart disease. Its importance lies not only in its hemodynamic effect but also in the fact that it is a strong and independent predictor of thromboembolism. Atrial fibrillation, which affects many patients and can easily be identified by clinical examination or electrocardiography, causes ineffective mechanical function of the atria. This leads to dilatation and low flow through both atria and their appendages. Theoretically, the underlying hemodynamic state, combined with the lack of mechanical function, determines the risk of thromboembolism. Conditions that cause enlarged atria with low flow have a higher risk for thromboembolism than do those conditions with normal left atrial size and normal or increased flow. Patients with rheumatic mitral stenosis and atrial fibrillation have a very high incidence of thromboembolism, whereas those with lone atrial fibrillation (no other cardiac disease including hypertension) have a very low incidence. In evaluating and treating patients with atrial fibrillation,

it is important to include diagnostic studies to identify cardiovascular abnormalities that affect atrial size and flow.

1. Rheumatic mitral stenosis—Patients with mitral stenosis and atrial fibrillation have a higher incidence of left atrial thrombus (frequently located in the left atrial appendage; Figure 28–2) than those with normal sinus rhythm.

These patients also have a high incidence of systemic embolism. Population-based studies have shown that the risk of systemic embolism, primarily stroke, increases almost 18 times for those with mitral stenosis and atrial fibrillation compared with age-, sex-, and hypertension-matched controls without these findings. This high risk of thromboembolism justifies anticoagulation, but no prospective studies have been performed to document the efficacy of this approach. Most studies of anticoagulation for the prevention of thromboembolism with rheumatic mitral stenosis and atrial fibrillation have been retrospective studies of secondary prevention in which a 50% reduction in subsequent thromboembolism was generally reported for patients

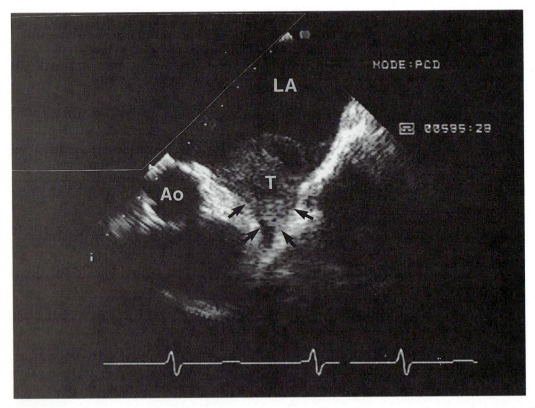

Figure 28-2. Short-axis transesophageal echocardiogram image at left atrial level, showing the left atrium and its appendage. A thrombus is present in the left atrial appendage. Ao = aorta; LA = left atrium; T = thrombus. Arrows outline the left atrial appendage.

who received anticoagulants. Long-term anticoagulation with warfarin to maintain an INR of 2.0–3.0 is therefore recommended for patients with atrial fibrillation and mitral stenosis; patients who have thromboembolism while on appropriate anticoagulant therapy should have their target INR raised to 2.5–3.5, receive 80–160 mg aspirin daily, or both.

2. Nonvalvular atrial fibrillation—This type of atrial fibrillation refers to patients with a wide variety of cardiovascular abnormalities but excludes those with rheumatic mitral valve disease. Patients with nonvalvular atrial fibrillation also have an increased incidence of stroke and systemic emboli (approaching 5% a year). The incidence of stroke or systemic emboli can be reduced with low-intensity long-term anticoagulation; the efficacy of aspirin is less well established (Table 28–3).

The underlying etiology and hemodynamic status of patients with nonvalvular atrial fibrillation vary; some favor thromboembolism, and three risk-stratification profiles have been proposed to aid clinical decisions for antithrombotic therapy (Table 28–4). These risk stratification schemes vary somewhat but share the common theme that thromboembolic risk increases with the severity of cardiovascular disease. The Atrial Fibrillation Investigators performed a meta-analysis of placebo-assigned patients from the first five randomized clinical trials of antithrombotic therapy and found age older than 65 years, hypertension, coronary artery disease, and diabetes as high-risk clinical features. When transthoracic echocardiographic parameters were also included from three of these clinical trials, moderate or worse left ventricular dysfunction was also an independent predictor of subsequent thromboembolism. The Antithrombotic Consensus Panel of the American College of Chest Physicians risk stratification scheme categorized patients with nonvalvular atrial fibrillation into high, moderate, and low risk for thromboembolism. High-risk factors included age >75, history of hypertension, and at least moderate left ventricular dysfunction on transthoracic echocardiography. Intermediate risks included age 65–75, diabetes, coronary artery disease, and thyrotoxicosis. Low-risk factors include age <65 years with no high- or intermediate-risk factors.

The SPAF investigators identified a clinical history of recent congestive heart failure (within 3 months) or left ventricular fractional shortening <25% on M-mode echocardiography, previous thromboembolism, systemic hypertension, and females older than 75 years of age as independent predictors of subsequent thromboembolism. Patients with one or more of these predictors had a thromboembolic event rate of 7.2% per year, whereas those with none had an event rate of only 2.5% per year. The results of SPAF-III prospectively verified this risk stratification scheme and the efficacy of anticoagulation for high-risk patients.

Table 28–3. Ischemic stroke and systemic embolus rates for placebo-controlled studies of antithrombotic therapy for NVAF.[a]

	AFASAK[b] n = 1007 (%)	SPAF-1[c] (n = 1330) (%)	BAATAF[d] (n = 420) (%)	CAFA[e] (n = 378) (%)	SPINAF[f] (n = 538) (%)
Placebo	5.5	6.3	3.07	4.6	3.9
Warfarin	2.2	2.3	0.4	3.0	1.0
Aspirin	4.7	3.6	NA	NA	NA
Hemorrhagic rate	0.5	1.5	0.8	2.5	1.3

[a] Intention-to-treat analysis.

[b] Data from Peterson P et al: Placebo-controlled, randomized trial of warfarin and aspirin for prevention of thromboembolic complications in chronic atrial fibrillation. The Copenhagen AFASAK Study. Lancet 1989;1:175.

[c] Data from Stroke Prevention in Atrial Fibrillation Investigators: Stroke prevention in atrial fibrillation study: Final results. Circulation 1991;84:527.

[d] Data from Boston Area Anticoagulation Trial for Atrial Fibrillation Investigators: The effect of low dose warfarin on the risk of stroke in patients with nonrheumatic atrial fibrillation. N Engl J Med 1990;323:1505.

[e] Data from Connolly SJ et al: Canadian atrial fibrillation anticoagulation (CAFA) study. J Am Coll Cardiol 1991;18:349.

[f] Data from Ezekowitz MD et al: Interim analysis of VA cooperative study: Stroke prevention in non-rheumatic atrial fibrillation (SPINAF). N Engl J Med 1992;327:1406.

NA = no information available.

Table 28–4. Published risk-stratification schemes for primary[a] prevention of thromboembolism in patients with nonvalvular atrial fibrillation.

Source	High Risk[b]	Intermediate Risk	Low Risk
Atrial Fibrillation Investigators	Age ≥ 65 years		Age <65 years
	History of hypertension		No high-risk features
	Coronary artery disease		
	Diabetes		
American College of Chest Physicians	Age >75 years	Age 65–75 years	Age <65 years
	History of hypertension	Diabetes	No risk factors
	Left ventricular dysfunction[c]	Coronary artery disease	
	More than one intermediate risk factor	Thyrotoxicosis	
Stroke Prevention in Atrial Fibrillation	Women >75 years	History of hypertension	No high-risk features
	Systolic BP >160 mm Hg	No high-risk features	No history of hypertension
	Left ventricular dysfunction[d]		

[a] Patients with AF and prior thromboembolism are at high risk of stroke, and anticoagulation is indicated for secondary prevention in such cases.

[b] Patients are classified on the basis of the presence or absence of any risk factor.

[c] Left ventricular dysfunction refers to moderate to severe wall motion to severe wall motion abnormality assessed globally by two-dimensional echocardiography, reduced ejection fraction, fractional shortening less then 0.25 by M-mode echocardiography, or clinical heart failure.

[d] Did not distinguish high-risk from intermediate-risk groups.

BP = blood pressure.

Source: Adapted, with permission, from Pearce et al: Assessment of these schemes for stratifying stroke risk in patients with nonvalvular atrial fibrillation. Am J Med 2000;109:45. © 2000, with permission, from Excerpta Medica, Inc.

For nonvalvular atrial fibrillation, long-term anticoagulation with warfarin to maintain an INR of 2.0–3.0 is recommended, particularly for those with clinical or echocardiographic predictors of high risk for thromboembolism. For those who are not candidates for anticoagulation, aspirin is a reasonable alternative. For patients with lone atrial fibrillation (<60 years old with no cardiopulmonary disease and no systemic hypertension), the risk of anticoagulation outweighs the potential benefit. These patients should receive either aspirin therapy alone or no specific antithrombotic therapy until aspirin efficacy data and the results of further risk-stratification profiles become available.

For nonvalvular atrial fibrillation patients who experienced thromboembolism while on anticoagulants with INRs in the therapeutic range, increasing the targeted INR to 2.5–3.5, adding aspirin (80–160 mg/day), or both should be considered.

3. Cardioversion of atrial fibrillation—Atrial fibrillation can be effectively treated with pharmacologic or electrical cardioversion. Conversion to normal sinus rhythm, however, can cause systemic embolism through two potential mechanisms. The first is embolization of existing left atrial or atrial appendage thrombus by reestablishing mechanical function. The second is development of left atrial or atrial appendage thrombus during the postconversion period when the atrium is mechanically stunned; embolization of the thrombus may then occur as mechanical function returns. Retrospective studies have shown a significantly higher risk of systemic embolization following cardioversion to normal sinus rhythm for patients who did not receive anticoagulants. The time necessary for thrombus formation in a fibrillating left atrium is unclear although it has been reported that patients can have embolic episodes within days of the onset of atrial fibrillation. Patients in atrial fibrillation longer than 48 h should receive anticoagulation before cardioversion. Two strategies of equal efficacy and safety have been developed for anticoagulant therapy for elective cardioversion. The first, or conventional, strategy is for anticoagulation with an INR 2.0–3.0 for at least 3 weeks before cardioversion. The second is TEE-guided cardioversion. For this strategy, anticoagulation with either unfractionated heparin (target PTT 1.5–2.5 times normal) or warfarin (INR 2.0–3.0) is given prior to TEE. Patients with no left atrial or atrial appendage thrombus may undergo cardioversion. Those with left atrial or atrial appendage thrombus are not cardioverted but rather continued on anticoagulant therapy with warfarin with a target INR or 2.0–3.0 and reevaluated with TEE in 3 weeks. Whether patients undergo conventional or TEE-guided cardioversion, both groups should continue on warfarin anticoagulation for 4 weeks following cardioversion with a target INR of 2.0–3.0.

The incidence of systemic emboli in patients cardioverted from atrial flutter to normal sinus rhythm appears to be low but there are few data to guide therapy. Patients with atrial flutter with or without atrial fibrillation should be treated as though they have atrial fibrillation and undergo conventional or TEE-guided cardioversion and undergo 4 weeks of anticoagulation following conversion.

C. Ischemic Heart Disease

1. Acute myocardial infarction not treated with thrombolytics—Postmortem findings of patients with acute myocardial infarction before the thrombolytic era indicated a high incidence of left ventricular thrombus, pulmonary and systemic embolism, and coronary artery thrombus. Left ventricular thrombi were common and although embolic events were uncommon, they were frequently devastating since most (>80%) were to the central nervous system (87% occur between days 5 and 21 following infarction). The risk of systemic embolism can be decreased with long-term oral anticoagulation, with a relatively low risk of hemorrhagic complications. Risk stratification to identify high- and low-risk groups for the development of thrombosis and embolism can improve the efficacy of anticoagulation following infarction.

Echocardiographic studies have shown thrombus formation to be more common in patients with anterior rather than inferior myocardial infarction. An even higher risk group can be identified by analysis of the left ventricular apex. Patients with anterior infarction and akinesia or dyskinesia of the apex are the most likely to develop thrombus. In addition, the larger the wall motion abnormality and the worse the global ventricular function, the higher the incidence of left ventricular thrombus. On the basis of these clinical and echocardiographic data, there appears to be good rationale for long-term (3 months) treatment with oral anticoagulants following anterior infarction in patients who did not receive or achieve reperfusion therapy. Patients receiving therapeutic doses of heparin following acute anterior infarction develop significantly fewer left ventricular thrombi and have fewer embolic episodes than those treated with low-dose or no heparin. Studies of long-term oral anticoagulation following infarction have documented that anticoagulant therapy reduces the incidence of stroke and systemic emboli, although most did not report results based on infarct location.

For patients with anterior infarction with apical akinesis or dyskinesis and reduced left ventricular function who have not received reperfusion therapy in the form of thrombolytic therapy or direct angioplasty, initial anticoagulation with heparin followed by warfarin to maintain an INR of 2.0–3.0 for a 3-month period in addition to low-dose aspirin (81–160 mg/day) is recommended because most systemic emboli occur during this interval. After that time, aspirin (325 mg/day) should be given as an antithrombotic, particularly if no intracardiac thrombus can be shown by echocardiography.

2. Acute myocardial infarction treated with thrombolytics or direct angioplasty—Stroke following thrombolytic therapy for acute infarction may be secondary to intracranial bleed or ischemic infarction. An intracranial bleed is a cause of very early stroke; ischemic stroke is a later complication. Although the incidence of an intracranial bleed is expectedly higher in patients treated with thrombolytics, the incidence of ischemic stroke appears to be low, for reasons that are unclear. A large anterior infarction is the only high-risk factor reported for ischemic stroke in patients receiving thrombolytics. It is possible that thrombolytic treatment reduces thrombus formation by decreasing stasis (because of more rapid recovery of function from earlier reperfusion) or by interfering with the earliest stages of thrombus formation at the endothelium-blood interface. Treatment protocols for continued antithrombotic treatment following acute thrombolytic therapy vary from no specific therapy to aspirin alone, heparin alone, or heparin and aspirin in combination.

Reperfusion therapy achieved with direct angioplasty may have the lowest rate of subsequent stroke. A lower rate of hemorrhagic stroke compared with thrombolytic therapy is intuitive, and a lower rate of ischemic stroke potential could be the result of more effective reperfusion with less regional and global myocardial dysfunction.

Because the incidence of ischemic stroke is so low in patients receiving reperfusion therapy, either with thrombolytic therapy or direct angioplasty, it is unclear whether the risk-benefit ratio favors oral anticoagulation therapy acutely and for the first 3 months following infarction. A reasonable approach is clinical evaluation and echocardiography before the patient is discharged from the hospital. Those with inferior infarction or anterior infarction without akinesia or dyskinesia of the apex and with good left ventricular function should be treated with aspirin alone. Patients with left ventricular thrombus are at high risk for thromboembolism and oral anticoagulation should be given for a period of 3 months to maintain an INR of 2.0–3.0. If the echocardiogram shows resolution of the thrombus at 3 months, anticoagulation can be discontinued.

3. Remote infarction with thrombus—Antithrombotic management of remote myocardial infarction (more than 3 months after the acute event) is controversial. Although traditional studies have not indicated a high risk of embolization, some reports indicate that thrombus detected at least 3 months following infarction still carries a risk for embolism. Patients with remote infarction and thrombus should be treated with warfarin to maintain an INR of 2.0–3.0 and reevaluated with echocardiography in 3 months.

4. Left ventricular aneurysm—Although an uncommon complication of myocardial infarction in the reperfusion era, left ventricular aneurysm provides the necessary substrate for thrombus. These aneurysms frequently contain thrombus, but systemic embolization is unusual. It has been hypothesized that the decreased incidence of systemic emboli found with left ventricular thrombus contained within a discrete aneurysm, compared with thrombus that complicates congestive cardiomyopathy, relates to a smaller surface area of the clot being exposed to circulating blood. It is unclear whether patients with left ventricular aneurysm warrant long-term anticoagulant therapy, particularly if the aneurysm contains flat thrombi. Documented systemic embolization, however, in patients with left ventricular aneurysm and thrombus should certainly prompt therapeutic anticoagulation to maintain an INR of 2.0–3.0. Recurrent embolization while receiving anticoagulants in this setting is an indication for left ventricular aneurysmectomy.

D. DILATED CARDIOMYOPATHY

Dilated cardiomyopathy may be the end result of many types of heart disease. Characteristically, generalized four-chamber cardiac enlargement is present with right and left ventricular dysfunction that can cause stasis in any cardiac chamber. These patients have a high incidence of intracardiac thrombi, particularly in the left ventricle, and a high incidence of systemic emboli. In one clinical study, atrial fibrillation was shown to be the only independent predictor for thromboembolism in dilated cardiomyopathy, and another study stressed the importance of severe depression of left ventricular function as a predictor.

The characteristics and embolic potential of left ventricular thrombi in dilated cardiomyopathy and those in left ventricular aneurysm seem to differ. In dilated cardiomyopathy, left ventricular thrombi have a tendency to protrude and thus expose a greater surface area to circulating blood. Several studies have indicated that thrombi that protrude (Figure 28–3) into the left ventricular cavity or demonstrate free intracavitary motion are associated with a high risk of embolic events. Thrombi in left ventricular aneurysms are frequently mural and contained within the aneurysm; exposure to circulating blood is minimal because of both their containment and their flat shape, and they are at low risk to embolize (Figure 28–4).

Unlike acute infarction, the natural history of left ventricular thrombus complicating dilated cardiomyopathy is unclear because no clinically apparent event marks the initiation of thrombus development. The studies of intracardiac thrombi complicating dilated cardiomyopathy have, in general, consisted of small numbers of patients, varying definitions of dilated cardiomyopathy, varying proportions of patients with coronary artery disease, and incomplete reporting of the anticoagulation status. Aggregate analysis of these clinical and echocardiographic studies indicates that anticoagulation can reduce the thromboembolic rate. Anticoagulation following a thromboembolic event also appears effective as a secondary preventive measure.

Patients with dilated cardiomyopathy are at highest risk if they have atrial fibrillation, severe left ventricular dysfunction with fractional shortening (shown by M-mode echocardiography) of less than 10%, previous thromboembolism, or left ventricular thrombus documented by imaging techniques. For patients with these high-risk characteristics, therapeutic anticoagulation is recommended to maintain an INR of 2.0–3.0.

E. SPECIAL CONDITIONS

1. Pregnancy—Oral anticoagulation during pregnancy represents a significant risk of both maternal and fetal complications. Warfarin is a small molecule that crosses the placenta and causes a specific embryopathy (the risk appears highest when warfarin is administered between the sixth and twelfth weeks of gestation). Fetal central nervous system abnormalities that are also associated with maternal warfarin use may occur after exposure in any trimester. Oral anticoagulation with warfarin presents a high risk to the fetus, and its use is not recommended during pregnancy.

Because heparin is a large molecule that does not cross the placenta, its use in pregnancy is safer for the fetus. Although maternal osteoporosis has been reported, this complication is uncommon and probably related to the dose. A retrospective study of 100 pregnancies receiving subcutaneous heparin (primarily for treatment or prevention of venous thromboembolism)

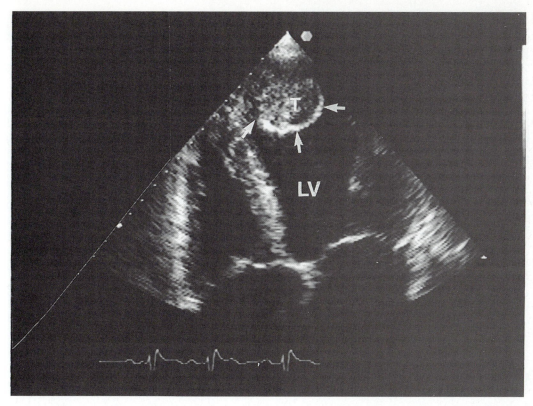

Figure 28-3. Apical four-chamber two-dimensional echocardiogram, demonstrating a protruding left ventricular thrombus. LV = left ventricle; T = thrombus. Arrows indicate the intracavitary margin of the thrombus.

showed adverse fetal outcomes similar to those in the normal population. The primary cardiac reason for continuous anticoagulation during pregnancy is a mechanical valve prosthesis, although other conditions may be encountered. As noted earlier, the incidence of thromboembolism with mechanical valve prostheses is significant without anticoagulation, and moderate doses of subcutaneous heparin twice daily to maintain an activated partial thromboplastin time 1.5–2.5 times control 6 h after administration are recommended. Because the numbers of patients reported receiving this regimen is small, conclusions cannot be made regarding its efficacy in this setting. A lower dosage of heparin (5000 units SQ, bid) has been reported to be ineffective in preventing prosthetic valve thrombosis.

It would be preferable to avoid anticoagulation during pregnancy because of the potential for fetal and maternal complications, including hemorrhage at the time of delivery. Women of childbearing age who have cardiovascular disease and are at risk for thromboembolism, especially those with mechanical heart valves, should be carefully and thoroughly informed of the risks of thromboembolism and anticoagulation prior to contemplating pregnancy. Women with native valve disease requiring intervention should be considered for valvular repair or replacement with biologic valves if they desire children.

2. Elective surgery—Interruption of anticoagulation may be necessary during a surgical procedure. Because no randomized trials have been performed to evaluate anticoagulation management, during surgery, clinical management must be dictated by the type of surgery and the need for anticoagulation. A pragmatic approach of temporarily discontinuing anticoagulation has been used, apparently with a reasonable degree of safety. Another regimen includes reversal of the warfarin effect with vitamin K while continuing anticoagulation with heparin until 4–6 h before surgery. After surgery, anticoagulation with heparin is resumed as soon as acceptable, followed by reinstitution of warfarin.

For emergency surgery, immediate reversal of warfarin anticoagulation with parenteral vitamin K and fresh frozen plasma is indicated. Resumption of anticoagulation with heparin should be dictated by the surgical procedure and clinical status.

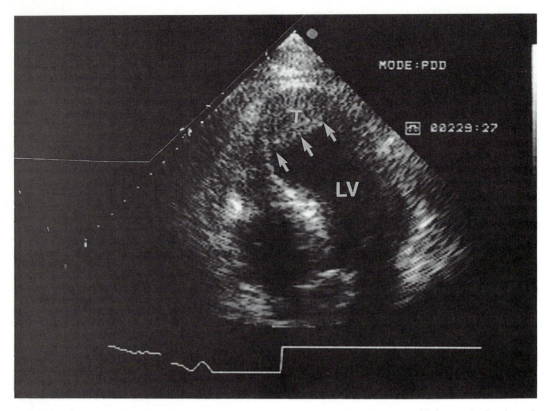

Figure 28-4. Apical four-chamber two-dimensional echocardiogram, showing a mural left ventricular thrombus. LV = left ventricle; T = thrombus. Arrows indicate the intracavitary margin of the thrombus.

3. Intracranial hemorrhage—Perhaps the most feared complication of long-term oral anticoagulation, intracranial hemorrhage may be encountered more frequently as the need for anticoagulation increases along with large populations who are older and have a high incidence of hypertension. Intracranial hemorrhage without anticoagulation usually presents suddenly, with rapid progression to the maximum neurologic deficit. Intracranial hemorrhage that occurs while on anticoagulants, however, is different, with continued bleeding and progressive neurologic deterioration. Anticoagulated patients who have intracranial hemorrhage require emergency reversal. Although this has traditionally been done with parental vitamin K and fresh frozen plasma, this approach requires time and may require administration of a significant intravascular volume. An alternative approach is to use prothrombin complex, which reverses anticoagulation more quickly and does not require a large volume load.

Altman R, Rouvier J, Gurfinkel E et al: Comparison of two levels of anticoagulant therapy in patients with substitute heart valves. J Thorac Cardiovasc Surg 1991;101:427.

Adjusted-dose warfarin versus low-intensity, fixed dose warfarin plus aspirin for high-risk patients with atrial fibrillation: Stroke Prevention in Atrial Fibrillation III randomized clinical trial. Lancet 1996;348:633-8.

Benavente O, Hart R, Koudstaal P et al: Antiplatelet therapy for preventing stroke in patients with nonvalvular atrial fibrillation and no previous history of stroke or transient ischemic attacks. In: Warlow C, Van Gijn J, Sandercock P, eds: Stroke module of the Cochrane Database of Systematic Reviews. Oxford: The Cochrane Collaboration; 1999. CD-ROM available from BMJ Publishing Group (London).

Boston Area Anticoagulation Trial for Atrial Fibrillation Investigators: The effect of low dose warfarin on the risk of stroke in patients with nonrheumatic atrial fibrillation. N Engl J Med 1990;323:1505.

Cannegieter SC, Rosendaal FR, Briët E: Thromboembolic and bleeding complications in patients with mechanical heart valve prostheses. Circulation 1994;89:635.

Connolly SJ, Laupacis A, Gent M et al: Canadian atrial fibrillation anticoagulation (CAFA) study. J Am Coll Cardiol 1991;18:349.

Diener HC, Lowenthal A: Antiplatelet therapy to prevent stroke: risk of brain hemorrhage and efficacy in atrial fibrillation. J Neuro Sci 1997;153:112.

Ezekowitz MD, Bridgers SL, James KE et al: Warfarin in the prevention of stoke associated with nonrheumatic atrial fibrillation: Veterans affairs stoke prevention in nonrheumatic atrial fibrillation investigators. N Engl J Med 1992;327:1406.

Falk RH, Foster E, Coats MH: Ventricular thrombi and thromboembolism in dilated cardiomyopathy: A prospective follow-up study. Am Heart J 1992;123:136.

Fredriksson K, Norrving B, Strömblad L: Emergency reversal of anticoagulation after intracerebral hemorrhage. Stroke 1992; 23:972.

Ginsberg JS, Brill-Edwards P, Kowalchuk G et al: Heparin therapy during pregnancy: Risks to the fetus and mother. Arch Intern Med 1989;149:2233.

Ginsberg JS, Hirsh J: Use of antithrombotic agents during pregnancy. Chest 1992;102:385S.

Gullov AL, Koefoed BG, Petersen TS et al: Fixed minidose warfarin and aspirin alone and in combination vs adjusted-dose warfarin for stroke prevention in atrial fibrillation: Second Copenhagen Atrial Fibrillation, Aspirin, and Anticoagulation Study. Arch Intern Med 1998;158:1513.

Hart RG, Benavente O, McBride R et al: Antithrombotic Therapy To Prevent Stroke in Patients with Atrial Fibrillation: A Meta-Analysis. Ann Intern Med 1999;131:492-501.

Hellemons BS, Langenberg M, Lodder J et al: Primary prevention of arterial thromboembolism in patients with nonrheumatic atrial fibrillation in primary care: Randomised controlled trial comparing two intensities of coumarin and aspirin. BMJ 1999;319:958.

Klein AL, Grimm RA, Murray RD et al: Use of transesophageal echocardiography to guide cardioversion in patients with atrial fibrillation. N Engl J Med 2001;344:1411-20.

Kopecky SL, Gersh BJ, McGoon MD et al: The natural history of lone atrial fibrillation: A population-based study over three decades. N Engl J Med 1987;317:669.

Laupacis A: Antithrombotic therapy in atrial fibrillation. Chest 1998;114(5 Suppl);579.

Maggioni AP, Franzosi MG, Santoro E et al: The Gruppo Italiano per lo Studio Della Sopravvivenza nell'Infarto Miocardico II (GISSI-2) and the International Study Group: The risk of stroke in patients with acute myocardial infarction after thrombolytic and antithrombotic treatment. N Engl J Med 1992;327:1.

O'Connor CM, Califf RM, Massey EW et al: Stroke and acute myocardial infarction in the thrombolytic era: Clinical correlates and long-term prognosis. J Am Coll Cardiol 1990;16:533.

Patients with nonvalvular atrial fibrillation at low risk of stroke during treatment with aspirin: Stroke Prevention in Atrial Fibrillation III Study. The SPAF III Writing Committee for the Stroke Prevention in Atrial Fibrillation Investigators. JAMA 1998;279:1273.

Peterson P, Boysen G, Godtfredsen J et al: Placebo-controlled, randomised trial of warfarin and aspirin for prevention of thromboembolic complications in chronic atrial fibrillation. The Copenhagen AFASAK Study. Lancet 1989;1:175.

Posada IS, Barriales V: Alternate-day dosing of aspirin in atrial fibrillation. Am Heart J 1999;138:137.

Resnekov L, Chediak J, Hirsch J et al: Antithrombotic agents in coronary artery disease. Chest 1989;95(Suppl):52S.

Risk factors for stroke and efficacy of antithrombotic therapy in atrial fibrillation. Analysis of pooled data from five randomized clinical trials. Arch Intern Med 1994;154:1449.

Saour JN, Sieck JO, Mamo LA et al: Trial of different intensities of anticoagulation in patients with prosthetic heart valves. N Engl J Med 1990;322:428.

Scati (Studio Sulla Calciparina nell'Angina e nella Trombosi Ventricolare nell'Infarcto) Group: Randomized controlled trial of subcutaneous calcium-heparin in acute myocardial infarction. Lancet 1989;2:182.

Secondary prevention in non-rheumatic atrial fibrillation after transient ischaemic attack or minor stroke. EAFT (European Atrial Fibrillation Trial) Study Group. Lancet 1993;342: 1255.

Stein PD, Alpert JS, Copeland J et al: Antithrombotic therapy in patients with mechanical and biological prosthetic heart valves. Chest 1992;102(Suppl):445S.

Stroke Prevention in Atrial Fibrillation Investigators: Patients with nonvalvular atrial fibrillation at low risk of stroke during treatment with aspirin: Stroke Prevention in Atrial Fibrillation III Study. The SPAF III Writing Committee for the Stroke Prevention in Atrial Fibrillation Investigators. JAMA 1998;279:1273–1277.

Stroke Prevention in Atrial Fibrillation Investigators: Predictors of thromboembolism in atrial fibrillation. I. Clinical features of patients at risk. II. Echocardiographic features of patients at risk. Ann Int Med 1992;116:1;6.

Stroke Prevention in Atrial Fibrillation Investigators: Stroke prevention in atrial fibrillation study: Final results. Circulation 1991;84:527.

Stroke Prevention in Atrial Fibrillation Investigators: Warfarin versus aspirin for prevention of thromboembolism in atrial fibrillation: Stroke prevention in atrial fibrillation II study. Lancet 1994;343:687.

Turpie AG, Gent M, Laupacis A et al. A comparison of aspirin with placebo in patients treated with warfarin after heart-valve replacement. New Engl J Med 1993;329:524.

Turpie AGG, Gent M, Laupacis A et al: Comparison of high-dose with low-dose subcutaneous heparin to prevent left ventricular mural thrombosis in patients with acute transmural anterior myocardial infarction. N Engl J Med 1989;320:352.

Vaitkus PT, Berlin JA, Schwartz JS et al: Stroke complicating acute myocardial infarction: A meta-analysis of risk modification by anticoagulation and thrombolytic therapy. Arch Intern Med 1992;152:2020.

Warfarin versus aspirin for prevention of thromboembolism in atrial fibrillation: Stroke Prevention in Atrial Fibrillation II Study. Lancet 1994;343:633.

Weinberg DM, Marcini GBJ: Anticoagulation for cardioversion of atrial fibrillation. Am J Card 1989;63:745.

Infective Endocarditis

Bruce K. Shively, MD

ESSENTIALS OF DIAGNOSIS

- *Fever*
- *Blood cultures positive for bacteria or fungi*
- *Cardiac lesions on echocardiography*

General Considerations

Infective endocarditis is one of several infections in which endothelium is the initial site of infection. Healthy endothelium possesses an effective system of defense against both hemostasis and infection. Infection of the endothelium of blood vessels occurs only at sites markedly altered by disease or surgery, such as the severely atherosclerotic aorta or the suture lines of vascular grafts. By contrast, infection of the cardiac valve leaflet endothelium (endocardium) is not rare and occurs even in the absence of identifiable preexisting valve disease.

Pathophysiology & Etiology

A. CARDIAC INFECTION—VEGETATIONS

1. Precursor lesion and bacteremia—Valve infection probably begins when minor trauma, with or without accompanying valve disease, impairs the antihemostatic function of valve endocardium. Infection usually first appears along the coapting surface of the leaflets, suggesting a role for valve opening and closing. This hypothesis is supported by the observation that the ranking of valves in order of frequency of infection corresponds to the ranking of valves according to the force acting to close the valve (mitral > aortic > tricuspid > pulmonic).

This minor trauma may cause the formation of a microscopic thrombus on the leaflet surface. A small noninfected thrombus on the leaflet is called **nonbacterial thrombotic endocarditis (NBTE)**. The next step is infection of the fibrin matrix of the thrombus by blood-borne organisms, which appear briefly in blood under many circumstances, such as brushing one's teeth and during diagnostic procedures. When transient bacteremia coincides with the presence of an NBTE lesion, organisms may adhere to the valve leaflet and begin to proliferate.

This theory for the pathogenesis of endocarditis is supported by observations regarding the circumstances under which endocarditis occurs and the particular organisms involved. Patients with endocarditis often tell of a preceding event that likely resulted in transient bacteremia. The common infecting agents are those that gain entry to the blood because they colonize body surfaces and are adapted for attachment and proliferation in the NBTE lesion (see Clinical Syndromes).

2. Growth of vegetations—Vegetations begin near the coaptation line of the leaflet on the side that contacts the opposite leaflet during valve closure. Mitral valve vegetations are typically attached within 1–2 cm of the leaflet tip on the left atrial side and prolapse into the left atrium during systole. Aortic valve vegetations usually occur on the left ventricular (LV) side of the mid or distal portions of the aortic cusps and prolapse into the LV outflow tract during diastole. A similar distribution of lesions occurs on the tricuspid and pulmonic valves.

Although the course of cardiac lesions in endocarditis varies, in a typical sequence of events (without treatment), the infection progresses by enlargement of the vegetation and extension of its region of attachment toward the base of the leaflet. Valve regurgitation almost always develops, as a result of either destruction of the leaflet tip or scarring and retraction of the leaflet. Erosion of the leaflet may lead to perforation (usually associated with clinically significant regurgitation). Weakening of the leaflet's spongiosum layer may result in a deformity called a leaflet aneurysm. Mitral or tricuspid chordal involvement may cause rupture and acute severe regurgitation. In rare cases (primarily in mitral bioprosthetic endocarditis; see Management of High-Risk Endocarditis) a large vegetation may cause hemodynamically significant valve obstruction.

3. Metastatic vegetations—These vegetations may form when the regurgitant jet of blood from an infected valve strikes an endocardial surface in the receiving chamber (wall or chordae), producing a small area of denuded endothelium. The thrombus that forms at this site also becomes infected, constituting a secondary vegetation. Such metastatic vegetations most often appear on the ventricular side of the anterior mitral leaflet where it is struck by a regurgitant jet from aortic valve endocarditis. Another common location is on the mitral chordae, also from aortic regurgitation. Metastatic lesions on the mural endocardium of the cardiac chambers can occur as well.

4. Abscess and fistula formation—Organisms eventually invade the valve annulus and adjacent myocardium. Abscess formation can take multiple forms and may occur with or without fistula formation. Aortic annular abscess is an infective mass that burrows into or around the outside of the annulus. The abscess may extend upward to the sinus of Valsalva or ascending aorta (a type of mycotic aneurysm). This extension may lead to a fistulous communication between the aorta and the left atrium or (rarely) the right atrium. In other patients, the abscess extends down through the fibrous trigone and forms a fistula to the LV outflow tract.

A band of fibrous tissue at the base of the anterior mitral leaflet (the intervalvular fibrosa) separates the aortic annulus from the left atrial wall. Infection extending down from the posterior aortic annulus may produce an aneurysm in this area, which may in turn fistulize to the left atrium, aortic root, or into the pericardial space. Infection extending down from the anterior aortic annulus may invade the septal myocardium, causing a block in the conduction system.

When mitral valve infection extends to the base of the anterior leaflet, abscess formation involving the fibrous trigone may track upward and become fistulous. Infection from the posterior leaflet may extend to form a myocardial abscess in the LV posterior wall or a fistula around or through the mitral annulus between the left atrium and left ventricle. Infection may even penetrate through to the pericardial space, producing purulent pericarditis.

B. Extracardiac Disease

At any time during cardiac infection, extracardiac complications may supervene and dominate the clinical picture. Although these manifestations are emphasized in the medical literature, it should be kept in mind that many patients with endocarditis do not have them, especially at the time of presentation. The extracardiac disease in endocarditis results from the shedding of bacteria and fragments of infected thrombus from the valve vegetations.

1. Immune disease—The bacteremia accompanying endocarditis persists over long periods of time and represents a prolonged antigenic challenge to the immune system. Various antibodies and immune complexes appear in the blood—more so with longer duration of illness. Rheumatoid factors (anti-IgG or IgM antibody) and the antibodies yielding a false-positive Venereal Disease Research Laboratory (VDRL) test are rarely of interest for their diagnostic value. Other antibodies, such as those that form circulating immune complexes and activate complement, are of major importance because they cause microvascular damage, most frequently glomerulonephritis and vasculitic skin lesions.

2. Systemic and pulmonary emboli—The embolization of fragments of vegetation is a frequent and potentially catastrophic complication of endocarditis. The clinical consequences are highly variable and depend on many factors, including the size of the embolus, the site at which it lodges in the vasculature, the type and quantity of organisms carried, the point during treatment at which embolism occurs, and the host response. Small emboli are likely to present as metastatic infection; the most dreaded of these is brain abscess. Septic embolization may also lead to abscesses in the kidney, liver, bone, and (from the right heart) lung.

Large emboli present with signs and symptoms of major vascular obstruction. For endocarditis of the left heart, the most frequent and serious extracardiac complication is embolism to the brain. Strokes from this cause tend to be large, complicating subsequent management and often causing death. Emboli may also cause infarction of the spleen, liver, kidney, and the myocardium itself. Embolism to large arteries of the extremities is unusual and occurs primarily in fungal endocarditis.

3. Mycotic aneurysms—When infection of the arterial wall results in localized dilatation and progresses to abscess formation, mycotic aneurysms can occur. The cause is thought to be embolization of vegetation that does not obstruct blood flow enough to present clinically as embolism. These lesions frequently occur at vessel branch points. The mycotic aneurysm may produce signs and symptoms many weeks after the diagnosis of endocarditis, and recognition may be difficult. Their effects are especially devastating in the central nervous system. Aneurysms may act as a protected site of infection and cause persistent fever or bacteremia despite appropriate antibiotic therapy. Alternatively, if antibiotic therapy has sterilized the aneurysm, it may present months or years later as unexplained hemorrhage.

C. Clinical Syndromes

Endocarditis can assume any of a wide variety of forms because of the many possible combinations of infecting organisms, portals of entry, and host factors such as immunity and concomitant diseases. Although the list of organisms capable of causing endocarditis is very long (and the list of possible combinations of organisms and host factors is even longer), there are several common and distinctive clinical syndromes.

A distinction between the acute and subacute forms of endocarditis has been found to be of some clinical value. The differing characteristics of patients with these two forms are shown in Table 29–1. Many patients with endocarditis cannot be easily placed into one or the other of these two categories, however. Because the mean interval from the onset of infection to presentation is now short (10 days), many patients fail to develop the clinical syndrome originally ascribed to the subacute syndrome, but also do not meet the criteria for acute endocarditis.

1. Viridans streptococcal endocarditis—The bacterial species classified as viridans streptococci account for approximately 30–40% of cases of endocarditis. These organisms can be divided into three groups: normal human oral flora (*Streptococcus mitis, S sanguis, S anginosus, S mutans, S salivarius,* and other nutritionally variant species), inhabitants of the lower gastrointestinal and genitourinary tracts (nonenterococcal group D organisms, of which *S bovis* is important), and *S pneumoniae,* or *pneumococcus,* which infrequently causes endocarditis—and causes a syndrome very different from the other viridans streptococci. The first two groups of streptococci cause almost no other disease in humans, except for endocarditis. This predilection appears to stem from bacterial cell wall proteins that bind to fibronectin, platelets, laminin, and other components of blood clots.

Viridans streptococci usually grow slowly, and the patient typically presents with a febrile illness of at least 10 days' duration and modest intensity; many cases fit the clinical syndrome of subacute bacterial endocarditis. Although valve destruction may be extensive, it is gradual, and abscess formation in the heart or elsewhere is uncommon. Infection of a normal valve by viridans streptococci is probably unusual. The renal disease accompanying endocarditis caused by these organisms is usually mild and rarely causes significant renal insufficiency. Viridans streptococcal endocarditis is therefore often treatable medically and has a relatively good prognosis if antibiotic treatment is begun before complications occur.

Endocarditis from *S bovis* is strongly associated with underlying colorectal disease, especially malignancy. Colonization of the gastrointestinal tract by this organism increases with age and with malignancy for reasons that are not well understood. After initial endocarditis treatment, a patient with this disease should undergo a barium enema and sigmoidoscopy. If these tests are negative, evaluation should be repeated in 6 months.

Extra vigilance for complications is needed when treating patients with endocarditis from certain other streptococci. *S anginosus* and *S milleri* tend to cause abscesses in the brain and other major organs, and nutritionally variant streptococci are associated with higher morbidity and mortality rates than are the other viridans organisms—again for reasons that are not understood.

Complications from viridans streptococcal endocarditis are almost never due to failure to sterilize vegetations. Nevertheless, the sensitivity of these organisms to penicillin is not uniform, and testing for resistance is essential for establishing an appropriate antibiotic regimen.

2. Staphylococcus aureus endocarditis—*Staphylococcus aureus* is a relatively common cause of endocarditis, accounting for approximately 25% of all cases. In hospitals serving a large population of intravenous drug users, this may be the most common cause of endocarditis. Although *S aureus* frequently enters the circulation from the skin or nares, a culprit lesion may not be apparent on examination of these areas. Fewer than one quarter of episodes of *S aureus* bacteremia in hospitalized patients are caused by endocarditis.

Unlike patients with streptococcal endocarditis, those with endocarditis from *S aureus* are likely to present soon after the onset of bacteremia, which generally produces a febrile illness with marked constitutional symptoms and often rigors. This picture is especially common in intravenous drug users. *S aureus* tends to cause valve destruction more rapidly than do other or-

Table 29–1. Characteristics of acute and subacute endocarditis.[a]

Acute	Subacute
Symptom onset to diagnosis: 1 week	Symptom onset to diagnosis: 4 weeks
Acute malaise	Weight loss
Shaking chills	Fatigue
	Night sweats
Fever (may be high)	Low or no fever
Leukocytosis	Normal white cell count or leukopenia
Normal gamma globulins	Elevated gamma globulins
Rheumatoid factor +	Rheumatoid factor +

[a] Elevated erythrocyte sedimentation rate and anemia common to both syndromes.

ganisms; approximately 30% of cases result in extensive left-heart valve involvement complicated by abscess or fistula formation or pericarditis. *S aureus* endocarditis of the aortic valve is the most common cause of aortic annular abscess, often signaled by the appearance of PR interval prolongation. Mitral annular and myocardial abscesses are also associated with this organism.

Central nervous system involvement is present in 20% or more of cases, as cerebral embolization, intracranial hemorrhage from mycotic aneurysm rupture, and microscopic or macroscopic brain abscesses. Other significant complications include septic arthritis, osteomyelitis, and major organ abscesses. Renal involvement, as indicated by an active urine sediment, is present in almost all cases, and frank renal impairment occurs in approximately 20%. The renal dysfunction caused by *S aureus* rarely progresses to dialysis or permanent renal failure.

S aureus is the most lethal of the organisms commonly causing endocarditis, with mortality rates of approximately 30% in non-intravenous-drug users and >50% in patients with prosthetic valves. Intravenous drug users have a much lower mortality rate (approximately 5%).

3. Enterococcal endocarditis—This form accounts for approximately 5–15% of cases of endocarditis—almost all from *Enterococcus faecalis*. Enterococcal endocarditis tends to occur in elderly men undergoing diagnostic manipulation or surgery involving areas colonized by this organism, such as the gastrointestinal and genitourinary tracts; in intravenous drug users; or in women following obstetrical procedures. Patients with enterococcal endocarditis may present with an acute or insidious syndrome, although the findings typical of subacute bacterial endocarditis are unusual.

Enterococcal endocarditis is especially difficult to treat due to antibiotic resistance (discussed later). It is markedly different from and far more serious than streptococcal endocarditis. Overall mortality is only slightly less than that for staphylococcal endocarditis, and the incidence of major complications and need for valve replacement is approximately 30–40%.

4. Endocarditis from gram-negative bacteria—Gram-negative bacteria rarely cause endocarditis, with the exception of three groups of organisms: *Pseudomonas aeruginosa*, the HACEK organisms (*Hemophilus* spp., *Actinobacillus*, *Cardiobacterium*, *Eikenella*, *Kingella*) and the enteric organisms (*Escherichia coli*, *Proteus*, *Klebsiella*, and *Serratia marcescens*). *Pseudomonas* and *Serratia* are occasional causes of endocarditis in intravenous drug users.

The HACEK organisms are relatively slow growing and usually cause a subacute clinical syndrome. Organisms such as *Hemophilus* and *Cardiobacterium* are thought to account for cases of culture-negative endocarditis. Despite the often mild symptoms and signs of endocarditis caused by these organisms, valve destruction may be extensive by the time of diagnosis. The HACEK organisms are associated with endocarditis that causes major vessel embolism from large vegetations. Enteric organisms tend to produce an acute clinical syndrome similar to that caused by *Pseudomonas*.

5. Fungal endocarditis—Fungal endocarditis is associated with settings of immune compromise and procedures that give the organism access to the bloodstream, such as surgery, IV catheter placement, and IV drug abuse. *Candida* species (especially *C albicans*), *Histoplasma capsulatum*, and *Aspergillus* account for approximately 80% of cases of fungal endocarditis. Other less common causative organisms include *Mucor* and *Cryptococcus*. Clinicians must recognize when patients are at risk for fungal endocarditis because the signs and symptoms of the disease often escape notice or lead to misdiagnosis. Risk factors are listed in Table 29–2. In most patients with fungal endocarditis of a native valve, the infection is related to a fundamental immune system impairment. Fungal superinfection should be considered when a patient with bacterial endocarditis relapses either late in the antibiotic course or after completing treatment. This observation is especially true for bacterial infection of a prosthetic valve. *Candida* species infection is usually nosocomial, whereas histoplasmosis may be a community-acquired infection. Fungal endocarditis in intravenous drug users is almost always due to non-*albicans* species of *Candida*.

The clinical syndrome of fungal endocarditis is more difficult to recognize than that of bacterial endocarditis. This may be due partly to the postsurgical state or multisystem disease common in these patients. It has also been suggested that fever and murmurs develop later in the course of fungal disease than in bacterial endocarditis and that leukocytosis and such peripheral manifestations as petechiae are less frequent. The development of symptoms is often insidious, extending over weeks or months. Cardiac involvement is generally limited to the development of vegetations; invasion of the

Table 29–2. Risk factors for fungal endocarditis.

History of an implanted cardiac device (eg, prosthetic valve, pacemaker, AICD)
Indwelling vascular catheter and prolonged hospitalization
Prolonged treatment with broad-spectrum antibiotics
Immunosuppression (eg, steroid or cytotoxic drugs, radiation, malnutrition, untreated malignancy)
Intravenous drug use

AICD = automatic implantable cardioverter-defibrillator.

Table 29–3. Native valve endocarditis: Causative organisms.

Organism	% of cases
Viridans streptococci	60
S sanguis	12
S mitior	15
S mutans	6
S bovis	15
S milleri	2
Other	10
Enterococci	5
Staphylococcus aureus	25
S epidermidis	3
Fungi	1
Pseudomonas	2
Other gram-negative bacteria	3
Other	1

myocardium occurs with a lower frequency than in bacterial endocarditis. The vegetations usually lead to leaflet destruction and valve regurgitation; they may be large and may occasionally cause valve orifice obstruction. The most likely complication of fungal infective endocarditis is embolism, including occlusion of large peripheral arteries from embolization. Table 29–3 lists the approximate frequency of causative organisms in native valve endocarditis.

6. Prosthetic valve endocarditis—The risk of developing endocarditis is higher with prosthetic heart valves than with severely diseased native valves, approximately 0.5% per patient-year. Despite some overlap, there is a clear difference between the causes of disease that develops within 2 months of implantation and that occurring later (Table 29–4). The difference is probably due to infection occurring during surgery in early prosthetic endocarditis, with organisms from the skin of the patient and operating room personnel (*Staphylococcus epidermidis* and *aureus*) accounting for more than half the cases. The incidence of early prosthetic endocarditis has been greatly reduced by the routine use of prophylactic antibiotics for several days after operation. Prosthetic infection after 2 months usually involves the same mechanism as does native valve endocarditis, except that the causative organisms are those adapted to nonbiologic material.

Infection of a bioprosthesis involves primarily the sewing ring. Vegetations similar to those of native valve endocarditis can occur when the prosthesis is biologic, but infection more often begins in the area of attachment of the sewing ring to the annulus. Vegetations may form in this area, but—most important—early in the disease abscesses often form along the suture line, resulting in fistulization, paravalvular regurgitation, and partial or complete detachment (dehiscence) of the prosthesis.

Infection of a mechanical prosthesis centers on the sewing ring. The inward growth of an infective mass from the ring frequently causes the occluder to become stuck in a partially open or closed position. The lesions caused by sewing ring infection of mechanical prostheses are otherwise similar to those of bioprostheses.

Two important differences distinguish prosthetic valve endocarditis from native valve infection. Prosthetic valve infection may be extensive without the

Table 29–4. Prosthetic valve endocarditis: Causative organisms.

Early (<60 days postsurgery)	%	Late (>60 days postsurgery)	%
Staphylococcus epidermidis	33	Streptococci	30
Gram-negative bacteria	19	*Staphylococcus epidermidis*	26
S aureus	17	*S aureus*	12
Diptheroids	10	Gram-negative bacteria	12
Candida albicans	8	Enterococci	6
Streptococci	7	Diptheroids	4
Enterococci	2	*Candida albicans*	3
Aspergillus	1		

clinical signs, such as a murmur of regurgitation, heart failure, or embolism, usually seen in advanced native valve infection. When prosthetic valve dysfunction does occur (especially in a mechanical prosthesis), it tends to be abrupt and severe, as when the occluder becomes fixed in a half-open position. (Other differences are discussed later in this chapter.)

7. Endocarditis in the intravenous drug user—The patient usually presents with an intense febrile illness of several days' duration, starting within 24–48 h of the last injection. The mode of infection is a needle contaminated by skin flora, and an IV injection site may show an abscess or thrombophlebitis. The most likely causative organism is *S aureus,* which, overall, causes 70% of endocarditis in intravenous drug users, and which in this setting has a benign prognosis with only 2–5% mortality. Many other organisms can cause endocarditis in intravenous drug users, including gram-negative bacilli, especially *Pseudomonas aeruginosa, C albicans,* enterococci, and *Serratia marcescens;* as well as viridans streptococci. The prevalence of specific causative organisms varies widely in different urban areas. Endocarditis from these organisms tends to be less acute than that caused by *S aureus,* but only rarely is it truly subacute.

Infection of the tricuspid valve is almost unique to IV drug abusers and occurs in approximately 60% of cases of endocarditis in this population. Significant tricuspid regurgitation may not be clinically apparent. In as many as 40% of cases, the left heart valves alone are infected. Despite its proximity to the portal of entry in intravenous drug users, the pulmonic valve is rarely involved, probably because of the low pressure gradient and low wear and tear of this valve. Chest pain and dyspnea should prompt consideration of septic pulmonary emboli, which occur in 30% of tricuspid valve endocarditis. This complication usually presents as chest pain accompanied by scattered fluffy pulmonary infiltrates. On serial chest films, these lesions may appear migratory because of simultaneous resolution of older infiltrates and appearance of new ones. Infiltrates may also progress to cavitation.

8. Endocarditis and HIV—HIV infection and AIDS do not increase the risk of infective endocarditis. The increased frequency of endocarditis in patients with HIV is due to the prevalence of intravenous drug use in this population. HIV/AIDS patients appear to have an increased susceptibility to *Salmonella* endocarditis, a relatively antibiotic-responsive infection. Otherwise, the types of causative organisms seen is not altered by HIV status. The clinical syndrome and natural history of the disease in HIV patients is also unchanged, except that patients with advanced AIDS (CD4 count <200) tend to have a more fulminant course and increased mortality rates.

9. Nosocomial endocarditis—Hospital-acquired endocarditis is uncommon; overall approximately 5% of positive blood cultures in hospitalized patients are due to infective endocarditis (exceptions include strep viridans and nutritionally variant streptococci). Prosthetic valves are at far greater risk than native valves: 15–20% of patients with prosthetic valves who become bacteremic have or will develop endocarditis. Nosocomial endocarditis is marked by an increased likelihood of the presence of unusual or antibiotic-resistant organisms and an infected indwelling catheter as the likely portal of entry. Endocarditis occurs only rarely in postsurgical patients, usually after prolonged sepsis.

The usual causative organisms are coagulase-negative staph, *S aureus, Enterococcus,* and enteric gram-negative organisms, such as *Pseudomonas* and *Serratia.* Fungi, especially *Candida,* and fastidious organisms should also be suspected when endocarditis occurs in debilitated, leukopenic patients and those previously treated with long courses of antibiotics. Nosocomial endocarditis should be suspected when a hospitalized patient develops fever and positive blood cultures without an apparent source. Potential culprit catheters should be removed and cultured, followed by transesophageal echocardiography (TEE) if an additional risk factor for endocarditis exists. Examples of risk factors in this setting include a prosthetic valve, native valve disease predisposing to infection, or *S aureus* bacteremia. If the TEE is negative, and other sources of infection have been ruled out, a short (2-week) course of antibiotics is usually appropriate. Surveillance blood cultures during and after treatment, and a repeat TEE, should be considered if uncertainty regarding the response to treatment persists. In the case of exposure of a prosthetic valve to bacteremia, blood culture surveillance should be extended for at least 2 months.

10. Pacemaker endocarditis—Pacemaker endocarditis is infection of the lead or of parts of the heart in contact with the lead (tricuspid valve, right ventricular endocardium). Mortality is high, up to 25%, and the diagnosis is often missed due to the indolent nature of the infection. The vast majority of cases are due to contamination at the time of implant; hematogenous infection of a lead is rare. Most cases have evidence of present or prior infection at the implant site. The delay from the most recent pacemaker procedure to the diagnosis of endocarditis may be as long as 2 years or as little as 6 weeks. In addition to fever and positive blood cultures, infection causes septic pulmonary emboli in about a third of cases. Transesophageal echocardiography is the diagnostic test of choice, with a sensitivity of over 90%. Transthoracic echocardiography is often falsely negative.

Staphylococci are the usual infecting organisms, with *S epidermidis* accounting for 70% of cases and *S aureus* for most of the rest. As with prosthetic valve endocarditis, early after implant, *S aureus* is the most likely culprit, whereas *S epidermidis* is more likely later. *Staphylococcus* species produce a slime-like "sleeve" along the lead that protects bacteria from host defense and antibiotics. Treatment requires removal of the lead, and usually the entire system. Lead removal can be accomplished percutaneously with reasonable safety if the mass(es) attached to the lead are small (<1 cm). Surgery is indicated if the lead is fixed, if a large mass (>1 cm) is present (with dislodgement likely to result in severe pulmonary embolism), or if tricuspid valve involvement is extensive. Lead removal is followed by 6 weeks of antibiotic therapy. The pacemaker-dependent patient is given an epicardial lead; reimplant of a transvenous system can be considered after 2 months with negative surveillance blood cultures.

Clinical Findings

A. Diagnostic Criteria

In the current era, with the availability of sensitive blood culture techniques and transesophageal echocardiography, the clinician will rarely need to rely on a formal schema for the diagnosis of endocarditis. Prior to these technical advances, "major" criteria (fever, positive blood cultures) were combined with "minor" criteria (skin lesions, emboli, serologic abnormalities) to reach a probable diagnosis. This approach was useful because of the low sensitivity and specificity of each feature by itself. Now TEE and blood cultures independently have a diagnostic sensitivity of greater than 90%, and TEE has a specificity of greater than 90%. Diagnostic uncertainty may arise when the result of TEE is ambiguous or when adequate blood cultures are not obtained before starting antibiotics. In many such situations a diagnosis can be reached by gathering more data. For example, if the TEE fails to show endocarditis-specific valve disease and the patient is doing well, discontinuing antibiotics in order to repeat cultures should be considered. Many of the common features of endocarditis—fever, a cardiac murmur, and a set of positive blood cultures—occur frequently in other diseases and are occasionally absent in patients with endocarditis. Other diseases frequently mimicked by endocarditis include malignancy, autoimmune disease, and septicemia. In addition, patients with endocarditis may come to the physician because of a complication of endocarditis so dramatic as to distract attention from the underlying infection. Typical settings in which this error occurs include heart failure, stroke, and myocardial infarction.

The recognition of possible **prosthetic valve endocarditis** may be difficult because the signs of infection may be very subtle. In early prosthetic endocarditis, the symptoms and signs may be incorrectly ascribed to other diseases. Fever and bacteremia during the first few weeks after prosthetic implantation should be considered to indicate prosthetic valve endocarditis until proven otherwise. This is especially important because early prosthetic valve endocarditis appears to follow a more fulminant course than either late prosthetic or native valve endocarditis. These patients often have other potential causes of bacteremia, however, and an effort to prove infection from another site should be pursued vigorously. Transesophageal echocardiography probably has a sensitivity of approximately 80% for prosthetic valve endocarditis and should be performed whenever an alternative explanation for fever or bacteremia is not readily apparent. If the TEE is negative but bacteremia persists (especially if the organism is a frequent cause of prosthetic endocarditis), prosthetic infection should be presumptively treated. Fluoroscopy to rule out dehiscence has been replaced by TEE.

Fungal endocarditis is also often difficult to diagnose. Blood cultures are negative in approximately half of cases from *C albicans,* the majority of histoplasmosis cases, and almost all cases caused by *Aspergillus.* Histologic examination and culture should be performed whenever possible on specimens of embolic material, oropharyngeal lesions (especially for histoplasmosis), skin lesions (for *Candida* species and *Aspergillus*), liver, bone marrow, and urine (for histoplasmosis). In addition, a careful eye examination should be performed in patients with suspected fungal endocarditis because of the high frequency of anterior uveitis and chorioretinitis.

Tricuspid valve endocarditis (as seen in IV drug users) produces a distinctive picture because of the frequent occurrence of septic pulmonary emboli. Scattered fluffy infiltrates seen on chest film are accompanied by pleuritic chest pain. Less often, the presentation may mimic pneumonia or include pleural effusion. The murmur of tricuspid regurgitation may be inaudible or soft because right-heart pressures are normally low, even when tricuspid infection is extensive. A loud holosystolic murmur at the left lower sternal border that increases with inspiration, *v* waves in jugular veins, and a pulsatile liver indicate the development of severe tricuspid regurgitation and pulmonary hypertension.

B. Symptoms and Signs

Constellations of certain symptoms should arouse suspicion of endocarditis. One combination of symptoms often seen is constitutional symptoms (eg, fatigue, malaise, headache, arthralgias or myalgias, nausea, anorexia, weight loss) and fever, which can range from mild feverish feelings and night sweats to shaking chills. When these symptoms are chronic or mild, other diagnoses are often considered, such as malignancy and autoimmune disease.

A high suspicion of endocarditis is warranted when this picture is associated with any symptom pointing to the circulatory system, such as complaints associated with left- or right-heart failure (dyspnea, orthopnea, cough, peripheral edema), vascular occlusion (stroke, systemic embolism), and chest pain (Table 29–5).

C. PHYSICAL EXAMINATION

The physical examination is not essential for the diagnosis of endocarditis. Most of the physical findings caused by endocarditis are not specific for this diagnosis and should be interpreted in the context of the overall examination and the patient's history. There are also no physical findings that, when absent, are useful for ruling out the diagnosis. A prominent murmur or skin lesion may arouse a clinical suspicion of endocarditis, but a murmur of valve regurgitation may be absent in patients with endocarditis. Vegetations may be present, but may cause only slight regurgitation.

The examination is absolutely essential, however, to the treatment of endocarditis patients. The initial examination assists the clinician in assessing the severity of the illness. During treatment (or observation for more definite evidence of endocarditis), serial physical examinations are vital for identifying important changes in the patient's status because physical findings may signal the need for surgery.

1. Fever—Fever is usually present when the patient comes to medical attention, although it may be intermittent or already resolved through inappropriate antibiotic treatment. It may be infrequently masked by severe comorbid conditions, such as alcoholic cirrhosis, leukopenia, or malnutrition. The diversity of endocarditis does not permit generalizations about the temporal pattern or degree of fever. Fever may be low grade (37.5–38.5°C) and accompanied by only malaise and anorexia, or it may be hectic with rigors, sweats, and temperature higher than 40°C. Recurrence of fever during treatment of endocarditis is a very important problem (see section on Failure of antibiotic therapy).

2. Cardiac examination—The cardiac examination in the patient with suspected or known endocarditis focuses on identifying which heart valves are infected, the hemodynamic severity of the resultant regurgitation (or

Table 29–5. Frequency of symptoms and signs in endocarditis.

Frequency	Symptom	Sign
High (>40% of patients)	Fever	Fever
	Chills	Murmur
	Weakness	Skin lesions or emboli
	Dyspnea	Petechiae
Moderate (10–40% of patients)	Sweats	Osler or Janeway lesions
	Anorexia/weight loss	Splinter hemorrhages
	Cough	Splenomegaly
	Stroke	Major complication: stroke, heart failure, pneumonia, meningitis
	Rash	
	Nausea/vomiting	
	Headache	
	Chest pain	
	Mylagias/arthralgias	
Low (<10% of patients)	Abdominal pain	New or changing murmur
	Delirium/coma	Retinal lesions
	Hemoptysis	Renal failure
	Back pain	

stenosis), and the adequacy of the patient's circulatory state.

At the time of initial evaluation of a patient with suspected endocarditis, the value of a detected murmur may be low because there may be no reliable information about the patient's prior cardiac condition. Systolic murmurs, for example, are common in the general population and very frequent in older or hospitalized patients; they are usually due to LV outflow or degenerative sclerosis of the aortic valve. Because endocarditis rarely causes valve stenosis, a systolic murmur related to endocarditis is almost always regurgitant.

Specific auscultatory features occasionally may be useful for determining how a valve has been damaged by infection. In mitral valve endocarditis, the examination may help identify which mitral leaflet has become partially flail. If the mitral regurgitant murmur radiates to the patient's back, the jet is likely to be directed posteriorly as a result of anterior leaflet prolapse into the left atrium. If the murmur radiates to the upper parasternal area (mimicking aortic stenosis), the posterior leaflet is likely to have lost its support.

It is essential that the examiner carefully note and document the cardiac findings as soon as the diagnosis of endocarditis is suspected. In addition to murmurs, the clinician should pay close attention to those aspects of the examination related to hemodynamic consequences of valvular dysfunction. Signs of pulmonary edema, dysfunction of either ventricle, and a low output state should be sought.

3. Skin and extremities—Assessment of the severity of extracardiac disease in endocarditis begins with a careful examination of the skin and peripheral circulation for evidence of vasculitis and emboli. Although these findings are not specific for the diagnosis of endocarditis, in the context of probable endocarditis, they strongly support that diagnosis. Their appearance during antibiotic therapy may signal the need for a change in the treatment plan.

a. Petechiae—Examine the soft palate, buccal mucosa, conjunctiva, and the skin of the extremities for petechiae, which are often transient, appearing in crops and fading in 2–3 days.

b. Splinter hemorrhages—These brown streaks are 1–2 mm in length and found under the fingernails and toenails. Lesions in the proximal nail bed are moderately specific for endocarditis, whereas similar lesions under the distal nails are commonly found in healthy persons who work with their hands.

c. Roth spots—Vasculitis affecting small arteries of the retina may, on rare occasions, produce retinal infarction. The resulting funduscopic lesion, usually seen near the optic disc, is a pale retinal patch surrounded by a darker ring of hemorrhage.

d. Osler nodes—These painful indurated nodules are 2–15 mm in diameter and appear on the palms and soles and often involve the distal phalanges. They are usually multiple and, like petechiae, tend to occur in crops and fade over 2–3 days. Osler nodes are thought to be caused by either vasculitis or septic embolization.

e. Janeway lesions—These painless, flat red macules are similar in size and location to Osler nodes that usually persist longer than a few days. Their pathogenesis is uncertain but is suspected to be either vasculitis or septic embolization.

f. Blue-toes syndrome—Embolization of small vegetation fragments may cause ischemia in the distal arterial distribution of an upper or lower extremity. The affected finger or toe is tender, mottled, and cyanotic; over a period of days to weeks, the area becomes black and develops dry gangrene. Management is usually conservative (see 3. Embolism, later in this chapter). Acute arterial occlusive ischemia of a larger portion of an extremity raises the possibility of fungal endocarditis and is usually managed by embolectomy.

4. Neurologic examination—Cerebral embolization in endocarditis signals a poor prognosis and has a major impact on the overall management approach. The neurologic examination is an integral part of the evaluation of any patient with known or suspected endocarditis. During antibiotic treatment, symptoms that may be of neurologic origin justify careful repeat examination, often with CT.

5. Abdominal examination—Splenomegaly occurs in patients with endocarditis as part of generalized hyperplasia of the reticuloendothelial system. Its presence usually indicates endocarditis of at least 10 days' duration. Marked splenomegaly may be accompanied by abdominal pain from splenic infarction.

D. Diagnostic Studies

1. Detection of blood-borne infection—Bacteremia or fungemia invariably occurs at some point during endocarditis (a role for viruses is unproven). The presence of the organism in the blood is generally of low grade and continuous because of the vegetations in the circulating bloodstream. Bacteremia may be intermittent or of variable intensity, however, especially if abscess formation has occurred or if the patient is under treatment.

The method of obtaining blood cultures depends on the severity of the patient's illness, as judged from the clinical syndrome and results of TEE. The preferred method in cases of suspected endocarditis is to obtain three to six sets of aerobic and anaerobic cultures, each from a separate venipuncture site, over a period of 24 h. This approach should be used if the suspicion of endocarditis is low, the patient appears well enough to tolerate a 24-h delay of antibiotic therapy, or the TEE is negative or inconclusive.

Initiation of antibiotic therapy, however, should not be delayed if the suspicion of endocarditis is high and the patient is acutely ill, with a temperature more than 40°C, tachycardia, discomfort, or hypotension; the TEE is positive; or complications of endocarditis, such as embolism or congestive heart failure, have already occurred. Under these conditions, the cultures should be obtained over 1–2 h, followed immediately by antibiotic therapy.

Blood cultures have been found positive for an infecting organism in 70–95% of cases of endocarditis reported in studies since 1970. Proper technique and timing of blood cultures can improve the positive yield. Potential causes of negative blood cultures in patients with endocarditis are shown in Table 29–6. When blood cultures remain negative at 24–48 h in a patient with probable endocarditis, the most important concern is infection from unusual organisms, such as the fungi, HACEK organisms, *Coxiella burnetii* (Q fever), *Chlamydia psittaci, Bartonella* and abiotrophia species (nutritionally variant streptococci). The laboratory should be notified of the suspected diagnosis, and infectious disease consultation obtained.

If antibiotics have already been started for another diagnosis, modification of the blood culture technique can increase the positive yield. The importance of recovering the causative organism may warrant stopping all antibiotics. (The use of antibiotic removal devices or specialized media have not proven to be useful for increasing the yield from blood cultures in this situation.) Blood cultures then should be drawn according to the routine outlined earlier, usually with an additional three blood cultures drawn over a second 24-h period. If the patient is acutely ill or the TEE demonstrates extensive infection, at least one set of blood cultures should be obtained promptly and empiric treatment begun (See section on Empiric antibiotic therapy).

Table 29–6. Causes of negative blood cultures in endocarditis.

Failure to obtain more than one set of blood cultures

Failure to hold blood cultures for longer than 1 week

Prior antibiotic prescription (normally within 2–3 days of culture)

Organism grows slowly in standard culture (eg, HACEK organisms, nutritionally variant streptococci)

Organism fails to grow in standard culture (eg, fungi, rickettsiae, Q fever, psittacosis, nutritionally variant streptococci)

Intermittent bacteremia or fungemia (rare)

If the suspicion of endocarditis remains moderate or high after the initial blood culture sets are drawn, empiric antibiotic therapy should also begin. The antibiotics should be changed according to the blood culture results as soon as these become available. If the initial blood cultures are negative after 24 h but endocarditis is still suspected, three more sets should be obtained and processed under the guidance of an infectious disease specialist. Hypertonic and nutritionally supplemented media are useful for detecting cell wall-deficient and nutritionally variant organisms, respectively. The lysis-centrifugation method of blood culture preparation also should be used in an attempt to detect fungi, and the microbiology laboratory should be notified to hold the cultures for 4 weeks. Serologic testing should be considered.

2. Serologic testing—Serologic testing can be helpful for identifying certain causes of endocarditis when blood cultures are negative. Histoplasmosis antigen is highly specific for systemic infection by this organism. Positive antibody titers for Q fever (*Coxiella burnetii*) or *Brucella* in a patient with culture-negative endocarditis identify these organisms as the cause. The usefulness of other serologic tests, such as that for *Candida albicans,* is highly dependent on the clinical situation.

Although not essential to the diagnosis of endocarditis, serologic testing is supportive and can be useful in certain situations. A positive rheumatoid factor, commonly found in patients with endocarditis of longer than 2 weeks' duration, and a false-positive VDRL, which is less frequent, signal the presence of high titers of antibodies (stimulated by the prolonged antigenemia occurring in endocarditis). These two laboratory abnormalities are not specific for endocarditis, however, and are found in other diseases that may imitate endocarditis, such as systemic lupus erythematosus. When blood cultures are positive but other evidence of endocarditis is lacking or equivocal, a positive rheumatoid factor or VDRL should prompt careful follow-up and retesting (eg, repeat TEE) for further evidence of endocarditis. Under some circumstances, these positive serologic tests may even warrant extension of antibiotic therapy to treat presumed endocarditis.

3. Echocardiography—

a. Transesophageal echocardiography—TEE should be performed within the first few hours after presentation of a patient with suspected endocarditis. With its detailed images of the heart valves and related structures, TEE is highly sensitive and specific for the diagnosis of endocarditis and is essential to defining the extent of disease. A positive TEE for a mass with the characteristics of a vegetation has a specificity of more than 90% for endocarditis (in the absence of a history of endocarditis, since it is difficult to distinguish between old and new vegetations). A negative TEE does not rule out endocarditis, but it has a negative predictive accuracy of at least 90%. Because false-negative TEE studies can occur, however, a patient with a negative study but a high clinical suspicion of endocarditis should be either observed carefully or treated, depending on the clinical severity of the illness. The TEE should be repeated if needed.

(1) Classification—Transesophageal echocardiographic studies in patients with suspected endocarditis may be classified according to the probability of the disease. A useful scheme is based on four categories: normal, possible, probable, and almost certain. In the **normal** category, no substrate for endocarditis or other abnormalities is present.

The TEE findings are classified as **possible endocarditis** in the presence of valve disease, such as a prosthetic heart valve, rheumatic or degenerative valvular sclerosis, or valve regurgitation likely to be pathologic, that predispose the patient to endocarditis—but without evidence of lesions. The classification of **probable endocarditis** is used when less specific lesions are found. Examples of such abnormalities include localized leaflet thickening or an nonmobile leaflet-related mass (especially if the lesion has the reflectance of soft rather than sclerotic tissue), mitral or aortic valve prolapse, chordal rupture, intracardiac thrombi, and paravalvular regurgitation in patients with prosthetic valves.

Patients with no history of endocarditis who have a lesion very strongly associated with infective endocarditis fall into the **almost-certain** category. In such cases, TEE shows an intracardiac mass with typical vegetation characteristics—a pedunculated mass attached near the leaflet tip and prolapsing during valve closure into the lower pressure chamber. Vegetations have soft-tissue reflectance (like myocardium) and vibratory or rotatory motion independent of the motion of the leaflet. Vegetations apparent on TEE vary in length from 1 or 2 mm to several centimeters.

Other lesions considered almost certain for endocarditis would be an abscess or fistula, a metastatic vegetation, and an aneurysm of the intervalvular fibrosa. An abscess appears on TEE as an echolucent space adjacent to a valve annulus or prosthetic sewing ring. The abscess often appears to be separated from adjacent structures by thin septa, and jets of blood flowing into the abscess during systole or diastole (depending on abscess location) may be shown by Doppler interrogation. The abscess is considered a fistula when there is communication with two or more adjacent cardiac chambers or blood vessels. Metastatic vegetations appear on echocardiography as vibratory or rotatory masses attached to an endocardial surface at a site with a regurgitant jet.

It should be noted that this classification scheme is appropriate for TEE only on patients with other reasons to suspect endocarditis (eg, unexplained fever, positive blood cultures) and no prior history of endocarditis.

(2) Diagnostic accuracy—Possible causes of a false-negative or false-positive TEE are shown in Table 29–7. Of particular importance is the possibility that a negative TEE may be due to endothelial infection in the vasculature rather than the heart. Because vascular infection is rare in the absence of prior vascular surgery, the diagnosis is usually suspected based on the patient's history. Nevertheless, the TEE examination in patients with suspected endocarditis routinely includes the thoracic aorta. Transesophageal echocardiography may identify severe atherosclerosis with mobile atheroma or thrombi. Although these abnormalities are not nearly as specific for infection as are intracardiac vegetations, the clinical picture may justify antibiotic treatment.

In general, fewer than 10% of positive TEE are false-positives. By causing thickened, prolapsing leaflets and ruptured chordae, a myxomatous mitral valve can closely mimic endocarditis. A benign leaflet tumor, called a **papillary fibroelastoma,** may give the appearance of a vegetation. Several other abnormalities seen by TEE have lower specificity for the diagnosis of endocarditis than do typical vegetations; examples include paraaortic cavities (potentially representing either an abscess or an aneurysm of the sinus of Valsalva) and paraprosthetic regurgitation. Clinical context is often crucial to the interpretation of these findings. The paraneoplastic syndrome of myxomas may mimic endocarditis, although usually location and morphologic features of myxomas distinguish them from thrombi or vegetations. Intracardiac thrombi may be innocent bystanders in a patient with a clinical syndrome sug-

Table 29–7. Causes of false-negative and false-positive results of transesophageal echocardiography.

False-Positives
  Myxomatous mitral valve disease
  Papillary fibroelastomas
  Partially flail leaflet
  Healed vegetations
  Mitral valve strands
  Nodules of Arantii (aortic valve)
  Lambl's excrescences (mitral valve)
False-Negatives
  Aortic valve prosthesis
  Mitral valve mechanical prosthesis (includes shadowing of acortic valve by a mitral prosthesis)
  Calcified aortic root shadowing tricuspid or pulmonic valves
  Mitral annular calcification
  Aortic atheroma or aneurysm infection
  Study done too early in disease course

gesting endocarditis, or they may be secondarily infected.

Lambl's excrescences are thin, strand-like structures extending 1–10 mm from the mitral leaflet margins. Because they prolapse a few millimeters into the left atrium and exhibit hypermobility, Lambl's excrescences can be mistaken for small vegetations. Nodules of Arantii are similar extensions, not more than a few millimeters in length, from the center of the aortic cusp margin. When the aortic valve is closed, they may be seen by TEE prolapsing from the center of the valve.

In addition to detecting vegetations, TEE usually provides a detailed picture of the extent of cardiac infection; it is very accurate at assessing the exact size and location of vegetations. Several complicated forms of cardiac involvement are usually identifiable by TEE. Because many of these complex lesions require surgery, TEE should be performed as soon as possible in a patient with a moderate of high suspicion of endocarditis.

Blood cultures should be drawn either before or 15 min after TEE to avoid the transient bacteremia that infrequently occurs during the procedure. Prophylaxis for endocarditis is not indicated prior to TEE.

b. Transthoracic echocardiography—The initial diagnostic value of transthoracic echocardiography (TTE) is limited in patients with possible endocarditis because of its low sensitivity: a large number of false-negatives occur, particularly in patients with prosthetic valves. On the other hand, a positive TTE showing typical vegetations is at least 90% specific for the diagnosis of endocarditis. Transthoracic echocardiography, however, cannot provide the detailed information regarding the anatomic extent of infection available from TEE.

Despite these limitations, TTE has a valuable ancillary role to play in patients with known endocarditis. It is well suited to assessing cardiac chamber dilatation, left and right ventricular dysfunction, and the patient's hemodynamic status. Presystolic closure of the mitral valve on TTE is a sign of elevated LV end-diastolic pressure and is an indication that the patient with aortic insufficiency should be considered for surgery. Similarly, right atrial and pulmonary artery pressures can be estimated by transthoracic Doppler examination. Additional Doppler data is essential to assessing the severity and hemodynamic sequelae of mitral regurgitation, including elevated left atrial pressure. Changes in the patient's clinical status during treatment often can be readily diagnosed by comparison of serial TTE studies. For these reasons it is advisable to perform transthoracic study at the same time as the initial TEE. One useful strategy is to discuss the results of TTE with the referring physician while the patient is still in the laboratory, and then proceed to TEE if appropriate.

4. Electrocardiography and chest radiography—The electrocardiograph (ECG) is occasionally useful in alerting the clinician to the severity of endocarditis. In patients with known or suspected aortic valve endocarditis, the PR interval should be followed closely for prolongation, an indication of aortic annular abscess formation. Less frequently, the ECG may show increased QRS voltage and a precordial strain pattern in patients developing either severe aortic or mitral regurgitation with marked LV enlargement. The chest radiograph is primarily useful in evaluating the patient with suspected endocarditis to assess the presence and severity of pulmonary edema and to detect septic pulmonary emboli in patients with possible right-heart endocarditis.

Management

A. INITIAL DECISIONS

Management of newly diagnosed endocarditis requires the physician to make two decisions promptly. The first is whether to initiate empiric antibiotic therapy based on available clinical information or to await the exact identity and antibiotic sensitivities of the infecting organism and then to select the optimal regimen. The second decision is whether valve surgery is indicated immediately or can be deferred to allow assessment of the patient's response to antibiotic therapy.

Both decisions depend on the extent of cardiac infection (usually characterized by TEE), the severity of the patient's symptoms and signs of infection, the patient's circulatory status, the seriousness of extracardiac complications, and the available data about the organism.

Once initial treatment is underway, the physician must maintain a high level of vigilance for evidence of an inadequate response to treatment or the development of complications that will require additional medical or surgical intervention.

B. ANTIBIOTIC THERAPY

The goal of antibiotic therapy is to sterilize vegetations. For most causative organisms, this is an achievable goal and will cure the patient if cardiac abscess and metastatic infection to other organs have not occurred. Vegetations, however, provide proliferating organisms with an environment that is protected against both the patient's immune system and antibiotics. Organisms grow under the surface of the vegetation where phagocytes cannot penetrate, and bacterial metabolism is slowed within the nutrient-poor vegetation, contributing to antibiotic resistance. For these reasons, antibiotic treatment is directed toward achieving bactericidal concentrations of drug within the vegetation over an extended period. It must be noted that certain important aspects of antibiotic dosing, especially in seriously ill patients, are beyond the scope of this text, and infectious disease consultation is advised.

1. Principles of antibiotic therapy—

a. **In vitro sensitivity testing**—For organisms with variable antibiotic sensitivity (eg, streptococci), the choice of drug and the dosage depend on in vitro sensitivity testing of the strain infecting the patient. An organism's sensitivity to an antibiotic is quantified by the minimum inhibitory concentration (MIC) and minimum bactericidal concentration (MBC). The MIC is defined as the minimum concentration of antibiotic that prevents proliferation of the organism in a standardized culture system. The MBC is the minimum concentration that kills 99.9% of the bacteria at 24 h in a similarly standardized system. These tests are widely used to guide treatment of endocarditis, as in the characterization of penicillin sensitivity of the multiple species of streptococci and staphylococci (Table 29–8).

MIC and MBC data are also used to identify organisms with antibiotic tolerance, which is defined as an MBC more than ten times higher than the MIC. In such cases, although the infecting organism is susceptible to the antibiotic, the rate of killing is not increased at higher antibiotic concentrations, as would be expected. The tolerance of *Enterococcus* for penicillin, for example, probably explains the substantial failure rate of medical therapy in diseases caused by this organism despite the use of a high-dose multidrug regimen. In all patients with enterococcal endocarditis, the organism's MIC for penicillin and vancomycin should guide the choice of which antibiotic to pair with an aminoglycoside. Resistance to gentamicin and streptomycin should be determined as well. *Staphylococcus aureus* is among the other potentially tolerant organisms that may require an alteration in the antibiotic regimen. Methicillin resistance, if present, requires pairing of vancomycin with an aminoglycoside.

b. **Drug combinations**—Combinations of drugs with additive, or synergistic, killing power are used frequently for treating endocarditis. A frequent combination (see Table 29–8) is a β-lactam antibiotic (the penicillins and cephalosporins) with an aminoglycoside. This combination is synergistic because the β-lactam drug damages the bacterial cell wall, which allows more rapid penetration of the aminoglycoside into the cell.

c. **Parenteral treatment**—Antibiotic treatment must be given parenterally to ensure high and consistent serum drug levels and compliance. Outpatient IV drug therapy can be undertaken only under specific conditions (See Section 3. Outpatient Treatment), and oral therapy is almost never sufficient.

d. **Prolonged treatment**—The duration of antibiotic administration is almost always for a month or more. Prolonged exposure of the patient to antibiotics can lead to frequent side effects and serious toxicity (monitoring antibiotic therapy is discussed in the following section).

2. Empiric antibiotic therapy—Empiric antibiotic therapy is the initiation of antibiotics for the purpose of treating endocarditis without identifying the causative organism. Ideally, empiric therapy is needed only briefly until culture and sensitivity data are available. It requires treating the patient for the worst-case organism and can subject the patient to the additional risk of receiving multiple antibiotics over a prolonged period. This approach should be avoided whenever the patient's clinical status allows waiting for blood culture results, and the physician should make every effort to draw blood cultures consistent with a tolerable delay in the initiation of appropriate therapy.

Empiric therapy may be necessary if the patient presents with the syndrome of acute endocarditis (see Table 29–1), appears with symptoms of significant toxicity, or shows signs of septic shock; if the patient presents with signs and symptoms of left-heart failure and is likely to need surgery in the near future; or if the patient's echocardiogram (preferably TEE) shows evidence of extensive cardiac involvement. Although data on the prognostic implications of specific TEE findings are still incomplete, extensive involvement probably includes a vegetation longer than 2–3 cm, valve dysfunction likely to be hemodynamically significant, more than one infected valve, leaflet perforation, annular abscess, and pericarditis. A history of endocarditis must be ruled out. The choice of antibiotic for empiric therapy may be guided by considering the most likely infecting organisms based on the patient's presentation. Table 29–9 shows a four-category scheme for the selection of empiric therapy.

3. Outpatient treatment—Outpatient parenteral antibiotic therapy, now widely used, can provide an excellent outcome. Careful patient selection and management are mandatory. The first 2 weeks of treatment should almost always be as an inpatient because complications are most likely during this time. If the patient has a low-virulence organism, if valve involvement is limited to vegetations attached to leaflets and vegetations are not large (<15 cm), and the first 2 weeks have been uncomplicated, then outpatient treatment should be considered. Endocarditis due to strep viridans and the HACEK group can be treated as an outpatient. At present, it is less certain that infection with *S aureus,* especially of the aortic valve, can be safely treated this way, due to the frequency of abscess and subvalve extension.

In addition to a specialized team of nurses managing the infusion and assessing the patient daily, a physician experienced in the treatment of endocarditis should be available for a same-day visit in the event of evidence of complications (discussed further under Section C. Management of Complications). The patient should live close to a hospital and have drug levels, blood cul-

Table 29–8. Antibiotic treatment of endocarditis.

Organism Category	Regimen	Penicillin-Allergic Regimen	Comments
Penicillin-sensitive streptococci (eg, *S miltis, S bovis,* β-hemolytic streptococci); (MIC < 0.1 μg/mL)	penicillin G 2 million units IV q6h × 4 w or 2 million units IV q6h × 2 w plus gentamicin 1 mg/kg (max 80 mg) IV q8h × 2 w	ceftriaxone 2 g IV q24h × 4 w or vancomycin 15 mg/kg IV q12h × 4 w plus gentamicin 1 mg/kg (max 80 mg) IV q8h × at least 2 w	Determine MIC in each patient; streptococci have variable sensitivity to penicillin. Complicated cases required extended or modified treatment. Check blood culture at 3–5 days. Not necessary to check MIC or MBC during treatment. Prosthetic-valve infection; penicillin × 6 w plus gentamicin × 2 w. Also treats *Meningococcus, Gonococcus,* and penicillin-sensitive *Pneumococcus.*
Penicillin-tolerant streptococci (eg, *S mutans*); (MIC >0.1 μg/mL, <0.5 μg/mL	penicillin G 2 million units IV q6h × 4 w plus gentamicin 1 mg/kg (max 80 mg) IV q8h × 2 w	vancomycin and gentamicin as above	
Penicillin-resistant streptococci (MIC ≥0.5 μg/mL) and enterococcus	penicillin G 4 million units IV q6h × 6 w plus gentamicin 1 mg/kg (max 80 mg) IV q8h × 4–6 w	vancomycin 15 mg/kg IV q12h × 6 w plus gentamicin 1 mg/kg (max 80 mg) IV q8h × 8 w	*Enterococcus* is often resistant to multiple antibiotics. Vancomycin resistance is an increasing problem in some regions and must be tested. In vitro sensitivity testing is mandatory. Careful attention to signs of drug toxicity is required for all regimens. β-lactamase-producing and highly penicillin resistant strains are usually treated with vancomycin plus an aminoglycoside.
Staphylococcus aureus	nafcillin 2 g IV q4h × 4–6 w plus gentamicin 1 mg/kg (max 80 mg) for initial 3–5 d If methicillin-resistant; vancomycin 15 mg/kg IV q12h × 4–6 w plus gentamicin 1 mg/kg (max 80 mg) IV q8h × 4–6 w	ceftriaxone 2 g IV q24h × 6 w plus gentamicin 1 mg/kg (max 80 mg) IV q8h × 4–6 w	If penicillin sensitive (very unusual), treat as for penicillin sensitive streptococci. Testing for methicillin resistance (resistance to penicillin, nafcillin, and all cephalosporins) is mandatory. Alternative regimens for special situations are available. Prosthetic valve infection; nafcillin or vancomycin plus an aminoglycoside and rifampin × 6 w Tricuspid valve endocarditis can be treated for 2 w if methicillin-sensitive, no cardiac or extra cardiac extension, and no HIV.
Pseudomonas aeruginosa	piperacillin 3 g IV q4h × 6 w plus tobramycin 1.7 mg/kg IV q8h × 6 w	imipenem 0.5–1 g IV q6h × 6 w plus tobramycin 1.7 mg/kg IV q8h × 6 w	Sensitivity testing is very important. Valve replacement is almost always required for cure. Imipenem is toxic at high doses.

(continued)

Table 29–8. Antibiotic treatment of endocarditis. (continued)

Organism Category	Regimen	Penicillin-Allergic Regimen	Comments
Pseudomonas aeruginosa	piperacillin 3 g IV q4h × 6 w plus tobramycin 1.7 mg/kg IV q8h × 6 w.	imipenem 0.5–1 g IV q6h × 6 w plus tobramycin 1.7 mg/kg IV q8h × 6 w	Sensitivity testing is very important. Valve replacement is almost always required for cure. Imipenem is toxic at high doses.
Enteric gram-negative bacteria (eg, *Escherichia coli*, *enterobacter, Serratia, Klebsiella*)	cefotaxime 2 g IV q8h × 4–6 w plus gentamicin 1.7 mg/kg q8h × 4–6 w	See comments.	Multiple alternatives to cefotaxime may be used in combination with aminoglycoside. These organisms are difficult to treat because of clinical setting (hospitalized, debilitated patient) and emergence of resistance during therapy. Serum bactericidal liters should be followed during treatment. Valve replacement almost always required for cure (especially *Serratia*).
Fungi (eg, *Candida albicans, histoplasma, Aspergillus*)	amphotericin B 1 mg/kg IV qid × 2 w, then lower dose as needed to achieve total dose of 40–50 mg/kg after 6–8 w plus flucytosine 150 mg/kg PO × 4 doses		Highly toxic regimen. Valve replacement mandatory after 1–2 w of full-dose amphotericin B. Flucytosine serum levels should be monitored and kept at 50–100 µg/mL. Hematologic toxicity can develop rapidly when amphotericin-induced renal dysfunction reduces flucytosine excretion.
Staphylococcus epidermidis	vancomycin 15 mg/kg IV q12h × 6 w plus rifampin 300 mg q8h × 6 w plus gentamicin 1 mg/kg (max 80 mg) IV q8h initial 2 w		Strongly associated with prosthetic valve infection, especially within 6 mon of implantation. Almost always methicillin resistent; if not, can be treated with nafcillin plus gentamicin.
Hemophillus	If β-lactamase; ampicillin 2 g IV q4h × 4 w plus gentamicin 1.7 mg/kg IV q8h × 4 w	If β-lactamase+; ceftriaxone, 1 g IV q12h plus gentamicin 1.7 mg/kg IV q8h 4 w	Other organisms in the HACEK group can be treated with this regimen.
Coxiella burnetii (Q fever)	tetracycline or trimethoprim sulfa plus rifampin for months or years		Surgery required but cure not usually possible, leading to long-term suppressive treatment. *Chlamydia* infection treated similarly.
Diphtheroids	penicillin G 2 million units IV q6h × 4–6 w plus gentamicin 1.7 mg/kg IV q8h × 4–6 w	vancomycin 15 mg/kg IV q12h × 6 w plus gentamicin 1.7 mg/kg q8h × 4–6 w	Testing for sensitivity to penicillin required; vancomycin can be substituted if necessary.

Note: In all treatment regimens, gentamicin dose must be adjusted according to blood levels. A once-daily dosing with 5.1 mg/kg q24h may become accepted practice.

Table 29–9. Empiric treatment for endocarditis.

Patient Presentation	Likely Organisms	Regimen	Duration
Subacute presentation, no IV drug use	*Streptococcus, Enterococcus*	penicillin G 4 million units IV q6h plus gentamicin 1 mg/kg (max 80 mg) IV q8h	4–6 w
Acute presentation, no IV drug use	*Staphylococcus aureus* (β-lactamase-producing)	nafcillin 2 g q4h IV plus gentamicin 1 mg/kg (max 80 mg) IV q8h	4–6 w
Acute presentation, IV drug use	*Staphylococcus aureus* (β-lactamase-producing)	vancomycin 7.5 mg/kg IV q6h	4–6 w
Prosthetic valve	*Staphylococcus aureus* and *epidermidis*	vancomycin 7.5 mg/kg IV q6h plus gentamicin 1 mg/kg (max 80 mg) q8h IV initial 2 w plus rifampin 300 mg q8h PO	6 weeks

Note: Treatment durations apply when blood culture data remain unavailable and clinical response is favorable. IV = intravenous; PO = by mouth.

tures, and other blood work monitored as with an inpatient.

4. Monitoring antibiotic therapy—

a. Drug levels—Monitoring the levels and effects of antibiotics is important in managing endocarditis because the patient's prolonged exposure to high doses of antibiotics increases the frequency of adverse drug effects. The use of aminoglycosides requires monitoring of serum levels at peak (1–2 h after infusion is started) and trough (immediately before the next dose). A peak level for gentamicin or tobramycin of less than 5 μg/mL is associated with treatment failure for many organisms and may warrant adjustment of the dose or the dosing interval. At a trough level of more than 2 μg/mL, gentamicin carries an increased risk of nephrotoxicity, and the dose should be reduced. Monitoring these levels assumes even greater importance in the setting of renal insufficiency, especially if renal function is changing. Although vancomycin and flucytosine levels should always be monitored for the same reasons, levels for β-lactam antibiotics are available but rarely needed.

b. Serum bactericidal titers—The efficacy of the antibiotic therapy can be estimated by testing the killing power of the patient's serum. (The serum bactericidal titer is defined as the greatest dilution of serum that kills an inoculum of the organism in a standardized system.) In general, a titer of 1:8 or greater is associated with cure; however, serum bactericidal titers provide no significant additional benefit over the use of standardized antibiotic regimens for most organisms. They are occasionally useful in assessing the adequacy

of treatment against unusual organisms or when an unconventional antibiotic regimen must be used.

c. Adverse effects—The most frequent adverse effects are a pruritic maculopapular rash and low-grade fever seen with β-lactam antibiotics. The rash may signify delayed hypersensitivity and may be accompanied by hepatic or renal dysfunction. Liver function tests (aspartate aminotransferase and alkaline phosphatase) and creatinine should be checked in this situation. If these tests are abnormal, substitution of another drug is required. If not, it is preferable to continue the antibiotic and treat the symptoms. Patients on β-lactam antibiotics should have a routine complete blood count every 3 or 4 days during therapy to detect anemia, thrombocytopenia, and leukopenia. The sodium content of β-lactam antibiotics may require diuretic therapy in patients with heart failure.

Patients on aminoglycosides should have the serum creatinine checked routinely at 3–4-day intervals. Equally useful for detection of renal dysfunction is the periodic examination of urine for white cell or granular casts. Ototoxicity is an idiosyncratic reaction unrelated to aminoglycoside levels that occurs in 10–20% of cases.

Diarrhea may occur during antibiotic therapy; this is usually due to overgrowth of gut organisms competing with those sensitive to the antibiotic (eg, *Clostridium difficile* colitis).

C. MANAGEMENT OF COMPLICATIONS

1. Failure of antibiotic therapy—Changes in the cardiac examination during antibiotic treatment are particularly important in detecting failure of medical therapy. Changes in a regurgitant murmur almost always indicate valve dysfunction, and the appearance of a new murmur may signal metastatic infection of another valve. Such new findings almost always warrant repeat echocardiography (usually TEE) and blood cultures. There may also be an increase in the resting sinus rate and the appearance of heart failure.

Failure of antibiotic therapy is usually heralded by persistent or recurrent fever. Persistent fever is that which continues more than a week during antibiotic treatment. Recurrent fever develops after an afebrile period of several days and occurs at least a week after initiation of antibiotics. Persistent infection is only one cause of fever in this setting; others include hypersensitivity to antibiotics and other drugs, phlebitis, silent emboli (especially pulmonary and splenic), intercurrent urinary or upper respiratory tract infection, or simply a delayed response to antibiotic therapy. Blood cultures should be obtained and efforts made to rule out these possibilities. If blood cultures are negative, and the patient shows no other evidence of deterioration, watchful waiting is appropriate.

Positive blood cultures after more than 1 week of antibiotic therapy strongly suggest persistent infection. The cause may be either antibiotic resistance or a protected site of infection. The site may be an intracardiac annular or myocardial abscess or an extracardiac site of metastatic infection, septic embolization, or mycotic aneurysm. Repeat TEE is strongly indicated. Careful comparison to the studies obtained at the time of initial diagnosis may detect intracardiac suppurative complications; there is a sensitivity range of 80–90%. If the TEE is positive, urgent surgery is indicated. If it is negative, a careful history and physical examination coupled with CT or a technetium, gallium, or indium scan will often reveal an infective focus.

2. Worsening valve dysfunction and heart failure—
At any time during the course of endocarditis, heart failure signs and symptoms may appear as a result of worsening regurgitation and failure of ventricular compensatory mechanisms. In fact, heart failure may appear despite effective antibiotic therapy—and even after bacteriologic cure. The onset of heart failure may be insidious and difficult to recognize, or it may be abrupt and catastrophic. Frequent appraisal of the patient's status by history and physical examination is the best way to ensure early detection of heart failure. Any change in the patient's regurgitant murmur during antibiotic therapy usually signifies progression of valvular dysfunction and the likely need for surgery. A persistent tachycardia or slowly increasing heart rate is a useful sign of impending heart failure prior to the appearance of the typical signs such as rales, S_3, and pulmonary vascular redistribution on chest x-ray film. In patients with aortic valve endocarditis, the appearance of a

widened pulse pressure usually indicates increased valve regurgitation.

Serial TTE or TEE is useful in confirming a suspected change in the patient's hemodynamic status; it may even identify the cause. Worsening of the mitral regurgitant lesion is suggested by an increase in size of the color-flow Doppler jet or an increase in the radius of the flow convergence region on the LV side of the regurgitant orifice. A rise in transmitral early filling velocity (E wave) and a fall in forward systolic pulmonary venous flow (S wave) may indicate a rise in mean left atrial pressure.

In the case of aortic regurgitation, jet enlargement over time is also a useful indicator of worsening regurgitation. Additional indications of severe aortic regurgitation include closure of the mitral valve on M-mode echocardiography prior to the onset of the QRS and shortening of the pressure half-time of the aortic insufficiency velocity, both from a rapid rise of LV pressure to a high level in late diastole. For either mitral or aortic regurgitation, the presence or development of a hyperdynamic left ventricle (increased ejection fraction, stroke volume, or both) and progressive LV dilatation on two-dimensional echocardiography are useful indirect indications of an excessive regurgitant burden. The appearance of pulmonary or right atrial hypertension, as estimated from tricuspid jet velocity and inferior vena caval dynamics, is another sign of hemodynamic decompensation. Transesophageal echocardiography has the additional major advantage of being able to detect the intracardiac complications accounting for the change in the patient's hemodynamic status.

If heart failure is mild, surgery should be deferred while diuretics, digoxin, and afterload-reducing drugs are given to optimize the patient's hemodynamic status. If the patient responds readily to therapy, surgery might be optional. In most cases, however, surgery should be undertaken as soon as feasible because it is almost certain that valve repair or replacement will be required eventually (for the hemodynamic lesion, if not for infection), and the patient's surgical risk is lowest at this early stage. One clear exception to surgery for mild heart failure is sodium overload (related to antibiotic therapy) and suspected valve dysfunction not confirmed by echocardiography.

If heart failure is moderate or severe, valve surgery should be undertaken immediately while drug therapy is used to stabilize the patient. Because of the difficulty in predicting the rate of progression of valve dysfunction, delaying surgery for hemodynamic optimization is ill-advised. Rapid development of heart failure may signal the occurrence of a major intracardiac complication, such as leaflet perforation, chordal rupture, or fistula formation. Preoperative or intraoperative TEE is usually helpful in guiding surgical planning in this setting.

3. Embolism—Embolism most often occurs early in the course of antibiotic therapy but can occur at any time, even after biologic cure. Suspected cerebral embolism should be evaluated immediately by CT; if necessary, cerebral angiography should be performed in order to rule out an intracranial mycotic aneurysm. Nonhemorrhagic infarcts may warrant measures to reduce cerebral edema.

If the patient is already on anticoagulant therapy prior to development of endocarditis, anticoagulation is usually continued. After cerebral embolism in a patient with endocarditis, however, anticoagulation therapy is usually discontinued (if possible) for 7–14 days to reduce the likelihood of massive intracerebral bleeding. If stroke occurs in mechanical prosthetic valve endocarditis, the balance of risks and benefits of continuing anticoagulation is unknown. In patients with stroke from endocarditis, serial neurologic examinations and (if a change is suspected) repeated CT scans are indicated to permit early detection of brain abscess.

Because no clinically useful means (including echocardiography) has been found to identify patients at high risk for embolism, valve surgery in endocarditis is not indicated to prevent embolism. Even the probability of embolism recurring after one episode is not necessarily high enough to warrant surgery for prevention. On the other hand, surgery may be advised if the patient has had more than one episode and has a persistent vegetation.

Peripheral embolization is managed conservatively and without anticoagulation whenever possible. Vascular surgery to restore the circulation may be indicated if major organ embolization becomes life-threatening. Embolectomy is generally indicated in culture-negative endocarditis in order to make an causative diagnosis; likely organisms include *Aspergillus, Candida,* and the HACEK group. Embolectomy is necessary, strictly for treatment, in fungal endocarditis in order to remove as much infection as possible from the circulation.

4. Mycotic aneurysm—A complaint of severe headache or visual disturbance (especially homonymous hemianopsia) in a patient with endocarditis should prompt an urgent CT scan for the possibility of an expanding intracranial mycotic aneurysm. This catastrophic complication may also present as a subarachnoid or intracerebral hemorrhage, usually massive. If the scan is negative, cerebral angiography is often necessary to confirm or rule out the diagnosis. Treatment is surgical removal as soon as the patient's condition will allow.

5. Myocardial infarction—Chest pain in the course of infective endocarditis is most likely due to myocardial infarction, pericarditis, or septic pulmonary embolization. Myocardial infarction during infective endocarditis is almost always caused by coronary embolization, although it may occasionally complicate purulent pericarditis or myocardial abscess. In the latter setting, inflammatory thrombosis of the artery probably occurs. Treatment is noninterventional. Anticoagulation is probably not indicated because its benefits for reducing myocardial ischemia in this setting are unknown and the risks of potential cerebral embolization are significant.

6. Pericarditis—The possibility of purulent pericarditis complicating infective endocarditis should be evaluated by TTE. If pericardial fluid is seen, prompt pericardiocentesis is needed. A transudate may be present; in this infrequent case management can be conservative. Usually a purulent exudate will be found, necessitating surgical drainage or pericardiectomy. Most important, purulent pericarditis may signal the presence of an intracardiac abscess. Transesophageal echocardiography is indicated, and if an abscess is found, surgical drainage and valve surgery should be performed. Fortunately, the treatment of these related problems can be performed in a single operation. If an underlying myocardial abscess is not found, a pericardial window may be sufficient therapy. Continued observation is indicated because of the risk of subsequent additional cardiac or pericardial suppurative complications.

D. MANAGEMENT OF HIGH-RISK ENDOCARDITIS

1. Prosthetic valve endocarditis—Far higher morbidity and mortality rates are associated with prosthetic valve endocarditis than with native valve endocarditis. Infection of a prosthesis by fungi carries a mortality rate of more than 90%, whereas prosthetic infection from streptococci has a mortality rate of approximately 30%. In addition, the mortality rate from prosthetic valve endocarditis early after implantation is around twice that of late infection (after 2 months). Survival is improved by early operation in most cases, when the patient's surgical risk is acceptable. Surgical replacement is necessary in 85% of cases of biologic valve endocarditis and in almost all cases of mechanical prosthetic infection. Indications for surgery in prosthetic valve endocarditis are summarized in Table 29–10.

Medical treatment can be attempted in mechanical valve endocarditis when the surgical risk is high and the only evidence of valve involvement (using TEE) is a vegetation in the area of the sewing ring. In such cases, frequent serial TEE may be useful to follow valve function and the response of the infected mass to treatment. Initial medical treatment of bioprosthetic endocarditis may be attempted when infection is due to a low-risk organism (such as *Streptococcus*) and involvement is limited to a vegetation on the either the prosthetic leaflets or sewing ring (see Table 29–9). Repeated TEE is very useful if the patient fails to respond to antibiotics. Blood cultures should be obtained every 4–7 days during treatment and weekly for a month following apparently successful treatment.

Table 29–10. Indications for surgery in prosthetic valve endocarditis.

Mechanical prosthesis (almost all cases)
Bioprosthesis if:
New paravalvular regurgitation or fistula
Sewing-ring abscess or dehiscence
Infection from *Staphylococcus epidermidis* or *aureus*,
Enterococcus, gram-negative bacteria, fungi
Blood cultures still positive after 1 week of antibiotics
Embolism or other major complication

Table 29–11. Indications for valve surgery in native valve endocarditis.

Absolute Indications
Intracardiac abscess or fistula
Left heart failure from severe regurgitation or (rarely)
obstruction
Endocarditis caused by fungi and resistant gram-negative
organisms
Relative Indications
Mild heart failure in otherwise uncomplicated case
Recurrent embolization with persistant vegetation
Purulent pericarditis
Bacteremia despite optimal antibiotic therapy
Recurrent life-threatening septic pulmonary emboli
Severe tricuspid regurgitation with a low output state

2. Fungal endocarditis—Overall mortality rates for fungal endocarditis are more than 80%; they are especially high in cases caused by *Aspergillus* and *Candida* species. Treatment requires the close collaboration of the primary physician, cardiologist, surgeon, and infectious disease specialist. Treatment is almost always a combination of valve replacement and a full course of amphotericin B (see Table 29–8). Late relapses are common and require prolonged surveillance for years following successful completion of antibiotic therapy. In addition to serologic tests and blood cultures, TEE is useful in monitoring the patient during and after treatment.

3. Endocarditis from gram-negative bacteria—*Pseudomonas* endocarditis carries a mortality rate of almost 80% because of the frequent inability to sterilize vegetations by medical treatment. Among the causes for this inability is the frequent emergence of antibiotic-resistant bacterial strains during therapy. Surgery is usually performed as soon as possible after the diagnosis of *Pseudomonas* endocarditis of the left-sided valves. Surgery is also frequently indicated in endocarditis caused by the HACEK organisms, but here the reason is extensive valvular destruction by the time of diagnosis. In contrast to *Pseudomonas,* infection from HACEK organisms is readily cured by antibiotics. The treatment of endocarditis from enteric gram-negative bacteria is similar to that for *Pseudomonas* in that antibiotic therapy may fail, leading to a need for valve replacement. In vitro antibiotic sensitivity testing is crucial to antibiotic therapy of gram-negative bacteria.

E. SURGERY

The indications for valve replacement or repair during infective endocarditis (discussed in the preceding section) are summarized in Table 29–11. The indications and timing of valve surgery are guided by several important principles. Surgical morbidity and mortality rates are much higher if the patient is in even mild heart failure, is hypotensive, or has a low cardiac output when sent to the operating room. Similarly, uncontrolled infection, with its attendant systemic stress and

peripheral dilatation, confers a higher surgical risk. In the absence of these factors, surgical risk generally is low despite active infective endocarditis. Surgery should not be delayed with the intention of prolonging preoperative antibiotic therapy. It has never been shown that either the risk of reinfection of the new prosthetic valve or surgical complications are reduced by longer preoperative antibiotic treatment.

The anatomic location and extent of valve involvement and other factors may allow valve debridement and repair rather than replacement. The advantages of valve repair are that future anticoagulation is not needed, and subsequent valve replacement carries a lower risk. The disadvantages of valve repair are the greater possibility of residual infected tissue and significant valve regurgitation. Valve repair is not considered in the presence of abscess or fistula near the valve or when significant leaflet erosion has occurred. As part of a repair, however, leaflet perforation can be patched and chordal support reconstructed. In general, valve repair is feasible when excision of the infected leaflet with a 2-mm margin of normal tissue will still leave enough normal leaflet to preserve valvular competence. Preoperative or intraoperative TEE is usually indicated for surgical planning and guidance.

F. FOLLOW-UP AFTER ENDOCARDITIS

Long-term survival of the patient following an episode of endocarditis is much lower than that of the general population. Overall survival following native valve endocarditis is approximately 80% at 5 years and 50% at 10 years. Survival is considerably lower after prosthetic valve endocarditis. The patient remains at risk for three consequences of the disease: relapse of the original infection, noninfective sequelae of the infection, and recurrent endocarditis.

Failure to eradicate infection completely is usually apparent within 15 days after antibiotics are discontinued, although relapse has been reported up to 6 months after apparently successful treatment. Relapse rates tend to be low with viridans streptococci (<5%), intermediate with enterococci (8–20%) and high with *Pseudomonas* and fungi (>20%). Relapse of *Staphylococcus aureus* endocarditis is not frequent (5%) but should prompt a search for an extracardiac source. Treatment of a relapse includes a reassessment of the extent of cardiac infection, and surgery warrants careful consideration. If antibiotic therapy is given a trial, the patient should be carefully monitored during therapy to determine the need for surgery.

After successful treatment of infection, the patient remains at risk for the development of heart failure, stroke, and rupture of a mycotic aneurysm. If the patient had moderate or severe valve regurgitation or an episode of heart failure prior to hospital discharge, the probability of late heart failure is greatly increased. The risk of embolic stroke is very low after the first 4 weeks of antibiotic treatment but may persist for an unknown length of time. Rupture of a mycotic aneurysm after treatment is also rare but should be considered when a patient with stroke has a history of prior endocarditis.

Although estimates vary, recurrent endocarditis, defined as a repeat episode after more than 6 months, occurs in approximately 5–8% of cases. Controversy exists regarding the tendency for the infecting organism and the involved valve to be similar to those of the original episode. The recurrent episode probably carries a higher mortality rate than does the original one. Risk factors for recurrent endocarditis include intravenous drug use, congenital heart disease, rheumatic and myxomatous disease, and (in one study) periodontitis.

Andrews MM, von Reyn CF: Patient selection criteria and management guidelines for outpatient parenteral antibiotic therapy for native valve infective endocarditis. Clin Infect Dis 2001;33:203.

Barnes PD, Crook DWM: Culture-negative endocarditis [Review]. J Infection 1997;35:209.

Bayer AS et al: Diagnosis and management of infective endocarditis and its complications. Circulation 1998;98:2936.

Dajani AS et al: Prevention of bacterial endocarditis. Circulation 1997;96:358.

Fang G et al: Prosthetic valve endocarditis resulting from nosocomial bacteremia. Ann Intern Med 1993:119:560.

Fowler VG et al: Role of echocardiography in evaluation of patients with staphylococcus aureus bacteremia, experience in 103 patients. J Am Coll Cardiol 1997;30:1072.

Klug D et al: Systemic infection related to endocarditis on pacemaker leads. Circulation 1997;95:2098.

Li JS et al: Proposed modifications to the Duke criteria for the diagnosis of infective endocarditis. Clin Infect Dis 2000;30:633.

Mylonkis E, Calderwood SB et al: Infective endocarditis in adults. [Review] N Engl J Med 2001;345(18):1318.

Wilson WR et al: Antibiotic treatment of adults with infective endocarditis due to streptococci, enterococci, staphylococci, and HACEK microorganisms. JAMA 1995;274:1706.

Cardiac Tumors

Edmond W. Chen, MD & Rita F. Redberg, MD

ESSENTIALS OF DIAGNOSIS

- *Positive imaging study for characteristic cardiac masses*
- *Positive biopsy of cardiac masses*

General Considerations

A. METASTATIC CARDIAC TUMORS

Metastatic cardiac tumors are about 40 times more common than primary tumors. Cardiac metastases occur in approximately 5% of patients who die of malignant tumors and are often present as pericardial effusions; myocardial, coronary, and intracavitary involvement occurs with less frequency. The tumors that most often metastasize to the heart are bronchogenic carcinoma and breast cancer (by direct extension or hematogenous spread) and lymphoma and leukemia (by lymphatic spread). Disseminated malignant melanoma has the highest predilection for cardiac metastases, which occur in 50–65% of afflicted patients. Rarely, adenocarcinoma of the colon can metastasize to the heart by lymphatic or hematogenous spread, usually affecting first the pericardium and then the myocardium. Cardiac metastases that occur in patients with colon cancer are usually preceded by involvement of other organs. Metastases to the endocardium have been reported in renal cell carcinoma, adenocarcinoma of the stomach, laryngeal carcinoma, pancreatic cancer, and mucinous adenocarcinoma of the cecum and of the ovary. However, rare metastases from other tumors such as pheochromocytomas have been reported. Renal cell carcinomas can extend into the inferior vena cava, and the tumor thrombus occasionally involves the right atrium (Figure 30–1).

B. PRIMARY TUMORS

Primary tumors of the heart are rare, with an incidence from 0.001% to 0.28% reported in unselected autopsy studies. Although myxoma is the most frequent tumor type in adults, rhabdomyomas represent the most common type in the pediatric population.

1. Benign—The majority (75–80%) of primary cardiac tumors are benign and therefore potentially curable (Table 30–1).

McAllister HA, Hall RJ, Cooley DA: Tumors of the heart and pericardium. Cur Probl Cardiol 1999;24:57–116.

a. Myxomas—These tumors account for approximately half of benign cardiac tumors and are usually found in patients between 30 and 60 years old, with a mean age of onset of 51 years. They occur predominantly in females; although most are isolated or sporadic, they can also be familial or complex. Fewer than 10% of myxomas are familial and are apparently transmitted in an autosomal-dominant pattern. Familial myxoma presents earlier in life, with a mean age of onset of 25 years. Complex cardiac myxomas or the familial Carney's complex may include such features as multiple pigmented skin lesions (lentigines), myxoid fibroadenomas of the breast, tumors of the pituitary and testes, and primary pigmented nodular adrenocortical disease. Carney's complex appears to be genetically heterogenous with gene localization on chromosome 2p16 and chromosome 17q24. The majority of Carney's complex appears to be caused by a mutation in the PRKAR1α gene that encodes the R1α regulatory subunit of the cyclic adenosine monophosphate-dependent protein kinase A (PKA). Patients with familial or complex myxomas are more likely than those with sporadic myxomas to have multiple (30–50%) and recurrent (12–22%) tumors. This occasional recurrence of myxomas and a few reported cases of invasion of surrounding tissue by the tumor suggest that myxomas have some low-grade malignant features.

Most myxomas (74%) occur in the left atrium, although they can occur in any chamber (right atrium, 18%; right ventricle, 4%; left ventricle, 4%) or on any valve. They arise from the endocardial surface of the cardiac chamber with a stalk attached to the interatrial septum close to the fossa ovalis. When a myxoma occurs in the ventricles, it almost always originates from the free wall. Although asymptomatic myxomas have

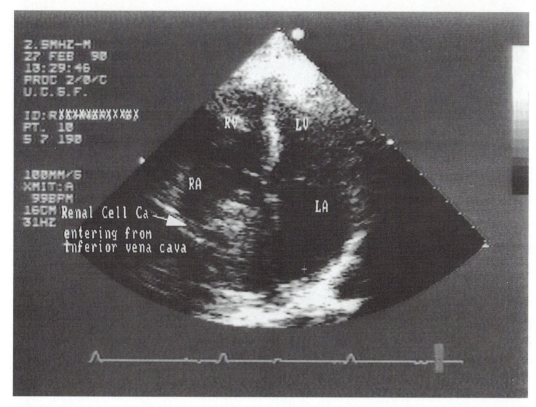

Figure 30–1. Transthoracic echocardiogram showing a large renal cell carcinoma with tumor thrombus (*arrow*) extending into the right atrium through the inferior vena cava. LA = left atrium; LV = left ventricle; RA = right atrium; RV = right ventricle.

been recognized, most patients experience one or more effects from the classical triad of constitutional, embolic, and obstructive manifestations. (For details, refer to the section on Clinical Findings.)

Goldstein MM, Casey M, Carney JA, Basson CT: Molecular genetic diagnosis of the familial myxoma syndrome (Carney complex). Am J Med Genetics 1999;86:62–65.

Table 30–1. Primary cardiac neoplasms.

Benign
  Myxoma
  Lipoma
  Papillary fibroelastoma
  Fibroma
  Rhabdomyoma
  Rare tumors
Malignant
  Sarcoma
  Lymphoma
  Rare tumors

Kirschner LS, Carney JA, Pack SD et al: Mutations of the gene encoding the protein kinase A type 1-a regulatory subunit in patients with the Carney complex. Nat Genet 2000;26: 89–92.

Vaughan CJ, Veugelers M, Basson CT: Tumors and the heart: Molecular genetic advances. Cur Opin Cardiol 2001;16:195–200.

b. Lipomas—These occur as circumscribed, encapsulated tumors. These usually solitary, intramuscular, subendocardial, or subepicardial tumors are often asymptomatic.

c. Papillary fibroelastomas—These tumors are rare, accounting for 7–8% of cardiac tumors. They are usually discovered postmortem, with an autopsy incidence of 0.002–0.33% although their premorbid detection rate is rising with the increasing use of echocardiography (Figure 30–2). A review of echocardiograms at the Mayo Clinic from 1980 to 1995 found 54 patients with a diagnosis of papillary fibroelastoma, representing 0.019% of all patients who underwent echocardiograms during this period. They are usually found in patients older than 60 years of age, although they have been reported in patients from 3 to 86 years old. A pro-

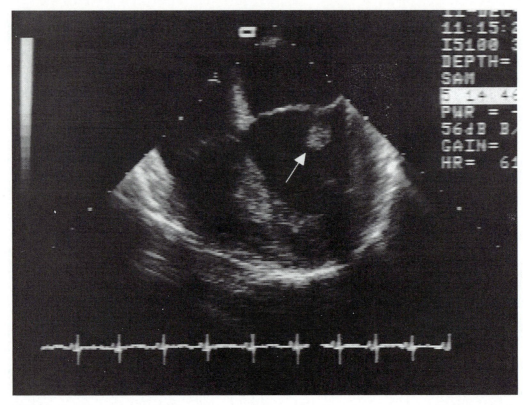

Figure 30–2. Transesophageal echocardiogram in horizontal-plane four-chamber view to define the attachment site of mitral valve papillary fibroelastoma (*arrow*), performed after incidental discovery of the tumor on transthoracic echocardiogram.

fusion of names—**cardiac papilloma, papillary fibroma, giant Lambl's excrescence,** and **papillary endocardial tumor**—have been used to describe what is properly a papillary fibroelastoma. These tumors (first described as small filiform projections on the cusps of aortic valves) have multiple papillary fronds and look like a sea anemone, attached to the endocardial surface of the valves by a small pedicle.

Papillary fibroelastomas can form a nidus for platelet and fibrin aggregation and lead to systemic or neurologic emboli. They are most commonly identified on the valves, arising on the left-sided valvular structures much more frequently than the right-sided ones. They have also been found on the chordae and papillary apparatuses, left ventricular septum, left ventricular outflow tract, left ventricular free wall, and the left atrium. Clinical manifestations include such conditions as cerebral embolism, myocardial infarction, sudden death, pulmonary embolism, and syncope. Surgical excision is generally recommended in symptomatic individuals.

Klarich KW, Enriquez-Sarano M, Gura GM et al: Papillary fibroelastoma: Echocardiographic characteristics for diagnosis and pathologic correlation. J Am Coll Cardiol 1997;30:783–790.

Sun JP, Asher CR, Yang XS, et al: Clinical and echocardiographic characteristics of papillary fibroelastomas: A retrospective and prospective study in 162 patients. Circulation 2001;103:2687–2693.

Shahian DM: Papillary fibroelastomas. Semin Thorac Cardiovasc Surg 2000;12:101–110.

d. Fibromas—Approximately three quarters of all fibromas occur in the pediatric population. The second most common benign tumor of childhood, they have been reported in patients from age 2 to 57 years. Almost always solitary, fibromas can occur in any chamber but are most commonly found in the ventricular myocardium—usually in the anterior wall of the left ventricle and interventricular septum—and in the right ventricle. These tumors are often large, between 4 and 7 cm in diameter, and exert a mass effect. They are also associated with ventricular arrhythmias and heart failure; when arising from the ventricular septum, they can be associated with sudden death. Their size can make complete excision difficult.

e. Rhabdomyomas—Rhabdomyomas also occur mainly in the pediatric population, and most cases present in the first year of life. There are frequently multiple tumors, occurring equally in the right and left ventricles or the atria; the valves are spared. They range in size from a few millimeters to a few centimeters and are white to yellow. Rhabdomyomas are often associated with tuberous sclerosis (Figure 30–3). Spontaneous regression is well established in the pediatric population. Unless the patient is symptomatic, surgical intervention is often unnecessary. In fact, an intracavitary mass discovered incidentally in a pediatric patient is suggestive of rhabdomyoma until proven otherwise.

f. Cardiac hamartomas (oncocytic cardiomyopathy)—Cardiac hamartomas have been found in the pediatric population. They occur in the left ventricle and are associated with ventricular arrhythmias. Although surgical resection is recommended to treat tachyarrhythmias, as many as 50% of cardiac hamartomas undergo involution with time, and recent data suggest that conservative management is appropriate. Control-

ling the arrhythmia medically, when possible, obviates the need for surgery.

g. Hemangiomas—Occurring in patients from age 2 weeks to 65 years old, hemangiomas can be isolated or associated with hemangiomas in other locations. They are located in any of the cardiac chambers; depending on their location, they have been associated with arrhythmias or sudden death (Figure 30–4).

Becker AE: Primary heart tumors in the pediatric age group: A review of salient pathologic features relevant for clinicians. Ped Cardiol 2000;21:317–323.

Freedom RM, Lee KJ, MacDonald C, Taylor G: Selected aspects of cardiac tumors in infancy and childhood. Ped Cardiol 2000;21:299–316.

2. Malignant—

a. Sarcomas—These the most common malignant cardiac tumors. They are a highly malignant group, afflicting men more commonly than women, at a rate of 65–75%. Angiosarcomas are the most common, followed by rhabdomyosarcomas, fibrosarcomas, and osteosarcomas. Because angiosarcomas usually occur in the right atrium or pericardium, most patients present with right-sided failure, pericardial disease, or vena

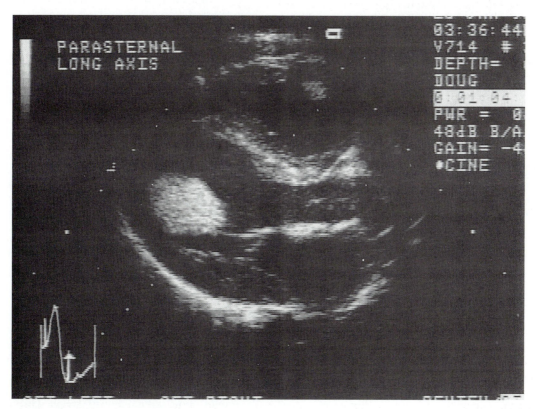

Figure 30–3. Transthoracic echocardiogram in parasternal long-axis view showing a rhabdomyoma in the left ventricle of a pediatric patient with tuberous sclerosis.

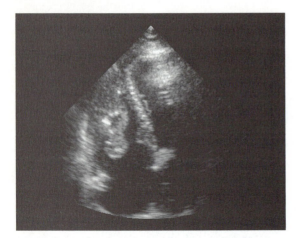

Figure 30–4. Transthoracic echocardiogram of a hemangioma in a 50-year-old woman who presented with a month history of palpitations. A four-chamber view showing the large right ventricular mass.

caval obstruction. The tumor is extensively infiltrative of cardiac structures, and metastatic spread at the time of diagnosis is high. The tumor can be diagnosed by lung biopsy if pulmonary metastases are present. Rhabdomyosarcomas have been reported in all age groups; there is a slight male predominance. Fibrosarcomas, which occur equally in the left and right heart, are often multiple and protrude into a cardiac chamber. A valve is affected in half the cases. Osteosarcomas have been found in patients ranging in age from 24 to 67 years. They usually originate in the posterior wall of the left atrium, near the entrance of the pulmonary veins, and can be intramural or intracavitary. Intramural infiltration leads to arrhythmia, conduction defects, and even asystole. Intracavitary tumors produce obstructive-type symptoms secondary to left ventricular inflow-tract obstruction. Osteosarcomas can metastasize to thyroid, skin, and lungs. Leiomyosarcomas have rarely been reported in the heart. When they do occur, they are found in an older age group (older than 55 years) and mainly in the atria. Primary cardiac liposarcomas occur in younger patients (28–37 years) and are found in the right atrium or left ventricle and on the mitral valve. Cardiac liposarcomas may also be metastatic in origin (Figure 30–5).

Ananthasubramaniam K, Farha A: Primary right atrial angiosarcoma mimicking acute pericarditis, pulmonary embolism, and tricuspid stenosis. Heart 1999;81:556–558.

Donsbeck AV, Ranchere D, Coindre JM et al: Primary cardiac sarcomas: An immunohistochemical and grading study with long-term follow-up of 24 cases. Histopathol 1999;34:295–304.

Zanella M, Falconieri G, Bussani R et al: Polypoid osteosarcoma of the left atrium: Report of a new case with autopsy confirmation and review of the literature. Ann Diagn Pathol 1998;2:167–172.

b. Lymphomas—Although cardiac involvement is seen (at autopsy) in 25% of lymphoma patients, primary cardiac lymphoma is extremely rare. It can involve any area of the heart; if the occurrence is intracavitary, it produces obstructive symptoms. The infiltrative nature of this disorder can lead to conduction abnormalities and even congestive heart failure symptoms from restriction.

Mejhert M, Muller-Suur R: Primary lymphoma of the heart. Scand Cardiovasc J 2000;34:606–608.

Tighe DA, Anene CA, Rousou JA et al: Primary cardiac lymphoma. Echo 2000;17:345–347.

c. Mesotheliomas—These malignant pericardial tumors are present with pericarditis or signs of pericardial effusion. There is a 2:1 male predominance, and adults are most frequently afflicted. Pericardial mesotheliomas usually cover most of the parietal and visceral surfaces encasing the heart, with only superficial invasion of adjacent myocardium. Unlike pleural mesotheliomas, pericardial mesotheliomas are not linked to asbestos exposure.

d. Malignant fibrous histiocytomas—These have been reported to occur in the heart, usually in the left atrium. These are very invasive tumors, with a high likelihood of recurrence after surgical resection.

Schena S, Caniglia A, Agnino A et al: Survival following treatment of a cardiac malignant fibrous histiocytoma. Chest 2000;118:271–273.

Vander Salm TJ: Unusual primary tumors of the heart. Semin Thorac Cardiovasc Surg 2000;12:89–100.

Clinical Findings

A. SYMPTOMS AND SIGNS

Cardiac tumors are challenging to diagnose because there are no specifically identifiable symptoms. The anatomic location of the tumor rather than the histopathology determines the clinical findings. Small tumors that cause obstruction of flow may produce symptoms earlier than would large, infiltrative tumors. They usually present in one of the following four ways. Table 30–2 shows a summary of general clinical manifestations related to cardiac neoplasm.

- The majority of patients present with cardiovascular symptoms, such as congestive heart failure or thromboembolism. Arrhythmias and interventricular conduction defects may occur if infiltration of the conduction system is present.

- Patients may present with constitutional symptoms, most commonly with weight loss, fatigue, fever, and arthralgias. Occasionally, there will be cachexia, malaise, Raynaud's phenomenon, rash,

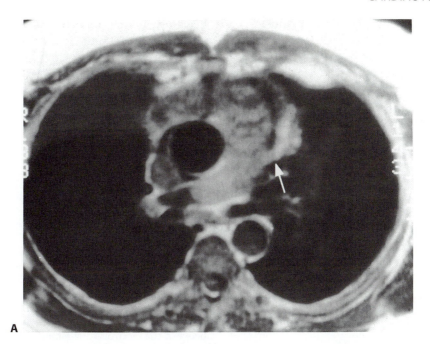

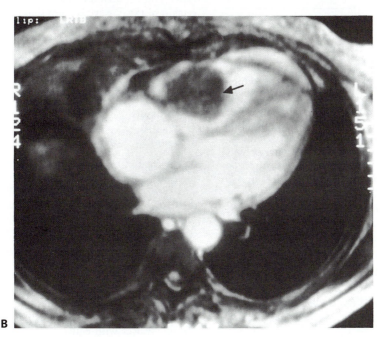

Figure 30–5. Transaxial spin-echo magnetic resonance image of the heart through the level of the main pulmonary artery and right pulmonary artery. **A:** An intermediate-signal-intensity mass (*arrow*) is seen filling both arteries. **B:** Transaxial gradient-echo magnetic resonance image of heart at the midventricular level in the same patient showing a mass in the right ventricle. This patient was found to have a metastatic liposarcoma to the heart from a primary tumor in the leg. *(Courtesy of G Caputo and C Higgins).*

Table 30–2. Clinical manifestations of cardiac neoplasms.

Endocardial
  Thromboembolism: Cerebral, coronary, pulmonary, systemic
  Cavitary obliteration or obstruction
  Valve obstruction and valve damage
  Constitutional manifestations
Myocardial
  Arrhythmias, ventricular and atrial
  Conduction abnormalities
  Electrocardiographic changes
  Radiographic enlargement
Congestive heart failure
Coronary involvement: angina, infarction
Pericardial
  Pericarditis and pain
  Pericardial effusion
  Arrhythmias
  Tamponade
  Constriction
Valvular
  Valvular damage, obstruction, or regurgitation
  Congestive heart failure
  Sudden death or syncope

clubbing, or episodic bizarre behavior. Constitutional manifestations occur in more than 90% of patients with myxomas. Patients may present with an acute febrile illness; the myxomas can simulate peripheral vasculitis or connective tissue disease, secondary to peripheral arterial myxomatous emboli to the skin. Laboratory evaluation may show a normochromic, normocytic, or low-grade hemolytic anemia; polycythemia; thrombocytosis; leukocytosis; and elevated sedimentation rate and immunoglobulin levels.

• Patients with known noncardiac malignancies may develop cardiac metastases with or without cardiovascular symptoms.

• Cardiac tumors can present as an incidental finding on an imaging study, such as a chest radiograph or echocardiogram.

1. Endocardial tumors—Endocardial tumors can lead to embolic events or events related to cardiac obstruction. Emboli may occur to the pulmonary, coronary, carotid, or peripheral circulation. Repeated embolization of right-sided tumors can cause cor pulmonale. Because of their endocardial attachment and mobility as well as the friability of the tumor, myxomas have an embolization rate of 30–40%. Half of these are cerebral emboli, which manifest themselves as transient ischemic attacks, cerebral vascular events, or seizures. The remaining emboli deposit in the spleen, kidneys,

bone, retina, skin, coronary vessels, or distal arterial tree. Embolic events in a young person without another source should raise the suspicion for a myxoma. Left atrial myxoma can cause obstruction by intermittently occluding left ventricular inflow and becoming evident as syncope. Myxomas sometimes prolapse into the mitral orifice and cause mitral regurgitation.

Right-sided tumors can lead to venous congestion and to progressive edema secondary to the obstruction. Rarely, endocardial tumors may produce an endocardial friction rub.

2. Myocardial tumors—These most commonly cause arrhythmias, or disturbances of conduction. For example, new atrioventricular conduction disturbances, such as complete heart block or asystole, can help diagnose a tumor near the atrioventricular node. Atrial fibrillation, atrial flutter, paroxysmal atrial tachycardia with or without block, junctional rhythm, premature ventricular contraction, ventricular tachycardia, and ventricular fibrillation may also be associated with cardiac tumors. Eighty percent of cases of malignant myocardial tumors show ST segment elevation. There is a close correlation between the electrocardiographic lead showing ST elevation and the anatomic location of the infiltration. Inversion of the T wave is a less sensitive and less specific marker of infiltration, occurring in 47% of such cases. When ST-T wave segments remain normal, the infiltration is generally limited to the right side of the heart. Unstable angina with persistent ST segment elevation from compression of the left main coronary artery is caused by metastatic lung cancer.

Krasuski RA, Hesselson AB, Landolfo KP et al: Cardiac rhabdomyoma in an adult patient presenting with ventricular arrhythmia. Chest 2000;118:1217–1221.

3. Pericardial tumors—Pericardial tumors can lead to pericardial pain, constriction, pericardial tamponade, and symptoms related to the invasion of contiguous mediastinal structures. Pericardial invasion occurs most often with the contiguous spread of metastatic breast and lung cancers. In patients with rhabdomyosarcoma involving the pericardium, systemic symptoms and pleuritic chest pain and dyspnea may be present.

Warren WH: Malignancies involving the pericardium. Semin Thorac Cardiovasc Surg 2000;12:119–129.

4. Valvular tumors—These tumors can affect any of the four valves with equal frequency, and the presence of symptoms is common. Mitral valve tumors are more likely than aortic valve tumors to produce serious neurologic symptoms or sudden death. The most common type of valve tumor is the papillary fibroelastoma.

B. PHYSICAL EXAMINATION

1. Left atrial tumors—Physical findings may include signs of pulmonary congestion, a loud, widely split S_1;

an S_4; a holosystolic murmur that is loudest at the apex; a diastolic murmur caused by the obstruction of the mitral valve orifice by the tumor, or a diastolic tumor "plop." The loud S_1 that occurs in patients with left atrial myxoma may be due to delayed mitral valve closure caused by prolapse of the tumor through the valvular orifice. This causes the left ventricular/left atrial pressure curves to intersect at a higher pressure, similar to what is seen in patients with mitral stenosis or a short PR interval. A marked spontaneous variation over short periods with changes in position is characteristic of the diastolic murmur associated with left atrial tumor. The tumor plop is thought to be created by the tumor hitting the endocardial wall or as the excursion of the tumor is halted. Although, in most cases, the plop occurs later than the opening snap of the mitral valve and earlier than the S_3, it can be difficult to distinguish these sounds. Physical findings consistent with mitral stenosis in a patient without a history of rheumatic fever should raise the possibility of a left atrial tumor.

Myxoma is the most common left atrial tumor, and the physical findings can mimic mitral stenosis. Myxomas are associated with a mitral diastolic murmur in 75% of cases; mitral regurgitation murmur in 50%; pulmonary hypertension in 70%; right heart failure in 70%; pulmonary emboli in 25%; anemia in 33%; elevated erythrocyte sedimentation rate in 33%; and a third heart sound (the tumor plop) in 33%.

2. Left ventricular tumors—These are often silent and do not become symptomatic until they grow to be quite large. Patients with infiltrative tumors can present with conduction disease and arrhythmias.

3. Right atrial tumors—Sometimes associated with elevated jugular venous pressure or right-heart failure, right atrial tumors are also often clinically silent and asymptomatic until they become quite large. Twenty percent of myxomas occur in the right atrium and can cause hemodynamic compromise from right ventricular inflow obstruction. Right atrial tumors can interfere with tricuspid valvular function, leading to elevated systemic venous pressure, which is manifested by hepatomegaly, peripheral edema, and ascites. An obstructed venous return leads to a low cardiac output and exertional dyspnea; syncope is often apparent and is probably related to movement of the tumor. A diastolic rumble that varies with respiration should raise the possibility of a right atrial tumor. New and rapidly progressive right-heart failure, with new murmurs and prominent a waves in the jugular venous pulse, also suggests a right atrial tumor.

Elevated right atrial pressure from obstructed blood flow can lead to the opening of a previously closed patent foramen ovale and right-to-left shunting. The arterial oxygen desaturation in these patients can be severe; it can be associated with polycythemia.

4. Right ventricular tumors—The obstruction caused by right ventricular tumors can lead to symptoms of venous congestion and progressive edema. Obstruction of the right ventricular outflow tract from metastatic disease is associated with congestive symptoms, systolic murmur, and right-axis deviation or a right bundle branch conduction abnormality. Acute cor pulmonale can be secondary to metastatic laryngeal carcinoma of the right ventricle, with subsequent tumor emboli to the pulmonary vasculature.

5. Pericardial tumors—Neoplastic pericardial effusions are often painless, although they can be associated with dyspnea and cough, especially if tamponade is present. Other physical findings suggestive of tamponade are tachycardia, tachypnea, narrow pulse pressure and pulsus paradoxus. Pericardial tumors can be associated with a pericardial friction rub or knock.

Kann BR, Kim WJ, Cilley JH Jr: Hemangioma of the right ventricular outflow tract. Ann Thorac Surg 2000;70:975–977.

C. Diagnostic Studies

Advances in noninvasive imaging techniques have facilitated the early diagnosis of cardiac tumors and increased the accuracy and complexity of information available to both the cardiologist and the cardiac surgeon. Angiocardiography and digital subtraction angiography have been replaced by these newer techniques; because routine chest radiographs have a low sensitivity and specificity for tumor detection, they are rarely useful.

1. Echocardiography—With its high resolution and dynamic imaging capability, echocardiographyhas had a major influence on the recognition and treatment of cardiac tumors and has become the diagnostic modality of choice. (It is also efficient, widely available, and cost-effective.) Its sensitivity is highest for endocardial lesions because the mass is easily distinguished from the echolucent chamber; the sensitivity is slightly lower for intramyocardial lesions and lowest for pericardial tumors. The increasing use of ultrasonic contrast can help improve the detection of suspicious masses on echocardiogram. Cardiac tissue characterization by echocardiography may aid in differentiating among thrombus, tumor, and normal tissue.

Transesophageal echocardiography using higher frequency transducers with better resolution provides even more detailed information than does surface echocardiography. It can localize the site of tumor attachment, the involvement of contiguous cardiac structures, and the morphologic features of the tumor. It is especially useful for patients with prosthetic valves, aortic pathology, or suboptimal transthoracic windows. It is also instrumental in differentiating between pathologic findings and normal—or variants of normal—anatomy. Increasingly, transesophageal echocardiography is used to aid cardiac biopsy. In addition, it can also be used as a guide during surgical intervention (Figure 30–6), helping to ensure that there is no residual tumor and that the repaired structures are free of defects. Intraoperative transesophageal echocardiography has proven extremely useful to the surgeon for guidance of tumor resection, particularly in cardiac sarcoma. Follow-up echocardiography is recommended after resection of a myxoma, because of a 5% recurrence rate. Although transesophageal echocardiography generally offers higher resolution imaging than transthoracic echocardiography, the advantage is especially evident when imaging posterior structures (eg, the left atrium) that are distant from the anterior chest wall. It can add useful information to transthoracic echocardiography, particularly for right atrial masses, lesions in the left atrial appendage, and extracardiac masses. In general, surface and transesophageal echocardiography are of similar sensitivity for diagnosing myxoma, but transesophageal echocardiography is superior in visualizing left atrial appendage thrombi, small and flat thrombi in the left atrial cavity, thrombi and tumors in the superior vena cava, and masses attached to the right heart and the descending thoracic aorta.

Dujardin KS, Click RL, Oh JK: The role of intraoperative transesophageal echocardiography in patients undergoing cardiac mass removal. J Am Soc Echocardiogr 2000;13:1080–1083.

Jurkovich D, de Marchena E, Bilsker M, et al: Primary cardiac lymphoma diagnosed by percutaneous intracardiac biopsy with combined fluoroscopic and transesophageal echocardiographic imaging. Catheter Cardiovasc Interv 2000;50:226–233.

Lo FL, Chou YH, Tiu CM et al: Primary cardiac leiomyosarcoma: Imaging with 2-D echocardiography, electron beam CT and 1.5-tesla MR. Eur J Radiol 1998;27:72–76.

2. Computed tomography—Conventional, nongated computed tomography (CT) is most useful in diagnosing paracardiac masses in the region of the pericardium. It can differentiate tissue types and help to identify the type of tumor and its extent within the lungs, mediastinum, pericardium, and cardiac chambers. It also can help in soft-tissue characterization, by using internal references of subcutaneous fat and normal myocardium. The lower intensity of fatty materials can be distin-

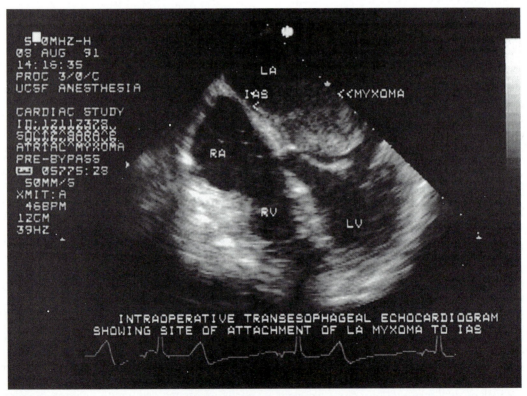

Figure 30–6. Intraoperative transesophageal echocardiogram in the horizontal-plane four-chamber view, showing clearly the site of attachment in the interatrial septum (*single arrowhead*) of a left atrial myxoma (*double arrowheads*). The echocardiogram helps guide the surgeon and evaluate completeness of the resection and postbypass valve integrity. IAS = interatrial septum; LA = left atrium; LV = left ventricle; MV = mitral valve; RV = right ventricle.

guished from the higher intensity of clots and myxomas and other tumors. This differentiation can be increased with contrast enhancement.

Computed tomography is useful in evaluating pericardial tumors, such as mesothelioma, lymphoma, and lipoma and in characterizing cardiac blastomas and rhabdomyosarcomas as well as large primary cardiac tumors that are incompletely visualized by echocardiography. Computed tomography is also superior in identifying tumor involvement of the pericardium when there is no pericardial effusion and in identifying nodular pericardial thickening. Computed tomography imaging may be useful when the mediastinum, pleura, and lungs must also be examined to provide therapeutic guidance and management of cardiac tumors. This modality can show a complete cross section of all cardiac, mediastinal, pulmonary, and thoracic structures (in contrast to angiocardiography), without the anatomic restrictions of echocardiography.

Ultrafast CT and more recently electron beam computed tomography (EB-CT), which are increasingly available, overcome the limitation caused by cardiac motion in conventional CT (the motion artifacts reduce the quality of the image) by using continuous high-speed scanning, with 50–100 ms exposures. This improves the detection of para- and intracardiac masses, and the images have excellent spatial and density resolution. The technique also allows a movie mode, adding information to the static images; because it avoids superimposition of other tissues, it is useful in evaluating multiple masses.

Araoz PA, Eklund HE, Welch TJ et al: CT and MR imaging of primary cardiac malignancies. Radiographics 1999;19:1421–1434.

Grebenc ML, Rosado de Christenson ML, Burke AP: Primary cardiac and pericardial neoplasms: radiologic-pathologic correlation. Radiographics 2000;20:1073–1103.

3. Magnetic resonance imaging—MRI is a three-dimensional imaging technique that can be used to supplement the information provided by echocardiography about cardiac masses. The high natural contrast between the blood pool and cardiovascular structures allows internal cardiac structures to be visualized by this technique. Magnetic resonance imaging's ability to characterize fat also makes it superior to CT for identifying lipomas and their relationship to coronary arteries (Figure 30–7). Its direct multiplanar imaging capability is advantageous in demonstrating vessels and vessel/mass relationships. This capability makes it superior to CT for such areas as the aortopulmonic window and subcarinal region and lesions at the cervicothoracic or thoracoabdominal junction. Magnetic resonance imaging can be useful for surgical planning in questions of chest wall invasion, brachial plexus involvement, and extension to the diaphragm, pericardium, or lung apex.

The coronal or sagittal format makes MRI useful in planning radiation therapy. Structures such as the trachea and the superior vena cava can be evaluated in their plane of anatomic orientation. Although MRI may be useful for detecting pericardial tumor involvement, its reconstruction imaging technique often makes small mobile tumors difficult or impossible to image.

Magnetic resonance imaging also has the potential for tissue characterization. It has been used with cardiac tagging to differentiate contractile from noncontractile tissue in neonates with congenital cardiac rhabdomyoma and can be useful in evaluating tumor response and recurrence in patients after radiation therapy. Fibrous tissue remains at low signal intensity on T_2-weighted images; tumors have an increased signal intensity, which can also serve as a guide to the appropriate site for biopsy to confirm recurrence. No imaging technique, however, can reliably distinguish between a benign and a malignant cardiac mass.

In a study of patients whose intracavitary tumors were first detected by transthoracic echocardiography, MRI offered important additional information—except in patients whose echocardiograms indicated myxomas (Figure 30–8). No study to date has compared MRI to transesophageal echocardiography for the evaluation of cardiac tumors.

Siripornpitak S, Higgins CB: MRI of primary malignant cardiovascular tumors. J Comput Assist Tomogr 1997;21:462–466.

Wintersperger BJ, Becker CR, Gulbins H et al: Tumors of the cardiac valves: Imaging findings in magnetic resonance imaging, electron beam computed tomography, and echocardiography. Eur Radiol 2000;10:443–449.

4. Cardiac catheterization—Coronary arteriography is indicated in patients older than 50 years before surgical tumor resection, if there is a high risk of coronary artery stenosis. Angiography can also help confirm a diagnosis of myxoma, by locating a tumor blush (caused by opacification of the tumor vasculature). Right-heart catheterization is contraindicated in patients with right ventricular outflow-tract obstruction because of adverse hemodynamic consequences.

Differential Diagnosis

The differential diagnosis of cardiac masses includes tumors, thrombus, nonbacterial thrombotic endocarditis, vegetations, flail or prolapsing valve leaflets, giant aneurysm of the coronary artery, pericardial cysts, and even diaphragmatic hernia. Clinical features that help suggest a diagnosis of tumors are a known primary malignancy, particularly breast or lung cancer; constitutional symptoms; and embolic phenomena. Left atrial thrombi are seen in the setting of mitral valve disease, enlarged left atrium, and atrial fibrillation, while ventricular thrombi are associated with cardiomyopathies or regional wall-motion abnormalities. Right atrial

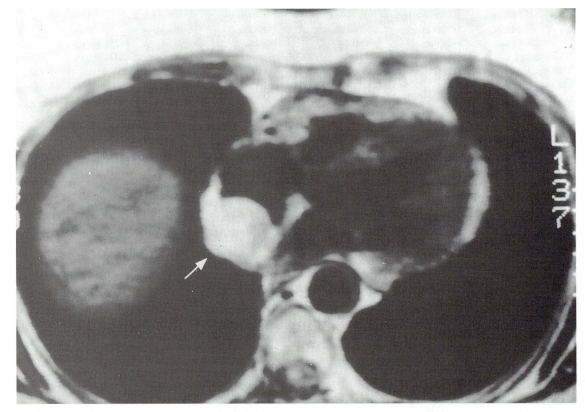

Figure 30–7. Transaxial spin-echo magnetic resonance image of the heart through the level of the right atrium. A high-signal-intensity mass (*arrow*) is adherent to the posterior aspect of right atrial wall. This signal intensity is characteristic of fat in this patient with a right atrial lipoma. *(Courtesy of G Caputo and C Higgins).*

thrombi are seen in the setting of indwelling central venous lines, pulmonary artery catheters or pacemaker wires (Figure 30–9).

Noninfective thrombotic endocarditis is found in debilitated patients with chronic, progressive diseases. The valvular vegetation of noninfective thrombotic endocarditis occurs on the left side of the heart in 90% of cases, unless a chronic indwelling right-sided catheter has been present. Pericardial cysts can be identified by their unilocular nature and their location in either the right or left costophrenic angle. They have a typical radiographic appearance; once diagnosed, they require no intervention. Diaphragmatic hernia can mimic a left atrial mass on transthoracic echocardiography. Transesophageal echocardiography, on the other hand, can help to diagnose the hernia by showing an extracardiac structure indenting the left atrium posteriorly and the swirling nonuniform echo densities within this structure caused by motion of the gastric contents.

Although lipomatous cardiac infiltration can mimic a tumor, it can be distinguished by its characteristic location (atrial septum) and dumbbell-shaped appearance (Figure 30–10). The shape is due to the thin fossa vallis that separates the lipomatous atrial septum on either side. The incidence of lipomatous septal hypertrophy increases with age and has some association with diabetes; its clinical significance is its association with atrial arrhythmias. Treatment is limited to controlling arrhythmias; surgical therapy is not warranted.

A number of normal variants of anatomic structures are occasionally confused with tumors. These include the Chiari network, a remnant of the sinus venosus seen in the right atrium (Figure 30–11); the eustachian valve (the valve of the inferior vena cava) and the septum spurium, both also seen in the right atrium; the thebesian valve; and the floor of the left superior pulmonary vein adjacent to the left atrial appendage. An aneurysm of the atrial septum, which can be quite large and mobile, may resemble a right atrial myxoma. It is important to recognize these as normal—or normal variants of—anatomic structures. Imaging features that favor a diagnosis of tumor are a mobile, pedunculated appearance and an associated pericardial effusion. Thrombi may also appear pedunculated, but their clin-

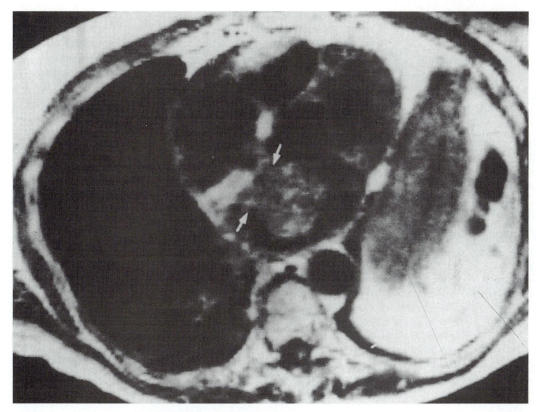

Figure 30–8. Transaxial spin-echo magnetic resonance image of the heart through the level of both atria. A pedunculated mass *(arrows)* is seen attached to the interatrial septum; its intermediate intensity is typical of left atrial myxoma. *(Courtesy of G Caputo and C Higgins).*

ical setting distinguishes them from tumors. Masses that cross anatomic planes—from myocardium to pericardium or endocardium—are likely to be tumors.

Treatment

A. Pharmacologic Therapy

Pharmacologic therapy can be an important adjunct or alternative therapy for malignant tumors and is essential in patients with primary cardiac tumors and extracardiac metastases. It is unknown whether adjuvant chemotherapy is beneficial in patients in whom so-called curative surgery has been performed. The results of treating cardiac sarcomas with the alkylating agents, dactinomycin, doxorubicin, and vincristine have been disappointing. A combination of several agents is thought to be more effective than single-agent therapy. Adjuvant chemotherapy overall has not been effective in malignant cardiac neoplasms.

Llombart-Cussac A, Pivot X, Contesso G et al: Adjuvant chemotherapy for primary cardiac sarcomas: the IGR experience. Br J Cancer 1998;78:1624–1628.

B. Radiation

Adjuvant radiotherapy can be helpful if total surgical excision is not successful or curative for malignant tumors. One review reports a more-than-twofold increase in survival, from 9.6 months to 22.7 months, with postoperative mediastinal radiation (the average course of radiation was 5220 rads over a 1-month period). Radiation (compared with repeated pericardiocentesis) may prolong life in patients with pericardial metastases; however, high doses of radiation can lead to cardiac damage.

Movsas B, Teruya-Feldstein J, Smith J et al: Primary cardiac sarcoma: A novel treatment approach. Chest 1998;114:648–652.

C. Surgery

Because of embolic complications and the limited capacity of the heart to tolerate space-occupying lesions, most cardiac tumors—benign or malignant—require prompt surgical removal.

1. Benign tumors—Myxomas should be removed expeditiously because of their high embolic potential.

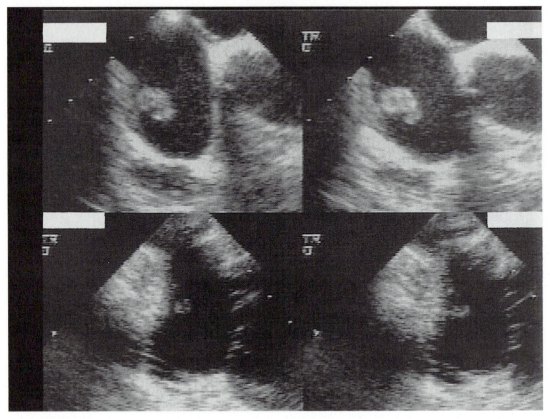

Figure 30–9. Serial transesophageal echocardiograms for evaluation of a right atrial mass in a 24-year-old woman with an indwelling central venous hyperalimentation line. The span between the top and bottom studies, showing a marked interval diminution in size, was 3 months. The size reduction, the mobility of this mass, the lack of myocardial invasion, the atypical location for a myxoma, and the clinical history support the diagnosis of right atrial thrombus. Signal strength of a cine-MRI in the same patient also favored a diagnosis of a clot.

Lipomas are often asymptomatic and do not require further treatment. Because large papillary fibroelastomas are a nidus for platelet aggregation, resection is recommended to prevent emboli. Small papillary fibroelastomas, such as Lambl's excrescences, on an elderly patient's aortic leaflets need not be resected. Present data suggest a conservative approach to treatment of rhabdomyomas in asymptomatic patients. A recent study showed resolution of 20 of 24 rhabdomyomas over a 2–15-year period. Although surgery is indicated for symptomatic patients (a large mass can cause inflow and outflow obstruction), it can be difficult because these tumors tend to be multiple, nonencapsulated, and embedded in the myocardium. Patients may need inotropic support in the postoperative period because of the extensive surgical dissection, which often involves the myocardium. Fibromas are often large (4–7 cm in diameter); prompt surgery is recommended. Excision may remove much ventricular myocardium.

Complete excision is recommended, because any fibroma that remains may be a focus for ventricular arrhythmias. Reconstructive surgery with a synthetic patch may be necessary.

2. Malignant tumors—Although total surgical resection for sarcoma is often impossible, surgery is done to relieve compressive or obstructive symptoms in some cases. Surgery is rarely performed to remove metastatic tumor masses unless a cure of the primary tumor is highly likely. In additional to high in-hospital mortality rate, surgery for malignant tumors remains palliative without effective adjuvant therapy. Prognosis of malignant cardiac tumor is overall extremely poor.

Almassi GH: Surgery for tumors with cavoatrial extension. Semin Thorac Cardiovasc Surg 2000;12:111–118.

Centofanti P, Di Rosa E, Deorsola L et al: Primary cardiac tumors: Early and late results of surgical treatment in 91 patients. Ann Thorac Surg 1999;68:1236–1241.

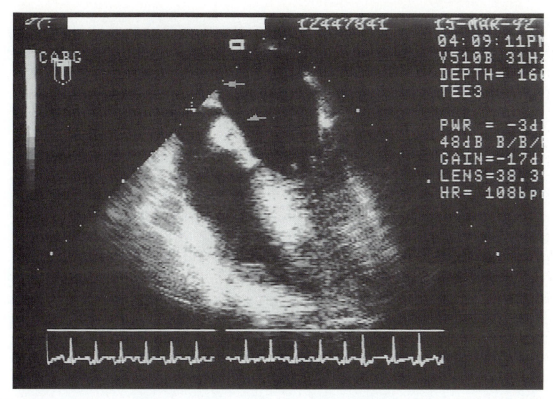

Figure 30–10. Transesophageal echocardiogram in the horizontal plane. Four-chamber view showing lipomatous hypertrophy of the interatrial septum (*arrows*). Note the dumbell-shaped appearance.

Schaff HV, Mullany CJ: Surgery for cardiac myxomas. Semin Thorac Cardiovasc Surg 2000;12:77–88.

D. PERICARDIOCENTESIS

Symptomatic neoplastic effusions, such those seen in metastatic breast or lung cancer, may require pericardiocentesis, and recurrent effusions may require partial pericardiectomy. Echocardiographic guidance is generally preferred. Instilling isotopes or sclerosing agents such as tetracyclines and chemotherapeutic agents in the pericardial space has been successfully used to prevent such recurrences; recurrence rates are 13–50% after pericardiocentesis for recurrent malignant pericardial disease. In one review of medical and surgical experience subxiphoid pericardiocentesis with intrapericardial sclerotherapy proved to be as effective as open surgical drainage for the management of malignant pericardial effusions. In a separate series of consecutive patients with malignant pericardial effusion at the Mayo Clinic, echocardiographically guided pericardiocentesis with extended catheter drainage appeared to be safe and effective

Other modalities for neoplastic pericardial effusion includes subxiphoid pericardiostomy, percutaneous balloon pericardiostomy, and more aggressive open procedure for drainage and pericardectomy. The therapeutic approach needs to be individualized. For example, a patient with recurrent pericardial effusion but with otherwise acceptable surgical risks may benefit from subxiphoid pericardiostomy, which has a recurrent rate generally of less than 5%. In the critically ill, percutaneous approach may be preferred. In loculated disease, open incision or drainage may be necessary.

Fiocco M, Krasna MJ: The management of malignant pleural and pericardial effusions. Hematol Oncol Clin North Am 1997; 11:253–265.

Girardi LN, Ginsberg RJ, Burt ME: Pericardiocentesis and intrapericardial sclerosis: Effective therapy for malignant pericardial effusions. Ann Thorac Surg 1997;64:1422–1427.

Tsang TS, Seward JB, Barnes ME et al: Outcomes of primary and secondary treatment of pericardial effusion in patients with malignancy. Mayo Clin Proc 2000;75:248–253.

E. CARDIAC TRANSPLANTATION

An increasing number of reports have cited the use cardiac transplantation as an alternative therapy for unresectable cardiac tumors, for example, when infiltration by fibroma is too extensive for excision. This approach remains experimental and is limited by the potential for posttransplant recurrence, which can theoretically be

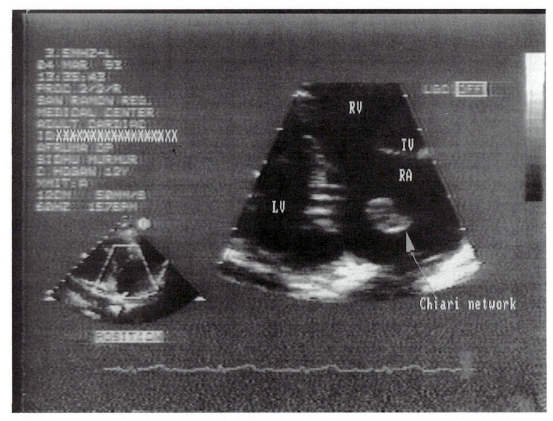

Figure 30–11. Transthoracic echocardiogram in a right ventricular inflow view showing a prominent Chiari network (*arrow*), a normal variant. RA = right atrium; RV = right ventricle; LV = left ventricle; TV = tricuspid valve.

accelerated by immunosuppressive therapy. In a review of 28 patients with cardiac neoplasms who underwent transplantation, the mean survival of patients with benign tumors was 46 months compared to 12 months for patients with malignant tumors.

Gowdamarajan A, Michler RE: Therapy for primary cardiac tumors: Is there a role for heart transplantation? Curr Opin Cardiol 2000;15:121–125.

Michler RE, Goldstein DJ: Treatment of cardiac tumors by orthotopic cardiac transplantation. Semin Oncol 1997;24:534–539.

Prognosis

A. METASTATIC TUMORS

The prognosis here depends on the pathology of the primary tumor, but it is generally poor.

B. PRIMARY TUMORS

Surgical resection usually results in cure of benign cardiac tumors. Approximately 1.5% of myxomas (12–22% in patients with familial or syndrome-related myxomas)

recur within 10–15 years. Because of this small risk of recurrence, patients should be followed with periodic echocardiography every 1–2 years for 15 years following the resection.

Long-term results for primary malignant tumors are disappointing, usually because of early metastatic or local spread or recurrence. Postoperative survival ranged from 2 to 55 months in one series, with a mean of 14 months.

CARDIAC TOXICITIES FROM ONCOLOGIC TREATMENTS

General Considerations

With improved survival of various oncologic conditions, more patients are surviving to present with early or especially late adverse cardiac effects related to the treatment. Fortunately, because of increasing recognition of some of these potential toxicities, modern treatment protocols have been modified to minimize side effects. Nevertheless, it is important to recognize some of the adverse outcomes related to earlier treatments because of living survivors. At the same time, one needs to be cognizant of potential late effects of contemporary therapy.

A. CHEMOTHERAPY

1. Anthracyclines—These drugs are all associated with cardiac toxicities. The most important offending anthracyclines include daunorubicin and doxorubicin. Clinical manifestations include arrhythmias, pericardial effusion, and myocardial dysfunction with the development of permanent cardiomyopathy. Myocardial dysfunction is by far the most important and can occur acutely, subacutely, or late (after years of treatment). The cardiac toxicity is dose-dependent. In one study, patients who received 550 mg/m^2 of doxorubicin, incidence of cardiac failure is 30%. This recognition led to the concept of a threshold cumulative dose to reduce cardiac toxicities. Older patients and patients with lymphoma are most at risk for adverse effects.

Baseline cardiac evaluation with echocardiography or radionuclide cardiac imaging to assess ventricular function is recommended in all patients. For patients who receive a cumulative dose of 300 mg/m^2, serial evaluation is required. The total cumulative dose is recommended at less that 450 mg/m^2. In patients with equivocal results on serial monitoring, endomyocardial biopsy may be necessary. Combination and cardioprotective agent are currently being used and undergoing evaluation to minimize side effects.

2. Cyclophosphamide—Cyclophosphamide can lead to endothelial capillary damage, resulting in hemorrhagic complications. Red cells can extravasate into cardiac and pulmonary tissues, leading to pericardial effusion, pulmonary edema, endocardial, and myocardial bleeding. In addition, systolic or diastolic dysfunction, restrictive cardiomyopathy have also been associated with cyclophosphamide use. In general pretreatment radionuclide left ventricular ejection fraction of less than 50–55% is correlated with increased incidence of cardiac toxicities. The most common complication is the development of small-to-moderate pericardial effusion. Pericardiocentesis is usually not necessary. Analgesics and steroids with serial echocardiographic monitoring are effective treatment.

3. Retinoic acid—Retinoic acid produces a syndrome in up to 25% of cases, with manifestations of fever, dyspnea, pleural and pericardial effusion, pulmonary infiltrates, peripheral edema, and transient myocardial dysfunction. This syndrome is usually responsive to steroid therapy.

4. Paclitaxel (Taxol)—Paclitaxel commonly leads to electrocardiographic (ECG) changes and cardiac rhythm disturbances. In a phase II study of ovarian cancer, sinus

bradycardia is seen in 29% of the patients. In addition, more progressive rhythm abnormalities such as atrioventricular conduction abnormalities, complete heart block, and even asystole have been reported. Fortunately, these conduction abnormalities are usually reversible with the termination of treatment. Thus, continuous ECG monitoring is advised during treatment.

5. 5-Fluorouracil—This drug is frequently associated with cardiotoxicity. In a study with continuous ECG monitoring, 68% of the patients exhibited ischemic ECG changes. Reported side effects include precordial pain (anginal or nonspecific), ST-T changes on ECG, rare myocardial infarction, arrhythmia, ventricular dysfunction, cardiac failure, pulmonary edema, cardiogenic shock, and sudden death. In general, ECG changes resolve following termination of treatment, and anginal symptoms are responsive to conservative medical treatment. More malignant cardiac abnormalities are far less common to rare. As such, careful monitoring of ECG and symptoms is generally recommended.

6. Other common agents—Other agents such as vincristine and vinblastine can lead to cardiac autonomic dysfunction with rate myocardial infarction or angina even in the absence of coronary artery disease. Mitomycin C can act to potentiate anthracycline toxicity. Cisplatin can lead to arrhythmia. Interferon is associated with the development of arrhythmia or congestive heart failure. Many other agents, such as mitoxantrone, amsacrine, and, more recently, trastuzumab, which are used in combination with anthracyclines in breast cancer, are also associated with cardiac toxicities.

Brockstein BE, Smiley C, Al-Sadir J et al: Cardiac and pulmonary toxicity in patients undergoing high-dose chemotherapy for lymphoma and breast cancer: prognostic factors. Bone Marrow Transplant 2000;25:885–894.

Feldman AM, Lorell BH, Reis SE: Trastuzumab in the treatment of metastatic breast cancer: Anticancer therapy versus cardiotoxicity. Circulation 2000;102:272–274.

Sparano JA: Doxorubicin/taxane combinations: Cardiac toxicity and pharmacokinetics. Semin Oncol 1999;26(Suppl):14–19.

B. RADIATION

Radiation-induced heart disease involves most structures of the heart (Table 30–3). Pericardial involvement is the most common cardiac toxicity. For patients who had undergone radiation to the chest, pericardial effusion was reported in 6–30% of the patients. In the past, acute pericarditis was seen in 10–15% of the patients with Hodgkin's disease. Today contemporary delivery of radiation has led to a dramatic decrease of pericardial disease estimated now at about 2–2.5% of patients. However, survivors of past treatment of radiation such as the Hodgkin's disease survivors are still at risk for late development of pericardial complications such as constrictive pericarditis. A history of past irradiation to the

Table 30–3. Clinical manifestations of radiation-induced heart disease.

Pericardial disease
  Acute pericarditis
  Delayed pericarditis
  Pericardial effusion
  Constrictive pericarditis
Myocardial disease
  Ventricular dysfunction
  Myocarditis
Valvular heart disease
  Predominantly mitral and aortic valves
Electrical conduction disturbances
Coronary artery disease

---

chest (especially with greater than 40 Gy) and unexplained signs or symptoms of constriction should raise the index of suspicion for constrictive pericarditis. Diagnosis may involve a combination of echocardiographic, MRI/CT, and invasive cardiac hemodynamics evaluations. Afflicted patients will often require pericardectomy.

Furthermore, radiation is associated with an increased incidence of early ischemic heart disease, the worsening of valvular heart disease, and the development of electrical abnormalities.

Gregor A: How to improve effects of radiation and control its toxicity. Ann Oncol 2000;3(Suppl):231.

Keefe DL: Cardiovascular emergencies in the cancer patient. Semin Oncol 2000;27:244.

Heart Disease in Pregnancy

Syed W. Bokhari, MD & Cheryl L. Reid, MD

ESSENTIALS OF DIAGNOSIS

- *Pregnancy*
- *History of heart disease*
- *Symptoms and signs of heart disease*
- *Echocardiographic evidence of heart disease*

General Considerations

Heart disease (most frequently congenital or valvular diseases) occurs in 1–4% of pregnancies, and the incidence is increasing. The unique hemodynamic changes associated with pregnancy make diagnosis and management of heart disease in pregnant patients a challenge to the physicians, who must consider not only the patient but also the risks to the fetus.

Danzell JD: Pregnancy and pre-existing heart disease. J La State Med Soc 1998;150(2):97.

Physiology & Etiology

A. CARDIOVASCULAR PHYSIOLOGY OF "NORMAL" PREGNANCY

Normal pregnancy is accompanied by significant physiologic changes, although underlying mechanisms remain virtually unknown (Table 31–1). The normal signs and symptoms associated with pregnancy may obscure the diagnosis of heart disease during that time. The clinician must, therefore, have a thorough knowledge of these normal changes and the aspects of the history and physical examination that suggest the presence of heart disease.

1. Blood volume—The increase in maternal blood volume begins as early as the sixth week of pregnancy, peaks at approximately 32 weeks of gestation, and stays at that level (40–50% higher than pregestational levels) until delivery. The plasma volume shows a more rapid and significant rise than the red blood cell mass, ac-

counting for the appearance of **physiologic anemia during pregnancy.** The increased blood volume is maintained until after delivery, when a spontaneous diuresis occurs. This rapid postpartum change in blood volume is a critical period for patients with underlying heart disease.

2. Cardiac function—Normal pregnancy is characterized by enhanced myocardial performance. Numerous studies have shown a gradual increase in left ventricular systolic function attributed to left ventricular afterload reduction due to the low-resistance runoff of the placenta. Then rise in left ventricular systolic function begins in early pregnancy, peaks in the twentieth week, and then remains constant until delivery.

3. Cardiac output—One of the most significant changes during pregnancy is the increase in cardiac output, which begins to rise during the first trimester and peaks at twenty-fifth and thirty-fifth weeks of gestation. Total cardiac output increases up to 50% over pregestational levels. Cardiac output is the product of stroke volume and heart rate. During the early part of pregnancy, the increase in cardiac output is predominantly the result of an increase in stroke volume, augmented by increased intrinsic myocardial contractility. As preg-

Table 31–1. Cardiovascular changes in normal pregnancy.

Increase	Decrease
Blood volume	Systolic arterial pressure
Heart rate	Diastolic arterial pressure
Stroke volume	Systemic vascular resistance
Cardiac output	Peripheral vascular resistance
Pulse pressure	
Left ventricular end-diastolic pressure	
Venous compliance and volume	

nancy advances, heart rate increases and stroke volume mildly decreases. The increased cardiac output in late pregnancy is maintained because of the increased heart rate.

A unique aspect of pregnancy is the hemodynamic changes induced by a change in a patient's position. When the patient is in the supine position, the gravid uterus induces profound mechanical compression of the inferior vena cava, decreasing venous return to the heart, and thus, cardiac output. A change from the supine to the left lateral position results in a 25–30% increase in cardiac output because of an increase in stroke volume.

4. Intravascular pressures and vascular resistance—Systolic and diastolic pressures drop during pregnancy. A small decrease in systolic blood pressure begins in the first trimester, peaks at midgestation, and returns to near prepregnancy levels at term. The diastolic blood pressure decreases more than the systolic blood pressure, due to a significant fall in systemic vascular resistance, and results in a wider pulse pressure. The systemic blood pressure increases during pregnancy with the patient's age and parity. It also varies with the patient's position. The highest levels are recorded early in the pregnancy when the patient is upright, and lowest when she is supine. During the latter part of pregnancy the effect of position on systemic blood pressure depends on the relative degrees of inferior vena cava and aortic compression. Total vascular resistance, including both the systemic and the pulmonary, decrease during pregnancy. The mechanism for the fall in resistances is poorly understood but is attributed to the low-resistance circulation of the pregnant uterus and to hormonal changes associated with pregnancy.

Thornburg KL, Jacobson SL, Giraud GD et al: Hemodynamic changes in pregnancy. Semin Perinatol 2000;24(1):11.

Gilson GJ, Samaan S, Crawford MH et al: Changes in Hemodynamics, ventricular remodeling, and ventricular contractility during normal pregnancy: A longitudinal study. Obstet Gynecol 1997;89(6):957.

Poppas A, Shroff SG, Korcarz CE et al: Serial assessment of the cardiovascular system in normal pregnancy. Role of arterial compliance and pulsatile arterial load. Circulation 1997;20; 95(10):2407.

B. ETIOLOGY AND SYMPTOMATOLOGY

1. Congenital heart disease—As medical and surgical treatment of such patients has improved, congenital heart disease is found more frequently during pregnancy. As a result, more women with either uncorrected or surgically corrected congenital heart diseases are surviving into the adulthood (Table 31–2).

Only a few conditions place a patient at a high risk to advise against pregnancy (Table 31–3). A majority of the patients with mild to moderate acyanotic congeni-

Table 31–2. Common congenital abnormalities found in pregnant women.

Uncorrected malformations
Acyanotic
Atrial septal defect
Patent ductus arteriosus
Pulmonic valve stenosis
Coarctation of aorta
Aortic valve disease
Cyanotic
Tetralogy of Fallot
Surgically corrected malformations

tal heart disease tolerate pregnancy, labor, and delivery well. Treatment should involve frequent counseling by the obstetrician and cardiologist. In severe cases, physical activity and salt intake limitation, early treatment of any infection, heart failure, and arrhythmia should be undertaken. Cesarean delivery should be reserved only for obstetric indications because most patients can be safely delivered vaginally.

High-risk patients with severe cyanotic congenital heart disease, decreased functional capacity, or Eisenmenger's syndrome should be advised against pregnancy. Antibiotic prophylaxis for bacterial endocarditis is recommended in most patients with congenital heart disease. The risk of fetal malformation in the offspring should be considered carefully.

a. Atrial septal defect—Secundum atrial septal defect is the most common congenital cardiac abnormality encountered during pregnancy. Patients with uncomplicated atrial septal defects usually tolerate pregnancy with little problem. Patients may not be able to tolerate the acute blood loss that can occur at the time of delivery because of increased shunting from left to right caused by systemic vasoconstriction associated with hypotension. The incidence of supraventricular arrhythmias may increase in older pregnant patients, which may result in right ventricular failure and venous stasis leading to paradoxical emboli. Low-dose aspirin, once daily after the first trimester until delivery may

Table 31–3. Relative contraindications to pregnancy.

1. Pulmonic vasoocclusive disease
2. Severe pulmonary hypertension
3. Marfan's syndrome with a dilated aortic root
4. Severe aortic stenosis
5. Eisenmenger's syndrome
6. Severe ventricular systolic dysfunction
7. Cyanotic heart disease

help prevent clot formation. Pulmonary hypertension from an atrial septal defect usually occurs late in life, past the childbearing years. Bacterial endocarditis prophylaxis is recommended only for ostium primum defect due to associated aortic valve abnormality. Vaginal delivery is preferred over cesarean. Risk in the offspring is about 2.5%.

b. Ventricular septal defect—Most isolated ventricular septal defects have closed by adulthood. Women with ventricular septal defects generally fare well in pregnancy. Congestive heart failure and arrhythmia are reported only in patients with decreased left ventricular systolic function prior to pregnancy. Endocarditis prophylaxis during delivery, preferably vaginal, is recommended.

c. Patent ductus arteriosus—Most patients with a patent ductus arteriosus undergo surgical repair in childhood. A normal pregnancy can be expected in patients with small-to-moderate shunts and no evidence of pulmonary hypertension. Patients with a large patent ductus arteriosus, elevated pulmonary vascular resistance, and a reversed shunt are at greatest risk for complications during pregnancy. The decreased systemic vascular resistance associated with pregnancy increases the right-to-left shunt and the intrauterine oxygen desaturation. Patients developing heart failure are treated with digoxin and diuretics. The preferred mode of delivery is vaginal in most patients with endocarditis prophylaxis and hemodynamic monitoring considered at the time of delivery. The risk in an offspring is about 4%.

d. Pulmonic stenosis—The natural history of pulmonic stenosis favors survival into adulthood even with severe obstruction to right ventricular outflow. Mild-to-moderate pulmonic stenosis (peak gradient ≤100 mm Hg) usually presents no increased risk during pregnancy. Patients with severe pulmonic stenosis may occasionally tolerate pregnancy without developing congestive heart failure. Vaginal delivery is tolerated well. Ideal treatment consisting of balloon valvuloplasty should be performed before gestation. The risk in the offspring is about 3.5%.

e. Coarctation of the aorta—In uncomplicated coarctation of the aorta, pregnancy is usually safe for the mother but may be associated with fetal underdevelopment because of the diminished uterine blood flow. The blood pressure may decrease slightly, as during normal pregnancy, but still remains elevated. Maternal deaths in these patients are usually the result of aortic rupture or cerebral hemorrhage from an associated berry aneurysm of the circle of Willis. Patients with the greatest risk during pregnancy are those with severe hypertension or associated cardiac abnormalities, such as bicuspid aortic valves, which increase the risk of endocarditis. Treatment consists of limitation of physi-

cal activity and maintenance of systolic blood pressure around 140 mm Hg for fetal circulation. Beta-blockers should be used preferably and continued through delivery. Most patients undergo vaginal delivery with endocarditis prophylaxis. Surgical treatment should be reserved for patients who develop complications, eg, aortic dissection, uncontrollable hypertension, and refractory heart failure.

f. Congenital aortic stenosis—Congenital bicuspid aortic valve is usually more common in men, but occasional cases of aortic stenosis may be encountered in pregnant women. In patients with congenital aortic stenosis, the outcome during pregnancy depends on the severity of the obstruction. Pregnancy is usually well tolerated in mild-to-moderate aortic stenosis. Patients with severe aortic stenosis with an area of <1.0 cm^2 and peak transvalvular gradients greater than 100 mm Hg may experience an increased risk of complications. The increased cardiac output and decreased systemic vascular resistance of pregnancy creates an additional hemodynamic instability in these patients. Syncope, cerebral symptoms, dyspnea, angina pectoris, and even heart failure may occur for the first time during pregnancy. Ideally, valvuloplasty in symptomatic patients should be performed before pregnancy. Valvuloplasty, if needed, is preferred over surgery during pregnancy. There is a 4% concordance rate in the offspring.

g. Tetralogy of Fallot—This is the most common cyanotic congenital heart disease found in pregnant patients. The syndrome consists of pulmonary stenosis, right ventricular hypertrophy, an overriding aorta, and a ventricular septal defect. The decrease in systemic vascular resistance, the increased cardiac output, and the increased venous return to the right heart augment the amount of right-to-left shunt and further decrease the systemic arterial saturation. Acute blood loss during postpartum hemorrhage is particularly dangerous because venous return to the right heart is impaired. The labile hemodynamics during labor and the peripartum period may precipitate cyanosis, syncope, and even death in surgically untreated women (see Table 31-3). Patients who have had good surgical repair may anticipate successful pregnancies. The risk in the offspring is approximately 4%.

2. Congenital heart disease that has been surgically corrected—The obstetrical care of patients who have had surgical correction of a congenital heart disease requires an understanding of the type of surgical procedure, the sequelae, and the hemodynamic consequences. Although atrial flutter may occasionally develop following surgical closure, the successful closure of an uncomplicated atrial septal defect results in no increased maternal risk during pregnancy. Surgical closure of a patent ductus arteriosus that is not associated with pulmonary hypertension is also not associated with maternal complications during pregnancy. In pulmonary hypertension that develops before surgical closure, the decrease in the pulmonary vascular resistance may not be complete, and complications during pregnancy will depend on its severity. Correction of congenital pulmonary stenosis with either surgery or balloon dilatation that leaves little or no transvalvular gradient presents no difficulty to pregnant patients. Surgical correction of coarctation of the aorta with complete relief of the obstruction decreases the development of associated hypertension and the risk of aortic rupture during pregnancy. Successful repair of tetralogy of Fallot with little residual gradient across the pulmonary outflow tract and relief of the cyanosis should result, with careful management, in a normal pregnancy. Pregnancy after repair of complex congenital heart disease is increasingly encountered. In such patients, the outcome depends on the mother's functional status, the type of repair, the sequelae, and the cardiovascular response to an increase in stress.

Schmaltz AA, Neudorf U, Winkler UH: Outcome of pregnancy in women with congenital heart diseases. Cardiol Young 1999; 9(1):88.

Colman JM, Sermer M, Seaward PG et al: Congenital heart disease in pregnancy. Cardiol Rev 2000;8(3):166.

3. Rheumatic heart disease—High rates of teenage pregnancies in combination with endemic prevalence of rheumatic fever in developing countries makes cardiac disease a serious comorbidity in pregnancy. The incidence of rheumatic heart disease is on the rise, and its prevalence in complicating pregnancy has been reported to be 0.7%. Mild rheumatic fever may be difficult to diagnose in pregnancy due to tachycardia, functional murmur, and anemia. The management of acute rheumatic fever is similar in pregnant and nonpregnant patients and consists of bed rest, anemia correction, and penicillin. In severe cases, vasodilators, positive inotropes, or even surgery may be required. Commonly encountered valvular lesions are mitral stenosis (90%), mitral regurgitation (7%), and aortic regurgitation.

4. Valvular heart disease—No randomized controlled trial data are available to guide decision making for pregnant women with valvular heart disease. However, many patients with valvular heart disease can be treated successfully through their pregnancy with conservative medical treatment, focusing on optimization of intravascular volume and systemic load. Ideally, symptomatic patients should be treated before conception. Drugs, in general, should be avoided whenever possible. Antibiotics for infective endocarditis prophylaxis for uncomplicated vaginal delivery are not indicated, although many practitioners routinely administer antibiotics for high-risk patients, eg, with prosthetic valves, history of endocarditis, or complex congenital heart disease (Table 31–4).

Table 31–4. Valvular disease associated with high maternal or fetal risk during pregnancy.

1. Severe aortic stenosis
2. Aortic regurgitation with NYHA class III-IV CHF
3. Aortic regurgitation in Marfan's syndrome
4. Mitral stenosis or regurgitation with NYHA class III-IV CHF
5. Aortic or mitral valve disease with severe pulmonary hypertension (PASP >75 mm Hg)
7. Aortic or mitral valve disease with left ventricular dysfunction (EF <40%)
8. Mitral valve prosthesis requiring anticoagulation

EF = ejection fraction; HF = heart failure; NYHA = New York Heart Association; PASP = pulmonary artery systolic pressure.

a. Mitral valve disorders—Mitral stenosis is not only the most common rheumatic valvular disorder, it is also most likely to develop serious complications. In critical mitral stenosis, due to a large diastolic gradient, even at rest, any demand of increased cardiac output results in a significant elevation in the left atrial pressure and pulmonary edema. The most common symptoms include dyspnea, fatigue, orthopnea, and dizziness or syncope. Signs and symptoms of mitral stenosis may develop for the first time during pregnancy. The greatest danger is in late pregnancy and labor due to increased heart rate and cardiac output, blood volume expansion, and intensified oxygen demand. Mild-to-moderate mitral stenosis can be managed safely with the use of diuretics to relieve pulmonary and systemic congestion and β-blockers to prevent tachycardia to optimize diastolic filling. Diuretics, β-blockers, digoxin, or DC cardioversion for atrial fibrillation should be instituted in cases of hemodynamic compromise, taking into consideration maternal safety. Refractory cases and patients with severe mitral stenosis with heart failure prompt mechanical relief, either by percutaneous balloon valvuloplasty or surgery, preferably before conception if the valve is anatomically suitable. Patients with a history of acute rheumatic fever and carditis should continue penicillin prophylaxis.

Mitral valve prolapse is the most common cause of **mitral regurgitation** in pregnant patients. Rheumatic mitral regurgitation is tolerated well during pregnancy. The decrease in systemic vascular resistance in pregnancy may reduce the amount of mitral regurgitation. Left ventricular dysfunction, if severe, may precipitate heart failure. Medical management includes use of diuretics and, in rare instances, surgery, preferably mitral valve repair, which is indicated for severe, acute regurgitation or ruptured chordae.

Mitral valve prolapse is also the most common heart disease encountered in pregnancy. Patients without comorbidity, such as a connective tissue, skeletal, or other cardiovascular disorders, tolerate pregnancy. The click and murmur become less prominent during pregnancy. No special precautions for isolated mitral valve prolapse are required. Selected use of endocarditis prophylaxis is recommended in mitral valve prolapse patients with a murmur of mitral regurgitation. The incidence of complications of the mitral valve prolapse (3%) is similar in pregnant and nonpregnant patients.

b. Aortic valve disorders—The most common cause of **aortic stenosis** in pregnant patients is congenital bicuspid valve. Mild-to-moderate obstruction with normal left ventricular function may be managed conservatively. Patients with severe obstruction a mean pressure gradient >50 mm Hg, or those who are symptomatic or have heart failure should undergo valvotomy or surgery, preferably before conception or labor (if diagnosed during pregnancy). A bicuspid aortic valve is associated with cystic medial necrosis, which may lead to aortic dissection in the third trimester.

Isolated **aortic regurgitation** can be managed medically with diuretics and vasodilators. Surgery is only indicated for patients with refractory (class III or IV) symptoms.

c. Pulmonic and tricuspid valve disorders—**Pulmonic valve stenosis** may occur in isolation or in combination with other heart lesions. Isolated pulmonic stenosis can be managed conservatively with valvotomy reserved for severe cases. **Tricuspid valve disease** may be congenital or acquired. Isolated tricuspid valve disease can be managed successfully with diuretics. Special care should be given to diuretic-induced hypoperfusion.

Mauri L, O'Gara PT: Valvular heart disease in the pregnant patient. Curr Treat Options Cardiovasc Med 2001;3(1):7.

Treelink JR, Foster E: Valvular heart disease in pregnancy. A contemporary perspective. Cardiol Clin 1998;16(3):573.

ACC/AHA guidelines for the management of patients with valvular heart disease. A report of the American College of Cardiology/American Heart Association Task Force on Practice Guidelines (Committee on Management of Patients with Valvular Heart Disease). J Am Coll Cardiol 1998;32:1486.

5. Prosthetic heart valves—Females with a prosthetic heart valve can usually tolerate the hemodynamic burden of pregnancy without difficulty. The function of the prosthesis can be evaluated and followed throughout the pregnancy with noninvasive Doppler echocardiography. Unfortunately, significant maternal and fetal risk of either hemorrhage or thrombosis with the accompanying use of warfarin or heparin remains a major problem. Maternal thromboembolism complicates 4–14% of pregnancies in women with mechanical valves despite therapeutic International Normalized Ra-

tio. The incidence of warfarin embryopathy has been estimated to be 4–10%. Contrary to the old belief of heparin being a preferred and safe anticoagulant, numerous recent studies have reported a 12–24% risk of fatal valve thrombosis in high-risk pregnant patients treated with subcutaneous heparin. High-risk cases may benefit from addition of low-dose aspirin. Risk of pregnancy in patients with prosthetic heart valves should be discussed in detail with the patient and the family prior to conception. Potential problems include increased hemodynamic load, hypercoagulability, enhanced degeneration of bioprosthetic valves, and fetal risks associated with cardiovascular drugs and anticoagulation.

In women of childbearing age who desire a pregnancy, a tissue valve may be inserted if there are no other indications for anticoagulation, and if the patient accepts the eventual need for replacement of the prosthesis. Also, the decision to use heparin during the first trimester versus warfarin should be made after a detailed discussion with the patient making her aware of the possible adverse events. A high rate of pregnancy loss in women with a mitral valve prosthesis has reportedly been associated with warfarin treatment throughout pregnancy, whereas heparin is associated with thromboembolic cardiac events. Infective endocarditis in these patients also remains a concern.

Bioprosthetic tissue valves may be selected for a pregnant patient to avoid anticoagulation, but increased deterioration of the valve during pregnancy requires a repeat operation within several years. Mechanical valves are indicated in pregnant patients with other coexisting heart disorders requiring anticoagulation, eg, atrial fibrillation, apical thrombus, rheumatic heart disease, or thromboembolism. Despite adequate anticoagulation, mechanical prosthetic valve thrombosis has been described in about 10% of the cases. The choice of prosthetic valve and the safe method of anticoagulation are therefore still of concern in the pregnant patients and need to be studied more.

Sadler L, McCowan L, White H, Stewart A et al: Pregnancy outcomes and cardiac complications in women with mechanical, bioprosthetic, and homograft valves. BJOG 2000;107(2):245.

Messmore HL, Kundur R, Wehrmacher W, Scanlon P: Anticoagulant therapy of pregnant patients with prosthetic heart valves: Rationale for a clinical trial of low molecular weight heparin. Clin Appl Thromb Hemost 1999;5(2):73.

6. Infective endocarditis—Underlying structural abnormalities of the heart predispose patients to the development of infective endocarditis. The most common cause is rheumatic heart disease, with others being mitral valve prolapse, intravenous drug abuse, and iatrogenic procedures. The estimated incidence of infective endocarditis during pregnancy is 0.005–1.0% of all pregnancies. Although it is rare, the development of infective endocarditis during pregnancy can have devastating consequences, with maternal and fetal mortality rates estimated to be 20% and 25%, respectively. The management of infective endocarditis in pregnancy is the same as for nonpregnant patients; however, special consideration must be given to the diagnostic and therapeutic approaches during pregnancy to reduce the risk to the fetus.

The most common organism to cause infective endocarditis during pregnancy is *Streptococcus viridans.* Streptococcal infection is often subacute, with symptoms present for months before the diagnosis is made. Acute infective endocarditis with symptoms present for only a few days to weeks is often due to *Staphylococcus aureus, Streptococcus pneumoniae,* and *Streptococcus pyogenes.* In patients with a history of intravenous drug abuse, the most common organism is *S aureus,* although polymicrobial infections may occur. Any organism capable of causing infective endocarditis in the nonpregnant state can also be a potential pathogen during pregnancy. Many organisms reported to cause infective endocarditis during pregnancy have also been cultured from the normal vagina and postpartum uterus.

Clinical diagnosis is made on the basis of the classic triad of fever, murmur, and anemia, along with positive blood cultures. The integumentary, renal, and neurologic systems are involved besides the cardiovascular.. The most frequently involved valve is the aortic, followed by the mitral. Echocardiography can be performed safely during pregnancy to delineate the valves and shunts. Treatment is determined by results of the organism culture and the safety of the antibiotics for both the pregnant patient and the fetus. The initial therapy of choice includes penicillin in combination with an aminoglycoside. Endocarditis prophylaxis is indicated in susceptible cases. The most common cause of death in infective endocarditis is heart failure, most often due to aortic valve regurgitation.

Wilansky S, Hare JY, Klima T: Staphylococcal endocarditis in pregnancy. Tex Heart Inst J 1998;25(3):222.

7. Myocarditis—This inflammatory process is either focal or diffused and involves the heart musculature. Of all the infectious and noninfectious causes, viral infection with Coxsackie B virus is the most common, accounting for nearly 50% of cases. Other important causes include **acquired immune deficiency syndrome (AIDS)** and **Chagas' disease** due to *Trypanosoma cruzi,* which is the most common cause in South and Central America. Only a few cases of myocarditis have been reported in pregnancy. Clinical manifestations range from incidental finding of silent myocarditis to overt heart failure with hemodynamic collapse. In the acute stage, the electrocardiogram is almost always abnormal, showing Q waves with ST and T wave changes, which

may mimic acute myocardial infarction. The erythrocyte sedimentation rate (ESR) and cardiac enzymes are usually elevated. Viral cultures may or may not be helpful. Noninvasive imaging studies may reveal regional wall motion abnormalities. Although endomyocardial biopsy is the "gold standard" for the diagnosis of myocarditis, a negative result does not rule it out. All pregnant women with a suspicion of myocarditis should be hospitalized. Therapy is supportive with bed rest, avoidance of strenuous activity, and treatment of heart failure with digoxin, diuretics, and vasodilators, avoiding angiotensin-converting enzyme (ACE) inhibitors because of the risk of fetal anomalies. Administration of steroids and immunosuppressive therapy has been controversial and has demonstrated no proven benefit. Potential complications of myocarditis include arrhythmia, heart blocks, and cardiogenic shock. Anticoagulation should be seriously considered, especially for patients with severe left ventricular dysfunction.

Shotan A, Bokhari SW, Elkayam U: Myocarditis in pregnancy. In Elkayam U, Gleicher N: *Cardiac Problems in Pregnancy,* 3rd ed. New York: Wiley-Liss, 1998.

8. Peripartum cardiomyopathy—This rare but distinct form of heart failure with left ventricular dysfunction occurs during pregnancy or postpartum. Its estimated incidence in the United States is 1 in 15,000. Its cause is unknown but is probably multifactorial. Histopathology reveals a dilated heart with pale myocardium, but myocardial biopsy is of little value. Because signs and symptoms of normal pregnancy resemble heart failure, peripartum cardiomyopathy is easily missed or diagnosed late in the course. Usually peripartum cardiomyopathy presents with dyspnea, cough, orthopnea, paroxysmal nocturnal dyspnea, fatigue, palpitations, and chest pain. The echocardiography is central to diagnosis. The echocardiogram demonstrates dilated left ventricle with marked overall impairment of systolic function. Right-sided catheterization should be considered for optimized treatment of these patients. Medical therapy is essentially supportive and similar to that for other forms of heart failure and includes sodium restriction, diuretics, digoxin, and after load reduction with hydralazine (the drug of choice). ACE inhibitors are contraindicated because of associated fetal CNS anomalies. Heparin should seriously be considered for treating possible thromboembolic phenomena in pregnant patients with congestive heart failure due to peripartum cardiomyopathy. In cases refractory to medical therapy, use of an intraaortic balloon pump for temporary stabilization and left ventricular assist device as a bridge to transplant are indicated. Approximately 20% of peripartum cardiomyopathy patients survive only because they get heart transplants. A majority of the patients recover partially or even completely. High mortality rates of 18–56% have been reported. A recent study demonstrated less than 10% mortality over a 4-year period in patients with peripartum cardiomyopathy, indicating improved therapeutic modalities for treating heart failure. Nevertheless, women with a history of peripartum cardiomyopathy have a significant risk of deleterious fetal and maternal outcome in subsequent pregnancies, even if their left ventricular function has returned to normal.

Elkayam U, Tummala PT, Rao K et al: Maternal and fetal outcomes of subsequent pregnancies in women with peripartum cardiomyopathy. N Engl J Med 2001;344(21):1567.

Pearson GD, Veille JC, Rahimtoola S et al: Peripartum cardiomyopathy: National Heart, Lung, and Blood Institute and Office of Rare Diseases (National Institutes of Health) Workshop recommendations and review. JAMA 2000;283(9):1183.

Futterman LG, Lemberg L: Peripartum cardiomyopathy: An ominous complication of pregnancy. Am J Crit Care 2000;9(5):362.

Heider AL, Kuller JA, Strauss RA et al: Peripartum cardiomyopathy: A review of the literature. Obstet Gynecol Surv 1999;54(8):526.

Brown CS, Bertolet BD: Peripartum cardiomyopathy: A comprehensive review. Am J Obstet Gynecol 1998;178(2):409.

9. Hypertrophic cardiomyopathy—This primary myocardial disease shows a characteristic hypertrophy of the left or right ventricular myocardium. The hypertrophy is asymmetrical and most commonly involves the intraventricular septum (asymmetric septal hypertrophy). Pathophysiologic mechanisms include presence of a hyperdynamic left ventricle, obstruction of left ventricular outflow tract, mitral regurgitation, and myocardial ischemia. Prevalence in young population (23–35 years) is 2 per 1000. A large number of patients are asymptomatic. Severe illness is manifested by poor functional capacity, heart failure, and sudden death.

Dyspnea is the most common symptom, with others being chest pain, dizziness, syncope, and palpitations. In younger patients, sudden death may be the first manifestation, with an annual incidence in the population being 6%. Physical examination varies from normal to characteristic findings in patients with high gradients. The auscultatory hallmark is a diamond-shaped, grade 3–4/6 systolic murmur, heard best at apex radiating to the left sternal border. The murmur increases in intensity during the strain phase of the Valsalva maneuver. Electrocardiogram shows ventricular hypertrophy, ST and T changes, and Q waves in inferolateral leads. Ventricular arrhythmias are commonly seen on Holter monitoring. Echocardiography diagnostically demonstrates asymmetric septal hypertrophy (with a ratio of septum to posterior wall thickening exceeding 1.5) and decreased septal motion.

High-risk pregnant patients with a higher likelihood of worsening symptoms during pregnancy include those who were symptomatic prior to pregnancy and asymptomatic patients with left ventricular dysfunction. Increased incidence of supraventricular as well as ventricular arrhythmia in pregnancy has been reported. Maternal hypertrophic cardiomyopathy does not influence fetal outcome, although in about half of the patients it is familial with autosomal-dominant inheritance. The risk in an offspring is approximately 8–14%. A detailed discussion regarding risks and a thorough evaluation of the patient is required prior to conception.

In asymptomatic patients, outcome is usually good, but close monitoring is recommended. Therapy needs to be individualized in symptomatic patients. Beta-blockers have been used most frequently and relatively safely in symptomatic patients but are not recommended for routine use. Of the calcium channel blockers, verapamil has been used sporadically in pregnant patients. Dual-chamber pacing for arrhythmia has been shown beneficial but is reserved for severely symptomatic cases refractory to medical therapy. Surgical myectomy has not yet been reported in pregnancy. Atrial fibrillation recurs in 10% of the patients, leading to an increased risk of systemic emboli and hemodynamic worsening. Sotalol, procainamide, and DC cardioversion have all been used to treat pregnant patients. Hemodynamic monitoring with a pulmonary catheter is recommended for clinical deterioration encountered during labor and delivery and should be considered even in asymptomatic patients. Fortunately, the strain of vaginal delivery is well tolerated in women with hypertrophic cardiomyopathy. Cesarean section is reserved for obstetric indications. Epidural anesthesia should be avoided. Magnesium should be used for tocolysis if needed. The American Heart Association does not recommend antibiotic prophylaxis, but it should be considered in patients with obstructive hypertrophic cardiomyopathy.

Wilansky S, Belicik T, Osborn R et al: Hypertrophic cardiomyopathy in pregnancy. The use of two-dimensional and Doppler echocardiography during labor and delivery: A case report. J Heart Valve Dis 1998;7(3):355.

10. Coronary artery disease—Coronary artery disease (CAD) is a leading cause of death in women in the United States. CAD kills more women than the next 16 common causes of death combined. The incidence of myocardial infarction (MI) during pregnancy has been estimated to be 1 in 10,000. CAD is being encountered more often in pregnancy due to older childbearing age. The mortality rate of 37–50% due to MI during pregnancy has been reported. A major problem in the diagnosis of MI during pregnancy is the failure to recognize its possibility. Smoking is recognized as a major risk factor, others being diabetes, hypertension, dyslipidemia, and a positive family history. The causes of MI in pregnancy include atherosclerosis, congenital lesions (anomalous origin of coronary artery), inflammatory diseases of coronary arteries (Kawasaki's disease), connective tissue or vasospastic disorders, and spontaneous coronary artery dissection.

The most common presentation is angina pectoris. Patients with high suspicion of index should undergo a stress test risk stratification. Left ventricular function needs to be assessed to determine the choice of therapy and predict likelihood of survival. The normal physiologic changes of pregnancy may precipitate myocardial ischemia and heart failure in women with left ventricular impairment caused by a MI. Troponin I remains the most useful marker for monitoring pregnant women for a myocardial injury because it is undetectable during normal labor and delivery. Aspirin and lipid-lowering therapies improve mortality rates in chronic, stable angina. Beta-blockers, nitrates, and long-acting calcium channel blockers reduce symptoms and improve exercise tolerance in nonpregnant females. The majority of MIs during pregnancy are anterior and transmural, involving the left anterior descending artery. Successful treatment of acute MI during pregnancy with thrombolytic therapy has also been reported. Revascularization procedures pose increased hazards to pregnant women. Beta-blockers are the mainstay of medical therapy. A maternal mortality rate of 45–50% has been reported if the infarction occurs during the third trimester, the patient is less than 35 years old, the delivery occurs within 2 weeks of the MI, or the patient undergoes a cesarean. Efforts should be made to limit myocardial oxygen consumption, particularly during late pregnancy and delivery, in women with known CAD.

Hameed AB, Tummala PP, Goodwin TM et al: Unstable angina during pregnancy in two patients with premature coronary atherosclerosis and aortic stenosis in association with familial hypercholesterolemia. Am J Obstet Gynecol 2000;182(5):1152.

Shivvers SA, Wians FH, Keffer JH et al: Maternal cardiac troponin I levels during normal labor and delivery. Am J Obstet Gynecol 1999;180(1 Pt 1):122.

Schumacher B, Belfort MA, Card RJ: Successful treatment of acute myocardial infarction during pregnancy with tissue plasminogen activator. Am J Obstet Gynecol 1997;176(3):716.

Webber MD, Halligan RE, Schumacher JA: Acute infarction, intracoronary thrombolysis, and primary PTCA in pregnancy. Cathet Cardiovasc Diagn 1997;42(1):38.

11. Arrhythmias—Most arrhythmias occurring during pregnancy are benign. Sinus tachycardia, sinus arrhythmia, sinus bradycardia, atrial premature beats, and ventricular premature beats are relatively common during pregnancy. These arrhythmias are hemodynamically insignificant and require no treatment, and the patient can be reassured of their innocence. The occurrence of more complex arrhythmias should, however, raise the suspicion of underlying cardiac disease. Symptomatic arrhythmias, which are rare during pregnancy, may develop during an otherwise uncomplicated pregnancy or in association with underlying cardiac disease. In fact, cardiac arrhythmias may be the first manifestation of cardiac disease during pregnancy.

a. Paroxysmal supraventricular tachycardia—The most common arrhythmia encountered during pregnancy is paroxysmal supraventricular tachycardia (PSVT); it has been estimated to occur in approximately 3% of pregnant patients. In patients with a previous history of PSVT, the frequency and severity of the episodes may increase during pregnancy. The symptoms of PSVT are dyspnea, lightheadedness, and anxiety in patients without underlying cardiac disease. In patients with underlying cardiac abnormalities, angina, heart failure, and syncope may occur as a result of myocardial ischemia and decreased cardiac output. Although there is concern about the effects of hypotension on the fetus during these episodes, women with PSVT do not have an increase in perinatal complications.

b. Atrial flutter and fibrillation—Atrial flutter, which is uncommon during pregnancy, and atrial fibrillation are usually found in patients with underlying cardiac disease. The hemodynamic consequences and the associated symptoms depend on the underlying cardiac status. During pregnancy, atrial fibrillation is most commonly found in association with mitral stenosis. The development of this arrhythmia in these patients may precipitate congestive heart failure and embolic events.

c. Wolff-Parkinson-White syndrome—This preexcitation syndrome usually occurs in patients without underlying cardiac disease. Patients with Wolff-Parkinson-White syndrome (WPW) may have recurrent arrhythmias—most commonly, atrioventricular (AV) reentry tachycardia, atrial fibrillation, or atrial flutter. The hemodynamic effects of the associated arrhythmias are related to the type of arrhythmia and the ventricular rate. Many patients with WPW are asymptomatic, but pregnancy is associated with an increased incidence of arrhythmias in women with this syndrome.

d. Premature ventricular complexes—Premature ventricular complexes (PVCs) are relatively common in pregnant women and are associated with complaints of palpitations. Pregnant women with PVCs and no underlying cardiac disease have an excellent prognosis and require no treatment. Reassurance to the patient is frequently all that is required, along with avoidance of such aggravating factors as smoking and stimulants.

e. Ventricular tachycardia—Defined as the occurrence of three or more consecutive ventricular complexes, ventricular tachycardia (VT) is a serious cardiac arrhythmia that, if sustained, can lead to death. Ventricular tachycardia is rare during pregnancy, but when it occurs, it is usually associated with underlying cardiac disease. The most common cardiac abnormalities associated with VT are mitral valve prolapse, valvular disease, and cardiomyopathy. The prognosis for patients with nonsustained VT (less than 30 s in duration) and no underlying cardiac disease is excellent. In such patients, the VT is catecholamine-sensitive, and extreme exercise should be avoided. In some patients, therapy with β-adrenergic blocking drugs may be indicated. Sustained VT (more than 30 s in duration) or hemodynamically significant VT is usually associated with underlying cardiac disease, and therapy with antiarrhythmics is usually indicated. Such patients should also undergo evaluation for such precipitating factors as myocardial ischemia, electrolyte imbalance, congestive heart failure, digitalis intoxication, stimulants, and hypoxia.

12. Heart blocks—First-degree heart block is evident as PR prolongation on the electrocardiogram (ECG) and results from an increased time of conduction through the AV junction. First-degree heart block is primarily associated with rheumatic heart disease or digitalis therapy and does not usually require therapy. Second-degree heart block can may be divided into two types: Mobitz type I (Wenckebach) and Mobitz type II. Mobitz type I is characterized by progressive lengthening of the PR interval until an impulse is blocked. It is a relatively benign disorder and occurs when vagal tone is increased. Treatment is seldom indicated. Mobitz type II is a sudden block of conduction without previous prolongation of the PR interval. It often precedes the development of complete heart block. It is rare during pregnancy but may occur in association with rheumatic heart disease or infections. If the ventricular rate is slow and the patient is symptomatic, treatment with permanent pacing is indicated.

Complete heart block can be congenital or acquired. Its onset is usually prior to the pregnancy, and it rarely progresses. Approximately half the cases of complete heart block occurring during pregnancy have an associated ventricular septal defect. Other causes include ischemic heart disease, myocarditis, and rheumatic heart disease. The need for pacemaker therapy depends on the ventricular escape rate. Symptoms are rare at a rate of 50–60 beats/min; if the rate suddenly slows, however, syncope may develop. Permanent pacing is indicated in such patients.

Wolbrette D, Patel H: Arrhythmias in women. Curr Opin Cardiol 1999;14(1):36.

13. Pericardial diseases—Pericarditis is usually a mild, self-limited disease. Its incidence, diagnosis, and treatment are similar in pregnant and nonpregnant patients. Most pregnancies, even the complicated ones, may be brought safely to term. Idiopathic pericarditis is the most common cause of pericardial disease, others being trauma, infections (viral, bacterial, fungal, tuberculosis), radiation, and collagen vascular diseases.

Sharp, stabbing chest pain that is exacerbated in the supine position and relieved by leaning forward is the most common complaint. Pathognomonic finding of pericardial friction rub is best heard with the diaphragm of the stethoscope over the second and fourth intercostal spaces in midclavicular line or the left sternal border, with the patient leaning forward and inspiring deeply. Characteristic ST segment elevations with upward concavity and upright T waves have been reported in 80% of patients with acute pericarditis. Only a chest roentgenogram would indicate suspicion of pneumonia in a pregnant patient. Echocardiography is an important diagnostic modality and may reveal thickened pericardium, pericardial effusion, and most importantly cardiac tamponade.

Pregnant patients with suspected pericarditis should be hospitalized for complete bed rest. Nonsteroidal antiinflammatory drugs (NSAIDs), aspirin and indomethacin, are effective analgesics. Steroids should be avoided in tuberculosis. Pericardiectomy is reserved for severe, relapsing pericarditis, refractory to medical treatment.

Asymptomatic pericardial effusion is frequently encountered in all trimesters, most commonly in the third, but resolves postpartum. Pericardial constriction has been rarely reported in pregnancy, although it could occur as a pericarditis sequel. Most patients present with dyspnea, marked edema, and ascites in the latter half of pregnancy. Diuretics, steroids, and pericardiectomy (reserved for refractory cases, and associated with reasonable maternal and fetal risk) have all been used to treat pericardial constriction in pregnant patients. Preterm delivery and fetal death have been reported.

14. Primary pulmonary hypertension—This uncommon though distinct entity is defined as *mean* pulmonary artery pressure of more than 30 mm Hg at rest, or more than 40 mm Hg during exercise, without a demonstrable cause. Primary pulmonary hypertension poses a significant risk to pregnant women, with mortality approaching 40%, warranting prevention of pregnancy or early therapeutic abortion. Although a number of potential mechanisms are postulated, the exact cause of primary pulmonary hypertension is still unknown. The most common presenting symptoms are dyspnea, fatigue, chest pain, palpitations, syncope or near syncope, and Raynaud's phenomenon. Characteristic physical findings are a result of markedly increased pulmonary pressures, leading to right ventricular hypertrophy and failure with decreased cardiac output. The echocardiogram reveals elevated pulmonary artery pressures, right atrial enlargement, right ventricular hypertrophy, and tricuspid regurgitation. A new onset or worsening of symptoms is commonly seen in the second and third trimesters.

Treatment with prostacyclin infusion for short periods to lower pulmonary artery pressure in pregnancy has been reported to be safe and effective. Incidents of premature labor and delivery are high. Patients should be laid in the left lateral decubitus position to improve cardiac output. Planned vaginal delivery seems to be safe in stable patients. Epidural anesthesia has been used in most reported cases. Patients should be monitored for 7–10 days postpartum prior to discharge to ensure stability. Due to its grave prognosis and a high incidence of maternal and fetal morbidity and mortality, pregnancy seems to be contraindicated in patients with primary pulmonary hypertension. Therapeutic abortion is indicated as soon as possible if pregnancy occurs. Adequate counseling should be provided to all of the patients regarding sterilization.

Elkayam U, Bokhari SW, Dave R: Primary pulmonary hypertension in pregnancy. In Elkayam U, Gleicher N: Cardiac Diseases in Pregnancy, 3rd ed. New York: Wiley-Liss, 1998.

Stewart R, Tuazon D, Olson G et al: Pregnancy and primary pulmonary hypertension: Successful outcome with epoprostenol therapy. Chest 2001;119(3):973.

15. Vascular disease—Marfan's syndrome, an inheritable connective tissue disorder of the fibrillin gene on chromosome 15, is an autosomal-dominant disorder. It involves ocular, skeletal, and cardiovascular systems. It predisposes patients to aortic dissection or actual rupture of the aorta most commonly originating in the ascending portion during pregnancy, most likely in the third trimester. High-risk patients are patients with significant associated cardiac abnormalities, such as mitral valve prolapse or regurgitation and an aortic root greater than 4.0 cm in diameter. All women with Marfan's syndrome planning to become pregnant should undergo a screening (transthoracic echocardiogram). High-risk patients should have elective surgery before conception. If the diagnosis is made during pregnancy, β-blockers are strongly recommended, with some authorities advocating prompt termination of pregnancy with aortic repair. Women at increased risk of complications during pregnancy should be advised against attempting a pregnancy that may be associated with a 50% maternal mortality rate. Stable patients can be treated medically and delivered vaginally. The risk of the offspring inheriting the disorder is 50%.

Clinical Findings

A. History

The evaluation of heart disease in pregnancy may become difficult due to the normal anatomic and physiologic changes of pregnancy. A careful history taking therefore becomes more important and should include a history of rheumatic fever, valvular disorder, arrhythmia, congenital heart disease, coronary risk factors or established coronary artery disease, and cardiac surgery.

Reduced exercise tolerance and fatigue are the most common symptoms reported in pregnant women, probably due to increased body weight and anemia. Dizziness, light-headedness, or even syncopal episodes may occur during the latter part of pregnancy because mechanical compression of the uterus on the inferior vena cava decreases venous return, and thus the cardiac output. Palpitations are also a frequent complaint but usually are not associated with a significant arrhythmia. Dyspnea and orthopnea, probably due to hyperventilation, are also reported.

B. Physical Examination

The physical examination of pregnant patients with normal cardiovascular systems changes because of the increased hemodynamic burden. The evaluation of patients with suspected heart disease during pregnancy requires a thorough knowledge of the normal physiologic changes.

A normal pregnant patient has a slightly fast resting heart rate, large pulse, slightly widened pulse pressure, and warm extremities. The jugular venous distention is seen from the twentieth week. Edema of the ankles and legs is commonly encountered in late pregnancy. A prominent but unsustained left ventricular impulse may be palpated in late pregnancy and may simulate the volume overload seen in aortic or mitral regurgitation. The auscultatory findings of normal pregnancy begin late in the first trimester and usually disappear 2–4 weeks after delivery. During cardiac auscultation, the first heart sound is loud and exhibits an exaggerated splitting. The second heart sound during late pregnancy is often increased and may exhibit persistent expiratory splitting, especially with the patient in the left lateral position. A third heart sound has been reported to be frequent in late pregnancy. However, because of its association with heart failure, the presence of a third heart sound should lead to further investigation of underlying heart disease, especially in women with symptoms and other signs suggestive of heart disease. A fourth heart sound is rarely heard during a normal pregnancy.

Systolic murmurs are common during pregnancy and result from the increased blood volume and hyperkinetic state. Most frequently they are innocent midsystolic murmurs, grade 1–2/6, that are best heard at the lower left sternal border and over the pulmonary area, radiating to the suprasternal notch or to the left of the neck. They usually represent vibrations created by ejection of blood into the pulmonary trunk. A cervical venous hum or mammary soufflé heard best in the right supraclavicular area in a supine position is a benign systolic, or a continuous, murmur occurring in late pregnancy. Diastolic heart murmurs are unusual and usually represent valvular abnormalities (Table 31–5).

1. Diagnostic difficulties—Problems in diagnosis encountered during physical examinations are often due to the normal physiologic changes of pregnancy. Cardiac auscultation may be particularly confusing in pregnant patients. Along with innocent systolic murmurs heard in many normal pregnant women, benign vascular murmurs are also heard. These murmurs can be differentiated from those of cardiac origin by their disappearance when pressure is applied with the stethoscope or when the patient sits upright, but they can be easily misinterpreted.

Although systolic murmurs are common, the finding of a diastolic murmur is rare during a normal pregnancy and should warrant further diagnostic evaluation. Both systolic and diastolic murmurs associated with cardiac disease can increase or decrease in intensity during pregnancy. The systolic murmurs of aortic or pulmonic stenosis usually increase in intensity because of the increased cardiac output and blood volume. The diastolic murmur of mitral stenosis is also increased and may even be first detected during pregnancy. The augmented blood volume and the increased heart rate of pregnancy shorten the diastolic filling period and increase the rate of blood flow across the mitral valve. In contrast, murmurs of mitral or aortic regurgitation may soften or even disappear during pregnancy as a result of the decrease in peripheral vascular resistance. The circulatory changes of pregnancy also affect the auscultatory findings in cardiac abnormalities, such as mitral valve prolapse and hypertrophic cardiomyopathy, which are dependent on volume. The increase in left ventricular

Table 31–5. Cardiovascular signs and symptoms in normal pregnancy.

Symptoms
 Fatigue
 Orthopnea
 Dyspnea
 Decreased functional capacity
 Dizziness
 Syncope
Physical signs
 Jugular venous distension
 Displaced left ventricular apical impulse
 Right ventricular heave
 Palpable pulmonary impulse
 Increased intensity of the first heart sound
 Persistent splitting of the second heart sound
 Systolic ejection murmur at the left lower sternal border or
  pulmonary area with radiation to the neck
 Cervical venous hum, mammary soufflé

volume during pregnancy may attenuate or abolish the click and late systolic murmur typical of mitral valve prolapse. The systolic murmur of hypertrophic obstructive cardiomyopathy may also decrease or disappear as the left ventricular volume increases during pregnancy. The diagnosis of infective endocarditis during pregnancy may be difficult. Fever is present in more than 95% of patients with endocarditis; however, the hemodynamic changes associated with pregnancy make cardiac murmurs common, and previously existing murmurs may diminish in intensity. A high index of suspicion is therefore necessary to make the diagnosis of infective endocarditis in pregnant patients. The most useful clinical findings are fever, murmur, evidence of preexisting cardiac disease, and positive blood cultures.

C. DIAGNOSTIC STUDIES

1. Chest radiography—The usefulness of chest films during pregnancy is limited because of the potential hazard to the fetus from radiation exposure. Whenever a chest film is believed necessary, the abdominopelvic area should be shielded with lead to minimize exposure. The normal cardiac changes of pregnancy, such as chamber enlargement and the horizontal position of the heart because of the elevation of the diaphragm, should not be misinterpreted as cardiac disease. Newer and more accurate techniques such as Doppler echocardiography have largely replaced chest films in the evaluation of cardiac structure and function.

2. Electrocardiography—The electrocardiogram is an important diagnostic technique that can indicate the presence of underlying cardiac abnormalities. Cardiac chamber hypertrophy, myocardial ischemia and infarction, pericarditis, myocarditis, conduction abnormalities, and the presence of atrial and ventricular arrhythmias may be detected by electrocardiography. In patients with suspected cardiac arrhythmias, ambulatory Holter monitoring may be indicated. During normal pregnancy, sinus tachycardia, a shift of the axis to the left or right may be observed, and transient ST abnormalities are common.

3. Echocardiography—Transthoracic echocardiography is an important diagnostic noninvasive study, which can be performed safely in pregnancy. The intracardiac structures can be evaluated for abnormalities of the great vessels, cardiac chambers, and heart valves. Chamber sizes and ventricular function can also be measured.

During the echocardiographic examination, the normal physiologic changes that occur with pregnancy should be kept in mind. When the patient is evaluated in the left lateral position, an increase in the diastolic dimensions of the right and left ventricles is common because of volume increases that occur with a normal pregnancy. Because of the increase in the left ventricular dimensions, mitral valve prolapse may improve or disappear during pregnancy. Right and left atrial dimensions may also increase slightly; these changes increase as the pregnancy progresses. Small pericardial effusions have been noted in late pregnancy in healthy women.

Two-dimensional echocardiography gives diagnostic information about the cause of the valvular abnormality and its associated effects on ventricular size and function. Doppler echocardiography provides reliable quantitative and qualitative information regarding the presence and severity of valvular stenosis and regurgitation. Doppler echocardiography can measure the valve area and gradients across stenotic valves. Small degrees of pulmonary, tricuspid, and mitral regurgitation have frequently been found in normal individuals, whether pregnant or not. In patients with congenital heart disease (corrected or uncorrected) Doppler echocardiography can detect the presence of intracardiac shunts and estimate the shunt ratios by determining the right and left cardiac outputs. It can measure pulmonary artery systolic pressure to assess the effects of the valvular lesions and intracardiac shunts on the pulmonary circulation.

Transesophageal echocardiography (TEE) provides superior images of the intracardiac structures and great vessels, providing the same detailed analysis of cardiac structure, function, and hemodynamic assessment possible with transthoracic echocardiography. TEE can be used for patients in whom the transthoracic examination is technically suboptimal and for those with suspected prosthetic or native valve dysfunction, infective endocarditis, congenital heart disease, or aortic dissection. Although experience with TEE during pregnancy has been limited, the procedure should be considered in pregnant patients for whom the risks are less than the possible benefit. The procedure should be performed by an experienced echocardiographer, and fetal monitoring, in addition to the routine monitoring of the patient, should be available (Table 31–6).

4. Exercise tolerance test—Little is known about the safety of an exercise test to establish ischemic heart disease in pregnancy. Fetal bradycardia, marked hypoxia, acidosis, and severe hypothermia at peak exercise have been reported. In light of these facts, the use of a submaximal stress test (approximately 70% of the maximal predicted heart rate) with close fetal monitoring is recommended, until more information regarding its safety is available. Maximal oxygen consumption, unchanged in pregnancy, could be used for the assessment of the functional status in cardiac patients during pregnancy.

5. Radionuclide studies—Myocardial perfusion scans and radionuclide ventriculography should be avoided, if possible, especially in the first trimester of pregnancy because of the risk of rare but possible fetal malformations. Also, in women of childbearing age, the inci-

Table 31–6. Diagnostic test findings in pregnancy.

Electrocardiogram
  Sinus tachycardia
  Increased incidence of arrhythmias
  QRS axis deviation
  Increased amplitude of R wave in lead V_2
  ST segment and T wave changes
  Small Q waves
Chest roentgenogram
  Increased lung markings
  Horizontal positioning of the heart
  Straightened left upper cardiac border
Echocardiogram
  Mildly increased biatrial size
  Increased biventricular dimensions
  Mildly increased left ventricular systolic function
  Small pericardial effusion
  Increased tricuspid valve diameter
  Mild tricuspid, pulmonic, and mitral regurgitation

dence of coronary heart disease is low and other noninvasive techniques, such as exercise echocardiography, can be used to assess coronary artery disease.

6. Pulmonary artery catheterization—Bedside hemodynamic monitoring can be performed with a balloon-tipped pulmonary artery catheter. In the majority of patients, inflating the balloon permits floatation of the catheter through the right heart without the need for fluoroscopy. With the catheter in the pulmonary artery, the balloon is inflated until it occludes a small vessel; the pulmonary artery wedge pressure obtained reflects the left ventricular end-diastolic pressure. Pulmonary artery pressures and cardiac output can also be measured. The placement of a balloon floatation catheter should be considered during the early stages of labor in any patient with cardiac disease who has been symptomatic during the pregnancy. Furthermore, because of postpartum hemodynamic changes, hemodynamic monitoring should be continued for up to 48 h following delivery.

7. Cardiac catheterization—In some patients with cardiac disease who decompensate during pregnancy, complete diagnostic information cannot be obtained by noninvasive methods alone. This is particularly important when surgical intervention is contemplated. Cardiac catheterization in these patients may need to be performed during pregnancy. Because the radiation required for the performance of this technique has potentially adverse effects on the fetus, cardiac catheterization should be performed only if the needed information cannot be obtained by any other means. Whenever possible, cardiac catheterization should be performed after major organogenesis has occurred (more than 12 weeks after the last menses). The brachial approach is the preferred method to minimize the risk of radiation exposure to the abdomen, which should be lead shielded. The exposure to x-rays should be reduced to a minimum; catheter position can be guided in some cases by Doppler and contrast echocardiography.

Treatment

A. DRUG TREATMENT IN PREGNANCY

Treatment of the pregnant patient with cardiac disease requires the collaborative consultation of the obstetrician and cardiologist at regular intervals during gestation and careful planning for delivery with the anesthesiologist. All cardiovascular drugs during pregnancy should be avoided, if possible, especially in the first trimester. Most cardiovascular drugs cross the placenta and are secreted into the breast milk, mandating a detailed evaluation of risk-to-benefit ratio (Table 31–7).

1. Heart failure—Treatment of heart failure is more challenging in pregnant patients than in nonpregnant women. Salt restriction and activity limitation are extremely important. In patients with pulmonary congestion, medical therapy should begin with digoxin. Although digoxin has been safely used during pregnancy for many years, blood levels should be monitored to avoid toxicity. Diuretics, although not teratogenic may cause impaired uterine blood flow and placental perfusion, and hence should only be used in severely symptomatic patients. Thiazide diuretics have been associated with neonatal thrombocytopenia, jaundice, hyponatremia, and bradycardia.

Afterload is already reduced during pregnancy, hence further reduction in afterload may only be beneficial in selected cases. Hydralazine, the most frequently used afterload-reducing agent during pregnancy, is a direct arteriolar dilator and has not been associated with adverse fetal effects. ACE inhibitors are contraindicated in pregnancy due to their associated increased risk of pre-

Table 31–7. Alphabetical list of the commonly used cardiovascular medications, their potential side effects, and overall safety.

Drugs	Potential Side Effects	Safety
ACEI	IUGR, prematurity, low birth weight, neonatal renal failure, bony malformations, limb contractures, patent ductus arteriosus, death	Contraindicated
ARB	Same as ACEI	Unsafe
Adenosine	Limited data (in first trimester only)	Safe
Amiodarone	IUGR, prematurity, hypothyroidism	Unsafe
Beta-blockers	Neonatal bradycardia, hypoglycemia, and apnea at birth, uterine contraction initiation	Safe
CCB	Maternal hypotension leading to fetal distress	Unsafe
Digoxin	Low birth weight	Safe
Disopyramide	Uterine contraction initiation	Safe
Diuretics	Hyponatremia, bradycardia, jaundice, low platelets, impaired uterine blood flow	Potentially unsafe
Heparin	None reported	Probably safe
Lidocaine	CNS depression due to fetal acidosis with high blood levels	Safe
Mexiletine	IUGR, fetal bradycardia, neonatal hypoglycemia, and hypothyroidism	Safe
Nitrates	Fetal bradycardia	Potentially unsafe
Nitroprusside	Thiocyanate toxicity	Potentially unsafe
Procainamide	None reported	Safe
Quinidine	Premature labor, fetal VIII cranial nerve damage with high blood levels	Safe
Warfarin	Embryopathy, In utero fetal hemorrhage, CNS abnormalities	Unsafe

ACEI = angiotensin-converting enzyme inhibitor; ARB = angiotensin receptor blockers; CCB = calcium channel blockers; CNS = central nervous system; IUGR = intrauterine growth retardation.

mature delivery, low birth weight, fetal hypotension, renal failure, bony malformations, persistent patent ductus arteriosus, respiratory distress syndrome, and even death. Angiotensin II receptor blockers have similar adverse reactions and are thus rendered unsafe. Data on nitrates are limited and require further evaluation.

2. Arrhythmias—During pregnancy any precipitating factors of arrhythmia should be avoided or corrected. In general, conservative treatment of cardiac arrhythmias is indicated. DC cardioversion is the treatment of choice in patients with hemodynamic compromise due to arrhythmia. Although no antiarrhythmic is completely safe during pregnancy, most are tolerated well and are relatively safe. Drugs with the longest record of safety should be used as first-line therapy. Digoxin, although one of the safest drugs for treating arrhythmia during gestation, may cause increased risk of prematurity and intrauterine growth retardation. Adenosine has been reported safe and successful in terminating supraventricular tachycardias during pregnancy.

Quinidine, with minimal fetal risk, has the longest record of being used safely and effectively in the treatment of both atrial and VT during pregnancy. When quinidine is indicated during pregnancy, blood levels should be closely monitored because of drug interactions with warfarin may develop excessively prolonged prothrombin time, with the potential for hemorrhage. Procainamide has also been used safely and is the drug of choice in the treatment of wide-complex tachycardias.

Amiodarone is associated with fetal hypothyroidism, smaller size at birth for date of gestation, and prematurity, and is also secreted in breast milk. Amiodarone is thus reserved only for treating life-threatening arrhythmias or those refractory to other medical therapy. Verapamil, although used during pregnancy, should be discontinued at the onset of labor to avoid dysfunctional labor and postpartum hemorrhage.

Beta-adrenergic blocking agents are relatively safe and have frequently been used in pregnant patients to treat arrhythmia, hypertrophic cardiomyopathy, and hyperthyroidism. Propranolol is a nonselective β-blocker that has been used frequently during pregnancy. Fetal and newborn heart rate, blood glucose levels, and respiratory status should be monitored closely.

Lidocaine may be used for VT, especially in the setting of an acute MI, but it requires close monitoring of blood levels.

3. Thrombosis and thromboembolism—Even though increased concentrations of clotting factors and platelet adhesiveness, and decreased fibrinolysis in pregnancy result in an overall increased risk of thrombosis and embolism, the actual incidence of venous thromboembolism during pregnancy is lower than previously reported. The gestational age at presentation appears to be equally distributed. Pulmonary embolism cases are reported to occur most commonly in the postpartum period and are strongly associated with a cesarean section. About 40% of asymptomatic patients with deep venous thrombosis may indeed have a pulmonary embolism.

The major indications for anticoagulants during pregnancy include the presence of mechanical heart valves and prophylaxis for recurrent pulmonary thromboembolism. Some patients with rheumatic heart disease with atrial fibrillation and cardiomyopathies may also be candidates for anticoagulation during pregnancy. The best method of anticoagulation in a pregnant patient is still controversial.

Warfarin has been associated with fetal wastage due to spontaneous abortion and stillbirths, optic nerve atrophy and blindness, microcephaly, mental retardation, and even death due to intracranial hemorrhage. Its use in the first trimester is associated with warfarin embryopathy in 4–10% of newborns, a syndrome comprising nasal bone hypoplasia and epiphyseal stippling. Warfarin poses significant risks to both the mother and the fetus during labor and delivery; however, breast-feeding women can be prescribed warfarin because it is not secreted in the breast milk.

Heparin is the drug of choice for anticoagulation in pregnant patients. As soon as pregnancy is diagnosed, oral anticoagulants should be discontinued and subcutaneous heparin, with a goal partial thromboplastin time (PTT) of twice normal, should be initiated. Complications of heparin administration include abdominal wall hematoma or abscess, thrombocytopenia, alopecia, and osteoporosis. At the thirty-sixth week of gestation subcutaneous heparin should be switched to intravenous route. To avoid the risk of bleeding during labor and delivery, heparin should be discontinued 24 h prior. Recent reports suggest that subcutaneous heparin, despite being in the therapeutic range, may not provide safe anticoagulation in high-risk patients.

Current recommendations are to discontinue warfarin early (as soon as the pregnancy is diagnosed) in the first trimester and start subcutaneous heparin to a goal PTT of twice normal. Alternatively, warfarin at low dose (<5 mg) could be continued in high-risk patients after obtaining an informed consent from the patient. In the second trimester warfarin is the treatment of choice, with International Normalized Ratio monitoring. Warfarin should then be discontinued at 36–38 weeks in the third trimester, and intravenous heparin should be instituted. Heparin should be stopped 24 h prior to expected labor and delivery. Anticoagulation should then be resumed 4 h after delivery (Table 31–8).

Low-molecular-weight heparin has mostly been used to treat deep venous thrombosis in the pregnant patient, but its long-term use requires further evaluation. Low-dose aspirin has been safely used in pregnancy. Dipyridamole should not be used in a pregnant

Table 31–8. Recommendations regarding anticoagulation during pregnancy.

During first trimester	Discontinue warfarin. SQ heparin (keep PTT > twice normal) OR Low-dose warfarin to be continued in high-risk patients after an informed consent obtained
During second trimester	Warfarin—drug of choice (Keep INR adjusted.)
During third trimester	Stop warfarin at 36–38 weeks. Start intravenous heparin. Stop heparin peripartum. Resume anticoagulation 4–6 h after uncomplicated delivery.

INR = international normalized ratio; PTT = partial thromboplastin time; SQ = subcutaneous.

patient. Thrombolytic therapy has been used safely and effectively but should be avoided whenever possible.

4. Endocarditis prophylaxis—The American Heart Association does not recommend prophylaxis for infective endocarditis in pregnant patients expected to have an uncomplicated course of pregnancy and labor and delivery. However, urinary catheter placement in established urinary tract infection, and vaginal delivery in vaginal infection are indications for intramuscular or intravenous antibiotics. The conservative approach is to administer endocarditis prophylaxis in pregnant patients with mechanical prosthetic heart valves, a history of infective endocarditis, those with most congenital heart disorders, obstructive hypertrophic cardiomyopathy, and those with mitral valve prolapse with mitral regurgitation who are undergoing interventions likely to cause septicemia.

Joglar JA, Page RL: Antiarrhythmic drugs in pregnancy. Curr Opin Cardiol 2001;16(1):40.

Chow T, Galvin J, McGovern B: Antiarrhythmic therapy in pregnancy and lactation. Am J Cardiol 1998;82(4A):581.

Witlin AG, Mattar FM, Saade GR et al: Presentation of venous thromboembolism during pregnancy: Am J Obstet Gynecol 1999;18(5 Pt 1):1118.

Tam WH, Wong KS, Yuen PM et al: Low-molecular-weight heparin and thromboembolism in pregnancy. Lancet 1999;353 (9156):932.

Ramin SM, Ramin KD, Gilstrap LC: Anticoagulants and thrombolytics during pregnancy. Semin Perinatol 1997;21(2):149.

B. SURGICAL TREATMENT IN PREGNANCY

Ideally, most cardiac diseases requiring surgical correction are diagnosed and treated before the patient be-

comes pregnant, so the data is anecdotal. In general, cardiac surgery in pregnant patients is not associated with significant maternal risk but may cause fetal wastage. Fetal risk has been reported to be as high as 33%. Pregnant women requiring cardiac surgery need utmost care, adequate valve selection, and anticoagulation to ensure a good outcome.

Surgery should be reserved for severely symptomatic patients and those who are refractory to medical therapy, and it should be avoided in the first trimester, if possible. Procedures not involving cardiopulmonary bypass are preferred because of associated risks of fetal bradycardia and hypoperfusion.

Vaska PL: Cardiac Surgery in special populations, Part 2: Women, pregnant patients, and Jehovah's Witnesses. AACN Clin Issues 1997;8(1):59.

C. LABOR AND DELIVERY

Labor and delivery are periods of maximal hemodynamic stress during pregnancy. Pain, anxiety, and uterine contractions all contribute to altered hemodynamics. Oxygen consumption is higher, and cardiac output is increased up to 50% due to stroke volume changes. Both systolic and diastolic pressures are increased significantly during uterine contractions, especially in the second stage. Anesthesia and analgesia during labor and delivery may affect oxygen consumption, but the do not reduce increased cardiac output secondary to uterine contractions.

Patients with preexisting cardiac disease may develop acute decompensation. This increase in preload and cardiac output can be devastating in a patient with limited cardiac reserve or an obstructive valvular lesion. Patients at greatest risk for complications during labor and delivery include those with significant pulmonary hypertension and those in New York Heart Association functional class III or IV.

The preferred method of delivery is vaginal, with careful attention paid to pain control by regional anesthesia to avoid tachycardia. Postpartum hemorrhage and excessive fluid intake should be prevented. Invasive hemodynamic monitoring may be needed in some cases to guide treatment rapidly during labor and delivery. In these patients, the monitoring should be continued for at least 24–48 h after delivery or until hemodynamic stability is ensured. Cesarean section should be performed only for obstetric indications because it can also create blood loss and fluid shifts. Regardless of the delivery method, however, effective pain control is absolutely essential. Antibiotic prophylaxis should be administered when indicated.

Prognosis

Maternal mortality and morbidity rates during pregnancy depend on the underlying cardiac lesion and the functional status of the patient (see Table 31–2). The greatest risk of maternal mortality (25–50%) is for patients with pulmonary hypertension, complicated coarctation of the aorta, and Marfan's syndrome with a dilated aorta. Pulmonary vascular disease prevents the adaptive mechanisms of normal pregnancy and makes labor, delivery, and the early postpartum period particularly problematic. Moderate-to-severe mitral stenosis, aortic stenosis, the presence of mechanical prosthetic valves, uncomplicated coarctation of the aorta, uncorrected congenital heart diseases, and Marfan's syndrome with a normal aorta are associated with a 5–10% mortality rate. Left-to-right shunts, pulmonary valve disease, corrected congenital heart disease, bioprosthetic valves, and mild-to-moderate mitral stenosis have a mortality rate of less than 1%.

The functional status of a patient should be classified according to the New York Heart Association classification system. Patients in class I or II can be expected to undergo pregnancy with a less than 0.5% risk of death. Patients in class III or IV have a higher expected mortality rate of approximately 7%.

Crawford MH: Pregnancy and the heart. In Alpert JS: The AHA Clinical Cardiac Consult. Philadelphia: Lippincott Williams & Wilkins, 2001;54.

Endocrinology and the Heart

32

B. Sylvia Vela, MD

Endocrinology involves the study of glands that secrete hormones into the circulation for effects at distant target sites. At present, more than 100 hormones are known to be released into the circulation, with more than 200 types of receptors on target cells in the human body. Many of these cells contain literally thousands of receptors on their surfaces. Because these hormone receptors are so ubiquitous throughout the body, the presence or absence of a single hormone can have multiple effects on one or more organ systems, including the cardiovascular system. This chapter considers most of the common and some uncommon endocrinopathies that can affect the heart, addressing specifically how they can be recognized and treated to best restore cardiovascular health.

THYROID AND THE HEART

Thyroid hormone has profound effects on the cardiovascular system, regulating vascular tone and contractility and the metabolic demands of the body. Thyroid disease often presents solely with cardiovascular manifestations, necessitating a thorough search for this potentially reversible cause of heart disease.

Thyroid hormone regulates oxidative and metabolic processes throughout the body, by directing cellular protein synthesis at the nuclear level. Both overproduction or underproduction of thyroid hormone can disrupt normal metabolic function. Under the control of pituitary release of thyroid-stimulating hormone (TSH), the thyroid gland secretes approximately 90 mg of 3,5,3′,5′-tetraiodothyronine (T_4) and 30 mg of 3,5,3′-triiodothyronine (T_3), mostly bound to plasma proteins. The free, or unbound, fraction of hormone negatively feeds back at the level of the hypothalamus and pituitary to suppress further release of thyroid-releasing hormone (TRH) and TSH. Steps necessary in the production of thyroid hormone include the trapping of iodine by the gland; organification, or iodination, of the tyrosyl residues within the prohormone thyroglobulin; and coupling of monoiodotyrosines and diiodotyrosines to form either T_3 or T_4.

1. HYPERTHYROIDISM

ESSENTIALS OF DIAGNOSIS

- *Suppressed TSH below the lower normal limits*
- *High free T_4, total T_4 and free thyroxine index, or high free T_3 or total T_3 radioimmunoassay in T_3 toxicosis*
- *High 24-h radioactive iodine uptake in Graves' disease or toxic multinodular goiter; low uptake in thyroiditis or exogenous cause*
- *Symmetric goiter (often with bruit) and exophthalmos in Graves' disease*

General Considerations

In hyperthyroidism, increased levels of thyroid hormone result in a hyperdynamic cardiovascular system. The enhanced diastolic and systolic performance is due to the effect of T_3 on the regulation of specific cardiac genes. These genes promote the expression of structural proteins of the contractile apparatus of the cardiac myocyte; the α and β-heavy chains. Changes in expression of these isoforms occur in thyroid disease. The fast α-myosin heavy-chain molecule, which has greater ATPase activity and thus augments cardiac contraction, is regulated by T_3. In the absence of thyroid hormone, the slow β-myosin heavy-chain isoform is expressed. In addition, thyroid hormone increases calcium-activated ATPase and decreases phospholamban in the sarcoplasmic reticulum, thereby regulating intracellular calcium concentration and increasing inotropism. The causes of hyperthyroidism are listed in Table 32–1.

In general, the hyperdynamic activity of the hyperthyroid cardiovascular system is similar to that of other conditions in which the sympathetic nervous system is activated with the release of catecholamines. There is

Table 32–1. Causes of hyperthyroidism.

Etiology	Comments
Graves' disease	Symmetric smooth goiter, ophthalmopathy, elevated/iodine-131I uptake, homogeneous uptake on thyroid scan, TSH-receptor antibodies
Toxic multinodular goiter	Nodular goiter, nonhomogeneous uptake on thyroid scan
Autonomous thyroid nodule	Single large "hot" nodule on thyroid scan, suppressing rest of thyroid tissue
Thyroiditis	
Subacute	Tender firm goiter, low 131I uptake, transient high ESR
Radiation	Tender goiter, low iodine-131 uptake, high ESR; occurs after iodine-131 therapy
Painless (silent)	Nontender goiter, low iodine-131 uptake, normal ESR
Postpartum	Nontender goiter, low iodine-131 uptake, antithyroid antibodies, transient; tends to recur with each pregnancy
Exogenous	
Amiodarone	Low or normal Iodine-131 uptake
Iatrogenic	Absent goiter, low serum thyroglobulin, low iodine-131 uptake
Factitious	Absent goiter, low serum thyroglobulin, low iodine-131 uptake
Iodine induced	Low iodine-131 uptake, high 24-h urinary iodide excretion; history of iodine ingestion or exposure (contrast agents)
Rare Causes	
Struma ovarii	Low iodine-131 uptake; may have palpable ovary
Trophoblastic tumor	Very high HCG
Metastatic follicular carcinoma	Usually obvious metastases on iodine-131 scan
TSH-producing adenoma	TSH not suppressed, tumor on CT or MRI of pituitary; consider if gland regrows post thyroidectomy or iodine-131 treatment

CT = computed tomography; ESR = erythrocyte sedimentation rate; HCG = human chorionic gonadotropin; MRI = magnetic resonance imaging; TSH = thyroid-stimulating hormone.

enhanced cardiac output, increased stroke volume, enhanced left ventricular contractility, decreased systemic vascular resistance, tachycardia with a wide pulse pressure, a hyperdynamic precordium, increased myocardial oxygen consumption, and increased coronary flow. Although systolic contraction and diastolic relaxation are augmented, the heart is functioning near capacity, with little cardiac reserve.

Surprisingly, catecholamine levels are low or normal in hyperthyroidism, and these catecholamine-like effects are believed to be due to a demonstrable increase in the responsiveness of β-catecholamine receptors as well as increases in the guanine-nucleotide-binding regulatory protein (G protein), an intermediate mediator of signal transduction. In addition, thyroid hormone may have direct effects on sinoatrial node automaticity

that are not mediated through the autonomic nervous system.

Clinical Findings

A. SYMPTOMS AND SIGNS

1. Systemic symptoms and signs—Patients with hyperthyroidism often complain of weight loss despite an increased appetite; this helps distinguish this condition from other wasting conditions such as cancer or acquired immune deficiency syndrome. Occasionally, the appetite may be so great as to result in weight gain. A fine resting tremor of the hands is noticed, along with nervousness, anxiety, insomnia, mood swings, and irritability. Heat intolerance and sweaty skin are seen. Proximal muscle weakness and muscle wasting may be prominent. An increased number of bowel movements or diarrhea is due to decreased transit time in the gut. Diplopia on lateral gaze is seen in Graves' ophthalmopathy as a result of extraocular muscle hypertrophy. Rarely, choreoathetosis and periodic paralysis occur.

2. Cardiovascular symptoms and signs—Frequently the patient has cardiovascular symptoms, including palpitations, dyspnea, and atypical chest pain. Cardiac arrhythmias are common, especially atrial premature contractions and atrial fibrillation. In the elderly, atrial fibrillation may be the only manifestation of thyrotoxicosis, a condition known as **apathetic hyperthyroidism.** Approximately 10–20% of patients with atrial fibrillation are thyrotoxic, and 10–20% of thyrotoxic patients have atrial fibrillation. The risk of arterial thromboembolism is increased in thyrotoxic patients with atrial fibrillation, as it is in other patients with atrial fibrillation. Other atrial dysrhythmias, such as paroxysmal atrial tachycardia and atrial flutter, are unusual. Ventricular arrhythmias usually indicate underlying cardiac disease.

Exercise intolerance and dyspnea on exertion can occur with or without left-sided heart failure. Heart failure is usually precipitated by atrial fibrillation, in which the rapid ventricular rate and the loss of the atrial kick impair diastolic filling. Most patients with heart failure have underlying cardiac disease that predisposes them to the development of ventricular dysfunction. High-output heart failure can also occur, but it is rare.

Often, thyrotoxicosis precipitates exacerbation of angina when the increased demands placed on the heart by the thyrotoxic state are accompanied by the underlying fixed atherosclerotic lesions of coronary artery disease. The angina improves once the thyrotoxicosis is treated, and frank myocardial infarction precipitated by thyrotoxicosis is rare.

B. PHYSICAL EXAMINATION

Stare, lid retraction, and lid lag are usually present because of the high catecholamine-like state. Exophthalmos, proptosis, and diplopia are only seen in Graves' disease and are caused by hypertrophy of the extraocular muscles. In most conditions a goiter is present; in Graves' disease, it is symmetric and smooth, often with an audible bruit. Multinodular goiters are usually asymmetric and lumpy and may extend behind the sternal notch into the thorax, or they may cause tracheal deviation. Absence of a goiter, especially in a young person, should raise the suspicion of factitious hyperthyroidism; elderly patients, however, may not have a palpable goiter in the presence of disease.

The precordium is hyperdynamic, with loud heart sounds reflecting accelerated atrioventricular flow. Systolic ejection murmurs may be heard, reflecting increased flow across the aortic and pulmonic valves. The pulse is rapid and bounding. The skin has an unusually soft and velvety texture and is often sweaty. There is proximal muscle weakness, with patients often having difficulty rising from a squatting position. Deep tendon reflexes are hyperreflexic, and a resting tremor is present. Dermopathy or localized edema may be present on the shins (pretibial myxedema). Acropachy (subperiosteal resorption of the distal digits) can look like clubbing of the fingers. Onycholysis (lifting of the nail from the nail bed) is a rare but very supportive finding of hyperthyroidism.

In younger patients, especially young women, Graves' disease is the most common cause of thyrotoxicosis. Graves' disease is an autoimmune disease in which antibodies to the TSH receptor stimulate both excessive thyroid growth and thyroid hormone production. These patients typically have a symmetric goiter (often with a bruit) with or without exophthalmos. In the elderly, especially those with apathetic hyperthyroidism, symptoms and signs may be absent. Toxic multinodular goiter is a more common diagnosis in patients over the age of 40. Usually these goiters are very large and nodular (as the name suggests). Iatrogenic or factitious thyrotoxicosis should always be considered; these patients typically have no goiter, and the thyroglobulin level is suppressed. Clinicians should suspect hyperthyroidism in patients with persistent sinus tachycardia and atrial fibrillation, unexplained congestive heart failure, or unstable angina.

C. DIAGNOSTIC STUDIES

1. Electrocardiography and echocardiography—Sinus tachycardia is usually present, although any supraventricular tachycardia can be seen. Atrial fibrillation occurs in 10–20% of hyperthyroid patients; its prevalence in the population at large is 0.4%. On echocardiography, a hypercontractile state is seen with rapid filling of a highly compliant ventricle. Increased left ventricular mass and cardiac hypertrophy can also be seen.

2. Laboratory findings—Diagnosis is made by measurement of thyroid function tests (Table 32–2). Thyroid-stimulating hormone should be suppressed below the lower limit of detection, and the free T_4 or free thyroxine index (FTI) should be elevated, confirming the diagnosis. If the free T_4 or FTI is normal, measurement of total or free T_3 is recommended to rule out a condition known as T_3 toxicosis, in which the serum T_4 level is normal, but the total or free T_3 is elevated. If the only abnormality is a suppressed TSH, subclinical hyperthyroidism versus a systemic nonthyroidal illness must be considered. Thyroid function tests should be repeated after any period of illness to determine whether the abnormal thyroid function

Table 32–2. Tests in hyperthyroidism.

Condition	T$_4$	T$_3$	TSH	Iodine-131 Uptake
Graves' disease	↑, N	↑	↓	↑↑↑
Multinodular goiter	↑, N	↑	↓	↑↑
Solitary nodule	↑, N	↑	↓	↑ or nl
Early subacute and silent thyroiditis	↑	↑	↓	↓
Exogenous T$_4$	↑	↑	↓	↓
Exogenous T$_3$	↓	↑	↓	↓
Iodine-induced	↑	↑	↓	↓
Ectopic	↑, N	↑	↓	↓
TSH-producing pituitary tumor	↑, N	↑	↑, N	↑

T$_4$ = tetraiodothyronine; T$_3$ = triiodothyronine.

tests have resolved and were due to nonthyroidal illness.

Other tests that may be helpful include measurement of antithyroid antibodies (antimicrosomal or thyroidperoxidase antibodies) or TSH receptor antibody, which are elevated in patients with Graves' disease. Thyroglobulin levels will be suppressed in patients with factitious or iatrogenic thyrotoxicosis. Before treatment with radioactive iodine, all suspected hyperthyroid patients should have a radioactive iodine uptake (RAIU) test to ensure that hyperthyroid patients with thyroiditis or exogenous hyperthyroidism are not mistakenly treated for these transient, reversible conditions. Elevated RAIU is seen in Graves' disease, toxic multinodular goiter, and occasionally in an autonomously functioning thyroid nodule. In contrast, a decreased RAIU is seen in thyroiditis and exogenous hyperthyroidism. Thyroid scans rarely add any useful information to a good physical examination in patients with diffusely enlarged thyroid glands. In Graves' disease, the scan typically shows an enlarged symmetric gland with homogeneous uptake. Thyroid scans are occasionally helpful in identifying an adenoma or multinodular gland, in which one or more cold spots are seen.

Treatment

Treatment is directed at rapidly improving symptoms and reducing demands on the heart. The mainstay of treatment is accomplished by preventing thyroid hormone synthesis and release with antithyroid drugs, followed by radioactive iodine thyroid ablation (Table 32–3). β-blockers are most commonly used to improve symptoms. If the tachycardia is considered to be significantly deleterious in patients with heart failure, esmolol, which has a rapid onset of action and short half-life, may be given intravenously; it should be stopped—with rapid reversal—if heart failure worsens. Tremor and tachycardia will improve almost immediately with β-blocker therapy although systolic and diastolic contractile performance will not change due to direct effects of thyroid hormone on cardiac muscle. Of the oral β-blockers, propranolol is preferred because it also prevents the peripheral conversion of T$_4$ to T$_3$. The dose should be titrated to the patient's pulse and is usually 20–80 mg qid. Occasionally, high doses (80–320 mg qid) of propranolol are required in thyroid storm.

Thionamides are used to prevent thyroid hormone release and synthesis, by blocking iodine oxidation, organification, and iodotyrosine coupling. Propylthiouracil (PTU) and methimazole are the thionamides used in this country. Because they deplete intrathyroidal stores of thyroid hormone, they circumvent the precipitation of thyroid storm that can result from radiation thyroiditis after radioactive iodine ablation. Doses typically begin at 50–100 mg tid of PTU and 10–30 mg daily of methimazole. Methimazole may be preferred because of its once-a-day dosing and lower incidence of side effects. These drugs are typically withdrawn 3–5 days prior to radioactive iodine ablation and restarted 3–5 days after ablation. Thionamides are known to cause nausea and rash and, of most concern, agranulocytosis in 10% of patients.

Other drugs, including lithium, iodides, and steroids, are usually reserved for the prevention of life-threatening conditions such as thyroid storm; occasionally, they are used for patients with severe congestive heart failure

Table 32–3. Agents used to treat hyperthyroidism.

Agent	Dose	Mechanism of Action
Thionamides		
Propylthiouracil	50–300 mg, PO tid	Inhibits thyroid hormone synthesis
		Inhibits T_4 conversion to T_3
Methimazole	10–60 mg, PO QD	Inhibits thyroid hormone synthesis
Beta-blockers		
Propranolol	10–80 mg, PO q6–8h	Decreases β-adrenergic activity; inhibits T_4 conversion to T_3
Atenolol	50–100 mg/day PO	Decreases β-adrenergic activity
Nadolol	80–160 mg/day PO	Decreases β-adrenergic activity
Metoprolol	100–200 mg/day PO	Decreases β-adrenergic activity
Iodides		
SSKI	5 drops PO q6–8h	Prevents thyroid hormone release
Lugol's	5 drops PO q6–8h	Prevents thyroid hormone release
Ipodate	3 g PO q2–3 days or 0.5 g/day	Prevents thyroid hormone release
Iodine-131	Calculated dose	Destroys overfunctioning thyroid
Other agents		
Lithium	300 mg PO tid (monitor blood levels)	Prevents thyroid hormone release
Hydrocortisone	50–100 mg IV q6–8h	Decreases peripheral conversion of T_4 to T_3; prevents thyroid hormone release

SSKI = saturated solution of potassium iodide; T_4 = tetriiodothyronine; T_3 = triiodothyronine.

or unstable angina secondary to thyrotoxicosis. Lithium prevents thyroid hormone release, and the dosage is determined by monitoring therapeutic serum levels. Iodides abruptly prevent the release of thyroid hormone. They **must** be used in conjunction with thionamides because rebound or escape occurs commonly. Doses are usually 3–5 drops of a supersaturated potassium iodide solution or Lugol's solution (50 mg of iodide per drop) every 6–8 h.

Parenteral glucocorticoids are usually given in stress doses for thyroid storm. Steroids inhibit thyroid hormone secretion and prevent peripheral conversion of T_4 to T_3. Doses are usually 50–100 mg of hydrocortisone every 6–8 h.

Radioactive iodine (^{131}-I) is the preferred and definitive treatment for thyrotoxicosis in patients with a high RAIU. Because thyroid tissue is the only tissue that requires iodine (for thyroid hormone synthesis), radioactive iodine is used for thyroid gland destruction. The advantages of radioactive iodine include the fact that usually only a single treatment is needed and that it is relatively safe and inexpensive. Because the treatment usually requires 3–6 months to resolve the hyperthyroidism, most patients will require interim therapy with thionamides during that time. The patient is usually rendered hypothyroid as a result of the treatment and is then treated with long-term thyroid hormone replacement.

Patients with multinodular goiters, who have lower RAIU (than do patients with Graves' disease), often have an inadequate response to ^{131}I, and may require retreatment or surgery. Pregnant patients should not receive ^{131}I and should therefore be treated with PTU, with or without β-blockers, or with subtotal thyroidectomy in the second trimester.

Aspirin, nonsteroidal antiinflammatory drugs, and—rarely—steroids are used if painful thyroiditis is present. Thyroiditis is reversible and requires short-term therapy only. Beta-blockers can be used temporarily to improve thyrotoxic symptoms.

Treatment of congestive heart failure and atrial fibrillation are essentially the same as for a euthyroid individual. Treatment should include use of a nonselective β-blocker (eg, propranolol) or a selective $β_1$-blocker (eg, atenolol) to normalize the heart rate. The physician should be aware, however, that treatment of atrial fibrillation is limited to control of the ventricular rate because cardioversion will not be successful as long as the thyrotoxicosis is present. In addition, patients may be relatively resistant to digoxin. Usually, sinus rhythm returns within 6 weeks with resolution of the thyrotoxic state. Older patients with underlying cardiac disease may not spontaneously revert and may require cardioversion. Anticoagulation should be considered until the patient is euthyroid and in sinus rhythm.

Once the patient becomes euthyroid, the hyperdynamic cardiovascular manifestations disappear. Atrial fibrillation should convert to normal sinus rhythm in more than 60% of patients, and angina should improve because of decreased demands on the heart.

Prognosis

The prognosis is generally excellent for most hyperthyroid conditions. Graves' disease and autonomously functioning thyroid nodules usually respond well to ^{131}I and do not recur. As noted previously, multinodular goiters may be relatively resistant to ^{131}I and may ultimately require subtotal thyroidectomy. Despite surgical treatment, multinodular goiters frequently recur.

Biondi B, Fazio S, Carella C et al: Cardiac effects of long term thyrotropin-suppressive therapy with levothyroxine. J Clin Endocrinol Metab 1993;77:334.

Giladi M, Aderka D, Zeligman-Melatzki L et al: Is idiopathic atrial fibrillation caused by occult thyrotoxicosis? A study of one hundred consecutive patients with atrial fibrillation. Int J Cardiol 1991;30:309.

Glikson M, Freimark D, Leor R et al: Unstable anginal syndrome and pulmonary oedema due to thyrotoxicosis. Postgrad Med J 1991;67:81.

Klein I, Ojamaa K: Cardiovascular manifestations of endocrine disease. J Clin Endocrinol Metab 1992;75:339.

Klein I, Ojamaa K: Thyrotoxicosis and the heart. Endocrinol Metab Clin North Am 1998;27(1):51.

Klein I, Ojamaa K: Thyroid hormone and the cardiovascular system. N Engl J Med 2001;344:501.

Ladenson PW: Recognition and management of cardiovascular disease related to thyroid function. Am J Med 1990;88:638.

Levey GS, Klein I: Catecholamine thyroid hormone interactions and the cardiovascular manifestations of hyperthyroidism. Am J Med 1990;88:642.

Mintz G, Pizzarello R, Klein I: Enhanced left ventricular diastolic function in hyperthyroidism: Noninvasive assessment and response to treatment. J Clin Endocrinol Metab 1991;73;146.

Toft AD, Boon NA: Thyroid disease and the heart. Heart 2000;84: 455.

Valcavi R, Menozzi C, Roti E et al: Sinus node function in hyperthyroid patients. J Clin Endocrinol Metab 1992;75:339.

Woeber KA: Thyrotoxicosis and the heart. N Engl J Med 1992; 327:94.

2. HYPOTHYROIDISM

 ESSENTIALS OF DIAGNOSIS

- TSH above the range of normal (primary hypothyroidism)
- Low free T_4 or low free thyroxine index

General Considerations

Hypothyroidism is the term given to any degree of thyroid hormone deficiency. The term **myxedema** is reserved for patients with thyroid hormone deficiency of such severity that profound hypothermia, hypoventilation, hypotension, and central nervous system signs are evident on physical examination. It is estimated that anywhere from 0.5% to 5.0% of the adult population of the United States has underlying hypothyroidism.

Hypothyroidism is associated with accelerated atherosclerosis, likely from the accompanying hyperlipidemia. The atherosclerosis is especially pronounced in the presence of hypertension; however, angina is uncommon and the incidence of myocardial infarction is not increased. This is probably due to the decreased metabolic demands placed on the heart in the hypothyroid state. More commonly, angina is precipitated or worsened by rapid thyroid hormone replacement.

Clinical Findings

A. SYMPTOMS AND SIGNS

1. Systemic symptoms and signs—Hypothyroidism is an insidious disease and may be subtle in its progression and presentation. Patients typically complain of weight gain (although morbid obesity does not occur), weakness, lethargy, fatigue, depression, muscle cramps, constipation, cold intolerance, dry skin, and coarse hair. Women often have menstrual disorders (most commonly amenorrhea), and men may have impotence or decreased libido.

2. Cardiovascular symptoms and signs—Cardiovascular findings are the opposite of those found in hyperthyroidism. There is a decrease in cardiac output because of a reduction in stroke volume and heart rate, reflecting the loss of inotropism and chronotropism characteristic of thyroid hormone. Congestive heart failure rarely occurs, because the decrease in cardiac output is usually matched by a decrease in metabolic demand. Myocardial oxygen consumption appears to be decreased below levels expected by the reduced workload to an extent that the hypothyroid heart can be thought of as being more efficient. Systemic vascular resistance is increased and blood volume is reduced, causing prolongation of circulation time and a decrease in blood flow to the periphery. In most tissues, this decrease in tissue perfusion is accompanied by decreased oxygen consumption, so that the mixed arteriovenous O_2 difference remains normal. The hemodynamic alterations resemble those of congestive heart failure except that pulmonary congestion does not occur, and pulmonary artery and right ventricle pressures are often normal. In addition, cardiac output and systemic vascular resistance increase normally in response to exercise, unlike heart failure from other causes.

Marked hypothyroidism must be present for several months before cardiovascular manifestations occur. Common complaints of hypothyroid patients are exertional dyspnea, decreased exercise tolerance, and easy fatigability. As the hypothyroidism worsens, congestive heart failure and pleural and pericardial effusions become prominent. Myxedematous heart failure can be distinguished from other causes in that it responds to exercise with an increased heart rate; improves with thyroid hormone replacement, but not digitalis and diuretics; rarely results in pulmonary congestion; and exhibits high protein content effusions.

B. Physical Examination

Hypothermia, bradycardia with weak arterial pulses, and mild hypertension are characteristic vital signs. The hypertension may be due to increased peripheral resistance related to an increased number of α-sympathetic receptors. Thyroid hormone replacement will normalize blood pressure in approximately one third of these patients. The patient may appear pale, with periorbital edema and facial puffiness. Hair and skin are usually coarse and dry. Goiter is present in patients with Hashimoto's thyroiditis, congenital enzyme deficiencies, iodine deficiency, and thyroid hormone resistance; it is also present in patients taking amiodarone and antithyroid drug therapy such as thionamides and lithium. Goiter is absent after thyroidectomy, successful ^{131}I therapy, thyroid dysgenesis, and panhypopituitarism.

Percussion of the chest may reveal pleural effusions from increased capillary permeability and the leakage of proteins into the interstitial space. Distant heart sounds are present, especially if a pericardial effusion is present. Reflexes are characteristically delayed in the return phase. Nonpitting edema may be present as a result of the deposition of mucopolysaccharides. Severe hypothyroidism can progress to myxedema coma, and anasarca may be present. In the presence of congestive heart failure, pitting edema may be superimposed on the nonpitting edema.

C. Diagnostic Studies

1. Electrocardiography and echocardiography— Electrocardiographic (ECG) changes include sinus bradycardia, prolonged PR and QT intervals, low voltage complexes, and flattened or inverted T waves. Atrial, ventricular, and intraventricular conduction delays are three times as likely in patients with myxedema as in the general population. Pericardial effusion is probably partly responsible for these ECG changes. Systolic time intervals are altered, the preejection period is prolonged, and the ratio of preejection period to left ventricular ejection time is increased.

Pericardial effusions occur in as many as 30% of all hypothyroid patients. Cardiac tamponade is unusual because of the slow accumulation of fluid, which does not increase pericardial pressure excessively. A reduced velocity of shortening, despite normal total shortening, can be seen on echocardiography. These studies have also revealed asymmetric septal hypertrophy and obstruction of the left ventricular outflow tract in a large percentage of patients. These findings disappear when the hypothyroidism is treated.

2. Laboratory findings—Asymptomatic hypothyroid individuals—such as the elderly—frequently go unrecognized. Therefore, all elderly patients and patients with premature atherosclerosis should be screened for primary hypothyroidism with a TSH. Although the most common cause of hypothyroidism is Hashimoto's thyroiditis, there are other causes of hypothyroidism (Table 32–4), such as lithium use or postsurgical or radioactive iodine ablation.

In primary hypothyroidism, TSH is elevated, and T_4, free T_4, and FTI are reduced. The absence of an elevated TSH indicates either nonthyroidal illness or hypothalamic-pituitary dysfunction. Severely ill patients are unlikely to have panhypopituitarism in the absence of other hormone deficiencies.

Occasionally TSH is mildly elevated in the face of a normal T_4. Subclinical hypothyroidism, as opposed to recovery from a nonthyroidal illness, must be considered. These patients are typically asymptomatic but are at intermediate risk of cardiovascular disease when compared with euthyroid or frankly hypothyroid individuals.

Antithyroid antibodies (antimicrosomal or thyroid peroxidase antibodies) are elevated in Hashimoto's thyroiditis. Creatine kinase isoenzymes are increased in hypothyroidism, although the isoenzyme pattern is usually MM and not MB. Hypothyroidism is a common cause of hyperlipidemia; 95% of hypothyroid individuals will have an elevated cholesterol, and 70% will have elevation in both cholesterol and triglycerides. Anemia of chronic disease may be seen, as may hyponatremia from impaired free-water clearance.

Treatment

Thyroxine therapy reverses all of the cardiovascular manifestations associated with hypothyroidism, including the subtle prolongation of contraction seen in sub-

Table 32–4. Causes of hypothyroidism.

Causes	Comments
Destructive	
^{131}I ablation	No palpable thyroid tissue
Thyroid surgery	Scar evident
External radiation to neck	History of malignancy
Infiltrative diseases	Diagnose by fine-needle aspirate
Autoimmune	
Hashimoto's thyroiditis	Goiter, antithyroid antibodies
Following Graves' disease	History of Graves'; may have ophthalmopathy
Hereditary or congential	
Congenital dyshormonogenesis	Goiter, usually diagnosed in childhood
Thyroid hormone resistance	Rare, familial
Iodine deficiency	Cretin if untreated; unusual in United States
Drug-induced	
Lithium	Goiter, on lithium, usually with underlying predisposition to thyroid disease
Thionamides	History of hyperthyroidism
Iodines	Wolff-Chaikoff effect
Pituitary/hypothalamic failure	Other hormone deficiencies usually apparent

clinical hypothyroidism. The most important consideration with thyroid hormone replacement therapy is the speed of rendering the patient euthyroid. Young patients without evidence of cardiac disease can be replaced with full doses of thyroxine. Patients over the age of 55 or patients with evidence or suspicion of cardiac disease require slow and judicious use of thyroid hormone replacement to prevent exacerbation of angina or precipitation of myocardial infarction. The typical regimen would begin with 25 μg (0.025 mg/day) or one fourth of a normal replacement dose, gradually increased over several months to normal replacement doses of approximately 100–150 μg (0.1–0.15 mg/day). Because the half-life of T_4 is 1 week, patients will notice alleviation of their symptoms in 1–2 months after reaching a typical replacement dose.

Patients with unstable angina and hypothyroidism are more difficult to treat because of the risk of exacerbating the angina. Very small doses of hormone should be used, and the dosage increments must be made slowly over a longer-than-usual time. If necessary, angioplasty or coronary artery bypass grafting (CABG) should be recommended, after which—if revasculariza-tion is complete—thyroid hormone replacement can occur at the usual dosage and rate. Angioplasty and CABG surgery can safely be done in a hypothyroid individual without significantly increasing morbidity and mortality. Adjustments in anesthesia and drug doses should be made because their decreased metabolic clearance makes hypothyroid patients very sensitive to these agents.

It is important to monitor therapy with TSH levels. TSH-suppressive doses of levothyroxine may cause or aggravate osteopenia, precipitate angina pectoris, increase left ventricular mass, and increase the incidence of atrial arrhythmias.

Treatment of myxedema coma is controversial. Many authors recommend high initial doses of intravenous T_4 (400 μg) to saturate receptors and replenish diminished stores, followed by 100 μg per day. Others prefer a more conservative approach of 50–100 μg IV per day. Stress doses of hydrocortisone should also be administered (100 mg IV every 6–8 h) because hypothyroidism and adrenal insufficiency frequently coexist, and thyroid hormone replacement may precipitate adrenal crisis.

Prognosis

In the absence of coexisting heart disease, treatment with thyroid hormone and restoration of a euthyroid status correct the hemodynamic, ECG, and serum enzyme alterations and restores heart size to normal. Therapy is lifelong, and relapses occur if the patient is noncompliant or taken off therapy for any reason.

Gottehrer A, Roa J, Stanford GG et al: Hypothyroidism and pleural effusions. Chest 1990;98:1130.

Hak AE, Pols HA, Visser TJ et al: Subclinical hypothyroidism is an independent risk factor for atherosclerosis and myocardial infarction in elderly women: The Rotterdam study. Ann Intern Med 2000;132:270.

Klein I, Ojamaa K: Cardiovascular manifestations of endocrine disease. J Clin Endocrinol Metab 1992;75:339.

Klein I, Ojamaa K: Thyroid hormone and the cardiovascular system. N Engl J Med 2001;344:501.

Ladenson PW: Recognition and management of cardiovascular disease related to thyroid dysfunction. Am J Med 1990;88:638.

Lee RT, Plappert M, Sutton MG et al: Depressed left ventricular systolic ejection force in hypothyroidism. Am J Cardiol 1990;65:526.

Monzani F, Di Bello V, Caraccio N et al: Effect of levothyroxine on cardiac function and structure in subclinical hypothyroidism: A double blind, placebo-controlled study. J Clin Endocrinol Metab. 2001;86:1110.

Polikar R, Kennedy B, Maisel A et al: Decreased adrenergic sensitivity in patients with hypothyroidism. J Am Coll Cardiol 1990;15:94.

Staub JJ, Althaus BU, Engler H et al: Spectrum of subclinical and overt hypothyroidism: Effect on thyrotropin, prolactin and thyroid reserve, and metabolic impact on peripheral target tissues. Am J Med 1992;92:631.

Tielens ET, Pillay M, Storm C, et al: Changes in cardiac function at rest before and after treatment in primary hypothyroidism. Am J Cardiol 2000;85(3):376.

Toft AD, Boon NA: Thyroid disease and the heart. Heart. 2000; 84:455.

3. EFFECT OF HEART DISEASE ON THYROID FUNCTION

Acute or chronic illness such as occurs with myocardial infarction, congestive heart failure and during the postoperative period of cardiopulmonary bypass can make the interpretation of thyroid function tests difficult. T_3 and T_4 levels can drop as much as 20–40%, the so-called nonthyroidal illness. TSH is inhibited centrally and can be suppressed further by use of drugs such as dopamine or steroids to undetectable levels. As recovery from the underlying illness occurs, the TSH may rise above normal into the hypothyroid range. Consequently, patients with significant cardiovascular disease in a coronary care unit are likely to have abnormal thyroid function tests. In general, thyroid function testing should not be requested unless suspicion of thyroid disease is great because of such symptoms as goiter, oph-

thalmopathy, or unexplained atrial fibrillation. Studies examining the effect of T_3 treatment in the immediate post-CABG period have shown mixed results. Treatment with thyroid hormone for nonthyroidal illness cannot be recommended at this time.

Klein I, Ojamaa K: Thyroid hormone and the cardiovascular system. N Engl J Med 2001;344:501.

Toft AD, Boon NA: Thyroid disease and the heart. Heart 2000; 84:455.

4. CARDIOVASCULAR DRUGS AND THE THYROID

Normally, the thyroid gland secretes approximately 20% of the T_3 that is in the peripheral circulation. The remaining 80% is produced from monodeiodination of T_4 by the enzyme 5′-deiodinase. Propranolol and amiodarone inhibit the deiodinase enzyme and prevent peripheral conversion of T_4 to T_3 (the more potent thyroid hormone). This leads to low T_3 levels, which stimulates transient TSH release from the pituitary and consequent T_4 release from the thyroid. The overall result is a transiently elevated TSH for the first 1–3 months, a slightly elevated T_4 with a low-normal T_3. Typically, the patient remains euthyroid. Iodine is a major component of amiodarone; constituting 37% of the compound by weight. Maintenance doses of amiodarone (200–600 mg) provide 75–225 mg of iodine daily. Because the normal optimal daily intake of iodine is considered to be 150–200 µg, amiodarone provides a massively expanded iodine pool. Normally, the thyroid gland adjusts to the increased iodine substrate; however, in some individuals thyroid dysfunction, that is, thyrotoxicosis and hypothyroidism may occur. Because the elimination half-life of amiodarone is so long (22–55 days) and due to tissue storage of the drug and its slow release, thyroid dysfunction has been reported to occur even after discontinuation of the medication.

Overall incidence of thyroid dysfunction in patients receiving amiodarone is estimated to be between 2–24%. Amiodarone-induced thyrotoxicosis (AIT) is more common in countries with low iodine uptake, and amiodarone-induced hypothyroidism in areas that are iodine replete.

Amiodarone-induced thyrotoxicosis may occur at any time during or even after amiodarone treatment, particularly in patients with an underlying predisposition to thyroid disease, who have a goiter. These patients may present with weight loss, weakness, tremor, or new or recurrent atrial tachyarrhythmias. Classic symptoms may be masked by the antiadrenergic effects of amiodarone. Biochemical diagnosis is straightforward if the T_3 or free T_3 is elevated and the TSH suppressed to undetectable levels.

Pathogenesis is complex and can involve excessive thyroid hormone synthesis from the iodine load (so called type I AIT), or destructive thyroiditis (type II AIT). Features of both types of AIT can be seen in Table 32–5.

Therapy for AIT is difficult and requires knowledge of the underlying pathogenesis. In type I AIT, thionamides should be used to block further organification of iodine and synthesis of hormones. Larger then usual doses are often required (methimazole 40–60 mg/d or propylthiouracil 600–800 mg/d) because the iodine-rich gland is resistant to thionamide therapy. Potassium perchlorate (800–1000 mg/d for 15–45 days), a drug that inhibits iodine uptake into the gland, can also be used although with caution because agranulocytosis, aplastic anemia, and nephrotic syndrome have occurred at doses >1.5 g. Discontinuation of amiodarone, although often difficult, may be recommended and necessary in some cases. Thyroidectomy can be undertaken in severe cases unresponsive to medical therapy.

Type II AIT can be treated with high-dose steroids (prednisone 30–40 mg/d or equivalent) for 3 months with a gradual slow taper to minimize recurrence. Discontinuation of amiodarone is usually not necessary because the thyroiditis resolves within several weeks to months and rarely recurs. If the two types of AIT cannot be distinguished, therapy with both steroids and antithyroid drugs should be started.

Radioactive iodine therapy is not helpful because the high iodine concentration in the plasma and thyroid gland prevents the uptake of radioactive iodine. In patients with a history of AIT who require restarting amiodarone, consideration of radioactive iodine ablation prior to reinstitution of the drug should be strongly considered.

Like amiodarone, radiologic contrast material containing iodine such as that used in cardiac catheterizations, has the potential for causing transient thyrotoxicosis and for potentially causing decompensation in a patient with coronary artery disease.

Amiodarone-induced hypothyroidism occurs more frequently in the United States than AIT due to iodine sufficiency of the population. Patients typically are older and frequently have an underlying predisposition to thyroid disease as evidenced by the presence of antithyroid antibodies. Diagnosis is confirmed by an elevated TSH in conjunction with a low T_4 or free T_4.

The proposed pathogenesis is continual inhibition of thyroid hormone synthesis from excess iodine; the so called Wolff-Chiakoff effect. Treatment is much simpler than that for AIT because thyroid hormone replacement can easily be given along with amiodarone therapy. The goal of therapy is to bring the TSH and T_4 or free T_4 to the upper range of normal or slightly above normal. This target mimics the range of thyroid function seen in euthyroid individuals who take amiodarone.

Daniels GH: Amiodarone induced thyrotoxicosis. J Clin Endocrinol Metab 2001;86:3.

Haraj KJ, Licata AA: Effects of amiodarone on thyroid function. Ann Intern Med 1997;126:63.

Martino E, Bartalena L, Bogazzi F et al: The effects of amiodarone on the thyroid. Endocrine Reviews 2001;22:240.

Newman CM, Price A, Davies DW et al: Amiodarone and the thyroid: A practical guide to the management of thyroid dysfunction induced by amiodarone therapy. Heart 1998;79:121.

Table 32–5. Features of amiodarone-induced thyrotoxicosis.

	Type I	Type II
Pathogenesis	Excess hormone synthesis due to excess iodine	Excess hormone release due to thyroid destruction
Goiter	Often present; multinodular or diffuse	Occasionally present; small diffuse, firm, may be tender
Autoantibodies	May be present	Usually absent
IL-6	Normal/elevated	Markedly elevated
Radioactive iodine uptake	Low or normal	Low or suppressed
Color-flow Doppler	Normal or increased flow	Decreased flow
Thyroid Ultrasound	Nodular, hypoechoic, large	Normal
Therapy	Methimazole or PTU, perchlorate may be necessary, thyroidectomy may be necessary	Steroids
Subsequent hypothyroidism	No, unless thyroidectomy performed	Possible

Il-6 = interleukin-6; PTU = propylthiouracil.

PARATHYROID AND THE HEART

Parathyroid hormone (PTH) is responsible for calcium, phosphate, and magnesium homeostasis throughout the body. Although PTH itself has few effects on the heart, an excess or deficiency of this hormone can affect the cardiovascular system indirectly through its regulation of calcium.

1. HYPERPARATHYROIDISM

ESSENTIALS OF DIAGNOSIS

- *Inappropriately normal or elevated PTH*
- *Serum calcium level more than 10 mg/dL when corrected for serum albumin, or ionized calcium level higher than upper limit of normal range*
- *Increased 24-h urine calcium (more than 200 mg)*
- *Elevated alkaline phosphatase*
- *Decreased phosphate*

General Considerations

Primary hyperparathyroidism is most commonly due to overproduction of PTH from a parathyroid adenoma. Rare causes include parathyroid hyperplasia in familial cases, often in the setting of a multiple endocrine neoplasia syndrome (MEN). Secondary hyperparathyroidism occurs in hypocalcemic states in which the lack of negative feedback of calcium to the parathyroid glands results in overproduction of PTH and is usually seen in the setting of chronic hypocalcemia, vitamin D deficiency, or renal failure. Tertiary hyperparathyroidism can occur when chronic overstimulation of the parathyroid gland (as in renal failure) causes the autonomous release of PTH.

When the disorder is detected in an outpatient setting, the most common diagnosis is primary hyperparathyroidism from a parathyroid adenoma. Although parathyroid hyperplasia is rare, it is usually found in the setting of MEN; a rare hereditary condition of multiple endocrine neoplasias. MEN I comprises hyperparathyroidism, pituitary adenoma, and pancreatic islet-cell tumor; MEN II consists of hyperparathyroidism, medullary thyroid carcinoma, and pheochromocytoma. Other considerations include benign familial hypercalcemia or familial hypocalciuric hypercalcemia; this condition looks like hyperparathyroidism except that urinary excretion of calcium is less than 200 mg in 24 h. Affected family members are asymptomatic, without the typical sequelae of hypercalcemia, and consequently do not require any treatment.

Granulomatous disease, such as tuberculosis or histoplasmosis, can cause hypercalcemia by increased 1-α-hydroxylase activity, which converts the inactive 25-hydroxy vitamin D to the active 1,25-dihydroxy vitamin D. All patients with hypercalcemia should be queried regarding calcium (including over-the-counter calcium carbonate antacids) and vitamin intake to rule out milk-alkali syndrome and vitamin D and A toxicity. Thyrotoxicosis can cause hypercalcemia because of increased bone turnover. Adrenal insufficiency is another cause of hypercalcemia.

When detected in an inpatient setting, hypercalcemia is usually the harbinger of malignancy and portends a poor prognosis. Malignancies associated with hypercalcemia include bone metastases, multiple myeloma, lymphoma, leukemia, and squamous cell cancers, primarily of the head and neck, which secrete PTH-related peptide. This can bind to PTH receptors and cause PTH-like effects.

The hyperparathyroid state, by altering serum calcium and PTH, has the potential to adversely effect the cardiovascular system. Hypertension; left ventricular hypertrophy (LVH); hypercontractility; arrhythmias; calcific deposits in the myocardium, aortic and mitral valves, and coronary arteries have all been described. Some but not all studies have demonstrated an increased incidence of cardiovascular death that seems to correlate with the degree and duration of disease.

Clinical Findings

A. SYMPTOMS AND SIGNS

1. Systemic symptoms and signs—Most patients with chronic hyperparathyroidism are asymptomatic and are detected through routine laboratory testing. Others complain of nonspecific symptoms such as fatigue and vague aches and pains. Nephrolithiasis, polyuria, polydipsia, constipation, osteoporosis, occasional pancreatitis and peptic ulcer, pruritus (from calcium phosphate deposits in the skin), and mental status changes now occur much less commonly among those whose symptoms are referable to the hyperparathyroidism.

Acute severe hypercalcemia (calcium levels higher than 15 mg/dL), which is not typically seen in primary hyperparathyroidism, can be due to the rare condition of parathyroid carcinoma or to other malignancies. These patients present with confusion, nausea, vomiting, volume depletion, depression, or psychosis; they need emergency treatment to survive.

2. Cardiovascular symptoms and signs—Arrhythmias are uncommon, but acute hypercalcemia can cause bradycardia and first-degree heart block. Acute elevation of calcium may cause hypertension, although this may be due to renal damage from nephrocalcinosis and elevated peripheral vascular resistance—a direct effect of calcium on the vascular smooth muscle cells. Left ventricular hypertrophy is noted in as many as 80% of patients referred for parathyroidectomy and can be reversible particularly in normotensive individuals. Valvular sclerosis on the other hand, does not appear to improve after parathyroidectomy but also does not appear to progress. Although European studies previously demonstrated an increased mortality rate from cardiovascular disease in patients with primary hyperparathyroidism, more recent data from the United States did not support this conclusion.

B. Physical Examination

Calcium deposition in the cornea, or band keratopathy, may be noted. In hyperparathyroidism secondary to renal failure, calcium and phosphate may precipitate in the soft tissues and in and around joints. These precipitants are usually readily seen on radiograph, palpated on physical examination, and, if severe, can limit mobility of the joints.

C. Diagnostic Studies

1. Electrocardiography and echocardiography—Hypercalcemia decreases the plateau phase of the cardiac action potential, reflected by a shortened ST segment and a reduced QT interval. The QT interval corrected for heart rate is probably the most reliable ECG index of hypercalcemia. With severe hypercalcemia (calcium level >16 mg/dL, or 4 mmol/L), the T wave widens, tending to increase the QT interval.

Echocardiography reveals a high incidence of LVH and calcification of aortic and mitral valves as well as the coronary tree and myocardium. Several studies have shown improvement after successful parathyroidectomy in subjects with symptomatic hyperparathyroidism. Cardiac abnormalities in the asymptomatic, mild hyperparathyroid patient are less demonstrable.

2. Laboratory findings—Typically, both serum calcium and ionized calcium are elevated, with an inappropriately normal or elevated PTH. Other causes of hypercalcemia are accompanied by a suppressed or low normal PTH. The 24-h urine calcium level is usually more than 200 mg. Phosphate levels are usually low or low normal because PTH has a phosphaturic effect on the kidney, and a hyperchloremic metabolic acidosis is present because of the bicarbonaturic effect of PTH. Alkaline phosphatase levels may be elevated, especially in the setting of hyperparathyroid bone disease.

Treatment & Prognosis

Parathyroidectomy is the definitive treatment for hyperparathyroidism and is indicated in all patients with symptoms as well as patients felt to be at high risk of progressive disease. Risk factors for progression include significant hypercalcemia (calcium level greater than

12 mg/dL) above the upper limit of normal, unexplained renal insufficiency, reduced cortical bone density at the one third distal forearm site (t-score <–2.5 SD) and relatively young patients <50 years of age. Additional considerations for surgical management include coexistent vitamin D deficiency, fracture, and perimenopausal status.

Successful parathyroidectomy normalizes calcium, phosphate, PTH, and alkaline phosphatase levels while improving bone density, slowing the progression of renal insufficiency, diminishing LVH, and improving symptoms. Hypertension may persist or progress in a percentage of patients, most likely the result of nephrocalcinosis and irreversible renal impairment. Postoperative hypocalcemia is common and may be transient or permanent. If it is permanent, the patient will require life-long calcium and vitamin D replacement.

Medical treatment is less preferable than surgery unless the patient has a contraindication to the latter. Current medical treatment is limited and includes administration of the bisphosphonates, pamidronate or risedronate (alendronate has not been studied), and estrogen in postmenopausal women. Estrogen doses are typically two to three times higher than the usual postmenopausal replacement doses (eg, 1.25 mg of Premarin to start) and will lower calcium by 0.5 mg/dL but not affect PTH. The bisphosphonates prevent bone resorption without inhibiting mineralization, therefore decreasing serum calcium levels. Unfortunately, bisphosphonates increase PTH levels, limiting their efficacy. Future medical therapy that holds significant promise includes use of calcimimetic agents that act as calcium receptor-agonists in parathyroid cells and inhibit parathyroid hormone secretion. For asymptomatic patients not felt to be at risk for progression of their disease, medical observation may be warranted.

Bilezikian JP: Primary hyperparathyroidism when to operate and when to observe. Endocrinol Metab Clin N Am 2000;29(3);465–478.

Consensus Development Conference on the Diagnosis and Management of Asymptomatic Primary Hyperparathyroidism. Ann Intern Med 1991;114:593.

Heath H: Primary hyperparathyroidism: Recent advances in pathogenesis, diagnosis and management. Adv Intern Med 1991;37:275.

Lind L, Jacobsson S, Palmer M et al: Cardiovascular risk factors in primary hyperparathyroidism: A 15 year follow-up of operated and unoperated cases. J Int Med 1991;230:29.

Piovesan A, Monineri N, Casasso F et al: Left ventricular hypertrophy in primary hyperparathyroidism. Effects of successful parathyroidectomy. Clin Endocrinol 1999;50:321-8.

Potts JT: Management of symptomatic hyperparathyroidism. J Clin Endocrinol Metab 1990;70;1489.

Silverberg SJ, Marriott TB, Bone III HG et al: Short term inhibition of parathyroid hormone secretion by a calcium receptor agonist in primary hyperparathyroidism. N Engl J Med 1997; 307:1506–1510.

Stefenelli T, Abela, C, Frank H et al: Cardiac abnormalities in patients with primary hyperparathyroidism: Implications for follow-up. J Clin Endocrinol Metab 1997;82:106-112.

ENDOCRINOLOGY AND THE HEART / **523**

Strewler G: Medical approaches to primary hyperparathyroidism. Endocrinol Metab Clin N Am 2000;29(3):523–39.

Wermers RA, Khosla S, Atkinson EJ et al: Survival after the diagnosis of hyperparathyroidism: A population-based study. Am J Med 1998;104:115-22.

2. HYPOPARATHYROIDISM

Hypoparathyroidism usually occurs in the postoperative setting after neck or thyroid surgery; it also occurs idiopathically. A functional hypoparathyroidism can occur in patients with magnesium deficiency because magnesium is a cofactor for PTH release. Patients usually complain of tingling around the mouth and in the hands and feet. Cardiovascular manifestations are insignificant although one case report has been published of ST segment elevation mimicking myocardial infarction in the setting of hypocalcemia presumably due to coronary spasm. The physical examination reveals positive Chvostek's and Trousseau's signs. Laboratory evaluation reveals a low serum calcium or ionized calcium with a low or inappropriately low normal PTH level. Hypoparathyroidism is associated with a prolonged QT interval on the ECG because of ST-segment lengthening; the T wave is usually normal. Occasionally, impaired left ventricular dysfunction is detected. Restoration of eucalcemia may improve cardiac function.

Csandy M, Forster T, Julesz J: Reversible impairment of myocardial function in hypoparathyroidism causing hypocalcaemia. Br Heart J 1990;63;58.

Kudoh C, Tanaka S, Marusaki S et al: Hypocalcemic cardiomyopathy in a patient with idiopathic hypoparathyroidism. Internal Med 1992;31:561.

Lehmann G, Deisenhofer I, Ndrepepa G et al: ECG changes in a 25-year-old woman with hypocalcemia due to hypoparathyroidism. Chest 2000;118:260-2.

ADRENAL AND THE HEART

1. PHEOCHROMOCYTOMA

ESSENTIALS OF DIAGNOSIS

- *Biochemical evidence of excess catecholamine*
- *Adrenal tumor or tumor along the sympathetic chain (paraganglioma)*
- *Headache, palpitations, sweating in conjunction with either hypertension (may be paroxysmal) or orthostatic hypotension*
- *Pressor response to anesthesia induction or to antihypertensive or sympathomimetic drugs*

General Considerations

Catecholamine-secreting neoplasms, or pheochromocytomas, can be life-threatening and cause hypertension, arrhythmia, and hyperglycemia. One case per 2 million persons is diagnosed annually in this country, accounting for less than 0.1% of underlying primary causes of hypertension. Despite the rarity of this condition, its importance cannot be overstated because correct diagnosis and treatment leads to cure, and a missed diagnosis can be fatal. Ninety percent of pheochromocytomas are located in the adrenals; 10% arise from extraadrenal chromaffin tissue along the sympathetic chain and are known as paragangliomas. Cardiac pheochromocytoma arising from the visceral autonomic paraganglia (atrium or interatrial septum) or branchiomeric paraganglia (branchial arch) are extremely rare, with only 31 cases reported in the literature to date. Approximately 10% are malignant, and recurrences can be seen in 6–23% of cases.

Most pheochromocytomas secrete predominantly norepinephrine; about 15% secrete mainly epinephrine. The majority of pheochromocytomas occur sporadically; occasionally (about 10% of cases) they are seen as part of a familial syndrome such as MEN IIa (hyperparathyroidism, medullary thyroid cancer, pheochromocytoma), MEN IIb (pheochromocytoma, medullary thyroid carcinoma, mucosal neuromas, marfanoid habitus), or von Hippel-Lindau disease (cerebelloretinal hemangioblastomas, pheochromocytoma, pancreatic islet cell tumors, renal cell cysts, testicular cysts). Affected family members may have only one manifestation of these syndromes. All members of the family should be screened for pheochromocytomas up until the age of 40 because of the potentially life-threatening nature of these tumors.

Clinical Findings

A. SYMPTOMS AND SIGNS

1. Systemic symptoms and signs—The release of catecholamines from the tumor is unpredictable and usually causes paroxysmal attacks of headache, palpitations, and sweating. Together with hypertension, these three symptoms when present have a diagnostic specificity of 94% and sensitivity of 91%. When this triad of symptoms is absent, pheochromocytoma can be excluded with 99.9% certainty. Patients may also complain of increased nervousness, irritability, and an impending sense of doom. Mild abdominal pain and constipation are relatively common. Pallor and hyperventilation may be noted on examination. The clinician should suspect a pheochromocytoma in any patient who develops a sudden elevation of blood pressure during anesthesia induction.

2. Cardiovascular symptoms and signs—The effects of catecholamines on the heart are mediated by β_1-

receptors and include increased heart rate, enhanced contractility, and augmented conduction velocity—all of which contribute to an increase in cardiac output. Eighty-five percent of patients will have hypertension, which can be either sustained, labile (with hypotension and hypertension) or paroxysmal. Patients without hypertension most likely secrete dopa or dopamine, which can be vasodilating. Orthostatic hypotension is often noted, and the combination of severe hypertension and orthostasis should suggest the possibility of pheochromocytoma. Light-headedness and syncope occur rarely.

Both dilated and hypertrophic cardiomyopathies and myocarditis have been described with pheochromocytoma, and exposure to high levels of catecholamines can cause contraction-band necrosis and fibrosis. The cardiomyopathy is reversible if the excessive catecholamine stimulus is removed early, before extensive replacement fibrosis takes place. Chest pain, angina, and acute myocardial infarction may occur in the absence of coronary artery occlusive disease. Catecholamine-induced increases in myocardial oxygen consumption, myocarditis, and coronary artery spasm likely contribute to the infarction. Cardiac arrhythmias such as atrial and ventricular fibrillation occur, especially in the setting of surgical resection of the tumor. Sudden death is not an uncommon presentation for patients with pheochromocytoma. Pulmonary edema and shock may also be presentations of such patients; shock may be associated with myocarditis or infarction, or it may follow a hypertensive crisis.

B. Physical Examination

Sustained or paroxysmal hypertension is common. Orthostasis is also often seen, and noncardiogenic pulmonary edema of obscure origin has also been described. Retinal hemorrhage or papilledema is a rare occurrence.

C. Diagnostic Studies

1. Electrocardiography and echocardiography— Electrocardiographic changes are common; nonspecific ST-T wave changes and prominent U waves may be seen. Sinus tachycardia, sinus bradycardia, and atrial and ventricular tachyarrhythmias have all been noted and may be associated with palpitations. Conduction disturbances, including right and left bundle branch block and ventricular strain patterns, sometimes occur. Clinically significant cardiomyopathy and increased left ventricular mass have been noted on echocardiography.

2. Laboratory findings—Elevations in plasma catecholamines or their metabolites are necessary for the diagnosis in addition to localization-imaging studies. The most useful tests are 24-h collections of urinary metanephrines, and free catecholamines. Most clinicians favor urinary or plasma metanephrines as the initial screening test. In general, if the results are equivocal, plasma catecholamines should be measured.

Plasma catecholamines must be collected after placement of an IV catheter for 30 min, with the patient resting supine, preferably in a quiet room to avoid release of catecholamines from pain or emotional arousal. False-positive results should be minimized by avoiding drugs, foods, and conditions that affect the tests (Table 32–6).

Occasionally, suppressive pharmacologic testing may be needed, if all prior testing is equivocal and clinical suspicion is high. The clonidine-suppression test is the most widely used. The test is performed by measuring plasma catecholamines at rest and 3 h after oral administration of 0.3 mg of clonidine. In patients with pheochromocytoma, catecholamines remain unchanged because tumor secretion is unaffected by the centrally acting clonidine. Patients with essential hypertension, on the other hand, will decrease their catecholamine levels to less than 500 pg/mL.

Treatment

Treatment involves the prevention of cardiovascular complications such as myocardial infarction, heart failure, hypertensive crisis and stroke, arrhythmias, and sudden death; it also involves surgical removal of the tumor. Recent advances in localizing studies (computed tomography, magnetic resonance imaging, metaiodobenzylguanidine) and the emergence of laparoscopic adrenalectomy along with proper preoperative medical preparation have reduced morbidity and mortality significantly. Preoperative α- and β-blockade is used to reverse the effects of excessive catecholamines and prevent crisis. Because most pheochromocytomas secrete norepinephrine, α-blockade should be given first to prevent aggravation of hypertension and precipitation of coronary spasm or pulmonary edema from unopposed α-receptor stimulation. The most frequently used combination of drugs is phenoxybenzamine, started at 20 mg/day and increasing to 80–100 mg/day, as tolerated, and propranolol or labetalol to control hypertension and arrhythmias. Phenoxybenzamine causes orthostasis and should be titrated according to the severity of the orthostasis before the β-blocker is added. Blood pressure control should be attempted for 2 weeks before surgery. Metyrosine is a drug that inhibits the rate-limiting step in catecholamine synthesis by 40–80%. It can be used in patients with inoperable pheochromocytoma, or it can be used preoperatively if the hypertension is difficult to control. Doses are 250 mg tid, increased by increments of 250–500 mg to a maximum of 4 g/day.

Prognosis

Nonmalignant surgically treated pheochromocytoma has a 5-year survival rate of 95%. In malignant disease,

Table 32–6. Drugs, foods, and conditions that artificially increase or decrease tests for pheochromocytoma.

Test	Increase	Decrease
Metanephrines, VMA	Sympathomimetics: amphetamines, ephedrine, nasal decongestants, bronchodilators	Large doses of ganglionic blockers: guanethidine, reserpine
Catecholamines	Levodopa	Fenfluramine
	Rapid clonidine withdrawal	Renal Insufficiency
	Excess banana ingestion	Malnutrition, dysautonomia, quadriplegia
	Nitroprusside, nitroglycerin	
	Theophylline, aminophylline	
	Severe stress	
	Diseases: intracranial lesions, psychosis, Guillain-Barré, lead poisoning, eclampsia, hypoglycemia, carcinoid, acute porphyria, acrodynia, quadriplegia, amyotrophic lateral sclerosis	
	Fluorescent substances: quinidine, chloral hydrate, tetracyclines, niacin, erythromycin, quinine, bretylium, methenamine, methocarbamine	
Catecholamines	Ethanol, isoproterenol, methyldopa, MAO inhibitors, phenothiazines, α-methyl p-tyrosine, methenamine, bilirubin, labetalol	
Metanephrines	Ethanol, methyldopa, MAO inhibitors, benzodiazepines, phenothiazines	Radiopaque media: renografin, Hypaque-M, Renovist, Cardiografin, Urografin, conray
VMA	Lithium, nalidixic acid, methocarbamol, glycerol guaiacolate, p-aminosalicylic acid, salicylates, mephenesin, sulfonamides, chocolate, citrus, tea, vanilla, coffee	Ethanol, MAO inhibitors, disulfiram, clofibrate, mandelamine, salicylates

MAO = monoamine oxidase; VMA = vanillylmandelic acid.

the 5-year survival is less than 50%. If a surgical cure is achieved before the cardiovascular system has been irreparably damaged, cardiovascular health will be completely restored. In 25% of patients hypertension persists due to underlying essential hypertension or irreversible vascular or renal damage but is usually well-controlled with standard antihypertensives. However, in this instance, a search for a second or residual tumor should be considered.

Benowitz NL: Pheochromocytoma. Adv Intern Med 1990;35:195.

Boutros AR, Bravo EL, Zanettin G et al: Perioperative management of 63 patients with pheochromocytoma. Cleve Clin J Med 1990;57:613.

Cryer PE: Pheochromocytoma. West J Med 1992;156:399.

Duh Q: Evolving surgical management for patients with pheochromocytoma. J Clin Endocrinol Metab 2001:86:1477.

Feldman JM: Diagnosis and management of pheochromocytoma. Hosp Prac 1989:145.

Green JP, Guay AT: New perspectives in pheochromocytoma. Urol Clin North Am 1989;16:487.

Klingler HC, Klingler PJ, Martin JK et al: Pheochromocytoma. Urology 2001;57:1025–1032.

Liao W, Liu CF, Chaiang CW et al: Cardiovascular manifestations of pheochromocytoma. Am J Emerg Med 2000;18: 622–625.

Malone MJ, Libertine JA, Tsapatsaris NP et al: Preoperative and surgical management of pheochromocytoma. Urol Clin North Am 1989;16:567.

Plouin P, Duclos JM, Sopppelsa F et al: Factors associated with perioperative morbidity and mortality in patients with pheochromocytoma: Analysis of 165 operations at a single center. J Clin Endocrinol Metab 2001;86:1480.

Sjoberg RJ, Simcic KJ, Kedd GS: The clonidine suppression test for pheochromocytoma. Arch Int Med 1992;152:1193.

Stein PP, Black HR: A simplified diagnostic approach to pheochromocytoma: A review of the literature and report of one institution's experience. Medicine 1991;70:46.

2. ADRENAL INSUFFICIENCY

ESSENTIALS OF DIAGNOSIS

- Inability to increase cortisol to more than 20 mg/dL in response to synthetic adrenocorticotrophic hormone (ACTH) during rapid ACTH stimulation testing
- Orthostatic hypotension, salt wasting, hyperkalemia in primary adrenal insufficiency (Addison's disease)
- Hyponatremia in both primary and secondary (pituitary) adrenal insufficiency
- Elevated ACTH in Addison's disease
- Hypovolemic shock, hypoglycemia, fever in adrenal crisis

General Considerations

Deficient production of glucocorticoids, mineralocorticoids, or both results in adrenal insufficiency. This is classified into two types: primary adrenal insufficiency, or Addison's disease, in which the adrenal cortex is destroyed; and secondary adrenal insufficiency, in which ACTH hyposecretion leads to decreased production of glucocorticoids from the zona fasciculata.

Today, the most common cause of Addison's disease is autoimmune destruction of the adrenal cortex. Adrenal hemorrhage, metastasis, acquired immunodeficiency syndrome, and granulomatous diseases such as tuberculosis and histoplasmosis are other etiologic considerations. Adrenal hemorrhage usually occurs in the setting of anticoagulation in adults or fulminant meningococcemia and *Pseudomonas* sepsis in children. The most common cause of secondary adrenal insufficiency is withdrawal of steroids, which suppresses the hypothalamic pituitary adrenal axis and therefore causes glucocorticoid deficiency. Because the zona glomerulosa, which produces mineralocorticoid, remains intact under the influence of the renin-angiotensin system in secondary adrenal insufficiency, these patients may not have hyperkalemia and hypotension.

Adrenal insufficiency is rare in the general population, with an incidence of <0.01%. However, the overall risk of adrenal insufficiency is increased in critically ill patients; especially those over the age of 55 who are hypotensive and require pressors. Estimates are that in this setting adrenal insufficiency is present in 30–40%.

Clinical Findings

A. SYMPTOMS AND SIGNS

1. Systemic symptoms and signs—Glucocorticoid deficiency causes fatigue, anorexia, nausea, vomiting (and therefore weight loss), hypotension, and hypoglycemia. Mineralocorticoid or aldosterone deficiency causes renal sodium and bicarbonate wasting, resulting in hyponatremia, hyperkalemia, acidosis, and profound dehydration. Acute adrenal insufficiency or crisis occurs when the patient is exposed to the stress of infection, trauma, surgery, dehydration, and the like and cannot compensate adequately with augmented steroid release.

2. Cardiovascular symptoms and signs—Hypotension, often orthostatic, is present in 90% of patients and may cause syncope. Chronic adrenal insufficiency is characterized by decreased systemic vascular resistance and decreased myocardial contractility. On the other hand, acute adrenal insufficiency can have variable cardiac function with low, normal or high systemic vascular resistance, cardiac output and capillary wedge pressure. Thus, in acute adrenal insufficiency—which can be superimposed on a setting of chronic adrenal insufficiency—the patient may present in hypovolemic shock, accompanied by fever, volume depletion, depressed mentation, nausea, vomiting, abdominal pain, and hypoglycemia. Patients often present as if they have an acute abdominal emergency and can mistakenly be taken for exploratory surgery—which can be lethal in this setting. Shock and coma can rapidly progress to death, if untreated. Adrenal crisis should be considered in any patient with unexplained hypovolemic shock.

B. PHYSICAL EXAMINATION

The classic physical examination finding for chronic primary adrenal insufficiency is hyperpigmentation of the skin and mucous membranes, especially over pressure points such as the knuckles, toes, elbows, and knees and also in scars, palmar creases, nail beds, areolae, and the perianal and perivaginal areas. The hyperpigmentation is caused by increased levels of ACTH, which are released along with melanocyte-stimulating hormone and stimulate the melanocyte receptor. Vitiligo is a clue that the adrenal insufficiency is autoimmune in nature. Calcification of the pinna and the loss of pubic and axillary hair from decreased production of adrenal androgens may also be seen. In secondary adrenal insufficiency, patients lack the hyperpigmentation; the presence of cushingoid features suggests glucocorticoid withdrawal.

C. DIAGNOSTIC STUDIES

1. Electrocardiography and echocardiography—Electrocardiographic findings include sinus bradycardia, sinus tachycardia, nonspecific T wave changes, peaked T waves if hyperkalemia is prominent, and low voltage and a shortened QT interval if hypercalcemia is present. Echocardiography reveals small cardiac chambers with normal function.

2. Laboratory findings—Hyponatremia, hyperkalemia, hypercalcemia, hypoglycemia, and acidosis are seen in Addison's disease. As noted earlier, patients with secondary adrenal insufficiency will not have hyperkalemia because their renin and angiotensin system is able to stimulate aldosterone production. A normocytic, normochromic anemia with lymphocytosis and eosinophilia is seen on the blood smear.

The rapid ACTH stimulation test is used to diagnose adrenal insufficiency. Administration of synthetic ACTH (cosyntropin) causes an elevation of cortisol within 30–60 min. Failure to increase cortisol to 20 mg/dL confirms the insufficiency. An ACTH level can help distinguish primary from secondary causes; hypersecretion is characteristic of primary adrenal insufficiency only.

In the setting of critical illness, the diagnosis of adrenal insufficiency is more problematic. Although it is well known that stress such as that seen with hypotension, inflammation, sepsis, or surgery results in elevated cortisol levels, the definition of adrenal insufficiency in this setting is less clear. Most authors believe that a stress cortisol level in critically ill patients (ie, those who are hypotensive, hypoglycemic, hypoxemic) should be >25 μg/dL. When the level of stress is uncertain, the low-dose corticotropin stimulation test (1 μg) can be used. Failure to increase stimulated cortisol to >25 μg/dL indicates the need for treatment with glucocorticoids.

Treatment

The treatment of adrenal crisis is lifesaving. If the patient is in serious shock, delay of treatment to make the diagnosis of adrenal crisis is both unwise and dangerous. Patients should receive stress doses of steroids, such as 100 mg of hydrocortisone IV every 6–8 h, starting immediately. Saline volume resuscitation along with glucose infusion is necessary to correct volume and electrolyte abnormalities. A search for the underlying precipitant, such as infection, should be undertaken and treated as necessary. Once the patient is safely over the crisis, steroids can be slowly withdrawn, and the diagnosis of adrenal insufficiency confirmed. An alternative approach would be to use dexamethasone, 2–4 mg IV initially, which does not interfere with the cortisol assay; perform the rapid ACTH stimulation test; and then switch to hydrocortisone.

The treatment of chronic Addison's disease involves both glucocorticoid and mineralocorticoid replacement. Glucocorticoid replacement can be in the form of hydrocortisone, cortisol acetate, or prednisone. Dexamethasone is not recommended because of its long half-life. Typical replacement doses are one tenth those of stress doses. Hydrocortisone is usually started at 20 mg in the morning and 10 mg in the evening to mimic the body's circadian secretion of cortisol. The lowest doses possible to render the patient asymptomatic, with normal electrolytes, are preferable; this regimen will avoid the long-term effects of glucocorticoid excess. Mineralocorticoid is given in the form of oral fludrocortisone (Florinef) in doses of 0.05–0.1 mg/day in patients with Addison's disease.

Johnson TL: Tuberculous Addison's disease. Postgrad Med 1991;90: 139.

Muir A, Schatz DA, Maclaren N: Autoimmune diseases of the adrenal glands, parathyroid glands, gonads, and hypothalamic pituitary axis. Endocrinol Metab Clin North Am 1991;20: 619.

Oelkers H, Diedrich S, Bahr V: Diagnosis and therapy surveillance in Addison's disease: Rapid ACTH test and measurement of plasma ACTH, renin activity and aldosterone. J Clin Endocrinol Metab 1992;75:259.

Pulakhandam U, Dincsoy HP: Cytomegalovirus adrenalitis and adrenal insufficiency in AIDS. Am J Clin Pathol 1990;93:651.

Rivers E, Gaspari M, Saad GA et al: Adrenal insufficiency in high-risk surgical ICU patients. Chest 2001;119:889–896.

Siu SC, Kitzman DW, Sheedy PF et al: Adrenal insufficiency from bilateral adrenal hemorrhage. Mayo Clin Proc 1990;65:664.

Stoffer SS: Addison's disease: How to improve patients quality of life. Postgrad Med 1993;93:265.

Zaloga GP, Marik P: Endocrine and metabolic dysfunction syndromes in the critically ill. Crit Care Clin 2001;17:25–41.

3. CUSHING'S SYNDROME

General Considerations

The term **Cushing's syndrome** refers to excess cortisol in the circulation. **Cushing's disease** is that state of hypercortisolemia caused by an ACTH-producing pituitary adenoma. Other causes of Cushing's syndrome are ectopic ACTH production from tumors, such as small cell carcinoma of the bronchus; primary adrenal disease, such as glucocorticoid-secreting adrenal tumors; or the exogenous use of steroids. **Pseudo-Cushing's syndrome** refers to patients who, on screening, appear to have hypercortisolemia but have relatively few physical signs. These patients typically are alcoholic or obese or have psychiatric conditions. Confirmatory testing for Cushing's syndrome is normal in pseudo-Cushing's.

Cushing's syndrome patients typically have central obesity, hypertension, hyperlipidemia, and hyperglycemia; it is not surprising that they are at risk for coronary artery disease. The longer the duration of the hypercortisolemia, the greater the risk of coronary disease; congestive heart failure can occur.

Diagnostic Considerations

Diagnosis requires three steps: screening, confirmation, and determination of the cause. Screening tests are a 24-h urine collection for free cortisol, or a 1-mg overnight dexamethasone-suppression test. Patient's with Cushing's or pseudo-Cushing's syndrome will have an elevated urinary free cortisol level, and 1 mg of dexamethasone will not suppress their cortisol to less than 5 mg/dL. Confirmation requires a low-dose (2 mg/day) dexamethasone-suppression test, with or without corticotropin-releasing factor testing. True Cushing's syndrome will not suppress with low-dose testing. To determine cause, an ACTH level, should be performed. Elevated ACTH indicates a pituitary tumor or ectopic production of ACTH. Low ACTH levels indicate adrenal disease. High-dose (8 mg) dexamethasone suppression testing and the cortisol-releasing hormone stimulation test are the main tests used to differentiate pituitary from ectopic sources of ACTH. Inferior petrosal sinus sampling should be reserved for patients with confusing hormonal testing who have a pituitary adenoma on imaging studies or in patients suspected of having an ectopic source of ACTH. Imaging should be done after the biochemical workup is completed.

Treatment

Treatment involves surgical removal of the pituitary tumor, with or without radiation, in Cushing's disease; removal of the adrenal tumor; or removal of the ectopic source of ACTH production. If these procedures are not feasible, medical treatment can be done, using adrenolytic therapy such as mitotane, or adrenocortical-blocking drugs such as aminoglutethimide, metyrapone, or ketoconazole.

Boscaro M, Barzon L, Sonino N et al: The diagnosis of Cushing's syndrome: Atypical presentations and laboratory shortcomings. Arch Intern Med 2000;160:3045–3053.

Findling JW, Mazzaferri EL: Cushing's syndrome: An etiologic workup. Hosp Prac 1992;27:107.

Flack M, Oldfield EH, Cutter GB Jr et al: Urine free cortisol in the high dose dexamethasone suppression test for the differential diagnosis of the Cushing's Syndrome. Ann Intern Med 1992;116:211.

Loriaux DL: The treatment of Cushing's syndrome and adrenal cancer. Endocrinol Metab Clin North Am 1991;20:767.

Miller JW, Crapo L: The medical treatment of Cushing's syndrome. Endocrine Reviews 1993;14:443.

Yanovski JA, Cutler GB Jr, Chrousos GP et al: Corticotropin releasing hormone stimulation test following dexamethasone administration: A new test to distinguish Cushing's syndrome from pseudo-Cushing's states. JAMA 1993;269:2232.

4. PRIMARY HYPERALDOSTERONISM

General Considerations

The increased and autonomous production of aldosterone by the adrenal gland is known as primary hyperaldosteronism. Consequences of excessive aldosterone production include sodium retention, with plasma volume expansion and hypertension; renal loss of potassium and bicarbonate, causing hypokalemia and alkalosis; and suppression of renin and angiotensin. Hyperaldosteronism was previously believed to account for 0.5–2% of all patients with hypertension; however, recent reviews suggest this is an underestimate and that as many as 12–20% of cases referred to hypertension clinics have primary hyperaldosteronism.

Patients usually come to medical attention because of hypertension and hypokalemia. The hypertension may be moderately severe, requiring several antihypertensives; malignant hypertension, however, is rare. Despite the sodium retention, edema is not a feature of hyperaldosteronism; the kidney can presumably compensate for the excess sodium. The heart is usually only modestly enlarged and heart failure is rarely seen. Electrocardiographic changes are those of mild LVH and hypokalemia.

Diagnostic Considerations

The diagnosis should be considered in any hypertensive patient with spontaneous hypokalemia, resistant hypertension, adrenal incidentaloma, or in patients suspected of having secondary hypertension. Basal plasma renin activity should be suppressed, with elevated plasma aldosterone and an elevated aldosterone/renin ratio. If this is the case, the diagnosis can be confirmed by demonstrating failure of the elevated aldosterone to suppress normally with salt or saline loading. The patient must discontinue any antihypertensives that affect the renin-angiotensin-aldosterone axis for 3–6 weeks before salt suppression testing; prazosin can be used to control blood pressure. The patient is typically placed on a high-salt diet (>120 mEq/day) with sodium chloride supplementation for 3–4 days to suppress aldosterone; on the last day of the high-salt diet, a 24-h urine is collected to test for aldosterone, sodium, and creatinine. If urinary Na is >200 mEq and aldosterone is >12 μg, unsuppressibility of aldosterone is documented. After confirmation of hyperaldosteronism, imaging of the adrenals should be performed with computed tomography to look for hyperplasia versus adenoma. In equivocal cases, adrenal vein sampling for aldosterone can be performed.

Treatment

Treatment for adenoma involves surgical resection. In as many as 70% of patients, this cures the hypertension and hypokalemia. The blood pressure, however, may require several months following surgery to return to normal. Medical therapy for patients who are not surgical candidates or those with hyperplasia includes the aldosterone-antagonist spironolactone (100–200 mg/day), amiloride (10–40 mg/day), and calcium channel blockers. For male patients, spironolactone has the troubling side effects of gynecomastia and impotence.

Biglieri EG: Spectrum of mineralocorticoid hypertension. Hypertension 1991;17:251.

Irony I, Kater CE, Biglieri EG et al: Correctable subsets of primary aldosteronism: Primary adrenal hyperplasia and renin responsive adenoma. Am J Hypertens 1990;3:576.

McKenna JT, Sequeira SJ, Heffernan A et al: Diagnosis under random conditions of all disorders of the renin-angiotensin-aldosterone axis, including primary hyperaldosteronism. J Clin Endocrinol Metab 1991;73:952.

Melby JC: Diagnosis of hyperaldosteronism. Endocrinol Metab Clin of North Am 1991;20:247.

Nomura K, Toraya S, Horiba N et al: Plasma aldosterone response to upright posture and angiotensin II infusion in aldosterone producing adenoma. J Clin Endocrinol Metab 1992;75:323.

Young WF Jr: Primary aldosteronism: A common and curable form of hypertension. Cardiol Rev 1999;7:2107–2114.

ACROMEGALY AND THE HEART

ESSENTIALS OF DIAGNOSIS

- *Elevated somatomedin C*
- *Inability to suppress growth hormone to less than 2 ng/mL during glucose tolerance test*
- *Pituitary adenoma found on magnetic resonance imaging*

General Considerations

Acromegaly is caused by the excessive secretion of growth hormone (GH) by a pituitary adenoma in an adult; gigantism occurs in children. It is characterized by bony overgrowth, organomegaly, and premature death, often due to cardiovascular, cerebrovascular, and respiratory dysfunction. In rare cases, carcinoid, small-cell, islet cell, and other tumors can secrete growth hormone-releasing hormone ectopically and cause acromegaly. The effects of GH are mediated through the insulin-like growth factor 1 (IGF-1 or somatomedin C) in the liver and its periphery.

Clinical Findings

A. SYMPTOMS AND SIGNS

1. Systemic symptoms and signs—Excessive GH causes bony, soft tissue, and visceral overgrowth. Patients may also complain of symptoms related to the lo-

cal expanse of the tumor such as headache or bitemporal hemianopsia. Impotence, galactorrhea, and amenorrhea may result from cosecretion of prolactin or the destruction of normal gonadotrophs by the tumor. Other symptoms include excessive sweating, hoarseness, carpal tunnel syndrome, polyuria, and polydipsia.

2. Cardiovascular symptoms and signs—Cardiac dysfunction and heart failure are a major cause of death in acromegalics. The older the patient and the longer the duration of disease, the more likely acromegalic cardiomyopathy will develop. The most striking clinical feature is concentric biventricular hypertrophy with inadequate filling capacity leading to both systolic and diastolic dysfunction. Histologic findings include interstitial fibrosis, collagen deposition, myofibrillar derangement, lymphomononuclear infiltration, and myocyte apoptosis resembling myocarditis.

Other factors can potentially contribute to the cardiac dysfunction. The coexistence of hypertension, diabetes, or both in this condition can accelerate the cardiac hypertrophy. Hypertension, the most common cardiovascular finding in acromegalics, is usually mild in nature and easily treated with antihypertensives. The mechanism of the hypertension may be due to increased sodium, extracellular fluid, and plasma volume. Aldosterone is usually suppressed as a result. Acromegalics also have increased sensitivity to angiotensin II. The presence of a circulating digitalis-like factor has been hypothesized; this might affect arterial smooth muscle tone and provide a rare basis for hypertension in this condition.

Because of the role of GH as a counterregulatory hormone for hypoglycemia, most acromegalics have either glucose intolerance or frank diabetes, which may explain their increased incidence of premature coronary artery disease. Untreated acromegaly is associated with hypertriglyceridemia and elevated levels of apoprotein A-1, apoprotein E, fibrinogen, and plasminogen activator-1 activity.

A rare disorder known as **Carney's syndrome** involves any three of the following: GH-secreting pituitary tumors, cardiac or cutaneous myxoma, Sertoli cell tumors, cutaneous hyperpigmentation, and pigmented nodular adrenocortical disease. The myxomas seen in Carney's syndrome are usually multiple and may involve more than one chamber. Family members should be screened with echocardiography.

B. PHYSICAL EXAMINATION

Because acromegaly is such an insidious disease, changes in the body occur gradually and usually go unnoticed until complications develop. Bitemporal hemianopsia may be detected on gross confrontation, indicating optic chiasm compression from the tumor. Thickened, oily skin, particularly of the face, and other facial changes, including thick lips, macroglossia, bulbous nose, frontal bossing, prominent cheek bones, hollow temporal fossa, and malocclusion with protrusion of the lower jaw, are usually seen. Synovial and periarticular swelling may be noted, and dorsal kyphosis, barrel chest, and spade-like hands with sausage-like digits are seen. The chest examination is most remarkable for galactorrhea. Abdominal exam may reveal generalized organomegaly.

C. DIAGNOSTIC STUDIES

1. Electrocardiography and echocardiography—Cardiomegaly is present, even in the absence of hypertension, suggesting a direct effect of GH on the myocyte. Both symmetric and asymmetric cardiac hypertrophy have been seen on echocardiography. In early disease, both ventricular dimension and wall thickness are increased; therefore, relative wall thickness remains unchanged. In later stages, impaired diastolic filling and cardiac dilatation occur, leading to congestive heart failure.

Electrocardiographic abnormalities include ST depression and nonspecific T wave changes, LVH, and intraventricular conduction defects. Cardiac arrhythmias often occur, with ventricular ectopias and atrial fibrillation or flutter being the most frequent.

2. Laboratory findings—Diagnostic tests includes random and glucose-suppressed GH levels, along with somatomedin C or insulin-like growth factor (IGF)-1 levels. Because GH secretion is episodic, a random level alone is rarely helpful. Normally, GH is suppressed to less than 2 ng/mL in response to glucose infusion. Other findings often associated with acromegaly include hyperglycemia, hyperphosphatemia, and hypertriglyceridemia.

Treatment

The goal in treating acromegaly is to normalize GH and somatomedin C concentrations in order to prevent early cardiovascular mortality. Treatment includes surgical removal of the pituitary adenoma with postoperative x-ray therapy, or medical therapy with octreotide (200–500 µg/day SQ) or bromocriptine (5–30 mg/day). Many authors have suggested that once control of the disease occurs, defined as a GH level of < 2 ng/mL and a normal age adjusted IGF-1 level, the progression of cardiac disease can be arrested and cardiovascular mortality reduced. The hypertension, heart failure, and arrhythmias are treated conventionally.

Bennett WS, Skelton TN, Lehan PH et al: The complex of myxomas, pigmentation, and endocrine overactivity. Am J Cardiol 1990;65:399.

Colao A, Marzullo P, Di Somma et al: Growth hormone and the heart. Clin Endocrinol 2001;54:137–154.

Fazio S, Cittadini A, Biondi B et al: Cardiovascular effects of short-term growth hormone hypersecretion. J Clin Endocrinol Metab 2000;85(1):179–182.

Frohman L: Therapeutic options in acromegaly. J Clin Endocrinol Metab 1991;72:1175.

Melmed S: Acromegaly. N Engl J Med 1990;322:966.

Salmela PI, Juustila H, Pyhtinen J et al: Effective clinical response to long term octreotide treatment, with reduced serum concentrations of growth hormone, IGF-1, and the amino terminal propeptide of type III procollagen in acromegaly. J Clin Endocrinol Metab 1990;70:1193.

Yen RS, Allen B, Ott R et al: The syndrome of right atrial myxoma, spotty skin pigmentation and acromegaly. Am Heart J 1992; 123:243.

GROWTH HORMONE DEFICIENCY

Unlike acromegaly, in which cardiac involvement has been appreciated for many decades, the cardiac abnormalities associated with adult growth hormone deficiency (GHD) have only recently been recognized. GHD is associated with abnormal body composition with increased fat mass, abnormal lipid metabolism, impaired capacity for exercise, decreased bone mineral density, decreased quality of life and a risk of increased mortality from cardiovascular disease that is approximately twice that found in the normal population. Myocardial infarction, cardiac failure, and cerebrovascular accidents are the main causes of death.

The precise mechanisms responsible for the increase in cardiovascular disease are unknown, but a characteristic hypokinetic syndrome has been described. In this syndrome, a decrease in left ventricular and septal wall thickness is noted on echocardiography along with low heart rate and blood pressure. One study using radionuclide angiography has noted decreased left ventricular ejection fraction (LVEF) compared with that in controls.

Most commonly, adult GHD results from childhood onset of GHD that continues throughout life. Thus, the patient with a history of pituitary or hypothalamic disease, childhood-onset GHD, cranial irradiation or trauma is a candidate for GHD testing. Testing consists of provocative stimulation with an insulin tolerance test. A biochemical diagnosis of adult GHD is determined by a subnormal response, for example, a peak level of GH <5 ng/mL. Testing should not be performed in patients with ischemic heart disease or seizure disorder. Treatment is initiated with a daily SQ injection of 2–5 µg/kg/day of GH and can be titrated to 10-12 µg/kg/day. Side effects are dose-dependent and consist of fluid retention and carpal tunnel syndrome.

Growth hormone therapy has been implicated in the health of the endothelium and increases nitric oxide production in in vitro studies. In humans with GHD, short-term treatment has been shown in various studies to increase cardiac mass, decrease carotid intimal medial thickness, reverse early atherosclerotic changes in major arteries, and possibly improve the vasodilatory function of the endothelium. However, the hypertrophic effect of long-term replacement with GH appears to subside over time. It remains to be seen if GH replacement therapy will reduce the prevalence of cardiovascular disease in this population.

Colao A, Marzullo P, Di Somma C et al: Growth hormone and the heart. Clin Endocrinol 2001;54:137–154.

Kleinberg DL, Melmed S: The adult growth hormone deficiency syndrome: Signs, symptoms and diagnosis. Endocrinologist 1998;8:8S–14S.

Pfeiffer M, Verhovec R, Zizek B et al: Growth hormone (GH) treatment reverses early atherosclerotic changes in GH-deficient adults. J Clin Endocrinol Metab 1999;84:453–457.

Rosen T, Bengtsson BA: Premature mortality due to cardiovascular disease in hypopituitarism. Lancet 1990;336:285–288.

ROLE OF GROWTH HORMONE IN CHRONIC HEART FAILURE

Animal studies have suggested that GH may be a useful therapeutic agent for treating idiopathic dilated cardiomyopathy, a condition in which compensatory cardiac hypertrophy is lacking. Most studies to date have been small, nonrandomized, and uncontrolled and have demonstrated mixed results. At this time, GH therapy cannot be recommended for routine treatment of chronic heart failure until large, randomized, placebo-controlled trials are performed to assess safety and long-term results.

Colao A, Marzullo P, Di Somma C et al: Growth hormone and the heart. Clin Endocrinol 2001;54:137–154.

Smit JWA, Janssen YJH, Lamb HJ et al: Six months of recombinant human GH therapy in patients with ischemic cardiac failure does not influence left ventricular function and mass. J Clin Endocrinol Metab 2001;86:4638–4643.

Volterrani M, Manelli F, Cicoira M et al: Role of growth hormone in chronic heart failure: Therapeutic implications. Drugs 2000;60(4):711–719.

CARCINOID TUMORS AND THE HEART

General Considerations

Carcinoid tumors are neuroendocrine tumors containing vasoactive secretagogues and are found in the gastrointestinal tract, urogenital tract, or the pulmonary bronchioles. Although these tumors can secrete a number of hormones, including ACTH and growth hormone-releasing hormone, they most commonly secrete serotonin and serotonin metabolites. The presentation of the patient depends on the location of the carcinoid; hence tumors are classified into foregut (respiratory tract, thymus, stomach and pancreas), midgut (small intestine, appendix, and right colon), and hindgut (transverse and descending colon, sigmoid, and rectum) tumors. Symptoms include flushing of the head and neck, diarrhea (with liver metastases), and bronchospasm (with pulmonary carcinoid).

A unique endocrine effect of carcinoid tumors is fibrotic plaque-like thickenings on the endocardium of the tricuspid and pulmonic valves, atria, and ventricles. Deposition may also be seen on the superior and inferior venae cavae, pulmonary artery, and coronary sinus. The right side of the heart is affected predominantly, and although left-sided heart disease may occur, it is of lesser significance. Thickening of the valves results in tricuspid regurgitation and pulmonic stenosis. If the tricuspid regurgitation is severe, right-sided heart failure and cardiomegaly result. Nearly one half of patients who die from carcinoid die from congestive heart failure.

Elaboration of serotonin by the tumor is felt to mediate the fibrosis; however, lowering serotonin levels does not cause regression of the plaques. Diagnosis is made by documenting more than 30 mg of 5-hydroxy indole acetic acid (a serotonin metabolite) in a 24-h urine collection. Normal individuals secrete less than 10 mg in 24 h, and values between 10 and 30 mg are equivocal. Testing must be done while the patient has been on a diet free of serotonin-rich foods for several days. Localization should be attempted with bowel series, computed tomography, somatostatin receptor scintigraphy, or positron emission tomography. All patients with carcinoid should have echocardiography to look for heart involvement.

Treatment

Treatment is surgical removal of the tumor if it has not metastasized. Synthetic somatostatin (octreotide) has been shown to shrink tumor metastases in addition to decreasing serotonin levels. Unfortunately, the heart disease does not improve with reduction of serotonin levels, and some patients will require valve replacement.

Ahlman H, Wangberg B, Theodorssone E et al: Aspects on diagnosis and treatment of the foregut carcinoid syndrome. Scand J Gastroenterol 1992;27:459.

Denney WE, Kemp WE, Anthony LB et al: Echocardiographic and biochemical evaluation of the development and progression of carcinoid heart disease. J Am Coll Cardiol 1998;32:1017.

Ganim RB, Norton JA: Recent advances in carcinoid pathogenesis, diagnosis and management. Surg Oncol 2000;9:173.

Fetherston GJ, Davis BB: Surgical management of carcinoid heart disease. Ann Thorac Surg 1991;51:493.

Lundin L: Surgical treatment of carcinoid heart disease. J Thorac and Cardiovasc Surg 1990;100:552.

Wynick D, Bloom SR: The use of the long acting somatostatin analog octreotide in the treatment of gut neuroendocrine tumors. J Clin Endocrinol Metab 1991;73:1.

DIABETES MELLITUS AND THE HEART

General Considerations

The incidence of coronary artery disease in diabetics is two to four times that for nondiabetics, with cardiovascular disease reigning as the number one cause of death. Two types of vascular disease are seen: macrovascular disease, causing atherosclerosis and arteriosclerosis; and microvascular disease, producing retinopathy, nephropathy, neuropathy, and possibly small artery occlusion in the heart as well. Macrovascular disease develops prematurely in diabetics and is usually severe, with a striking predominance in diabetic women. Diabetics with no history of coronary heart disease (CHD) have identical risk for cardiovascular death to patients with myocardial infarction. Consequently, the Adult Treatment Panel III has designated diabetes as a CHD risk equivalent.

A large body of evidence now links endothelial dysfunction to microangiopathy and atherosclerosis in diabetes. The evidence is particularly striking in type 1 diabetics with microalbuminuria and proteinuria; however, endothelial dysfunction also occurs in patients with type 2 diabetes and normal urinary albumin excretion as well as in patients with insulin resistance who are normoglycemic. Once established, endothelial dysfunction induces changes in vascular tone, reactivity, and function that contribute to the progression of vascular disease. Insulin sensitizers, hypolipidemic therapy, and angiotensin-converting enzyme inhibitors have all been shown to improve endothelial function.

Hyperinsulinemia and insulin resistance have been postulated to relate directly to both hypertension and CHD in type 2 diabetes. The so called metabolic syndrome, a constellation of metabolic risk factors that includes obesity, insulin resistance, elevated triglycerides, low high-density lipoprotein, hypertension, hyperuricemia, and fasting hyperglycemia, enhances the risk for CHD at any given low-density lipoprotein level. To achieve maximum benefit from risk factor modification, the underlying insulin resistant state must be a primary target of therapy.

Clinical Findings

Angina and myocardial infarction in diabetics are often manifested by atypical symptoms. Painless infarction is common, and unusual pain patterns may delay diagnosis. Diabetics have a high mortality rate from myocardial infarction; recurrence is frequent, and the long-term prognosis is poor, with a higher incidence of congestive heart failure and ventricular rupture. Diabetic men have a 2.4-fold increase in heart failure, but diabetic women have a particularly high incidence: 5.1 times that of nondiabetics. Diabetic cardiomyopathy occurs even in the absence of epicardial vessel disease, causing some investigators to hypothesize a preponderance of small-vessel disease. Autonomic neuropathy frequently occurs and results in sympathetic denervation manifested by a fixed tachycardia with subsequent parasympathetic damage that

results in lowering of the heart rate. Complete autonomic cardiac denervation finally occurs, resulting in a heart rate that is no longer responsive to such physiologic stimuli as standing.

Echocardiographic studies show abnormal systolic and diastolic function, with impaired diastolic filling as one of the earliest manifestations of diabetic cardiomyopathy. Various studies have shown diabetics to have a delayed opening of the mitral valve, a longer preejection period, and a shorter left ventricular ejection time, resulting in decreased filling and contractility. Other studies have shown an increase in contractility in patients with diabetes of recent onset. The cause of the left ventricular dysfunction is probably multifactorial, reflecting the effects of both hypertension and coronary atherosclerosis.

Treatment

Diet, oral hypoglycemics, insulin sensitizers, and insulin remain the mainstay of therapy for hyperglycemia. Recent studies have illustrated that tight glucose control decreases the progression and development of diabetic microvascular complications. Only one of several trials thus far examining tight glucose control has shown a substantial reduction in macrovascular disease. The DIGAMI trial, which studied intensive therapy for 3 months versus standard diabetes care, showed large differences in cardiovascular mortality rates at 1 year. Whether tight glucose control influences CHD risk is still unclear and is being studied in the ongoing Diabetes VA cooperative trial expected to yield results in 2008. To prevent microvascular disease, target hemoglobin A_1C levels should be less than 7%, which corresponds with mean glucose levels of 150 mg/dL.

Current trial evidence suggests that aggressive treatment of hypertension and hyperlipidemia results in large and statistically significant reductions in cardiac event rates for patients with type 2 diabetes. Most studies have shown that cardiovascular benefits begin to accrue 2–4 years from the onset of treatment. Early and vigorous antihypertensive therapy with angiotensin-converting enzyme inhibitors or angiotensin receptor blockers should be first-line therapy. Beta-blockers, calcium antagonists, and diuretics in low dose are second-line therapy, with the goal being a systolic and diastolic blood pressure of less than 130/80. Diabetic patients require more antihypertensive therapy to reach this goal; the majority needing two to three drugs concomitantly, but these patients also reap more benefit in terms of reduction in cardiovascular mortality rate per millimeter of mercury reduction of blood pressure compared with non diabetic hypertensives.

The benefits of aggressive lipid-lowering therapy in patients with type 2 diabetes and CHD has been demonstrated in four major secondary prevention trials with simvastatin and pravastatin (4S, CARE, LIPID Heart Protection Study). A primary prevention trial using lovastatin (AFCAPS/TexCAPS) showed a decreased risk of CHD in the small number of diabetics studied. The VA-HIT trial demonstrated improvement in CHD risk with triglyceride lowering from gemfibrozil use in type 2 diabetes. Target lipid levels are similar to those for patients with established CHD and include an low-density lipoprotein of <100 mg/dL, triglycerides <150 mg/dL, high-density lipoprotein >45 mg/dL in women and >55 mg/dL in men. Statin therapy is preferred as first-line therapy unless triglycerides are markedly elevated above 500 mg/dL, necessitating use of fibrates as first-line therapy.

Treatment of CHD for diabetics is similar to that for nondiabetics with some important caveats. Endothelial dysfunction and the platelet and coagulation disturbances characteristic of type 2 diabetes have been postulated to affect morbidity and mortality in the setting of unstable angina, non ST segment elevation myocardial infarction, and after percutaneous transluminal coronary angioplasty (PTCA), stenting, and CABG. Diabetics have higher rates of adverse outcomes and restenosis in these settings.

Given the known hemostatic disturbances associated with type 2 diabetes, current evidence supports antiplatelet therapy. A recent meta-analysis of glycoprotein IIb/IIIa inhibitors in acute coronary syndromes suggests that active treatment is associated with a 26% reduction in mortality rates in patients with diabetes but not their nondiabetic counterparts. A prior meta-analysis pooling data from the PCI, EPIC, EPILOG, and EPISTENT trials demonstrated a 44% decrease in 1-year mortality rates with abciximab in diabetic patients at the time of PTCA and stenting.

The optimal therapeutic modality of diabetic patients with multivessel disease is controversial. The BARI trial and, to a lesser extent, the BARI registry have shown that diabetics with multivessel disease have a marked decrease in cardiovascular mortality rates when compared with patients who receive PTCA. Not all trials however, have shown the superiority of CABG. Superiority has been demonstrated for internal mammary artery grafts when CABG is performed compared with saphenous vein grafts.

Overall, diabetics with multivessel disease appear to do better with CABG using the internal mammary artery than with PCTA coronary intervention, but there are still many unanswered questions. Some of these questions will be addressed in the NIH-funded BARI II trial, which will examine the type of revascularization with or without aggressive medical therapy as well as tight glucose control on mortality and cardiac events. A randomized trial of percutaneous coronary interventions with glycoprotein IIb/IIIa inhibitors versus CABG in patients with diabetes would also be valuable.

Until future trial results become available and new technologies and medical therapies emerge, aggressive secondary prevention and ongoing management of CHD in the setting of diabetes will continue to pose a challenge.

American Diabetes Association: Management of dyslipidemia in adults with diabetes position statement. Diabetes Care 2002; 25:S74–S77.

Arayz-Pacheco A, Raskin P: Management of hypertension in diabetes. Endocrinol Metab Clin North Am 1992;21:371.

Bhatt DL, Marso SP, Lincorr AM et al: Abciximab reduces mortality in diabetics following percutaneous coronary intervention. J Am Coll Cardiol 2000;35:922–928.

Brooks RC, Ketre KM: Clinical trials of revascularization therapy in diabetes. Curr Opin Cardiol 2000;15(4):287–292.

Calles-Escandon J, Cipolla M: Diabetes and endothelial dysfunction: A clinical perspective. Endocr Rev 2001;22:36.

Downs JR, Clearfield M, Wies S et al: Primary prevention of acute coronary events with lovastatin in men and women with average cholesterol levels: results of AFCAPS/TexCAPS. Air Force/Texas Coronary Atherosclerosis Prevention Study. JAMA 1998;279:1615–1622.

Goldberg IJ: Diabetic dyslipidemia: Causes and consequences. J Clin Endocrinol Metab 2001;86:965

Hammoud T, Tanguay JF, Bourassa MG: Management of coronary artery disease: Therapeutic option in patients with diabetes. J Am Coll Cardiol 2000;36:355–365.

Huang ES, Meigs JB, Singer DE: The effect of interventions to prevent cardiovascular disease in patients with type 2 diabetes mellitus. Am J Med 2001;111:633–642.

Long-term Intervention with Pravastatin in Ischaemic Disease (LIPID) study group: Prevention of cardiovascular events and death with pravastatin in patients with CHD and a broad range of initial cholesterol levels. The long-term Intervention with Pravastatin in Ischaemic Disease (LIPID) Study Group. N Engl J Med 1998;339:1349–1357.

Malmberg K, Ryden L, Hamsten A et al, on behalf of the DIGAMI study group: Effects of insulin treatment on cause-specific one year mortality and morbidity in diabetic patients with acute myocardial infarction. Eur Heart J 1996;17: 1317–1344.

McFarlane SI, Banerji M, Sowers JR: Insulin resistance and cardiovascular disease. J Clin Endocrinol Metab 2001;86:713.

Nathan DM: Long-term complications of diabetes mellitus. N Engl J Med 1993;328:1676.

National Cholesterol Education Program (NCEP) Expert Panel on Detection, Evaluation and Treatment of High Blood Cholesterol in Adults (Adult Treatment Panel III): Executive summary of the third report of the National Cholesterol Education Program (NCEP) Expert Panel on Detection, Evaluation and treatment of high blood cholesterol in Adults (Adult Treatment Panel III). JAMA 2001;285:2486–2497.

Pyorala K, Pedersen TR, Kjeksus J et al: Cholesterol lowering with simvastatin improves prognosis of diabetic patients with coronary heart disease: A subgroup analysis of the Scandinavian simvastatin study (4S). Diabetes Care 1997;20:614–620.

Roffi M, Chew DP, Mukherjee E et al. Platelet glycoprotein IIb/IIIa inhibitors reduce mortality in diabetic patients with non-ST segment elevation acute coronary syndromes. Circulation 2001;104:2767–2771.

Rubins HB, Robins SJ, Collins D et al: Gemfibrozil for the secondary prevention of CHD in men with low levels of high-density lipoprotein cholesterol. Veterans Affairs High-Density Lipoprotein Cholesterol Intervention Trial Study Group. N Engl J Med 1999;341:410–418.

Sacks FM, Pfeffer MA, Moye LA et al for the Cholesterol and Recurrent events trial investigators: The effect of pravastatin on coronary events after myocardial infarction in patients with average cholesterol levels: Cholesterol and Recurrent Events Trial Investigators. N Engl J Med 1996;335:1001–1009.

Sowers JR, Epstein M, Frohlich ED: Diabetes, hypertension, and cardiovascular disease: An update. Hypertension 2001;37:1053.

UK Prospective Diabetes Study Group: Tight blood pressure control and risk of macrovascular and microvascular complications in type 2 diabetes: UKPDS 38. BMJ 1998:317:703–713.

Vega GL: Obesity, the metabolic syndrome, and cardiovascular disease. Am Heart J 2001;142:1108–1116.

ESTROGENS AND THE HEART

1. HORMONE REPLACEMENT THERAPY

A great deal of interest has recently focused on estrogens and coronary artery disease. There is a strong link between menopause and increased CHD in women. Postmenopausal status or premature menopause without hormone replacement therapy (HRT) was previously considered a risk factor for coronary artery disease by the Adult Treatment Panel II based on several observational studies, such as the Nurses' Health Study, which suggested that current users of HRT had a 40% lower risk for CHD. This observation was supported by mechanistic studies of cellular and molecular actions of estrogen on lipids, hemostasis, endothelial function, and vascular reactivity.

The Adult Treatment Panel III deleted postmenopausal status without HRT as a CHD risk factor after unexpected results from the first prospective, blind, placebo-controlled, randomized trial of HRT in secondary prevention were released in 1998; the Heart and Estrogen/progestin Replacement Study, or HERS, trial. HERS found no benefit from 4 years of treatment with HRT in women with prior CHD.

Importantly, HERS demonstrated a 52% increased risk of major coronary events within the first year of the trial. During the second year risk was equal in the two groups, and by years 4–5 risk was higher in the placebo group. The early increase in risk suggests that HRT may predispose to thrombosis, arrhythmia, or ischemia.

The Estrogen Replacement on the Progression of Coronary Artery Atherosclerosis (ERA) trial demonstrated that postmenopausal HRT is not beneficial in the short term (3 years) in preventing progression or inducing regression of coronary atherosclerosis in women with established CHD who undergo angiography.

It should be noted that both HERS and ERA were designed to examine the role of HRT in secondary prevention. The Women's Health Initiative is the first trial examining the effect of HRT in primary prevention and was terminated in early 2002 due to increased risk of invasive breast cancer. Rates of CHD, stroke, deep venous thrombosis, and pulmonary embolism were higher in women on HRT. Therefore, postmenopausal HRT cannot be recommended solely for prevention of CHD.

Cole PL: Coronary artery disease in women: Differences in diagnosis therapy and prognosis. Coron Artery Dis 1993;4:595.

Grady D, Rubin SM, Pettiti DB et al: Hormone therapy to prevent disease and prolong life in postmenopausal women. Ann Intern Med 1992;117:1016–1037.

Herrington DM, Reboussin DM, Brosnihan KB et al: Effects of estrogen replacement on progression of coronary artery atherosclerosis (ERA). N Engl J Med 2000;343:522–529.

Hulley S, Grady D, Bush T et al: Randomized trial of estrogen plus progestin for secondary prevention of coronary heart disease in postmenopausal women. JAMA 1998;280:605–613.

LaRosa JC: Estrogen: Risk vs. benefit for the prevention of coronary artery disease. Coron Art Dis 1993;4:588.

Mendelsohn ME, Karas RH: The protective effects of estrogen on the cardiovascular system. N Engl J Med 1999;340:1801–1811.

Nabulshi AA, Folsom AR, White A et al: Association of hormone replacement therapy with various cardiovascular risk factors in postmenopausal women. The Atherosclerosis Risk in Communities Study Investigators. N Engl J Med 1993;328:1069.

Psaty BM, Herbert SR, Atkins D et al: A review of the association of estrogens and progestins with cardiovascular disease in postmenopausal women. Arch Intern Med 1993;153:1421.

Soma MR, Osnago-Gadda I, Paoletti R et al: The lowering of lipoprotein(a) induced by estrogen plus progesterone replacement therapy in postmenopausal women Arch Intern Med 1993;153:1462.

Tolbert T, Oparil S: Cardiovascular effects of estrogen. Am J Hypertension 2001;14:186S–193S2.

Writing group for the women's health initiative investigators: Risks and benefits of estrogen plus progestin in healthy postmenopausal women: Principle results from the Women's Health Initiative randomized controlled trial. JAMA 2002; 288:321–333.

ORAL CONTRACEPTIVES

Oral contraceptives have long been touted as risks for deep venous thrombosis, myocardial infarction, and stroke. The high risk reported in early studies was increased among women who were cigarette smokers. Women who had stopped taking oral contraceptives did not appear to be at increased risk, suggesting a coagulation rather than a progressive atherosclerotic effect of these agents. Most of these studies used high-dose estrogen preparations. Current-day oral contraceptives are low-dose estrogen (≤50 mg) and some are progestin only; they are generally safe. Otherwise healthy women who are not diabetic or hypertensive and do not smoke have no excess risk.

Gaspard UJ, Lefebvre PJ: Clinical aspects of the relationship between oral contraceptives, abnormalities in carbohydrate metabolism, and the development of cardiovascular disease. Am J Obstet Gynecol 1990;163:334.

Rosondaal FR, Helmerhorst FM, Vandenbroucke JP: Female hormones and thrombosis. Arterioscler Thromb Vasc Biol 2002; 22:201–210.

Tanis BC, Van Den Bosch MA, Kemmeren JM et al: Oral contraceptives and the risk of myocardial infarction. N Eng J Med 2001;345:1787–1793.

Connective Tissue Diseases and the Heart

Carlos A. Roldan, MD

The connective tissue diseases are immune-mediated inflammatory diseases, primarily of the musculoskeletal system; however, they frequently also involve the cardiovascular system. The most important of these diseases are systemic lupus erythematosus, rheumatoid arthritis, scleroderma, ankylosing spondylitis, polymyositis/dermatomyositis, and mixed connective tissue disease. They affect the pericardium, myocardium, valve leaflets, conduction system, and great vessels with different rates of prevalence and degrees of severity. Although heart involvement in patients with connective tissue diseases contributes significantly to their morbidity and mortality rates, there is a large discrepancy between clinically recognized heart disease and postmortem series. Furthermore, the pathogenesis, natural history, and effects of therapy are poorly understood. Increased awareness and better understanding of the cardiovascular disease associated with connective tissue diseases may lead to earlier recognition, treatment and, perhaps, increased longevity.

SYSTEMIC LUPUS ERYTHEMATOSUS

ESSENTIALS OF DIAGNOSIS

- *Musculoskeletal and mucocutaneous manifestations of systemic lupus erythematosus (SLE)*
- *Acute pericarditis with antinuclear antibodies detected in the pericardial fluid*
- *Libman-Sacks vegetations, atrioventricular (AV) valve regurgitation, myocarditis, vascular thrombotic disease, and SLE*
- *Infective endocarditis or cardioembolism and SLE*

General Considerations

Systemic lupus erythematosus is a multisystem chronic or recurrent inflammatory disease of unknown origin that affects predominantly the musculoskeletal and mucocutaneous systems. Patients present with fatigue, myalgias, arthralgias or arthritis, photosensitivity, and serositis. The prevalence of SLE varies widely, from 4 to 250 cases per 100,000 persons. It is more frequent in a patient's relatives than in the general population and is three times more frequent in blacks than in whites. SLE is predominantly seen in females, with a female-to-male ratio of 10:1. The pathophysiology of the disease, although still uncertain, is probably related to the multiorgan deposition of circulating antigen-antibody complexes and activation of the complement system, leading to humoral- and cellular-mediated inflammation.

Although SLE affects the cardiovascular system with varied frequency and degrees of severity, cardiovascular disease is the third most important cause of death in SLE patients (after infectious and renal diseases). The most significant SLE-associated heart diseases are valvular heart disease, pericarditis, myocarditis or cardiomyopathy, and arterial or venous thrombosis and systemic thromboembolism. Coronary artery disease (CAD), cardiac arrhythmias or conduction disturbances are less common.

The pathogenesis of SLE-associated cardiovascular disease is also uncertain. It is believed, as it is for the primary disease, that the immune complex deposition and complement activation lead to an acute, chronic, or recurrent inflammation of the vascular endothelium, pericardium, myocardium, endocardium, conduction system, or valve leaflets. The presence in these tissues of immune complexes, complement, antinuclear antibodies, lupus erythematosus cells, mononuclear inflammatory cells, necrosis, hematoxylin bodies, and deposits of fibrin and platelet thrombi support this theory. Some studies suggest that antiphospholipid antibodies (eg, anticardiolipin, lupus anticoagulant) may cause cardiovascular injury. These antibodies, present in as many as half of SLE patients, are IgG, IgM, or IgA immunoglobulins directed against negatively charged phospholipids present in the membrane of endothelial cells. Although these antibodies have been clearly associated with venous and arterial thrombosis and systemic thromboembolism, their primary pathogenetic role in SLE-associated heart diseases is still controversial. As of now, no immune marker has been definitely identified as indicative or predictive of heart disease in SLE patients.

1. VALVULAR HEART DISEASE

General Considerations

Valvular heart disease is the clinically most important and frequent of the SLE-associated cardiovascular manifestations. Valvular heart disease is associated with an increased morbidity and mortality of SLE patients. It has been categorized as masses or vegetations (Libman-Sacks endocarditis), leaflet thickening, valve regurgitation, and, infrequently, valve stenosis. The actual prevalence of clinically recognized valve disease is unknown, but rates are higher in patients who have had SLE for more than 5 years, probably also in those treated with corticosteroids, and those older than 50 years of age. The activity or severity of SLE disease and the duration or dosage of steroid therapy are *not* associated with higher prevalence rates or more severe forms of valve disease.

A. VALVE MASSES, OR LIBMAN-SACKS ENDOCARDITIS

Considered pathognomonic of SLE-associated valve disease, valve masses are almost exclusively seen on the mitral and aortic valves. The majority are located on the basal portions of the leaflets, on the atrial side for the mitral, and the aortic vessel side for the aortic valve. The valve masses are usually less than 1 cm^2 in size, have irregular borders and heterogeneous echodensity, and have no independent motion (Figures 33–1 and 33–2). Most valves with masses have associated thickening or regurgitation. Although, valve masses have been more commonly seen in younger subjects (younger than 40 years), their association with SLE activity, severity, duration, and therapy has been recently questioned.

The pathogenesis of SLE-associated valvular heart disease is still uncertain. Current data suggest that subendothelial deposition of immunoglobulins and complement lead to an increased expression of $\alpha_3\beta_1$-integrin on the endothelial cells; increased amounts of collagen IV, laminin, and fibronectin; proliferation of blood vessels; inflammation; thrombus formation; and finally fibrosis. Antiphospholipid antibodies (ie, IgG and IgM anticardiolipin antibodies, lupus anticoagulant, and a false-positive result for the Venereal Disease and Research Laboratories [VDRL] test) have also been proposed to play a role. However, their primary pathogenic role is still debatable because patients with valvular disease can have low levels of these antibodies; those with normal valves have elevated antibodies; and those without antibodies also have valvular disease.

Pathological examination reveals that active Libman-Sacks vegetations have central fibrinoid necrosis with fibroblastic proliferation and fibrosis, surrounded by mononuclear and polymorphonuclear cellular infiltration, small hemorrhages, and platelet thrombus. Healed vegetations have central fibrosis, minimal or no inflammatory cell deposition, and no or hyalinized and endothelialized thrombus. Active, healed and mixed vegetations can be seen in the same valve.

B. VALVE THICKENING

With or without abnormal mobility or calcification, valve thickening may be seen in up to half of patients; it is generally diffuse, with greater involvement of the middle and tip portions. When leaflet thickening is localized, the basal, middle, and tip portions are equally affected. Valve thickening predominantly affects the mitral and aortic valves and is commonly associated with valve regurgitation, valve masses, or both.

C. VALVE REGURGITATION

This most frequent abnormality is predominantly mild in severity and therefore usually clinically silent. Although the prevalence of regurgitation is similar for the mitral, tricuspid, and pulmonic valves (about 50–75%) and the lowest for the aortic valve ($\leq 25\%$), the mitral and aortic valves are those most commonly associated with complications.

Mitral or aortic tricuspid valve stenosis associated with respective valve regurgitation has been described in rare cases.

Clinical Findings

Unless it is severe or associated with complications, valvular heart disease is generally asymptomatic or overshadowed by the musculoskeletal and systemic inflammatory symptomatology. Complications, such as severe valvular regurgitation due to recurrent or acute valvulitis, leaflet perforation including bioprosthetic leaflets, noninfective mitral valve chordal rupture, infective endocarditis, need for valve replacement, congestive heart failure, or cardioembolism, occur in 20–25% of patients with valvular disease. SLE-associated valve masses can manifest with systemic thromboembolism before symptoms or signs of severe valve dysfunction occur.

It is important to note that infective endocarditis can mimic, accompany, or trigger a flare of SLE and lead to severe valvular dysfunction, heart failure, and death from septicemia. Similarly, a flare of SLE can mimic infective endocarditis (pseudo-infective endocarditis). A low white count, elevated antiphospholipid antibodies, and negative or low C-reactive protein indicate active SLE.

A. PHYSICAL EXAMINATION

The physical findings of musculoskeletal and mucocutaneous disease generally predominate in SLE patients, even in those with cardiovascular disease. If moderate-to-severe mitral or aortic regurgitation or stenosis is present, the auscultatory findings found on physical examination will be typical. Less significant degrees of re-

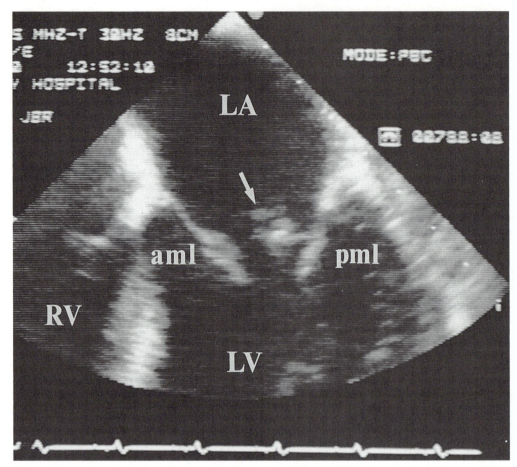

Figure 33–1. Mitral valve thickening and a mass in a patient with systemic lupus erythematosus. This transesophageal four-chamber view shows diffuse thickening predominantly of the middle and tip portions of the anterior (aml) and posterior (pml) mitral leaflets. An irregular mass *(arrow)* is evident on the atrial side of the posterior mitral leaflet. Moderate mitral regurgitation was present. LA = left atrium; LV = left ventricle; RV = right ventricle.

Reprinted, with permission, from Roldan et al: Systemic lupus erythematosus valve disease by transesophageal echocardiography and the role of the antiphospholipid antibodies. J Am Coll Cardiol 1992;20:1127.

gurgitation (these are the majority) may not be clinically detected or may be mistaken for functional murmurs. These functional murmurs are believed to be related to the frequent presence of fever, anemia, hypertension, or volume overload in SLE patients.

B. Diagnostic Studies

1. Electrocardiography—Results of ECG studies are nonspecific. Left atrial abnormality and left ventricular hypertrophy can be seen in patients with chronic and severe aortic or mitral regurgitation.

2. Chest radiography—Cardiomegaly with left ventricular and atrial enlargement may be seen in the presence of significant mitral or aortic regurgitation.

3. Echocardiography—Transthoracic color-flow Doppler echocardiography is the most commonly applied technique for the diagnosis of SLE-associated valve disease. This technique accurately determines the presence and severity of valve regurgitation or stenosis and abnormal leaflet thickening or masses. The prevalence of Libman-Sacks vegetations by transthoracic echocardiography is less than 10%. Color-flow Doppler echocardiography will also detect associated increased wall thickness, chamber enlargement, and ventricular systolic dysfunction. Transesophageal echocardiography (TEE) is superior to transthoracic echocardiography (TTE) in detecting and characterizing SLE-associated valve masses and leaflet thickening. This technique detects valve masses in up to 30% of patients. By serial TEE Libman-Sacks vege-

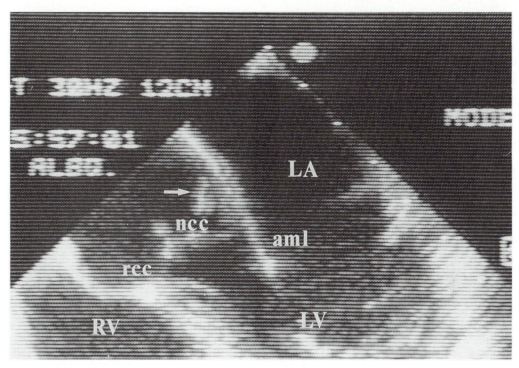

Figure 33–2. Aortic valve mass in a patient with systemic lupus erythematosus. This transesophageal longitudinal view shows a mass *(arrow)* of irregular borders and irregular echogenicity located at the base of the noncoronary cusp (ncc) and posteromedial aortic root wall. No aortic regurgitation was present. LA = left atrium; LV = left ventricle; rcc = right coronary cusp; RV = right ventricle. Reprinted, with permission, from Roldan et al: Systemic lupus erythematosus valve disease by transesophageal echocardiography and the role of antiphospholipid antibodies. J Am Coll Cardiol 1992;20:1127.

tations resolve, appear de novo, or change their morphology over time independently of SLE activity, severity, duration, or therapy. However, this technique is indicated for those patients with a focal neurologic defect, to exclude sources of cardioembolism, and for patients with suspected complicating infective endocarditis.

Treatment

A. SPECIFIC ANTIINFLAMMATORY THERAPY

Currently, no available prospective data indicate that corticosteroids or immunosuppressive therapy are either beneficial or harmful in treating SLE-associated valve disease.

B. LONG-TERM ANTICOAGULATION

The effect of long-term anticoagulation in patients with antiphospholipid antibodies and Libman-Sacks vegetations is controversial.

C. OTHER THERAPY

Diuretics, vasodilators, or prosthetic valve replacement are indicated in patients with severe symptomatic valve

disease, including those whose conditions are complicated by infective endocarditis. The mortality rate associated with valve replacement in SLE patients is twice that for patients without SLE.

2. PERICARDITIS

General Considerations

Pericarditis, with or without effusion or pericardial thickening, is common in postmortem series. The clinical diagnosis of pericarditis, however, is made less frequently.

Clinical Findings

Symptomatic pericarditis is generally acute and uncomplicated and is most commonly seen during flare-ups of the disease. Asymptomatic pericardial disease may be present in some patients. It is manifested by incidentally detected small effusions in most cases and far less frequently by pericardial thickening found on echocardiography. Asymptomatic pericardial disease is generally seen in patients with stable disease that is either mildly active or in remission. Cardiac tamponade may complicate acute pericarditis in a few patients. Occasionally, acute pericarditis, cardiac tamponade, or both may be the initial manifestation of SLE. Chronic constrictive pericarditis is rare. Although infectious pericarditis is extremely rare, it should be considered. About ten cases of infectious pericarditis have been reported, with the majority caused by *Staphylococcus aureus*. The presence of pericardial effusion in SLE patients may also be secondary to severe uremia or nephrotic syndrome.

A. PHYSICAL EXAMINATION

Because it is frequently symptomatic, acute pericarditis is the SLE-related cardiovascular disease most often detected clinically. It presents with fever, tachycardia, pleuritic chest pain and, on auscultation, the presence of a pericardial rub. If a large effusion is present, decreased heart sounds, jugular venous distention, facial edema, ascites, and pulsus paradoxus may be noted.

B. DIAGNOSTIC STUDIES

1. Electrocardiography—The ECG most frequently shows no abnormalities or nonspecific ST segment and T wave changes. The characteristic diffuse ST segment elevation with upward concavity and PR segment depression of acute pericarditis is occasionally seen. Low voltage or electrical alternans may also be seen if a large pericardial effusion is present.

2. Chest radiography—The chest roentgenogram is generally of little diagnostic value because the majority of patients with acute pericarditis have no—or only small—pericardial effusions. If a large pericardial effusion is present, cardiomegaly with a characteristic water-bottle shape may be seen.

3. Echocardiography—In the majority of cases, echocardiography will demonstrate small pericardial effusions, or none. Small, asymptomatic pericardial effusions have been found in up to 20% of SLE patients hospitalized with active disease. The absence of such effusions on echocardiography does not exclude a clinically suspected pericarditis, however. In cases of pericarditis with large pericardial effusion and clinically suspected cardiac tamponade, echocardiography may have complementary diagnostic value by demonstrating right atrial or ventricular diastolic collapse and significant respiratory variability of the mitral or tricuspid Doppler inflows, indicating the need for therapeutic pericardiocentesis. Echocardiography is less useful in detecting pericardial thickening or calcification in cases of suspected chronic pericardial constriction.

4. Computed tomography and nuclear magnetic resonance imaging—Although both techniques are less available and more expensive than echocardiography, they are superior in assessing pericardial thicken-

ing and calcification in patients with suspected pericardial constriction.

5. Laboratory findings—Pericardial fluid is generally exudative. The presence of antinuclear antibodies in the pericardial fluid is considered pathognomonic of SLE-associated pericarditis.

Treatment

A. MEDICAL THERAPY

1. Specific antiinflammatory therapy—The treatment of acute symptomatic pericarditis consists of bed rest and nonsteroidal antiinflammatory drugs (NSAIDs), such as indomethacin or aspirin. If symptoms are refractory to this therapy, low-dose prednisone at 10–20 mg/day for 7–14 days is indicated.

2. Other therapy—Pericardiocentesis should be performed when large effusions are unresponsive to medical therapy and when cardiac tamponade or complicating infectious pericarditis with effusion are suspected.

B. SURGICAL THERAPY

Pericardiectomy has been performed in isolated cases of SLE-associated chronic pericardial constriction.

3. MYOCARDITIS OR CARDIOMYOPATHY

General Considerations

Myocardial disease in SLE patients has three principal causes: (1) A primary acute, chronic, or recurrent myocarditis is the most frequent. (2) The second most common cause is myocardial ischemia or infarction caused by coronary arteritis, coronary atherosclerosis, coronary thrombosis, or coronary embolism. (3) Third is heart failure resulting from severe mitral or aortic regurgitation. Myocarditis can be seen in autopsy series in up to 80% of SLE patients; by contrast, only 20% of cases can be clinically detected. The presence of the cellular-antigen Ro (SSA) antibody is highly associated with myocarditis.

Clinical Findings

Acute myocarditis typically manifests with fever, tachycardia, chest pain, and, rarely, with symptoms of heart failure, arrhythmias, or conduction disturbances. The myocarditis is generally mild and usually does not cause left ventricular systolic dysfunction. However, up to one third of young patients with active SLE have asymptomatic diastolic dysfunction. Occasionally, severe dilated cardiomyopathy is seen; this is due to a single, acute, and severe myocarditis or to recurrent myocarditis, which leads to myocardial necrosis and fibrosis. Myocardial dysfunction secondary to coronary arteritis, coronary atherosclerosis, small-vessel vasculitis, or severe valvular heart disease is infrequent (<6%). Acute coronary thrombosis without underlying atherosclerosis and coronary embolism from aortic or mitral valve masses is rare.

A. Physical Examination

If diastolic or systolic dysfunction is present, tachycardia, third and fourth heart sounds, pulmonary rales, and edema may be found.

B. Diagnostic Studies

1. Electrocardiography—Nonspecific ST segment and T wave abnormalities and atrial or ventricular ectopic complexes are common. Rarely, atrial or ventricular tachyarrhythmias can be detected.

2. Chest radiography—Cardiomegaly may be present if dilated cardiomyopathy has developed.

3. Echocardiography—Generally, no abnormalities are detected in acute myocarditis. When the myocarditis is severe, diffuse or regional wall motion abnormalities may be observed. Evidence of ventricular systolic or diastolic dysfunction may also be seen. Diastolic dysfunction as determined by Doppler echocardiography can be demonstrated in 15–35% of young patients with active SLE, normal epicardial coronary arteries, and myocardial perfusion defects. These data suggest subclinical myocardial or small-vessel coronary artery disease. In patients with dilated cardiomyopathy, chamber enlargement and biventricular systolic dysfunction are present. Increased wall thickness and left ventricular mass secondary to hypertension also may be demonstrated.

4. Radionuclide ventriculography—Either first-transit or gated-acquisition radionuclide angiography also can be used to assess ventricular systolic and diastolic dysfunction, wall motion abnormalities, and chamber enlargement. In up to one third of SLE patients, this technique has shown an abnormal ventricular function response to exercise, as evidenced by a fall or subnormal rise in ejection fraction and the appearance of new or worsened wall motion abnormalities indicative of myocarditis or CAD. Reversible, fixed, or mixed myocardial perfusion defects can be seen in patients with normal epicardial coronary arteries.

5. Endomyocardial biopsy—Tissue samples may demonstrate SLE-associated myocarditis or cardiomyopathy when a clinical or serologic diagnosis cannot be made.

Treatment

A. Specific Antiinflammatory Therapy

Acute myocarditis is treated with high-dose oral prednisone (1 mg/kg/day). The exact duration of treatment has not been established, but a course of 7–14 days is generally recommended.

B. Other Therapy

Symptomatic therapy with NSAIDs or other analgesics, bed rest, and electrocardiographic monitoring for the detection of arrhythmias are indicated. If symptomatic dilated cardiomyopathy is present, diuretics, vasodilators, and digoxin therapy are used.

4. THROMBOTIC DISEASES

Clinical Findings

A. Physical Findings

Deep vein thrombosis and pulmonary emboli and peripheral or cerebral arterial thrombosis are frequent in SLE patients. Acute coronary thrombosis in the absence of angiographic CAD has also been reported. Both arterial and venous thrombotic events have been frequently associated with the presence of antiphospholipid antibodies. These antibodies, it is suggested, are directed against phospholipids present on the membrane of the endothelial cells. This produces endothelial dysfunction with decreased production of prostacyclin and endothelial relaxing factor, leading to increased vasoconstriction, platelet aggregation, and thrombus formation. SLE cerebrovascular disease can be due to cardioembolism from Libman-Sacks endocarditis, chronic or acute vasculitis, or left ventricular or atrial thrombi.

Although acute pleuritic chest pain and tachycardia could be related to the presence of pericarditis, pleuritis, or pneumonitis, they should prompt the suspicion of pulmonary emboli and deep vein thrombosis. Focal transient or permanent neurologic deficits are due to vasculitis, cerebritis, or cardioembolism from valvular or myocardial disease.

B. Diagnostic Studies

1. Transesophageal echocardiography—TEE may be indicated in SLE patients with focal neurologic deficits or peripheral arterial thrombosis to exclude cardioembolism, rather than vasculitis or in situ thrombosis, as their cause.

2. Doppler echocardiography, plethysmography, scintigraphy, or venogram—These imaging methods of the lower extremities should be performed if deep vein thrombosis is suspected.

3. Pulmonary ventilation-perfusion scan—This method should be considered if pulmonary embolism is clinically suspected.

4. Laboratory findings—Although the presence of antiphospholipid antibodies in the form of IgG, IgM, or IgA anticardiolipin antibodies; lupus anticoagulant; and, less frequently, a false-positive VDRL test are highly associated with venous or arterial thrombotic events, the antibodies can also be present in SLE patients without thrombosis. They are also found, although infrequently, in non-SLE patients. Therefore, routine measurement of antiphospholipid antibodies to identify patients at high thrombotic risk and as a basis for prophylactic anticoagulant therapy is not currently indicated.

Treatment

A. SPECIFIC ANTIINFLAMMATORY THERAPY

No therapeutic role has been determined for steroids or immunosuppressives in SLE patients with antiphospholipid antibodies and thrombosis or thromboembolism.

B. OTHER THERAPY

If no contraindications exist, anticoagulation with warfarin for 6 months or more is the treatment of choice.

5. CORONARY ARTERY DISEASE

General Considerations

Postmortem studies in SLE patients have demonstrated up to a 25% prevalence of CAD, but clinically evident disease or arteritis is uncommon. The low prevalence of CAD may likely relate to the predominance of young females with SLE. However, young women (35–44 years old) are 50 times more likely to have an MI than women of similar age without SLE. Risk factors for CAD in SLE patients are a longer mean duration of the disease, a longer mean duration and dose of prednisone therapy, a cholesterol level greater than 200 mg/dL, systemic hypertension, and obesity. Patients with inactive or active SLE have high levels of very low density lipoproteins and triglycerides and low levels of high-density lipoproteins. Antiphospholipid antibodies are also associated with CAD. They produce peroxidation of low-density lipoproteins and endothelial dysfunction leading to vasoconstriction and thrombosis by release of platelet-derived growth factor and thromboxane A_2 and decrease production of prostacyclin and prostaglandin I. Angina, MI, and left ventricular dysfunction rarely result from coronary arteritis, in situ thrombosis, or embolization to a coronary artery.

The clinical or angiographic differentiation of coronary arteritis and coronary atherosclerosis is difficult. Rarely, acute coronary obstruction of angiographically normal coronaries may result from embolism of a Libman-Sacks vegetation or from the in situ formation of intracoronary thrombi. Intramural CAD is more frequent than epicardial coronary disease in postmortem series.

Clinical Findings

A. PRESENTATION

The presentation of CAD in SLE patients is not unique and involves stable or exertional angina, unstable angina, acute transmural or nontransmural MI or, rarely, heart failure from ischemic left ventricular dysfunction. In addition, fatal MI can occur in SLE patients, and some data suggest an increased risk of myocardial rupture after MI in SLE patients treated with steroids. Coronary arteritis should be suspected in a young patient with an acute ischemic syndrome, active SLE, and evidence of vasculitis affecting other organs. Coronary embolism or in situ thrombosis warrant consideration when an MI occurs in association with a cardioembolic substrate or a procoagulant state.

B. DIAGNOSTIC STUDIES

Electrocardiography, exercise testing with or without perfusion scanning, echocardiography, and coronary angiography can be used with SLE patients suspected of having CAD. The diagnostic value of these techniques is similar to that in the general population. None of these techniques, including angiography, can reliably differentiate coronary arteritis from common coronary atherosclerosis.

Treatment

A. SPECIFIC ANTIINFLAMMATORY THERAPY

If coronary arteritis is suspected, high-dose corticosteroids (1 mg/kg/day) are used. The duration of therapy is still uncertain, and it may be contraindicated in patients with recent transmural MI.

B. OTHER THERAPY

Except for the use of steroids in suspected arteritis, the treatment of CAD is not different from that in the general population. Both angioplasty and bypass surgery have been successfully performed in SLE patients.

6. CARDIAC ARRHYTHMIAS & CONDUCTION DISTURBANCES

General Considerations

The prevalence of these abnormalities is unknown. Although they are common with myocarditis and highly associated with the presence of anti-Ro antibodies, no primary pathogenetic role of these antibodies has been demonstrated. Atrial fibrillation or flutter may be seen during episodes of acute pericarditis. Rarely, ventricular arrhythmias or conduction disturbances may be associated with acute myocarditis. Chronic conduction disturbances may be due to the inflammation and fibrosis of the conduction system frequently found at autopsy. *Electrocardiography* is the most valuable technique for detecting arrhythmias and conduction disturbances.

Treatment

A. SPECIFIC ANTIINFLAMMATORY THERAPY

Although experience is limited, up to one third of acute high-degree AV blocks may resolve with the use of high-dose steroids.

B. OTHER THERAPY

Temporary pacing is an alternative treatment for acute AV blocks. Permanent pacemakers should be used in cases of symptomatic high-grade AV blocks that are unresponsive to steroids.

Prognosis

The overall survival rate of SLE patients is about 75% over 10 years. If the heart, lung, kidney, or central nervous system is clinically involved, the prognosis is worse. Cardiovascular disease is the third major cause of mortality in SLE patients, after infectious and renal diseases. Valvular, myocardial, or CAD are now known to decrease the survival of SLE patients. The prognostic implications of clinically or echocardiographically detected pericardial disease, however, is unknown. The quality of life and survival of SLE patients with significant valvular heart disease or CAD is significantly improved following surgical correction of the defect.

Afek A, Shoenfeld Y, Manor R et al: Increased endothelial cell expression of alpha$_3$beta$_1$ integrin in cardiac valvulopathy in the primary (Hughes) and secondary antiphospholipid syndrome. Lupus 1999;8:502.

Borba EF, Bonfa E: Dyslipoproteinemia in systemic lupus erythematosus: Influence of disease activity and anticardiolipin antibodies. Lupus 1997;6:533.

Espinola-Zavaleta N, Vargas-Barron J, Colmenares-Galvis T et al: Echocardiographic evaluation of patients with primary antiphospholipid syndrome. Am Heart J 1999;137:973.

Kalke S, Balakrishanan C, Mangat G et al: Echocardiography in systemic lupus erythematosus. Lupus 1998;7:540.

Lagana B, Schillaci O, Tubani L et al: Lupus carditis: Evaluation with technetium-99m MIBI myocardial SPECT and heart rate variability. Angiology 1999;50:143.

Manzi S, Meilahn EN, Rairie JE et al: Age-specific incidence rates of myocardial infarction and angina in women with systemic lupus erythematosus: Comparison with the Framingham Study. Am J Epidemiol 1997;145:408.

Nesher G, Ilany J, Rosenmann D et al: Valvular dysfunction in antiphospholipid syndrome: Prevalence, clinical features, and treatment. Semin Arthritis Rheumatol 1997;27:27.

Oshiro AC, Derbes SJ, Stopa AR et al: Anti-Ro/SS-A and La/SS-B antibodies associated with cardiac involvement in childhood systemic lupus erythematosus. Ann Rheum Dis 1997;56:272.

Rangel A, Lavalle C, Chavez E et al: Myocardial infarction in patients with systemic lupus erythematosus with normal findings from coronary arteriography and without coronary vasculitis—case reports. Angiology 1999;50:245.

Rhaman P, Urowitz MB, Gladman DD et al: Contribution of traditional risk factors to coronary artery disease in patients with systemic lupus erythematosus. J Rheumatol 1999;26:2363.

Roldan CA, Shively BK, Crawford MH: An echocardiographic study of valvular heart disease associated with systemic lupus erythematosus. N Engl J Med 1996;335:1424.

Tikly M, Diese M, Zannettou N et al: Gonococcal endocarditis in a patient with systemic lupus erythematosus. Br J Rheumatol 1997;36:270.

Zonana-Nacach A, Barr SG, Magder LS et al: Damage in systemic lupus erythematosus and its association with corticosteroids. Arthritis Rheum 2000;43:1801.

RHEUMATOID ARTHRITIS

 ESSENTIALS OF DIAGNOSIS

- *Clinical evidence of rheumatoid arthritis*
- *Pericarditis and myocarditis with granuloma on biopsy*
- *Granulomatous valve disease, predominantly of the mitral and aortic valves*

General Considerations

Rheumatoid arthritis is an immune-mediated chronic inflammatory disease characterized by morning stiffness, arthralgias, or arthritis, predominantly of the metacarpophalangeal or proximal interphalangeal joints; rheumatoid nodules; serum IgM or IgG rheumatoid factor; and articular erosions seen on x-ray film. The disease prevalence is about 1%, and it affects females more than males with a ratio of from 2–4:1. The natural history of the disease is such that the median life expectancy is reduced by 7 years in men and 3 years in women. The most common causes of death are articular and extraarticular complications such as atlantoaxial subluxation, cricoarytenoid synovitis, sepsis, cardiopulmonary complications, and diffuse vasculitis. Rheumatoid arthritis patients with the worst prognosis are those with positive rheumatoid factor, nodular disease, and male gender.

Rheumatoid cardiovascular disease is produced by a nonspecific immune inflammation, vasculitis, or granulomatous deposition on the pericardium, myocardium, heart valves, coronary arteries, aorta, or the conduction system. Clinically apparent rheumatoid heart disease occurs in one third of patients, compared with up to 80% in autopsy series. Rheumatoid heart disease may appear as pericarditis, myocarditis, valvular heart disease, conduction disturbances, coronary arteritis, aortitis, or cor pulmonale.

Predictors for clinically apparent cardiovascular disease include male sex, advanced age at the onset of the disease, hypertension, corticosteroid therapy early in the disease, long-standing disease; active extraarticular, erosive polyarticular, and nodular disease; systemic vasculitis; and high serum titers of rheumatoid factor. Also, those patients who experience cardiovascular events have higher erythrocyte sedimentation rates (ESR) and higher levels of haptoglobin, von Willebrand factor, and plasminogen activator inhibitor than patients who do not have cardiovascular disease. These findings suggest an inflammatory and prothrombotic processes leading to cardiovascular disease.

1. RHEUMATOID PERICARDITIS

The prevalence of pericarditis is higher in hospitalized patients with active disease. Pericarditis generally follows the diagnosis of rheumatoid arthritis by about 20 years. There is a high association between pericarditis and IgG or IgM rheumatoid-factor positivity, rheumatoid nodular disease, and ESR of >55 mm/h. Rheumatoid pericarditis occurs by three mechanisms: a nonspecific immune inflammatory process, vasculitis, and, less frequently, granulomatous or nodular disease.

Clinical Findings

A. Presentation

Rheumatoid pericarditis is generally uncomplicated and most commonly is evidenced by typical pleuritic pain, atrial fibrillation or flutter, or both. About one third of patients are asymptomatic. On physical examination most will have a pericardial rub. Rarely, complicating cardiac tamponade or constrictive pericarditis may occur, generally in adult patients with active and severe disease of a longer duration and in those with extraarticular involvement. Dyspnea and orthopnea, edema, jugular venous distention, rales, pulsus paradoxus, Kussmaul's sign, and hepatojugular venous distention are common when cardiac compression is present.

B. Diagnostic Studies

1. Electrocardiography—ECG commonly shows nonspecific ST segment and T wave changes; a classic diffuse ST segment elevation can be seen. Low voltage or electrical alternans may be seen with large pericardial effusions.

2. Chest radiography—The chest film is generally normal. Cardiomegaly is seen in patients with large pericardial effusions. Pericardial calcifications are rarely seen.

3. Echocardiography—This is the most important diagnostic technique for rheumatoid pericardial disease. The most common echocardiographic findings are pericardial effusion and pericardial thickening. Right atrial or ventricular diastolic compression may be seen with large pericardial effusions; this generally indicates tamponade hemodynamics. The presence of pericardial thickening and calcification without significant effusion, and the presence of symptoms or signs of cardiac compression, suggest constrictive pericarditis, which can be confirmed by cardiac catheterization. It is im-

portant to note that the absence of pericardial abnormalities on echocardiography does not exclude the presence of pericarditis in a patient with typical symptoms or a pericardial rub.

4. Computed tomography or magnetic resonance imaging—CT or MRI is useful in detecting pericardial thickening and calcification in patients with chronic constrictive pericarditis.

5. Laboratory findings—Findings commonly associated with rheumatoid pericarditis include an ESR of more than 55 mm/h and positive antinuclear antigen (ANA). Pericardial fluid is exudative and serosanguineous, with a high protein content and high lactate dehydrogenase (LDH) but a characteristically low glucose level, and may contain rheumatoid factor. The cellular content is usually more than 2000, predominantly neutrophils. On pericardial biopsy (by immunofluorescence), granular deposits of IgG, IgM, C3, and C1q are seen in the interstitium and blood vessel walls of the pericardium.

Treatment

Bed rest and NSAIDs are recommended for mild, uncomplicated rheumatoid pericarditis. Steroids are frequently successful in treating unresponsive or severe cases. If large pericardial effusions or tamponade are present, pericardiocentesis or pericardiotomy is indicated. For chronic constrictive pericarditis, pericardiectomy is generally performed. The use of intrapericardial steroids at the time of pericardiocentesis is controversial.

Prognosis

The prognosis of rheumatoid arthritis in the presence of pericardial disease is unaltered when the pericardial involvement is mild. Large pericardial effusions with tamponade or chronic constrictive pericarditis, however, increases the morbidity and mortality rates among rheumatoid patients.

2. RHEUMATOID VALVULAR HEART DISEASE

General Considerations

Rheumatoid valvular heart disease is produced by a nonspecific acute, chronic, or recurrent inflammatory process, vasculitis, or deposition of granulomata on the valve leaflets. The inflammatory process consists of infiltration with plasma cells, histiocytes, lymphocytes, and eosinophils that lead to leaflet fibrosis, thickening, and retraction. The valve granulomata, which resemble rheumatoid nodules, are present inside any portion of the four valves, valve rings, papillary muscle tips, and atrial or ventricular endocardium. The aortic and mitral valves are most often affected. The granulomata are most commonly located at the basilar attachment of the valves; usually focal, and generally do not produce valve dysfunction.

Rheumatoid mitral or aortic valve disease is usually mild and asymptomatic, whether it is acute or chronic; rarely does valve disease progress to severe forms. Occasionally, acute and severe valvulitis or the rupture of a valve granulomata will lead to severe regurgitation and heart failure. In rare cases, aortitis may lead to aortic root dilatation and aortic regurgitation. Rheumatoid aortic regurgitation is more rapidly progressive than is that from other causes. Rheumatoid valve disease occurs in patients with long-standing rheumatoid disease and severe cases with erosive polyarticular and nodular disease, systemic vasculitis, and high levels of rheumatoid factor.

Clinical Findings

A. PHYSICAL EXAMINATION

The physical examination in rheumatoid valve disease may not be revealing because in the majority of cases the disease is mild. In the rare cases of severe chronic or acute aortic or mitral regurgitation, classic auscultatory findings and associated signs of left or biventricular failure may be present.

B. DIAGNOSTIC STUDIES

1. Electrocardiography and chest radiography— The ECG and chest film have limited diagnostic value. Both techniques may show chamber enlargement in cases of severe valve disease.

2. Transthoracic color-flow Doppler echocardiography—TTE color-flow Doppler is the most used test for detecting and assessing the severity of rheumatoid valve disease. Mitral or aortic valve leaflets, the most commonly involved, may show either diffuse or localized nodular thickening, with or without calcification. On TEE, mitral and aortic regurgitation of any degree are seen in up to 80% and 33%, respectively, of patients. Rheumatoid valve nodules appear as small (<0.5 cm^2), oval masses with homogeneous reflectance, usually single and on any portion of the leaflet. The adjacent leaflet appears normal or mildly sclerotic. Granulomatous valve disease, is probably unique to rheumatoid arthritis (Figure 33–3).

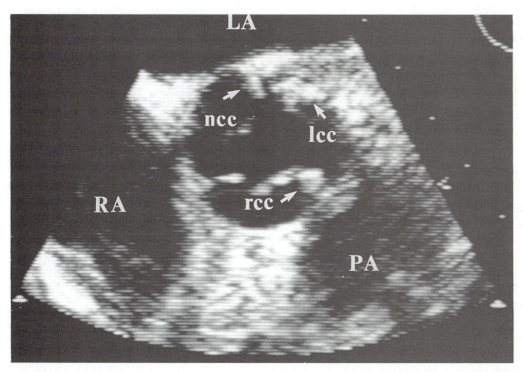

Figure 33–3. Granulomatous aortic valve disease in a patient with rheumatoid arthritis. This transesophageal basilar short-axis view shows multiple irregular, localized nodularities predominantly at the bases (*arrows*) of the left, right, and noncoronary cusps. Mild aortic regurgitation was detected. lcc = left coronary cusp; LA = left atrium; ncc = noncoronary cusp; PA = pulmonary artery; RA = right atrium; rcc = right coronary cusp.

Treatment

No specific antiinflammatory therapy for rheumatoid valve disease has been established. The use of steroids or other immunosuppressives in a few cases of acute severe valvulitis has resulted in significant improvement. Mitral or aortic valve replacement has been successfully performed in acute or chronic severe regurgitation. A homograft root-and-valve replacement has been successfully performed in severe aortitis and aortic regurgitation.

3. RHEUMATOID MYOCARDITIS

General Considerations

Rheumatoid myocarditis is observed in as much as 30% of patients in postmortem series but is rare in clinical and echocardiographic reports. Rheumatoid myocarditis is more common in patients with active and extraarticular disease, highly positive rheumatoid factor, and ANA, and in those with systemic vasculitis. Rheumatoid myocarditis may result from autoimmunity, vasculitis, or granulomata deposition; rarely, it is due to amyloid infiltration. Unless granulomata are present, rheumatoid myocarditis is difficult to differentiate on histopathology from eosinophilic, toxic, or infectious myocarditis.

Clinical Findings

The clinical presentation of rheumatoid myocarditis is similar to that for myocarditis from other causes. Most commonly it is mild, asymptomatic, and clinically unrecognized. When it is symptomatic, nonspecific symptoms of fatigue, dyspnea, palpitations, and chest pain may be present. The chest pain is usually pleuritic and probably reflects the presence of myopericarditis. Rarely, severe acute myocarditis with left ventricular dysfunction may present as congestive heart failure or symptomatic atrial or ventricular arrhythmias.

A. PHYSICAL EXAMINATION

Fever and sinus tachycardia are common. First and second heart sounds are normal; a third or fourth heart sound may rarely be present. Functional systolic murmurs are common. If myopericarditis is present, a pericardial rub may be detected.

B. DIAGNOSTIC STUDIES

1. Electrocardiography—ECG generally shows non-specific ST segment and T wave abnormalities. Atrioventricular conduction disturbances and atrial or ventricular ectopy can be detected.

2. Echocardiography—may show segmental wall motion abnormalities or diffuse left ventricular contractile dysfunction and chamber dilatation in cases of severe focal or diffuse myocarditis. This technique exhibits no abnormalities in the majority of patients with mild myocarditis, however.

3. Radionuclide scanning—Scanning with indium-111, gallium-67, or technetium-99 may show focal patchy or diffuse myocardial uptake indicative of myocardial inflammation, necrosis, or both.

4. Laboratory findings—In severe cases, mild elevation of myocardial isoenzymes, such as creatine phosphokinase-myocardial band (CPK-MB) or LDH_1 may be seen.

Treatment & Prognosis

Few data are available about the treatment of rheumatoid myocarditis. Few patients have shown benefit with high oral or IV doses of steroids in severe cases. The value of cytotoxics is undefined. Nonspecific therapy includes bed rest, analgesics, and cardiac monitoring for at least 48–72 h. The natural history and prognosis of rheumatoid myocarditis are unknown.

4. RHEUMATOID CORONARY ARTERY DISEASE

General Considerations

The prevalence of CAD in postmortem series of rheumatoid arthritis patients is about 20%. Of the two etiologic types, the most common is coronary atherosclerosis, probably accelerated by steroid therapy and recurrent episodes of coronary arteritis. The second—and rarely described form—is coronary arteritis itself. Patients with coronary arteritis generally have rheumatoid nodules, overt vasculitis, rapidly progressive rheumatoid disease, high titers of rheumatoid factor, and increased cardiovascular mortality.

Clinical Findings

The majority of rheumatoid arthritis patients with CAD are asymptomatic. Atherosclerotic coronary disease will manifest as chronic stable angina, unstable angina, or acute MI, whereas coronary arteritis is more commonly seen as unstable angina and, rarely, acute MI.

A. PHYSICAL EXAMINATION

Findings during acute ischemic syndromes include tachycardia, third or fourth heart sounds, and pulmonary rales if left ventricular failure is present.

B. DIAGNOSTIC STUDIES

1. Electrocardiography—ECG will show diagnostic Q waves indicative of previous MI, ST elevation or depression suggestive of epicardial or subendocardial ischemic injury, or T wave inversion suggestive of ischemia.

2. Echocardiography—During severe ischemia, echocardiography may show segmental wall motion abnormalities or myocardial scars if previous infarction has occurred. This technique will also determine the presence (or absence) of left ventricular dysfunction and its severity.

3. Other tests—Myocardial isoenzymes such as CPK-MB, troponin, and LDH_1 may be elevated if myocardial necrosis has occurred. Exercise treadmill testing, with or without radionuclide scanning or echocardiography, can be used to detect suspected CAD. Coronary angiography should be performed to confirm the diagnosis when there is a high suspicion of CAD or an abnormal exercise treadmill test and incapacitating symptoms. The diagnosis of coronary arteritis can be suspected if multiple stenotic lesions are found in the epicardial coronary arteries.

Treatment

Although experience in this area is limited, suspected severe and symptomatic coronary arteritis can initially be treated with high doses of steroids and cyclophosphamide in conjunction with heparin, aspirin, nitrates, and calcium channel or β-blockers. No data are available about percutaneous coronary angioplasty in coronary arteritis. Symptomatic coronary atherosclerosis should be treated medically or with coronary revascularization as appropriate.

5. CONDUCTION DISTURBANCES

General Considerations

The prevalence of AV or intraventricular conduction disturbances in patients with rheumatoid arthritis may not be different from that in age-matched controls in the general population. Possible mechanisms include acute inflammation of the AV node or His bundle (related to pancarditis), vasculitis of the arterioles supplying the conduction pathway, granulomata deposition in the conduction system, and amyloid infiltration.

Clinical Findings

A. PHYSICAL FINDINGS

The mean age of patients with conduction disturbances is generally more than 60 years, and the majority of these have severe forms with nodular disease, requiring steroid therapy. The conduction disturbances are generally mild, asymptomatic, and incidentally diagnosed by electrocardiography. In extremely rare cases, high-degree AV block may be evidenced with tiredness, dizziness, presyncope, or syncope. Although it is uncommon, complete AV block may be asymptomatic because the joint disease severely limits the patient's activity. Rarely, AV block is transient and can be reversed with antiinflammatory therapy.

B. DIAGNOSTIC STUDIES

The best diagnostic methods are routine electrocardiography, 24-h electrocardiographic monitoring, or both.

Treatment

The treatment of severe and symptomatic high-degree AV or intraventricular blocks associated with acute myocarditis or valvulitis consists of temporary pacing and high-dose steroids. Patients who are unresponsive to this therapy should receive permanent pacemakers.

6. RHEUMATOID PULMONARY HYPERTENSION

General Considerations

The possible causes of pulmonary hypertension with normal pulmonary venous pressure include serum hyperviscosity, interstitial fibrosis, obliterative bronchiolitis, and pulmonary vasculitis. The prevalence of these diseases is uncertain, but low. Severe pulmonary hypertension may lead to right ventricular hypertrophy, enlargement, and dysfunction (cor pulmonale) and produce the symptoms and signs of right heart failure.

Clinical Findings

Dyspnea is a common manifestation of pulmonary hypertension and cor pulmonale. However, moderate pulmonary hypertension not associated with cor pulmonale can be asymptomatic.

A. PHYSICAL FINDINGS

Findings include a parasternal heave, split second heart sound with loud pulmonic component, tricuspid regurgitation, right-sided S_3 gallop, and, rarely, hepatomegaly and edema.

B. DIAGNOSTIC STUDIES

1. Electrocardiography—ECG may show right atrial and ventricular enlargement and right bundle branch block.

2. Color-flow Doppler echocardiography—Color-flow Doppler may show right atrial and ventricular enlargement, hypertrophy or dysfunction, tricuspid regurgitation, and evidence of high pulmonary artery systolic pressure.

3. Open-lung biopsy and bronchoalveolar lavage—These methods should be done if severe pulmonary vasculitis or bronchiolitis obliterans is suspected as the cause of pulmonary hypertension.

Treatment & Prognosis

The treatment of pulmonary hypertension from pulmonary vasculitis is immunosuppressives or steroids, but the prognosis is poor, and most patients die within one year of diagnosis.

Guedes C, Bianchi-Fior P, Cormier B et al: Cardiac manifestations of rheumatoid arthritis: A case-control transesophageal echocardiography study in 30 patients. Arthritis Rheumatism 2001; 45:129.

Kvalvik AG, Jones MA, Symmons DP: Mortality in a cohort of Norwegian patients with rheumatoid arthritis followed from 1977 to 1992. Scand J Rheumatol 2000;29:29.

Nossent H: Risk of cardiovascular events and effect on mortality in patients with rheumatoid arthritis. J Rheumatol 2000;27: 2282.

Shimaya K, Kurihashi A, Masago R, Kasanuki H: Rheumatoid arthritis and simultaneous aortic, mitral, and tricuspid valve incompetence. Int J Cardiol 1999;71:181.

Wallberg-Jonsson S, Johansson H, Ohman ML, Rantapaa-Dahlqvist S: Extent of inflammation predicts cardiovascular disease and overall mortality in seropositive rheumatoid arthritis. A retrospective cohort study from disease onset. J Rheumatol 1999;26:2562.

Wallberg-Jonsson S, Cederfelt M, Rantapaa Dahlqvist S: Hemostatic factors and cardiovascular disease in active rheumatoid arthritis: An 8 year followup study. J Rheumatol 2000;27:71.

Wislowska M, Sypula S, Kowalik I: Echocardiographic findings and 24-h electrocardiographic Holter monitoring in patients with nodular and non-nodular rheumatoid arthritis. Rheumatol Int 1999;18:163.

SCLERODERMA

 ESSENTIALS OF DIAGNOSIS

- *Sclerotic skin, esophageal dysfunction, Raynaud's phenomenon*
- *Heart failure*
- *Multisegmental myocardial perfusion abnormalities*
- *Cor pulmonale*

General Considerations

Scleroderma, or systemic sclerosis, is a generalized disorder characterized by excessive accumulation of connective tissue; fibrosis; and degenerative changes of the skin, skeletal muscles, synovium, blood vessels, gastrointestinal tract, kidney, lung, and heart. Raynaud's phenomenon, esophageal dysfunction, and sclerotic skin characterize the disease and are present in more than 90% of patients. The two major clinical variants are diffuse cutaneous (20% of cases) and limited cutaneous disease (80%). The less common diffuse type is characterized by skin thickening of the distal and proximal extremities and the trunk, with frequent involvement of the kidney, lung, or heart. In the more common limited type, which includes the CREST syndrome (calcinosis, Raynaud's phenomenon, esophageal dysfunction, sclerodactyly, and telangiectasia), the skin changes are limited to the face, fingers, and distal portions of the extremities. A third, uncommon variant is the overlap syndrome that includes scleroderma in association with other connective tissue disease.

The incidence of scleroderma is 10–20 per million population per year. The disease affects all races, is three times more common in women than in men, and usually occurs between the ages of 30 and 50 years. The diffuse cutaneous type has a poorer prognosis than does the limited type. The overall cumulative survival rates after 3, 6, and 9 years are 86%, 76%, and 61%, respectively. The prognosis is worst for males who are older than 50 years with kidney, lung, or heart disease. Pulmonary disease, including pulmonary hypertension, and renal diseases are the major causes of mortality; these are followed by heart disease, with a cumulative survival of only 20% at 7 years. The major causes of cardiac death are ischemic heart disease, followed by refractory heart failure, sudden death, and pericarditis. Scleroderma cardiac disease manifests predominantly as CAD, myocarditis, and pulmonary hypertension with or without cor-pulmonale. Pericarditis, conduction disturbances, and arrhythmias are less common. Clinically overt scleroderma heart disease is reported in fewer than one fourth of patients; the rate rises to as high as 80% in autopsy series. Scleroderma heart disease is generally less frequent and less severe in the limited type than in the diffuse type.

1. CORONARY ARTERY DISEASE

Pathophysiology

Although the epicardial coronary arteries are usually normal, intramural coronary arteries and arterioles frequently show narrowing, fibrosis, fibrinoid necrosis, and intimal hypertrophy. Immune-mediated endothelial cell injury, stimulation of fibroblasts, collagen deposition, and increased production of platelet-derived growth factor may impair the endothelial responses to thrombosis, inflammation, and vasodilation. In addition, mast cell degranulation of vasoactive constituents such as histamine, prostaglandin D_2, and leukotrienes C_4 and D_4 may cause coronary vasospasm. The common finding on autopsy of myocardial contraction-band necrosis (necrotic myocardial cells with dense eosinophilic bands) is likely related to intermittent intramyocardial coronary spasm or intramyocardial Raynaud's phenomenon. Furthermore, almost all patients with evidence of intramyocardial CAD have peripheral Raynaud's phenomenon.

Clinical Findings

A. PRESENTATION

Chest pain is uncommon; when present, it is related more commonly to pericarditis or esophageal reflux than to myocardial ischemia. Most patients, even with resting or stress-induced myocardial perfusion imaging defects or wall motion abnormalities, are asymptomatic. Although intramyocardial coronary vasospasm is the rule, severe vasospasm of the epicardial coronary arteries leading to transmural MI has rarely been reported.

B. DIAGNOSTIC STUDIES

1. Electrocardiographic exercise testing—This method has limited sensitivity because the prevalence of epicardial CAD in patients with scleroderma is low.

2. Radionuclide studies—Resting or exercise-induced multisegmental perfusion abnormalities are common; they are frequently reversed or improved with nifedipine or dipyridamole, which suggests recurrent vasospastic episodes leading to myocardial ischemia or fibrosis. Cold-induced reversible or partially reversible myocardial perfusion defects detected during thallium-201 scintigraphy and corresponding segmental wall motion abnormalities observed on echocardiography further support coronary vasospasm. On exercise thallium-201 scintigraphy, the majority of patients show fixed defects and some show reversible defects or both fixed and reversible defects (Figure 33–4). Most patients have nor-

mal left ventricular function at rest despite the high frequency of perfusion defects, but almost half have an abnormal left ventricular response (a failure to increase the ejection fraction more than 5% from baseline) during exercise radionuclide ventriculography. Irreversible or partially reversible perfusion defects or corresponding wall motion abnormalities are consistent with MI with fibrosis and periinfarct ischemia, respectively.

3. Echocardiography—Findings typical for transmural MI are generally absent. Instead, patients usually present with left ventricular diastolic or global systolic dysfunction. Occasionally, a transmural MI due to epicardial coronary vasospasm can occur, and its echocardiographic diagnosis relies on the same findings as those of atherosclerotic disease. The cold pressor test with simultaneous echocardiography frequently demonstrates transient wall motion abnormalities.

4. Coronary angiography—Coronary angiography usually shows normal epicardial coronary arteries, a slow dye flow indicative of increased intramyocardial coronary resistance, and impaired coronary sinus blood flow indicative of abnormal coronary flow reserve.

Treatment

Although calcium channel blockers such as nifedipine and nicardipine have clearly demonstrated short-term improvement in the number and severity of perfusion defects, their long-term benefit is unknown. Captopril has shown similar beneficial effects.

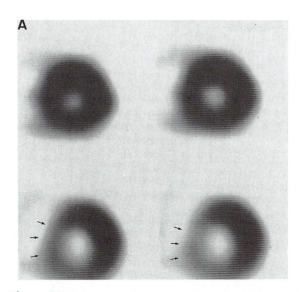 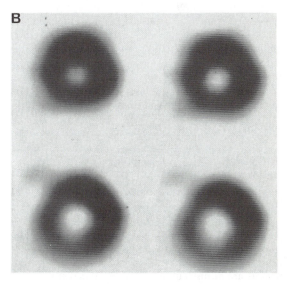

Figure 33-4. Intramural coronary artery disease in a patient with scleroderma. **A:** This short-axis postexercise perfusion scan of the left ventricle shows septal and inferoseptal wall ischemia (*small arrows*) that resolve on the resting images. **B:** This patient had normal epicardial coronary arteries.

2. MYOCARDITIS

General Considerations

Two types of scleroderma myocardial disease are described. The most common is due to recurrent intramyocardial ischemia leading to fibrosis; the second, rarely described and of unknown pathogenesis, is an acute inflammatory myocarditis. Recently, it has been demonstrated that scleroderma patients with active skeletal myopathy have up to a 21% prevalence of myocardial disease, compared with only 10% of those patients without peripheral myopathy. Myocardial disease is also more frequent and severe in scleroderma patients with diffuse cutaneous disease, anti-Scl70 antibodies, and older than 60 years.

Clinically apparent myocarditis is rare, but postmortem series report a high prevalence. Focal or diffuse myocardial fibrosis and contraction-band necrosis are common. Contraction-band necrosis typical of transient coronary occlusion and reperfusion is common but not pathognomonic. These pathologic findings differ from atherosclerotic myocardial disease by their lack of relation to coronary arteries and their frequent involvement of the right ventricle and subendocardium.

Clinical Findings

A. PHYSICAL EXAMINATION

Focal or diffuse myocardial fibrotic disease may result in significant left ventricular diastolic or systolic dysfunction, arrhythmias, and conduction disturbances. Patients with skeletal myopathy and those with myocarditis more commonly have clinical heart failure that is often intractable. Insidious symptoms of dyspnea, orthopnea, and peripheral edema are the most common symptoms; acute symptoms of heart failure and sudden death rarely occur. Physical examination may demonstrate cardiomegaly, S_3 or S_4 gallops, systolic murmurs, decreased-intensity heart sounds, pulmonary rales, and peripheral edema.

B. DIAGNOSTIC STUDIES

If clinical or laboratory evidence of myositis is present, diagnostic screening for asymptomatic cardiac involvement is warranted.

1. Electrocardiography—A septal infarction pattern is seen in some patients, correlating with septal or anteroseptal thallium perfusion abnormalities, despite the presence of normal epicardial coronary arteries. This presumably represents septal fibrosis.

2. Echocardiography—Preserved left ventricular systolic function is evident on the echocardiogram in the majority of patients. Regional or global left and, less commonly, right ventricular wall motion abnormalities

can be found and are more commonly seen in patients with clinically evident heart disease. Normal left ventricular systolic function with hypertrophy, left atrial enlargement, and abnormal mitral Doppler diastolic velocities in patients with symptoms of heart failure suggest the presence of diastolic dysfunction. Ultrasonic myocardial videodensitometry in patients younger than 50 years of age who are not hypertensive and not diabetic demonstrate low cyclic variation indexes that may represent primary myocardial fibrosis or microvascular disease rather than changes related to aging or hypertension.

3. Radionuclide studies—Radionuclide angiography demonstrate abnormal resting ejection fraction in 15% of patients. Myocardial perfusion scanning is a sensitive method for diagnosis and follow-up of the myocardial disease and for assessing therapeutic responses.

4. Endomyocardial biopsy—This technique has been used occasionally to diagnose scleroderma myocardial disease; however, the heterogenous and nonspecific pattern of involvement limit the sensitivity and specificity of this technique.

Treatment

Calcium channel blockers may abolish or decrease the frequency and severity of episodes of ischemia and thereby of myocardial fibrosis, but this hypothesis has not been longitudinally tested. When asymptomatic left ventricular systolic dysfunction is present, the treatment is nonspecific and consists of diuretics, digitalis, and vasodilators. The use of intravenous methylprednisolone in acute inflammatory myocarditis is controversial.

Prognosis

The presence of an S_3 gallop is indicative of left ventricular systolic dysfunction and increases the risk of death by more than 500%. Patients with heart failure have a 100% mortality rate at 7 years, with the highest number (82%) occurring during the first year after diagnosis.

3. CONDUCTION DISTURBANCES & ARRHYTHMIAS

General Considerations

Conduction defects occur in up to 20% of scleroderma patients; the highest prevalence is seen in those patients with demonstrated myocarditis or myocardial perfusion defects. Fibrous replacement of the sinoatrial (SA) and AV nodes, bundle branches, and surrounding myocardium is seen on postmortem series of patients with conduction disturbances.

Clinical Findings

A. PHYSICAL FINDINGS

Arrhythmias are common and frequently associated with active myocarditis. Atrial or ventricular premature contractions, supraventricular tachycardias, and nonsustained ventricular tachycardia are also common. Ventricular and supraventricular arrhythmias are more common in patients with diffuse cutaneous disease than in those with the limited type. Palpitations occur in 50% of patients. Syncope (Stokes-Adams attacks) can occur and is related to either high-degree AV block or ventricular arrhythmias; it may occasionally be the primary manifestation of scleroderma. Syncope can also occur in patients with severe pulmonary hypertension. From 40 to 67% of cardiac deaths in scleroderma patients who have active skeletal myopathy and myocarditis may be sudden and related to ventricular arrhythmias.

B. DIAGNOSTIC STUDIES

1. Electrocardiography—The majority of patients have a normal electrocardiogram (ECG), which is highly predictive of normal left ventricular function. The presence of left or right bundle branch block or bifascicular block generally correlates with resting or exercise-induced left ventricular systolic dysfunction. Also, left ventricular potentials on signal-averaged electrocardiography, complex atrial and ventricular arrhythmias, or conduction abnormalities on electrocardiography have been noticed with increased frequency. These findings correlate with left ventricular dysfunction or myocardial perfusion defects.

2. Electrophysiologic studies—EPS show a high prevalence of abnormal SA and AV nodes and His-Purkinje function and conduction. These studies, however, are recommended only for patients with syncope of undefined origin, for those with sustained ventricular tachycardia, or for survivors of sudden cardiac death.

Treatment

A pacemaker is indicated for symptomatic high-grade conduction disturbances, and antiarrhythmic therapy is appropriate for symptomatic arrhythmias. Whether suppression of arrhythmias reduces the risk of sudden cardiac death in scleroderma patients is unknown.

Prognosis

The presence on ambulatory ECG of frequent ventricular and supraventricular arrhythmias predicts a mortality risk two to six times higher than that of patients without arrhythmias. Because these arrhythmias are strong independent predictors of sudden cardiac death, 24-h ambulatory electrocardiographic monitoring should be performed in all patients with scleroderma to identify patients at high risk of sudden cardiac death. Cardiac conduction defects on the resting ECG also indicate a poor prognosis: the mortality rate is 50% by 6 years following diagnosis.

4. PERICARDITIS

General Considerations

The pathogenesis of scleroderma pericardial disease is unknown and is usually clinically silent. Acute symptomatic pericarditis is uncommon, in contrast to the high prevalence of pericardial disease in postmortem series. Fibrinous pericarditis, chronic fibrous pericarditis, pericardial adhesions, and pericardial effusion are the pathologic types described. Pericardial disease is more common in patients with the limited cutaneous form of the disease.

Clinical Findings

A. PRESENTATION

Clinically evident pericardial disease occurs in 5–15% of patients and more commonly in those with the limited cutaneous type. The most common clinical presentation is a chronic pericardial effusion with dyspnea, orthopnea, and edema; it is less frequently seen as an acute pericarditis with fever, pleuritic chest pain, dyspnea, and pericardial rub. Cardiac tamponade or chronic constrictive pericarditis is rare.

B. DIAGNOSTIC STUDIES

1. Echocardiography—Echocardiography commonly shows asymptomatic small pericardial effusions and thickening. It can also confirm clinically suspected cardiac tamponade.

2. Computed tomography and magnetic resonance imaging—CT and MRI are important diagnostic adjuncts to echocardiography. They aid in the further assessment of the presence of pericardial effusion and pericardial thickening or calcification in patients with suspected chronic constriction (Figure 33–5).

3. Other tests—Pericardial fluid aspirates are usually exudative without autoantibodies, immune complexes, or complement depletion. Antiphospholipid antibodies may be associated with pericardial disease.

Treatment

Symptomatic pericarditis or significant pericardial effusions can be treated with NSAIDs. If tamponade is suspected, pericardiocentesis or pericardiotomy is usually successful. Steroids are not effective in patients with large, chronic pericardial effusions.

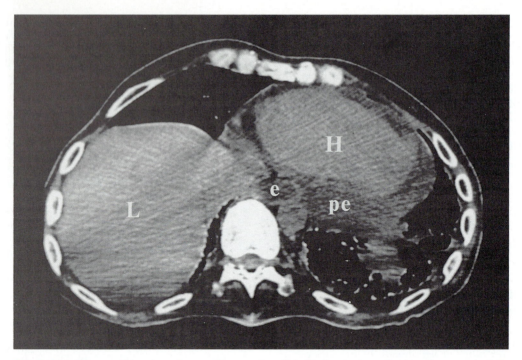

Figure 33-5. This CT scan of the chest shows a large pericardial effusion (pe) predominantly posteriorly located in a patient with scleroderma and pericarditis. No pericardial thickening or calcification was detected. Esophageal (e) dilatation is noted. H = heart; L = liver.

Prognosis

Patients with pericarditis and moderate pericardial effusion have a cumulative survival of only 25% after 6–7 years, with the highest mortality rates the first year after diagnosis. No clear explanation is available for this association, but it is believed to be related to complicating or accompanying progressive renal failure in patients with chronic pericardial effusions and to sudden death in those with associated acute myopericarditis or myocarditis.

5. VALVULAR HEART DISEASE

The true prevalence of this is unknown: it is rarely recognized clinically. Postmortem series report a prevalence of up to 18%. Systemic embolism in association with echocardiographically defined noninfective mitral valve vegetations, similar to those of SLE, has been described. One echocardiographic series reported a 67% frequency of mitral regurgitation in scleroderma patients, compared with only 15% in controls. Nonspecific thickening of the mitral or aortic valves without significant regurgitation also can be seen. In addition, a disproportionately high clinical and echocardiographic prevalence of mitral valve prolapse has been described in patients with either diffuse or limited scleroderma.

6. SECONDARY SCLERODERMA HEART DISEASE

Secondary causes of scleroderma heart disease are related to pulmonary and systemic hypertension. Pulmonary fibrosis can occur in up to 80% and pulmonary hypertension with cor pulmonale in up to 40–50% of patients. Pulmonary hypertension secondary to inflammatory vasculopathy or pulmonary vasospasm is less common and more commonly associated with the limited cutaneous type and overlap syndrome. Abnormal pulmonary function tests, abnormal lung uptake of gallium and technetium-99m Sestamibi, and radiographic abnormalities often precede cor pulmonale on echocardiography. Pulmonary hypertension is associated with a 50% mortality at 8 years. Oxygen, calcium channel blockers, and ACE inhibitors have provided long-term benefits. Selected patients with severe scleroderma related lung disease can undergo lung transplantation with similar morbidity and mortality to that of patients without scleroderma. Hypertension and hypertensive heart disease are generally related to renovascular disease. The prognosis is related to the severity of the heart disease.

Banci M, Rinaldi E, Ierardi M et al: 99mTc SESTAMIBI scintigraphic evaluation of skeletal muscle disease in patients with systemic sclerosis: Diagnostic reliability and comparison with cardiac function and perfusion. Angiology 1998;49:641.

Byers RJ, Marshall DA, Freemont AJ: Pericardial involvement in systemic sclerosis. Ann Rheum Dis 1997;56:393.

Ferri C, Di Bello, Martini A et al: Heart involvement in systemic sclerosis: An ultrasonic tissue characterisation study. Ann Rheum Dis 1998;57:296.

Handa R, Gupta K, Malhotra A et al: Cardiac involvement in limited systemic sclerosis: Non-invasive assessment in asymptomatic patients. Clin Rheumatol 1999;18:136.

Hata N, Kunimi T, Matsuda H et al: Cardiac disorders associated with progressive systemic sclerosis. J Cardiol 1998;32:397.

Morelli S, Sgreccia A, De Marzio P et al: Noninvasive assessment of myocardial involvement in patients with systemic sclerosis: Role of signal averaged electrocardiography. J Rheumatol 1997;24:2358.

Murata I, Takenaka K, Shinohara S et al: Diversity of myocardial involvement in systemic sclerosis: An 8-year study of 95 Japanese patients. Am Heart J 1998;135:960.

ANKYLOSING SPONDYLITIS

ESSENTIALS OF DIAGNOSIS

- *Characteristic lumbar spine and sacroiliac arthritis*
- *Positive HLA-B27 assay*
- *Aortic root sclerosis and dilation, leaflet thickening, and subaortic bump on echocardiography*
- *Aortic regurgitation*

General Considerations

Ankylosing spondylitis, also known as Marie-Strümpell, or Bekhterev's disease, is an inflammatory disorder of unknown origin that affects predominantly the vertebral and sacroiliac joints. It manifests itself as chronic low back pain and limitation of back motion and chest expansion. Less frequently, it affects the peripheral joints and extraarticular organs such as the heart. The disease is estimated to affect 1 in 2000 of the general population, predominantly white men less than 40 years old; the male-to-female ratio is 3–12:1. More than 90% of patients are characteristically positive for the histocompatibility antigen HLA-B27. Although the manifestations of the cardiovascular disease generally follow the arthritic syndrome by 10–20 years, they sometimes precede it. The most important cardiovascular manifestations of the disease are aortitis, with or without aortic regurgitation; conduction disturbances; mitral regurgitation; myocardial dysfunction; and pericardial disease. The clinical prevalence of cardiovascular disease in ankylosing spondylitis varies widely. The rates are higher in patients with more than 20 years of disease duration, in those who are older than age 50, and in those with peripheral articular involvement.

1. AORTITIS & AORTIC REGURGITATION

General Considerations

The pathogenesis of aortitis is unknown. Increased platelet-aggregating activity and platelet-derived growth factor are believed to be pathogenetic factors in the characteristic proliferative endarteritis of aortic root disease. The inflammatory process also is mediated by plasma cells and lymphocytes. It occurs in the intima, media, and adventitia of the proximal aortic wall and sinus of Valsalva and results in a marked fibroblastic reparative response, fibrous thickening, and calcification, especially of the adventitia and intima. This process extends proximally to the aortic annulus, valve cusps, and adjacent commissures. The consequent dilatation and thickening of the aortic root and annulus and the thickening or retraction of the aortic valve cusps cause aortic regurgitation generally of mild to moderate degree. Severe aortic regurgitation is rare. The mitral valve is frequently involved by downward extension of the aortic root fibrosis into the intervalvular fibrosa and base of the anterior mitral leaflet. This often results in localized fibrotic thickening at the base of the anterior mitral leaflet forming the characteristic "subaortic bump."

Clinical Findings

The most common and characteristic manifestation of ankylosing-spondylitis-associated heart disease is proximal aortitis, with or without aortic regurgitation. Associated mitral valve disease is also common. Aortitis and aortic regurgitation are generally mild to moderate, clinically silent, and chronic. In rare cases, severe aortic regurgitation from severe acute or chronic aortitis or valvulitis or complicating infective endocarditis occurs. It should be noted that clinically silent aortic root or valve disease, with or without aortic regurgitation, can be present in one third of patients before the joint disease manifests itself. Although it happens rarely, severe aortic regurgitation may present with mild or no articular disease.

A. PHYSICAL EXAMINATION

The most common and salient clinical findings in patients with ankylosing spondylitis will be those of the articular disease because cardiac disease when present is generally mild to moderate and asymptomatic. Although aortic root disease and valve regurgitation may be shown by echocardiography in up to 60% of patients, because it is generally mild to moderate, it is clinically detected in few of them.

B. DIAGNOSTIC STUDIES

1. Chest radiography—The appearance of the cardiac silhouette and great vessels is usually normal. If severe aortic root disease or aortic regurgitation is present, the ascending aorta may appear dilatated or elongated, and left ventricular and atrial enlargement may be noted.

2. Color-flow Doppler echocardiography—By TEE, aortic root thickening, increased stiffness and dilatation is seen in 60%, 60%, and 25% of patients, respectively. Aortic valve thickening detected in 40% of patients is manifested mainly as nodularities of the aortic cusps. Mitral valve thickening seen in 30% of patients manifests predominantly as basal thickening of the anterior mitral leaflet, forming the characteristic "subaortic bump" (Figure 33–6). Valve regurgitation seen in almost 50% of patients is moderate in one third of them. Aortic root disease and valve disease is related to the duration of ankylosing spondylitis but not to its activity, severity or therapy. The presence of left ventricular enlargement, hypertrophy, and systolic or diastolic function can also be assessed by this method.

3. Radionuclide ventriculography—This method can assess left ventricular systolic or diastolic function, left ventricular enlargement, and aortic or mitral regurgitant fractions.

Treatment

A. MEDICAL THERAPY

1. Specific antiinflammatory therapy—No data are available regarding the role of corticosteroids in the aortic root and valve disease associated with ankylosing spondylitis.

2. Other therapy—Diuretics and vasodilators can be used in patients with significant aortic regurgitation. Antibiotic prophylaxis for infective endocarditis is indicated if aortic valve disease with regurgitation is present.

B. SURGICAL THERAPY

Aortic valve replacement has been successfully performed in patients with severe and symptomatic aortic regurgitation.

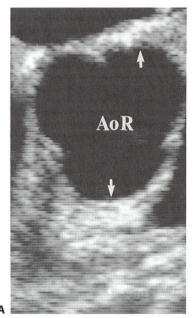

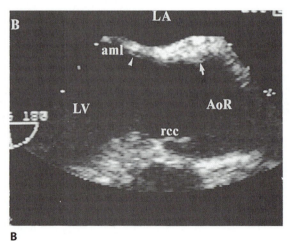

Figure 33-6. Aortic root and valve disease in a patient with ankylosing spondylitis. **A:** This transesophageal basilar short-axis view shows marked aortic root thickening, predominantly of the posterolateral and anteromedial walls (*arrows*). Mild aortic root dilation is present. **B:** Transesophageal basilar longitudinal close-up view of the aortic root also shows the marked thickening of the posterior wall (*arrow*) extending to the basilar portion of the anterior mitral leaflet (subaortic bump; *arrowhead*). Mild localized thickening of the right coronary cusp tip is noted. Moderately severe aortic regurgitation was detected on color-flow mapping. The distance between the dots at the edge of the image is 1 cm. aml = anterior mitral leaflet; AoR = aortic root; LA = left atrium; LV = left ventricle; rcc = right coronary cusp.

2. CONDUCTION DISTURBANCES

Conduction disturbances are the second most common characteristic of ankylosing-spondylitis-associated heart disease, although their pathogenesis is unknown. Although the prevalence of HLA-B27 is increased in patients with ankylosing spondylitis who have implanted pacemakers for heart block, it may be absent in these patients. Furthermore, because HLA-B27 may be present in 6% of normal patients, it cannot be implicated as a primary pathogenetic factor in ankylosing-spondylitis-associated conduction disturbances. Conduction disturbances can be the result of the subaortic fibrotic process extending to the basilar septum, leading to destruction or dysfunction of the atrioventricular node, the proximal portion of the bundle of His, bundle branches, and fascicles. In fact, echocardiographic studies have demonstrated an association of conduction disturbances with aortic root thickening and subaortic bump.

Clinical Findings

The prevalence of conduction disturbances varies greatly, but is at least 20%. Atrioventricular blocks (first, second and, rarely, third degree) are most frequent, followed by sinus node dysfunction (sinus arrhythmias, sinoatrial block, sinus arrest, and sick sinus syndrome) and bundle branch or fascicular block.

In terms of aortic disease, patients with conduction disturbances are generally asymptomatic and can be detected before clinically manifested in fewer than one fifth of patients. The conduction disturbances can occasionally be transient, and symptomatic patients can be treated with temporary pacing. The prevalence of aortic root disease and valve regurgitation is high in the presence of conduction disturbances, in contrast to the small number of cases of aortic regurgitation in patients without conduction disturbances. Occasionally, severe conduction disturbances that are associated with symptoms of dizziness, presyncope, or syncope and require cardiac pacing may precede the diagnosis of ankylosing spondylitis. Therefore, unrecognized ankylosing spondylitis should be considered in patients with unexplained conduction disturbances or aortic regurgitation.

A. PHYSICAL EXAMINATION

Severe bradyarrhythmias will be clinically detected if patients are symptomatic; otherwise, conduction disturbances are generally incidentally detected with electrocardiography.

B. DIAGNOSTIC STUDIES

Electrocardiography, including 24-h ambulatory monitoring, can easily detect the presence of previously described conduction disturbances.

Treatment

A. SPECIFIC ANTIINFLAMMATORY THERAPY

Antiinflammatory therapy has not proved beneficial in patients with conduction disturbances.

B. OTHER THERAPY

Permanent pacing has been successfully performed. The most common indications for pacing are complete heart block and sick sinus syndrome.

3. MITRAL VALVE DISEASE

The prevalence of mitral valve disease is about 30%, but it is generally not significant and therefore frequently unrecognized. Mitral valve disease is generally asymptomatic and frequently incidentally detected by echocardiography. The pathogenesis of mitral valve disease is related to the extension of the aortic root fibrosis into the subaortic basilar portion of the anterior mitral leaflet, producing the characteristic subaortic bump. Mitral regurgitation results from either the decreased anterior leaflet mobility caused by the basilar subaortic bump or, less frequently, from ventricular dilatation caused by aortic regurgitation. Only few cases of mitral regurgitation severe enough to require valve replacement have been reported. Except for antibiotic prophylaxis for infective endocarditis in patients with evidence of mitral regurgitation, no other therapy is currently recommended.

4. MYOCARDIAL DISEASE, PERICARDIAL DISEASE, & BACTERIAL ENDOCARDITIS

Primary myocardial disease is rare. Although its pathogenesis is unknown, it is caused by a diffuse increase in the myocardial interstitial connective tissue and reticulum fibers. It may manifest as left ventricular systolic dysfunction and dilatation in up to one fifth of patients. Abnormal left ventricular diastolic function assessed by Doppler echocardiography and radionuclide ventriculography has been reported in as many as 50% of patients. Diastolic dysfunction is unrelated to age, disease duration, or disease activity. Secondary myocardial dysfunction relates to chronic volume overload of aortic or mitral regurgitation. If significant left ventricular systolic or diastolic dysfunction is present, third or fourth heart sounds and pulmonary rales may be present. Echocardiography is the best diagnostic method to show primary or secondary left ventricular dysfunction. No specific therapy is available for primary myocardial disease.

Although the true prevalence of **pericardial disease** is unknown, it is rare in ankylosing spondylitis, and its pathogenesis is also obscure. It is generally asymptomatic and not hemodynamically significant. It is usually incidentally detected by echocardiography as pericardial thickening or small pericardial effusions. No specific therapy is available. **Bacterial endocarditis** as a complication of primary aortic or mitral valve disease and cor pulmonale secondary to pulmonary fibrosis has been described rarely.

Prognosis

The overall prognosis of patients with ankylosing spondylitis is good and almost comparable to that of a general population. In the past, the presence of severe cardiovascular disease significantly decreased the survival of these patients. Currently, improved diagnostic technologies, pharmacotherapy, and surgical and pacing techniques have allowed early diagnosis, appropriate follow-up, and proper timing of valve replacement or pacemaker implantation in patients with cardiovascular disease. These factors have made the prognosis of ankylosing spondylitis with cardiovascular disease more benign.

Angulo J, Espinoza LR: The spectrum of skin, mucosa, and other extra-articular manifestations. Baillieres Clin Rheumatol 1998;12:649.

Crowley JJ, Donnelly SM, Tobin M et al: Doppler echocardiographic evidence of left ventricular diastolic dysfunction in ankylosing spondylitis. Am J Cardiol 1993;71:1337.

Roldan CA, Chavez J, Weist P et al: Aortic root disease and valve disease associated with ankylosing spondylitis. J Am Coll Cardiol 1998;32:1397.

POLYMYOSITIS/DERMATOMYOSITIS

ESSENTIALS OF DIAGNOSIS

- *Muscle weakness, characteristic skin lesions*
- *Arrhythmias or conduction disturbances and myocarditis*
- *Pericarditis, coronary arteritis, valve disease*

General Considerations

Polymyositis or dermatomyositis is an acquired, chronic, inflammatory myopathy of unknown cause that presents clinically as symmetric proximal muscle weakness of the extremities, trunk, and neck. Dermatomyositis differs from polymyositis by the presence of a rash on the face, neck, chest and extremities, most commonly over the extensor surfaces, especially the dorsum of the hands and fingers. The incidence of polymyositis and dermatomyositis is estimated to be one to five new

cases per million population per year in the United States. Overlap syndrome is the association of polymyositis/dermatomyositis with other connective tissue diseases such as scleroderma, systemic lupus erythematosus, and rheumatoid arthritis. Rarely, polymyositis or dermatomyositis can be associated with the antiphospholipid antibody syndrome. Adults in the fourth to sixth decades are most commonly affected. Both childhood polymyositis/dermatomyositis and that with malignancy are less common. Females, especially black females, are predominantly affected. A cumulative survival rate of one half to three fourths after 6–8 years has been reported. The major causes of mortality (in descending order) are malignancy, sepsis, and cardiovascular disease. Poor prognostic indicators of the disease include an age older than 45 years, cardiopulmonary disease, and cutaneous necrotic lesions.

Clinical Findings

A. PHYSICAL FINDINGS

Polymyositis/dermatomyositis-associated heart disease is not uncommon and is manifested predominantly as arrhythmias or conduction disturbances and myocarditis. Dilated cardiomyopathy, pericarditis, coronary vasculitis, pulmonary hypertension with cor pulmonale, mitral valve prolapse, and hyperkinetic heart syndrome have also been reported. Clinically overt heart disease is less common than that found in postmortem series. Clinical heart disease is more common in polymyositis and overlap syndrome than in dermatomyositis or in malignant and childhood polymyositis/dermatomyositis. The presence of heart disease does not correlate with age, disease activity, severity, or duration and does not differ between men and women.

1. ARRHYTHMIAS & CONDUCTION DISTURBANCES

Nonspecific ST segment and T wave abnormalities are present in as many as half of patients. Other disorders include right bundle branch block, left anterior fascicular block, bifascicular blocks, nonspecific intraventricular conduction delay, left bundle branch block, first-degree AV block, and high-degree AV block. Occasionally, conduction disturbances can progress to more severe forms, despite remission of the disease, and permanent pacing has been required in a few cases.

The prevalence of arrhythmias varies. The most common arrhythmias are premature ventricular and atrial beats. Supraventricular tachyarrhythmias and ventricular tachycardia are rare. Sudden cardiac death may occur in a small number of patients. Active myocarditis or residual myocardial degeneration and fibrosis extending to the sinoatrial, AV nodal, and bundle branches explain the arrhythmias and conduction abnormalities.

2. MYOCARDITIS

Myocarditis is characterized at postmortem by diffuse interstitial and perivascular lymphocytic infiltration, contraction-band necrosis, and fibrosis. In one postmortem series, myocarditis was seen in half the patients, manifested equally as active myocarditis or focal myocardial fibrosis. Approximately 10–20% of them have dilated cardiomyopathy. Acute myocarditis as the principal manifestation of polymyositis has been reported in only two cases, one case mimicking acute MI, and the second case leading to fatal cardiac arrhythmias. A high correlation has been demonstrated between myocarditis and active myositis. About half of patients with peripheral myositis, as indicated by uptake of technetium-99m pyrophosphate, also have myocardial uptake. Increased myocardial uptake is also frequently associated with depressed ejection fraction and abnormal wall motion (shown by radionuclide ventriculography), which is further supportive of myocardial inflammation. Myocarditis may manifest itself clinically as congestive heart failure or as dilated cardiomyopathy.

3. CORONARY ARTERITIS

The clinical prevalence is unknown. One postmortem series demonstrated the presence of coronary arteritis in 30% of patients, manifested as active vasculitis with intimal proliferation or as medial necrosis with calcification. A history of MI has been reported.

4. VALVULAR HEART DISEASE

Except for a higher prevalence of mitral valve prolapse in more than half of patients, no other specific valve disease has been reported. The cause of mitral prolapse has not been determined.

5. PERICARDITIS

Acute uncomplicated pericarditis with small-to-moderate pericardial effusions has been described; acute pericarditis with cardiac tamponade and chronic constrictive pericarditis have rarely been reported. Pericarditis affects fewer than 20% of adults and slightly more than that in children. Echocardiography, however, shows a prevalence of pericardial effusion, usually small, in up to 25% in adults and up to 50% in children. One large series reported a higher prevalence of pericarditis in overlap syndrome than in isolated polymyositis or dermatomyositis. Only rarely does pericarditis form part of the initial clinical presentation of polymyositis/dermatomyositis. Cardiac tamponade and constriction are rare.

6. PULMONARY HYPERTENSION, COR PULMONALE, & HYPERKINETIC HEART SYNDROME

Both pulmonary hypertension secondary to interstitial lung disease and primary pulmonary vasculopathy leading to cor pulmonale have been found. In hyperkinetic heart syndrome, abnormally increased left ventricular performance, determined by increased mean velocity of circumferential fiber shortening and fractional shortening has been demonstrated in up to one third of patients with polymyositis. The cause of this asymptomatic abnormality is unknown.

Treatment & Prognosis

Corticosteroid therapy to treat the inflammatory myopathy has not shown a beneficial effect in patients with conduction disturbances, myocarditis, or pericarditis. Available data are limited about the natural history, effect of therapy, and prognosis in polymyositis/dermatomyositis-associated heart disease.

Spiera R, Kagen L: Extramuscular manifestations in idiopathic inflammatory myopathies. Curr Opin Rheumatol 1998;10: 556–561.

MIXED CONNECTIVE TISSUE DISEASE

 ESSENTIALS OF DIAGNOSIS

- Raynaud's phenomenon, sclerodactyly
- Myopathy with high titers of ribonucleoprotein antibodies
- Pericarditis, pulmonary hypertension
- High RNP antibody titers

General Considerations

Patients with mixed connective tissue disease are those with clinical findings of SLE, rheumatoid arthritis, scleroderma, and polymyositis. Characteristically, these patients have high titers of antibodies to nuclear ribonucleoprotein (RNP) and speckled antinuclear antibodies. Rheumatoid agglutinins also occur in more than half of patients. The disease occurs at all ages, affecting predominantly females (80%). Its prevalence is similar to that of scleroderma—more common than polymyositis but less than SLE. This disease has no particular racial or ethnic predominance. Primary cardiac involvement in mixed connective tissue disease is infrequent and less common than in other connective tissue diseases.

Clinical Findings

A. Physical Findings

Pericardial disease manifested as pericarditis, small pericardial effusions, or pericardial thickening is the most common. Pericarditis is more common in children, affecting almost half of patients. In rare cases, pericarditis is the initial presentation of the disease. Mitral valve prolapse has also been reported in this disease, with an unusually high prevalence (32%). Verrucous thickening of the mitral valve and regurgitation have been infrequently detected and are indistinguishable from those of SLE. Infrequently, supraventricular or ventricular arrhythmias and conduction disturbances have been reported. Although intimal hyperplasia of coronary arteries and perivascular and myocardial leukocytic infiltration have been described on postmortem examination, clinical coronary arteritis or myocarditis is rare. One case of fatal myocarditis complicated by congestive heart failure has been reported. Because of the high frequency of pulmonary disease (80%) in patients with mixed connective tissue disease, pulmonary hypertension associated with pulmonary fibrosis or proliferative pulmonary vasculopathy of the small and medium-sized pulmonary arteries can occur, especially in patients with features of scleroderma.

The clinical manifestations of primary cardiac disease, pulmonary hypertension, and cor pulmonale associated with mixed connective tissue disease do not differ from the other connective tissue diseases.

B. Diagnostic Studies

The methods used to diagnose cardiac disease associated with mixed connective tissue disease are the same used for other connective tissue diseases.

Treatment

Little data are available about the treatment of heart disease associated with mixed connective tissue disease. Pericarditis generally responds well to corticosteroids. Nifedipine, 30 mg/day, has demonstrated both acute and sustained reduction in pulmonary vascular resistance in patients with pulmonary hypertension.

Prognosis

The overall mortality rate of patients with mixed connective tissue disease is 13% at 6–12 years. The prognostic implications of cardiac disease associated with mixed connective tissue disease are unknown.

Alpert MA et al: Acute and long-term effects of nifedipine on pulmonary and systemic hemodynamics in patients with pulmonary hypertension associated with diffuse systemic sclerosis, the CREST syndrome and mixed connective tissue disease. Am J Cardiol 1991;68:1687.

Beier JM, Nielsen HL, Nielsen D: Pleuritis-pericarditis: An unusual initial manifestation of mixed connective tissue disease. Euro Heart J 1992;13:859.

Suzuki M, Hamada M, Sekiya M et al: Fatal pulmonary hypertension in a patient with mixed connective tissue disease: Report of an autopsy case. Intern Med 1992;31:74.

The Athlete's Heart

34

J. V. Nixon, MD

ESSENTIALS OF DIAGNOSIS

- *History of athletic training and performance*
- *Enhanced exercise ability (VO₂ max > 40 mL/kg/min)*
- *Resting bradycardia*
- *Increased left ventricular mass by echocardiography*

General Considerations

The concept of the athlete's heart is one that has been postulated for almost 100 years, promulgating the idea that myocardial hypertrophy could be a purely physiologic phenomenon. Although the concept has been relatively slow to gain acceptance, recent media attention to the sudden deaths of widely known athletes has helped to refocus attention on the important distinction between pathologic cardiac hypertrophy and physiologic hypertrophy and the upper limits of the latter.

The adaptations of the human body to physical training involve (but are not confined to) the cardiovascular system. The exercise-related changes in other organ systems influence the cardiovascular response to exercise. It is important for the physician to be familiar with the physiologic responses to physical training in order to distinguish them from similar changes that can occur with cardiovascular disease.

Different forms of exercise produce a number of physiologic responses, and cardiovascular responses to acute training and prolonged training differ. Exercise generally takes two basic physiologic forms—dynamic and static, or isometric, exercise—although most athletic activities are a variable combination of them. Dynamic exercise constitutes an alteration in the length of skeletal muscle with comparatively little change in muscle tension. Static exercise is essentially the reverse—that is, a marked alteration in skeletal muscle tension with little or no change in muscle length. Distance running is a classic example of dynamic exercise; weight lifting is a classic example of static exercise.

The morphologic and physiologic consequences of dynamic and isometric exercise are significant and may simulate changes associated with cardiac disease. The normal limits of changes that are due to athletic conditioning require careful identification. Awareness of these limits improves the physician's ability to determine the end-points at which normal anatomy and physiology become clinical disease.

Physiology of Exercise Training

The acute cardiovascular responses to exercise are specific and vary with different forms of exercise. There are also specific adaptive responses to exercise, particularly to dynamic exercise. In particular, the adaptive change in heart rate from an alteration in vagal parasympathetic tone defines the normal physiologic range; as noted earlier, this may be initially misinterpreted as representative of cardiovascular disease. (A classic example is the resting heart rate of 22 bpm of the winner of the 1993 Tour de France bicycle race.)

A. ACUTE RESPONSES TO EXERCISE

1. Dynamic exercise—Several acute cardiovascular responses to dynamic exercise are typical (Figure 34–1). As would be anticipated in meeting the demands of aerobic exercise, oxygen consumption increases because of an increase in both cardiac output and the arteriovenous oxygen difference. The increase in arteriovenous oxygen difference results from an increase in the oxygen extraction, or demand, by the exercising skeletal muscle and the increase in muscular capillary blood flow. Oxygen consumption is linearly related to the workload achieved during dynamic exercise. Maximal oxygen consumption (VO₂max) is a highly reproducible measure of aerobic capacity and thus dynamic exercise performance. Aerobic capacity varies with training, lean body mass, age, and gender and is significantly influenced by the individual's genetic characteristics. In children, gender differences are seen only after puberty, when the aerobic capacity of girls and young women tends to be approximately 30% less than that of boys and young men of the same age. Although incompletely explained, these differences are felt to be multi-

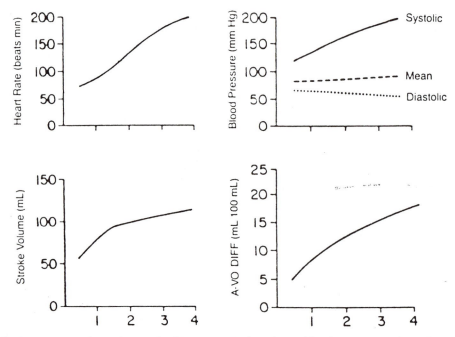

Figure 34–1. Responses to dynamic exercise: Heart rate, stroke volume, blood pressure, and arteriovenous oxygen difference in relation to VO₂ (oxygen uptake) during dynamic exercise. Reprinted, with permission, from Crawford MH: Physiologic consequences of systematic training. Cardiovasc Clin 1992;10:209.

factorial; females, for example, have a lower lean body mass and a lower hemoglobin level. Maximal oxygen consumption (VO$_2$max) diminishes with increasing age, as a result of such factors as the gradual detraining effect of age, an alteration in cardiac stiffness, and a reduction in β-adrenergic responsiveness that produces an attenuated heart rate response to exercise. Although it may be improved by dynamic training in older individuals, this improvement may well be due to an increased arteriovenous oxygen difference as much as to an increase in cardiac output and stroke volume. Furthermore, the improvement in VO$_2$max is relative when the overall decline in fitness is taken into account.

Oxygen consumption is also linearly related to cardiac output during dynamic exercise. The increase in cardiac output results principally from an increase in heart rate. Some increase in stroke volume takes place, resulting from the increase in venous return produced by the increasing skeletal muscle activity. The increase in left ventricular stroke volume during dynamic exercise is larger in an upright than in a supine posture, but the absolute stroke volume at peak exercise is greatest in the supine position. Other hemodynamic responses contribute to the increased stroke volume. Intrathoracic pressure is reduced, left ventricular filling pressure rises, the mitral valve orifice enlarges, and the left ventricular

end-diastolic volume increases. The net effect of these changes is activation of the Frank-Starling mechanism during the early initial and lower levels of dynamic exercise. Subsequently, at higher levels of exercise, sympathetic activation augments the Frank-Starling response in increasing stroke volume by increasing myocardial contractility and reducing end-systolic volume.

Resting heart rate is determined by vagal tone coupled with the level of sympathetic reflex activation. In the upright (versus supine) position, for example, resting heart rate is higher because of a mildly increased level of sympathetic activation. The initial increase in heart rate during exercise is due to a reduction in vagal tone, a central nervous system response mediated by stimulation of mechanoreceptors in the activated skeletal muscles. The heart rate increase is subsequently maintained by sympathetic activity and increased circulating catecholamines.

Systolic blood pressure increases during dynamic exercise, with a minimal increase in either diastolic or mean arterial pressure. The magnitude of the responses is determined by the size of the activated muscle mass. Thus, the response during large muscle or leg exercise is greater than during small muscle or arm exercise. There is a greater increase in pulmonary arterial pressure than in systemic pressure during exercise because the change in vascular resistance is less in the pulmonary vasculature. This relative increase in pulmonary pressures is believed to augment pulmonary oxygen transport during exercise.

2. Static exercise—In static exercise, intramuscular pressure increases dramatically, with a resultant reduction or obliteration of exercising skeletal muscle blood flow (Figure 34–2). Static exercise is sustained by anaerobic mechanisms, and the consequent increases in oxygen consumption and cardiac output are much less than during dynamic exercise. Furthermore, oxygen consumption and cardiac output increase after static exercise, presumably because of an immediate increase in blood flow to the involved muscles to rectify the oxygen debt acquired by anaerobic mechanisms during the static exercise.

The increase in cardiac output during static exercise is due mainly to the increase in heart rate; stroke volume remains almost unchanged. Systolic blood pressure increases significantly during static exercise. Because stroke volumes and systemic vascular resistance change only minimally, this increased arterial pressure

is due to the effects of increased muscle contraction on arterial pressure waves. Although arteriovenous oxygen difference remains unchanged during static exercise, an increase does take place immediately following release as a result of increased blood flow to the muscle bed.

B. EFFECTS OF SYSTEMATIC EXERCISE TRAINING

As previously stated, VO_2max is an accurate and reproducible measure of aerobic capacity and thus becomes an objective measure of dynamic fitness. In normal men, VO_2max ranges from 25 to 40 mL/kg/min, with the lower values occurring in the older individuals. More than 50 mL/kg/min is considered representative of an elite level of fitness (the level may go as high as 80 mL/kg/min), reflecting an increase in maximal cardiac output and arteriovenous oxygen difference.

1. Dynamic exercise training—This type of training decreases resting heart rate because of an adaptive increase in vagal tone; it also decreases the heart rate response at any level of exercise. The heart rate response

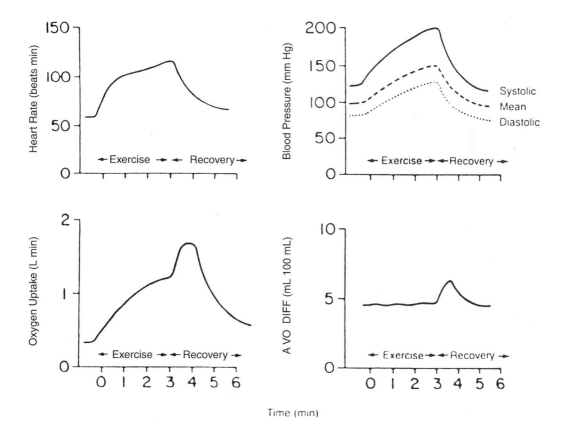

Figure 34–2. Responses to static, or isometric, exercise: Heart rate, oxygen uptake, blood pressure and arteriovenous oxygen differences during isometric exercise and recovery. Reprinted, with permission, from Crawford MH: *Physiologic consequences of systematic training. Cardiovasc Clin* 1992;10:209.

to maximal exercise, however, is identical in both the trained and untrained individual. Therefore, the increase in maximum cardiac output associated with dynamic training is due to increased stroke volume. It should also be noted that these physiologic adaptive changes to dynamic training occur in association with morphologic and physiologic changes in the heart.

2. Static exercise training—This type of training does not produce the same degree of VO_2max as does dynamic training. It is probable that the use of anaerobic rather than aerobic mechanisms to generate muscle energy requires a lower increase in cardiac output. Although morphologic changes do occur, the hemodynamic response to static exercise is similar in trained and untrained individuals.

3. Cross training—Dynamic training improves the response to static exercise in that the increased stroke volume at a lower heart rate allows the subject to sustain a greater cardiac pressure load and thus improve isometric performance. Static exercise training does not improve dynamic performance, however, except in areas or activities where greater strength or power is required (eg, pole vaulting).

4. Cardiovascular response—The frequency, intensity, and duration of exercise all affect the cardiovascular response. To obtain a significant training effect requires 30 min of dynamic exercise at 60–80% of maximal VO_2 three times per week. Little effect is seen unless rates of more than 130 bpm are achieved for prolonged periods. Although lower levels and less frequent episodes of training may create a training effect, cessation of exercise produces a rapid detraining effect—which is complete within 3 weeks.

Measurement of the heart rate provides a good index of training. As discussed earlier, the alteration in resting heart rate is said to be due to an increase in vagal parasympathetic tone rather than a decrease in sympathetic tone or lower circulating catecholamine levels. In trained athletes, circulating levels of both epinephrine and norepinephrine are lower during dynamic and static exercise, with a lower heart rate response to the relative intensity of both forms of exercise.

Systematic training has some effects on other organ systems. Total blood and plasma volumes increase with dynamic training; these changes are thought to be related to increases in renin activity and serum albumin levels. Higher hemoglobin levels lead to an increase in both maximal oxygen consumption and endurance. Well-trained athletes use oxygen more efficiently, and the vascular conductance of skeletal muscle changes, resulting in a greater arteriovenous oxygen difference during dynamic exercise. Dynamic exercise training also increases high-density lipoprotein levels and decreases low-density lipoprotein and very-low-density lipoprotein levels, as well as body weight.

C. Morphologic Responses to Training

Physiologic hypertrophy is a prominent feature of the athlete's heart. The morphologic adaptations to the increased stroke volume induced by exercise conform to the principles of Laplace's law, which relates the wall tension to intracavitary size and pressure. The increase in wall thickness in the setting of volume and pressure overload tends to normalize wall stress in both dynamic and isometric exercise.

The advent of two-dimensional and Doppler echocardiography and radionuclide ventriculography has stimulated attempts to assess the mechanics of systolic and diastolic function in the trained athlete. The value of these technologies, although substantial, is limited by the inability to directly measure changes in intracardiac pressures, making absolute conclusions regarding detailed adaptive changes more difficult. Nevertheless, when compared with matched controls (age, gender, and body surface area), any relative changes in parameters of systolic or diastolic function are valid. It is also evident that the functional changes are consequences of the adaptive morphologic changes of the dynamically and isometrically trained athlete. Noninvasive parameters of systolic function in trained athletes usually fall with accepted normal limits. The occasional abnormal findings may be satisfactorily explained as secondary to the adaptive morphologic changes associated with the different types of training. Similarly, noninvasive parameters of diastolic function usually fall within a normal range of values at rest, irrespective of the type of training.

Echocardiography, especially M-mode echocardiography, allows the cardiac anatomy to be detailed in a noninvasive serial manner; it is particularly useful in finding and documenting changes in cardiac morphology in athletes. Changes in cavity sizes, left ventricular wall thickness, and left ventricular mass have been documented in a number of studies of athletes undergoing both dynamic and static exercise training. Furthermore, a study of 947 athletes of both sexes established acceptable limits of normal values in trained athletes (Figure 34–3 and Table 34–1).

1. Left ventricular cavity—A consistent finding in dynamically trained athletes is an increased left ventricular end-diastolic dimension, which is present irrespective of body surface area, height, or gender. Compared with sedentary control subjects, the left ventricular end-diastolic dimension is increased by approximately 10%, which represents an increase in end-diastolic volume of approximately 33%. In the study mentioned earlier, 98% of the dynamically trained athletes had an end-diastolic dimension of 60 mm or less. In contrast, left ventricular end-diastolic dimension is not altered with static exercise training, whether expressed in absolute values, or normalized by body surface area,

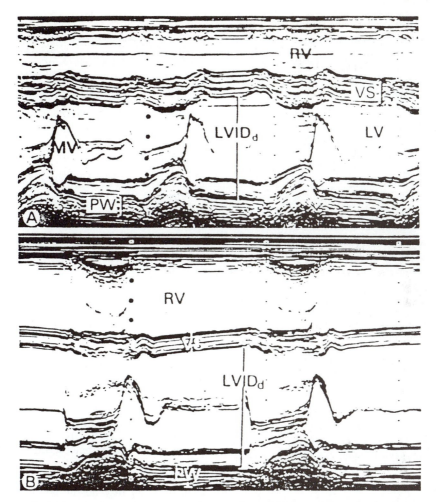

Figure 34–3. Morphologic responses to training. Examples of two athlete's response to dynamic exercise training. **A:** Thickened interventricular septum (VS) and posterior left ventricular wall (PW) and slightly enlarged left ventricular diameter (LVID$_d$ = 56 mm). **B:** A significantly enlarged left ventricular cavity (LVID$_d$ = 60 mm) with normal VS and PW thickness. LV = left ventricle; MV = mitral valve; RV = right ventricle. Reprinted, with permission, from Maron BJ: The structural features of the athletic heart as defined by echocardiography. J Am Coll Cardiol 1986;7:190.

weight, or lean body mass. This difference is felt to reflect the pressure, rather than volume load, on the left ventricle that is created by isometric training. The end-systolic dimension and volume remain within normal limits in the endurance athlete, producing the increase in stroke dimension and volume associated with dynamic exercise training.

2. Left ventricular wall thickness—Concomitant with the increase in left ventricular cavity size in the dynamically trained athlete, left ventricular posterior wall and interventricular septal thickness increase. The increase (compared with sedentary controls) in left ventricular posterior wall thickness is as high as 19%; in the 947-athlete study, 98% had a left ventricular posterior wall thickness of 12 mm or less. Isometric exercise produces septal wall thicknesses of up to 16 mm. These increased values fall within an acceptable range when normalized for body surface area, weight, or lean body mass.

Although septal hypertrophy is a characteristic of hypertrophic cardiomyopathy, the increase in septal thickness in athletes is rarely above 16 mm and the septal-posterior wall thickness ratio does not increase above 1.2:1. Furthermore, there is no evidence in the literature that primary hypertrophic cardiomyopathy may develop with training.

Table 34–1. Morphologic responses to training.

	Untrained	Dynamic Training		Isometric Training	
	Normal Range	Range	Increase above Normal	Range %	Increase above Normal %
LVEDD (mm)	35–37	36–60	10	35–37	0
LVWT (mm)	6–11	6–12	19	6–17	33
IVST (mm)	6–11	6–16	14	6–16	14
LVM (g)	155–260	240–370	45	225–400	45
RVD (mm)	9–26	11–33	24	9–26	0
LAD (mm)	19–40	19–42	12	19–44	14

IVST = interventricular septal thickness; LAD = left atrial dimension; LVM = left ventricular mass; LVED = left ventricular end-diastolic; LVWT = left ventricular wall thickness; RVD = right ventricular diameter.

Source: Data from Maron BJ: Structural features of the athletic heart as defined by echocardiography. J Am Coll Cardiol 1986; 7:190.

3. Left ventricular mass—Estimates of left ventricular mass incorporate measurements of intraventricular septum and posterior wall thickness, both of which increase significantly in trained athletes. It is therefore reasonable to expect a significant increase in left ventricular mass in both dynamically and isometrically trained athletes. An increase of as much as 45% is found, even after normalization for body surface area.

4. Right ventricular cavity—Increases of up to 24% in right ventricular cavity dimensions may be seen in trained athletes.

5. Left atrial cavity—Increases in left atrial cavity size are also found in trained athletes and appear to be related to both the intensity and duration of the exercise.

D. ELECTROCARDIOGRAPHY

Any type of athletic training in any form can alter the normal electrocardiogram (Table 34–2). In a recent survey of 1005 trained athletes, 40% of electrocardiograms (ECG) were abnormal. It is important to know the effects of normal training on the ECG as well as the ECG abnormalities that warrant further investigation. The ECG reflects the morphologic adaptive changes of the heart—sinus bradycardia and voltage criteria for left ventricular hypertrophy (LVH)—that are due to the nature of the training. In the dynamically trained athlete in particular, the sinus bradycardia, which can be profound, reflects the adaptive increase in left ventricular cavity size that delivers large stroke volumes at rest and during exercise. Sinus bradycardia is usually due to high vagal tone, which may also be associated with sinus arrhythmia, sinoatrial block, multifocal atrial rhythms, junction rhythms, first-degree atrioventricular block, and Mobitz I second-degree atrioventric-

ular block. All these abnormalities disappear during exercise. The P wave of the ECG may be notched and increased in amplitude. Interventricular conduction abnormalities are common in athletes. The ST segment may be elevated and the T wave increased in amplitude. Occasionally in trained athletes, the ST segment may be depressed and the T wave biphasic or inverted, all of which correct during exercise. These latter findings at rest are characteristic of ischemic heart disease, however, and their existence in the athlete warrants further investigation.

Distinguishing between physiologic and pathologic LVH by ECG may not be possible, particularly in a young athlete. The adaptive development of LVH and sinus bradycardia is characteristic of the trained athlete, as is the loss of these adaptive characteristics as a detraining effect. In the older athlete, where the preva-

Table 34–2. Effects of dynamic and isometric exercise and training on the electrocardiogram.

Notched P waves
Voltage criteria for LVH
Interventricular conduction abnormalities
Symmetrical peaked T waves
Sinus bradycardia
Sinus arrhythmia
Sinoatrial block
Multifocal atrial rhythm
Junctional rhythm
First-degree atrioventricular block
Mobitz I second-degree AV block

AV = atrioventricular; LVH = left ventricular hypertrophy.

lence of ischemic heart disease is much higher, voltage criteria for LVH, ST- and T-wave abnormalities, and repolarization abnormalities of the QRS complex are more common. The threshold for pursuing further investigation of abnormal ECG findings should be much lower in these older athletes.

E. RACIAL DIFFERENCES IN RESPONSE TO TRAINING

No detailed studies addressing the adaptive responses to training in the black athlete have yet been completed. Circumstantial evidence, however, would suggest that these responses may differ in black athletes. It is known that LVH is more prevalent in a black hypertensive population than in a white population, given similar levels of blood pressure elevation. Because a racial difference appears to exist in the blood pressure response to both dynamic and isometric exercise, the potential for an increased prevalence and greater degree of LVH appears to exist among black athletes. In a study of 260 black collegiate athletes, more than 30% had an interventricular septal thickness of more than 13 mm. A separate study of 500 white athletes found only 3% with similar increases in thickness. These factors, coupled with the occurrence of sudden death in athletes—including black athletes—clearly indicate the need for studies of trained black athletes as well as comparative studies of black and white athletes.

F. DETRAINING

The adaptive responses to both dynamic and isometric exercise training persist only if the training continues with sufficient duration and intensity. Cessation of the training activity results in a temporal regression of these adaptive changes: the detraining effect. Although this effect is consistent despite age, gender, or the overall duration or type of training, the time course appears to be influenced by these factors. Following cessation of training, a regression of physiologic hypertrophy of up to 60% takes place within 7 days, so-called left ventricular remodeling. Both posterior left ventricular wall thickness and interventricular septal thickness regress equally, and the septal-posterior wall thickness ratio remains unchanged. The left ventricular end-diastolic dimension decreases within 7 days, with little change thereafter. The detraining effect is also associated with a reduction in VO_2max. After 12 weeks of inactivity (cessation of training), VO_2max decreases up to 16%, with half of this loss occurring in the first 3 weeks. Maximal cardiac output during exercise is also reduced by up to 8% in the first 3 weeks of detraining.

Sudden Death in Athletes

The publicity attached to the sudden deaths of high-profile collegiate and professional athletes has raised the general awareness of sudden death in young athletes and led to a reappraisal of the validity and extent of a preparticipatory medical examination. It should be noted, however, that despite the publicity, the incidence of sudden death in athletes is very low, irrespective of age. In one study of male joggers age 30–55 years, only one death occurred per year for every 7620 joggers. When those with a documented history of coronary disease were excluded, the incidence was one death per year for every 152,440 joggers. In a separate study of joggers age 25–75 years, there was one death per year for every 18,000 joggers. The death rate during exercise in U.S. Air Force recruits is one per year for every 750,000 men. Clearly, the incidence of sudden death is low; in young athletes, it is rare. The incidence increases with age and an increased prevalence of coronary artery disease (see); however, it remains very low. Little data exist on the incidence of sudden death in female athletes.

The causes of sudden death in athletes appear to be related to age and the nature of the trained athlete population (Table 34–3). Athletes younger than 35 years are likely to die of hypertrophic cardiomyopathy (about 50%) or coronary artery anomalies. In hypertrophic cardiomyopathy, sudden deaths occur during exercise rather than at rest and are thought to be due to ventricular arrhythmias, particularly in individuals with ventricular arrhythmias documented prior to death. One study has shown exercise-induced ischemia as a prodromal feature of sudden death in hypertrophic cardiomyopathy. It should be noted, however, that the prevalence of hypertrophic cardiomyopathy in young athletes is very low and has been shown not to warrant routine Doppler echocardiographic surveys. The prevalence increases in individuals with symptoms of exertional or postexertional syncope or arrhythmias, or with a family history of similar symptoms or sudden death. Furthermore, the magnitude of LVH appears to be directly related to the risk of sudden death. A variant of hypertrophic cardiomyopathy as a cause of sudden death is idiopathic LVH. These individuals have normal myocardial histology and LVH and thus changes consistent with the training activity of the individual.

Table 34–3. Causes of sudden death in athletes.

Hypertrophic cardiomyopathy
Coronary artery disease
Arrythmogenic right ventricle
Congenital coronary anomalies
Marfan syndrome
Congenital aortic stenosis
Preexcitation syndrome
Prolonged QT syndrome

Among athletes older than 35, the most common cause of sudden death is coronary artery disease. Furthermore, older athletes tend to jog rather than engage in group sports activities. Risk factors for cardiovascular disease are usually present in those older than 35 years who have exercise-related sudden death; they also show prodromal features of angina or unusual fatigue. Retrospective reviews of these individuals often show a history of hypertension, cigarette smoking, and hyperlipidemia, and a family history of ischemic heart disease.

The second most common cause of sudden death for athletes younger than 35 years is a coronary artery anomaly, which invariably precipitates death during exercise (all coronary anomalies may predispose to sudden death). Both angina and syncope have retrospectively been identified as prodromal features of this condition; these symptoms should prompt an immediate evaluation of a young athlete. Right ventricular dysplasia and Uhl's anomaly are rare causes of sudden death in young athletes, who may have a history of syncope, palpitations, or ventricular tachycardia. There is a small literature of sudden death following anabolic steroid use, usually in weight lifters. Accelerated atherosclerosis in young subjects has been reported at autopsy in these individuals. Other rare causes of sudden death in athletes are listed in Table 34–3.

The Preparticipation Physical Examination

All athletes—of any age—should undergo a preparticipation cardiac examination and subsequent regular periodic examinations. These should be done in a closed setting, providing time for a detailed history and physical examination, rather than in an assembly-line atmosphere. Knowledge of the subject and the subject's family history are essential. The history should detail any information regarding congenital heart disease in the subject or family members as well as sudden death of any family members. Symptoms such as exercise intolerance, syncope at rest or during exercise, dyspnea, angina or its equivalents, and palpitations need to be recorded. In older athletes, close attention should be paid to the existence of cardiovascular risk factors as well as the symptoms and manifestations of coronary artery disease.

Physical examinations should exclude Marfan syndrome. Arterial blood pressure should be measured accurately. Auscultation of the heart should be comprehensive, keeping in mind that both S_3 and S_4 sounds are common in athletes, as are pulmonary arterial flow murmurs in young athletes and aortic valve flow murmurs in older athletes. The cardiac examination should be carried out in the upright position to lessen innocent murmurs and intensify the murmur from hypertrophic cardiomyopathy. Because of the significance of hypertrophic cardiomyopathy, when a systolic murmur

is auscultated, its features during squatting and during and after the Valsalva maneuver should be characterized.

Further testing is not routinely required, unless warranted by an abnormal feature of the history or physical examination. Furthermore, should a cardiovascular test be carried out, the limitations of the procedure as well as the altered normal ranges of parameters evaluated by the procedure must be kept in mind. The extent of any evaluation beyond the history and physical examination depends on any abnormality that emerges. The routine use of electrocardiography, exercise testing, and echocardiography is precluded on a cost-benefit basis because of the very low prevalence of sudden death in the trained athlete population. It is possible that the threshold for a diagnostic echocardiogram may be lower for an older or masters athlete, again emphasizing its indication is provided by any potential abnormality emerging from the detailed history and physical examination.

There are other relevant reasons for forgoing expensive cardiovascular tests. The morphologic changes produced by the various forms of athletic training often produce changes in certain tests (particularly the echocardiogram) that would be abnormal in a normal, sedentary, age-matched population. It must be remembered that the normal range of values for athletes varies considerably from the accepted normal ranges of left ventricular cavity size, posterior wall and interventricular septal thickness, and left ventricular wall mass. The same applies to routine ECGs in this population, in that abnormal ECG findings may be normal variants in a group of trained athletes. In addition, the incidence of false-positive exercise stress tests appears to be higher in a population of trained athletes. Although these observations do not completely preclude the use of cardiovascular tests, they reinforce the conclusion that they need not be done routinely.

Burke AP, Farb A, Virmani R et al: Sports-related and non-sports related sudden death in young adults. Am Heart J 1991;121: 568.

Colan SD, Sanders SP, Borow KM: Physiologic hypertrophy: Effects on left ventricular systolic mechanics in athletes. J Am Coll Cardiol 1987;9:776.

Glover DW, Mason BJ: Profile of preparticipation cardiovascular screening for high school athletes. JAMA 1998;279,1817.

Lewis JF, Mason BJ, Diggs JA et al: Participation echocardiographic screening for cardiovascular disease in a large predominantly black population of collegiate athletes. Am J Cardiol 1989;64:129.

Maron BJ: Structural features of the athletic heart as defined by echocardiography. J Am Coll Cardiol 1986;7:190.

Maron BJ: Sudden death in young athletes. N Engl J Med 1993; 329:55.

Maron BJ, Proujo CG, Thompson PD et al: Recommendations for preparticipation screening and the assessment of cardiovascular disease in masters athletes. Circulation 2001;103,327.

Nixon JV, Wright AR, Porter TR et al: Effects of exercise on left ventricular diastolic performance in trained athletes. Am J Cardiol 1991;68:945.

Pellicia A, Maron BJ, Spataro A et al: The upper limit of physiologic cardiac hypertrophy in highly trained elite athletes. N Engl J Med 1991;324:295.

Pellicia A, Maron BJ, Culasso F et al: Clinical significance of abnormal electrocardiographic patterns in trained athletes. Circulation 2000;102,278.

Pfister GC, Puffer JC, Maron BJ et al: Preparticipation cardiovascular screening for U.S. collegiate student athletes. JAMA 2000;283,1597.

Phillips M, Robmowitz M, Higgins JR et al: Sudden cardiac death in Air Force recruits. JAMA 1986;256:2696.

Rahrenback MC, Thompson PD: The preparticipation sports examination. Cardiovasc Clin 1992;10:319.

Spirito P, Bellone P, Harris KM et al: Magnitude of LVH and risk of sudden death in hypertrophic cardiomyopathy. N Engl J Med 2000;342,1778.

Zehender M, Meinertz T, Keul J et al: EKG variants and cardiac arrhythmias in athletes: clinical relevance and prognostic importance. Am Heart J 1990;119:1378.

Thoracic Aortic Dissection

Jorge A. Wernly, MD

ESSENTIALS OF DIAGNOSIS

- *Usually middle-aged or elderly hypertensive men; occasionally, young patients with history of Marfan's syndrome, other connective tissue disorder. Rarely, young women in late pregnancy or labor*
- *Acute chest pain, frequently with hemodynamic instability*
- *Possible appearance of shock but normal or elevated blood pressure*
- *Various neurologic symptoms, such as Horner's syndrome, paraplegia, and stroke*
- *Absent or unequal peripheral pulses*
- *Aortic regurgitation*
- *Widened mediastinum on chest radiograph*
- *Confirmatory aortic imaging study*

General Considerations

Acute dissection is the most frequent catastrophic illness involving the aorta, occurring in an estimated 10–20 cases per million people per year. Acute aortic dissection is at least twice as common as ruptured abdominal aneurysm, but it is not recognized nearly as frequently. Expedient confirmatory diagnosis and prompt therapy are crucial in achieving a successful outcome. Problems with both the accuracy and the timeliness of the diagnosis or treatment are a common cause for litigation.

Acute aortic dissection is a sudden event in which blood penetrates the aortic wall through an intimal tear and creates a false channel by dissection of the media; the process is usually rapid. Propagation of the dissection depends on the pulse-wave force. *Dissecting aneurysm* is a misnomer that should not be used to describe the acute phase of the aortic dissection. This term should be reserved to describe late development of aneurysms in previously dissected arteries or, more rarely, the devel-

opment of dissection in an already established aneurysm of other origin.

More than three quarters of the patients are older than 40. Acute aortic dissection occurs two to three times more frequently in men between the ages of 50 and 70 than in women of the same age. It is rare in young patients, except for those with familial predisposition, Marfan's syndrome, other connective tissue disorders, or congenital lesions such as bicuspid aortic valve or coarctation of the aorta. Below age 40 the distribution is nearly equal between men and women, with half the dissections in women occurring during pregnancy. The association of aortic dissection with pregnancy is poorly understood; the event may be partially related to the increase in blood volume and systemic blood pressure observed late in pregnancy.

Two types of aortic pathology different from classic aortic dissection have been recognized in the last decade. Penetrating aortic ulcer (PAU) and intramural hematoma (IMH) were virtually unknown before the widespread use of high-resolution imaging techniques for the diagnosis of aortic dissection. Even though the exact pathologic mechanisms of these conditions is being debated there is enough evidence to support the concept that they are different clinical entities that, in some cases, can progress to aortic dissection.

Classification

The two most commonly used classifications are the DeBakey and the Stanford systems. DeBakey's classification categorizes patients with aortic dissection into three groups, based on the location and extent of the dissection. In **type I** (70%), the ascending, transverse, and descending aorta are involved by the dissection. In **type II** (5%), only the ascending aorta is involved, and the dissection stops proximal to the innominate artery. In **type III** (25%), the dissection involves the descending thoracic aorta (IIIa) and commonly extends into the abdominal aorta (IIIb). Occasionally, it involves the ascending aorta by retrograde dissection, producing an anatomic type I.

The natural history of the lesion depends almost exclusively on whether the ascending aorta is involved (see the section on the Natural History of Untreated Patients, later in this chapter). The Stanford clinical classification system is far simpler and is based solely on whether the ascending aorta is involved, irrespective of the site of the primary intimal tear and the distal extent of the dissection. All dissections that involve the ascending aorta, regardless of the site of entry, are defined as type A (DeBakey's types I and II). All other dissections that do not include the ascending aorta are defined as type B. This includes all dissections of the descending thoracic aorta (DeBakey's type III) and the aortic arch (Figure 35–1).

Pathophysiology & Etiology

Aortic dissection has often been related to structural changes in the media. Such histopathologic changes as medionecrosis, cystic medial necrosis, fibrosis, and fragmentation of elastin fibers have been considered specific for this disease. Studies of undissected aortas indicate that these changes occur as part of the aging process; they are not specific to dissection, and they seem to be accentuated in patients with hypertension. The terms *cystic medial necrosis* and *medionecrosis* are probably also misnomers because there are no true cystic lesions in the former, and actual necrosis is rare in both.

Lesions involving elastin and collagen have been found predominantly in people under 40 years of age and in patients with Marfan's syndrome and other connective tissue disorders. These defects in the extracellular matrix cause a severe loss of integrity of the vessel wall. Clinical dissection in patients with these type of abnormalities often develops in the absence of hypertension. Degenerative changes in the smooth muscle cells have been found more commonly in older patients. Without associated defects in the extracellular matrix, these cause a less marked loss of aortal integrity than do the collagen and elastin lesions. Hypertension has been identified as a major predisposing factor in these patients.

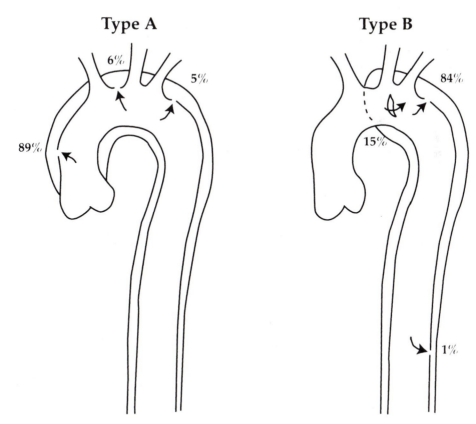

Figure 35–1. Stanford classification system. Reprinted, with permission, from Daily PO, Trueblood HW, Stinson EB et al: Management of acute aortic dissection. Ann Thorac Surg 1970;10:244.

Bicuspid aortic valves are nine times more frequently associated with acute dissection than are tricuspid aortic valves; associated congenital anomalies of the aortic wall may occur in these patients. Similarly, aortic coarctation has also been associated with an increased incidence of aortic dissection. This is most likely due to arterial hypertension and the frequent association with a congenital bicuspid aortic valve, however, and not directly related to the coarctation. The role of pregnancy remains unsolved. Other causes of dissection include trauma, cardiac catheterization, intraaortic balloon valvuloplasty, cannulation for cardiopulmonary bypass, and other surgical manipulations of the ascending aorta.

The true distribution of the different types of aortic dissection can best be inferred from autopsy series performed before the era of contemporary medical and surgical management. Most of the patients (60–70%) had an ascending aorta dissection, and almost one third had a descending aorta dissection. In approximately 90% of patients with ascending dissections, the entry tear was located in the ascending aorta; 6% of the patients had an arch tear; and 5%, a tear in the descending aorta. Most of the patients with descending dissections had the tear in the descending aorta; 15% had a tear in the arch.

The process of dissection involves an initial phase, during which the intimal tear occurs, and a second phase, in which the dissection propagates. Several hemodynamic factors as well as intrinsic properties of the aortic wall determine the propensity to develop primary tears. The greatest external flexion and motion occurs in the ascending aorta with each ventricular ejection. The pulsatile load—as determined by the contractility of the heart, the stroke volume, arterial wall compliance, and blood pressure—appears to be greatest in the ascending aorta. The upper descending thoracic aorta is also subjected to a significant amount of torsion and flexion with each cardiac cycle. At this place the aortic arch joins the relatively immobile descending thoracic aorta.

Experimental evidence suggests that propagation of the dissection is affected by the rate of rise of the blood pressure (dP/dt). The false channel develops and propagates rapidly, usually involving one half to two thirds of the circumference. The walls of the branches of the aorta may be involved by the dissection or may be sheared off from the true lumen creating reentry points between the two lumens. The avulsed branch may stay open, connected only to the false channel, or it may be closed by the dissection. The extent of the involvement of peripheral arteries helps explain the extreme variability of symptoms and signs found on presentation.

The dissection is initially contained by the thin outer layer of the media and the adventitia of the aorta. The false channel usually ruptures into the pericardium or the left pleural space. Before the rupture, in many cases, blood extravasates and forms large mediastinal hematomas. Thrombosis of the false channel is rare. In most of the patients who survive the acute dissection, the false lumen enlarges and reaches aneurysmal proportions; late rupture may eventually occur.

Clinical Presentation

The dissection is considered acute if the time from clinical onset of the dissection is less than 2 weeks and chronic if this period exceeds 2 weeks. The predisposing conditions leading to dissection will vary, depending on whether the ascending or descending aorta is involved. Patients with type A dissection tend to be younger (an average age of 49 years, versus 60 years for those with type B) and are less likely to have a history of hypertension (30%, versus 71% with type B). Patients with type A dissection are also more likely to have associated congenital defects (eg, bicuspid aortic valve, Marfan's syndrome) predisposing to dissection.

Contrary to common opinion, in most cases, no specific activity precedes the dissection; only a small group of patients have reported strenuous physical exertion before the onset of dissection. It is of interest in this connection that the acute hypertension seen in weight lifters has been associated with acute dissection.

A. SYMPTOMS AND SIGNS

The clinical presentations of aortic dissection include shock, hypertension, various neurologic symptoms, and sudden death (within 15 min of the onset of the dissection). Sudden death may be caused by free rupture or by one of the coronary arteries shearing off from the aorta. A significant number of the patients who present with aortic dissection are in shock, including hypovolemic shock, from blood loss in the channel and soft pericardial tissues, or cardiogenic shock from acute aortic valve regurgitation, myocardial infarction, or cardiac tamponade. Many patients who are sweaty and clammy and appear to be in shock are actually hypertensive, as are more than half the patients reaching the hospital. The picture may be further confused by peripheral vasodilation, which possibly results from an autosympathectomy of the dissected arterial wall.

Although the acute dissection produces no significant symptoms and goes unnoticed in a few patients, pain is the most frequent symptom. The onset of pain is sudden and unremitting in most patients. Patients with acute dissection present in obvious discomfort, and the fear of death is common. Localization of the pain varies, and a spectrum of presentations is seen. Although the localization of the pain may not indicate the site of the intimal tear, the type of pain occasionally suggests the extent of the process. For example, pain in the flank usually indicates involvement of the renal arteries.

The pulse may be diminished or absent in one or more extremities (usually the left leg). Oliguria or anuria suggests involvement of the renal arteries. New cardiac murmurs can also be heard. A diastolic murmur of aortic regurgitation, suggesting involvement of the ascending aorta, is present in more than 50% of cases. Systolic bruits may be heard over partially occluded arteries. A pericardial rub is infrequent but is an ominous symptom when present because it indicates leakage of blood into the pericardial space.

In approximately 40% of patients, diverse neurologic findings are present, ranging from Horner's syndrome to syncope, paraplegia, and stroke. Symptoms of neurologic origin may be temporary and related to the location of the dissection. The reappearance of pulses and wandering paralysis usually indicates either reentry of the false channel or intermittent occlusion of the vessel by an intimal flap. Table 35–1 summarizes the most common clinical features of aortic dissection.

B. Diagnostic Studies

The variability and nonspecific nature of the presenting symptoms requires a confirmatory diagnosis to institute immediate therapy. The diagnosis of dissection is based on direct signs (visualization of a double lumen or an intimal flap) and indirect signs (compression of the true lumen, abnormalities and thickening of the aortic wall, abnormalities of branch vessels, and aortic regurgitation; Figure 35–2).

1. Electrocardiography—Changes of chronic left ventricular hypertrophy from long-standing hypertension are often present. Acute ischemic changes can oc-

Table 35–1. Clinical features of acute aortic dissection.

Male-to-female ratio 3:1
Sudden, excruciating, migrating chest pain (90%)
Hypertension: type B (70%)
              type A (30%)
Between 11% and 35% of patients admitted to hospital die undiagnosed or misdiagnosed
Pulse deficits, bruits
Neurologic symptoms
  Focal deficits (20%)
  Syncope, paraplegia, stroke
  Hoarseness, Horner's syndrome
Myocardial ischemia or infarction (10%)
Aortic incompetence (25% overall, 60% type A)
Fatal outcome if undiagnosted and untreated
  Mortality rate = 1–3%/hour during first 24–48 h
  More than 90% of pateints dead at 3 months

cur when the dissection involves the coronary arteries. Because the dissection most commonly involves the right coronary artery, inferior wall changes are more common.

2. Chest radiograph—Plain films of the chest may show several changes suggestive of dissection: widening of the superior mediastinum, double shadow of the aortic wall, and disparity in size of the ascending and

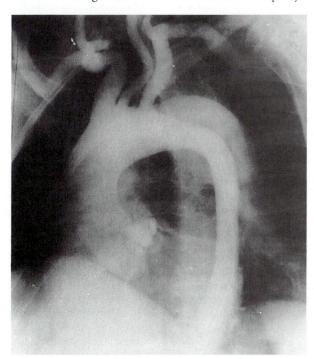

Figure 35–2. Angiogram showing flap separating two lumens of aortic dissection in descending aorta.

descending aorta. Cardiomegaly secondary to pericardial effusion or signs of pleural effusion, particularly in the left chest are sometimes present. In many patients, no mediastinal enlargement is visible in the early phases of acute dissection.

3. Retrograde aortography—This method was for a long time considered the gold standard in aortic dissection; however, its sensitivity was difficult to assess. Newer imaging techniques have revealed that aortography is not as sensitive as previously thought. Aortographic findings in aortic dissection include visualization of the false lumen in 80–90% of cases, the intimal flap in 70%, and the site of entry in approximately 50%. False-negative studies can occur in several situations: equal opacification of both lumens, flap not tangential to the x-ray beam, or tears proximal to the tip of the catheter. Retrograde aortography has a number of other disadvantages, such as the usual risks of any invasive procedure and the time necessary to perform the study. It is also the most expensive of the imaging procedures.

4. Computerized tomographic scanning—CT equipment is readily available in most hospitals, and the procedure is rapid and noninvasive. The two lumens with a visible intimal flap are visualized by CT in 80% of cases (Figure 35–3). CT is also helpful in identifying other causes of aortic widening such as periaortic hematomas, abnormal mediastinal fat, or adjacent tumor. Although CT scanning in the diagnosis of aortic dissection shows a sensitivity of from 83% to almost 100% and a specificity of 90–100%, it cannot reliably identify aortic regurgitation, detect the entry site or the involvement of branch vessels, or delineate coronary arteries.

Spiral CT or ultrafast CT are significantly faster and more accurate than conventional scanners. Spiral CT allows complete imaging of the thoracic aorta after a single injection of contrast material in less than 1 min. Imaging is performed with optimal contrast enhancement, giving a better definition of intimal flaps, entry points, and proximal coronary arteries. Ultrafast CT, which is technically complex and not generally available, also permits very rapid imaging with enhanced resolution.

5. Magnetic resonance imaging—MRI provides high-quality images in multiple planes (transverse, coronal, sagittal, and oblique) and better definition of the location and extent of the dissection, while requiring no use of intravenous contrast (Figure 35–4). Dissection is best seen when there is flow in both the true and the false lumens. Slow flow can sometimes resemble thrombosis. In such cases, it may be difficult to distinguish the dissection from an aortic aneurysm with mural thrombosis. A recent advance, cine MRI, supplies images that simulate real-time cardiac imaging. It can identify valvular regurgitation by identifying areas of turbulent flow.

Recent studies of MRI efficacy in diagnosing aortic dissection show sensitivity and specificity of almost 100%. Identification of the entry site was also quite high (sensitivity 85%, specificity 100%). The presence of aortic regurgitation was assessed with cine MRI, with 85% sensitivity and 100% specificity.

Although MRI is a very accurate method of diagnosing aortic dissection, several disadvantages limit its use in unstable patients. The time necessary to perform the test (significantly longer than that of CT scan and echocardiography) and the relatively limited access to the patient during imaging make MRI less than ideal for these patients, who are frequently intubated and receiving vasoactive drugs intravenously and are therefore in need of close monitoring. In addition, in many hospitals MRI scanners are located in decentralized special facilities that complicate the issues of patient transport.

6. Echocardiography—Echocardiography is an excellent test for patients with suspected aortic dissection because it is widely available and easily performed at the bedside. It is noninvasive and it does not require radiation or contrast agents.

Numerous echocardiographic criteria have been proposed for diagnosing dissection. The most definitive finding is the identification of the intimal flap in several views. When the false lumen is thrombosed, the central displacement of intimal calcification is considered evidence of a dissection. Echocardiography also provides useful additional information in establishing alternative diagnoses when aortic dissection has been ruled out; these include pericardial effusion, valvular abnormalities, and wall motion abnormalities.

a. Transthoracic echocardiography (TTE)—The effectiveness of TTE in diagnosing aortic dissection has been extensively evaluated; this technique has been found to have a sensitivity of 60–80% and a specificity of 63–96%. Its sensitivity is highest for dissection of the ascending aorta (78–100%). For descending aortic dissection, its sensitivity is significantly lower (30–50%). Although not very accurate for diagnosing dissection, TTE is a good complementary test that provides valuable additional information in terms of myocardial function, pericardial effusion, and valvular involvement in patients with suspected ascending aortic dissection. The sequential use of TTE and CT is extremely powerful in clarifying difficult cases.

b. Transesophageal echocardiography (TEE)—Because of the proximity of the probe to the cardiac and aortic structures, TEE overcomes many of the difficulties and technical limitations of TTE. Excellent visualization is possible because of the multiple planes that can be scanned as the probe is advanced and rotated. The procedure is very quick: at only 5–18 min long, it

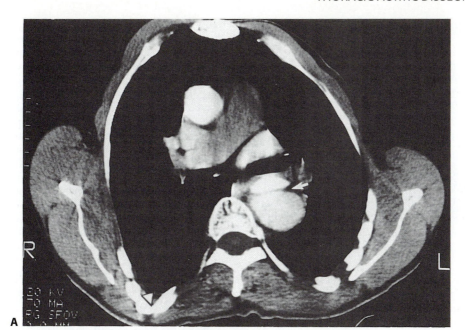

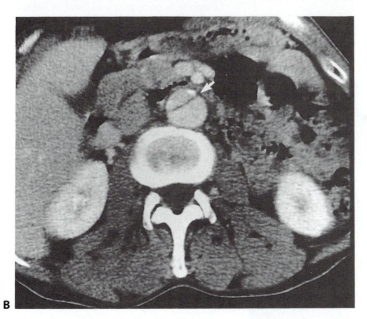

Figure 35–3. **A:** CT scan following bolus of contrast material, showing an internal flap in the descending aorta (*arrow*). **B:** CT scan through abdomen (in same patient) showing that flap extends into abdominal aorta *(arrow).* CT = computed tomography.

can be rapidly and safely performed in the emergency room, ICU, and other clinical environments. TEE plays an increasingly important role in the evaluation of aortic disease and has several advantages in the diagnosis of acute aortic dissection. It requires minimal preparation of the patient, avoids the need for contrast media and x-ray exposure associated with CT and angiography, and eliminates the delays and practical difficulties of MRI (Figure 35–5). One limitation of single-plane TEE is the difficulty in imaging the proximal aortic

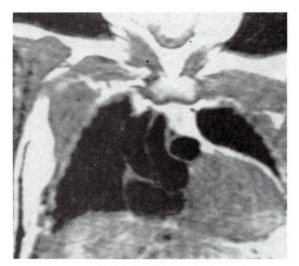

Figure 35–4. Coronal T₁-weighted MRI showing dissection involving aorta in patient with Marfan's syndrome. MRI = magnetic resonance image.

arch because of the interposition of the airways. The interposition of the trachea creates a blind spot that obscures portions of the distal ascending aorta, superior

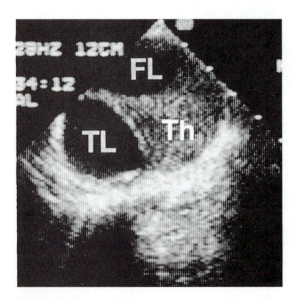

Figure 35–5. Short-axis transesophageal echocardiographic view of the descending aorta: image shows small true lumen (TL) and false lumen (FL) partially filled with thrombus (Th). Reprinted, with permission, from Shively BK: Transesophageal echocardiography is the diagnosis of aortic disease. Semin in Ultrasound, CT, MRI 1993;14:114.

transverse arch and, occasionally, the origin of the great vessels. This problem has been largely overcome by the newer biplane and omniplane probes.

Safety of the examination depends on adequately monitoring the patient and minimizing anxiety and pain. In the majority of cases, the esophagus can be intubated with minimal distress, using sedation or light general anesthesia. The incidence of complications during TEE is less than 1%. A number of studies examining the clinical value of TEE in diagnosing aortic dissection have demonstrated a sensitivity of 87–100% for identifying an intimal flap and 77–87% for identifying the site of entry. These studies also reported a specificity for the diagnosis of aortic dissection of 82–95%, a sensitivity of 92–100%, a positive predictive value of 80–96%, and a negative predictive value of 97–100%.

False-positive tests are usually the result of reverberations from sclerotic or calcific aortic disease. To minimize the possibility of false-positive examinations, the intimal flap should be visualized in more than one plane. Biplanar and multiplanar probes provide improved diagnostic accuracy and are extremely helpful in resolving the issue of artifactual flaps. Also, color-flow Doppler is particularly helpful in identifying these suspicious linear structures because it permits the recognition of different blood flow patterns in the true and false lumen and the identification of entry and reentry points into the false lumen.

TEE can readily identify complications of aortic dissection such as aortic regurgitation and pericardial effusion as well as rupture. In addition, TEE provides detailed morphologic information about involvement of the proximal coronary arteries; false-negative results are unusual. This compares very favorably with aortography in diagnosing proximal dissection of the coronary arteries. Assessment of distal coronary arteriosclerosis, however, requires coronary angiography.

Another advantage of TEE is that imaging can be easily performed in the operating room without affecting the performance of the operation. Intraoperative imaging by TEE can eliminate any uncertainty as to which structures are involved in the dissection and can provide critical information for the surgeon's management of the operation.

c. **Intraoperative epicardial echocardiography (IEE)**—Scanning of the aorta can be supplemented by intraoperative epicardial echocardiography. This imaging modality permits a larger number of acoustic windows and eliminates uncertainty regarding the involvement of the ascending aorta. IEE also can be helpful in the intraoperative treatment of the patient with dissection, permitting precise evaluation of potential aortic cannulation sites. Intraoperative epicardial Doppler echocardiography as well as TEE can be used during cardiopulmonary bypass to confirm that the retrograde flow from the femoral artery is actually delivered to the arch branches. Recognition of abnormal flow patterns at the initiation of cardiopulmonary bypass may force the surgeon to modify surgical strategy. In addition, IEE and TEE can be used immediately after repair of the ascending aorta to ensure that no residual flap or other tear is compromising antegrade flow to one of the great vessels and to assess the competence of the aortic valve after surgical repair.

7. Intravascular ultrasound imaging—IVUS provides precise visualization of both the lumen and wall of the aorta and is able to accurately determine the perfusion of visceral arteries. In addition, IVUS is used as a guide for new endovascular interventional procedures, such as stent-graft implantation across the entry point, stents in distal arteries involved in the dissection, and percutaneous fenestration of obstructing dissecting flaps.

8. Selecting the imaging method—Each of the aortic imaging methods has advantages and disadvantages in the diagnosis of aortic dissection. Proper understanding of the accuracy, limitations, and relative merits of each of the diagnostic procedures is paramount. The ideal test should rapidly and safely confirm or exclude the diagnosis of dissection, determine whether the dissection involves the ascending aorta, and identify the anatomic features of the dissection (presence of pericardial effusion, sites of entry and reentry, extension of the dissection, and severity of aortic regurgitation). The accuracy of the information must be considered. A false-negative diagnosis might lead to death; a false-positive test, to unnecessary surgery carrying a significant risk. The physician must carefully assess the clinical condition of the patient, which will of course influence the selection of the imaging method. The availability of the equipment, the need for transportation, the length of time necessary to perform the procedure, and its overall safety must also be considered.

Aortography, once considered the gold standard for the diagnosis of dissection, is seldom recommended. It is the most expensive of the imaging techniques, it takes a significant length of time, and has the inherent risk of any invasive procedure that (among other risks) requires the use of intravenous contrast agents.

CT scanning, although readily available, fast, and noninvasive, does require transport of the patient and is less accurate than the other imaging techniques. MRI, which is unsuitable for unstable patients, is not as readily available as CT scanning and is both quite expensive and time-consuming; it also requires transport and makes monitoring the patient during the test more difficult. TEE can be performed in a relatively short time at the bedside and is readily available. Biplane and multiplane probes are very accurate. When findings are unclear, a low threshold for repeat imaging of the same or complementary type is paramount to achieve a correct diagnosis. A simple diagnostic algorithm is suggested in Figure 35–6. In the final analysis, physicians should determine which is the best diagnostic approach for aortic dissection on the basis of their own experience and the resources available in each institution.

Armstrong WF, Bach DS, Carey LM et al: Clinical and echocardiographic findings in patients with suspected acute aortic dissection. Am Heart J 1998;136:1051.

Coady MA, Rizzo JA, Elefteriades JA et al: Pathologic variants of thoracic aortic dissection. Cardiol Clin 1999;17:637.

Gara PT, DeSanctis RW: Acute aortic dissection and its variants: Towards a common diagnostic and therapeutic approach. Circulation 1995;92:1376.

Harris KM, Braverman AC, Gutierrez, FR et al: Transesophageal echocardiographic and clinical features of aortic intramural hematoma. J Thorac Cardiovasc Surg 1997;114:619.

Lansman SL, McCullough JN, Nguyen KH et al: Subtypes of acute aortic dissection. Ann Thorac Surg 1999;67l:1975.

Nienaber CA et al: The diagnosis of thoracic aortic dissection by noninvasive imaging procedures. N Engl J Med 1992;328:1.

Nienaber CA, von Codolitsch Y: Diseases of the aorta. Cardiol Clin 1998;16:295.

Roman MJ, Devereaux RB, Kramer-Fox R et al: Two-dimensional echocardiographic aortic root dimensions in normal children and adults. Am J Cardiol 1989;67:507.

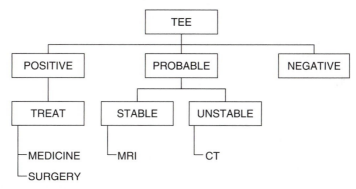

Figure 35–6. Diagnostic algorithm for diagnosis of aortic dissection.

Westaby S: Aortic dissection in Marfan's syndrome. Ann Thorac Surg 1999;67:1861.

Zeebregts CJ, Schepens MA, Hameeteman TM et al: Acute aortic dissection complicating pregnancy. Ann Thorac Surg 1997; 64:1345.

Differential Diagnosis

Acute aortic dissection is the great clinical masquerader that can be misdiagnosed like almost any other acute medical or surgical illness. A high clinical index of suspicion is therefore imperative. Acute dissection should be considered any time there is simultaneous acute involvement of multiple diverse organ systems without an obvious common explanation.

Careful evaluation of the presenting symptoms and signs permits an accurate differential diagnosis, including diseases as varied as myocardial infarction, cerebrovascular accident, pulmonary embolus, and acute surgical abdomen. Of paramount importance is distinguishing between cases of aortic dissection and those of myocardial infarction because administering thrombolytic agents to patients with acute dissection can be catastrophic.

Management

A. PREVENTION

Acute dissection may be preventable in many patients by proper treatment of systemic hypertension and by careful surveillance of patients with known risk factors for dissection. Patients with Marfan's syndrome, other connective tissue disorders, and bicuspid aortic valve can develop acute dissection, with or without hypertension. These patients must be followed carefully for aortic dilation. Several general recommendations that have emerged from the follow-up of patients with Marfan's syndrome are probably applicable to all patients with connective tissue disorders. Because the risk of developing acute dissection is three times higher in patients with a hereditary history of dissection and a dilated aortic root (in the range of 50–60 mm), Marfan's patients should undergo a cardiologic evaluation, including TTE, at least annually. When the aortic root diameter reaches a ratio of 1.3 above normal dimension, the evaluation interval should be shortened to 6 months. Patients with a ratio greater than 1.5 should be considered for elective surgical repair because the high risk of dissection.

The relationship between dilatation of the aortic root and the potential for dissection may also be extrapolated to all patients undergoing cardiac surgical procedures for other indications. In such cases, the surgeon should consider replacing the ascending aorta if it is significantly dilated. With current improvements in surgical techniques and myocardial protection strategies, the elective replacement of the aorta in this circumstance should not add a significant risk to the heart operation.

B. TREATMENT

Optimal treatment of patients with aortic dissection requires that the diagnosis and the extent of the process be identified as soon as possible. Advances in treatment over the last few decades have produced a remarkable improvement in the prognosis of patients affected by this highly lethal disease (see Prognosis). Rapid initiation of medical therapy followed by prompt surgical therapy when indicated is associated with a significant improvement in survival. Most patients with type A dissection require urgent surgical repair, whereas those with uncomplicated type B dissections can usually be treated successfully with medical therapy alone. The best treatment for patients with type B dissection with complications is debatable.

1. Acute management—All patients suspected of having aortic dissection should be evaluated and treated emergently. The initial goal is to stabilize the propagation of the dissection and prevent rupture. Regardless of the location of the dissection, all patients should receive pharmacologic therapy as soon as possible: An hour of delay in initiating treatment means another 6000 unmodified ventricular systoles on the already torn aorta. In our opinion, patients who present at a hospital without appropriate facilities should be transferred to a tertiary hospital with a cardiac surgery service as expeditiously as possible. Transfer should not be delayed for confirmatory diagnosis. Patients suspected of having aortic dissection should immediately be admitted to an ICU for the monitoring of arterial and venous pressure, urinary output, and electrocardiographic changes. Patients suspected of having type A dissections with pericardial effusion should probably be moved directly to the operating room where, if necessary, the diagnosis can be confirmed by TEE.

Acute reduction of arterial pressure is effectively accomplished by the administration of sodium nitroprusside (2–10 mg/kg/min IV). The dose is titrated against the blood pressure response. Blood pressure is reduced to the lowest level compatible with normal cerebral, renal, and cardiac function. Because nitroprusside alone can increase dP/dt, adequate simultaneous β-adrenergic blockade is routinely used. Intravenous propranolol (1–2 mg q 5 min, until the response is satisfactory) is administered to maintain heart rate in the range of 65–70 bpm. Alternatively, labetalol (20–40 mg IV q 2–4 h) can be used. Other agents to reduce blood pressure and decrease dP/dt include trimetaphan and reserpine. While this stabilization is accomplished, preparations should be made for aortic imaging and consultation with a cardiovascular surgeon.

2. Medical treatment—This is generally considered the primary treatment for dissection that involves the descending thoracic aorta as well as the aortic arch (type B). Occasionally, medical therapy is the only appropriate mode of therapy for patients with ascending aortic dissection who have serious associated medical conditions that contraindicate surgery (discussed in section 3a(1) Indication for acute type A dissection).

It is advisable to restrict patients to IV nutrition for the first day after medical treatment, in case surgery becomes necessary. Many patients have an ileus, and a nasogastric tube may be required. When the condition of the patient stabilizes after 2 or 3 days of treatment, oral feedings may be started. Antihypertensive medications are gradually switched to the oral route by the third day. Patients without complications can be moved out of the intensive care area and ambulation begun. Approximately 85–90% of patients with medically treated uncomplicated type B dissection can be discharged from the hospital in 7–10 days. Patients who develop complications usually have a prolonged course of treatment requiring endotracheal intubation, dialysis, and other therapies. Acute renal failure, other organ dysfunction, and neurologic deficits are common. Few patients with complications will survive.

3. Surgical treatment—The goal of surgical treatment is to prevent death from aortic rupture and to reestablish blood flow to arteries occluded by the dissection. In cases of ascending aortic dissection, a secondary goal is to correct aortic regurgitation when present. With the exception of a few patients with very localized dissections, the operation does not remove the entire false channel. Only areas of actual or impending rupture are excised.

a. Indications—

(1) Acute type A dissection—Emergency surgical intervention is the treatment of choice in essentially all patients; exceptions, which should be based on individual judgment, include the very old (aged 85 years or older) and those with other severe, chronic, or life-threatening illnesses. Serial aortic imaging and close clinical follow-up are mandatory if patients are not operated on immediately.

(2) Acute type B dissection—The optimal management of acute type B dissection is controversial. In most centers, patients with type B dissections are treated medically. This recommendation is based on the high morbidity and mortality rates associated with surgical resection and the observation that medical management achieves stabilization of the dissection process and prevents death in most of the patients. (Figure 35–7).

Surgery is reserved for patients with complications such as aortic expansion or rupture, compromise of distal organs, persistence or recurrence of intractable pain, uncontrollable hypertension, or progression of dissection during medical treatment. Several other conditions should prompt strong considerations for surgery but

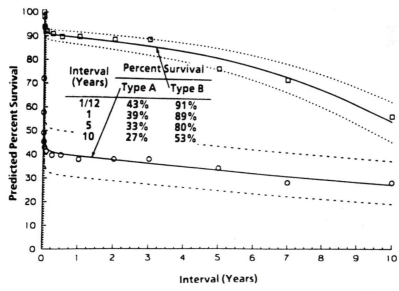

Interval (Years)	Percent Survival	
	Type A	Type B
1/12	43%	91%
1	39%	89%
5	33%	80%
10	27%	53%

Figure 35–7. Survival after nonsurgical treatment after acute aortic dissection, according to whether the dissection involves the ascending aorta with or without the arch (type A), or only the descending aorta beyond the left subclavian artery (type B). Reprinted, with permission, from Kirklin JW, Barrett-Boyes BG: Cardiac Surgery, 2nd ed. New York: Churchill Livingstone, 1993.

have not yet been accepted universally: Marfan's syndrome, a large localized aneurysm or diffuse enlargement of the aorta (more than 5 cm) and, in very carefully selected patients, involvement of the aortic arch.

When medical treatment fails, the outcome is usually catastrophic. The prognosis in such cases is dismal even if emergency operation is performed. It is paradoxical that the indications for operation are precisely those factors associated with increased surgical risk.

Early operative intervention for selected low-surgical-risk patients with uncomplicated acute type B dissection may reduce the incidence of distal false aneurysm and redissection and decrease the incidence of late death from aortic rupture. In some centers, urgent surgery is recommended as the treatment of choice for selected patients with acute type B dissections, even if uncomplicated. With this approach, surgical mortality rates with uncomplicated type B dissection have improved significantly and can now be as low as 10%. However, elderly patients and those with uncomplicated acute type B dissections who have severe pulmonary, cardiac, renal, or central nervous system disease, have a better prognosis if treated medically.

b. Surgical procedures—Current surgical management recommends local, conservative procedures. This approach prevents most deaths and is associated with the lowest operative risk. The operation is designed to resect a limited segment of aorta containing the worst damage (including the intimal tear, if exposed). If a primary intimal tear cannot be exposed and resected (eg, type A dissection with a tear in the descending thoracic aorta or aortic arch; type B dissection with a tear in the arch), early and late survival rates are not affected adversely, but the subsequent reoperation rate is higher.

The native aortic valve should be preserved whenever possible. Valve reconstruction can be performed in approximately 75–80% of patients with acute type A dissection and in 50% of patients with chronic dissection. When the native valve is structurally normal, aortic regurgitation is due to valve leaflet prolapse because of loss of commissural support. This conservative surgical approach, however, should not be used in patients with Marfan's syndrome, Ehlers-Danlos syndrome, or other connective tissue disorders because of the limited durability of aortic valve reconstruction.

One of the most important controversies in surgical treatment of acute dissection that involves the aortic arch is whether the arch should be included in the repair. If the tear can be visualized in the proximal arch through the open aorta, it should be included in the repair but we do not recommend including in the repair tears that extend distally because the operative risk for a complete arch replacement is significantly increased. This more aggressive approach may be reserved to selected low-risk younger patients in whom the risk of the operation is in the range of 10–15%. If the arch has

ruptured, concomitant arch replacement is mandatory, but the operative risk is substantially higher (25–50%).

c. Surgical results—The operative mortality risk for all patients with acute aortic dissection currently ranges from 5% to 30%. The current operative mortality rate for patients with acute type A dissection is 7% ± 5%; for uncomplicated acute type B dissection, it is 13% ± 12%. The mortality rate has been much higher (25–60%) for type B patients with complications. Most deaths that occur shortly after operations for acute dissection are secondary to hemorrhage, heart failure, brain damage, or respiratory failure.

Independent determinants of operative risk for type A dissections are renal failure, tamponade, and renal or visceral ischemia. Concomitant arch replacement or coronary artery bypass is a risk factor for early death. For type B dissections, the determinants of risk include an older age, rupture, renal or visceral ischemia, and infarction. The incidence and types of postoperative complications appears to be similar for both type A and type B dissections. The most significant exception to this is the development of new paraplegia after repair of descending thoracic aortic dissection; this is quite rare after type A dissection but can occur in approximately 4% of patients after type B dissection repair.

d. Endovascular therapies—These procedures represent the most dramatic recent advance in the management of acute dissection. For instance, in acute type B dissection, the use of endovascular stent-grafts permits the coverage of the primary tear with redirection of blood flow into the true lumen. Reperfusion of obstructed peripheral branches and thrombosis of the false lumen is achieved in most of the cases. Residual branch vessel obstruction, which is not completely relieved by redirection of flow into the true lumen, should be treated with placement of stent-grafts or uncovered stents in the affected branch. Additionally, in special situations the creation of catheter fenestrations in obstructing flaps can improve malperfusion syndromes.

Presently, stent-grafting of the entry point of descending aortic dissection is recommended in patients with an indication for surgical repair and with suitable anatomic characteristics: accessible primary tear distal to the subclavian artery, ileofemoral access free of dissection and no substantial tortuousity. Several investigators have shown that in selected patients, endovascular therapy of type B is technically successful in most cases and is associated with a mortality rate between 15% and 30%. Of significant interest is the observation that paraplegia has not been associated as a complication of this procedure as with conventional surgical repair.

The role of endovascular grafts in type A dissection is quite limited. In some special situations, retrograde propagation from a distal tear into the ascending aorta can be treated successfully by endograft coverage of the primary tear.

Ergin MA, Spielvogel D, Apaydin A et al: Surgical treatment of the dilated ascending aorta: When and how? Ann Thoracic Surg 1999;67:1834.

Fann JI, Smith JA, Miller DC et al: Surgical management of aortic dissection during a 30-year period. Circulation 1995;92 (Suppl II):113.

Sabik JF, Lytle BW, Blackstone EH et al: Long-term effectiveness of operations for ascending aortic dissections. J Thorac Cardiovasc Surg 2000;119:946.

Scholl FG, Coady MA, Davies R et al: Interval of permanent nonoperative management of acute type A aortic dissection. Arch Surg 1999;134:402.

4. Long-term management—All patients surviving acute dissection should be medically treated for life. In many postoperative patients and almost all medically treated patients, the false channel persists, frequently leading to complications and death. Aortic complications account for one third of late deaths. Progressive expansion of the dissected segment of the aorta is common and occurs in 25–40% of patients. Effective control of blood pressure and dP/dt should be continued after the initial episode, even if the patient is normotensive. Maximal blood pressure response to exercise should be assessed with treadmill testing. In one study, aneurysms developed in 45% of patients without good blood pressure control, compared with only 17% of patients with satisfactory control. The ideal drug should have a negative inotropic as well as hypotensive effect (eg, β-blockers, clonidine, reserpine, methyldopa). Pure vasodilator drugs such as hydralazine and minoxidil increase dP/dt and should be used only in the presence of adequate β-blockers. It should also be recognized that nonselective β-blockers can increase peripheral resistance, negating the favorable effects on dP/dt. Calcium channel blockers and angiotensin-converting enzyme inhibitors are potentially beneficial for the long-term management of aortic dissection (as a supplement to the traditional β-blocker agents). Their clinical value, however, remains to be assessed.

Accurate knowledge of the extent of the dissection at the time of discharge is mandatory for proper follow-up. The aortic size and the status of the false lumen should be monitored periodically. Aortic imaging should be performed on a regular basis to evaluate the involved and uninvolved aorta after treatment and to detect extension of the dissection or asymptomatic enlargement of distal false aneurysmal segments before complications occur.

Recommendations for follow-up after discharge of patients with aortic dissection include regular examinations and chest radiographs every 3 months during the first year and every 6 months thereafter. Aortic imaging should initially be performed at 3 months and then at 6 months, but for patients with significantly dilated aortas, the intervals should remain at 3 months. If the aorta is not significantly dilated and no clinical or anatomic changes develop between imaging studies, the studies can be done at 6-month intervals and then annually. It is probably not safe to exceed 1 year between examinations.

Early recognition of distal aortic pathology permits both prevention of aortic rupture and timely reoperation. It has been shown that the rate of late death from aortic rupture can be reduced if elective operations for progressive expansion of a persistent false lumen are carried out electively.

Prognosis

A. NATURAL HISTORY OF UNTREATED PATIENTS

The risk of death during the initial phase of acute dissection is very high. It is generally believed that approximately 10–15% of the patients die suddenly in the first 15 min. Approximately 50% of the patients are alive 48 h later, and only 10% of patients are alive after 3 months. These statistics, however, ignore the clear difference in prognosis between acute dissections involving the ascending aorta and those involving only the descending aorta. Without treatment, only 8% of patients with ascending dissection survive for more than a month, whereas almost 75% may survive after dissection of the descending thoracic aorta.

B. LONG-TERM PROGNOSIS AFTER TREATMENT

The prognosis of patients with acute aortic dissection has improved significantly as a result of earlier and more accurate diagnosis, more effective medical therapy, and better surgical techniques. In the last two decades the annual mortality rate for aortic dissection in the United States has declined steadily by more than 50%.

Information about the long-term survival of medically treated patients is limited. As mentioned earlier, a clear difference in early prognosis exists between patients with acute dissections involving the ascending aorta and those involving only the descending thoracic aorta. In a recent series of medically treated patients only 43% of patients with type A dissection were alive 1 month after the dissection, compared with 91% of patients with type B dissection (see Figure 35–6). Interestingly enough, for survivors of the acute episode, the difference in prognosis between type A and type B dissections disappears after the first month. The 5-year survival rate for patients who survived an acute dissection followed by medical treatment alone showed no difference between type A and type B dissections. Several factors may adversely affect the long-term prognosis of medically treated patients; these include age, presence of serious early complications before therapy was instituted, and large diameter of the descending aorta (more than 5 cm).

Although patients who survive the acute dissection continue to be at a significantly greater risk of death than the general population, their long-term survival after surgical treatment shows a relatively satisfactory prognosis. In the Stanford experience, the 5-year actuarial survival rate of patients with acute type A dissection showed a slightly (yet significantly) lower life expectancy at 10 years than that of the general United States population, matched for age and sex. For patients with acute type B dissection, the 5-year actuarial survival rate was not significantly different from that of the general population.

A recent report focusing on the long-term outcome of all types of dissections showed that 18% of late deaths were caused by rupture of another region of the aorta, 38% were cardiovascular in nature, and 24% were sudden and not defined. Even considering that many patients had cardiovascular disease, some (if not many) of these sudden deaths may have been due to aortic rupture. These results underscore the importance of indefinite clinical follow-up. The surgical nature of the late sequelae suggest that surveillance should ideally be performed by the surgeon—that is, the physician who must decide when to reoperate.

Reoperations are quite common in patients with treated aortic dissections. In the Stanford experience the incidence of reoperation was 13% ± 4% at 5 years and 23% ± 6% at 10 years (linearized rate, 3.1% per patient year). The type of dissection has no significant influence on the probability of reoperation, which is more likely in younger patients and in those with Marfan's syndrome. In addition, reoperations are more frequently necessary when the tear is in the arch.

Intramural Aortic Hematoma

The term *intramural aortic hematoma* was introduced to describe a localized area of aortic dissection without intimal disruption. It is thought to begin with the rupture of the vasa vasorum of the aortic wall, which results in a mural collection of blood around the lumen of the aorta. In its early stages, the extravasated blood does not communicate with the aortic lumen; therefore, it does not show enhancement with contrast administration nor does it show blood flow into the space on TEE. The absence of an intimal tear has been confirmed in several surgical and autopsy studies. Whereas IMH can develop in any location of the aorta, more than two-thirds of the patients have involvement of the descending aorta.

Echocardiographic findings suggestive of the diagnosis of IMH include a typical reflection pattern of loculated blood in the wall of the aorta, eccentric lumen, and displaced intimal calcium. Due to the nonspecific nature of these findings, a second imaging modality is frequently necessary after TEE in order to confirm the diagnosis. On CT images, IMH is identified as a nonenhancing circular or crescent-shaped thickening of the aortic wall without evidence of an intimal flap. A fresh hematoma has a higher density than that of the aortic wall. Thrombosis is identified by a multilayered pattern. On MRI, acute IMH is demonstrated as a circular or crescent-shaped thickening of the wall without evidence of an intimal flap and absence of blood flow in the false lumen. Different signal intensity between T1- and T2-weighted images permits the characterization of the age of the hematoma.

Nontraumatic IMH affects patients with longstanding hypertension and present with severe chest or back pain similar to that of classic dissection but without the signs and symptoms of arterial branch compromise. Pleural and pericardial effusions are not uncommon and represent impending rupture. Spontaneous progression of IMH to dissection may occur, characterizing IMH as a precursor of dissection.

Because of poor results with medical treatment, IMH of the ascending aorta should be managed surgically like ascending aortic dissection. On the other hand, patients with descending aortic IMH can probably initially be treated medically. Follow-up imaging to rule out progression should be carried out in 2–4 days. If expansion or progression to dissection are demonstrated, surgery should be performed to prevent rupture. Otherwise, patients may continue to be treated conservatively. Several patients have shown involution of the hematoma over time.

Penetrating Aortic Ulcers

Penetrating aortic ulcer is a rather unusual pathologic event that is quite different from the simple ulceration of an arteriosclerotic lesion and has special prognostic and therapeutic implications. They are atheromatous plaques that ulcerate and penetrate the internal elastic lamina, burrowing deeply into the aortic media and beyond. Depending on the degree of local inflammation and fibrosis, the plaque may precipitate a localized IMH within the aortic wall. Otherwise, the PAU may break through into the adventitia to form a pseudoaneurysm or may rupture freely into the mediastinum.

The clinical presentation is quite similar to that of classic aortic dissection, but the signs secondary to peripheral arterial obstruction are lacking. Most patients are significantly older than those with aortic dissection. Accurate differentiation between penetrating ulcers (PAUs) and classic aortic dissection is critical because the prognosis for PAUs may be more serious than with classic dissection due to a higher risk of rupture. This is of great clinical significance for those patients thought to have an uncomplicated type B dissection who are being treated conservatively. A high level of awareness and a correct diagnosis are paramount. The diagnosis of PAU can be made by most imaging techniques with the demonstration of a contrast material-filled outpouching of the aorta in the absence of a dissection flap or false lumen.

Regardless of the location of a PAU, patients should undergo immediate medical treatment to control pain and prevent rupture. PAUs of the ascending aorta should be treated as aortic dissection requiring urgent operation. Uncomplicated ulcers in the descending aorta may be managed medically with a high index of suspicion of potential expansion and rupture. Follow-up studies should be repeated at 3–5 days in order to confirm the safety of this approach. Persistent pain, hemodynamic instability, and radiographically demonstrated expansion are indications for surgical treatment. Although resection and graft interposition of the affected area is the preferred operation, in some situations patch repair and external wrapping of the aorta can be life-saving in moribund patients. Endovascular stent-grafting is emerging as a less invasive alternative to conventional operations with a progressive greater role in the treatment of selected patients with PAU. In some cases, the severity of the atherosclerotic disease and the tortuousity of distal arteries limit its application.

Coady MA, Rizzo JA, Hammond GL et al: Penetrating ulcer of the thoracic aorta: What is it? How do we recognize it? How do we manage it? J Vasc Surg 1998;27:1006.

Dake MD, Kato N, Mitchell RS et al: Endovascular stent-graft placement for the treatment of acute aortic dissection. N Engl J Med 1999;340:1546.

Detter C, Mair H, Klein HG et al: Long-term prognosis of surgically treated aortic aneurysms and dissections in patients with and without Marfan syndrome. Eur J Cardiothorac Surg 1998; 13:416.

Genoni M, Paul M, Jenni R et al: Chronic β-blocker therapy improves outcome and reduces treatment cost in chronic type B aortic dissection. Eur J Cardiothorac Surg 2001;19:606.

Hagan PG, Nienaber CA, Isselbacher EM et al: The international registry of aortic dissection (IRAD): New insights into an old disease. JAMA 2000;283:897.

Vilacosta I, San Roman JA, Ferrerios J et al: Natural history and serial morphology of aortic intramural hematoma: A novel variant of aortic dissection. Am Heart J 1997;134:495.

Thoracic Aortic Aneurysms

36

John A. Elefteriades, MD

ESSENTIALS OF DIAGNOSIS

- *Ascending aortic diameter >4 cm on imaging study*
- *Descending aortic diameter >3.5 cm on imaging study*

General Considerations

A. LOCATION AND CONFIGURATION OF THORACIC AORTIC ANEURYSMS

In the ascending aorta, aneurysms tend to take on three common patterns, as indicated in Figure 36–1. These include the supracoronary aortic aneurysm, annuloaortic ectasia, and diffuse tubular enlargement.

The most common pattern is that of supracoronary dilatation of the ascending aorta. In this pattern of disease, the short segment of aorta between the aortic annulus and the coronary arteries remains normal in size. We say that the sinuses are "preserved," meaning that

the aorta indents normally, forming a "waist," near the level of the coronary arteries. For this type of aneurysm, a supracoronary tube graft suffices.

In the second type, annuloaortic ectasia, the aortic annulus itself becomes dilated, giving a shape to the aorta like an Erlenmeyer chemistry flask. In this type of disease, the segment of aorta between the annulus and the coronary arteries is diseased, dilated, and thinned. We say that the sinuses are "effaced," meaning that the normal indentation, or waist, is lost. When surgery is required, the entire aortic root must be replaced.

In the third type of ascending aortic disease, the configuration is midway between the previous two patterns, that is, there is some dilatation of the annulus and root and some effacement of the sinuses, but these elements are not dramatic. The overall appearance is that of a large tube, rather than a flask. For such aortas, either supracoronary tube grafting or aortic root replacement may be appropriate.

The Crawford classification (Figure 36–2) is used to categorize the appearance of an aneurysm in the descending aorta and thoracoabdominal aorta. This classification is based on the longitudinal location and extent of aortic involvement and has implications for

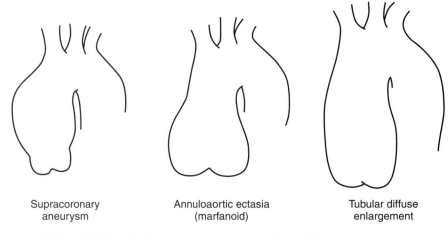

| Supracoronary aneurysm | Annuloaortic ectasia (marfanoid) | Tubular diffuse enlargement |

Figure 36–1. The three common patterns of ascending aortic aneurysm

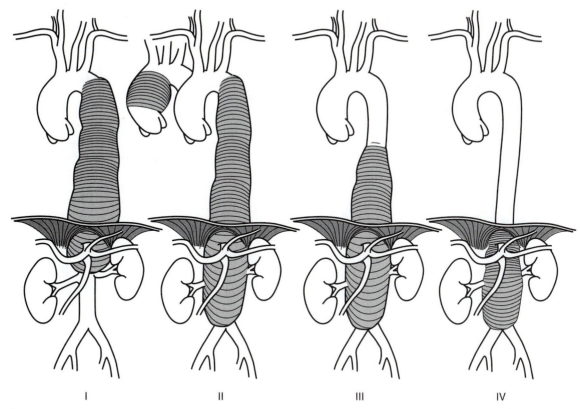

I   II   III   IV

Figure 36–2. The Crawford classification of descending and thoracoabdominal aneurysms. See text for description of each type. Reprinted, with permission, from Edmunds LH Jr, ed: Cardiac Surgery in the Adult. New York: McGraw-Hill, 1997.

surgical strategy and affects the risk of perioperative complications.

Type I aneurysms involve most of the thoracic aorta and the upper abdominal aorta. Type II aneurysms, the most extensive and most dangerous to repair, involve the entire descending and abdominal aortas. Type III aneurysms involve the lower thoracic and abdominal aortas. And Type IV aneurysms are predominantly abdominal, but involve thoracoabdominal exposure because of the proximity of the upper border to the diaphragm.

Etiology

The genetics of Marfan's disease, a well-known cause of aneurysms of the thoracic aorta, have been well delineated, with over 85 mutations identified at one locus on the fibrillin gene.

Increasingly, it is being appreciated that non-Marfan's patients also manifest familial clustering of thoracic aortic aneurysms and dissections. Aneurysm patients often answer one or both of the following questions affirmatively: "Do you have any family members with aneurysms anywhere in their bodies? Did any of your relatives die suddenly or unexpectedly of apparent cardiac causes?" Detailed construction of family trees on 200 of our 1200 patients have indicated that 21% of our aneurysm probands have a first-order relative with a known or likely aortic aneurysm. The true number is certainly much higher, as these estimates are based only on family interview and not on head-to-toe imaging of relatives. Figure 36–3 shows the 21 positive family trees of the first 100 families analyzed. The most likely pattern of inheritance appears to be autosomal-dominant with incomplete penetrance. Detailed genetic investigations are underway aimed at determining the specific genetic aberrations responsible for these family clusterings.

Clinical Findings

A. NATURAL HISTORY

The Yale computerized database now contains information on over 1200 patients with thoracic aortic

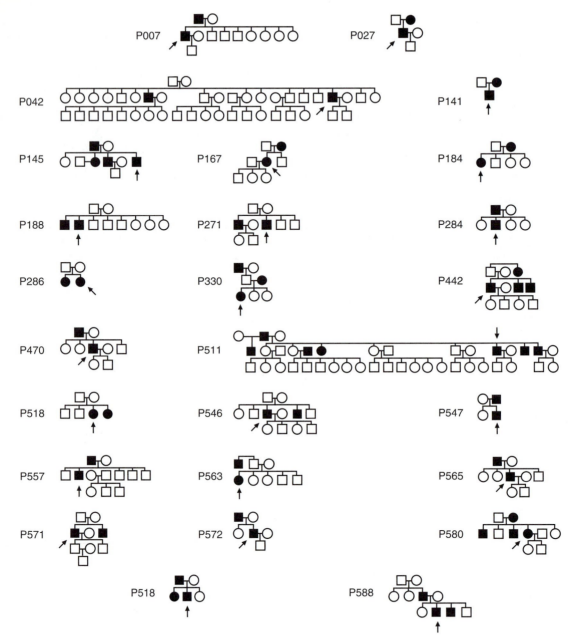

Figure 36–3. The 21 positive family trees among the first 100 patients assessed for genetic patterns of thoracic aortic disease.

aneurysm, including over 3000 tabulated serial imaging studies and over 3000 patient-years of follow-up. This database and these methods of analysis have permitted assessment of multiple fundamental topics and questions regarding the natural behavior of the thoracic aorta and have shed light on appropriate criteria for surgical intervention.

1. How fast does the thoracic aorta grow?— Calculation of growth rate of the aorta is more complicated than simply subtracting the original size of the aorta from the current size and dividing by the length of follow-up. Different modalities [echocardiography, computed tomographic (CT) scan, and magnetic resonance imaging (MRI)] may give different values. In addition, some interobserver variability may occur in size assessment. And, most importantly, some scans may show smaller size than original measurements. (This does not imply that the aorta gets smaller, but rather that variability in measurement can happen, especially in huge samples of data.) If these negative changes are truncated, falsely high growth rates result. Via specifically developed statistical methods designed to account for these potential sources of error, we have found that the aneurysmal thoracic aorta grows, on average, 0.12 cm/year. The descending aorta grows faster than the ascending aorta, at 0.19 versus 0.07 cm/year. Also, the larger the aorta becomes, the faster it grows.

2. At what size does the aorta dissect or rupture?—
Critical to decision-making in aortic surgery is an understanding of when complications occur in the natural history of unrepaired thoracic aortic aneurysms. In the case of the thoracic aorta, the two complications that are vitally important are rupture and dissection. Knowing when these complications are likely would permit rational decision-making regarding elective, preemptive surgical intervention to prevent them.

Size criteria apply *only* to asymptomatic aneurysms. Symptomatic aneurysms should be resected regardless of size. The usual symptom produced by an aortic aneurysm is pain. For ascending aneurysms, this pain is usually felt anteriorly, under the breastbone. For descending thoracic aneurysms, the pain is usually felt in the interscapular region of the upper back. For thoracoabdominal aneurysms, the pain is usually felt lower in the back and in the left flank. Other symptoms may occasionally be produced by thoracic aortic aneurysms, including bronchial obstruction, esophageal obstruction, and phrenic nerve dysfunction, and also constitute indications for surgical intervention.

Our initial statistical analysis revealed sharp "hinge points" (Figure 36–4) in aortic size at which rupture or dissection occurred. For the ascending thoracic aorta, the hinge point occurs at 6.0 cm. By the time aortas reach this size, 31% have ruptured or dissected. For the descending aorta, the hinge point is located at 7.0 cm. By the time descending aortas reach this size, 43% have ruptured or dissected.

If a surgeon were to wait for the aorta to achieve the median size at time of complications in order to intervene, by definition rupture or dissection would have occurred in half of the patients (Figure 36–5). Accordingly, it is important to intervene before the median value is attained. The following recommendations take this factor into account, permitting preemptive surgical extirpation before rupture or dissection in the majority of patients.

Our current recommendations are as indicated in Table 36–1 and are based on the hinge points noted in Figure 36–4. It is well-known that patients with Marfan's disease are prone to unpredictable dissection at an early size. For this reason, we intervene earlier in Marfan's patients, as indicated in Table 36–1.

For patients with a positive family history, but without Marfan's disease, we apply the same criteria as for Marfan's disease because our data indicate malignant behavior for these patients as well.

If the patient has a positive family history, and if an afflicted family member has suffered rupture, dissection, or death, preemptive surgical extirpation is carried out earlier than otherwise.

Studies of aortic anatomy increasingly recognize that patients with a bicuspid aortic valve also have inherently deficient aortas. We use the lower intervention dimensions for bicuspid patients as well. Table 36–2 indicates that a bicuspid aortic valve is actually a more common cause of aortic dissection than Marfan's disease. Table 36–2 compares the general incidence of

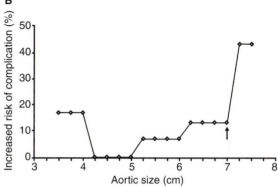
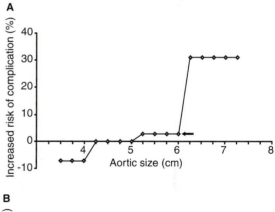

Figure 36–4. The "hinge-points" (*arrows*) in the cumulative, life-time incidence of complications (rupture or dissection) of thoracic aortic aneurysms, based on size. By the time the aorta reaches the dimensions on the *x*-axis, the percentage of patients shown on the *y*-axis has already incurred rupture or dissection. **A:** Curve for the ascending aorta. **B:** Curve for the descending aorta.

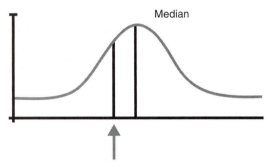

Figure 36–5. A schematic representation of the importance of selecting a criterion for intervention before complications (rupture or dissection) commonly occur. Utilization of the median as the criterion level would allow half the population to realize a devastating complication before preemptive intervention. Accordingly, a criterion below the median is selected *(arrow),* to allow preemptive intervention before a large proportion of patients have suffered a complication.

Marfan's disease with that of bicuspid aortic valve. Although the incidence of dissection is 40% for Marfan's patients and 5% for bicuspid patients, bicuspid valve disease is so much more common that bicuspid causes more total cases of dissection than Marfan's disease. This factor must be taken into account in planning surgical repair of the ascending aorta of the patient with a bicuspid aortic valve when the aorta is still in the aneurysmal stage, and not yet a dissection.

3. What is the yearly rate of rupture or dissection for thoracic aortic aneurysms?—The preceding data indicate the cumulative *lifetime* rates of dissection or rupture by the time the aorta reaches a certain size. Determining the *yearly* risk of complications from the natural history of thoracic aortic aneurysm is more challenging because it requires extremely robust data. Such data must produce enough hard end-points to permit analysis within a year's time for different size strata). Dr. Randall Griepp and his group at Mount Sinai Hospital in New York were able to accomplish this goal, el-

Table 36–1. Size criteria for surgical intervention for asymptomatic thoracic aortic aneurysm.

	Non-Marfan's (cm)	Marfan's (or familial) (cm)
Ascending	5.5	5.0
Descending	6.5	6.0

Table 36–2. Aortic manifestations of connective tissue disease.

	Incidence (%)	Likelihood of Aortic Dissection (%)
Marfan's syndrome	0.01	40.0
Bicuspid aortic valve	1–2	5.0

egantly producing an equation which permits calculation of the yearly rate of rupture:

$$\ln \lambda = -21.055 + 0.0093\ (age) + 0.842\ (pain) + 1.282\ (COPD) + 0.643\ (diameter\ of\ descending\ aorta) + 0.405\ (diameter\ of\ abdominal\ aorta)$$

Our group, as well, has recently been able to produce calculations of yearly rates of rupture or other complications based on size of the aorta. We have chosen to express these as yearly rates based simply on the size of the aorta (Table 36–3).

These data all point to a diameter of 6 cm as a very dangerous size threshold. At or above this size, the yearly risk for rupture is about 4%, the yearly risk of dissection is about 4%, and the risk of death is about 11%. (Death is often directly related to catastrophic complications from the aneurysm.) The chance of any one of these phenomena occurring—rupture, dissection, or death—is a full 14%/year. As a mnemonic point of reference, we often indicate that a 6 cm aneurysm is about the diameter of a soft-drink can. When a thoracic aortic aneurysm reaches the diameter of a soda can, it has certainly reached the point where it poses a major risk to the patient.

These analyses should permit accurate decision making when seeing a patient during an office visit and considering preemptive surgical extirpation of thoracic aneurysms. These data allow the physician to form a reasonable estimate of the individual patient's risk of dissection, rupture, or death for each future year of life, if the aorta is not resected. The risk of rupture, dissection, or death based on aortic size is presented graphically in Figure 36–6.

B. SYMPTOMS AND SIGNS

Most thoracic aortic aneurysms are asymptomatic and are detected fortuitously during imaging of other thoracic structures. When they are symptomatic, deep visceral pain in the upper anterior chest or interscapular back can occur. This pain differs from angina pectoris because it is not necessarily precipitated by exertion nor relieved by rest or nitroglycerin. Often it is rather constant and not influenced by body motion or position. All

Table 36–3. Yearly complication rates as a function of aortic size.

Yearly Risk	Aortic Size			
	>3.5 cm (%)	>4 cm (%)	>5 cm (%)	>6 cm (%)
Rupture	0.0	0.3	1.7	3.6
Dissection	2.2	1.5	2.5	3.7
Death	5.9	4.6	4.8	10.8
Any of above	7.2	5.3	6.5	14.1

patients with chest pain should have a screening chest radiograph. Rupture of a thoracic aneurysm usually causes excruciating pain, accompanied by profound dyspnea as the chest fills with blood, and quickly results in shock. A large ascending aortic aneurysm occasionally may result in dysphagia or stridor due to esophageal or large airway obstruction. Rarely a large aneurysm may cause bone pain due to pressure against thoracic skeletal structures.

C. PHYSICAL EXAMINATION

Physical examination is usually unremarkable. The presence of a murmur of aortic regurgitation should raise the suspicion of ascending aortic aneurysm, as should features suggestive of Marfan's syndrome or related conditions. Rarely, an abnormal pulsation will be felt due to a large aneurysm contacting the chest wall.

1. Imaging of thoracic aortic aneurysms—The remarkable strides made in recent decades in three-dimensional body imaging have dramatically advanced the diagnosis and treatment of thoracic aortic aneurysm. Echocardiography (especially transesophageal), CT scan, and MR imaging all yield beautiful representations of the thoracic aorta, clarifying presence, location, size, and extent of aneurysmal disease. An example of the precise imaging afforded by MRI is indicated for a specific, very extensive aneurysm in Figure 36–7.

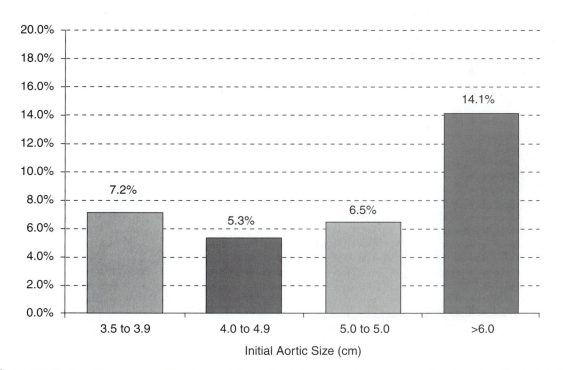

Figure 36–6. Graphic representation of cumulative natural risks posed by aneurysms of various sizes. Yearly risk of rupture, dissection, or death.

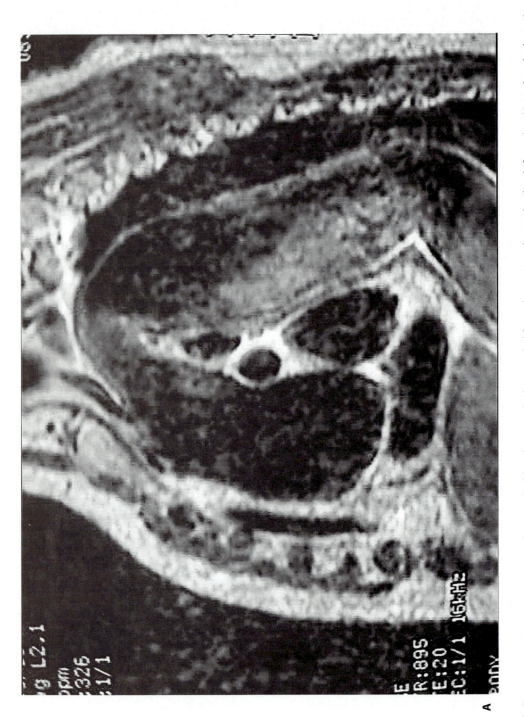

Figure 36–7. A: Magnetic resonance scan of massively dilated aorta, which extended from the aortic valve to the iliac bifurcation. Note that the heart is compressed to a small shadow crushed between the elongated aorta and the diaphragm. This aneurysm was successfully resected in two stages. **B:** Postoperative angiogram. Note that massive subclavian aneurysms have developed bilaterally.

(continued)

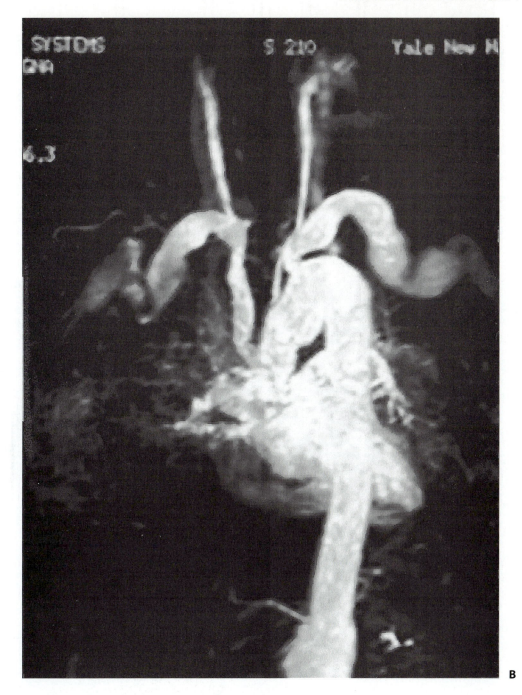

Figure 36–7. (cont.)

In this era of specialized 3D imaging, it is important not to forget the plain chest x-ray film, which can often yield significant information about the thoracic aorta. An example is provided in Figure 36–8. Ascending aortic aneurysm presents as a bulge beyond the right hilar border. Arch aneurysm produces enlargement of the aortic knob. Descending thoracic aneurysm is often easily seen as a deviation of the stripe of the descending aorta, which normally runs parallel to and just left of the vertebral column.

Treatment

A. RISKS OF AORTIC SURGERY

It is certainly helpful to know numerically and statistically the cumulative and yearly rates of rupture, dissection, and death imposed by an aortic aneurysm of a specific size. On the other hand, the equation is incomplete without consideration of the risks inherent in elective, prophylactic surgical extirpation of the thoracic aorta. We have recently published reports on both mortality rates and rates of other complications after aortic surgery. For the most experienced operators at our institution, in the present era, these rates are as indicated in Table 36–4.

These rates are typical of those at other centers with a focused interest and a specific program in thoracic aortic diseases. It should be noted that stroke can complicate not only ascending and arch operations, but also descending aortic operations.

B. INDICATIONS AND CONTRAINDICATIONS

By considering the rates of natural rupture, dissection, and death from the thoracic aneurysm itself versus the

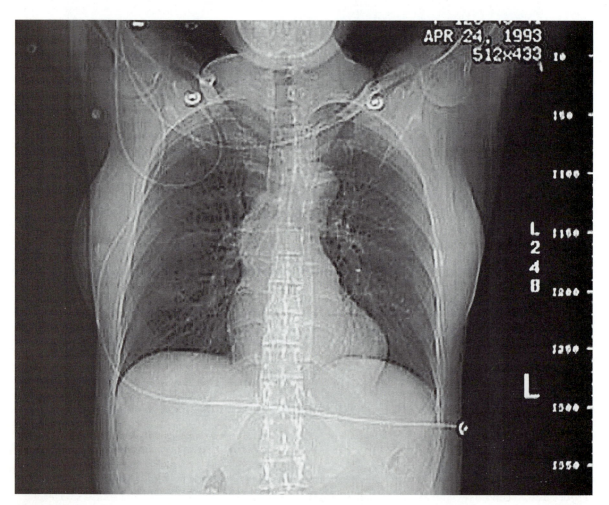

Figure 36–8. An exemplary plain chest x-ray film indicating that significant information about the aorta can be gleaned from this simple test. Note the bulge of the ascending aorta to the right of the upper mediastinal border. This young patient with Marfan's disease suffered dissection at an ascending aortic dimension of 4.8 cm.

Table 36–4. Current risks of thoracic aortic surgery.

	Mortality (%)	Stroke (%)	Paraplegia (%)
Ascending/arch	2.5	8.3	0
Descending/thoracoabdominal	8.2	4.1	2.0[a]

Data are for all comers. Percentages for elective patients would be lower.
Data are for the most experienced institutional surgeon, for the most recent 3-year period.
[a] Paraplegia rate not representative due to relatively small sample size in the time period analyzed.

risks of operation, the physician can make an informed recommendation about elective, preemptive surgery. Patients and their families, once provided natural history and surgical risk data, often have strong opinions of their own. Some families are reluctant to undergo major surgery, with its significant attendant risks, for an asymptomatic problem. Most families, however, seem to feel they will never be comfortable until the threatening aneurysm is resected.

One more very important general point needs to be considered. Once the aorta has dissected, the prognosis is thereafter adversely affected. This is illustrated in Figure 36–9. Patients who required emergency surgery not only had a higher rate of early mortality, but their survival curve was dramatically poorer. The patients who elected for surgery showed a survival rate very similar to that of a normal population. The poor long-term outlook for patients who required emergency surgery is due largely to the fact that, even after surgical replacement of portions of the aorta, the remainder of this vital organ will forever remain dissected. Because the aortic wall was deficient to start with, at half-thickness, after dissection, it is rendered even more vulnerable to subsequent enlargement and rupture.

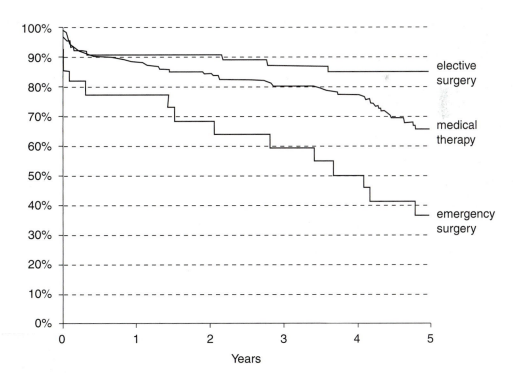

Figure 36–9. Long-term survival rates based on treatment. Medically treated patients had, of course, smaller and less symptomatic aneurysms. Note particularly that patients having emergent surgery not only manifested a higher likelihood of perioperative mortality, but also had a poorer long-term outlook. On the other hand, patients who receive elective surgery, showed excellent survival rates, comparable to an age and sex-matched normal population.

C. SURGICAL TECHNIQUES

As discussed, the type of operation for the ascending aorta is based on the pattern of aneurysmal pathology. For many patients, a supracoronary tube graft suffices (Figure 36–10). For others, a composite graft, including both a valve and a graft, with obligate coronary artery reimplantation, is appropriate. New valve-sparing aortic replacement procedures are being pioneered by David and Yacoub. Their appropriate application will become clearer as more patients are followed into the medium term and as more centers accumulate experience with these innovative techniques.

The main debate regarding the procedure for ascending aortic operations and those on the aortic arch concerns the optimal means of protecting brain function during the time that anastomoses in the vicinity of the aortic arch are performed. Deep hypothermic circu-

latory arrest—a state of suspended animation, which is generally safe for 30–45 min or longer—is preferred by many surgeons, for its simplicity and effectiveness. Retrograde cerebral perfusion—via the superior vena cava—has its advocates, although the actual amount of effective brain perfusion achieved by this means has been questioned. Direct perfusion of the head vessels—usually via a cannula in the innominate artery or cannulas in both the innominate and the left carotid artery—also has its supporters, despite its added complexity. No technique has been demonstrated conclusively superior over the others. Some recent attempts have been made to develop a solution and technique for "cerebroplegia," taking a cue from the paralyzing cardioplegia used to protect the heart.

For descending and thoracoabdominal operations, the technique of left atrial to femoral artery bypass has

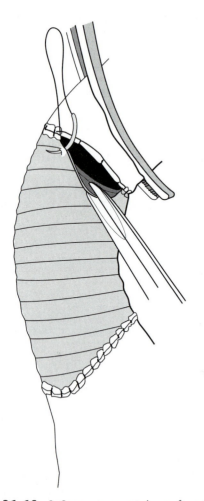

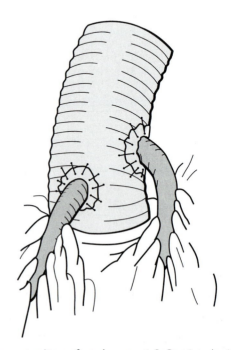

A   B

Figure 36–10. **A:** Supracoronary tube graft replacement and **B:** composite graft replacement. **A:** Reprinted, with permission, from Cooley DA, Wukasch DC: Techniques in Vascular Surgery. Philadelphia: WB Saunders, 1979.

become extremely popular. This method takes strain off the heart by diverting blood away from the left ventricle. This approach mitigates the effect of high aortic cross-clamping on cardiac afterload. It also perfuses the lower body, especially the extremely vulnerable spinal cord. Despite decades of concerted attention, paraplegia from descending and thoracoabdominal aortic replacement continues to be a major clinical problem. The cause is multifactorial, with clamp time, air and particulate embolism, and disconnection of critical intercostal branches all playing a role. Besides the benefits of left atrial to femoral artery perfusion, most authorities feel that routine spinal fluid drainage and deliberate maintenance of a strong postoperative blood pressure (to encourage collateral blood flow) are also effective adjuncts against the dreaded complication of postoperative paraplegia.

D. SPECIFIC CLINICAL SCENARIOS AND ISSUES

1. Patient with pain, but aneurysm smaller than criteria—The answer to whether such an aorta should be replaced is a resounding yes. The dimensional criteria are specifically intended for asymptomatic patients. Any and all symptomatic aneurysms need to be resected because symptoms are a precursor to rupture. Aneurysm pain represents stretching or irritation of the aortic adventitia, the adjacent chest wall, the mediastinal pleura, or some other structure impinged on by the expanding aneurysm. Even an aorta smaller than the criterion can rupture or dissect. Such a patient is of extreme concern, and preemptive resection is needed. In one case, a patient presented with typical pain of an ascending aortic aneurysm. The aorta was 5.0 cm. Because the medical team felt this was too small for resection, they underestimated the symptoms at presentation. The aorta subsequently ruptured and the patient died within 48 h. This point cannot be overemphasized: The size criteria are explicitly intended only for asymptomatic patients; *all symptomatic aneurysms need to be resected.*

2. Differentiating aneurysm pain from musculoskeletal pain—This very important point is not always easy to determine, even in the most experienced hands. The patient usually has a good sense of whether the pain is originating from muscles and joints. The clinician usually gets an additional understanding by asking the following questions:

a. Is the pain influenced by motion or position? (If so, it is probably musculoskeletal.)

b. Do you have a history of lumbosacral spine disease or chronic low back pain? (If so, the symptoms may not be aortic in origin.)

c. Do you feel the pain in the interscapular back? (An affirmative answer indicates an almost certain relationship to thoracic aortic aneurysm.)

Presume that the pain is aortic in origin if no other cause can be conclusively established. This is the only approach that can prevent rupture.

3. Appropriate interval for serial aortic imaging—Patients with a thoracic aortic aneurysm should be followed indefinitely. Stable, asymptomatic patients can have imaging about once every 2 years, remembering that the aneurysmal aorta grows at a relatively slow 1 mm/year. In case of new onset of symptoms, we image promptly, regardless of the interval from the prior scan. For new patients, for whom only one size data point is available, we often image at short intervals until we understand their aortic behavior. We may even image every 3–6 months for new patients with moderately large aortas. Remember to compare the present scan with the patient's *first* scan, not with the last prior scan. That is the way to detect growth. Many a patient has suffered because his scans were only compared with the last prior scan, and major growth went undetected.

4. Choice of imaging modality for serial follow-up—Three quality imaging techniques are currently available: echocardiography, CT scan, and MRI. If echocardiography is chosen, it is important to remember that a standard transthoracic echocardiogram cannot see the distal ascending aorta, the aortic arch, or the descending aorta with conclusive accuracy because of intervening air-containing lung tissue. Supplement such studies with a periodic CT scan or MRI, which can visualize the entire aorta. The choice between CT and MRI may depend on ease of availability and radiologic expertise in a particular environment. Both modalities can image the entire aorta extremely well. Elevated creatinine or contrast allergy may contraindicate CT and instead favor MRI. The need to evaluate complex aortic lesions in multiple imaging plains would also favor MRI. Of course, indwelling metallic foreign objects, such as pacemakers or metal artifacts from previous surgery, may make CT the necessary choice instead of MRI.

5. Evaluation of family members—The data on familial inheritance has become strong enough that the treating physician is obligated to recommend that family members be evaluated. Physicians of family members should be made aware that aneurysm disease has been diagnosed in the family. We recommend a CT scan for adult males and for females beyond child-bearing age. For children and for females of child-bearing age, we recommend echo of the ascending aorta and abdominal aorta. We hope soon to identify humoral markers or genetic aberrations that can be used for familial screening of the aneurysm trait.

6. Activity restrictions—We recommend continuing any and all aerobic activities, including running, swimming, and bicycling. Serious weight lifters, at peaks of exertion, can elevate systolic arterial pressure to 300 mm Hg.

This type of instantaneous hypertension is, of course, not prudent for aneurysm patients. We recommend that weight lifters limit themselves to one-half their body weight. We proscribe participation in contact sports or those that might produce an abrupt physical impact, such as tackle football, snow skiing, water skiing, and horseback riding.

7. Role of stent grafting—A word of caution is appropriate concerning stent grafts. All three thoracic stent products previously in clinical trials are officially on FDA recall at the present time. Owing to the very high need for subsequent conventional surgery after abdominal aneurysm stent placement, the recent large, multicenter Eurostar study questioned the very efficacy and advisability of stent grafting. Endoleak, stent dislodgement, and aneurysm expansion or rupture were disturbingly widespread in medium-term follow-up. It should be remembered that stents were designed to keep tissue from encroaching on the vessel lumen, not to keep the vessel from expanding. One noted authority feels that the aneurysmal aorta essentially "ignores" the stent graft, dilating regardless of the stent, at its own pace. (Personal communication, Dr. L. Svennson.) Also remember that the natural history of the thoracic aorta is to grow only slowly, and that hard end-points (rupture, dissection, and death) take years to be realized. For this reason, short-term stent studies are nearly meaningless. Long-term studies are needed. This new modality should be approached with caution. Its advent should not at this point influence overall intervention strategy.

Conclusion

We might liken elective, preemptive resection of an asymptomatic thoracic aortic aneurysm to refinancing a mortgage that has a high interest rate with one with a lower rate. Each has initial costs. The mortgage has points and closing costs. The aneurysm has the risks associated with major surgery. However, both refinancing and aneurysm resection have major, long-term benefits. The refinanced mortgage provides a lower long-term interest rate. Preemptive resection virtually eliminates the risk of rupture and early death from the aneurysm. Both decisions must be based on strong empirical data.

Preemptive aortic surgery to treat large aneurysms has a mortality rate less than (or for ascending and arch, *much* less than) 1 year's natural history of rupture, dissection, or aneurysm-related death.

Birks EJ, Webb A, Child A et al: Early and long-term results of a valve-sparing operation for Marfan syndrome. Circulation 1999;100(19 Suppl)II: 29.

Coady MA, Davies RR, Roberts M et al: Familial patterns of thoracic aortic aneurysms. Arch Surg 1999;134:361.

Coady MA, Rizzo JA, Elefteriades JA: Pathologic variants of thoracic aortic dissections: Penetrating atherosclerotic ulcers and intramural hematomas. Cardiol Clin 1999;17:637.

Coady MA, Rizzo JA, Hammond GL et al: What is the appropriate size criterion for resection of thoracic aortic aneurysms? J Thorac Cardiovasc Surg 1997;113:476.

Coselli JS, LeMaire SA, Koksoy C et al: Cerebrospinal fluid drainage in thoracoabdominal aortic aneurysm repair: Results of a randomized clinical trial. J Vasc Surg 2002 Apr;35(4): 631.

David TE: Aortic valve-sparing operations for aortic root aneurysm. Semin Thorac Cardiovasc Surg 2001;13:291.

Davies RR, Goldstein LJ, Coady MA et al: Yearly rupture/dissection rates for thoracic aortic aneurysms: Simple prediction based on size. Ann Thorac Surg 2002;73(1):291–294.

Davies RR, Rizzo JA, Kopf GS, Elefteriades, JA: Safety of thoracic surgery in the present era. Circulation 2001;(Suppl II):643.

Fann JI, Miller DC: Endovascular treatment of descending thoracic aortic aneurysms and dissections. Surg Clin North Am 1999;79:551–574.

Goldstein LJ, Davies RR, Rizzo JA et al: Stroke in thoracic aortic surgery: Incidence, etiology, and prevention. J Thorac Cardiovasc Surg 2001;122:935.

Griepp RB, Ergin MA, Galla JD et al: Natural history of descending thoracic and thoracoabdominal aneurysms. Ann Thorac Surg 1999;67:1927.

Laheij RJ, Buth J, Harris PL et al: Need for secondary interventions after endovascular repair of abdominal aortic aneurysms. Intermediate-term follow-up results of a European collaborative registry (EUROSTAR). Brit J Surg 2000;81:1666.

Lynch RJ, Cole PE, Tittle LS et al: Mid-term follow-up penetrating ulcer and intramural hematoma of the aorta. J Thorac Cardiovasc Surg 2002;123(6):1051–1059.

Svensson LG, Nadolny EM, Penney DL et al: Prospective randomized neurocognitive and S-100 study of hypothermic circulatory arrest, retrograde brain perfusion, and antegrade brain perfusion for aortic arch operations. Ann Thorac Surg 2001; 71:1905.

Evaluation and Treatment of the Perioperative Patient

37

Helge U. Simon, MD, Alvin S. Blaustein, MD & Laura F. Wexler, MD

PREOPERATIVE RISK ASSESSMENT

General Considerations

It is common for internists, family physicians, and cardiologists to be asked to determine a patient's suitability to undergo noncardiac surgery. However, the frequently used term medical clearance is a misnomer because a complete perioperative evaluation should serve three purposes:

1. Assessing the patient's incremental risk of death or serious morbidity as a consequence of (potentially not yet diagnosed) cardiovascular conditions during surgery or the postoperative period

2. Minimizing the risk of these adverse cardiovascular events through medical, behavioral and (rarely) invasive measures

3. Using the opportunity to alter cardiovascular risk and disease progression, independent of the upcoming surgery

Risk—the possibility that the patient might die or experience serious complications—must be balanced against benefit—the expectation of significant improvement from the surgery.

A careful history and physical examination paying special attention to signs of valvular disease, vascular disease, and heart failure and a review of electrocardiograms and other clinical data (especially details of prior complete or incomplete coronary revascularization, coronary angiograms, ventricular function studies, and stress testing) are essential for the nonemergency evaluation. Unstable or unexplained symptoms or recent significant events are often indicators for additional preoperative tests and, often, for changes in medical therapy. The history alone is remarkably good at providing insights into the severity or stability of coronary artery disease or heart failure.

By convention, the term perioperative risk refers to the 30-day period after surgery and is traditionally divided into an early (0–48 h), a middle (postoperative days 3–8), and a late period. Morbid or mortal events

during this time are considered to be a result of the surgery, although preexisting medical conditions are critical determinants of outcome.

A. CARDIOVASCULAR DISEASE AND SURGICAL RISK

Cardiovascular disease is most prevalent in the segment of the population most likely to undergo surgery of any type. About 20–25% of all Americans have cardiovascular disease (including hypertension), accounting for almost 40% of the mortality from all causes in this country. The prevalence of cardiovascular disease and the death rate associated with it rises sharply after age 45, an age when the incidence of noncardiac surgeries is also increasing; and a significant percentage, perhaps one third, of the 25 million surgical procedures done annually are performed in patients with cardiovascular diseases. From several large studies, we can estimate that cardiac deaths and nonfatal myocardial infarction (MI) occur in about 0.2% of all cases of general anesthesia and surgery, about 500,000 events yearly. Cardiac death accounts for approximately 40% of all perioperative mortality, the same proportion as sepsis—although in many cases the cause of death is multisystem organ failure. These figures underestimate the total effect of cardiovascular diseases because another 500,000 persons a year suffer nonfatal MI, unstable angina, or congestive heart failure (CHF) perioperatively, prolonging both their time in the intensive care unit and the total hospital stay.

It is likely that the overwhelming majority of the 1 million patients suffering perioperative cardiac morbidity or mortality come from the 7–8 million who could potentially be identified as having predisposing factors. However, exhaustive and indiscriminate preoperative testing of even this group would be unacceptably costly, especially given the considerable controversy about the extent to which such risks can be modified by aggressive preoperative intervention. Coronary revascularization therapy by surgery or percutaneous intervention (PCI) carries its own morbidity and mortality risks. It is therefore the current approach to perform stress testing, coronary angiography and revascularization only on those patients who would have been treated the same way regardless of the impending surgery, that is, those for whom revascularization will decrease long-term risk or relieve symptoms.

B. CAUSES OF PERIOPERATIVE CARDIAC EVENTS

Despite the risks we might expect during general anesthesia, including myocardial depression, transient hypotension, and tachycardia, very few cardiac events occur during the surgery itself. The incidence of perioperative cardiac complications actually peaks between 2 and 5 days postoperatively. These data imply that factors activated during or following surgery, and not only the surgery itself, are crucial in determining adverse outcomes.

1. Metabolic and physiologic changes—A number of metabolic and physiologic changes occur after surgery that adversely influence the balance between cardiac oxygen supply and demand. In the first 48–72 h after surgery, activity of the sympathetic nervous system is increased, and a further increase may accompany pain, anxiety, hemorrhage, hypoxia, or infection. Disturbances of intravascular and interstitial volume regulation—associated with both changes in hormonal regulation of salt and water balance and altered capillary permeability—commonly result in volume overload. In addition, banked blood transfused does not reach optimum oxygen-delivering capacity immediately.

2. Other causes—Pneumonitis and microatelectasis produce ventilation-perfusion mismatch, and sedation or analgesia may cause respiratory depression and interfere with coughing. Together, these factors may contribute to marginal arterial oxygen saturation. Thrombocytosis and a generalized hypercoagulable state, caused by increased fibrinogen and activators from the damaged tissue, favor thrombosis. At the same time, sympathetically mediated increases in heart rate, blood pressure, and contractility combine with increased intracardiac volume (and therefore increased wall stress) to increase myocardial oxygen consumption, whereas thrombotic tendencies, anemia, and arterial desaturation impede oxygen delivery to the myocardium. In a patient with underlying coronary artery disease, this situation may lead to myocardial ischemia or infarction. The imbalance may be further exaggerated because antihypertensive or anginal medications are often withheld. By the third or fourth postoperative day, the patient is hypermetabolic, with negative nitrogen and potassium balances. A natriuresis follows, which can produce hypovolemia and further activate the sympathetic nervous system.

C. IDENTIFYING AND EVALUATING PATIENTS AT RISK

From the data obtained through the history, physical examination, review of prior objective data (radiographs, electrocardiographs [ECGs], laboratory values,

etc), and other diagnostic tests, the physician can determine the status of any comorbid factors and can generate a short list of clinical characteristics, several of which allow the identification of patients whose perioperative risk is likely to be high.

Table 37–1 provides weighted risk factors based on recently published AHA/ACC guidelines. Active disease processes require more attention than dormant ones.

Table 37–1. Clinical predictors of increased perioperative cardiovascular risk (myocardial infarction, congestive heart failure, death).

Major
  Unstable coronary syndromes:
    Acute (within 7) or recent MI (within 30 days)[a] with evidence of important ischemic risk by clinical symptoms or noninvasive study
    Unstable or severe[b] angina (Canadian class III or IV)[c]
    Decompensated congestive heart failure
  Significant arrhythmias:
    High-grade atrioventricular block
    Symptomatic ventricular arrhythmias in the presence of underlying heart disease
    Supraventricular arrhythmias with uncontrolled ventricular rate
    Severe valvular disease

Intermediate
Mild angina pectoris (Canadian class I or II)
Previous MI by history or pathological Q waves
Compensated or prior congestive heart failure
Diabetes mellitus (particularly insulin-dependent)
Renal insufficiency

Minor
Advanced age
Abnormal ECG (left ventricular hypertrophy, left bundle-branch block, ST-T abnormalities)
Rhythm other than sinus (eg, atrial fibrillation)
Low functional capacity (eg, inability to climb one flight of stairs with a bag of groceries)
History of stroke
Uncontrolled systemic hypertension

---

[a] American College of Cardiology National Database Library defines recent MI as greater than 7 days but less than or equal to 1 month (30 days); acute MI is within 7 days.

[b] May include "stable" angina in patients who are unusually sedentary.

[c] Campeau L: Granding of angina pectoris. Circulation 1976; 54:522.

ECG = electrocardiogram; MI = myocardial infarction.

Source: Reproduced from Eagle KA, et al: ACC/AHA Guideline Update for Perioperative Cardiovascular Evaluation for Noncardiac Surgery: A Report of the American College of Cardiology/American Heart Association Task Force on Practice Guidelines. Circ 2002;105:1251.

A variety of risk scales have been developed in the past, acknowledging both the surgery type and patient factors contributing to the risk (ASA-Dribbs, Goldman Cardiac Risk Index, Detzky Multifactorial Risk Index). Although a better predictive value can be achieved with introduction of an increasing number of variables, the risk is often overestimated (probably because of referral bias to undergo elective surgery and improved surgical and anesthesiologic technique). On the other hand, adverse cardiovascular events still do occur in the lower risk groups, and certain types of vascular and orthopedic surgery may have higher risks than predicted. If published perioperative risk scales are used, they should be validated in the respective institution.

Recently, a simpler risk stratification score based on the presence of ischemic heart disease, cerebrovascular disease, heart failure, creatinine > 2 mg%, type 2 diabetes mellitus, and anticipation of high-risk surgery (eg, abdominal aneurysm or other vascular surgery) has been developed and validated. Risk predicted by this index was substantially lower than that anticipated using the traditional indices.

Lee TH, Marcantonio ER, Mangione CM et al: Derivation and prospective validation of a simple index for prediction of cardiac risk of major noncardiac surgery. Circulation 1999;100: 1043.

1. Patients with low perioperative risk—Between 80% and 95% of the 25 million patients undergoing noncardiac surgery in this country will be at low risk, defined here as less than 5% chance of morbidity and mortality. For the majority of patients and procedures, the low-risk patients can be identified using common sense and one of the cardiac risk-factor scales that weigh age, type and intensity of surgery, patient's functional capacity, risk for and activity of coronary atherosclerosis, cardiac failure, and serious comorbid diseases.

a. Risk factors—As might be expected, left ventricular (LV) dysfunction, past MI, and advanced coronary disease—which multiply yearly mortality rates—are the factors that have the greatest effect on surgical complication rates.

(1) Left ventricular dysfunction—When patients have clinically overt congestive heart failure (CHF) preoperatively, or exhibit an S_3 gallop or jugular venous distention, postoperative heart failure occurs in roughly one third. Even in those with compensated heart failure, pulmonary congestion will occur in about 6%. The link between left ventricular ejection fraction (LVEF) and postoperative complications is more tenuous, partly because no prospective blind studies have examined surgical outcome in relation to preoperative ejection fraction. Although reduced LVEF is known to be associated with increased long-term mortality rates following vascular surgery, ejection fraction is less useful than perfusion scanning in predicting perioperative events in vascular surgery patients. Even if ejection fraction is normal, coronary disease can pose a significant and unsuspected risk.

(2) Coronary artery disease—Even with stable mild-to-moderate symptoms, coronary artery disease (CAD) has been shown to affect life expectancy independently of the influence of LVEF. However, it should be remembered that the studies commonly cited were performed 20–25 years ago and do not reflect the use of current invasive techniques or medical therapy. These studies therefore probably overestimate mortality and morbidity rates. In patients with mild-to-moderate angina, the current yearly mortality rate is 1–1.5%/year; with more severe stable angina the figure is 2–3%/year. In patients who also have LV dysfunction, mortality rates are much higher. Patients at low risk who do not require further testing even if CAD is suspected or known to be present include those who are physically active and asymptomatic or have mild stable symptoms and those who have been completely revascularized within the last 5 years and are without recurrent symptoms. Patients who would not be candidates for revascularization should also not be routinely tested unless a high risk result would change the plan to procede with the elective surgery.

Generally, elective surgery should be undertaken cautiously in patients who have had an MI within the last 6 weeks, if not 6 months. An analysis of thousands of patients between 1960 and 1975 revealed that, when patients had an MI within 3 months of planned noncardiac surgery, their reinfarction rate was 30%; if the infarction occurred 4–6 months preoperatively, the chances of infarction were still about 15%. Better methods of early detection, more aggressive monitoring after surgery, and closer attention to hemodynamic abnormalities and pain control have contributed to a decline in reinfarction rates to 6% at 3 months and 2% after 4–6 months. The associated mortality is still high when preoperative infarction has occurred: 33% after Q wave and 20% after non-Q wave MI. Stable angina, diabetes mellitus, and hypertension have in various studies appeared to identify patients with higher complication rates, but the association has been sporadic and these features are common even in low-risk groups, which minimizes their prognostic usefulness.

Gerson MC, Hurst JM, Hertzberg VS et al: Prediction of cardiac and pulmonary complications related to elective abdominal and noncardiac thoracic surgery in geriatric patients. Am J Med 1990;88:101.

If a patient presents with atypical symptoms or some functional disability limits his or her activity so that ischemic symptoms cannot be assessed, noninvasive testing with either physical or pharmacologic stress may be indicated. It is necessary to assess the ischemic threshold (ie, the level of oxygen consumption that surpasses oxygen supply), the amount of myocardium that is potentially ischemic, and resting ventricular function.

Knowledge of the coronary anatomy permits further stratification because mortality rates are highest in those with narrowing of the left main coronary artery or in the distribution of all three major coronary arteries. Identifying those patients is one of the major aims of noninvasive stress testing. In these categories, yearly mortality rates in medically treated patients range from about 5% if the LVEF is >0.50; 13% if the LVEF is <0.35. Frequently, the coronary anatomy is unknown, but the symptomatic status and the results of a stress test and radionuclide perfusion scan are known. Reversible defects indicating ischemia or regional deficits in perfusion can show which patients are more likely to suffer coronary events (infarction or death). In patients with symptoms of coronary atherosclerosis, a positive radionuclide perfusion scan increases the likelihood three- to fourfold that the patient will have an ischemic event over the next several years. The estimates are higher in patients with prior MI or LV dysfunction. A patient whose scan is free of reversible defects has a cardiac event rate of only 1–2%/year, similar to the rate for patients with mild-to-moderate stable angina and no high-risk features on exercise testing.

(3) Peripheral vascular disease—Because atherosclerosis is a generalized disease, peripheral vascular disease (PVD) is often associated with comorbid CAD. Peripheral vascular disease may mask the presence of CAD by decreasing functional status and being associated with silent ischemia in diabetics. Even in the absence of coronary symptoms, the presence of claudication alone increases the risk of cardiac death by a factor of 3.5 above the baseline. If peripheral vascular obstructions are confirmed by objective testing, the cardiovascular mortality rate is roughly five times higher. This translates into an annualized death rate of 5–6%, compared with less than 1% in those with no evidence of peripheral vascular obstruction. Moreover, if evidence of PVD precedes MI, subsequent mortality rates are greater both immediately and over an extended period.

Rihal CS, Sutton-Tyrrell K, Guo P et al: Increased incidence of periprocedural complications among patients with peripheral vascular disease undergoing myocardial revascularization in the Bypass Angioplasty Revascularization Investigation. Circulation 1999;100:171.

(4) Functional capacity—Even in the absence of a recent stress test, the functional status of a patient supplies information about surgical risk. Functional capacity can be standardized in metabolic equivalent (MET) levels: a resting 40-year-old male consumes about 3.5 mL O_2/min/kg. By convention, this $\dot{V}O_2$ equals one MET. Excellent functional capacity (>10 MET) like that achieved during strenuous sport activities carries an excellent prognosis. In contrast, patients able to perform only tasks less than 4 MET (baking, golfing with a cart, walking 3 mph) are at much higher risk of surgical complications. Exercise testing is much more reliable in assessing functional capacity than questioning and can be combined with nuclear or echocardiographic imaging.

Reilly DF, McNeely MJ, Doerner D et al: Self-reported exercise tolerance and the risk of serious perioperative complications. Arch Intern Med 1999;159:2185.

b. Risk of different surgical procedures—Cardiovascular complications are exceedingly rare in ophthalmologic procedures, even if performed in patients with known CAD. In contrast, lung resection surgery or transplant surgery of lung, kidney, liver, and pancreas carry measurable perioperative risk, and exercise or pharmacologic imaging stress testing have been shown to predict patients with the highest risk. Vascular surgery procedures are commonly associated with a high incidence of cardiovascular complications, with infrainguinal arterial revascularization probably being the procedure with the highest associated risk (Table 37–2).

Backer CL, Tinker JH, Robertson DM et al: Myocardial reinfarction following local anesthesia for ophthalmic surgery. Anesth Analg 1980;59:257–262

Eagle KA, Rihal CS, Holmes DR et al: Cardiac risk of noncardiac surgery: Influence of coronary disease and type of surgery in 3368 operations. CASS Investigators and University of Michigan Heart Care Program. Coronary Artery Surgery Study. Circulation 1997;96:1882.

Table 37–2. Cardiac risk stratification for noncardiac surgical procedures according to ACC guidelines.

High (Reported cardiac risk often greater than 5%)
    Emergent major operations, particularly in the elderly
    Aortic and other major vascular surgery
    Peripheral vascular surgery
    Anticipated prolonged surgical procedures associated with large fluid shifts and/or blood loss
Intermediate (Reported cardiac risk generally less than 5%)
    Carotid endarterectomy surgery
    Head and neck surgery
    Intraperitoneal and intrathoracic surgery
    Orthopedic surgery
    Prostate surgery
Low (Reported cardiac risk generally less than 1%)
    Endoscopic procedures
    Superficial procedure
    Cataract surgery
    Breast surgery

ACC = American College of Cardiology.

Source: Reproduced from Eagle KA, et al: ACC/AHA Guideline Update for Perioperative Cardiovascular Evaluation for Noncardiac Surgery: A Report of the American College of Cardiology/American Heart Association Task Force on Practice Guidelines. Circ 2002;105:1251.

Fleisher LA, Eagle KA, Shaffer T et al: Perioperative and long-term mortality rates after major vascular surgery: The relationship to preoperative testing in the Medicare population. Anesth Analg 1999;89:849.

Mistry BM, Bastani B, Solomon H et al: Prognostic value of dipyridamole thallium-201 screening to minimize perioperative cardiac complications in diabetics undergoing kidney or kidney-pancreas transplantation. Clin Transplant 1998;12:130.

2. Cardiac testing prior to noncardiac surgery— The ACC/AHA makes the algorithm shown in Figure 37–1 available on the Internet to guide preoperative

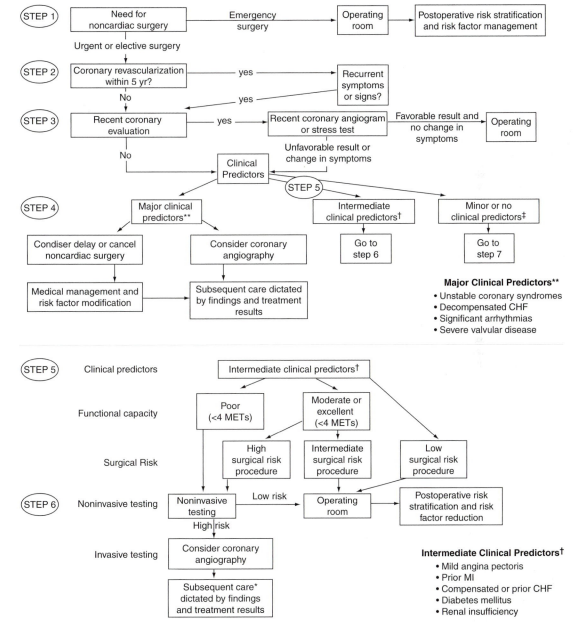

Figure 37–1. American Heart Association/American College of Cardiology guidelines for preoperative evaluation prior to noncardiac surgery.

(continued)

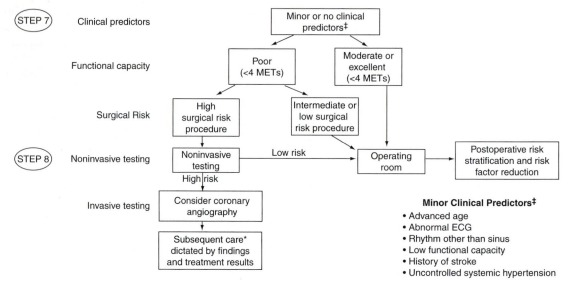

STEP 7 Clinical predictors

Minor or no clinical predictors‡

Functional capacity

Poor (<4 METs)

Moderate or excellent (<4 METs)

Surgical Risk

High surgical risk procedure

Intermediate or low surgical risk procedure

STEP 8 Noninvasive testing

Noninvasive testing — Low risk → Operating room → Postoperative risk stratification and risk factor reduction

High risk

Invasive testing

Consider coronary angiography

Subsequent care* dictated by findings and treatment results

Minor Clinical Predictors‡
• Advanced age
• Abnormal ECG
• Rhythm other than sinus
• Low functional capacity
• History of stroke
• Uncontrolled systemic hypertension

Figure 37–1. (cont.)

evaluation. Tests employed, in addition to the history and physical exam, include 12-lead ECG, noninvasive tests to assess the presence of prior infarction or inducible ischemia, and tests to image cardiac function and coronary angiography.

Eagle KA, Berger PB, Calkins H et al: ACC/AHA guideline update for perioperative cardiovascular evaluation for noncardiac surgery update: A report of the American College of Cardiology/American Heart Association Task Force on Practice Guidelines (Committee to Update the 1996 Guidelines on Perioperative Cardiovascular Evaluation for Noncardiac Surgery). 2002. American College of Cardiology Web site. Available at: http://www.acc.org/clinical/guidelines/perio/update/periupdate_index.htm

a. Twelve-lead electrocardiogram—In patients with known or likely CAD (multiple risk factors) or patients with diabetes mellitus, a recent (within the past 4 weeks) 12-lead resting ECG should be available. Left ventricular hypertrophy or ischemic ST depression are associated with increased surgical risk and long-term reduced life expectancy. Although a completely normal electrocardiogram makes significant LV dysfunction unlikely, extensive Q waves predict a long-term increased rate of mortality and give a rough estimate of LV systolic function. However an abnormal resting ECG fails to identify patients at increased risk undergoing low-risk surgery.

Landesberg G, Einav S, Christopherson R et al: Perioperative ischemia and cardiac complications in major vascular surgery: Importance of the preoperative twelve-lead electrocardiogram. J Vasc Surg 1997;26:570.

Schein OD, Katz J, Bass EB et al: The value of routine preoperative medical testing before cataract surgery. Study of Medical Testing for Cataract Surgery. N Engl J Med 2000;342:168.

b. Stress testing—Stress testing should be considered in patients with known CAD and recent change in symptoms or acute coronary syndrome for whom no initial or recent stress test has been performed for the purpose of evaluating the adequacy of medical, interventional, or surgical treatment.

If the patient's resting ECG is normal and, based on the criteria in Table 37–3, a stress test is indicated to stratify risk, simple exercise treadmill testing is able to identify patients with low risk (target heart rate is achieved and ischemia not detected or only at high workload). If an adequate test is performed (at least intermediate-level workload and target heart rate are

Table 37–3. Shortcut to noninvasive ischemia testing in preoperative patients if any two factors are present.

1. Intermediate clinical predictors (see Table 37–1) are present.
2. Poor functional capacity (less than 4 MET)
3. High-risk surgical procedure (emergency major operations; aortic repair or peripheral vascular surgery; prolonged surgical procedures with large fluid shifts or blood loss)

MET = metabolic equivalent level.
Source: Adapted, with permission, from the ACC Guidelines.

achieved), stress testing is able to accurately predict patients who are at low risk of cardiac events and those with a high likelihood of multivessel or left main disease who would be at highest risk (Table 37–4).

If the baseline ECG is abnormal (left bundle branch block [LBBB], left ventricular hypertrophy [LVH] with repolarization changes, digoxin effect), interpretation of stress-induced ECG repolarization abnormalities is not predictive. Either echocardiography or nuclear perfusion imaging should be added to standard exercise stress testing.

Patients who are unable to exercise or with pre-existing left bundle branch block should be risk-stratified by using either potent coronary vasodilators, such as dipyridamole and adenosine, or the "exercise mimic," dobutamine. These techniques have extended coronary perfusion imaging to patients whose exercise capacity is limited by comorbid (eg, neurologic, vascular, pulmonary, orthopedic) conditions. Stress echocardiography is an alternative to nuclear imaging for detecting potentially dangerous coronary lesions. Studies have shown that patients older than 65 years who are unable to exceed a heart rate of 99 bpm with exercise have a higher rate of perioperative cardiac events. Other factors, including ejection fraction and cardiac risk indices, are less predictive. These patients should have more extensive evaluation, usually with tests that detect jeopardized myocardium. Imaging tests can theoretically be helpful by predicting a low perioperative mortality risk to 0.5–1.5% when there is no evidence of ischemia and by identifying high-risk patients with a significant amount of jeopardized (potentially ischemic) myocardium.

(1) Nuclear stress imaging—By disclosing functional abnormalities in coronary flow, nuclear perfusion imaging identifies patients likely to suffer cardiac events, especially following transmural MI. Its use in preoperative evaluation is predicated on a similar theory because the inability of many of the patients awaiting surgery to exercise adequately reflects vascular insufficiency (stroke or claudication), heart failure, or chronic lung disease—all of which share risk factors with coronary atherosclerosis. In early studies of patients undergoing major vascular surgery, scans were positive in about one third to one half the group. When the scans were positive for nuclear redistribution, signifying viable but jeopardized myocardium, 4–20% of the patients experienced perioperative cardiac events; infarction, or unstable angina more often than cardiac death. Newer data indicate a lower event rate but probably reflect the current practice that patients with scans indicating high risk undergo revascularization procedures and receive increased medical attention.

Risk can be stratified in patients undergoing general surgical procedures by clinical evaluation; routine stress imaging for all patients is of questionable value and not particularly cost-effective. Nuclear perfusion scanning can be used in high-risk patients. In patients deemed to be at high risk based on the presence of diabetes, ECG evidence of LVH or LBBB, one-fourth of those with multiple reversible defects are at risk for cardiac complications. Although a patient with a positive scan with a mild defect and low clinical risk has only a mildly increased surgical risk, as the defect size increases to more than 20% of the LV, risk sharply increases. Few of those with fixed defects or normal scans will have perioperative cardiac problems, but a fixed defect does predict long-term risk of cardiac events. Increasing number and size of reversible defects, transient ischemic cavity dilation, increase in the ratio of lung-to-heart thallium-201 uptake, ischemic ECG changes during dipyridamole infusion are markers for high risk, often indicating left main or multivessel CAD. Patients undergoing abdominal aortic surgery with such markers but a normal perfusion scan have an event rate of 2%, which is comparable to

Table 37–4. Prognostic gradient of ischemic responses during an electrocardiographically monitored exercise test in patients with suspected or proven coronary artery disease.

High risk

Ischemia induced by low-level exercise[a] manifested by one or more of the following:

    Horizontal or downsloping ST depression greater than 0.1 mV

    ST segment elevation greater than 0.1 mV in noninfarct lead

    Five or more abnormal leads

    Persistent ischemic response greater than 3 min after exertion

    Typical angina

Intermediate risk

Ischemia induced by moderate-level exercise[b] manifested by one or more of the following:

    Horizontal or downsloping ST depression greater than 0.1 mV

    Typical angina

    Persistent ischemic response greater than 1–3 min after exertion

    Three to four abnormal leads

Low risk

No ischemia or ischemia induced at high-level exercise[c] manifested by:

    Horizontal or downsloping ST depression greater than 0.1 mV

    Typical angina

    One or two abnormal leads

[a] Less than 4 METs or heart rate less than 100 bpm or less than 70% age predicted.

[b] 4–6 METs or heart rate 100–130 bpm (70–85% age predicted).

[c] Greater than 7 METs or heart rate greater than 130 bpm (greater than 85% age predicted).

MET = metabolic equivalent level.

Source: Adapted, with permission, from the ACC guidelines.

those without clinical risk markers. Use of ECG-gated single-photon emission computed tomography imaging, allows assessment of global and regional systolic function while the perfusion pattern is being assessed.

In general, approximately 100 scans are required to identify accurately the two or three patients who might die; another eight to ten would have other cardiac complications.

Mangano DT, Londo MJ, Tubau JF et al: Dipyridamole thallium-201 scintigraphy as a preoperative screening test: A reexamination of its predictive potential. Circulation 1991;84:493.

Roghi A, Palmieri B, Crivellaro W et al: Preoperative assessment of cardiac risk in noncardiac major vascular surgery. Am J Cardiol 1999;83:169.

Shaw LJ, Eagle KA, Gersh BJ et al: Meta-analysis of intravenous dipyridamole-thallium-201 imaging (1985 to 1994) and dobutamine echocardiography (1991 to 1994) for risk stratification before vascular surgery. J Am Coll Cardiol 1996;27:787.

Vanzetto G, Machecourt J, Blendea D et al: Additive value of thallium single-photon emission computed tomography myocardial imaging for prediction of perioperative events in clinically selected high cardiac risk patients having abdominal aortic surgery. Am J Cardiol 1996;77:143.

(2) Stress echocardiography—Dobutamine stress echocardiography, is also used for risk stratification especially in patients undergoing vascular surgical procedures. Unlike pharmacologic stress agents that induce selective coronary vasodilation, which overrides local and neurohormonal regulatory mechanisms that balance flow with resting demand, dobutamine increases pressure and contractility, much as exercise does. In some cases, chronically ischemic (hibernating) or stunned regions may show transitory improvement of resting abnormalities during the low-dose infusion indicating viable myocardium as opposed to scar. The sensitivity and specificity of dynamic echocardiography are similar to those of thallium perfusion imaging when used in this way. Its advantages over nuclear scanning include reduced imaging time and cost and applicability to patients who are theophylline-dependent and therefore cannot undergo dipyridamole testing or who have severe reactive airway disease.

During preoperative risk stratification, when dobutamine stress echocardiography reveals large areas of jeopardized myocardium at low ischemic threshold, the patient is at higher risk for cardiac complications, both short and long term. As with nuclear scanning, the absence of detectable jeopardized myocardium confers a low perioperative risk, but the positive predictive value of an abnormal test in an individual patient is still low.

Bigatel DA, Franklin DP, Elmore JR et al: Dobutamine stress echocardiography prior to aortic surgery: Long-term cardiac outcome. Ann Vasc Surg 1999;13:17.

Davila-Roman VG, Waggoner AD, Sicard GA et al: Dobutamine stress echocardiography predicts surgical outcome in patients with an aortic aneurysm and peripheral vascular disease. J Am Coll Cardiol 1993;21:957.

Poldermans D, Arnese M, Fioretti PM et al: Sustained prognostic value of dobutamine stress echocardiography for late cardiac events after major noncardiac vascular surgery. Circulation 1997;95:53.

(3) Limitations of preoperative stress testing— As noted earlier, tests designed to detect ischemic myocardium can stratify patients into extremely low- and high-risk groups; the amount of myocardium at risk refines the analysis further. While stratifying indexes and tests give valuable information about short- and long-term prognosis, the specificity of risk—that is, the ability to predict perioperative complications in an individual patient—remains low, especially because patients with positive tests usually undergo more extensive treatment to modify the risk

c. Coronary angiography—Most patients may be risk-stratified and effectively prepared to undergo surgery with noninvasive testing. The criteria for coronary angiography are the same as those in the general patient population, namely when noninvasive testing has demonstrated high risk for adverse outcomes, when stable angina cannot be controlled with medical management, and when unstable angina is present, especially prior to intermediate- or high-risk surgery. When the results of noninvasive testing are equivocal in patients facing intermediate- or high-risk surgery, one also might proceed with angiography.

Patients undergoing urgent noncardiac surgery who have recently suffered an MI should also be considered for angiography unless the urgency of the surgery would preclude any treatment by percutaneous intervention or bypass grafting.

Treatment of Perioperative Patients

A. RISK STRATIFICATION

It is clear that CAD, as well as other cardiovascular disorders, multiplies the risk of cardiac complications during or after surgery. Therefore, the clinician who is asked to "clear" a patient for noncardiac surgery must balance the risk that a cardiac event will either complicate the surgery or have an independent effect on longer term mortality rates against the surgery's expected benefit. It is important to advise the patient and the surgeon of the possible consequences, especially if the surgery is elective rather than life-saving. If the procedure is considered worth the risk, the risk-assessment data will guide the surgeon and anesthesiologist in making decisions regarding the choice of anesthetic, the need for intensive monitoring during and after surgery, and the appropriate use of cardiac medications during the procedure.

The consulting physician must also determine whether definitive therapy of the cardiac disorder before the planned noncardiac surgery is likely to reduce the risk of complications. Before recommending additional invasive and expensive tests, the consultant must consider the risks of delayed surgery and successive diagnostic procedures. If the only reason for recommending definitive correction of the cardiac disorder is to protect the patient during the planned noncardiac surgery, it must be clear that the combined risk of both procedures would be less than the risk of doing the procedure without correction—even with the best available monitoring and medical therapy.

B. REDUCING PREOPERATIVE RISK

1. Ischemic heart disease: Protection by preoperative revascularization therapy—

a. Coronary artery bypass surgery—A strategy of recommending coronary revascularization prior to noncardiac surgery to reduce perioperative cardiac complications is based on the data associating perioperative mortality with the status of underlying CAD, especially in patients undergoing repair of an abdominal aortic aneurysm. Although no randomized trial has compared optimal medical management with preopertive bypass surgery to prevent ischemic surgical complications and reduce mortality, data from the CASS registry in the 1970s suggested that coronary artery bypass grafting (CABG) prior to noncardiac surgery involving the vasculature, thorax, abdomen, head, and neck reduced significantly postoperative deaths (1.7% vs 3.3%) and MIs (0.8% vs 2.7%). This protective effect was mostly evident in patients with multivessel or left main CAD. In contrast, retrospective data suggest that patients with CAD who have not undergone bypass surgery and need orthopedic, breast, urologic, eye, or skin surgery have a very low risk (<1%) for perioperative mortality. A series of retrospective studies demonstrating that perioperative mortality rates among patients with CABG prior to noncardiac surgery were comparable to those among patients free of manifest CAD have also been cited to support the concept of preoperative revascularization. The series implied that "prophylactic" CABG might be protective. In evaluating surgical revascularization as a preoperative strategy to protect high-risk patients with CAD, however, the mortality (and morbidity) rates associated with the revascularization procedure itself must be taken into account. In patients older than 65, the mortality rate of elective CABG may be as high as 3–18%, depending on the presence of other surgical risk factors and the experience at the institution performing the cardiac surgery. It is also worth considering that the majority of MIs occur as a result of acute plaque rupture of noncritical lesions; that is, minor blockages that would not have warranted revascularization prior to the event, thus limiting the use of elective bypass as a means of reducing the risk of perioperative infarction.

It is reasonable that patients who are candidates for revascularization should undergo it prior to elective surgery, regardless of the anticipated noncardiac surgical procedure. An exception would be patients in whom the noncardiac surgery would offer risk reduction prior to revascularization (eg, patients with severe carotid artery stenosis at high risk for stroke during CABG). Here, local preferences and a critical discussion including the patient, surgeon, and anesthesiologist will establish the course of action.

b. Percutaneous coronary intervention—No controlled trials have assessed the value of preoperative percutaneous coronary intervention (PCI), but the rapidly improving technique and equipment make PCI comparable, if not preferable, to CABG in a large number of patients. Introduction of glycoprotein IIb/IIIa receptor antagonists and thienylpyridines to prevent early stent thrombosis have improved safety and reduced the restenosis rate after the procedures, and preliminary data suggest that the introduction of brachytherapy and drug-eluting stents further significantly reduce the restenosis rate.

Available data suggest a low mortality and perioperative MI rate in patients undergoing major vascular surgery after PCI, but as with CABG, the risk of procedure-related morbidity and mortality has to be weighed against a possible benefit.

If a PTCA is performed prior to elective surgery, it is advisable to delay surgery at least 1–2 weeks after the procedure to allow healing of the vessel, thereby preventing thrombosis. Even more time is advisable in patients having undergone a stent implantation because it takes 4–8 weeks for the endothelium to cover the stent struts. During the first 4 weeks, the patient is required to prevent stent thrombosis by taking a theinylpyridine either (clopidogrel or ticlopidine), which may increase the risk of bleeding during and after noncardiac surgery. After 4 weeks, stent thrombosis is exceedingly rare. Therefore it is useful to perform elective surgery 4 weeks after a stent implantation but before 8 weeks, when significant restenosis might have already occurred. It may take 1 week for the effects of the thienylpyridines on platelet aggregation to disappear, therefore holding off surgery for a week after completion of that therapy often is requested by the surgery team.

Available data within the last 4 years (from the BARI registry that was performed prior to introduction of routine coronary artery stenting) suggest that in patients amenable to either procedure, PCI has similar outcomes to CABG prior to noncardiac surgery in terms to perioperative MI and death.

Eagle KA, Rihal CS, Mickel MC et al: Cardiac risk of noncardiac surgery: Influence of coronary disease and type of surgery in 3368 operations. CASS Investigators and University of Michigan Heart Care Program. Coronary Artery Surgery Study. Circulation 1997;96:1882.

Fleisher LA, Eagle KA, Shaffer T et al: Perioperative and long-term mortality rates after major vascular surgery: The relationship to preoperative testing in the Medicare population. Anesth Analg 1999;89:849.

Gottlieb A, Banoub M, Sprung J et al: Perioperative cardiovascular morbidity in patients with coronary artery disease undergoing vascular surgery after percutaneous transluminal coronary angioplasty. Cardiothorac Vasc Anesth 1998;12:501.

Hassan SA, Hlatky MA, Boothroyd D et al: Outcomes of noncardiac surgery after coronary bypass surgery or coronary angioplasty in the Bypass Angioplasty Revascularization Investigation (BARI). Am J Med 2001;110:260.

Massie MT, Rohrer MJ, Leppo JA et al: Is coronary angiography necessary for vascular surgery patients who have positive results of dipyridamole thallium scans? J Vasc Surg 1997;25:975.

2. Medical management of ischemic heart disease— Patients with symptomatic CAD who are not candidates for preoperative revascularization should be treated with optimal antianginal therapy and careful attention to exacerbating factors, such as tachycardia, hypertension, hypoxia, and anemia in the postoperative period. Antianginal therapy should not routinely be interrupted following surgery. Intravenous (IV) preparations of β-blockers, calcium blockers, and nitrates are available if the patient cannot take oral drugs.

a. Beta-blockers—Several studies have shown that perioperative β-blockade improves outcome in patients with CAD, reducing severe arrhythmia, ischemia, and heart failure. Perioperative β-blockade in high-risk patients undergoing high-risk procedures attenuates cardiovascular morbidity and mortality. Continuous monitoring has shown that the amount of ischemic episodes in the perioperative period are reduced. Keep in mind that careful up-titration of the β-blocker was used in these studies, and that they were done mostly on high-risk patients, although in patients with the highest ischemic burden, a protective effect of β-blockade was not demonstrable. However, perioperative β-blockade should be used (unless there is a contraindication to its use) in patients with known or highly likely ischemic CAD. In patients not tolerating β-blockade, central α-agonists such as mivazerol can be considered: They have been proven to reduce cardiac mortality rates in general and both MI and death rates independently in vascular surgery patients. Whether the studies using bisoprolol and esmolol for the β-blockers and mivazerol for the α-agonists represent a class effect is unknown. Clonidine has also been shown to reduce the incidence of myocardial ischemia in the perioperative period.

Bayliff CD, Massel DR, Inculet RI et al: Propranolol for the prevention of postoperative arrhythmias in general thoracic surgery. Ann Thorac Surg 1999;67:182.

Boersma E, Poldermans D, Bax JJ et al: Predictors of cardiac events after major vascular surgery: Role of clinical characteristics, dobutamine echocardiography, and beta-blocker therapy. JAMA 2001;285:1865.

Oliver MF, Goldman L, Julian DG et al: Effect of mivazerol on perioperative cardiac complications during non-cardiac surgery in patients with coronary heart disease: The European Mivazerol Trial (EMIT). Anesthesiology 1999;91:951.

Poldermans D, Boersma E, Bax JJ et al, for the Dutch Echocardiographic Cardiac Risk Evaluation Applying Stress Echocardiography Study Group: The effect of bisoprolol on perioperative mortality and myocardial infarction in high-risk patients undergoing vascular surgery. N Engl J Med 1999;341:1789ff.

Poldermans D, Boersma E, Bax JJ et al, for the Dutch Echocardiographic Cardiac Risk Evaluation Applying Stress Echocardiography Study Group: The effect of bisoprolol on perioperative mortality and myocardial infarction in high-risk patients undergoing vascular surgery. N Engl J Med 1999;341:1789.

Raby KE, Brull SJ, Timimi F et al: The effect of heart rate control on myocardial ischemia among high-risk patients after vascular surgery. Anesth Analg 1999;88:477.

Wallace A, Layug B, Tatoeo I et al, for the McSPI Research Group: Prophylactic atenolol reduces postoperative myocardial ischemia. Anesthesiology 1998;88:7.

Yeager RA, Moneta GL, Edwards JM et al: Reducing perioperative myocardial infarction following vascular surgery: The potential role of beta-blockade. Arch Surg 1995;130:869.

b. Nitroglycerin—Although little data are available, IV nitroglycerin is commonly used to prevent myocardial ischemia intraoperatively. It should be considered in high-risk patients, especially if they needed nitrates preoperatively to control anginal symptoms. It has to be used cautiously because it acts synergistically with various anesthetic agents to reduce vascular tone and blood pressure. No studies have demonstrated yet a reduced rate of MI or death by their use.

Thomson IR, Mutch WA, Culligan JD: Failure of intravenous nitroglycerin to prevent intraoperative myocardial ischemia during fentanyl-pancuronium anesthesia. Anesthesiology 1984; 61:385.

Gallagher JD, Moore RA, Jose AB et al: Prophylactic nitroglycerin infusions during coronary artery bypass surgery. Anesthesiology 1986;64:785.

3. Congestive heart failure—Optimal management of CHF prior to surgery does appear to improve outcome. All appropriate drugs—β-blockers, vasodilators (angiotensin-converting enzyme inhibitors or angiotensin receptor antagonists if the patients are unable to tolerate angiotensin-converting enzyme inhibitors), hydralazine plus nitrates (in patients with cough or angioedema, hyperkalemia, or significant renal impairment), and diuretics (especially spironolactone in patients with severe LV dysfunction)—should be used, paying special attention to avoiding hyperkalemia or hypokalemia and hypervolemia or hypovolemia. A period of preoperative invasive monitoring can be helpful in patients who need urgent surgery but are discovered to have hemodynamically challenging conditions such as severe LV dysfunction, severe hypertrophic cardiomyopathy, and aortic or mitral stenosis. Monitoring and careful application of combined diuretic and afterload-reduction therapy to patients with dilated cardiomyopathy and high pulmonary capillary wedge pressures can reduce elevated filling pressures to normal or near normal with maintenance (or improvement) in cardiac output. Although this has not been specifically tested as a preoperative strategy, it seems likely that such patients would be less susceptible to volume overload-related postoperative heart failure during the obligatory volume mobilization in the postoperative period.

4. Valvular heart disease—With the exception of significant aortic stenosis, valvular heart disease that is either asymptomatic or compensated on medical therapy does not appear as a risk factor for major noncardiac surgery in any of the published risk indexes. Patients with mitral or aortic regurgitation or mild-to-moderate mitral stenosis can usually be monitored during surgery with a Swan-Ganz catheter (see later in this chapter) and treated with appropriate drugs. Patients with severe mitral stenosis who are in need of urgent noncardiac surgery may be successfully treated with percutaneous mitral valvuloplasty, thus avoiding the prolonged recuperation period and the dilemma of anticoagulation associated with mitral valve replacement. In these patients the avoidance of tachycardia with consequential shortening of diastolic filling time is crucial.

Patients with **symptomatic severe aortic stenosis** are at increased risk and ideally should undergo valve replacement prior to elective noncardiac surgery. Aortic valvuloplasty, which initially seemed a potentially low-risk noninvasive alternative to surgical valve replacement, has universally proven to be disappointing with respect to long-term results and carries the risk of severe aortic insufficiency especially in the elderly patient with calcified aortic valve. Aortic valvuloplasty may be of merit to at least temporarily reduce the transvalvular gradient in elderly patients undergoing urgent or emergent nonvascular surgery when aortic valve replacement prior to noncardiac surgery is not feasible.

Such instances would include surgery for conditions that would, if uncorrected, pose a substantial risk of prosthetic valve infection; surgery for malignancy, when long-term survival is very uncertain; elderly patients undergoing high-risk surgical procedures in which the outcome is uncertain; urgent surgery in which the months-long delay required for recovery from aortic valve replacement would substantially compromise outcome; and emergency surgery.

Little information is available on the risks of noncardiac surgery for patients who have asymptomatic hemodynamically significant aortic stenosis. Data from several centers support the general practice of not recommending valve replacement to truly asymptomatic patients with normal LV function, regardless of the severity of aortic stenosis (measured by valve gradient). Although few data are available on the risks associated with major surgery in such patients, available information suggests that careful perioperative monitoring makes surgery safe. Stress testing may be considered to ensure that patients are truly asymptomatic from their valvular disease and did not tailor their activity level to the severity of the valvular lesion.

Torsher LC, Shub C, Rettke SR et al: Risk of patients with severe aortic stenosis undergoing noncardiac surgery. Am J Cardiol 1998;81:448.

5. Hypertension—In contrast to the data that indicate an improved outcome from optimal control of preoperative CHF, the zealous treatment of preoperative stage 1 and 2 (systolic blood pressure <180 mm Hg) hypertension probably does not improve the outcome. The incidence of postoperative exacerbation of hypertension does not correlate with the degree of control attained preoperatively. Most anesthetic agents lower blood pressure during induction, and, given the wide array of agents available for blood pressure titration during the perioperative period, delaying surgery to fine-tune moderate hypertension is probably not worthwhile. However, because a large number of patients are not enjoying adequate blood pressure treatment, and in fact the ratio of adequately treated patients is decreasing, the physician should use the preoperative encounter to

a. Screen for organic causes and sequelae of hypertension

b. Initiate adequate treatment in the perioperative period without delaying the surgery. The distinctive benefit of certain blood pressure drugs in patients with coronary disease has been extensively discussed elsewhere.

Most chronically administered antihypertensive drugs should be maintained until just prior to surgery and resumed as soon as possible postoperatively, substituting parenteral (or transcutaneous) drugs in patients who cannot take oral drugs for extended periods.

Some experts have expressed concern about intraoperative myocardial depression or blunted stress response in patients on high-dose β-blockers for hypertension (or angina). Not only has this risk not been validated, but there is evidence that the abrupt withdrawal of β-blockers may be distinctly harmful. Prolonged β-blockade leads to gradual increase in β-receptors. Abrupt withdrawal results in a state of hyperadrenergic stimulation with tachycardia and hypertension, which may precipitate acute ischemia in patients with previously stable CAD. This rebound effect has been documented with oral propranolol but not with other oral β-blockers, presumably because of their longer tissue half-life, which allows an effective gradual withdrawal and down-regulation of β-receptors. Patients with ischemic heart disease or severe hypertension, previously treated with propranolol, who cannot resume it orally within 24 h after surgery should probably be treated with IV propranolol or an ultra-short-acting IV preparation.

Oral clonidine and guanabenz are antihypertensives also associated with rebound hypertension after abrupt withdrawal. Clonidine is available as a transcutaneous patch, which can be used during the perioperative period.

Severe postoperative hypertension in a patient with long-standing underlying hypertension is usually best managed with a short-acting vasodilator such as nitroprusside and with prompt reinstitution of the patient's preoperative medication regimen.

6. Arrhythmias and conduction-system disease—

a. Atrial fibrillation—There is no evidence that prophylactic digitalis will prevent atrial fibrillation or other supraventricular arrhythmias after general or vascular surgery, although some data support its use in patients undergoing heart surgery. Rapid ventricular response during or after surgery in patients with preexisting atrial fibrillation can be easily and quickly controlled with IV digitalis or, as is often more appropriate, with IV β-blockers or calcium channel blockers (verapamil or diltiazem); thus, there is no indication for preoperative oral loading of digitalis. Beta-blockers have been shown to lead to a more rapid conversion of postoperative supraventricular tachycardias to normal sinus rhythm than occurs with diltiazem.

Balser JR, Martinez EA, Winters BD et al: Beta-adrenergic blockade accelerates conversion of postoperative supraventricular tachyarrhythmias. Anesthesiology 1998;89:1052.

b. Ventricular arrhythmias—Although ventricular ectopic beats and nonsustained ventricular tachycardia are frequently encountered in patients with underlying heart disease, preoperative ectopy does not predict postoperative cardiac complications. In the absence of evidence of MI, isolated ventricular ectopy probably does not require specific perioperative treatment. However their appearance may be prevented by use of perioperative β-blockade. Sustained and symptomatic ventricular tachycardia should be suppressed by using amiodarone, lidocaine, or procainamide.

Bayliff CD, Massel DR, Inculet RI et al: Propranolol for the prevention of postoperative arrhythmias in general thoracic surgery. Ann Thorac Surg 1999;67:182.

c. Conduction disorders—Asymptomatic patients who have conduction system disease detectable by ECG but who do not fulfill criteria for the insertion of a therapeutic pacemaker do not require prophylactic temporary transvenous pacemakers during surgery. In patients with bifascicular block (right bundle branch block plus left-axis deviation), even with a prolonged PR interval (implying trifascicular block), the risk of developing complete heart block during surgery appears to be less than 1%.

Patients with extreme degrees of bradycardia should be assessed before surgery for their ability to increase heart rate appropriately (chronotropic competence). This assessment can be done by having the patient exercise. The use of a pacemaker should be considered when there is failure to raise the heart rate with a decline in blood pressure or the development of symptoms suggesting impaired cardiac output. The decision depends on the type of surgery planned and the likelihood of major fluid shifts, reflex vasodilatations, fever, or other conditions that might significantly increase cardiac demand. Obviously, before the insertion of a pacemaker, it is advisable to reevaluate the need for and dosage of any drugs that might produce bradycardia.

Patients who require pulmonary artery pressure catheters for perioperative monitoring are at some risk for developing transient right bundle branch block during insertion of the Swan-Ganz catheter. This is estimated to occur in approximately 5% of insertions and is of concern only in patients with underlying LBBB, who would be at risk for complete heart block. A transvenous pacemaker system (and a person skilled in its insertion) should be available during pulmonary artery catheterization in patients with LBBB. An external (transcutaneous) pacing system is an acceptable alternative, and some right-heart catheters have pacing electrodes.

Patients with permanent pacemakers require no special treatment during the perioperative period except for caution regarding the use of electrocautery devices. Prolonged application may inhibit the pacemaker, and electrical interference may obscure the loss of pacing impulse on the ECG monitor. Therefore, in patients who are likely to be pacemaker-dependent, electrocautery should be applied in brief bursts and radial or other hemodynamic pulse-rate monitoring should be used in addition to the ECG.

d. Treatment of patients with an of automatic implantable cardioverter defibrillator—There is a small risk that prolonged electrocautery could trigger, reprogram or inadvertently offset an automatic implantable cardioverter defibrillator (AICD), interfere with pacemaker output and that anesthetic agents interfere with pacing thresholds. Some manufacturers have recommended that the device be inactivated during surgery. Supraventricular tachycardias, which are fairly common in the postoperative period, may exceed the rate threshold of the AICD and cause inappropriate shocks to be delivered. Automatic implantable cardioverter defibrillators should be interrogated prior to surgery to assess underlying rhythm and frequency of discharges. In pacemaker-dependent patients the rate response feature should be tuned off. The AICD defibrillation capacity should be disengaged just prior to and resumed until directly after surgery, and an external defibrillating device with personnel able to handle it should be close to the patient at all times during the period that the AICD is off. Of note, an anteroposterior lead placement of the external pacer paddles away from the device pocket is required in the event of external cardioversion or defibrillation.

Madigan JD, Choudhri AF, Chen J et al: Surgical management of the patient with an implanted cardiac device: Implications of electromagnetic interference. Ann Surg 1999;230:639.

7. Endocarditis—Endocarditis is a potential risk for patients with prosthetic heart valves or with acquired or congenital structural cardiac lesions that alter blood flow and create turbulence. It has been standard practice to treat such patients with antibiotics prior to procedures that entail a significant risk of bacteremia. In the absence of controlled trials of antibiotic prophylaxis, the American Heart Association has regularly published recommendations after reviewing the available literature on the incidence of infective endocarditis associated with specific cardiac conditions and the frequency of bacteremia with various diagnostic and therapeutic procedures. Recommendations published in 1997 included several significant changes. Oral amoxicillin has replaced penicillin as the drug of choice for dental and upper respiratory procedures, for example; this change is based on data showing higher blood levels, longer plasma half-life, and less protein binding with the former. Usually only one preoperative dose of 2 g is required. Oral antibiotics are now approved for high-risk patients with prosthetic valves who were previously considered to require parenteral antibiotics prior to dental or upper respiratory procedures. Clindamycin, first-generation cephalosporins, or azithromycin are considered an acceptable alternative to amoxicillin. Parenteral antibiotics are still favored for patients who cannot take oral drugs. The recommendation for high-risk patients (especially those with prosthetic valves) undergoing genitourinary or gastrointestinal procedures continues to be parenteral antibiotics (ampicillin or vancomycin plus gentamicin), but oral amoxicillin is now approved in low-risk patients.

A number of procedures that are commonly performed and have rarely (if ever) been implicated in infective endocarditis have been removed from the list of those requiring antibiotic prophylaxis, although it remains optional in high-risk patients. These procedures include endotracheal intubation, fiberoptic bronchoscopy, injection of local anesthetic into the gum, gastrointestinal endoscopy (with or without biopsy) and transesophageal echocardiography (TEE). Prophylaxis is not recommended in patients with mitral valve prolapse unless a murmur of mitral regurgitation is present.

Dajani AS, Taubert KA, Wilson W et al: Prevention of bacterial endocarditis: Recommendations by the American Heart Association. Circulation 1997;96:358.

8. Chronic anticoagulation—When and how to discontinue chronic anticoagulation during the perioperative period depends on the original need for the agent and the potential seriousness of a bleeding complication during or after surgery. Ideally, patients undergoing procedures in which even minor bleeding would be disastrous (neurologic or ophthalmologic surgery) should have all anticoagulant substances, including aspirin, stopped well in advance of elective surgery. This should be done in sufficient time for clotting parameters to return to normal (10–14 days for aspirin and ticlopidine; 5 days or longer for warfarin), with documentation of normal prothrombin time prior to surgery. Patients who have prosthetic heart valves with high thrombotic potential (any mechanical prosthesis in the mitral position) or a history of life-threatening or recurrent thromboembolic events should be withdrawn from warfarin 3 days prior to surgery and given heparin (during the withdrawal period) until 6 h prior to surgery. Patients with less severe indications for warfarin, such as stroke prophylaxis in patients with chronic atrial fibrillation or dilated cardiomyopathy, can stop taking warfarin (without interim heparin) 2–3 days prior to surgery, restarting it when the risk of postoperative bleeding has abated.

9. Other cardiovascular drugs—Altered metabolism and variable renal and hepatic function in a patient with a complex, prolonged, or unstable perioperative course may lead to serious drug toxicity in previously stable patients on digoxin, class Ia antiarrhythmics, or theophylline; for this reason, drug levels of all three should be carefully monitored. Arrhythmias associated with digitalis toxicity may also be precipitated by fluctuations in pH or serum electrolyte levels.

C. OTHER MEASURES TO REDUCE RISK DURING AND AFTER SURGERY

1. Maintenance of body temperature—Hypothermia is common during the perioperative period in the absence of active warming of patients. In a retrospective analysis of a prospective randomized trial comparing two different anesthetic techniques for infrainguinal revascularization surgery, hypothermia was associated with an increased risk of myocardial ischemia compared with patients who had a core temperature greater than 35.5°C in the postanesthesia care unit. Several methods of maintaining normothermia are available in clinical practice, the most widely studied being forced-air warming.

2. Choice of anesthetic agent—Although the specific choice of anesthetic agent is the responsibility of the anesthesiologist, the consulting cardiologist is often asked whether general or regional (eg, spinal, epidural) anesthesia is safer in a patient with underlying cardiac disease. Although regional anesthesia avoids myocardial depression, vasodilatation causing hypotension does occur as a result of the blockage of sympathetic outflow. A patient who is awake and receiving a regional block while undergoing a major surgical procedure can potentially experience greater anxiety than the patient under general anesthesia. Given that potential and the lack of any greater protection from hypotension, general anesthesia with careful monitoring would seem to be the best choice in patients whose primary perioperative risk factor is ischemia. However, despite all theoretical consideration favoring the one or the other approach, all five trials performed so far suggest no superiority for either regional or general anesthesia in the high-risk patient. Desflurane should be avoided in patients with CAD because it has been implicated as a cause of ischemia in patients undergoing CABG. The importance of adequate analgesia resulting in reduction of sympathetic output in the postoperative period (when most major complications occur) needs to be emphasized.

Baron JF, Bertrand M, Barre E et al: Combined epidural and general anesthesia versus general anesthesia for abdominal aortic surgery. Anesthesiology 1991;75:611.

Bois S, Couture P, Boudreault D et al: Epidural analgesia and intravenous patient-controlled analgesia result in similar rates of postoperative myocardial ischemia after aortic surgery. Anesth Analg 1997;85:1233.

Christopherson R, Beattie C, Frank SM et al: Perioperative morbidity in patients randomized to epidural or general anesthesia for lower extremity vascular surgery: Perioperative Ischemia Randomized Anesthesia Trial Study Group. Anesthesiology 1993;79:422.

3. Perioperative monitoring—

a. Continuous ECG monitoring—This method is the standard practice for patients undergoing major surgical procedures—or any procedure requiring general anesthesia. The purpose is to detect arrhythmias and allow the early detection of myocardial ischemia (ST depression or elevation). Computerized analysis is superior to physician surveillance. Algorithms for ischemia detection differ between commercially available systems and number of leads uses: Leads II and V_5 detect only 80% of perioperative ischemia compare with a 12-lead ECG recording. In low-risk patients this ST segment monitoring has poor specificity, however in high-risk patients it detects silent ischemia with a specificity of 74%. Postoperative ST depression carries a worse long-term prognosis, however use of continues ST segment monitoring has not been prospectively demonstrated to decrease short-term morbidity and mortality rates.

Fleisher LA, Zielski MM, Schulman SP et al: Perioperative ST-segment depression is rare and may not indicate myocardial ischemia in moderate-risk patients undergoing noncardiac surgery. J Cardiothorac Vasc Anesth 1997;11:155.

b. Hemodynamic monitoring—Continuous intracardiac pressure monitoring by pulmonary artery catheter has been suggested for those patients undergoing major surgery in whom anticipated changes in volume status, blood pressure, or systemic or pulmonary vascular resistance are unlikely to be well tolerated. This group includes patients with moderate-to-severe mitral stenosis who must maintain a fairly narrow range of left atrial filling pressures in order to achieve adequate cardiac output and avoid pulmonary edema; patients with severe LVH or outflow obstruction (eg, aortic stenosis) who may also be very volume-sensitive; and patients with very severe LV dysfunction, especially when associated with functional mitral regurgitation, in whom a modest degrees of volume overload will cause pulmonary edema. Paradoxically, prospective studies and case control analysis have revealed an increased incidence of heart failure in patients monitored by pulmonary artery catheterization to optimize perioperative fluid management. Sensitivity and specificity to detect ischemia-induced elevations in pulmonary capillary wedge pressure is also very poor. Although this may partially result from inadequately trained physicians relying on inaccurate data to liberally giving fluid and electrolyte solutions perioperatively, it casts at least some doubt on the concept of invasively monitoring fluid management. Physicians need to be optimally trained in the interpretation of the pressure volume relations of cardiac function and need to use invasively obtained numbers as an adjunct but not a substitute for careful clinical assessment.

Iberti TJ, Fischer EP, Leibowitz AB et al, for the Pulmonary Artery Catheter Study Group: A multicenter study of physicians' knowledge of the pulmonary artery catheter. JAMA 1990; 264:2928.

Polanczyk CA, Marcantonio E, Goldman L et al: Impact of age on perioperative complications and length of stay in patients undergoing noncardiac surgery. Ann Intern Med 2001;134:637.

Ziegler DW, Wright JC, Choban PS et al: A prospective randomized trial of preoperative "optimization" of cardiac function in patients undergoing elective peripheral vascular surgery. Surgery 1997;122:584.

c. Transesophageal echocardiographic monitoring—The detection of a new wall motion abnormality by TEE during surgical procedures is probably the most sensitive indicator of myocardial ischemia. Although it is predictive of an increased likelihood of adverse outcome, in fact, it is probably oversensitive. It is unclear whether TEE adds significantly to preoperative clinical data when combined with standard two-lead intraoperative monitoring. At present, TEE is not commonly used during general surgery but is used more often during cardiac surgery, when it can be useful in assessing the adequacy of valve repair or coronary revascularization. Whether it is an important adjunct in vascular surgery, especially abdominal aorta repairs, during which the aorta is cross-clamped, is unclear. Routine use of TEE during noncardiac surgery is not cost-effective or particularly useful.

Practice guidelines for perioperative transesophageal echocardiography: A report by the American Society of Anesthesiologists and the Society of Cardiovascular Anesthesiologists Task Force on Transesophageal Echocardiography. Anesthesiology 1996;84:986.

D. REDUCING RISK IN THE POSTOPERATIVE PERIOD

Most cardiac complications associated with noncardiac surgery occur in the first 3–5 postoperative days, not during the operation itself. The consulting physician should continue to follow high-risk patients during this period, even if no untoward events occur during the operation. It is important to remember that many conditions specific to the postoperative state will markedly increase myocardial oxygen demand (tachycardia, pain, fever, increased sympathetic tone, volume overload) at the same time that oxygen delivery may be limited by anemia, hypoxia, and enhanced thrombotic potential secondary to a hypercoagulable state. The treatment of cardiac complications (MI, CHF, angina, arrhythmias) after major surgery differs little from the routine care of such conditions (these are discussed elsewhere in this book). Continued hemodynamic monitoring with judicious use of analgesics, oxygen, β-blockers, aspirin, calcium channel blockers, afterload-reducing agents, and nitrates should be carried out as needed to minimize myocardial work, maximize oxygen delivery and coronary blood flow, and relieve pulmonary congestion. In patients without known CAD and no signs of angina or perioperative myocardial dysfunction, a perioperative MI does not need to be "ruled out." In patients with known or suspected CAD, serial ECGs at baseline and daily for 2 days after surgery is cost-effective and sufficiently sensitive to detect silent MI. Monitoring for silent MI should also include use of biomarkers. Elevations in postoperative troponin T or I, drawn on days 1 and 4, or prior to discharge, (whichever comes first) have a higher specificity for diagnosing MI and predicting future cardiac events than myocardial muscle creatine kinase isoenzyme. After a perioperative MI, risk stratification as outlined in Chapter 5, including an evaluation of ventricular function, should be performed prior to discharge.

Adams JE III, Sicard GA, Allen BT et al: Diagnosis of perioperative myocardial infarction with measurement of cardiac troponin I. N Engl J Med 1994;330:670.

Lopez-Jimenez F, Goldman L, Sacks DB et al: Prognostic value of cardiac troponin T after noncardiac surgery: Six-month follow-up data. J Am Coll Cardiol 1997;29:1241.

Metzler H, Gries M, Rehak P et al: Perioperative myocardial cell injury: The role of troponins. Br J Anaesth 1997;78:386.

Myocardial infarction redefined: A consensus document of The Joint European Society of Cardiology/American College of Cardiology Committee for the redefinition of myocardial infarction. J Am Coll Cardiol 2000;36:959.

Index

Note: Page numbers followed by *t* and *f* indicate tables and figures, respectively.